Cancer

FOURTH EDITION

Cancer

DIAGNOSIS, TREATMENT, and PROGNOSIS

Lauren V. Ackerman, M.D.

Professor of Surgical Pathology and Pathology, Washington University School of Medicine, St. Louis, Mo.; Surgical Pathologist in Chief to Barnes and Affiliated Hospitals and St. Louis Children's Hospital, St. Louis, Mo.; Consultant, Ellis Fischel State Cancer Hospital, Columbia, Mo.; Consultant, Armed Forces Institute of Pathology; Visiting Professor of Surgical Pathology, University of Witwatersrand, Johannesburg, R.S.A. (1969)

Juan A. del Regato, M.D.

Director, Penrose Cancer Hospital, Colorado Springs, Colo.; Clinical Professor of Radiology, University of Colorado School of Medicine; Member, National Advisory Cancer Council; Member, Board of Chancellors, American College of Radiology; Member, Advisory Commission on Biology and Medicine, Puerto Rico Nuclear Center; Member, Committee on the Genito-Urinary System, National Academy of Science–National Research Council

With 783 text figures and 4 color plates

FOURTH EDITION

THE C. V. MOSBY COMPANY

St. Louis   1970

To
ELIZABETH AND INEZ

Preface

Our purpose in writing this book has been to provide a text that will bring general information to the student, to the general practitioner, and to those specialists involved in the diagnosis and treatment of malignant tumors. Some articles in the current literature, often devoted to treatment, assume that the correct diagnosis has been established and may not even mention the clinical evolution or differential diagnosis. Others, devoted to histopathology, may give no information on incidence or prognosis. Our intention is to present an integrated view of all of these aspects and to point the way toward a more thorough basis of knowledge of malignant neoplasms.

Chapters 1 through 5 are devoted to subjects of general interest. *Dr. Michael Shimkin,* Professor of Community Medicine and Oncology, School of Medicine, University of California at San Diego, has written the chapter on *cancer research* for all four editions. *Dr. Harvey R. Butcher, Jr.,* Professor of Surgery, Washington University School of Medicine, has contributed the chapter on *surgery of cancer* to this edition and to the previous edition. The introductory chapter and the chapters on *pathology of cancer* and *radiotherapy of cancer,* written by us, complete this portion of the book.

Chapters 6 through 18 are organized according to systems or organs and are subdivided as necessary. Use of the word *cancer* in the chapter titles indicates that malignant tumors of different origin are included; the term *carcinoma* is used when only malignant epithelial neoplasms are considered, and the rarer tumors of the same area are included in the discussion on differential diagnosis; the word *tumor* is used whenever the frequency or the seriousness of the benign tumors, the difficulties of their differential diagnosis, or the importance of their treatment justifies a joint consideration.

Chapters 19 and 20 are devoted to *Hodgkin's disease* and *leukemia,* respectively, since these two important manifestations of neoplasia justify separate consideration.

The length of some chapters is neither commensurate with the importance of the subject nor with the incidence of the tumor under consideration. This disparity has been deliberate, for we have been guided rather by the desirability of information in certain rare subjects and by the necessity of greater knowledge on some aspects of the more curable forms of cancer. Important recent developments have also received priority on space.

The subject matter in Chapters 6 through 20 is presented under the following headings: anatomy, epidemiology, pathology, clinical evolution, diagnosis, treatment, and prognosis.

Under *anatomy* is included a short description of the relevant structures, with emphasis on details pertinent to the development of cancer, its symptoms and treatment. Also, a detailed discussion of the *lymphatics* of the organ or region is featured because of the unquestionable importance of these vessels in the understanding of the spread and the treatment of malignant tumors.

Under *epidemiology* is gathered whatever useful information is available concerning incidence, ethnic or racial predilections, sex and age ratios, and known or suspected causes. For much of this information we are indebted to *Dr. John C. Bailar III*, and to the members of the staff of the Demography Section of the National Cancer Institute.

Under *pathology* particular attention has been given to the *gross pathology* because of its importance to the clinician as well as to the surgeon and the radiotherapist. In general, the *microscopic pathology* is deliberately brief except when emphasis is deemed necessary. The *metastatic spread* of malignant tumors and the manner and frequency of this spread have been given special consideration.

In our opinion, an understanding of the clinical course and symptomatology of malignant tumors is of cardinal importance. Details are given under the heading of *clinical evolution.*

Under *diagnosis* are outlined the basic required procedures that lead to the recognition and identification of tumors. Included in the discussion of *differential diagnosis* are the various other pathologic entities that may offer difficulties in diagnosis. Rare tumors, not justifying an individual chapter or subdivision, have been listed and their details summarized when they are considered in the differential diagnosis of other more common tumors.

Under *treatment,* the reader will find the various accepted therapeutic procedures, unencumbered by details of technique, dosage, etc. which are of interest only to the informed specialist. The treatment of choice is stressed. We consider ourselves above suspicion of bias, but our choice may be disputed. The fact that our own opinions have undergone changes rather proves that they are not yet petrified. The skeptical reader may find among our comprehensive references a kindred soul who may agree with him.

An effort has been made to offer an idea of the *prognosis.* Under this heading have been included details of the natural history of a particular tumor, the results of various treatments, and the general mortality rates. For some of this information, we are indebted to *Dr. Sidney J. Cutler* and his staff at the End-Results Section of the National Cancer Institute.

We want to thank *Dr. Morton Smith* for his help on the chapter on *cancer of the eye* and *Dr. Frederick T. Kraus* for his constructive review of the chapter on *cancer of the female genital organs.*

A considerably greater number of articles have been consulted than are listed in the *references.* Because of the limitations of space, many of the older references were deleted to accommodate recent ones. The student seeking a chronologic panorama of the literature may consult the references in previous editions of this book.

The text is accompanied by 124 tables, four color plates, and 783 text figures, including clinical photographs, photographs of gross specimens, photomicrographs, and drawings. The quality of the drawings is a credit to Mrs. V. S. (Ackerman) Samter, Mrs. I. (Schubart) Gentile, and Miss E. M. Schubart. Always with the student in mind, we have endeavored to improve the quality of our illustrations.

Throughout the four editions of this work we have received valuable help and advice from numerous colleagues, associates, and students, all of whom have molded our opinions. Without the cooperation of our librarians and present and past secretaries, from whose dedicated efforts we have benefited, this book could not be presented to the medical profession. To all of them, we wish to extend our sincere expression of gratitude.

This book is affectionately dedicated to our wives, *Mrs. Elizabeth F. Ackerman* and *Mrs. Inez G. del Regato,* who have contributed their help as well as their interest and encouragement through the years.

Cancer is in ascendancy throughout the world. More than ever before, research is being done in all possible aspects leading to hoped-for solutions. Clinical research has opened new doors to early and more discriminating diagnoses as well as to more adequate modalities of treatment. To choose from the stream of increasingly cumulative cancer literature is in itself an almost insurmountable task. We have tried our best to add creditably new knowledge to each successive edition. In this endeavor, it is always easier to add than to substitute. Since we believe that the usefulness of this book would be hampered if it were to be published in two volumes, this fourth edition is presented in a new two-column format to conserve space and thus preserve the work in one volume.

Thousands of patients everywhere are depending on the judgment, knowledge, and skill of their various physicians. Although some forms of cancer remain incurable, there is no room for temporizing guesswork, amateurish approaches, or defeatist attitudes. Success depends entirely on intelligent understanding, skillful treatment, and a hopeful, compassionate attitude.

Lauren V. Ackerman

del Regato

Contents

Color plates

Cancer

FOURTH EDITION

Chapter 1

Introduction

Cancer is a generic term used for a large number and wide variety of malignant neoplasms, possibly related to as many different causes, that arise from any of the tissues of the human body (as well as from tissues of other animals) and result in deleterious effects on the host due to their invasive and metastasizing character. Since, in this book and in other medical publications on cancer, the words incidence, prevalence, occurrence, distribution, frequency, and mortality are used, it is important that their meanings be understood.

Incidence expresses the number of new cases diagnosed during one year in some well-defined population. The word incidence is incorrectly used unless it is related to total population. *Incidence rate* is the ratio of incidence to population, usually expressed as the number of new cases per 100,000 persons. Since some malignant tumors occur only in men or in women, their incidence may be expressed in terms of the total male or female population (i.e., as *sex-specific incidence rates*). Since some forms of cancer have a predominance for subjects within a given age group, their frequency may be given in terms of *age-specific rates* to conform to the actual population within such limits.

Prevalence is the number of cases (old or new) known to have been present during a given year and may be expressed as a *prevalence rate* per 100,000 population.

Often what is expressed, without relation to total population or time, is the *frequency* of cases of cancer in a community. Reports of hospital registration of cases and their classification according to organ, histopathology, age, sex, etc. is not incidence but frequency. *Relative frequency* is the percentage of cases of one form of malignant tumor in reference to all cases of cancer.

Mortality rates are expressed as number of patients dead of cancer within one year per 100,000 population.

Incidence rates, prevalence rates, and mortality rates are often calculated for the purpose of comparisons among different areas or populations. If the populations vary markedly in age or sex composition, it may be difficult to interpret any difference in rates unless they are *adjusted* to a single common population. The most usual standard for these conversions in the United States is the composition of the population in the census of 1950.

The *total incidence* of cancer in the different countries of the world may vary considerably for various reasons. One important variant influencing incidence is the average life span of the individuals in a nation, for as the public health improves and life expectancy is increased, cancer becomes a greater problem. The *relative incidence* of certain forms of cancer may vary from one country to the other for specific reasons of race, culture, habits, varied environmental differences, etc. which may hold a clue as to the cause or causes that bring them about (Dunham and Bailar[12]).

Some characteristically high incidences of given malignant tumors can be uncovered only if demographic and diagnostic facilities and information are available for proper evaluation (Marcial[37, 38]). Mortality rates do not give a correct idea of these differences nor of the relative frequency of all tumors. For one thing, mortality statistics disregard the relative curability of the various malignant tumors which differs from one area to another. For another, the diagnosis on death certificates is often based on clinical assumption and seldom verified histologically. In a study of 1,000 autopsies of cases clinically diagnosed as cancer, Willis[66] found that 310 were misdiagnosed as to point of origin and that no cancer was present in fifty-seven. The proportion of errors was greater for deep-seated primary tumors of the stomach, kidney, pancreas, etc. The true

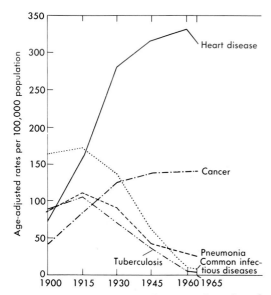

Fig. 1. Age-adjusted mortality rates for selected causes of death in United States in twentieth century. (Courtesy Dr. John C. Bailar, III, and Staff of Demography Section, Biometry Branch, National Cancer Institute.)

trend of cancer mortality can only be evaluated in the light of representative samples of cancer incidence (Levin[33]; Levin et al.[34]).

In 1900 there were in the United States 13 million persons over 45 years of age. By 1948 there were 39 million, in 1958 some 50 million, and in 1968 59 million. Since cancer is prevalent among aged individuals, the number of cases of cancer has increased by virtue of this increase in the relatively aged population alone. More than half of the cancer risk in men is due to cancer of the skin, lung, prostate, and intestine, whereas more than half of the risk in women is due to cancer of the breast, cervix, skin, and intestines. During a lifetime, 1 in every 5 men and 1 in every 4 women may be expected to develop cancer (Goldberg et al.[19]). The 1948-1949 survey of the National Cancer Institute revealed a cancer incidence rate of 40 per 100,000 individuals under 25 years of age, 475 per 100,000 for those under the age of 50 years, and 1900 per 100,000 for those under 75 years of age.

In 1966, with a total population of nearly 200 million in the United States, the estimated numbers of new cases of cancer and

of cancer deaths, for all sites, were 600,000 and 300,000, respectively (National Impact of Cancer[43]). The outstanding recent changes observed are as follows:

1 A considerable decrease in the incidence of cancer of the stomach
2 A marked decrease in the incidence of invasive carcinoma of the cervix
3 A progressive increase in the incidence of acute leukemia
4 A remarkable continued increase in the incidence of carcinoma of the bronchus (Foote et al.[16])

Cancer of the colon and rectum, in both sexes, leads in incidence. Cancer of the breast and uterus remain the most frequent in women and cancer of the lung and prostate are the most frequent in men. The gap between the greater probability of cancer in women than in men is closing due mainly to the persistent greater incidence of cancer of the lung in men. A study of cancer mortality rates of immigrants in the United States shows an excess mortality for cancer of the esophagus and stomach (Haenszel[23, 24]).

The mistaken concept that cancer is the curse that accompanies civilization has been dispelled by the increasing evidence that the incidence of certain forms of cancer is remarkably elevated in underdeveloped populations. Significant differences in the incidence of some malignant tumors are evident, but it is not explained whether they are due to racial or environmental differences in the various countries. Considering their relationship to environment, Higginson[27] proposes that the studied forms of cancer be divided into:

1 Cultural (oral cavity—betel nut)
2 Industrial (bladder—dyes)
3 Idiopathic (marked geographic variations—no evident etiology)
4 Miscellaneous (mostly occurring in children—no geographic variations)

The outstanding observed high incidences are cancer of the *nasopharynx* in China, primary cancer of the *liver* in the South African Bantu, cancer of the *stomach* in Japan, cancer of the *esophagus* in Puerto Rico, certain areas of South Africa, and Japan, and cancer of the *lung, colon, rectum,* and *endometrium* in the United States, United Kingdom, and Denmark (Fig. 4).

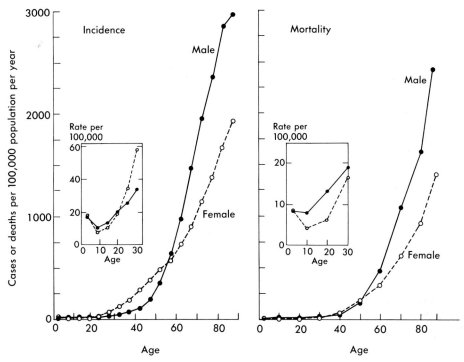

Fig. 2. Cancer incidence and mortality rates for males and females according to age. (Courtesy Dr. John C. Bailar, III, and Staff of Demography Section, Biometry Branch, National Cancer Institute.)

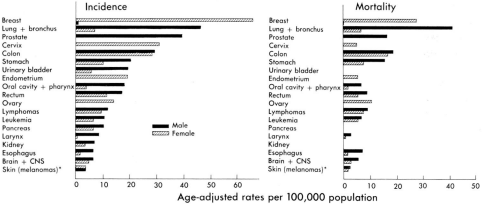

*Excludes skin cancers other than melanomas

Fig. 3. Age-adjusted cancer incidence and mortality rates for major forms of cancer in United States. (Courtesy Dr. John C. Bailar, III, and Staff of Demography Section, Biometry Branch, National Cancer Institute.)

The distribution of patients with cancer admitted to different hospitals varies with the economic, racial, and age composition of the clientele as well as with the type of institution (Table 1). Hospitals devoted to the treatment of aged, rural, indigent patients show a preponderance of cancer of the skin and lip (Modlin[39]). Urban general hospitals, on the other hand, report greater numbers of cancer of the gastro-

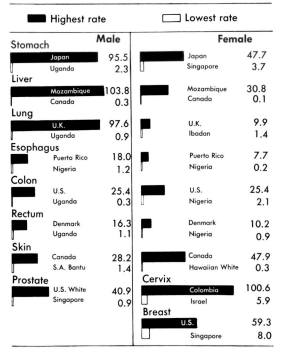

Fig. 4. Highest and lowest observed age-adjusted rates of incidence for selected cancer sites. Wide differences considered to indicate variations in exposure to environmental agents. (From Higginson, John: Annual Report, International Agency for Research on Cancer, World Health Organization, 1968.)

intestinal tract, with autopsy series revealing predominantly deep-seated or rare forms of cancer which motivated post-mortem examination (Saxton et al.[54]).

A knowledge of the relatively greater or lesser incidence of the different forms of cancer in the different age groups is important in clinical practice (Fig. 5). Leukemia, and tumors of the eye, brain, bone, and kidney predominate in patients of both sexes under 15 years of age, whereas cancer of the colon and rectum, cancer of the lung and prostate in men, and cancer of the breast and uterus in women show a relatively higher incidence among those 65 years of age or older. The high cancer death rate in children (Fig. 6) relative to other causes is worthy of note (Paterson[46]). Considering the major forms of cancer, the present yield of diagnosis, the results of treatments, and the mortality, one might estimate arbitrarily the size of the educational and research problems (Table 2) as suggested by Steiner[59].

Diagnosis

The results of the treatment of certain forms of cancer are, to some extent, influenced by the time interval that elapses

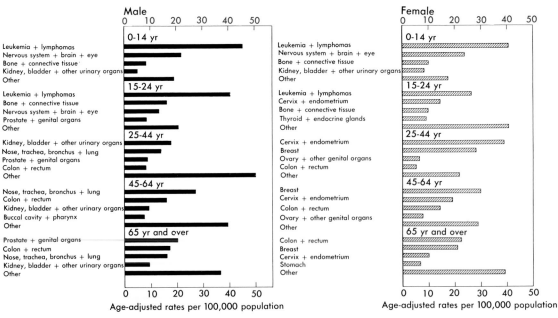

Fig. 5. Cancer incidence rates in broad age groups. (Courtesy Dr. John C. Bailar, III, and Staff of Demography Section, Biometry Branch, National Cancer Institute.)

between the genesis of the lesion and its diagnosis, and the patient is too often blamed for any delay. Large amounts of money have been expended and considerable attention given to the education of the laity as to the early signs and symptoms of cancer in an effort to get them to seek attention promptly. Such education of the public, which should be extended to high school youngsters, is limited by the educational level of population groups and can improve only with the betterment of

Table 1. Comparison of most common forms of cancer reported in patients admitted to a rural cancer hospital and observed at autopsy in a city hospital

Ellis Fischel State Cancer Hospital Columbia, Mo.*			St. Louis City Hospital St. Louis, Mo.†	
% of all cases of cancer	Organ	Rank	Organ	% of cancer autopsies
36	Skin	1	Large bowel	20
13	Breast	2	Lung	15
12	Cervix	3	Stomach	13
7	Lips	4	Prostate	9
6	Large bowel	5	Cervix	8
2.3	Endometrium	6	Breast	7
1.9	Stomach	7	Bladder	6.8
1.8	Melanocarcinoma	8	Esophagus	6.5
1.6	Prostate	9	Pancreas	6.2
1.5	Ovary	10	Brain	6.1

*Data from Modlin, J. J.: Five-year results of treatment, Ellis Fischel State Cancer Hospital, Proceedings of the Thirty-fourth Annual Clinical Congress, American College of Surgeons, pp. 38-41, 1948.
†Data from Saxton, J. A., Jr., Handler, F. P., and Bauer, J.: Cancer and ageing, Arch. Path. (Chicago) **50:**813-827, 1950.

Table 2. Comparison of present control with educational and research problems in cancer

Rank	Primary site of cancer	Number of deaths	% of cancer deaths	Five-year relative survival rate (%)	Estimates of	
					Size of educational problem (%)	Size of research problem (%)
	All malignant neoplasms	303,736	100.0	—	—	—
1	Lung and bronchus	51,348	16.9	8	62	30
2	Colon and rectum	43,474	14.3	45	10	45
3	Breast	27,533	9.1	61	19	20
4	Stomach	17,623	5.8	13	7	80
5	Pancreas	16,360	5.4	1	0	99
6	Prostate	15,941	5.2	49	31	20
7	Lymphatic system	15,802	5.2	30	35	35
8	Leukemia	14,012	4.6	20	5	75
9	Uterus (cervix and endometrium)	13,396	4.4	65	25	10
10	Ovary	9,041	3.0	30	5	65
11	Urinary bladder	8,136	2.7	57	18	25
12	Brain	5,881	1.9	25	15	60
13	Kidney	5,841	1.9	36	14	50
14	Esophagus	5,505	1.8	1	0	99
15	Liver	5,261	1.7	1	0	99
16	Skin (including melanoma)	4,560	1.5	98	1	1
17	Gallbladder and ducts	4,471	1.5	7	0	93
18	Pharynx	2,797	0.9	25	25	50
19	Larynx	2,623	0.9	57	23	20
20	Bone	1,792	0.6	35	15	50
21	Tongue	1,629	0.5	33	17	50
22	Connective tissue	1,318	0.4	51	10	39
23	Thyroid gland	1,008	0.3	78	12	10
	All other sites	28,384	9.3	—	—	—

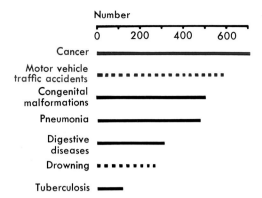

Number

0   200   400   600

Cancer

Motor vehicle
traffic accidents

Congenital
malformations

Pneumonia

Digestive
diseases

Drowning

Tuberculosis

Fig. 6. Cancer in relation to certain other causes of death in children 1 to 14 years of age, England and Wales, 1955. (From Paterson, E.: Malignant tumours of childhood, J. Fac. Radiol. 9:170-174, 1958.)

the standards of general education and general medical care. The American Cancer Society has made a worthwhile effort to make the public conscious of the importance of early diagnosis.

Considerable betterment may be derived from implementation of what we already know: "The vast majority of the cancer patients of today are far from receiving the benefits of knowledge, facilities and skills which have been available for decades; they have benefitted only a few. From early diagnosis to successful treatment the cancer patient is subject to a venturous course. The varied hurdles include: wishful thinking (to which physicians are not immune), geography, luck, misinformation (lay and professional), organization, luck, facilities, skills and a great deal of luck. In short, *too few make it where many could.* In practically every instance of failure there are several physicians, with varied skills, who did their diagnostic and therapeutic best: their very best was not equal to the needs of the case."*

It has long been recognized that one of the best means of obtaining an early diagnosis in certain forms of cancer is the periodic physical examination of symptomless patients (Regaud[51]). These periodic screening examinations, however, must be performed by examiners well trained in

the diagnosis of early cancer. Otherwise, they may convey a sense of false security to the patient. L'Esperance, McFarlane, Schram, and others were pioneers in developing a series of cancer screening clinics in the United States, the function of which was the examination of apparently healthy individuals in an attempt to detect cancer in its early stages. By 1950, there were 251 cancer screening centers in the United States. Levin[33] estimated that only in individuals past 55 years of age will these examinations be capable of yielding more than five cases of cancer for every 1000 individuals examined, because 75% of all cancer in men and 60% of all cancer in women occur past this age. Such "yield" may be considered worthwhile from a public health standpoint, but the cost of finding a case of cancer has been estimated by Newell[44] to be between $7,000 and $10,000.

The approach of cancer detection centers to the problem of early diagnosis has definite shortcomings. The time, personnel, effort, and facilities required make the attempt necessarily limited to a fraction of the population. In some centers, registrants have been obliged to wait from six to twelve months for an examination. Yet, such examinations should be repeated at least once annually if they are to render full usefulness. Further, such centers must, of necessity, undertake to advise patients when diseases other than cancer are discovered. Also, after centers have been in operation for some time, an ever-increasing number of patients are seen who have had a diagnosis of cancer but seek a confirmation of the diagnosis (Garland[17]). The increasing demands make the undertaking limitless, and the activities must be curtailed.

If a great number of individuals are to receive periodic examinations for the detection of symptomless cancer, the procedure should be reversed, with the effort and expense directed toward the aim of making *every doctor's office a cancer detection center.* We endorse MacDonald's statement:

"Detection centers as currently operated contribute little directly to education, lay or professional, and render a minimum service because of the small number of ex-

---

*From del Regato, J. A.: The community cancer hospital (1969 presidential address, American Radium Society), Amer. J. Roentgen. **108**:3-8, 1970.

aminees and their failure to continue periodic examinations."*

Little is accomplished by the early diagnosis of cancer if the proper therapeutic skill and facilities are not made available to the patient. The patients with cancer discovered in "cancer detection" centers are, as a rule, returned to their family physicians, and a large proportion of them are not subsequently followed. Under these circumstances, the very purpose of early diagnosis, the institution of adequate treatment, fails to culminate the effort. This paradox leaves little room for satisfaction, for a cancer that has been diagnosed early is as hopeless in unskilled hands as an advanced lesion. It would therefore seem more logical to devote more attention to the education of the practicing physician. Also, it may be justly considered whether the effort and expense cannot be put to better service in increasing and sponsoring facilities for the training of specialists (tumor pathologists, radiotherapists, and surgeons) on whose skills the therapeutic results will greatly depend. Such facilities provide the best means for improving medical cancer knowledge which unquestionably results in earlier diagnosis and treatment.

Treatment

If the prognosis of a patient with cancer depends in part upon the early diagnosis, the perfection of the treatment, whether it be surgical or radiotherapeutic, is decisive for cure or for death. Surgeons, radiotherapists, or medical oncologists who undertake to treat patients with cancer assume a heavy responsibility, for the life of the patient may be at stake. The constant thought of any physician should be to seek what is best for his patient rather than to impose on him the limitations of his own medical specialty.

It is imperative that the fundamental choice of method and execution of treatment of patients with cancer be entrusted only to those who are adequately trained and qualified. With the advent of radiotherapeutic methods in the beginning of this century, it became more and more

clear that a concerted effort was necessary in the fight against this disease and that such effort was better coordinated within special institutions. The Radium Institute of the University of Paris, The Radium-hemmet of Stockholm, the Memorial Hospital for Cancer and Allied Diseases in New York, and others made the first efforts toward an appropriate organization of facilities and toward the training of workers in this field. In 1929, a special committee of the American Society for the Control of Cancer (Ewing et al.[15]) reported upon the question of therapeutic cancer centers as follows:

". . . We have been forced to conclude that the treatment of many major forms of cancer can no longer be wisely entrusted to the unattached general physician or surgeon, or to the general hospital as ordinarily equipped, but must be recognized as a specialty requiring special training, equipment and experience in all arms of the service. We feel that the futher development of cancer therapeutics will develop along the lines of concentration, organization and specialization. . . . It is well known that the most conspicuous work in the treatment of cancer has long been accomplished by specialists. . . .

"We recommend, as an ideal well within the possibility of accomplishment, the establishment of a limited number of cancer institutes. They should be located in large cities, be prepared to give the best modern treatment, and offer facilities for research and education in the field of cancer."*

To recognize this triple aim of treatment, research, and education is to recognize that cancer institutions be exceptionally well staffed. It would indeed be dangerous to entrust these responsibilities to amateur specialists or to those who have only an incidental or sentimental interest in the disease not only because the results of treatment would suffer considerably, but also because of the unquestionable danger of a spirit of defeat that they would spread among the members of the medical profession. The accumulation of clinical and

---

*From MacDonald, I. Cancer detection, Arizona Med. **10:**1-10, 1953.

*From Ewing, J., Greenough, R. B., and Gerster, J. C. A.: The medical service available for cancer patients in the United States, J.A.M.A. **93:**165-169, 1929.

pathologic data in such institutions creates the background for training additional personnel. Thus the institutions fulfill not only a therapeutic service, but also the much broader service of educating and training specialists upon which the most immediate hope of cancer control depends.

In establishing a cancer institute or hospital, the most important step is choosing the staff. "The staff of the institute must be chosen with the realization that upon this selection alone depends the success or failure of the project; that neither the building nor the size of the endowment but the background, training, experience, spirit, imagination and idealism of the leaders and their associates will be the determining factors.

"The growth of the institute must be controlled and limited solely by its scientific contributions and accomplishments."*

Statewide cancer control campaigns usually include the establishment of a series of small centers for diagnosis and treatment strategically placed throughout the territory. Although it is desirable to bring the diagnostic centers closer to the patients, a dissemination of therapeutic facilities requires equal dissemination of capable personnel that is not generally available. If such centers are created, they should be planned for the purpose of diagnosis and screening of patients and to assist in the posttherapeutic follow-up. At any rate, their creation should never be contemplated in the absence, or to the detriment, of a central institution. In an initial stage of cancer control it is preferable to finance the transportation of indigent patients from their homes to the therapeutic center rather than to create multiple small centers where chances of a permanent cure will be extremely reduced.

The creation of cancer hospitals anywhere, by private institutions or by the state, should not be undertaken without securing the support and wholehearted cooperation of the state medical society. Members of the medical profession have become appreciative of these cancer institutions, and experience shows their growing support for them.

In the United States, the progressive dispersion of medical facilities has limited the development of large full-time staff cancer institutions. Moreover, the work of full-time cancer hospitals must be limited, for the most part, to the indigent population, which constitutes a small part of the cancer problem. *Open-staff cancer hospitals,* working in conjunction and sharing facilities with a general hospital, are a practical answer (Regato[50]). They will preserve the private practice of medicine while concentrating the necessary surgical, pathologic, and readiotherapeutic skills and facilitating the highly needed training of young physicians and continued postgraduate education of the practicing staff. The economics of such small-sized cancer hospitals are not prohibitive. Well-trained specialists participate in the work rendered and the education of residents in training, thus sharing in the work and in the credit of the institution, without losing their individuality and freedom of practice. The institution makes available to the medical community a measure of full-time skills in diagnosis, treatment, and follow-ups, as well as teaching and research facilities, which reinforce the strength of the participating staff.

In 1930 the Board of Regents of the American College of Surgeons,[2] on the advice of its Committee on the Treatment of Malignant Diseases, announced a new policy. Cancer institutes "require very considerable endowments or such generous annual appropriations as can be obtained usually only from the state or national government. They are undoubtedly the most effective method of dealing with the cancer problem but their cost is such that their number will inevitably be somewhat restricted. . . . Where funds sufficient for the maintenance of cancer institutes, research laboratories, or special cancer hospitals are not available, the demand for improved service for cancer cases has resulted in the organization of special cancer clinics in existing general hospitals and of cancer diagnostic clinics in many places in the country in the past few years."* It

---

*From Cutler, M.: Cancer, Illinois Med. J. **71:** 413-419, 1937.

*From American College of Surgeons: Organization of service for the diagnosis and treatment of cancer, Surg. Gynec. Obstet. **51:**570-574, 1930; by permission of Surgery, Gynecology & Obstetrics.

became the policy of the American College of Surgeons to help the development, inspection, and approval of these clinics when they complied with specified minimum standards.

This policy has resulted in the formation of hundreds of tumor clinics in the United States and Canada. The purpose of these clinics in general hospitals is to provide a workable system for close affiliation of the surgeon, pathologist, and radiotherapist to provide a more efficient service for the diagnosis and to place the treatment of cancer in the hands of the most capable few. By the creation of a special cancer service in a general hospital, those members of the staff who are interested in devoting their energies to cancer work can be brought into close cooperation with benefit to the patient, to the hospital, and to the scientific study of cancer. The American College of Surgeons has established a minimum standard for recognition of these clinics (Crowell[7]). Unfortunately, in many instances, a minimum of interest or of capability is not available to fulfill the praiseworthy aims of a tumor clinic. Some tumor clinics have fallen far short of their duties because of the biased attitude of the members, which is most often due to the lack of proper knowledge and experience (Simmons[57]).

Much has been said, though little has been written, about the proper qualifications for the ideal training of men who undertake to treat cancer. There is no question but that a skilled general surgeon may undertake the surgical removal of certain malignant tumors and that his background of general surgery is an asset in this undertaking. It is also true that general radiologists often have taught themselves the difficult art of radiotherapy of cancer and that their worthwhile effort has contributed countless good results. There are also numerous examples of general pathologists who have excelled in the field of tumor pathology. In recent years, hematologists have become interested in chemotherapy of tumors and have become part of the team as so-called medical oncologists.

Generally speaking, however, there is little harmony when these various specialists are obliged to work together. The finely integrated work of a tumor clinic or a cancer hospital may be the best example of scientific cooperation when each member, regardless of his own discipline, has been trained in a background of cancer pathology in an atmosphere of cancer research. It would consequently be desirable that those who undertake cancer work be trained in special institutions where surgeons would become acquainted with the rational possibilities and limitations of radiotherapy, where radiotherapists would look upon surgery as a necessary companion rather than as a competitor, where chemotherapists do not regard all malignant tumors as hopeless cases of acute leukemia, and where the tumor pathologists would become acquainted with the clinical and therapeutic aspects of the disease in addition to its gross and microscopic appearance. "The clinician who neglects to call, instruct, and learn from the pathologist is a bad clinician and the pathologist who avoids the clinic is apt to grow in ignorance with the years."[*]

This view is further reinforced by the fact that the greatest progress yet to be made in cancer control lies in the creation of a greater number of specialists and in the realization that the undertaking of such training cannot be entrusted to those whose interest in cancer is only incidental. There is little incentive for the long training that is necessary in the different disciplines of cancer work, and for this reason the number of specialists actually trained lags far behind the future need for their services. The fellowships that were founded at the Memorial Hospital for Cancer and Allied Diseases in New York by the Rockefeller Foundation in 1926 set a good example. Since 1937, the National Cancer Institute has devoted a great deal of attention to the selection and appointment of trainees in pathology and radiotherapy as well as in surgery of cancer. Thanks in great part to the training grants of the National Cancer Institute, the number of trainees in therapeutic radiology in the United States rose from twenty-five in 1960 to 180 in 1970 (Regato[50a]). The National Cancer

*From Stewart, F. W.: The importance of pathologists in the cancer program, Cancer Teaching Day, New York State Department of Health, Division of Cancer Control 3:55-66, 1943.

Institute Act, to which ninety-four of the then ninety-six members of the United States Senate attached their names, recognized cancer as a medico-socio-economic health problem (Spencer[58]). The National Cancer Institute has become one of the outstanding centers of basic research in cancer, and its hospital in Bethesda, Maryland, has made its own attempt toward clinical research. The vast extramural program of research, including cooperative clinical trials, has contributed beyond expectation to the stimulation and support of cancer research in a variety of directions. The evolution of these plans is a credit to the painstaking efforts of the devoted staff of the National Cancer Institute and to the wise policies of the National Advisory Cancer Council.

Results

"Papers which purport to decide the relative efficacy of different therapeutic procedures in the cancer field on the basis of statistics are often open to suspicion, especially when they deal with small numbers of patients, when the differences in reported cure rates are small, when there is reason to question the correctness of pathologic evaluation of material, and when the individual who reports the series is, from the very nature of his professional accomplishment, not beyond the suspicion of bias."*

It is indeed unfortunate that there is little uniformity in the reporting of clinical results, together with great disregard of essential statistical factors. A common error is the elimination of large numbers of patients lost to follow-up. Another is that of reporting survivals of three months to fifteen years, resulting in an "average" of 4.5 years! Reports of results based on few patients and short follow-up are, of course, of no value. Accuracy of histopathologic diagnosis is crucial. A surgeon whose pathologist calls cancer many lesions that would be diagnosed by others as intraductal papillomas, carcinoma in situ, and adenomatous polyps would appear to obtain better results. A discriminating surgeon

---

*From Stewart, F. W.: The importance of pathologists in the cancer programs, Cancer Teaching Day, New York State Department of Health, Division of Cancer Control 3:19-29, 1943.

who operates only on patients with very early lesions may have a greater "percentage" of cures but may not actually benefit as many patients as his colleague who extends his limits of operability. Comparison of two groups of patients requires not only that they have equal or approximate proportions of disease in different stages (with lymph node involvement, etc.), but also that they be approximately of the same age. Otherwise, two series are not comparable. Differences in histologic varieties may explain differences in results. A series of cases of carcinomas of the breast with a large proportion of intraductal, mucinous, medullary, and highly differentiated tumors will yield better results than one that contains a larger proportion of undifferentiated tumors.

It is conventional to report results of treatment by reference to the five-year survival. In carcinoma of the skin a shorter survival report is not only permissible but more accurate, but in other tumors the proportion of recurrences and metastases may still be high after five years. It may be better to report all cases on a cumulative basis and to compare survival of the patients with that of a similar group of individuals of the same age and sex who do not have cancer. After a given period of time, the annual death rate in both groups will become the same, and it is at this point that patients may be said to be cured.

Berkson and Gage[3] expressed the calculated survival rate as a percentage of the survival rate for normal individuals of similar age and constitution. Thus, if the survival rate for the cancer group is 60% and that of a normal comparable group is 90%, the relative survival rate would be 67% of normal. Ederer et al.[14] studied all the patients with cancer of the large bowel in the state of Connecticut between 1935 and 1954. The annual relative survival rate increased from less than 40% after one year to 90% after the fifth year, but the cancer group showed an excess mortality until the tenth year, when the two groups leveled off.

The differences in the survival curves of two groups of patients may be attributable to differences in the treatment or to differences in the distribution of parameters affecting the life expectancy of those in both groups. True differences can be established only when the frequency of these factors is presented for both groups. If no significant differences exist in the frequencies of such factors, the two groups may be said to be truly comparable, and differences in survival may be ascribed to differences in treatment. The Society of Head and Neck Surgeons has proposed a form for presenting end results (MacComb[35]) and concluded that a modified Berkson-Gage (actuarial) presentation of end results is ideal (Table 3).

There may be natural unavoidable differences among given series of cases. In addition, faulty or biased staging or clinical classification can cause artificial differences, as in carcinoma of the cervix. The same series of cases can be arranged in a number of different ways so that the survival rates may vary widely (Table 4). Unskillful histopathology may force an artificial grouping of patients with and without adenopathy, as in carcinoma of the breast.

Differences in the performance of surgery and radiotherapy are difficult to scrutinize from statistical tables, but the man who wields the knife and the one behind the powerful source of radiations are more decisive than the means that they use. Thus, the reader of medical reports must be discriminating to an extreme and must ask these questions:

1 Are all reported cases histopathologically proved?
2 Are all pertinent factors (age, sex, pathology, etc.) clearly stated?
3 Is the adopted staging clearly defined?
4 Are the pertinent details of the treatment clearly stated?
5 Is any selection or exclusion of material well accounted for?
6 Is there a cumulative follow-up of all patients?

When these facts are available, the reader may be able to arrange the material and estimate relative and absolute survivals in his own fashion. Most modalities of treat-

Table 3. Modified Berkson-Gage presentation of end results*

Interval years after admission	Alive at beginning of interval	Died of cancer during interval	Died of other causes during interval	Lost to follow-up study during interval	With-drawn alive during interval	Effective number exposed to risk	% dying	% surviving in interval	Cumulative % of survivors
1	340	29	21	1	13	322.5	9.0	91.0	91.0
2	276	9	13	1	29	254.5	3.5	96.5	87.8
3	224	10	7	—	37	202.0	5.0	95.0	83.4
4	170	1	9	—	25	153.0	0.7	99.3	82.8
5	135	1	8	—	24	119.0	0.8	99.2	82.1
6	102	1	5	—	21	89.0	1.1	98.9	81.2
7	75	—	5	1	12	66.0	0.0	100.0	81.2
8	57	—	2	1	18	46.5	0.0	100.0	81.2
9	36	—	2	—	7	31.5	0.0	100.0	81.2
10	27	—	1	1	8	22.0	0.0	100.0	81.2

*From MacComb, W. S.: Reporting end results, Amer. J. Surg. 114:486-488, 1967.

Table 4. Cancer of the rectum—five-year survival and cure rates (based on records of twenty-seven general hospitals in Connecticut, 1935-1945)*

Cases	Total cases	Survival rates (%)	Cure rates (%)
Total admissions	735	12.8	7.9
Total proved cases	515	16.5	11.2
Proved cases with known results	503	16.9	11.5
Total resections	237	25.3	15.6
All resections except cases with remote metastases	214	26.6	17.3
All survivals	178	32.0	20.8
Survivals without remote metastases	161	35.4	23.0

*From Ottenheimer, E. J.: Cancer of the rectum, New Eng. J. Med. 237:1-7, 1947.

ment capitalize on minor differences. Yet, considering the small clinical samples on which they are based, only large differences or persistent trends are significant. The trend of clinical comparisons on the basis of unbiased cooperative randomized experiments of a wide scope, although pregnant with difficulties of their own, is the present promise of accurate evaluation of certain forms of treatment. Yet, one should be careful not to allow old prejudices to be given the false dignity of randomized studies which have been inadequately planned and conducted.

REFERENCES

1 Ackerman, L. V.: A program for the control of cancer in Texas, Dedicatory Proceedings, M. D. Anderson Foundation for Cancer Research, 1944.

2 American College of Surgeons: Organization of service for the diagnosis and treatment of cancer, Surg. Gynec. Obstet. 51:570-574, 1930.

3 Berkson, J., and Gage, R. P.: Survival curve for cancer patients following treatment, J. Amer. Statist. Ass. 47:501-515, 1952.

4 Clemmesen, J., and Nielsen, A.: Comparison of age-adjusted cancer incidence rates in Denmark and the United States, J. Nat. Cancer Inst. 19:989-998, 1957.

5 Collins, V. P.: Time of occurrence of pulmonary metastasis from carcinoma of colon and rectum, Cancer 15:387-395, 1962.

6 Cramer, W.: Cancer statistics for morticians and for clinicians, Surg. Clin. N. Amer. 24:1255-1268, 1944.

7 Crowell, B. C.: The role of the cancer clinic in cancer control, Radiology 40:539-542, 1943.

8 Cutler, M.: Cancer, Illinois Med. J. 71:413-419, 1937.

9 Denoix, P. F.: La mortalité par cancer en France en 1959, Bull. Inst. Nat. Hyg. 15:1043-1074, 1960.

10 Denoix, P. F., and Schlumberger, J. R.: Le cancer chez le noir en Afrique française, Monographie de l'Institut National d'Hygiène, no. 12, Paris, 1957.

11 Dorn, H. F., and Cutler, S. J.: Morbidity from cancer in the United States, Pub. Health Monogr. 56:1-208, 1958.

12 Dunham, L. J., and Bailar, J. C.: World maps of cancer mortality rates and frequency ratios, J. Nat. Cancer Inst. 41:155-203, 1968.

13 Ederer, F.: A simple method for determining standard errors of survival rates with tables, J. Chronic Dis. 11:632-645, 1960.

14 Ederer, F., Cutler, S. J., and Eisenberg, H.: Survival of patients with cancer of the large intestine and rectum, Connecticut 1935-1954, J. Nat. Cancer Inst. 26:489-510, 1961.

15 Ewing, J., Greenough, R. B., and Gerster, J. C. A.: The medical service available for cancer patients in the United States, J.A.M.A. 93:165-169, 1929.

16 Foote, F. M., Eisenberg, H., and Honeyman, M. S.: Trends in cancer incidence and survival in Connecticut, Cancer 19:1573-1577, 1966.

17 Garland, L. H.: The case against diagnostic centres, Med. Press, pp. 653-657, July 9, 1958.

18 Gerhardt, P. R., Goldberg, M. P. H., and Levin, M. L.: Incidence, mortality and treatment of breast cancer in New York State, New York J. Med. 55:2945-2951, 1955.

19 Goldberg, I. E., Levin, M. L., Gerhardt, P. R., Handy, V. H., and Cashman, R. E.: The probability of developing cancer, J. Nat. Cancer Inst. 17:155-173, 1956.

20 Greenwood, M.: The natural duration of cancer, Rep. Pub. Health Med. Subj. (London), no. 33, 1926.

21 Griswold, M. H., Cutler, S. J., and Eisenberg, H.: Improvements in cancer survival rates, New Eng. J. Med. 254:1062-1068, 1956.

22 Griswold, M. H., Wilder, C. S., Cutler, S. J., and Pollack, E. S.: Cancer in Connecticut, 1955, Connecticut State Department of Health, Hartford, Conn.

23 Haenszel, W.: Cancer mortality among the foreign-born in the United States, J. Nat. Cancer Inst. 26:37-132, 1961.

24 Haenszel, W.: Report of the working group on studies of cancer and related diseases in migrant populations, Int. J. Cancer 4:364-371, 1969.

25 Handy, V. H., and Goldberg, I. D.: The occurrence of malignancies in children, New York J. Med. 56:258-260, 1956.

26 Heyman, J.: Presentation of results of treatment of cancer, Acta Radiol. (Stockholm) 33:1-8, 1950.

27 Higginson, J.: Environment and cancer, Practitioner 198:621-630, 1967.

28 Higginson, J., and Oettle, A.: Cancer incidence in the Bantu and "Cape Colored" races of South Africa; report of a cancer survey in the Transvaal (1953-1955), J. Nat. Cancer. Inst. 24:589-671, 1960.

29 Hueper, W. C.: Recent developments in environmental cancer, Arch. Path. (Chicago) 58:360-399, 475-523, 645-682, 1954.

30 Kutner, B., and Makover, H.: Delay in the diagnosis and treatment of cancer; a critical analysis of the literature, J. Chronic Dis. 7:95-120, 1958 (extensive bibliography).

31 Leach, J. E., and Robbins, G. F.: Delay in the diagnosis of cancer, J.A.M.A. 135:5-8, 1947.

32 L'Esperance, E. S.: The progress in cancer prevention clinics, Med. Woman's J. 52:25-28, 1945.

33 Levin, M. L.: Some epidemiological features of cancer, Cancer 1:489-497, 1948.

34 Levin, M. L., Haenszel, W., Carroll, B. E., Gerhardt, P. R., Handy, V. H., and Ingraham, S. C., II.: Cancer incidence in urban and rural areas of New York State, J. Nat. Cancer Inst. 24:1243-1257, 1960.

35 MacComb, W. S.: Reporting end results, Amer. J. Surg. 114:486-488, 1967.

36 MacDonald, I.: Cancer detection, Arizona Med. 10:1-10, 1953.

37 Marcial, V. A.: Socioeconomic aspects of the incidence of cancer in Puerto Rico, Ann. N. Y. Acad. Sci. **84**:981-988, 1960.

38 Marcial, V. A.: Cancer morbidity in Puerto Rico, Acta Un. Int. Cancr. **16**:1539-1550, 1960.

39 Modlin, J. J.: Five-year results of treatment, Ellis Fischel State Cancer Hospital, Proceedings of the Thirty-fourth Annual Clinical Congress, American College of Surgeons, pp. 38-41, 1948.

40 Nathanson, I. T., and Welch, C. E.: Life expectancy and incidence of malignant disease. I. Carcinoma of the breast, Amer. J. Cancer **28**:49-53, 1936.

41 Nathanson, I. T., and Welch, C. E.: Life expectancy and incidence of malignant disease. III. Carcinoma of the gastrointestinal tract, Amer. J. Cancer **31**:457-466, 1937.

42 Nathanson, I. T., and Welch, C. E.: Life expectancy and incidence of malignant disease. V. Malignant lymphoma, fibrosarcoma, malignant melanoma and osteogenic sarcoma, Amer. J. Cancer **31**:598-608, 1937.

43 The National Impact of Cancer: Estimated cancer incidence and deaths for 1966, CA **16**: back cover, 1966.

44 Newell, R. R.: Some thoughts concerning cancer detection clinics, News Letter of American College of Radiology **3**:no. 7, 1947.

45 Ottenheimer, E. J.: Cancer of the rectum, New Eng. J. Med. **237**:1-7, 1947.

46 Paterson, E.: Malignant tumours of childhood, J. Fac. Radiol. **9**:170-174, 1958.

47 Paterson, R., and Tod, M.: The presentation of the results of cancer treatment, Brit. J. Radiol. **23**:146-150, 1950.

48 Pedersen, E., and Magnus, K.: Cancer registration; the incidence of cancer in Norway, 1953-1954, Cancer Registry of Norway, Monograph no. 1, 1959, pp. 1-183.

49 Quisenberry, W. B., Tilden, I. L., and Rosengard, J. L.: Racial incidence of cancer in Hawaii; a study of 3,257 cases of malignant neoplastic disease, Hawaii Med. J. **13**:449-451, 1954.

50 del Regato, J. A.: The community cancer hospital (1969 presidential address, American Radium Society), Amer. J. Roentgen. **108**:3-8, 1970.

50a del Regato, J. A.: The training of therapeutic radiologists (editorial), Radiology **95**:703-704, 1970.

51 Regaud, C.: What is the value and what should be the organization and equipment of institutions for the treatment of cancer by radium and x-rays? Surg. Gynec. Obstet. **44** (suppl. II): 116-136, 1927.

52 Robbins, G. F., Conte, A. J., Leach, J. E., and McDonald, M.: Delay in diagnosis and treatment of cancer, J.A.M.A. **143**:346-348, 1950.

53 Saxen, E., and Korpela, A.: Cancer incidence in Finland, 1954, Ann. Chir. Gynaec. Fenn. **47**(suppl. 79):1-32, 1958.

54 Saxton, J. A., Jr., Handler, F. P., and Bauer, J.: Cancer and ageing, Arch. Path. (Chicago) **50**:813-827, 1950.

55 Shimkin, M. B.: Duration of life in untreated cancer, Cancer **4**:1-18, 1951.

56 Shimkin, M. B.: The epidemiology of cancer (symposium on cancer), Mod. Med., pp. 81-87, 1960.

57 Simmons, C. C.: Survey of state-aided cancer clinics, New Eng. J. Med. **227**:458-462, 1942.

58 Spencer, R. R.: The place of the National Cancer Institute in the cancer program, Radiology **42**:493-498, 1944.

59 Steiner, P. E.: An evaluation of the cancer problem, Cancer Res. **12**:455-464, 1952.

60 Steiner, P. E.: Cancer and race; with emphasis on the American and African Negroes and on the Mexican, Acta Un. Internat. Cancr. **13**: 959-966, 1957.

61 Steiner, P. E.: Cancer research in Trans-Saharan Africa, Cancer Res. **18**:489-490, 1958.

62 Stewart, F. W.: What may be logically expected from pre- and post-operative radiation in mammary cancer, Cancer Teaching Day, New York State Department of Health, Division of Cancer Control **3**:19-29, 1943.

63 Stewart, F. W.: The importance of pathologists in the cancer program, Cancer Teaching Day, New York State Department of Health, Division of Cancer Control **3**:55-66, 1943.

64 Welch, C. E., and Nathanson, I. T.: Life expectancy and incidence of malignant disease. II. Carcinoma of the lip, oral cavity, larynx and antrum, Amer. J. Cancer **31**:238-252, 1937.

65 Wells, H. G.: Cancer statistics as they appear to a pathologist, J.A.M.A. **88**:399-403, 477-482, 1927.

66 Willis, R. A.: Pathology of tumours, St. Louis, 1948, The C. V. Mosby Co., pp. 66-91.

Chapter 2

Cancer research

Michael B. Shimkin, M.D.*

The aim of cancer research is to find new knowledge relating to the causes, diagnosis, and treatment of cancer and to translate this knowledge to effective application in man. The target of cancer research is to reduce the impact of neoplastic diseases, which in the United States alone account every year for 600,000 new cases and 300,000 deaths among a population of 200 million.

Cancer research, by definition, is research directed toward the solution of a major medical problem. It must draw its sustenance from all sciences and utilize their advances. In turn, it generates discoveries that are of profound importance to the basic biomedical sciences.

The National Cancer Institute Act of 1937 is a dedication of United States resources toward the solution of the cancer problem. It is ably supported by public participation through the American Cancer Society and other voluntary health agencies. Endeavors toward the solution are of wide international scope as well. Great Britain, the Soviet Union, Germany, Japan, and many other countries also have impressive cancer research programs.

The main trends in cancer research throughout the world continue to be on the viral causation of cancer, chemical carcinogenesis, biochemistry, chemotherapy, and epidemiology. It is also becoming realized that the effective application of research findings, as well as of established procedures, to actual use by man involves research on human motivation and systems of delivery of preventive and curative methods to populations.

It is both inevitable and heartening that any review of cancer research that can be

written is outdated by the time it is published, for such reviews can be only transient progress reports.

Historical aspects

Clinical observations, classifications, and theories of cancer extend to the dawn of medical history (Wolff[80]). But it was not until the flowering of biology and pathology in the nineteenth century that a scientific approach to neoplastic diseases became feasible.

The foundation of oncology rests upon the compound microscope and the use of this tool in the study of normal and diseased tissues, facilitated by the techniques of preparation and staining of tissues for histologic examination. It was shown that the neoplastic diseases are characterized by an abnormal proliferation of cells that infiltrate, destroy contiguous tissues, and transplant to distant sites and grow there as metastases. In general, these neoplastic cells resemble those of the tissues in which they arise or some developmental stage of the cells of such tissue.

Johannes Müller, Leydig, Virchow, Cohnheim, and Ribbert were among the many illustrious students of the nineteenth century who laid the foundations of our present knowledge of neoplastic diseases. Their labors led to the description and classification of tumors, to differential diagnosis, and to the description of the course of the neoplastic processes. The observations were so exhaustive that few fundamental additions have been made to the gross and microscopic morphology of neoplastic diseases since their time. The limiting factor was the power of the microscope. Another great period of morphology is now upon us with the use of the electron microscope.

Progress in science depends, to a great

---

*Professor of Community Medicine and Oncology, School of Medicine, University of California at San Diego, La Jolla, Calif.

extent, upon data derived from observations of the effects of various controllable and reproducible environments upon a relatively stable material. In the biologic sciences, this material is most often some animal in which the condition to be studied can be reproduced. Experimental work on neoplastic diseases could not be undertaken on a significant scale until suitable material became available. Novinsky, in 1876, successfully transplanted tumors in dogs. In 1889, Hanau transplanted a carcinoma from rat to rat, and a few years later Moreau performed similar experiments with mice. It was not until 1903, however, when Jensen's systematic work on transplantable tumors became widely known, that the true value of their contributions was realized. A favorable experimental material had been found, and cancer research began in earnest (Oberling[55]).

The early investigators working with neoplasms arising in mice and other animals had to establish that the tumors were neoplastic in nature. Demonstrations of the development of metastases, recurrent growth, and infiltration and careful histologic observations left no doubt that these tumors were closely similar to malignant neoplasms in man (Woglom[79]). The validity of using tumors in animals in cancer research is now taken for granted. This does not, however, imply that the processes involved in the genesis of such tumors are identical. Indeed, it is dangerous to extrapolate from one species to another and even from one type of neoplasm to others in the same species. Until much more is known about cancer, it is best considered as a group of diseases rather than as one disease entity.

Nature of cancer

Cancer is a disease of the cell that is transferred to the descendants of the cell. It is recognized by the behavior of a population of abnormal cells within a normal tissue, as manifested by varying degrees of morphologic disorientation, aggressive growth, and invasion, with ultimate destruction of the normal cell population (Shimkin[66]).

The evidence that cancer is a characteristic of individual cells is based upon extensive experiments on the transplantation of tumors since the turn of this century. The investigations culminated in the work of Furth and Kahn,[21] who succeeded in transmitting leukemia in mice with a single cell. With the advent of reproducible methods of tissue culture and of heterotransplantation of tumors, some cancer cells of human origin have been grown in tissue culture, carried in the tissues of a laboratory rodent, and retransplanted into the species of origin with the maintenance of morphologic and biochemical characteristics. Insofar as the postulates of Koch regarding bacterial diseases can apply to a dissimilar situation, the postulates have been fulfilled for cancer cells.

The development of sarcomas from fibroblasts grown in tissue culture was convincingly documented by the research groups of Earle[16] and of Gey.[23] Several cell lines were developed from a single isolated fibroblast (Sanford et al.[60]). One cell line produced sarcomas in almost all mice that were inoculated with it, two lines produced no tumors, and another line gave rise to very few sarcomas unless the mice were irradiated. In these experiments, one type of mammalian cell was converted into neoplastic cells entirely removed from the systemic reactions of the original host and in an entirely heterologous culture medium.

The basic characteristics of neoplasms are autonomy and anaplasia. Both are relative terms distinguishing cancer quantitatively from normal processes of growth and differentiation.

Autonomy is the disregard by cancer for normal limitations of growth. The penetration of normal tissue boundaries by cancer and the occurrence of metastasis still represent the best evidence of malignancy. Neoplasms show a wide variation in the degree of autonomy. Some transplantable tumors in animals grow in practically every site of inoculation and in almost every strain of the species. Others survive and proliferate under specialized conditions. Similar relative autonomy is encountered in man, such as the partial dependence of some prostatic and mammary cancers upon the hormonal substrate of the host. Some tumors will grow under specific conditions in unrelated hosts, such as in the anterior chamber of the eye, on embryonated eggs

(Murphy[53]), or in cortisone-prepared rodents (Toolan[73]).

Anaplasia refers to loss of organization and of useful function. There is a wide spectrum, from tumors closely resembling normal tissue and continuing to perform some functions of the normal counterparts to neoplasms so disorganized that no guess can be made regarding the tissue of origin. The chief activity of most neoplasms appears to be self-propagation. They have characteristics that no longer fit them into the body physiology, which depends upon intricate and well-balanced adjustments, but obey their own laws of unbridled initiative at the expense of the well-being of the host. This departure from normal growth, including embryonic growth, may represent either the acquisition of new properties or the loss of control mechanisms present in normal cells. The rate of growth alone is not a criterion of neoplasia, since many normal growth processes exceed the growth rate of many tumors.

The neoplastic process is not a single event that endows cells with immutable, full-blown malignant characters. The stepwise, slow development of many neoplastic entities in man, as well as in animals, has been amply demonstrated. Furth[20] showed such stages in the evolution of several induced tumors of the endocrine system in rodents, and Berenblum[4] introduced the concept of successive developmental stages of carcinogenesis and cocarcinogenesis of the skin. In man, the transition of carcinoma in situ of the uterine cervix to the invasive neoplasm represents an analogous gradual acquisition of new characters by cell populations.

Cancer as a continued growth depends not only upon the characteristics of the abnormal cells, but also upon the existence of environmental conditions compatible with survival. Tumor cells can be demonstrated in distant organs of animals within a short time after implantation of tumors subcutaneously, yet few such cells lead to eventual gross metastases.

Fully established neoplasms maintain their appearance and other characteristics recapitulating their cellular properties through fission. They reproduce "true to type" in metastatic sites and upon transplantation into compatible hosts. Alterations in structure and behavior occur, of course, usually as "dedifferentiation" toward decreased organization. Occasional regression and disappearance of established malignant neoplasms are usually attributable to interruption of their nutrition, such as by vascular occlusion, rather than to loss of neoplastic properties or to other alterations in the neoplastic cells themselves (Everson and Cole[18a]). In heterozygous hosts, lack of growth or survival of tumors is attributable to immune reactions to foreign tissue.

Numerous observers have attempted to find specific morphologic differences between normal and neoplastic cells. Since any tissue is susceptible to neoplastic transformation and since tumors often closely resemble such tissues of origin, it is not surprising that no such universal characteristic has been found. Significant changes are detectable, however, when specific neoplasms are compared with their tissue of origin. Cancer cells tend to be larger than normal cells. There is an alteration in the nucleus-cytoplasm relationship, and chemical studies have shown increased amounts of ribonucleic acid in neoplastic cells, suggesting that the heterochromatic region of the chromatin is significantly altered. The nucleolus is usually more prominent, or more than one is often observed. A greater proportion of the cells appear to be in normal or abnormal mitosis. Chromosomal aberrations are frequently seen in neoplasms, including irregularity, suppression of the spindle, and alterations in number, size and shape.

Biochemical studies on cancer, aimed at discovering the molecular basis for neoplasia, have been extensive but inconclusive. If neoplasia is basically an alteration of deoxyribose nucleotides that carry the codes of identity and heredity, it would represent a change in perhaps a hundred molecules of multimillion-molecule structures. Techniques now available are yet inadequate to distinguish such subtle differences, except as they may be manifested by enzymatic and other functions.

Findings of systematic biochemical studies, such as those of Greenstein,[26] correlate in biochemical terms the general biologic properties of tumors.

The loss of organization and function

(i.e., anaplasia) is demonstrated by reduction or loss of specific enzymatic systems of specialized tissues of origin. There is usually a diminution in respiratory enzymes such as cytochrome and cytochrome oxidase.

Neoplasms as a whole tend to converge toward a common biochemical class, showing less diversity than normal tissues. This general conclusion is based upon studies with transplantable tumors that are highly selected, fairly homogeneous as to cell type, and usually rapidly growing. The observations suggest that tumors may form a separate type of tissue regardless of etiology or histogenesis. Data on enzyme systems or vitamin content in neoplasms in man show as great a diversity of values in neoplasms as in normal tissues, but such data are seldom corrected for the stromal elements of the tumor. Glutamine and asparagine are split faster by hepatoma than by liver extracts, and there is much greater incorporation of certain amino acids into hepatoma slices than into liver slices. The increased rate of protein synthesis by hepatoma may be related to decrease in activity of certain proteolytic mechanisms, so that the decreased rate of catabolism may be an important feature in the progressive growth of tumors.

Glycolysis under aerobic and anaerobic conditions, established by Warburg,[76] remains as one of the most constant and significant differences between neoplastic and most normal tissues. Most normal tissues accumulate lactic acid in the absence of oxygen, but most neoplasms accumulate lactic acid under aerobic as well as under anaerobic conditions. Glycolysis and lactic acid production can no longer be considered characteristic of neoplasia in view of recent work by Weinhouse on the "minimal deviation" hepatomas developed by Morris. In these well-differentiated tumors the enzymes for the metabolism of glucose are lost or decreased, and the energy needed by the tumor is derived from fats through other enzyme systems (Adelman et al.[1]).

Searches for specific abnormal constituents in neoplastic tissue that are absent in normal tissues are being actively pursued. Newer methods of fractionation and analysis of tissue components, combined with sensitive immunochemical reactions, show that some neoplasms contain specific antigens that distinguish them from normal tissues. Particularly intriguing are reports of immunologic detection of a viral component in human sarcomas (Morton et al.[51a]) and of circulating carcinoembryonic antigen in patients with colorectal cancer (Thomson et al.[72a]).

Distribution of cancer

Neoplasms of many different sites and tissues occur in all species of animals that have been studied in sufficiently large numbers for a sufficiently long time. They occur in lower forms such as amphibia and fish (Schlumberger and Lucke[62]), and many plants develop a cellular reaction that appears to be analogous to cancer (Braun[8]). This wide occurrence of neoplasms in nature excludes specific constituents of diets and other environmental exposures that man has developed in the process known as civilization from general implication as the only or the main factor responsible for cancer.

Practically every type of neoplasm that is seen in man has also been observed to occur in the mouse. The most common tumors in unselected mouse populations are the adenocarcinoma of the breast and the adenomatous pulmonary tumor. In rats, the most common tumors are fibroadenoma of the breast and leukemia. In dogs, mammary, testicular, and adrenocortical tumors are among the most frequent types of neoplasia. Monkeys develop but few malignant tumors. Leukemia in fowl, adenocarcinoma of the kidney in frogs, and a melanotic tumor in fish are among the so-called spontaneous tumors that have been studied in lower forms of animals. "Spontaneous tumor" merely implies that such neoplasms appear without a known stimulus or agent being applied to the animal. In other words, they are tumors of unknown etiology.

Neoplastic diseases are found in all human populations that have been adequately studied. There are some striking racial and regional differences in the occurrence of specific types of cancer, although data are insufficient to conclude what proportion of such differences is genetic and what proportion is attributable to environmental factors such as diet and habits.

In comparison with the white population of the United States, the following differences in the occurrence of cancer are noteworthy:

1 High incidence of cancer of the stomach in Scandinavia, Iceland, and Japan
2 High incidence of primary cancer of the liver in south and west Africa
3 High incidence of cancer of the nasopharynx in China
4 High incidence of cancer of the urinary bladder in Egypt
5 Low incidence of cancer of the breast in Japan
6 Low incidence of cancer of the uterine cervix in Israel and in Jewish women elsewhere
7 Low incidence of cancer of the skin in Negroes
8 Low incidence of cancer of the prostate in Japan and China (Segi[63])

Role of heredity

One of the first observations made on neoplasms in animals was that they occurred more frequently in certain cages or groups of animals. It was demonstrated that cancer was not contagious in the ordinary sense of the term and that the distribution was determined primarily according to family relationships. Attention was thus directed toward the hereditary or genetic aspects.

The earlier work attempted to explain occurrence of tumors on the basis of simple recessive or dominant inheritance. With more experience in complex characters such as tumors, it became evident that no simple interpretation was possible and that susceptibility to tumors is not a character with alternative (all-or-none) expression but is expressed in degree. The data also indicate that all tumors could not be grouped as a single character. As early as 1913, Lathrop and Loeb[43] were able to show that different mouse families had characteristic types of tumors, and with highly inbred strains it was possible to demonstrate that different types of tumors are inherited as separate characters.

A major obstacle in the early work on tumor inheritance was that of heterogeneous stocks. The development by geneticists of homozygous strains marks one of the major contributions of cancer research. Inbreeding per se does not influence the development of neoplasms other than concentrating by segregation a particular type of tumor within the strain.

There are over seventy strains of homozygous mice available in various laboratories throughout the world. The most commonly used strains include the following:

1 Strain A, developing a high percentage of pulmonary adenomatous tumors, and, in breeding females, of mammary tumors
2 Strain C3H, developing a high incidence of mammary tumors and of hepatomas
3 Strain BALB/c, developing a high incidence of pulmonary tumors and of lymphatic leukemia
4 Strain dba, developing a high percentage of mammary tumors
5 Strain C57 black, a tumor-resistant strain that develops very few mammary or pulmonary tumors (Green[25])

Analysis of the genetic factors involved in the susceptibility to these tumors by means of hybridization experiments with homozygous mice has been made most extensively with mammary tumors and pulmonary tumors. Females resulting from the matings of high-tumor strain females to low-tumor strain males developed mammary tumors in approximately the same incidence as that of the high-tumor strain, but when the reciprocal cross was made (i.e., when low-tumor strain females were mated with high-tumor strain males), the tumor incidence in the hybrid offspring was that of the low-tumor strain. Bittner[6] found that the extrachromosomal factor that was involved was transmitted through the milk (Moulton[52]). The agent in the milk is now established to be a virus.

Pulmonary tumors in mice are especially under the control of genetic factors. The incidence and the number of tumors in the lungs can be increased by numerous chemical agents. Such carcinogens increase and speed up the neoplastic reaction in the degree of susceptibility possessed by the animals. The genetic factors influencing susceptibility are multiple and are associated with at least five known genes (Heston[32]).

Noncontroversial information on genetic factors involved in neoplasia in man is extremely limited, particularly because of the heterogeneity of the species. A number of neoplasms and precancerous conditions, particularly xeroderma pigmentosum, retinoblastoma, and multiple polyposis of the colon, have strong hereditary factors. In addition, cancer of the breast, uterus, and rectum and leukemia may show hereditary tendencies. There is also an association between blood group A and gastric cancer and between mongolism and acute granulocytic leukemia. Many tumors may be inherited as characteristics showing incomplete dominance, although the possibility of multiple-factor inheritance cannot be excluded. The tendency to tumor localization also has suggestive hereditary bases. The association of Wilms' tumor and several congenital malformations (Miller et al.[49]) may have either genetic or extrachromosomal explanation.

Role of environment

The development of cancer in a species is influenced by a wide variety of changes in the internal and external environments of the host. The degree of effect on the development of neoplasms may be correlated roughly with the degree or extent of such changes. The aspects of internal environment that have been studied most thoroughly are the hormonal status and nutrition.

Hormonal inbalance in mice leads to the appearance of at least five types of tumors in tissues especially dependent upon hormonal secretions in their physiology (Shimkin[64]). Excessive estrogenic stimulation, endogenously or exogenously supplied, leads to the development of mammary, testicular, pituitary, or uterine tumors in appropriate strains of animals. Oophorectomy, causing gonadal deficiency and pituitary hyperfunction, reduces the number of mammary tumors but in one strain of mice induces adrenal cortical carcinomas that, in turn, can be prevented by an exogenous supply of estrogen. Ovarian tumors in rats or mice can be produced by the ingenious technique of transplanting ovaries into the spleen of castrate animals, thus producing gonadal deficiency through deactivation of estrogens by the liver and compensatory production of gonadotropic pituitary hormones.

The age of the animal at the time of exposure to a carcinogen profoundly influences the carcinogenic reaction. Neonatal rodents are more susceptible than adults, perhaps due to the underdevelopment of inducible detoxifying enzymes and to relative immune incompetence. When rats of certain strains are given single oral doses of 7,12-dimethylbenz[a]anthracene, the material can be recovered within six hours from every tissue in the body. Yet in mature female rats, mammary cancer is the predominant neoplastic response. In the mature male, few breast cancers appear, but cancers of the skin and sebaceous glands become prominent. In very young rats, subcutaneous sarcomas are elicited. Thus, the susceptibility of the end-organs to carcinogenesis varies with age and sex, and the limited responses suggest specific, dynamically changeable reaction sites.

In general, the incidence of tumors in mice can be lowered by placing the animals on restricted diets (Tannenbaum and Silverstone[72]). Reduction of the ad libitum caloric consumption by one-third practically eliminates the appearance of mammary carcinoma. Reduction in specific dietary constituents also influences the incidence and time of appearance of certain neoplasms. The incidence of methylcholanthrene-induced leukemia is lower in mice on a low-cystine diet than in those on a full diet. The effectiveness of azo dyes in producing hepatomas in rats appears to parallel their effectiveness in lowering hepatic riboflavin, and certain diets are protective against the carcinogenic effect in relation to their riboflavin content.

The incidence and time of appearance of neoplasms can be affected by other environmental factors. For example, mammary tumors appear at an earlier age in mice kept in isolation than in animals sharing the same restricted quarters (Andervont[2]). It is evident that the number of such influences is almost limitless and that they may be interrelated. One factor may produce secondary effects, such as the influence of diet on hormonal metabolism or the influence of isolation on food intake and temperature. Moreover, the hormonal and nutritional physiology are also affected by the genetic background of the organism.

Hormonal and nutritional factors are

also associated with certain tumors in man. Breast cancer is more frequent in nulliparous than in multiparous women, whereas carcinoma of the uterine cervix is more frequent among women with active reproductive experiences than among abstinent women. Iodine deficiency may be a factor in the genesis of thyroid cancer. Deficiency of proteins and of vitamins may be implicated in the development of pharyngeal cancer among individuals with the Plummer-Vinson syndrome.

Carcinogenic agents

Induced neoplasms are tumors that can be evoked at will in animals exposed to certain chemical and physical substances. The agents that are capable of eliciting a neoplasm are usually designated as carcinogenic. By usage, the term is not restricted to the induction of carcinoma but includes all neoplasms. Direct causative relation between the agent employed and the neoplasm produced is not implied. All that can be said is that following the injection or exposure to a certain procedure, certain tumors arise in significantly higher incidence than in untreated animals. The same considerations apply to industrial and general environmental carcinogens that have been established to increase the risk to cancer in human populations.

Several carcinogenic agents were known from clinical experience long before the extension of the investigations to the laboratory. Perhaps the first was the description by Percival Pott,[57] in 1775, of scrotal carcinoma in men exposed to constant contact with soot. In 1915, Yamagiwa and Ichikawa[81] reported that continuous painting of rabbits' ears with tar led to the appearance of carcinoma. The observation was rapidly extended to the rat and mouse, and the simplicity of the method led to its extensive use in cancer research. The histologic and gross changes following cutaneous application, subcutaneous injection, and introduction into other sites were meticulously described. The influence of dosage, length of exposure, variants in the tar, and the conditions of the animals and their environment were carefully studied. It was established that not all tars were equally efficacious in eliciting neoplasms and that some were entirely devoid of activity.

Polycyclic hydrocarbons

The successful search for the specific constituent that was active in tar was the achievement of the British group under the leadership of Kennaway and Cook. The active ingredient was found to be benzpyrene (Fig. 7). As a matter of fact, the first carcinogenic polycyclic hydrocarbon compound to be described, in 1930, was dibenzanthracene (Kennaway[39]). Further modifications of the benzanthracene nucleus led to the synthesis and biologic testing of numerous related compounds. Particular interest was aroused when one of the most active of the carcinogenic hydrocarbons, methylcholanthrene, was synthesized from bile acids. The structural molecular resemblance between the carcinogenic hydrocarbons, cholesterol, bile acids, and the steroid hormones that were also being isolated and synthesized during this period developed high hopes that a common molecular structure and the physiologic elaboration of the body of compounds similar to the hydrocarbons could clarify the cancer problem.

The carcinogenic hydrocarbons are usually painted on the skin, which evokes cutaneous carcinomas, or injected subcutaneously, which induces sarcomas at the site of injection. Carcinoma of the kidney and the stomach, brain tumors, and rhabdomyosarcomas have also been elicited upon injection into appropriate tissues. The feeding of carcinogenic hydrocarbons evokes intestinal adenocarcinomas in mice, and intravenous injection increases the number of pulmonary tumors. The action is not limited to the site of application. Pulmonary tumors appear following subcutaneous injection, and mammary tumors and leukemia are evoked in certain strains of mice.

Subcutaneous, cutaneous, and brain tumors are also produced in the rat, and, with somewhat larger doses, fibrosarcomas and liposarcomas appear in guinea pigs at the site of injection. Other species such as dogs and monkeys that have been tested are much more resistant.

It was soon found that even in mice the carcinogenic reaction was influenced by so many factors that only a relative definition is feasible of the property of carcinogenesis of any chemical. Limitations are

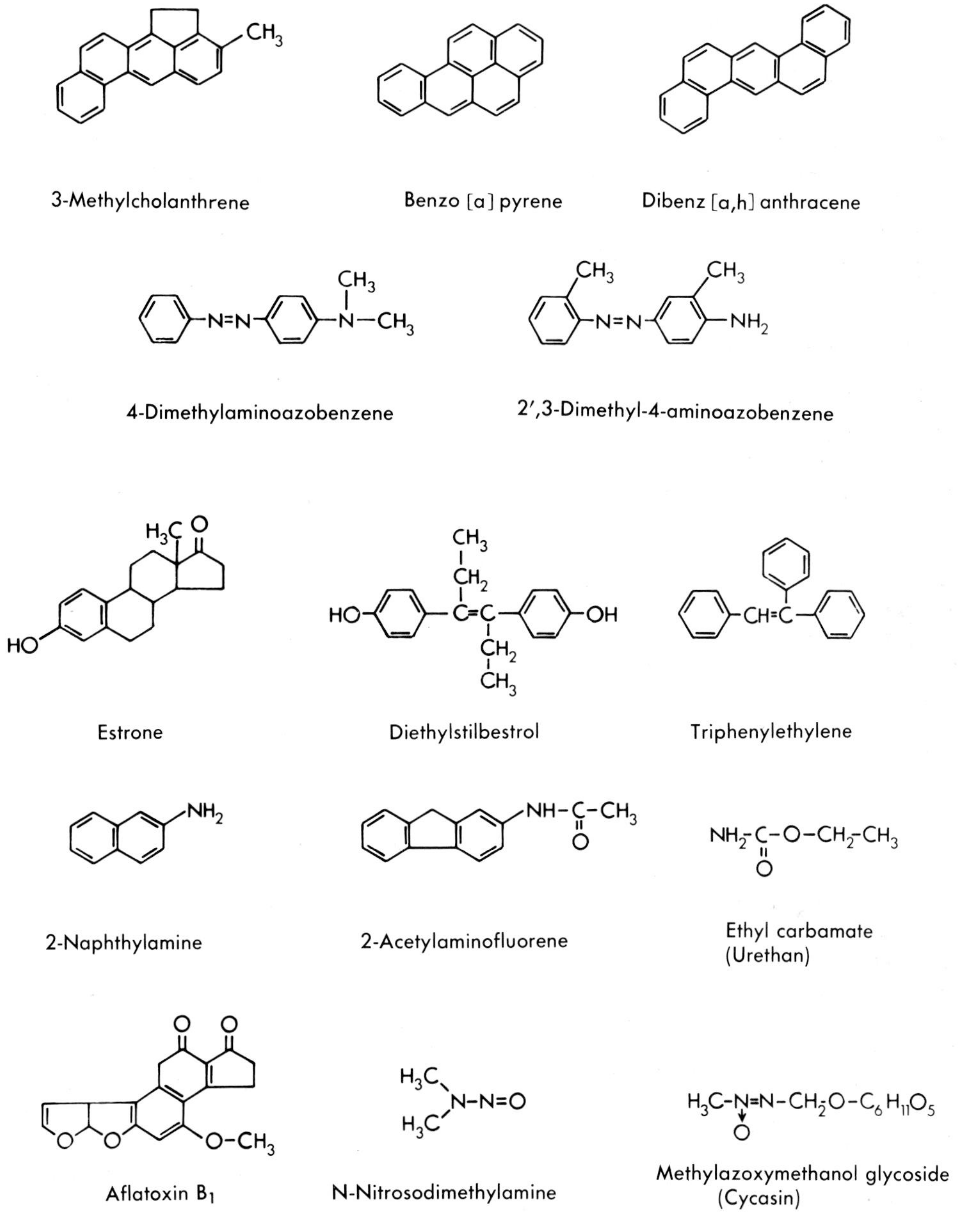

Fig. 7. Some carcinogenic chemicals. **First row,** Polycyclic hydrocarbons. **Second row,** Amino-azo dyes. **Third row,** Estrogenic compounds. **Fourth and fifth rows,** Other important carcinogens.

imposed by the strain of animal and its age and condition, by the site, method, and dose of injection, and by the physical state of the preparation.

Sarcomas in mice at the site of injection of nonsaponifiable lipid fractions of human livers and other tissues may be due to some endogenously produced carcinogens perhaps related to the polycyclic hydrocarbons (Schabad[61]). Smegma has been shown to be carcinogenic to the skin of the mouse.

In man, exposure is usually to crude mixtures of materials, so that incrimination of single chemicals is difficult. Nevertheless, compounds of the polycyclic hydrocarbon type are probably the active carcinogens in the industrial skin cancers of workers with coal tar, pitch, soot, asphalt, shale, petroleum, and paraffin oils (Hueper[36]). Similar compounds are also important in the production of cancer of the lung, larynx, and oral cavity among tobacco smokers (United States Surgeon General's Advisory Committee on Smoking and Health[75]) and in the increased incidence of respiratory cancers among city dwellers exposed to atmospheric pollutants.

Estrogens and other hormones

Among the chemical compounds whose carcinogenic action is limited to certain specific tissues are the estrogens, a generic term that encompasses synthetic chemicals such as diethylstilbestrol and triphenyl ethylene (Fig. 7), as well as physiologically produced chemicals with estrogenic activity.

The relationship of hormones to cancer was one of the earliest areas of interest in cancer research. Leo Loeb in 1918 demonstrated that breast cancer could be prevented in female mice if the ovaries were removed. Cancer of the breast could be induced in male mice, which do not develop breast cancer, if they were castrated and had ovaries implanted under the skin. With the advent of pure estrogenic compounds, Lacassagne[41] of France, in 1932, reported that these also would evoke breast cancer in male mice of susceptible strains. Subsequent research showed that breast cancer in mice required the presence of three biologic complexes: genetic susceptibility, hormonal milieu, and the Bittner virus.

The amounts of estrogenic hormones necessary for mammary carcinogenic action depend upon the physiologic potency and the dose of the compounds. Treatment must be prolonged if preparations of relatively short duration, such as oily solutions, are employed. A single subcutaneous implantation of pellets producing constant, prolonged absorption of the chemicals is sufficient to elicit mammary tumors at doses calculated to be not above those physiologically produced by mice.

The injection of estrogens into experimental animals has led to the appearance of several other types of tumors (Gardner[22]). These include, in certain strains of mice, pituitary adenoma, interstitial cell tumors of the testis, carcinoma of the uterine cervix, and leukemia. Fibromyomatous overgrowths are produced in the subserosa or myometrium of guinea pigs. These growths appear throughout the abdominal cavity, and although they invade contiguous organs, the tumors regress when estrogenic treatment is discontinued.

The carcinogenic effects of estrogens in rodents have not been demonstrated conclusively in man. The extensive use of estrogens and other hormones since their introduction into clinical practice thirty years ago has not led to an increase in the occurrence of breast cancer in women or in men. Earlier reports of breast cancer in men treated with estrogens for prostatic cancer may have been metastases from the prostate rather than primary lesions of the breast. Nevertheless, the carcinogenic activity of estrogens in rodents remains a relevant consideration in the use of such compounds in man.

Azo dyes and other compounds

The occurrence of cancer of the bladder in workers of the aniline dye industry led to the study of various chemicals in this group. Prolonged subcutaneous injection of 2-naphthylamine (Fig. 7) compound in dogs led to the appearance of papillomas and carcinomas of the bladder (Hueper[35]).

A similar site specificity had been determined for a group of azo dyes (Miller and Miller[48]). Incorporated into the diet and fed to mice or rats, aminoazotoluene and dimethylaminoazobenzene (Fig. 7) produce cirrhotic changes and eventually carcinoma of the liver. The latter compound is much more active for the rat than the mouse, whereas aminoazotoluene is more effective in the mouse. The specificity for the liver is only relative, however, since the incidence of pulmonary tumors is increased, and hemangioendotheliomas in subcutaneous and intraperitoneal sites are induced in some strains of mice.

The nitroso compounds (Fig. 7), such as nitrosamine, are a new group of chemicals with potent carcinogenic activity (Magee and Barnes[46]) and are of potential industrial and other environmental hazard to man. The alkylating agents (Fig. 8) used in cancer chemotherapy are also carcinogenic (Shimkin et al.[67]). They induce pulmonary tumors in mice and have been implicated as carcinogenic for man.

Hepatomas in mice can be induced also by protracted feeding of carbon tetrachloride or ethionine and, in rats, with diets containing selenium. These chemicals first elicit conspicuous cirrhosis in the liver, and the neoplasms arise subsequent to the cirrhotic changes, although cirrhosis is not an essential precursor to the neoplastic reaction. A compound initially proposed as an insecticide, 2-acetylaminofluorene (Fig. 7), not only induces hepatomas in rats, but also induces mammary carcinoma, carcinoma of sweat glands, and carcinoma of the kidney (Weisburger and Weisburger[77]). Propylthiouracil and other goitrogens produce thyroid adenomas and carcinomas in rats (Morris[50]).

Urethan (ethyl carbamate; Fig. 7) produces pulmonary tumors and hepatomas in mice and rats. It is also an "incomplete" carcinogen for the skin in that it will evoke skin carcinoma if the site is also painted with croton oil, an irritant with little or no carcinogenic activity (Roe and Salaman[58]).

Among chemical materials that have demonstrated carcinogenic properties following subcutaneous implantation in mice and rats, the synthetic plastics and polymers are particularly interesting. The mode of action of these "solid state" carcinogens may lead to some understanding of endogenous chemical factors (Bischoff and Bryson[5]).

A number of inorganic chemicals are incriminated in the production of cancer in man. These include arsenic, which produces cancer of the skin following extended medicinal or industrial exposures; chromates, which produce bronchogenic carcinoma upon inhalation; and nickel, which increases the occurrence of bronchogenic carcinoma and carcinoma of the nasal cavity (Hueper[36]). Sarcomas have now been elicited in rodents with chromate and nickel compounds, but arsenic remains to be demonstrated convincingly as carcinogenic in animals (Hartwell[30]).

Carcinogens from natural sources

Increasing interest and attention are being given to carcinogens from natural sources, such as plant foodstuffs, and contaminants thereof. Typical and pivotal have been the discoveries of aflatoxin and of cycasin (methylazoxymethanol glycoside).

In 1961, there occurred in England an outbreak of killing hepatatoxicity among turkey poults, ducklings and chickens. The epidemic was quickly traced to food sources, and thence to contamination of the food by a common fungus, *Aspergillus flavus*. Food containing the toxic material was fed to rats and produced hepatomas. A group of fluorescent lactones, the aflatoxins, were isolated chemically (Fig. 7). Based on molecular weight, they are by far the most active known hepatocarcinogens and also produce sarcoma at the site of injection in rats.

Concurrently, an outbreak of hepatomas in rainbow trout occurred in northwestern United States. The disease was also associated with sources of food on which the fish were raised. It was found that the food became contaminated with *Aspergillus flavus*, which grows luxuriously on many high-protein foods kept under humid conditions. Aflatoxin content in the food was correlated with the occurrence of trout hepatoma (Wogan[78]).

Recent investigations in Africa show correlation between the prevalence of hepatoma in man with aflotoxin levels in food, suggesting that aflatoxinosis may be an important carcinogenic factor in man.

Cycasin is a natural product of the *Cycas circinalis* nut, a nutritional source in Guam and other tropical regions. When it was fed to rats, cancers of the liver and kidney were induced (Laqueur et al.[42]). The active chemical is a glycone and is not carcinogenic unless the glycone portion of the molecule is first split off by intestinal flora, yielding the absorbable aglycone, methylazoxymethanol (Fig. 7).

The alkaloids of *Senecio jacobaea,* an edible plant of Africa, induces liver cancer in rats. Bracken fern, *Pteridium aquilina,* when ingested by cows over protracted periods, leads to hematuria and cancer of the bladder.

Roentgen and ultraviolet radiations

The fact that roentgen rays and radium are carcinogenic was first shown by the tragic skin carcinomas in physicians and other workers within ten years of the discovery of roentgen rays. Clunet[11] reproduced the process in rats by repeatedly exposing them to roentgen rays.

Ionizing radiations, whether delivered from external sources or administered in the form of fission products, have carcinogenic properties. Single exposures of mice up to 700 R lead to an increase and earlier appearance of leukemia and to the appearance of ovarian tumors. Chronic exposure to up to 8.8 R per day results in increased incidence of mammary carcinoma and sarcoma, ovarian tumors, and pulmonary tumors. Local fibrosarcomas and osteosarcomas are obtained in mice, rats, and rabbits with parenteral administration of radioactive fission products and of plutonium. Thorotrast also has produced sarcomas after its subcutaneous injection into rats and mice. Radium implanted into long bones has produced osteosarcomas in monkeys.

The appearance of leukemia in rodents exposed to ionizing radiations is attributable to the exteriorization of leukemogenic viruses (Kaplan[38]) and is an excellent example of the interplay of several factors in carcinogenesis.

The tragedy of Hiroshima established that ionizing radiations are also leukemogenic in man. Whether a viral entity is also involved remains conjectural. Therapeutic and even diagnostic doses of radiations increase the risk of leukemia, indicating that this may become an increasingly important source of carcinogenic exposure for the populations of the future (Glucksmann et al.[24]). Osteogenic sarcoma was produced in girls who ingested mesothorium in the process of preparing luminous watch dials.

The induction of skin cancer following exposure to ultraviolet radiations was first suspected on the basis of clinical experience and subsequently reproduced experimentally in mice. The effective wavelength was found to be in the 2900 to 3200 Å range. The production of tumors depends upon the quantity of radiant energy applied rather than upon its intensity, and a quantitative relationship has been established between the dose of radiations and the neoplastic reaction (Blum[7]). That a different type of action may be involved in the induction of neoplasia by ultraviolet radiations and carcinogenic hydrocarbons is indicated by investigations showing that the action of these two agents is not additive.

Parasites

The increased incidence of cancer of the urinary bladder in Egypt is associated with infestation by *Schistosoma haematobium* (Ferguson[19a]; Mustacchi and Shimkin[54]). In rats, infestation with *Cysticercus crassicollis* leads to the appearance of sarcomas of the liver. Sarcomas of the peritoneum can be produced by ground-up larvae, and the active principle is associated with the calcium carbonate fraction of the parasite (Dunning and Curtis[14]).

The causation of neoplasia in animals by bacteria or fungi has been rather conclusively disapproved, but the discoveries of aflatoxin and cycasin have renewed research on more indirect roles for microorganisms in the neoplastic process. In a variety of plants, overgrowths of abnormal cells that invade and destroy contiguous tissues and that disseminate to other portions of the organism and grow as metastases can be induced by *Agrobacterium tumefaciens*, a bacterium first described by Smith.[69] Metastases may be free of the organism, and the tumors may be thus transplanted without further intermediation of the bacterium. Whether crown gall of plants is identical with cancer of animals is unknown, but this interesting cellular reaction has not attracted the attention it deserves from scientists concerned with cellular physiology of neoplastic diseases.

Viruses

Investigations at the turn of the century failed to prove bacterial etiology of cancer, and experiments on transplantation of tumors indicated that such transfer is effected only by means of living cells. This led to early conclusions that cancer was not an infectious disease.

Rous,[59] in 1911, showed that certain spontaneous tumors of chickens could be transferred by cell-free filtrates. One of these neoplasms was the source of the Rous sarcoma. At the same time, Japanese workers also reported a filterable myxosarcoma in the fowl. Subsequent work established beyond doubt that these were neoplasms and that the transmission of living cells could be excluded.

Injection of the active filtrates results in the appearance of sarcomas at the site of injection or at sites of injury, such as the needle tract or a distant area that is wounded. The tumors appear much quicker than with chemical carcinogenic agents. The inciting agent is recoverable from the tumors, and, since its activity is not diluted out on serial passage, it must be self-reproducing or must cause the production by the body of additional quantities of the agent.

The chicken produces antibodies to the Rous virus, but neither active immunity nor passive imunity conferred by injection of immune sera from other species protects against the transplantation or growth of established sarcomas. The Rous virus, as are the tumors induced by it, is species specific under usual conditions. Duran-Reynals[15] showed that it can be transmitted successfully to other birds, such as ducks and turkeys, by intravenous injection into newly hatched animals. The tumors that appear within a month after the introduction of the agent can be returned to the chicken, but in later tumors the agent maintains its adaptation for the duck.

Also, hemorrhagic lesions rather than tumors may appear, and the tumors may localize in tissues different from those in the chicken, such as in bones.

Among the viral-induced tumors in fowl are at least five forms of leukemia, one of which was described by Ellerman and Bang[18] even before the investigations of Rous. However, at that time, leukemia was not usually included among the neoplastic entities, and this appeared even more distant to human diseases than chicken sarcomas.

Shope,[68] in 1933, discovered that a papilloma occurring in wild rabbits could be transferred by glycerolated tissue or filtered tissue extracts. In domestic rabbits, many of these lesions became frank carcinomas. The agent cannot be recovered from the lesions in the domestic rabbit, but its presence is signified by the appearance of antibodies in the blood as the tumor develops.

An active interest in the viral etiology of cancer was renewed by the demonstration by Gross[27] that mouse leukemia was transmissible by cell-free filtrates injected into newborn animals. Even greater impetus was created by description of another

Table 5. Some oncogenic viruses*

Nucleic acid	Group of viruses	Neoplasms evoked	Size (mμ)	Site of formation
RNA	Avian leukosis	Rous sarcoma Lymphomatosis Erythroblastosis Myeloblastosis	70-110	Cytoplasm
	Murine leukosis	Leukemias Sarcoma	100	Cell membrane
	Bittner	Mouse mammary cancer	100	Cell membrane
DNA	Polyoma	Multiple in mice, rats, hamsters, and rabbits	45	Nucleus
	SV-40	Hamster sarcoma	45	Nucleus
	Papilloma	Human, canine, rabbit, and bovine papilloma	50-55	Nucleus
	Adenoviruses	Hamster sarcoma Human types 12, 18, 31, and others Bovine type 3 Chicken (CELO)	80	Nucleus
	Poxviruses	Rabbit fibroma Squirrel fibroma Yaba monkey tumor	200-250	Cytoplasm

*Data from Howatson, A. F.: Architecture and development of tumor viruses and their relation to viruses in general, Fed. Proc. **21**:947-953, 1962, and from Macpherson, I.: Recent advances in the study of viral oncogenesis, Brit. Med. Bull. **23**:144-149, 1967.

filterable agent of the mouse, polyoma virus, that produced parotid gland tumors, sarcomas, kidney tumors, and many other neoplastic reactions.

There is now an impressive list of benign and malignant neoplasms in which a viral entity plays a causal role (Table 5).

Some viruses appear to be specific in evoking one type of neoplasm in one species. An example of this may be the Bittner virus, which produces mammary adeno-carcinoma in mice. Other viruses, partic-ularly the polyoma virus, evoke no less than twenty types of neoplastic reaction in the mouse, hamster, rat, and rabbit, so that it is neither tumor specific nor species specific (Stewart and Eddy[70]). Conversely, a similar neoplastic reaction in one species can be produced by a number of distinctly different viruses. Leukemia in the mouse is produced by at least five viruses that belong to a group composed of ribonucleic acids (Gross[28]).

Of particular importance was the demon-stration by Eddy et al.[17] of the carcino-genic activity in hamsters of SV-40, a virus recovered from kidney tissue of the Rhesus monkey. This was followed by the dis-coveries by Trentin et al.[74] and by Huebner et al.[34] of similar activity of human adeno-viruses, especially types 12, 18, and 31. It is now evident that oncogenic viruses do not comprise a single group but are dis-tributed widely among the kingdom of these entities at the interphase of life (Table 5).

Progress is being recorded at an im-pressive rate in the morphologic and im-munologic characterization of the viral entities, as well as in procedures of vac-cination and immunization against such agents.

Electron microscopic studies reveal viral-like particles in several human neoplasms, especially leukemia, Hodgkin's disease, breast cancer, and rectal polyps. Progress in the clarification of human neoplasms is impeded by the lack of biologic tests of activity of the cell-free fractions, and this is an area of intense research developments. No malignant neoplasm in man has been demonstrated as yet to be due to a viral entity. Acute leukemia and the Burkitt lymphosarcoma may be the first of such demonstrations.

Carcinogenic process

The continued reproduction of cells in neoplasia, the transmission of characters from one cell to another for an almost limitless number of generations, is in agree-ment with the view that cancer is a mani-festation of a genetic difference from nor-mal cells or a genetic alteration of normal cells. In order to assume that normal cells can acquire neoplastic properties through genic processes, some mechanism of action leading to a mutation is necessary. The cytoplasmic transmission of self-reproduc-ing entities, viruses, is the only nongenetic explanation that seems reasonable at pres-ent as an alternative. This may not repre-sent a conflicting view, since some viruses are now known to become intimately in-volved with the genetic material of the host cell (Macpherson[45]).

The number of carcinogenic chemicals is apparently limited only by patience of chemists to synthesize or to isolate them and of the biologist to test them on a suf-ficient number of animals of various species by various routes of administration. In 1951, Hartwell[30] collected data on 1329 chemicals that have been tested. Of these, 322 were reported to be carcinogenic. Since then, several hundred other compounds have been added to the list. The search for a correlation between molecular archi-tecture and the property of carcinogenesis seems futile except within the narrow con-fines of definite chemical groups. Nor does there seem to be any common general physiologic action that can be attributed to all carcinogenic chemicals.

A wide variety of chemical carcinogens also have the property of being able to induce germinal mutations and teratogene-sis. Some twenty compounds were assayed by Demerec[12] for mutagenic properties, using Drosophila exposed to aerosol mists containing the chemicals. Teratogenic cor-relations of carbamates and teratogenesis were studied by DiPaolo and Ellis.[13] There was surprisingly good correlation between carcinogenicity and teratogenicity in mice and mutagenicity in fruit flies.

In most situations in which the external stimulus leading to cancer appears to be well understood, such stimulation has to take place over a protracted period. This is true of carcinogenic hydrocarbons that evoke sarcomas upon single subcutaneous injection, for the material remains at the site for a long time. However, this is not true of some neoplastic reactions. For example, the pulmonary tumor of strain A mice is evoked by a single injection of urethan. The chemical is excreted within a day's time, and the tumors seem to have practically no latent period, their recognition as tumors being dependent upon a minimal number of cellular divisions to achieve an identifiable mass. Many neoplastic reactions have to proceed through a series of progressive changes, and different stimuli can be used during the early stages and in stages that complete the reaction. An alternate explanation is that the cancer reaction in individual cells is completely evoked by a few applications of the carcinogen and that the cocarcinogenic stimulus acts only on the surrounding stroma so that the dormant cells can begin to proliferate.

Studies are available on the distribution, metabolic conversion, and elimination of polycyclic hydrocarbons, azo dyes, and acetylaminofluorene. The techniques of detection by chemical or spectrographic methods have been extended by the use of radioactive tracers incorporated into their structure. Dibenzanthracene is metabolized by the mouse into at least four substances and is rapidly eliminated, largely through the feces. These compounds show reduced carcinogenic activity. Metabolites of the azo dyes and aminofluorenes are excreted chiefly in the urine. The metabolites, especially the N-hydroxylation products, show increased carcinogenic activity. The understanding of the metabolism of carcinogens contributes essential information and may cast some light upon the process of neoplastic transformation. Miller and Miller[48] showed that dimethylaminoazobenzene, upon ingestion by the rat, binds tightly with proteins and nucleic acids of the liver. Bound dye is not present in rat tissues in which tumors are not induced. No binding occurs in several species in which liver tumors are not induced. The fact that hepatomas no longer have the property of binding with the azo dye indicates that an essential cellular alteration has occurred.

It is possible, of course, that some single biophysical or biochemical reaction is produced by all carcinogens—chemical, physical, or viral. The search for such mechanisms and the postulations that lead to further investigations are to be encouraged (Haddow[29]). However, it would be surprising indeed if the great diversity of stimuli, the tremendous range of reactions and metabolic pathways available to cells, and the dissimilar end products of neoplasia all could be accounted for by one mechanism. Neoplastic diseases probably represent as great a class of diseases as the infections, and overall theories of their origin may be more restrictive than helpful at this stage of our knowledge.

Tumor-host relationships

The development and the growth of a neoplasm in an animal produces many profound effects not only at the site of the tumor, but also in tissues and systems distant to the tumor itself. Cachexia, anemia, and the hepatic dysfunction in patients with gastrointestinal cancer are examples frequently encountered clinically. There are profound effects of tumor growth upon the nitrogen metabolism of the host (Mider[47]). In animals, the catalase activity is lowered in the liver and kidneys, the red blood cells and hemoglobin decrease, the blood proteoses increase, the tissue and blood aldolase increases, the serum and tissue esterase decreases, and fatty material is lost from the suprarenal cortex. These effects are seen with a variety of neoplasms and may be reversed upon the removal or regression of the tumor. Although most of them become detectable when the tumor weight is an appreciable fraction of the body weight of the host, some are not correlated simply to the size of the neoplasm or to the degree of general debility of the host. Although none is established as unique for tumor growth, the effects are not due merely to the presence of growing tissue (Greenstein[26]).

There are numerous isolated studies on specific constituents or enzyme systems of urine or blood in patients with cancer. Electrophoretic observations on plasma proteins suggest an elevation of an acid protein component. A serum polysaccharide appears to be elevated in the presence of tuberculosis and of cancer. Blood from patients with carcinoma has a higher inhibition of hyaluronidase activity than normal blood. Mucoproteins are isolated in larger quantities from cancerous blood than from normal blood. In the presence of cancer, as well as in other disease states, there is disturbance in the proteins of the blood and diminution in its reducing power, probably due to lowering of the sulfhydryl content. Blood lactic dehydrogenase is often elevated in the presence of cancer.

In contrast with the systemic effects of neoplasms in general, certain definite effects are produced by specific neoplasms as a result of hyperfunction maintained from their tissue of origin. Manifestations of hormone-producing abnormalities are seen with tumors derived from hormonal tissues: hyperinsulinism with tumors of the islands of Langerhans, hyperepinephrinism with pheochromocytoma, increased 17-ketosteroid excretion with suprarenal tumors, excessive gonadotropins with choriocarcinoma, and masculinizing effects with arrhenoblastoma of the ovary. Determination of serum acid phosphatase in disseminated prostatic carcinoma, of serum alkaline phosphatase in osteogenic tumors, of serotonin in carcinoids, and of melanin in patients with metastatic melanoma are additional diagnostic procedures of considerable value in specific cases.

Chemotherapy of cancer

The overwhelming impetus for research on the chemotherapy of cancer is the fact that, with presently available methods, only one-third of all patients with cancer survive over five years. The earliest application of therapeutic measures to all patients may increase the salvage to 50%. Thus one-half of all cancer patients would still be destined to die of the disease.

The first chemotherapeutic agent for neoplastic disease was potassium arsenite in leukemia, described by Lissauer in 1865. The modern era of investigations can be timed from the introduction of nitrogen mustard under the cloak of wartime secrecy from 1942 to 1945 (Stock[71]). The next important step was the introduction of folic acid antagonists for acute leukemia (Farber[19]). The inhibition of breast cancer by altering the hormonal status of the host dates to Beatson's report of 1896.[3] In 1941,

this important field was revived by Huggins' work[37] on the effect of castration on prostatic cancer.

Since 1945, systematic programs in chemotherapy have been developed in the United States and several other countries. As a result of these efforts, over 250,000 chemicals and crude materials have been tested on transplanted tumors in mice, and over 300 materials have gone through clinical evaluation.

The only curative effects of chemotherapy are thus far recorded in women with choriocarcinoma, as Hertz et al.[31] showed with the use of methotrexate and actinomycin D. Similar effects are suggested in a small proportion of patients with acute leukemia and Burkitt's lymphoma. With these exceptions, the role of clinical cancer chemotherapy is either palliative or experimental. Most of such chemicals should be used under controlled experimental conditions and only after clinical considerations that include surgery and radiotherapy.

There are four main types or groups of chemicals that have shown activity against some of the neoplastic diseases of man:

1 The alkylating chemicals, of which the nitrogen mustards and their analogues are examples (Fig. 8). These agents display marked inhibiting effects upon hemic, lymphatic, and gonadal tissues. They resemble ionizing radiations in some of the effects and have been termed "radiomimetic." Such effects include carcinogenicity and mutagenicity. The clinical usefulness of the agents is found in lymphomas and leukemias.

2 The "antimetabolites" or chemical analogues of vitamins, purines, and amino acids that compete or interfere with the metabolic processes of the cell by mimicking but not fulfiling the requirements of the essential constituents. In this conceptually attractive field, the best examples to date are the antifolic acid compounds and 5-fluorouracil (Fig. 8). The former has clinical usefulness in acute leukemia, particularly in children, and the latter in some tumors such as colorectal and mammary carcinoma.

3 The steroid hormones, particularly chemicals with estrogenic or andro-

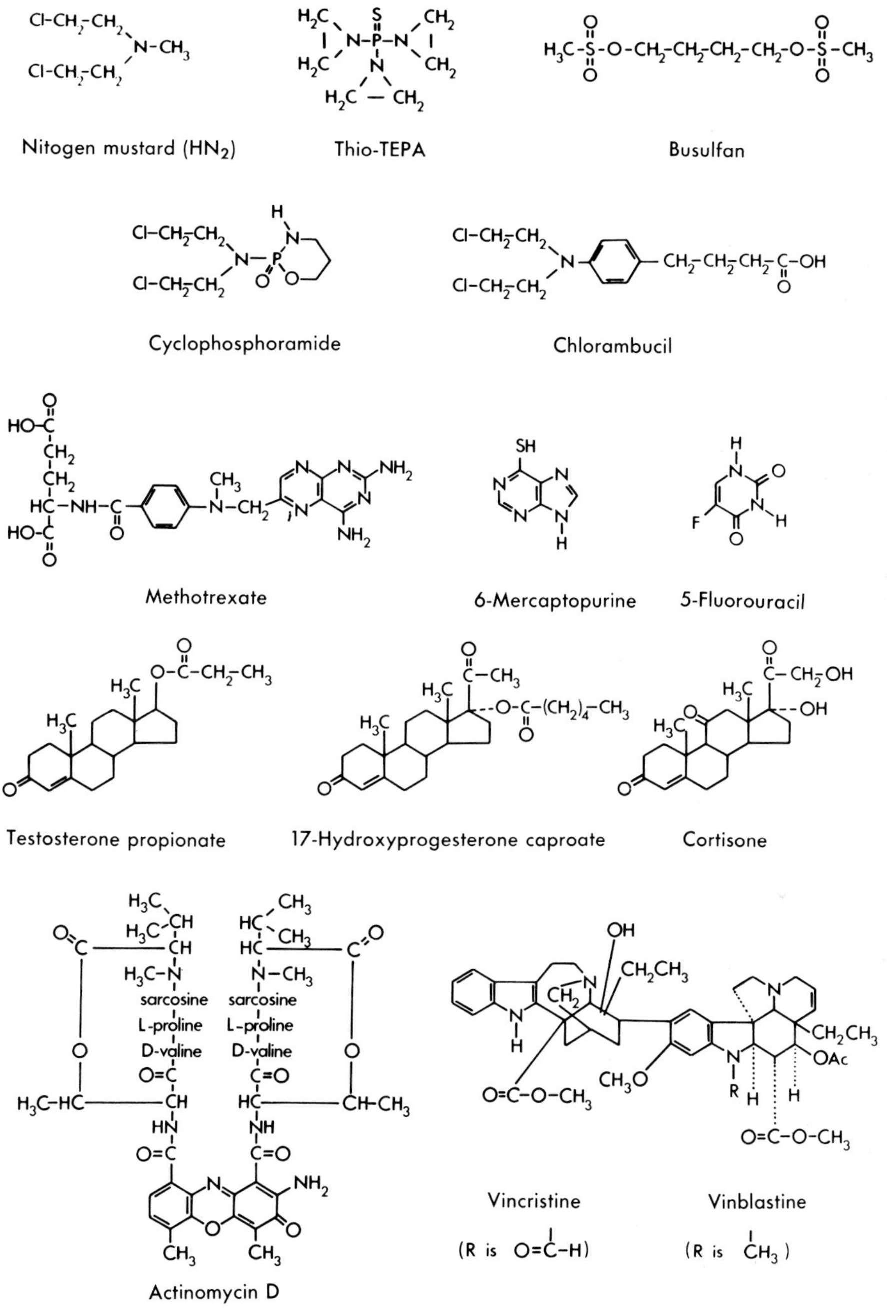

Fig. 8. Some chemicals that have shown effects on certain neoplasms in man. **First and second rows**, Alkylating agents. **Third row**, Antimetabolites. **Fourth row**, Hormones. **Fifth row**, Fungal and plant derivatives.

genic activity, which are useful in disseminated cancer of the breast. Estrogens, as well as castration, are useful in cancer of the prostate. Corticosteroids have some benefits in acute leu-

kemia and other lymphomas. Progestational compounds inhibit carcinoma of the endometrium. Hormones probably act by modifying the milieu upon which these partly hormone-dependent neoplasms are growing. Surgical ablation of the testis and the pituitary or adrenal glands as another means of modifying the hormonal status of patients is included by usage under this aspect of chemotherapy.

4 A number of antibiotics and other products of microbial and plant origin which have exhibited antitumor effects in animal systems and in man. Actinomycin D, isolated by Waksman, and mitomycin C, isolated by Hata from species of Streptomycetes, are examples. These highly toxic materials have clinical effects in some cases of lymphoma and sarcoma, especially in children. Vincristine and vinblastine (Fig. 8), isolated from the periwinkle plant *(Vinca rosea)*, are useful in Hodgkin's disease and other leukoses.

The reader is referred to recent reviews and to the periodical Cancer Chemotherapy Reports, issued by the National Cancer Institute for current information on this adventure in medical research.

Conclusion

Scientific progress depends not only on the acquisition of new knowledge, but also on the correction of errors, no matter how authoritative and traditional these errors may be. Progress against cancer requires not only research, but also the application of the research findings. And these applications, in turn, require research in order to advance from the laboratory to the clinic and from the clinic to the whole community of people (Shimkin[65]).

Among the few procedures that do, in fact, detect cancer at biologically curable stages is the vaginal cytology test developed by Papanicoloau and Traut. What logistic systems, in terms of cost, facilities, and personnel, as well as technologic developments of automatic cytoanalyzers, are required to provide this procedure annually to 50 million women of the United States?

Among the few important preventive procedures in cancer is the cessation of tobacco habit, especially cigarette smoking. What motivational approaches, regulations, and economic readjustments are necessary to reduce the tragic neoplastic and cardiovascular cost from this inane addiction?

Over one-half of all patients with cancer are doomed to die of their disease, often after long expensive treatment that debilitate the purses and the hearts of their families. What systems of medical and psychologic care can be developed to reduce these costs until research can include neoplastic diseases among its victories?

The scientific method is applicable to these technologic, sociologic, and economic questions. There is recent movement in these directions, as exemplified by the tasks imposed by the regional programs on cancer, heart disease, and strokes.

Cancer research has no place for fixed concepts, for vested interests, for orthodoxy, for artificial limitations to its objectives. But we can stand firm on this: cancer is a solvable problem within the capabilities of human intelligence using a human thought-and-action process that we call scientific research.

REFERENCES

1 Adelman, R. C., Morris, H., and Weinhouse, S.: Frucktokinase, triokinase and aldolases in liver tumors of the rat, Cancer Res. 27:3108-3113, 1967.
2 Andervont, H. B.: Influence of environment on mammary cancer in mice, J. Nat. Cancer Inst. 4:579-581, 1944.
3 Beatson, G. T.: On the treatment of inoperable cases of carcinoma of the mamma, Lancet 2:104-107, 162-165, 1896.
4 Berenblum, I.: Carcinogenesis and tumor pathogenesis, Advances Cancer Res. 2:129-176, 1954.
5 Bischoff, F., and Bryson, G.: Carcinogenesis through solid state surfaces, Progr. Exp. Tumor Res. 5:85-133, 1964.
6 Bittner, J. J.: Some possible effects of nursing on the mammary gland tumor incidence in mice, Science 84:162, 1936.
7 Blum, H. F.: Carcinogenesis by ultraviolet light, Princeton, N. J., 1959, Princeton University Press.
8 Braun, A. C.: Recent advances in the physiology of tumor formation in the crown-gall disease of plants, Growth 11:325-337, 1947.
9 Burkitt, D., Hutt, M. S. R., and Wright, D. H.: The African lymphoma; preliminary observations on response to therapy, Cancer 18:399-410, 1965.
10 Burmester, B. R., Prickett, C. O., and Belding, T. C.: Filterable agent producing lymphoid tumors and osteropetrosis in chickens, Cancer Res. 6:189-196, 1946.
11 Clunet, J.: Recherches experimentales sur les tumeurs malignes, Paris, 1910, G. Steinheil.
12 Demerec, M.: Genetic potencies of carcinogens, Acta Un. Int. Cancr. 6:247-251, 1948.
13 DiPaolo, J. A., and Elis, J.: The comparison of teratogenic and carcinogenic effects of some

carbamate compounds, Cancer Res. **27**:1696-1701, 1967.

14 Dunning, W. F., and Curtis, M. R.: Multiple peritoneal sarcoma in rats from intraperitoneal infection of washed ground taenia larvae, Cancer Res. **6**:668-670, 1946.

15 Duran-Reynals, F.: The infection of turkeys and guinea fowls by the Rous sarcoma virus and the accompanying variations of the virus, Cancer Res. **3**:569-577, 1943.

16 Earle, W. R.: Production of malignancy in vitro, J. Nat. Cancer Inst. **4**:165-248, 1943.

17 Eddy, B. E., Borman, G. S., Berkeley, W. H., and Young, R. D.: Tumors induced in hamsters by injection of Rhesus monkey kidney cell extracts, Proc. Soc. Exp. Biol. Med. **107**:191-197, 1961.

18 Ellermann, V., and Bang, O.: Experimentelle Leukamie bei Huhnern, Cbl. Bakt. Abt. 1 (Orig.) **46**:595-609, 1908.

18a Everson, T. C., and Cole, W. H.: Spontaneous regression of cancer, Philadelphia, 1966, W. B. Saunders Co.

19 Farber, S.: Chemotherapy in the treatment of leukemia and Wilms' tumor, J.A.M.A. **198**:826-836, 1966.

19a Ferguson, A. R.: Associated bilharziosis and primary malignant disease of the urinary bladder, J. Path. Bact. **16**:76-94, 1911.

20 Furth, J.: Conditioned and autonomous neoplasms; a review, Cancer Res. **13**:477-492, 1953.

21 Furth, J., and Kahn, M. C.: The transmission of leukemia of mice with a single cell, Amer. J. Cancer **31**:276-282, 1937.

22 Gardner, W. U.: Hormonal aspects of experimental tumorigenesis, Advances Cancer Res. **1**:173-232, 1953.

23 Gey, G. O.: Some aspects of the constitution and behavior of normal and malignant cells maintained in continuous culture, Harvey Lect. **50**:154-229, 1954-1955.

24 Glucksmann, A., Lamerton, L. F., and Mayneord, W. V.: Carcinogenic effects of radiation. In Raven, R. W., editor: Cancer, vol. 1, London, 1957, Butterworth & Co., Ltd., pp. 497-539.

25 Green, E. L., editor: Biology of the laboratory mouse, ed. 2, New York, 1966, Blakiston Division, McGraw-Hill Book Co.

26 Greenstein, J. P.: Biochemistry of cancer, ed. 2, New York, 1954, Academic Press, Inc.

27 Gross, L.: "Spontaneous" leukemia developing in C3H mice following inoculation, in infancy, with AK-leukemic extracts, or AK-embryos, Proc. Soc. Exp. Biol. Med. **76**:27-32, 1951.

28 Gross, L.: Oncogenic viruses, New York, 1961, Pergamon Press, Inc.

29 Haddow, A.: The chemical and genetic mechanisms of carcinogenesis. In Homburger, F., and Fishman, W. H., editors: The physiopathology of cancer, New York, 1953, Hoeber Medical Division, Harper & Row, Publishers, pp. 451-551.

30 Hartwell, J. L.: Survey of compounds which have been tested for carcinogenic activity, ed.

2, Washington, D. C., 1951, Federal Security Agency, United States Public Health Service.

31 Hertz, R., Lewis, J., and Lipsett, M. B.: Five years' experience with the chemotherapy of metastatic choriocarcinoma and related trophoblastic tumors in women, Amer. J. Obstet. Gynec. **82**:631-640, 1961.

32 Heston, W. E.: Genetics of cancer, Advances Genet. **2**:99-128, 1948.

33 Howatson, A. F.: Architecture and development of tumor viruses and their relation to viruses in general, Fed. Proc. **21**:947-953, 1962.

34 Huebner, R. J., Rowe, W. P., and Lane, W. T.: Oncogenic effects in hamsters of human adenovirus types 12 and 18, Proc. Nat. Acad. Sci. **48**:2051-2058, 1962.

35 Hueper, W. C.: Occupational tumors and allied diseases, Springfield, Ill., 1942, Charles C Thomas, Publisher.

36 Hueper, W. C.: Environmental factors in the production of human cancer. In Raven, R. W., editor: Cancer, vol. 1, London, 1957, Butterworth & Co., Ltd., pp. 404-496.

37 Huggins, C.: Prostatic cancer treated by orchiectomy; five-year results, J.A.M.A. **131**:576-581, 1946.

38 Kaplan, H. S.: On the natural history of the murine leukemias, Cancer Res. **27**:1325-1340, 1967.

39 Kennaway, E.: The identification of a carcinogenic compound in coal-tar, Brit. Med. J. **2**:749-752, 1955.

40 Knox, W. E.: The enzymatic pattern of neoplastic tissue, Advances Cancer Res. **10**:117-161, 1967.

41 Lacassagne, A.: Apparition de cancers de la mamelle chez la souris mâle, soumise a des injections de folliculine, C. R. Acad. Sci. (Paris) **195**:630-632, 1932.

42 Laqueur, G. L., McDaniel, E. G., and Matsumoto, H.: Tumor induction in germ-free rats wtih methylazoxymethanol (MAM) and synthetic MAM acetate, J. Nat. Cancer Inst. **39**:355-372, 1967.

43 Lathrop, A. E. C., and Loeb, L.: The incidence of cancer in various strains of mice, Proc. Soc. Exp. Biol. Med. **11**:34-38, 1913.

44 Lucké, B.: Carcinoma in the leopard frog; its probable causation by a virus, J. Exp. Med. **68**:457-568, 1938.

45 Macpherson, I.: Recent advances in the study of viral oncogenesis, Brit. Med. Bull. **23**:144-149, 1967.

46 Magee, P. N., and Barnes, J. M.: Carcinogenic nitroso compounds, Advances Cancer Res. **10**:163-246, 1967.

47 Mider, G. B.: Some tumor-host relationships, Canadian Cancer Conference, vol. 1, New York, 1955, Academic Press, Inc., pp. 120-137.

48 Miller, J. A., and Miller, E. C.: The carcinogenic aminoazo dyes, Advances Cancer Res. **1**:340-396, 1953.

49 Miller, R. W., Fraumeni, J. F., Jr., and Manning, M. D.: Association of Wilms's tumor with aniridia, hemihypertrophy and other congenital malformations, New Eng. J. Med. **270**:922-927, 1964.

50 Morris, H. P.: The experimental development and metabolism of thyroid gland tumors, Advances Cancer Res. 3:51-115, 1955.

51 Morris, H. P.: Development, biochemistry and biology of experimental hepatomas, Advances Cancer Res. 9:227-302, 1965.

51a Morton, D. L., Malmgren, R. A., Hall, W. T., and Schidlovsky, G.: Immunologic and virus studies with human sarcomas, Surgery 66: 152-161, 1969.

52 Moulton, F. R., editor: A symposium on mammary tumors in mice, pub. no. 22, Washington, D. C., 1945, American Association for the Advancement of Science.

53 Murphy, J. B.: Transplantability of tissues to the embryo of foreign species, J. Exp. Med. 17:482-493, 1913.

54 Mustacchi, P. O., and Shimkin, M. B.: Cancer of the bladder and Schistosoma hematobium, J. Nat. Cancer Inst. 20:825-842, 1958.

55 Oberling, C.: The riddle of cancer (translated by W. H. Woglom), New Haven, Conn., 1944, Yale University Press.

56 Oppenheimer, B. S., Oppenheimer, E. T., and Stout, A. P.: Sarcomas induced in rodents by imbedding various plastic films, Proc. Soc. Exper. Biol. Med. 79:366-369, 1952.

57 Pott, P.: Chirurgical observations relative to the cataract, the polypus of the nose, the cancer of the scrotum, the different kinds of rupture, and the mortification of the toes and feet, London, 1775, L. Hawes, Clarke and R. Collins.

58 Roe, F. J. C., and Salaman, M. H.: Further studies on incomplete carcinogenesis, Brit. J. Cancer 9:177-203, 1955.

59 Rous, P.: Transmission of a malignant new growth by means of a cell-free filtrate, J.A.M.A. 56:198, 1911.

60 Sanford, K. K., Likely, G. D., and Earle, W. R.: The development of variations in transplantability and morphology within a clone of mouse fibroblasts transformed to sarcoma-producing cells in vitro, J. Nat. Cancer. Inst. 15: 215-237, 1954.

61 Schabad, L. M.: Nouvelles donnees relatives a l'obtention experimental des tumeurs par un extrait benzenique du foie d'un cancereus; a propos des substances blastogenes endogenes, C. R. Soc. Biol. (Paris) 126:1180-1184, 1937.

62 Schlumberger, H. G., and Lucke, B.: Tumors of fishes, amphibians and reptiles, Cancer Res. 8:657-753, 1948.

63 Segi, M.: Cancer mortality for selected sites in 24 countries (1950-1957), Tohoku University School of Medicine, Sendai, Japan, 1960.

64 Shimkin, M. B.: Hormones and neoplasia. In Raven, R. W., editor: Cancer, vol. 1, London, 1957, Butterworth & Co., Ltd., pp. 161-213.

65 Shimkin, M. B.: Changing concepts concerning cancer, Proceedings of the fourth National Cancer Conference, Philadelphia, 1961, J. B. Lippincott Co., pp. 7-18.

66 Shimkin, M. B.: Science and cancer, United States Public Health Service, pub. no. 1162, Washington, D. C., 1964, U. S. Government Printing Office.

67 Shimkin, M. B., Weisburger, J. H., Weisburger, E. K., Gubareff, N., and Suntzeff, V.: Bioassay of 29 alkylating chemicals by the pulmonary-tumor response in strain A mice, J. Nat. Cancer Inst. 36:915-935, 1966.

68 Shope, R. E.: Infectious papillomatosis of rabbits, J. Exp. Med. 58:607-624, 1933.

69 Smith, E. F.: Studies on the crown-gall of plants; its relation to human cancer, J. Cancer Res. 1:231-310, 1916.

70 Stewart, S. E., and Eddy, B. E.: Tumor induction by S E Polyoma virus and the inhibition of tumors by specific neutralizing antibodies, Amer. J. Public Health 49:1493-1496, 1959.

71 Stock, C. C.: Experimental cancer chemotherapy, Advances Cancer Res. 2:426-492, 1954.

72 Tannenbaum, A., and Silverstone, H.: Nutrition in relation to cancer, Advances Cancer Res. 1:452-505, 1953.

72a Thomson, D. M. P., Krupey, J., Freedman, S. D., and Gold, P.: The radioimmunoassay of circulating carcinoembryonic antigen of the human digestive system, Proc. Nat. Acad. Sci. U.S.A. 64:161-167, 1969.

73 Toolan, H. W.: Transplantable human neoplasms maintained in cortisone-treated laboratory animals: H.S. #1; H.Ep. #1; H.Ep. #2; H.Ep. #3; and H.Emb.Rh. #1, Cancer Res. 14:660-666, 1954.

74 Trentin, J. J., Yabe, Y., and Taylor, G.: The quest for human cancer viruses, Science 137: 835-841, 1962.

75 United States Surgeon General's Advisory Committee on Smoking and Health: Smoking and health; report of the Advisory Committee to the Surgeon General of the Public Health Service, Washington, D. C., U. S. Department of Health, Education and Welfare, Public Health Service, Princeton, N. J., 1964, D. Van Nostrand Co., Inc.

76 Warburg, O.: The metabolism of tumours (translated by F. Dickens), London, 1930, Constable & Co., Ltd.

77 Weisburger, E. K., and Weisburger, J. H.: Chemistry, carcinogenicity, and metabolism of 2-fluorenamine and related compounds, Advances Cancer Res. 5:333-432, 1958.

78 Wogan, G. N., editor: Mycotoxins in foodstuffs, Cambridge, Mass., 1965, M.I.T. Press.

79 Woglom, W. H.: The study of experimental cancer; a review, George Crocker Special Research fund, no. 1, New York, 1913, Columbia University Press.

80 Wolff, J.: Die lehre von der Krebskrankheit (4 vols.), Jena, 1907-1928, Gustav Fischer.

81 Yamagiwa, K., and Ichikawa, K.: Experimental study of the pathogenesis of carcinoma, J. Cancer Res. 3:1-29, 1918.

Chapter 3

Pathology of cancer

Pathologist's responsibility

The pathologist has definite limitations of responsibility. He is responsible for the proper handling of tissue after it reaches his laboratory. He, however, can diagnose only the tissue submitted. If this tissue is poorly selected and does not reveal tumor, it is not his responsibility. If a negative report is given, then a false sense of security may be engendered in the physician who submitted the inadequate material.

The pathologist who not only has adequate material but also has all the pertinent data regarding the patient on whom the biopsy has been made will give the best diagnosis. He should know the name, age, and sex of the patient, the duration of the disease, the exact location of the lesion, its size, and all details of previous treatment (surgical or radiotherapeutic). The hospital chart should be available for consultation, the patient should be examined if necessary, and the results of other laboratory examinations should be available for inspection. There are definite limitations to diagnosis on the basis of morphology.

Biopsy

It is imperative that pathologic verification of malignant tumors be present before any therapy is instituted (Figs. 9 and 10). Grievous errors can be made if this is not done. An apparently typical epithelioma may be treated by radiotherapy and continue to increase in size instead of regressing. Histopathologic examination may then show a melanocarcinoma that is notoriously refractory to radiation therapy. Lesions thought to be inflammatory may instead be malignant, whereas lesions thought to be malignant may be inflammatory. The latter can occur in indolent ulcers of the leg.

Some of the hyperkeratotic lesions of the lip look like epidermoid carcinoma, but histopathologic examination will show only marked chronic inflammation. Fat necrosis of the breast, with its firmness and adherence to the skin, has admittedly been mistaken for typical carcinoma and radical mastectomy been done. If the patient has a basal cell carcinoma rather than a squamous carcinoma, then this will be of value in follow-up, for basal cell carcinomas practically never metastasize.

The foregoing examples serve only to emphasize why biopsy should always be compulsory.

Dangers. Formal biopsy entails little danger for the vast majority of tumors. The risk of infection, bleeding, or spread of the neoplasm is minimal.

Carcinoma of the breast is one tumor about which it has been said that metastases occur if biopsy is done. In a series of patients in whom the lesion was biopsied and a period of not less than two months elapsed before operation, we could not prove that any harmful results occurred (Lockhart and Ackerman[47]). In another series reviewed by Greenough,[31] there was no difference in prognosis between those in whom the lesion was biopsied before operation and those in whom the diagnosis was made at operation.

It has never been demonstrated that skin biopsies cause tumor spread. It has been said that biopsy of melanocarcinoma is dangerous, but the information gained by incisional biopsy in a doubtful case in which immediate radical incision would imply deformity outweighs any supposed danger of spread of the tumor.

Reliability of microscope in determining whether given lesion is benign or malignant. The microscopic diagnosis of cancer is not a black and white decision. It is true that in a high percentage of cases the pathologist can look at a given lesion microscopically and say whether it is benign or malignant. The usual cancer shows pronounced cellular proliferation, deviation

33

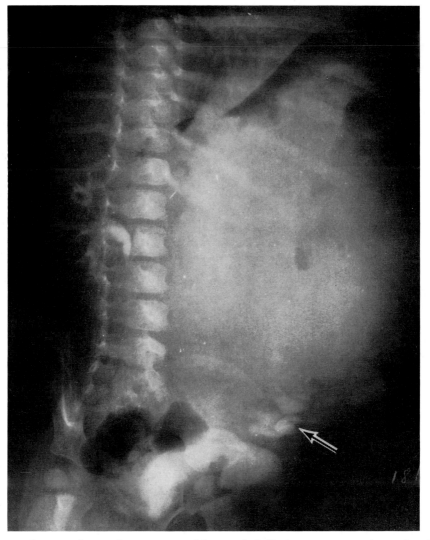

Fig. 9. Pyleogram showing huge mass in abdomen of child. Arrow points to dye within displaced kidney. Clinically and roentgenographically, lesion was thought to be Wilms' tumor, and preoperative radiotherapy was given. (WU neg. 61-1873.)

from the normal pattern with great variation in size and shape of cells, numerous mitotic figures, some atypical, and invasion of the surrounding tissue. Such lesions have the capacity to metastasize. In every organ, however, there are borderline lesions that are extremely difficult to evaluate, and the clinician must realize that in some it is impossible to make a definitive decision. Furthermore, proliferation of all types of tissue, often related to inflammatory lesions or other causes, may mimic patterns of cancer quite successfully.

The pseudoepitheliomatous proliferation that occurs within the oral cavity, overlies a granular cell myoblastoma, or is associated with fungal disease can be mistaken for cancer. Profound proliferation of cells within a lymph node related to infection, toxoplasmosis, rheumatoid arthritis, or other conditions requires considerable experience to differentiate from lymphoma. There are innumerable lesions that can mimic sarcoma, such as fasciitis, fibromatosis of children, and atypical fibroxanthoma (Fig. 11). There are instances in which the individual cells of a tumor and its pattern appear benign. On pathologic examination

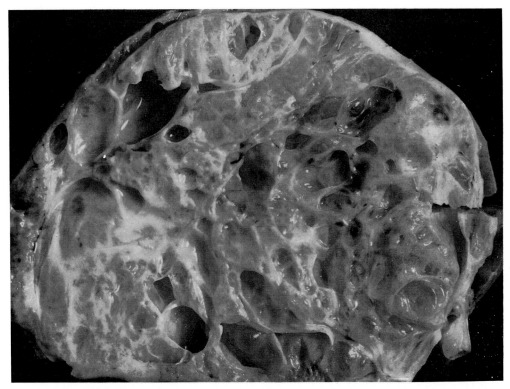

Fig. 10. Transected gross specimen of lesion shown in Fig. 9 demonstrating cystic process replacing and displacing renal parenchyma. Microscopically, lesion was perfectly benign. (WU neg. 61-1804.)

of the biopsy specimen it is not rare for a chondrosarcoma to show relatively normal-appearing cartilage cells, and yet the patient may have a lesion that may necessitate hemipelvectomy (Fig. 12). On relatively rare occasions, cancer of the thyroid gland may metastasize, and sections of the metastasis may look exactly like normal thyroid tissue.

The pathologist must always take into consideration the life history of a given neoplasm or lesion in determining its potentialities. Failure to do this has resulted in many errors.

Sclerosing adenosis of the breast was frequently called cancer because of its bewildering microscopic appearance, but follow-up of patients with this lesion, treated conservatively, always revealed cure. Its true nature as a benign proliferative, rather than a malignant, neoplastic condition was established. Certain types of cancer may have an innocuous microscopic pattern, and if the pathologist pays attention only to the pattern, it would seem unreasonable to designate the lesions as cancer. Such types of cancer occur in the thyroid gland, kidney, bone, liver, and other organs. Proof of their malignant nature is the fact that they metastasize and cause the death of the patient.

The pathologist wishing to make as accurate a diagnosis as possible as to whether or not a given lesion is malignant cannot do so just by looking at the slides. He must have all other relevant information and a knowledge of the life history of neoplasms presenting recognizable patterns.

Techniques. In extremely vascular tumors, preparation should be made to control any bleeding that may ensue from biopsy, and the endotherm knife probably should be used in order to avoid hemorrhage. Unfortunately, however, this knife dehydrates and chars tissue, thus making material unsatisfactory for histologic interpretation.

The techniques of obtaining a biopsy

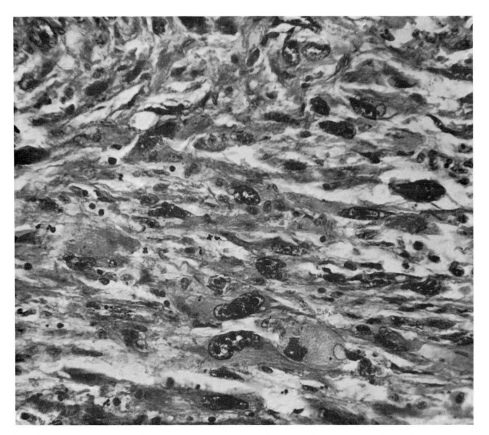

Fig. 11. Atypical fibroxanthoma showing extreme pleomorphism with atypical mitotic figures. (High power; WU neg. 60-5509.)

naturally vary with the location of the primary lesion. There are certain obstacles to securing specimens, and it should be emphasized and remembered that *only tissue submitted can be examined and diagnosed.* It is up to the clinician to choose a representative area for biopsy. Accessibility of lesions for biopsy varies.

In skin lesions, the section should be thin and deep rather than broad and superficial. It is best to take a biopsy from the margin of the tumor so that both abnormal and normal tissue are obtained, for if the section is taken from an area of central ulceration, there may be no tumor or only necrotic tumor present. If the biopsy is not carried deep enough, definite invasion of the base may be missed. Also, if the biopsy is cut tangentially, it may be mistaken microscopically for carcinoma because of the bizarre pattern revealed.

In the very friable tumors, biopsy should be taken from the cleanest zone near the tumor. It is preferable to introduce both branches of the open forceps into the tumor and then close and withdraw the instrument. The cutting forceps has its best indications for very firm or nodular tumors such as those that arise from the cervix or tongue. At times, several biopsies from different areas will be necessary. It is important to know, however, that epidermoid carcinoma may originate within the cervical canal, and external biopsy may be negative.

Diagnosis of tumors within the oral cavity is often difficult, and, as for lesions of the lip, biopsy should be deep. Special instruments are needed for malignant tumors of the nasopharynx, and repeated biopsies are often necessary for positive results.

Incisional biopsies are necessary in many instances in which aspiration biopsy has yielded insufficient material or is not indicated for reasons that will be elaborated

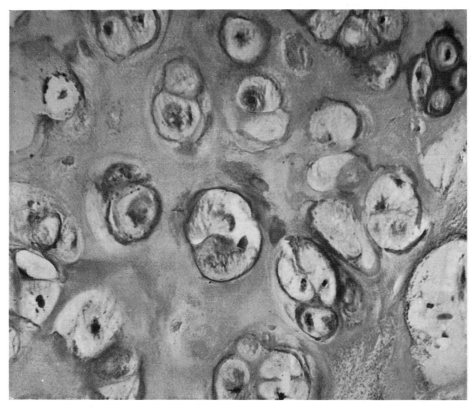

Fig. 12. Extremely well–differentiated chondrosarcoma. It is difficult to diagnose this as malignant cartilaginous tumor microscopically, but patient had huge tumor of ilium that necessitated hemipelvectomy. (×310; from Ackerman, L. V.: Is it cancer? Will it become cancer? In Proceedings of Fourth National Cancer Conference [1960], Philadelphia, 1961, J. B. Lippincott Co.; WU neg. 60-5515.)

upon later. Incisional biopsy should be done on all tumors easily accessible with ulcerated surfaces, such as those of the skin, lip, tongue, and alveolar ridge. The diagnosis of tumors of the breast, soft tissue, and bone is frequently difficult, and it is imperative that material be obtained from the area in which pathology is most likely to be demonstrated. Adequate material must be obtained so that more complete study by special stains can be made. Incisional biopsy on breast tumors should be done with a sharp scalpel under scrupulous surgical technique so that infection can be minimized. Upon exposure, the tumor should be handled very delicately to minimize the possibility of spread.

Biopsy of lymph nodes. The pathologic changes found in lymph nodes are often confusing. It is extremely important, therefore, that entire nodes be obtained when-ever possible and that they be carefully fixed and meticulously stained. Lymph node imprints stained by Wright-Giemsa stain preparations may supplement tissue diagnosis of lymph nodes.

When a node is to be removed in the presence of generalized lymphadenopathy, the inguinal nodes, although easily accessible, should not be chosen since they are almost invariably complicated by infection and consequently may present a confusing pathologic picture.

It is the rule to remove nodes in the operating room, for the removal of the supraclavicular or axillary nodes may take on the aspect of a major surgical procedure. Lymph nodes that feel superficial may actually be deep and elusive.

Biopsy of curettings. Curettings are best handled not by frozen section but by proper fixation and careful staining.

Endoscopic specimens. Endoscopic specimens are usually small, and these specimens, like others obtained in the operating room, should be quickly placed in fixative before dehydration occurs. Such small specimens should be cut at various levels. Three slides should encompass about thirty sections. Tumor may be found at one level and not at another.

Bronchoscopic, esophagogastroscopic, cystoscopic, and protoscopic approaches may be necessary to obtain biopsies from the bronchus, esophagus, upper portion of the stomach, bladder, rectum, and sigmoid. Needless to say, not only is special technical training necessary to perform these procedures, but also considerable experience is essential in order that biopsy be done in the proper area. Exploratory operations such as an exploratory laparotomy or a thoracotomy may also be necessary to obtain tissue.

Staining methods

The conventional stain, hematoxylin and eosin, is probably the most satisfactory routine stain for a surgical pathology department. This stain is technically easy, and technicians of even little experience can make good slides under proper direction. This stain is also the one used in most pathology departments for teaching purposes, and therefore the house staff and visiting physicians are most familiar with it.

Special stains require special techniques. The fibroglia fibrils of fibrosarcoma are revealed with accuracy with a phosphotungstic acid and hematoxylin stain. The fat globules within a liposarcoma are shown with clarity with a sudan IV stain. At times, an iron stain may be of differential importance in deciding whether or not a tumor is a melanocarcinoma. There are now elaborate histochemical methods that are beyond the scope of this book.

Specialized procedures
Aspiration biopsy

The attitude toward aspiration biopsy varies in application from absolute rejection to overenthusiasm and overapplication of the procedure. We feel that it has definite value in certain specific instances, that it is simple, rapid, and harmless, and that it is a valuable adjunct to diagnosis (Godwin[27]). The technique is simple and requires only a large syringe, usually 20 ml or 50 ml, an 18-gauge needle 5 cm to 12 cm long, a Bard-Parker knife (#11), and Novocain. The needle must be sharp, for if the tumor contains a great deal of fibrous tissue, it should be able to cut out a small wedge of tumor.

The skin is cut with the knife in order to avoid carrying infection or squamous epithelium into the body. The needle is then inserted into the tumor and is *moved around during the procedure* while vacuum is constantly kept in the syringe. *The material thus obtained is placed on filter paper in the usual fixative and treated as a paraffin section.* This is in contradistinction to the method of smearing the material and then immediately staining it. This smear method, while it can be used by very well trained pathologists, does have several disadvantages. All architectural detail is, of necessity, lost. Consequently, the diagnosis must be made on the basis of cellular detail alone. We therefore use the first method because, in reality, it provides a small specimen that retains architectural detail and the normal relationships and differs from the usual specimen only in size (Meatheringham and Ackerman[54]).

Indications and limitations. At all times there must be sympathetic cooperation between the surgeon and the pathologist (Stewart[96]). Aspiration biopsy is *restricted to hospitals in which men experienced in its technique and interpretation are available.* In no other biopsy is it so necessary for the pathologist to have an intimate knowledge of the patient's clinical history and the physical findings. Often it might be wise for him to question and examine the patient. The palpation of the tumor with the needle may reveal the thickness of a capsule, the consistency of the tumor, the presence of bone, or the depth of the lesion.

There is no doubt that while aspiration biopsy has its place, it should not be extended to cover all situations. Its use should be limited to those cases in which formal biopsy is difficult or impossible and those in which it can perhaps be substituted for a major surgical procedure such as a thoracotomy or an exploratory laparotomy.

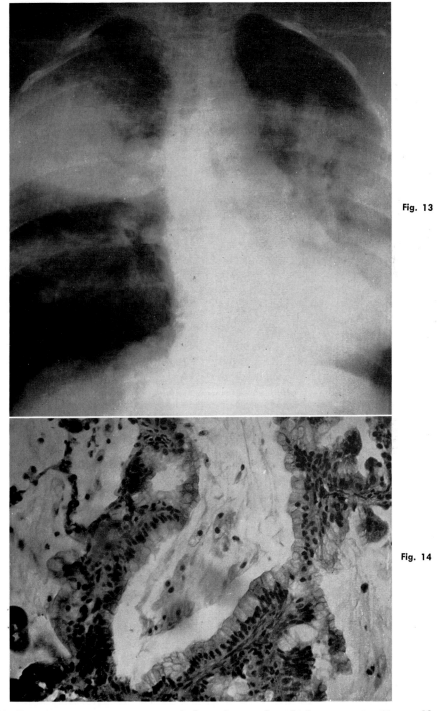

Fig. 13. Posteroanterior roentgenogram of chest showing bronchiolar cancer in 47-year-old woman. Note extensive bilateral involvement. (WU neg. 61-1874.)

Fig. 14. Needle biopsy specimen clearly demonstrating bronchiolar cancer. (×250; WU neg. 61-1769.)

Aspiration of metastatic nodules in the liver, soft tissue masses, particularly sarcomas, and even bone tumors can be accomplished easily, and the complication of leaving tumor implants along the tract of the aspirating needle has occurred only once in our experience following aspiration biopsy of a lymph node in the neck.

Lymph nodes. A formal biopsy of nodes in lymphomas should certainly be done, for the diagnosis is difficult enough with an incisional biopsy and would usually be impossible with an aspiration specimen. It is most valuable in diagnosing other lymph node lesions, particularly those suspected of containing carcinoma (Fig. 16). In practically all of these instances, the primary lesion will already have been diagnosed.

Difficulty in aspirating inguinal, cervical, and axillary nodes increases in the order listed. Inguinal nodes are easily found, and the biopsy material from them is of particular value in aged patients with carcinoma of the penis or vulva on whom a radical groin dissection is contemplated. Cervical nodes are a bit harder to locate, but the biopsy is advantageous for determining whether accessible ones contain tumor, particularly when there is a primary lesion within the oral cavity. If an enlarged cervical node is considered metastatic, it is imperative that proof of tumor within the node be shown so that treatment by radiotherapy may be given credit if cure is effected; if the node is only inflammatory, it is still just as important that proof be obtained. The axillary lymph nodes are located in a large volume of fat and loose tissue, and it is often difficult to isolate small nodes in this area.

Breast. Needle biopsy of breast lesions is well indicated when the cancer is advanced and radiotherapy is to be given. If the lesion is large, such a biopsy may save operating time. It is of less value in small lesions. If the needle biopsy is negative, then obviously formal biopsy has to be done. In a series of cases reported by Saltzstein,[78] no delay in therapy could be ascribed to false negatives at needle biopsy.

Lungs. Aspiration biopsy of the lung is only rarely indicated, but it can be done without difficulty and without complications. We feel that the risk of spread along the needle tract has been overemphasized.

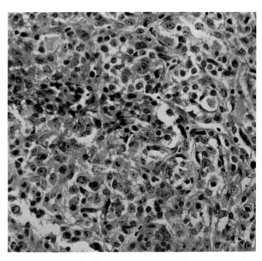

Fig. 15. Needle biopsy specimen of recurrent undifferentiated osteogenic sarcoma in soft tissues. Note preservation of architectural pattern. (Moderate enlargement.)

If a patient has a peripheral lesion of unknown etiology in the lung and if other procedures such as bronchoscopic examination and cytologic examination of the sputa render negative results, it is still imperative that the patient have an exploratory thoracotomy. At the time of exploratory thoracotomy, the lesion can be locally resected. Diagnosis by frozen section can then determine whether any further treatment is indicated. In advanced inoperable peripheral carcinoma of the lung, aspiration biopsy may be done to obviate exploratory thoracotomy. The same reasoning applies to tumors of the mediastinum. In bilateral lesions of the lung of unknown etiology in which all other laboratory methods have failed, material obtained by needle biopsy may be diagnostic (Figs. 13 and 14). Exploratory thoracotomy is a better procedure (Grant and Trivedi[29]).

Bone. When cortical bone has been destroyed and there is a pathologic lesion of bone, aspiration through the area of destruction is performed easily and adequate material is obtained (Fig. 15). This is of particular value in lesions of the mandible and antrum. Needle biopsy of lesions actually within the bone can be done (Schajowicz[83]). Such a procedure is particularly valuable for vertebral lesions.

Liver. Aspiration of masses within the abdomen can also be done if some common sense is used in the selection of patients. Aspiration biopsy of the liver can be done usually with little risk, and the approach recommended is at the midclavicular line just below the right costal border. If there is any question as to whether the intestine is firmly adherent to the liver, however, and if danger of perforation of intestine is present, aspiration should not be attempted. On the other hand, if the liver is nodular and close to the abdominal wall, aspiration of liver masses can be done with no difficulty. In 500 aspiration biopsies reported by Gillman and Gillman,[26] in only one instance did intraperitoneal hemorrhage occur, and this was not due to a capsular tear but to puncture of a large artery. They believed that aspiration biopsy was indispensable for the diagnosis of lesions that showed hepatic enlargement. We have made the diagnosis of both primary and secondary malignant tumors and by so doing have at times saved the time and cost of an exploratory laparotomy.

Interpretation. The interpretation of aspiration biopsy depends upon the experience of the pathologist and the cooperation he receives from the surgeon. This interpretation will be enhanced when all available information is at hand.

The diagnosis of squamous carcinoma or adenocarcinoma within lymph nodes is made with no difficulty. If keratinized material is obtained from a lymph node, there can be no doubt that this represents metastatic squamous carcinoma (Fig. 16). It is usually impossible to make a diagnosis of Hodgkin's disease or lymphosarcoma or related entities from aspiration material; in these instances, formal incisional biopsy is indicated. The diagnosis of the adenocarcinoma within a lymph node (e.g., within an inguinal lymph node representing metastasis from an adenocarcinoma of the endometrium) presents no difficulty. Soft tissue lesions such as sarcoma present considerable difficulty in diagnosis at times, and it is frequently impossible to classify them exactly, although one is usually able to state that it is a sarcoma. In both soft tissue sarcomas and bone tumors a microscopic diagnosis through incisional biopsy may be necessary for exact classification.

We have been using needle biopsy for

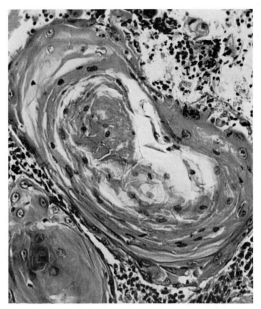

Fig. 16. Needle biopsy specimen of submaxillary lymph node containing metastatic epidermoid carcinoma. Primary tumor arose from lower lip. Note epithelial pearls. (High power.)

bone tumors increasingly. It has proved particularly valuable in lesions of the vertebrae and, when properly planned before surgery, reduces the risk of implantation (Schajowicz and Derqui[84]).

Electron microscopy

Electron microscopy is a valuable tool in biologic research, but it has been generally considered to have little or no value in diagnosis. Certainly, it could not be used as a routine method. In the past, special fixation was considered to be necessary. However, in a number of cases, even with material fixed in 10% formalin (4% reagent grade formaldehyde) in phosphate buffer at pH 7.4, it has provided a definitive diagnosis. Naturally, the cases were selected with considerable care. For instance, an enlarged axillary lymph node removed from a 64-year-old man was found to be replaced by undifferentiated malignant tumor. When examined under the electron microscope, the cytoplasm of many of the tumor cells showed numerous round and ovoid organelles averaging 500 mμ in diameter. They were limited by a single membrane and had a finely granular matrix. The morphology of these organelles

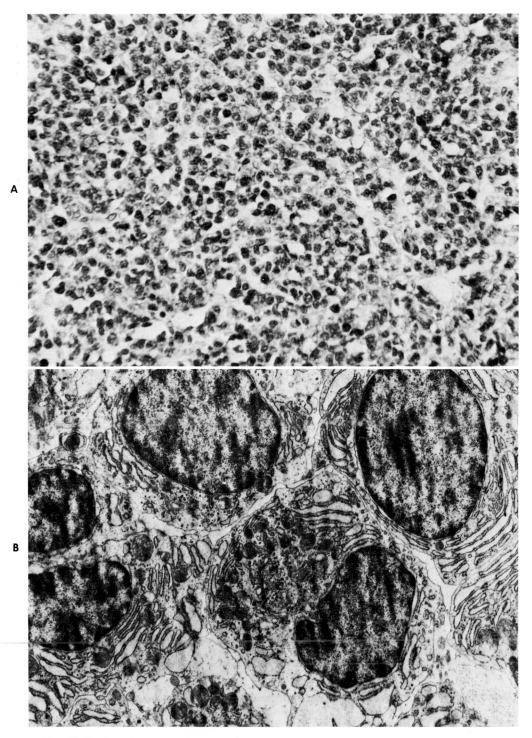

Fig. 17. For legend see opposite page.

was consistent with that of premelanosomes and, therefore, the diagnosis was amelanotic malignant melanoma. In another case, a firm diagnosis of plasma cell myeloma was made (Rosai and Rodriguez[76]) (Fig. 17).

Many other examples can be given, and other investigators have been using this method in diagnosis (Ashworth and Stembridge[7]; Lynn et al[49]).

Exfoliative cytology

There has been extensive investigation of exfoliative cytology as a method of diagnosis of cancer (Koss[43]). Secretions from every orifice have been looked at, and attempts have been made to diagnose practically every type of tumor. Overenthusiasm has now been replaced by a more judicious attitude toward this method of examination.

The organization of a laboratory of exfoliative cytology is difficult, and it is important that this laboratory be under the supervision of a pathologist. The training of personnel is extremely time consuming. It is impractical for the pathologist to attempt to screen all specimens submitted, and such screening can be done by a cytologist with a minimum of one year's training. However, it must always be the responsibility of the pathologist to see all suspicious specimens, and the responsibility of making the final diagnosis of cancer rests with him.

Exfoliative cytology can be used as a screening procedure. As such, however, it has extremely limited value in most instances because it is time consuming and extremely expensive. It finds its greatest usefulness in the detection of cancer of the cervix or endometrium in asymptomatic women. It has been demonstrated by Erickson et al.[22] that exfoliative cytology is a valuable screening procedure when

used for this purpose. It is even within the realm of possibility that, with adequate personnel, cancer of the cervix, for all practical purposes, could be eliminated. Cervical cancer is a highly curable disease in its early clinical phase (p. 78).

It must be stressed that a negative cytologic examination indicates only that cancer cells were not present on the slide. *It does not necessarily indicate that the patient does not have cancer.* Moreover, it is not practical to do a cytologic examination on excretions from organs in which a diagnosis can be made much more simply by biopsy (skin surface, oral cavity, bladder). Also, there are limitations of accuracy that make the cytologic diagnosis in some organs impractical. For instance, in cancer of the prostate it is often too difficult.

Cytologic examination, however, has proved to be *extremely valuable in certain organs in which clinical signs and symptoms suggest cancer but in which a positive histopathologic diagnosis cannot be made.* The procedure has proved to be of great value in diagnosing cancer of the lung and in detecting early cancer of the endometrium and cervix. Further, with its use the diagnosis of cancer of the stomach has now reached a level of high accuracy (Raskin et al.[68]; Schade[82]). In certain instances, it is also valuable as a follow-up procedure in detecting recurrence of cancer, as in treated lesions of the cervix, endometrium, and lung.

The methods of reporting a diagnosis made on exfoliative cytology have great practical significance. It is true that the pathologist may have considerable difficulty in making a definite diagnosis, but it does not do any good for the pathologist to transfer his uncertainty to the clinician. The pathologist should be content to stay within his limitations. Otherwise, false positives will occur. If false positives occur,

Fig. 17. A, Photomicrograph of bone tumor. It is composed of regular, round cells growing in diffuse fashion. **B,** Low-power electron micrograph of tumor cells. Note eccentric nucleus with clumped chromatin, prominent perinuclear Golgi apparatus, and numerous parallel cisternae of granular endoplasmic reticulum. From these changes, a diagnosis of plasma cell myeloma was made. Uranyl acetate–lead citrate. (**A,** Hematoxylin and eosin; ×350; WU neg. 68-949; **B,** ×2500; WU neg. 67-8449; **A** and **B,** from Rosai, J., and Rodriguez, H. A.: Application of electron microscopy to the differential diagnosis of tumors, Amer. J. Clin. Path. **50:**555-562, 1968; © 1968, The Williams & Wilkins Co., Baltimore, Md., U.S.A.)

they invalidate the procedure. We have found that the best method of reporting the tests is in four categories:

1 Material submitted inadequate
2 No evidence of cancer
3 Cells present that appear suspicious (this indicates only that more material is needed for examination and that cancer may or may not be present)
4 Diagnosis of cancer

In the latter instance, we must have confidence in our report. For instance, in the lung, with clinical signs and symptoms suggesting cancer but with no histo-pathologic diagnosis obtainable, the positive cytologic report swings the balance to pulmonary resection. The percentage of positive findings in a given number of malignant tumors from any particular organ depends on many factors, including the method of collection of the specimens, their preparation, the completeness of the examination, the training of the cytologist and the pathologist, and whether or not repeated examinations are done. Such factors and percentages will vary from organ to organ.

There is no doubt that the cytologic method of examination in the diagnosis of cancer is here to stay, and the pathologist must take the responsibility for the proper organization of the laboratories and must be ready and capable of examining material sent to him. The indications for, and limitations of, exfoliative cytology will be discussed in more detail in the various chapters as exfoliative cytology is applicable.

Examination of pleural and peritoneal fluid

If cancer is suspected and either pleural or peritoneal fluid develops, this fluid can be aspirated and then examined for the presence of malignant cells by two methods: (1) the fluid can be centrifuged and stained smears made of the sediment or (2) the sediment can be prepared in the same fashion as a biopsy and paraffin sections made.

Mesothelial cells are frequently inaccurately diagnosed as cancer because they can arrange themselves in a pseudoglandular formation, may have multiple nuclei, and are not too rarely seen in mitoses (Takagi[98]). The presence of single cells showing great variation in size of the nuclei with prominent nucleoli and the presence of atypical mitotic figures are positive evidence of a malignant tumor. False positive reports should be rare. The percentage of false negatives that occur depends on the thoroughness of the examination, the experience of the examiner, the method of preparation of the specimens, and other factors.

Frozen section

Frozen section diagnosis is a rapid method of taking fresh tissue and cutting and staining it for microscopic examination so that a number of slides can be examined in a short period of time. It is a highly accurate method of diagnosis. There is only one purpose in doing a frozen section and that is *to make a therapeutic decision*. This method achieves its highest accuracy when it is the result of cooperation between an experienced surgeon with an interest in pathology and a pathologist with a clinical point of view.

With present refinements in technique, there are few difficulties in making an exact histologic diagnosis. The cryostat is now being used widely. Sections can be cut at 5μ, and the quality of the preparations is just as high as in the conventional sections. Errors occur only because of failure to select the proper area for sectioning or because of intellectual failure on the part of the examining pathologist. The latter would make the same error on the permanent sections. In any event, pathologists can usually say if a given lesion is a malignant neoplasm, a benign neoplasm, or a nonneoplastic process. It is on the basis of these broad diagnoses that major therapeutic decisions are made.

There are certain statements that are still being made that are no longer true. It is often said that diagnoses of thyroid and lymphoid lesions are impossible by frozen section. In sixty-three consecutive frozen sections of thyroid lesions, we had no false positives and two false negatives. In 143 consecutive frozen sections of lymph nodes, we had no false positives and three false negatives (Ackerman and Ramirez[3]). The pathologist, of course, must do his best to reach a decision in order that the proper treatment can be given without delay. Such a decision is very important when the surgeon is operating within the thoracic cage and abdomen and is of less importance during surgery for lesions of the breast. Over 95% of the time a definite decision can be made. In the series of 3000 consecutive cases reported by Nakazawa et al.,[60] there was an accuracy of 98.6% when deferred diagnoses were excluded.

False positive diagnosis must not be made. Rarely, such errors will occur, but they should be few and far between. Otherwise, the procedure is invalidated. False negative errors are of much less importance than false positives. Naturally, if such an error is made, it may be necessary to do a second surgical procedure.

There is always a risk of implantation of cancer if frozen section is done. Such a risk will vary from organ to organ. Of course, if the lesion can be completely excised at the time of frozen section, the risk will be reduced to practically zero. Thyroid nodules can be excised in their entirety, and this implies lobectomy. Frozen section of a lesion of the breast carries with it little risk because the entire area is excised at the time of definitive procedure. In other areas, risk is always present because it is necessary to incise the area. This occurs in the stomach, pancreas, and gastrointestinal tract.

In some instances, because of the location of the lesion, definitive surgery can be done without benefit of frozen section. In other instances, because of high mortality and morbidity, together with low possibility of cure of the cancer, the risk of the procedure is outweighed by the information gained by the frozen section. This situation occurs in patients with cancer of the head of the pancreas. With increasing experience, the pathologist learns his limitations and works with the surgeon for the best interests of the patient.

Tissue culture

There are certain specialized tests that are valuable in the diagnosis of tumors. It is realized that the microscopic study of tumors is often not satisfactory because it is a static rather than a dynamic discipline.

Tissue culture as a method of identification of certain specific types of tumors has

been proved fruitful in the hands of Murray et al.[58, 59] They have been able to identify definitely such tumors as neuroblastomas, synovial sarcomas, liposarcomas, etc. by comparing the cultural characteristics of the tumor type in question with those of the normal tissue to which it is thought to be related. Goldstein et al.[28] have also demonstrated the value of tissue culture in tumors of the sympathetic nervous system. Marcuse[53] used short-term tissue culture methods in 600 cases of benign and malignant tumors. The speed at which tumor appeared in the culture bore no relation to whether it was benign or malignant.

Tissue culture complements the study of tissue sections and smears made from exfoliative material.

Gross description of surgical specimens

The tumor should be described in relation to other structures, with its exact size, color, and consistency noted. All lymph nodes or large vessels should be found and carefully charted. The blood vessels should be opened and tumor invasion looked for. The diagnosis in some tumors is grossly obvious. The chalky streaks of a carcinoma of the breast, the polypoid, well-delineated carcinoma of the rectum, the serous cystadenocarcinomas of the ovary with their papillary projections and cysts, and the bright yellow of the kidney carcinomas are clearly evident on inspection.

There are a number of standardized surgical procedures such as radical mastectomy, abdominoperineal resection for cancer of the large bowel, neck dissection, pneumonectomy, etc. These extensive surgical procedures have necessitated the creation of a manual to ensure that certain minimum information is always recorded for each type of specimen and the preparation of diagrams that can be used with various types of specimens (Fig. 18). If the instructions are followed in describing the specimen and if certain required sections are taken using the diagram, the body of uniform information obtained will be of tremendous value in analyzing the effectiveness of treatment in groups of cases.

Lymph node metastases

The prognosis of many tumors is directly dependent upon the presence or absence

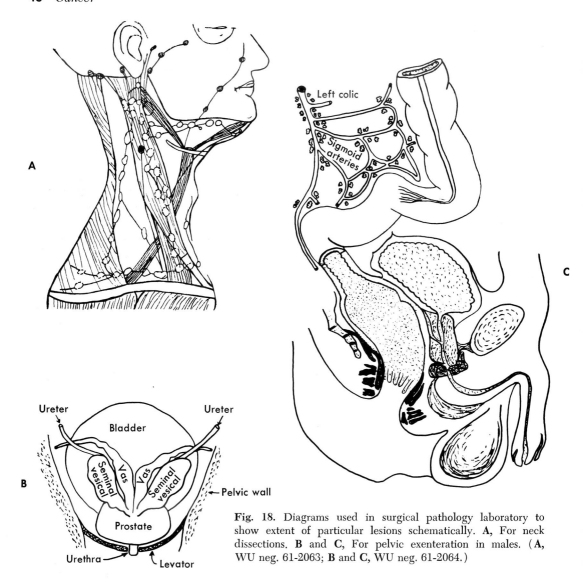

A

B

Ureter — Bladder — Ureter

Vas — Seminal vesical — Vas — Seminal vesical

Pelvic wall

Prostate

Urethra — Levator

C

Left colic

Sigmoid arteries

Fig. 18. Diagrams used in surgical pathology laboratory to show extent of particular lesions schematically. **A,** For neck dissections. **B** and **C,** For pelvic exenteration in males. (**A,** WU neg. 61-2063; **B** and **C,** WU neg. 61-2064.)

of lymph node metastases. Many series of cases report either the presence or the absence of spread, but seldom is it clear by what methods the nodes are proved negative. If the nodes are positive microscopically, there is indeed no challenge. When the nodes are stated to be negative, however, there should be further verification.

When recording information about metastatic lymph nodes, the number, distribution, and respective involvement should be diagrammatically portrayed after gross and microscopic examination of the specimen (Fig. 18). It is obviously of greater significance in carcinoma of the breast when the

high point of the axilla is involved than when the lower part alone is involved.

The number of involved nodes also has prognostic significance. There is no doubt that if refined methods of clearing are used, large numbers of nodes will be found. However, we do not think that clearing has practical value. Coller et al.[15] found an average of thirty in the stomach, and Grinnell[32] found an average of fifty-two in the rectum. Upon careful examination and without clearing of surgical specimens, we have found an average of thirty-one lymph nodes in axillary dissections for cancer of the breast, thirty in abdominoperineal resections for cancer of the large bowel, and forty-nine in neck dissections for head and neck cancer.

Harvey and Auchincloss[37] reviewed a large number of patients who had had surgery for various types of cancer and were apparently cured. In considering only the problem of lymph node metastases in patients with carcinoma of the stomach, rectum, breast and colon, 72% of the survivors had no lymph node metastases, 94% had metastases in three or fewer lymph nodes, and less than 3% had metastases in more than five nodes.

The dissection of lymph nodes from any surgical specimen is a meticulous and time-consuming procedure, but the rewards are gratifying. For instance, in carcinoma of the breast, it is not unusual to find that only one of perhaps thirty axillary nodes is replaced by tumor. A few negative nodes, therefore, are of much less consequence than are fifty negative nodes.

Frequently, small, soft, grossly negative lymph nodes are replaced by tumor in the same surgical specimen in which there are negative, large, fairly firm, homogenous gray nodes. When infection accompanies the primary tumor, the nodes may be hard, homogeneous, enlarged, and gray on cross section but still be negative. The large, obviously involved nodes show focal zones of grayish yellow tumor. The reason that cure is not effected by surgery in some patients with carcinoma of the breast, penis, vulva, and other organs in spite of apparent negative regional nodes may revert back to an initial examination that was not thorough.

Blood vessel invasion

Invasion of blood vessels usually is not noted grossly in surgical specimens. Certain tumors removed surgically should be closely examined grossly for evidence of such invasion. This applies particularly to carcinoma of the thyroid gland and other lesions of the upper neck, kidney, and large bowel.

Gross blood vessel invasion will be seen as tumor that has grown directly within the vein. In certain metastatic lesions of the neck, a lymph node may break into a jugular vein, and tumor may be present there. It is extremely important that evidence of blood vessel invasion be searched for in tumors of the thyroid gland. In kidney neoplasms, the prognosis will depend on whether the renal vein is invaded. Rarely, such gross blood vessel invasion will be noted in malignant tumors of the large bowel and lung.

Microscopic description of surgical specimens

The microscopic description should be as brief as possible. Some mention should be made of the degree of differentiation. Any evidence of blood vessel or nerve sheath invasion should be indicated, for this may very well be of prognostic significance. Frequently, special sections are taken to determine whether the excision has been adequate, and careful statements should be made concerning them. Detailed descriptions may be necessary in rare tumors.

At the end of the microscopic description of any of the large surgical specimens, such as a neck dissection, radical mastectomy, or tissue obtained from radical resection of large bowel and stomach, it is worthwhile to summarize the pertinent gross and microscopic findings and to attempt to relate them to the prognosis.

Precancerous lesions

We later discuss the possibility of a benign tumor becoming malignant and indicate the tremendous change of attitude on this point. This whole problem of a precancerous lesion has to be reviewed with certain concepts in mind (Ackerman[2]). Clinical and pathologic opinion are changing rapidly about many of these lesions. The chronic ulcer of the stomach used to be considered a serious precancerous lesion. It is now doubtful if a cancer ever arises from a preexisting ulcer of the stomach. The senile keratoses do become cancer, but this is a relatively minor problem, and such lesions can be removed, depending upon their location, number, and appearance.

To give an example of the looseness of thought that is used in speaking of precancerous lesions, we need only to mention leukoplakia. Leukoplakia occurs in many areas. It is said to be precancerous and must be removed. The evidence for this is based on tenuous grounds. Usually the observer states that a certain number of carcinomas of the vulva or oral cavity were associated with leukoplakia, therefore inferring that the cancer arose from the leukoplakia. Also, frank but superficial and multicentric carcinomas may produce the clinical appearance of leukoplakia. If we look at this problem from another angle and take 100 patients with leukoplakia of the oral cavity, in how many with the passage of time would such a lesion become cancer? It has now been shown by careful follow-up studies that the number of times that leukoplakia progresses to cancer is minimal (Renstrup[71]; Shafer and Waldron[88]).

Other possible cancerous lesions such as chronic cystic disease and cancer of the breast and polyps and cancer of the colon, as well as numerous other lesions, will be discussed in the appropriate chapters.

The therapist must consider the potentiality of a given lesion based on follow-up of a group of patients and must decide whether the operative procedure contemplated will prevent enough cases of cancer to justify its use at this particular moment. Certain cancers and congenital defects occur together more often than can be attributed to chance (Miller[55]).

Growth rate of cancer

On occasion, it has been stated that cancer grew with appalling speed during the last few weeks of a patient's life. On the other hand, there is the patient who has, say, a cancer of the breast removed and then after a long latent period, perhaps even more than fifteen years, there will be recrudescence of the breast cancer in the surgical scar. Was the cancer in the first patient really growing with appalling speed during the last few weeks of life? In the second patient, did the cancer remain dormant and then was it stimulated by some hormonal influence, or why did it recur?

We now have information that at least provides a partial answer to these questions. We believe that cancer cells divide at a randomly steady rate and that the growth of cancer obeys the compound interest law: that the increase in size of a malignant tumor at any moment is proportional to the size it has already attained.

The mean length of time required for the division of all the cancer cells has been designated as the *doubling time* (Spratt and Ackerman[93]). Collins et al.,[16] using roentgenographic mensuration, found that the doubling time of pulmonary metastases from rectal cancer varied between 49 and 123 days. We believe that the doubling time of neoplasms in different organs or of different carcinomas of the same microscopic type of the same organ may have entirely different doubling times. For instance, we have measured primary pulmonary malignant neoplasms and have found varying doubling times from 8 to 763 days.

By referring to Fig. 19, it can easily be seen that there is an extremely long time period before a lesion becomes visible. It takes thirty doubling times for a lesion to reach a centimeter in diameter. After it has reached a certain size, then the volume of tissue is so great that the tumor *appears to grow* with appalling speed yet it is still obeying its doubling time, which remains at a constant rate.

Let us say further that we have a cancer of the breast that has an extremely slow doubling time and that we remove all the cancer at surgery except a small cluster of cells. Therefore, if there is a long latent period before the cancer clinically reappears, this can be explained by a small residual number of cancer cells plus a slow doubling time (Baserga et al.[8]). The term "early cancer" in the sense that the lesion is small as seen radiographically or noted on palpation is an extremely inadequate statement. It appears certain that most carcinomas are present three to four times as long in their preclinical period as in their clinical time period. Furthermore, in our studies of certain malignant tumors, the size of the tumors as we have measured them, as in cancer of the large bowel (Spratt and Ackerman[93]) and cancer of the lung (Spjut et al.[92]), bears no relation to prognosis.

Differentiation between benign and malignant tumors

The differentiation between the benign and malignant tumor is usually not difficult. A typical benign tumor is usually encapsulated, and the capsule is made up of connective tissue. On section, it usually

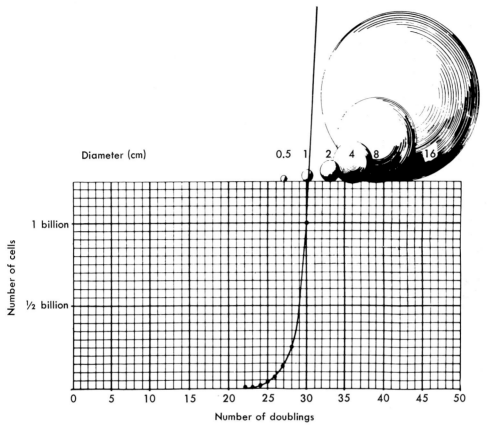

Fig. 19. Growth curve of hypothetical tumor on arithmetic coordinates. Note how many doubling times it takes before tumor becomes any appreciable size. (From Collins, V. P., et al.: Observations on growth rates of human tumors, Amer. J. Roentgen. **76**:988-1000, 1956; WU neg. 60-988.)

reveals a relatively homogeneous appearance if it is made up of the same type of tissue. At times, the encapsulation may be rather poorly defined, as in a lipoma.

Degenerative and regressive changes occur much less frequently in benign tumors than in malignant tumors. However, if a benign tumor has been present long enough, has grown large enough, or has had some impairment of its blood supply, then changes can take place. For instance, hemorrhage may occur in a lipoma, calcification in a leiomyoma of the uterus, or a necrosis in a benign ovarian cyst with a twisted pedicle. Microscopically, the pattern of these tumors is *orderly*. Individual cells all appear the same. Mitotic figures may occur in fairly rapidly growing cellular benign tumors, and they should not be construed as evidence of malignancy.

Benign tumors do not metastasize, but if they are located in a strategic position, they may cause major pathologic alterations. For instance, a large leiomyoma may partially block the ureters, resulting in kidney insufficiency. A benign tumor growing in the bronchus may result in partial occlusion of the bronchus with secondary infection in the lung and sequential changes that may lead to death.

Transformation of benign to malignant tumor

It should be mentioned that, at times, a benign tumor may be transformed into a malignant one. In order to prove this, it is necessary to demonstrate that a benign tumor has been present for a period of time and that, upon its removal, cancer was found in one portion of the lesion and the benign tumor in the other. Preferably, there should be a good transition from the benign tumor to the malignant neoplasm. Furthermore, it is necessary that the cancer have the capacity to metastasize.

If a patient has had a tumor for a number of years and it is removed and proved to be entirely cancer, there is no way of proving that it ever arose from a preexisting benign neoplasm. We know that some carcinomas can exist for exceedingly long time periods. A good example of the change in thinking is reflected in the attitude toward neoplasms of the thyroid gland. It was frequently stated in the past (even in this book) that three out of four carcinomas of the thyroid gland arose from preexisting adenomas. We now know that practically all carcinomas of the thyroid arise de novo and that only rarely will one arise from a preexisting adenoma.

Most malignant tumors arise de novo. A liposarcoma does not arise from a lipoma, a fibrosarcoma from a fibroma, or synovial sarcoma from nodular synovitis. Probably leiomyosarcomas of the uterus do not arise from preexisting leiomyomas. It is possible that, in rare instances, a malignant schwannoma could arise from a neurofibroma, and we know that on rare occasion mixed tumors of the salivary gland become malignant. However, in the past, the transition of a benign tumor to a malignant tumor was greatly exaggerated. This problem will be considered as it relates to different organs.

The reasons for removing a benign tumor are usually motivated by (1) the changes produced by a benign neoplasm because of its critical position or (2) the inability to identify it clinically as being either a benign or a malignant tumor.

The malignant tumor usually does not have a capsule or, if the capsule is present, it is incomplete. Grossly, extension into the surrounding tissues or evidence of involvement of blood vessels or contiguous lymph nodes may be observed. On section, the tumor may be homogeneous and, if very cellular, grayish yellow in color. The malignant tumor frequently shows areas of necrosis that are manifested as yellowish zones or areas of hemorrhage, recent or old.

Microscopically, the malignant tumor invariably has a *disorderly pattern*. Mitotic figures may or may not be present, and if abnormal forms are seen with asymmetrical spindles or giant forms, then the probability of malignancy is high. The microscopic search may reveal tumor within veins, lymphatics, or perineural spaces. Malignant tumors metastasize, but at the time of examination some tumors still remain localized.

There is no doubt that it is extremely difficult to determine whether certain tumors are benign or malignant. This is particularly true in some well-differentiated tumors of salivary gland origin, in certain cartilaginous tumors, and in some breast neoplasms. These borderline lesions require considerable study and much experience in tumor pathology before a decision can be made as to whether they should be treated as a benign or a malignant tumor.

Carcinomas
Epidermoid carcinoma

In 1890, von Hansemann[34] originated the idea of grading certain tumors, and this was popularized by Broders.[11] In our practice, we have given the squamous or epidermoid carcinoma only three grades, for further division seems impractical.

Grade I presents uniform cells, many epithelial pearls, and rare or no mitotic figures (Fig. 20). Grade II shows some tendency to variation in cell size and has

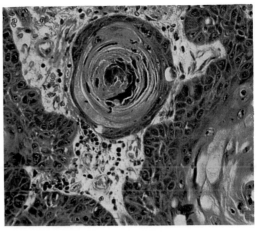

Fig. 20. Well-differentiated epidermoid carcinoma with epithelial pearls and intercellular bridges. (Moderate enlargement.)

occasional mitotic figures, few epithelial pearls, and a moderate tendency to keratinization. At times, particularly in the cervix, it may take a plexiform pattern (Fig. 21). Grade III has a most disorderly pattern with many mitotic figures, some of which are abnormal, and no tendency to keratinization (Fig. 22).

Adenocarcinoma

The adenocarcinomas can be divided into three grades. Further division does not seem practical.

Grade I shows glands arranged in a very orderly pattern with only a few mitotic figures. The individual acini appear almost normal. Early, the cells of the glands show loss of nuclear polarity and stratification of cells. Grade II shows only moderate tendency to glandular formation, numerous mitotic figures, and tendency to a fairly irregular pattern. Grade III is so very undifferentiated that it is scarcely recognizable as an adenocarcinoma. There are numerous mitotic figures, some of which are abnormal.

Törnberg[99] described a method of grading breast carcinoma which emphasizes the margins of the tumors. The presence of pushing borders and a mantle of lymphocytes diminishes the frequency of metastases (Hultborn and Törnberg[39]). Pushing borders have also been well described in cancer of the stomach (Urban and Mc-Neer[101]) and in cancer of the larynx (Mc-

Gavran et al.[50]), and we have found them to be important in cancer of the large bowel.

Carcinoma in situ

The term carcinoma in situ has been applied to true epithelial tumors of both glandular and squamous character. It has become apparent that carcinoma of all types in many organs may undergo focal changes in which atypical alterations do not show evidence of breakthrough of their basement membranes. In the squamous type of epithelium, we have seen these changes not only in the cervix, where they have been described by many investigators, but also in other areas such as the skin, oral cavity, esophagus, and bronchus. We have also seen focal alterations in glands in early carcinoma of the stomach, endometrium, and large bowel. In both instances, there is a disorganization of the epithelium.

In organs lined by squamous epithelium, the transition consists of thickening of the epidermis with disorganization and increase of mitotic activity (Fig. 23). In organs lined by glandular epithelium, the changes consist of atypical glands, stratification of nuclei, and loss of nuclear polarity with interglandular budding. It is not known how long such lesions may remain in situ before becoming invasive carcinoma. It has been shown in carcinoma of the cervix that the time interval can be

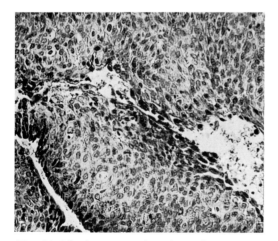

Fig. 21. Plexiform type of epidermoid carcinoma, fairly well differentiated. (Moderate enlargement.)

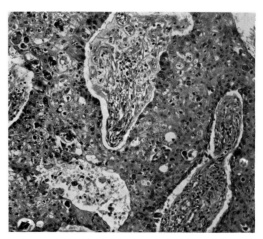

Fig. 22. Very undifferentiated epidermoid carcinoma showing innumerable mitotic figures and nuclear monstrosities. (Moderate enlargement.)

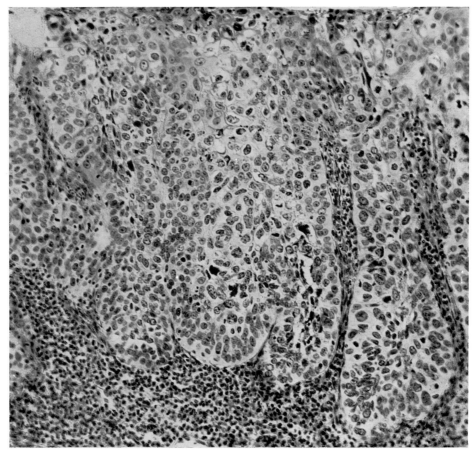

Fig. 23. Carcinoma in situ with intact basement membrane, disorganization of pattern, and innumerable mitotic figures throughout all layers. (High power.)

years. However, if such changes are found, they may be associated with invasive carcinoma. The decision as to the proper treatment of carcinoma in situ may be extremely difficult.

Multiple foci of origin. It is a fundamental principle of pathology of cancer to consider the frequency of multiple foci of origin of a given neoplasm in a given organ. It seems certain that the extrinsic and intrinsic influences acting on a given type of tissue may make it susceptible to the development of cancer. For some reason, one particular zone shows obvious changes first. This area may be controlled by therapeutic measures, and then, at a later time, evidence of carcinoma may appear elsewhere in the same organ. In the past, many of these carcinomas were considered local recurrences but now they are often considered new tumors.

As the treatment of cancer becomes more successful locally, the incidence of such multiple primary lesions in a given organ is bound to increase. We all know of the frequency of multiple carcinomas in the farmer whose skin has been altered because of many years' exposure to sunlight. It appears to be a certainty that if a patient has one cancer of the oral cavity, there is an increased chance of another developing. We have also seen simultaneous development of multiple carcinomas within the oral cavity. Further, by the use of multiple biopsies, we have demonstrated in situ changes over discontinuous areas within the oral cavity. Such changes have also been seen in the esophagus, bronchus, vulva, breast, and bladder. This concept of multiple foci of origin may modify consideration of the treatment. In addition, it is helpful in directing attention to the increased risk to the patient with a particular form of cancer so that he will be followed with special care.

Value of grading

The grading of a tumor may often be overemphasized and overrated, for it may be an unimportant feature. If, for instance, one found a Grade I adenocarcinoma of the endometrium that had extended out to the peritoneal surface, the extension of the tumor would certainly be of much more significance than its grade. If the tumor were a small Grade III adenocarcinoma localized to the endometrium, it would still be curable, and the grade would not be of too great significance. In large groups grading is of importance for determining end results, but in individual tumors its value is diminished. The more undifferentiated the tumor, the greater the incidence of metastases and the more rapid the clinical course.

There is no doubt that squamous carcinomas in certain locations such as lip, penis, vulva, and skin have a tendency to be well differentiated, whereas those in the cervix, hypopharynx, nasopharynx, and esophagus are less differentiated. This characteristic is important when the possibility of metastases is being considered.

An epidermoid carcinoma of the lower lip usually spreads only to a submaxillary or a submental lymph node, where it tends to grow slowly and remain localized. However, when it is undifferentiated, it may spread to involve many groups of lymph nodes in the neck. In the highly undifferentiated squamous carcinomas, it can be said with some certainty that the chances of distant metastases and rapid spread of the tumor are very high. Usually these highly anaplastic carcinomas make up only a relatively small percentage of the total group. This certainly applies to carcinomas of the cervix. On the contrary, when the tumor is extremely well differentiated and a Grade I carcinoma, then it will tend to remain localized for long periods of time. Individual squamous carcinomas in this category have been reported from the esophagus and the bronchus.

Sarcomas

Sarcomas of the soft tissues make up a smaller percentage of malignant tumors than the carcinomas. They arise from mesoderm and derive their names from their parent tissue. Each type, whether it be fibrosarcoma, liposarcoma, or rhabdomyosarcoma, arises wherever its primary type of tissue is available. Their individual characteristics are the subject of a special chapter (Chapter 17).

Lymphosarcoma is often seen first as a generalized process, but a certain unknown but increasing proportion of cases have been reported with a definite focus of origin. Regato[69] reported that lymphosarcoma frequently arose from the region of Waldeyer's ring (nasopharynx, tonsil, base of the tongue). The second most common site of origin is the gastrointestinal tract—the stomach, the large bowel, or the small bowel. Lymphosarcomas have been reported to arise from many other areas, and in some of these lymphatic tissue has been minimal in amount. The lacrimal gland (Perera[63]), dura (Abbott and Adson[1]), breast (Harrington and Miller[35]), vulva (Saxton[81]), testis (Dockerty and Priestley[20]), lung (Saltzstein[79]), and bladder (Moloney[56]) are some of the zones in which lymphosarcomas have apparently been primary.

It may be questioned whether lymphosarcoma ever originates in lymph nodes (Regato[70]). This may be a purely academic question, but it is a worthwhile concept to stimulate search for a primary focus when lymphosarcoma is discovered first in the lymph nodes.

The following classification of lymphomas is certainly easily defined and acceptable:

1 Lymphocytic
   a Well differentiated (nodular or diffuse)
   b Poorly differentiated ("lymphoblastic")
2 Mixed, lymphocytic and histiocytic
3 Histiocytic
4 Undifferentiated

The lymphocytic type of lymphosarcoma in a lymph node biopsy cannot be distinguished from a lymphocytic leukemia. A differential diagnosis would have to be made on the basis of hematologic findings and bone marrow studies. The reticulum cell sarcoma has large cells with extremely prominent nucleoli and pale pink cytoplasm. It makes up a relatively small percentage of the total group (Stout[97]; Oberling[61]). The giant follicle or nodular lymphoma is a stage of lymphoma in which the clinical evolution is relatively slow, although eventually all cases merge into other forms of lymphoma. The differential diagnosis between this form of lymphoma and a nonneoplastic lymph node may be difficult, and the differential diagnosis has been beautifully described by Rappaport et al.[67]

Patients with lymphoma, particularly of the well-differentiated type (lymphocytic), usually have generalized lymphadenopathy and splenomegaly and usually are in good general condition. There is a rough correlation between duration of the disease and differentiation of pattern (Rappaport et al.[67]). This type of lymphoma eventually becomes disseminated and culminates in lymphocytic leukemia, diffuse lymphosarcoma, and reticulum cell sarcoma. Treatment of this type is by radiotherapy, and often the duration of the disease is many years. When the patients die, in a few instances a pattern of giant follicle (nodular) lymphoma may be maintained in the various organs, and it may be particularly striking in the spleen. There may be bone involvement.

General properties of malignant tumors

Malignant tumors have certain general properties. They are sometimes abundantly supplied with blood vessels and accordingly may give rise to profound hemorrhage when biopsy is performed. The growth of the tumor may be so rapid that the blood supply is affected, and necrosis may ensue. When there is a profuse blood supply, fragments of tumor cells may reach the circulating bloodstream. The tumor may be very hard because of dense hyalinized connective tissue stroma (breast), but the amount of stroma varies with each tumor and even in different parts of the same tumor. The cellularity of a tumor may also determine its hardness. A papillomatous tumor of the large bowel may be soft because it is made up almost entirely of epithelial cells with a very delicate connective tissue framework.

Various degenerative processes may take place within the tumor. Some tumors form mucin and consequently are very soft and gelatinous. This occurs particularly in carcinomas of the gastrointestinal tract, breast, pancreas, and gallbladder. Mucin production does not occur in carcinoma of the thyroid gland, but small amounts may be produced in carcinomas of the prostate, liver, and kidney (Foster and Levine[25]). This finding may be helpful in determining the site of origin of a metastatic cancer. Granulosa cell tumors of the ovary may cause feminizing changes and, conversely, cortical tumors of the suprarenal gland may initiate virilizing changes in a woman.

An ever increasing number of new syndromes and new patterns of neoplasms are being reported and will be discussed in detail in the appropriate chapters (Lipsett[46]; Greenberg et al.[30]). We have known for a long time of functioning islet cell tumors of the pancreas and the rare functioning tumors of the thyroid gland. Serotonin-producing carcinoid tumors of the gastrointestinal tract and bronchus also occur. Patients with carcinomas of various organs such as the kidney and lung may have a profound hypercalcemia of unknown cause in the absence of metastases (Plimpton and Gellhorn[64]). Potassium-losing villous tumors of the large bowel may cause clinical abnormalities. Hematologic disorders may be associated with tumors of the ovary, kidney, and thymus. Peripheral neuropathy of sensory motor type may also be associated with malignant disease (Croft et al.[19]). Pluriglandular syndromes involving functioning endocrine tumors of numerous endocrine organs have been reported. Certainly, innumerable other syndromes and abnormalities associated with cancer remain to be identified by the alert clinician.

It has become increasingly important to study neoplasms by more sophisticated methods. To do this, the surgeon and the pathologist must obtain material at the time of operation which can be properly fixed for electron microscopic and histochemical examination. It also may be necessary to freeze material for further study. Only by doing this can it be shown that a given tumor is producing ACTH, parathyroid hormone, glucagon, etc. The study by McGavran et al.[51] is a model of what can be done in demonstrating the unique properties of a tumor—a glucagon-producing alpha cell cancer of the pancreas.

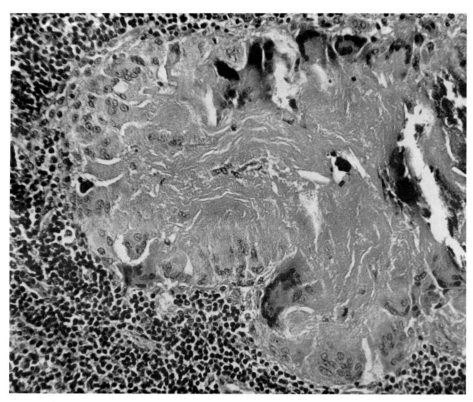

Fig. 24. Photomicrograph of all that remains of metastatic squamous cancer in cervical lymph node of patient with carcinoma of pyriform fossa. Patient had surgical resection of cancer of pyriform sinus in continuity with radical neck dissection. There had been no treatment of lymph nodes by radiotherapy and no chemotherapy. Serial section of this involved node showed no evidence of viable tumor, yet changes were identical with those produced by radiotherapy. There is no explanation at present for this evidence of spontaneous regression.

Death rarely is caused by a malignant tumor alone but rather by the effects of the tumor on the contiguous organs. Tumors of the oral cavity, particularly carcinoma of the tongue, pharynx, and larynx, are especially prone to interfere with deglutition, and necrotic infected tumor in the oral cavity is prone to be aspirated into the respiratory tract. Carcinoma of the cervix and, to a lesser degree, of the ovary, rectum, and prostate may obstruct the ureters and cause death from a combination of obstruction and pyelonephritis. Other tumors, primarily in the gastrointestinal tract, may cause intestinal obstruction, perforation, or hemorrhage.

There are undoubted instances of spontaneous regression of cancer in the absence of treatment or in the presence of inadequate therapy (Fig. 24). Some of these cases have a permanent regression, but in others recrudescence of the disease appears. Everson[23] collected 119 biopsy-proved cases, including neuroblastoma (twenty-five), renal cell cancer (fourteen), choriocarcinoma (thirteen), malignant melanoma (ten), soft tissue sarcoma (nine), and carcinoma of the bladder (seven). The remainder included osteosarcoma, breast carcinoma, and numerous others. Spontaneous regression is often permanent with neuroblastoma.

Correlation of morphologic changes with radiosensitivity

The pathologist is often asked by the clinician whether the tumor that he sees under the microscope is radiosensitive. The problem of radiosensitivity is mainly dealt with in the chapter on radiotherapy. The pathologist cannot determine whether any particular tumor is radiosensitive or not.

It is true that certain types of tumors arising in certain locations will melt under radiation therapy. Therefore, if the pathologist sees a lymphosarcoma, a so-called lymphoepithelioma of the nasopharynx, or a seminoma, generally speaking he might say that this tumor is radiosensitive. Usually, the more undifferentiated the tumor, the more sensitive it is to radiations, and if the pathologist examines a very poorly differentiated squamous carcinoma of the cervix, he might believe that this tumor would be sensitive to radiations. However, such statements would be made rather on his knowledge of the evolution of that particular tumor and on the radiotherapist's experience than on what he saw under the microscope.

There is no doubt that there are many tumors that appear to be similar microscopically and that arise from the same organ but whose response to radiotherapy may be diametrically different. The pathologist cannot predict this. It is the pathologist's duty to describe and diagnose the tumor, but it is outside of his province to determine radiosensitivity on the basis of morphologic changes.

Spread of tumors

The dissemination of neoplastic cells throughout the body is often intricate and capricious and may take diverse forms. Tumor may directly invade contiguous organs, spread by implantation, and reach distant organs by lymphatics and veins. Chance can play a pertinent role in the transfer of tumor cells. A very small tumor breaking into a large blood vessel may result in widespread metastases, whereas another may reach a huge size and still remain confined to its capsule. Its rate of growth, its degree of differentiation, the presence or absence of barriers to spread, and biologic and unknown factors all play a variable role in the spread of a tumor. For instance, the ability of a malignant tumor to spread as contrasted to that of a benign tumor is probably related to the lack of cohesiveness in the malignant tumor, together with its ameboid character (Coman[17]).

A thorough knowledge of anatomy and a familiarity with tumor pathology are prerequisites for understanding the spread of tumors. The dissection of the tumor should be in experienced and careful hands. Autopsy examination, which is an important basis of medical learning and teaching, is more or less fruitless when the knowledge of possible metastases is limited.

Direct extension

Direct extension of tumor is influenced by anatomic location. Bone, periosteum, cartilage, and dense connective tissue capsules are natural barriers against spread. To some extent, muscle resists invasion, and, within bone, tumor grows through the periosteum with difficulty. Tumor extending around an organ may be barred from invading it by its dense capsule. Retroperitoneal tumors often grow around but do not invade the kidney. Carcinoma of the endolarynx remains localized not only because of the sparsity of lymphatics, but also because of the cartilaginous, almost avascular enclosure.

Lymphatics

By far the most noteworthy method of spread of malignant tumors is via the lymphatics. Consequently, an intimate knowledge of the lymphatic system is essential for treating tumors. Some tumors metastasize early and others late, and some, for no apparent reason, may remain localized for years without metastases.

Spread by lymphatics is usually a matter of emboli rather than permeation. It is only when the lymph nodes are completely filled with tumor that retrograde permeation takes place (Fig. 25). For instance, in carcinoma of the rectum, the nodes *distal* to the tumor are never involved unless the *proximal* nodes are completely replaced by disease.

Zeidman and Buss[109] and Zeidman et al.[110] demonstrated that a carcinoma does not contain lymph channels. This information has some practical value for, in the absence of lymph channels within a carcinoma, Au^{198} cannot penetrate it. Cancer spreads to lymphatics by embolization and appears first in the subcapsular sinus (Fig. 26). In the examination of surgical specimens, the involvement of lymph nodes appears to be an orderly one and follows usually without bypassing a chain of lymph nodes. In their experimental work, Zeidman and Buss[109] and Zeidman et al.[110] found that there has to be considerable involvement of a draining lymph node before the next node in the chain is implicated.

These results emphasize that lymph nodes, at times, do act as temporary barriers to the further spread of cancer. Tumor may grow within a node and gradually replace it, continue growing and enlarge it to as much as 10 cm in diameter, and still be confined to it. It is not unusual for a metastatic lymph node to be the first indication that a neoplasm exists. Breast carcinoma may be first suggested by an enlarged axillary node, a nasopharyngeal carcinoma by an enlarged cervical node, and a melanocarcinoma by an enlarged inguinal node.

After node replacement and enlargement, the tumor may break through the capsule and begin to grow in the surrounding loose fat and connective tissue. After it has grown outside of the capsule, further dissemination by direct extension, replacement of soft tissue, and invasion of the small veins can occur. The involved nodes thus become fixed.

Each organ varies in the number and distribution of its lymph vessels; this variation naturally influences the extent of possible metastases from it. The thoracic duct is a significant ally for metastasizing tumors below the diaphragm because this duct empties into large veins leading to the right side of the heart. Tumor brought to the lungs by the thoracic duct often multiplies, breaks into the pulmonary veins, and reaches the left side of the heart and thus the systemic circulation. Young[108] dissected the thoracic duct in 150 consecutive cases of cancer at autopsy and found involvement in 37% of the carcinomas and 71% of the lymphomas (Fig. 28).

Perineural space invasion by carcinoma is much more common than suspected and should be searched for in every tumor. It is positive proof that cancer is present. We

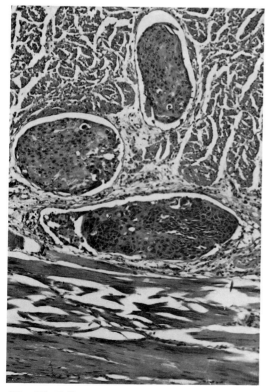

Fig. 25. Diffuse permeation of lymphatics in cancer of esophagus. (×85; WU neg. 61-78.)

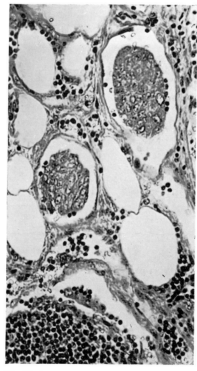

Fig. 26. Early metastatic carcinoma in peripheral sinuses of axillary lymph node from primary carcinoma of breast. (Low-power enlargement.)

have found such invasion in cancer of the prostate, rectum, breast, gallbladder, pancreas, stomach, lung, penis, tongue, salivary glands, skin, esophagus, cervix, and vulva (Fig. 29). In certain of the very well-differentiated carcinomas of the prostate, it may be the only sure sign of malignancy and may extend over a distance of several centimeters (Warren and Meyer[105]).

Nerve invasion may be accompanied by intractable pain in carcinoma of the pancreas, prostate, cervix, and large bowel, invariably severe in carcinoma of the body and tail of the pancreas.

After surgical removal of a rectal car-

cinoma in which nerve invasion is present, the incidence of local recurrence is high (Seefeld and Bargen[86]). Worthy of mention also is that with nerve invasion lymph node metastases are usually existent and the disease is advanced. Large nerves can also be involved. The facial nerve can be affected by malignant tumors of the pa-

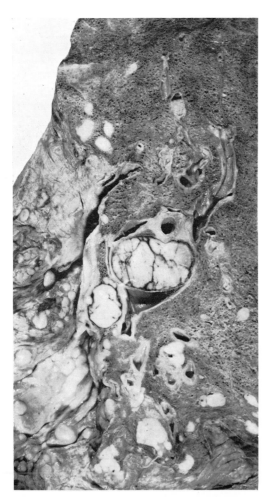

Fig. 27. Lymphangitic metastases in lung from carcinoma of breast. Grayish white areas represent tumor within lymphatics along path of blood vessels. There were also metastases to hilar lymph nodes.

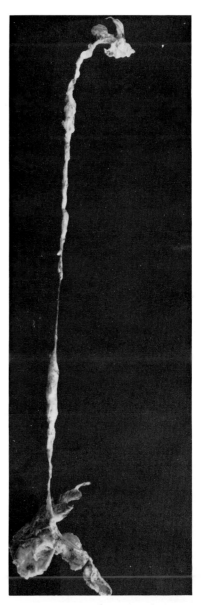

Fig. 28. Extensive involvement of cisterna chyli by cancer of jejunum. Retroperitoneal and supraclavicular lymph nodes also demonstrate involvement. (From Young, J. M.: The thoracic duct in malignant disease, Amer. J. Path. 32:253-269, 1956.)

rotid gland, the vagus nerve by carcinoma of the esophagus, and the phrenic nerve by carcinoma of the bronchus. The recurrent laryngeal nerve is commonly involved in carcinoma of the bronchus and even by metastatic disease from the breast.

There is some question as to whether there are lymphatics within the perineurium. Larson et al.[44] have demonstrated that this is probably a myth. The major lymphatics, however, lie in or near the neurovascular bundle but have no association with the nerve except that of proximity.

It was once an accepted truism that sarcomas metastasized only by the bloodstream. Statistics now show, however, that about 5% to 10% of the soft tissue sarcomas (exclusive of melanocarcinoma and

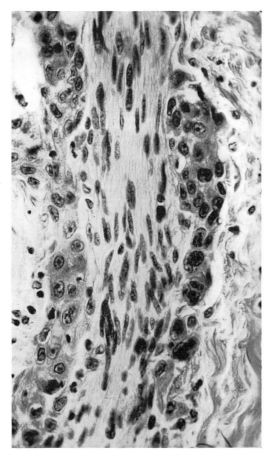

Fig. 29. Perineural space involvement by undifferentiated epidermoid carcinoma. (High-power enlargement.)

lymphosarcoma) metastasize by lymphatics (Warren and Meyer[105]; Willis[106]).

Lymphangiography has been helpful in demonstrating the anatomic distribution of the lymph nodes (O'Brien et al.[62]). It was often thought that tumor reaching the lymph nodes did not reach the venous system. However, communications between the lymphatic and venous systems have been demonstrated by several investigators (Rusznyak et al.[77]; Blalock et al.[10]; Pressman et al.[65] Furthermore, if tumor involves a group of lymph nodes, then, because of block, other pathways become available and metastases occur in bizzare locations (Ariel and Resnick[6]). The tumor may also drain directly into the thoracic duct.

Veins

Spread of tumors through the bloodstream is common and is as important as spread by lymphatics. Tumor may grow into a vein and form a thrombus from which tumor emboli disperse (Fig. 30). If a patient develops a tumor thrombus, the malignant cells enmeshed within the thrombus may be protected from chemotherapeutic agents and may be nourished by the host, enabling them to penetrate the endothelium and to establish a successful metastasis (Wood et al.[107]). From the lung, tumor frequently invades the pulmonary veins and thus reaches the left side of the heart. It can practically destroy the wall of a vein and compress it so that thrombi form in the retarded bloodstream. It can also invade the lumen and form a thrombus. This may be followed by a complete destruction of the wall and the formation of a true tumor thrombus. Metastatic disease may also invade veins.

It should be emphasized that proof of vein invasion by tumor can be determined only by special histologic study. Stains to demonstrate the smooth muscle of the vein (phosphotungstic acid and hematoxylin) and its elastic tissue (Verhoeff–van Gieson) are necessary. Otherwise, lymphatics may be mistaken for veins. The degree of tumor vascularity is also a factor inasmuch as retrograde flow through veins without valves can occur with the production of unusual metastases. Tumor cells lying free within the veins do not represent acceptable evidence of true vein invasion.

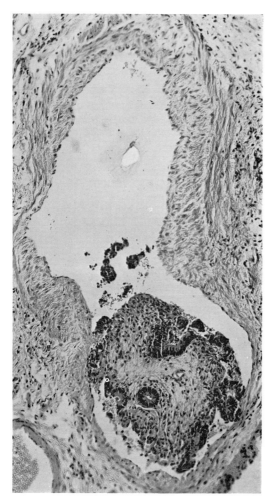

Fig. 30. Blood vessel invasion by carcinoma. Note adherence to vein wall.

Some tumors only occasionally invade the blood vessels, and this is true for lesions in the upper neck, where the jugular vein can be secondarily invaded. This can occur through metastatic carcinoma, particularly from oral cavity lesions. After the tumor invades the jugular vein, it carriers tumor cells to the lung through the right side of the heart. Rather rarely, carcinoma of the breast, after it has metastasized to the axilla, can invade branches of the axillary vein and reach the right side of the heart. Metastatic tumor within the abdomen can directly involve the inferior vena cava and iliac veins. Tumor lying in the peribronchial lymph nodes can also involve bronchial veins.

Some tumors almost exclusively metasta-

size by the bloodstream. This is partially explainable on the basis of anatomy, but in certain tumors it cannot be explained on this basis.

The sarcoma group is the one that predominantly spreads through the bloodstream. Chondrosarcomas, in particular, may propagate for long distances. In two cases reported, a tumor thrombus extended from the femoral vein all the way to the right side of the heart and then to the pulmonary arteries (Warren[104]; Kósa[42]).

Carcinomas of the kidney predominantly spread through the bloodstream, and evidence of such spread is usually observed in the surgical specimen or it may be the first clinical manifestation. This blood vessel invasion can often be a determining factor in prognosis. Other tumors, such as carcinoma of the rectum, may spread through the bloodstream as well as by the lymphatics. If blood vessel invasion can be demonstrated, this may indicate the presence of liver metastases (Brown and Warren[12]). It is also well known that carcinoma of the thyroid gland as well as involving nodes, frequently involves the bloodstream, and the presence or absence of blood vessel invasion is important in prognosis.

The trajectory of tumor emboli through the bloodstream will vary somewhat according to the vein system that the tumor involves. If tumor invades the veins of the upper neck, it quickly empties into the right side of the heart. If the tumor empties into the inferior vena cava, the emboli also reach the heart and then the lungs. After tumor reaches the lungs, it is not infrequent for this tumor to break secondarily into branches of pulmonary veins and thus be released to the systemic circulation, where tumor may lodge in viscera or go to the brain. Also, if the tumor invades the portal vein system, then it ends in the liver, where secondarily it may involve the veins and thus again reach the right side of the heart.

Vertebral vein plexus

Batson's studies[9] of the vertebral vein plexus have been of great value in explaining the bizarre distributions of metastases. The vertebral vein plexus has no valves and communicates with all major vein systems. When pressure changes occur within the abdominal or pleural cavity, metastases to unexpected organs appear.

If opaque material is injected into the dorsal vein of the penis, it can reach the vertebral vein system. It is certainly by this method that carcinoma of the prostate reaches the vertebrae, pelvis, and upper ends of the femur without evidence of disease in any other organ. This pattern of spread of carcinoma of the prostate duplicates the anatomic picture of the vertebral vein plexus. When abdominal pressure is increased (by cough or other means) when tumor cells lie within veins, it is by this same system that metastatic foci in apparently unrelated organs may be explained.

A cancer of the breast may be transported directly to the dorsal vertebra without evidence of disease within the lung. With cough a carcinoma of the lung located in the area drained by the posterior bronchial vein may metastasize through this vein into the vertebral vein plexus and thence to the brain.

The high incidence of metastases in the lung, liver, and bones of the skeletal axis is probably related to venous pathways available, and no doubt the vertebral vein plexus plays a major role.

Arteries

Although tumor often grows in the nodes along the aorta, it rarely invades it. In rare instances, it may involve the adventitia but, because of the barrier of elastic tissue and smooth muscle, it does not penetrate the media. Carcinoma of the midesophagus that is firmly fixed to the aorta can, at times, ulcerate into its lumen.

Metastatic carcinoma in cervical lymph nodes can ulcerate into the carotid artery in the same fashion that metastatic carcinoma within the inguinal lymph nodes can erode the femoral artery.

It has been shown that tumor cells are more often arrested in arterioles than in capillaries or thin-walled veins (Willis[106]).

Implantation

In a few tumors, particularly those arising in the ovary, the favorite method of spread is by implantation. The mucinous cystadenocarcinoma may fill the entire abdomen and grow luxuriantly on the peritoneum. With further growth, it tends to invade contiguous structures. It is not unusual for tumor to recur in a surgical wound even many years after a removal of a mucinous carcinoma of the ovary. The serous cystadenocarcinoma of the ovary also implants itself on the peritoneal surface, and sometimes following surgery the satellite nodules regress spontaneously.

Neoplasms associated with mucin production primarily in the pancreas, stomach, and gallbladder may implant on the surface of the bowel, encircle, invade, and compress it, and cause symptoms suggesting primary gastrointestinal carcinoma. These implants customarily are most prominent in the pelvic peritoneum.

In rare instances, fragment of tumor within the oral cavity may break away and implant in the tracheobronchial pathways. This is conceivably the method of spread in some ameloblastomas (Schweitzer and Barnfield[85]).

The practical importance of this knowledge in surgery and radiotherapy is obvious. For instance, tumors arising from the vocal cord remain localized for long periods of time mainly because the lymphatics of the endolarynx are sparse. On the other hand, because of the rich lymphatic plexus of the hypopharynx, in practically every instance by the time the diagnosis of tumor in that region is made, dissemination has already taken place. If it is known that the subcutaneous lymphatics of both inguinal regions communicate with each other, then it can readily be understood why bilateral rather than unilateral groin dissection is indicated in a carcinoma of the vulva or penis. If it is known that there are communications between the lymphatics on one side of the aorta and those on the other side, it is easily comprehended why radical dissection of lymph nodes of just one side (for carcinoma of the testicle) is of little practical value and consequently why radiotherapy should be used and directed to both sides. If it is known that tumors of the breast located in the inner upper quadrant may metastasize directly to the supraclavicular nodes or anterior mediastinum, then clinical attention will be given to these zones.

Most autopsies done on patients who die of malignant tumors are, for the most part, a routine procedure with no or only little attempt to find out how the particular tumor spreads. Thorough knowledge of the spread and its various manifestations is of utmost importance in doing intelligent autopsies. Willis[106] eloquently proved the value of this hypothesis in his book on the spread of tumors.

Implantation of cancer and tumor cells in circulating blood

The problems of implantation and tumor cells in the bloodstream are related. It has been known for some time that cancer cells may be present on the surgeon's knife and gloves and that such cancer cells can be implanted at the time of the surgical procedure. The number of times this occurs is limited, and there are numerous factors and conditions involved in the question of whether a given cancer will be implanted at surgery. The growth characteristics of a cancer, the size of the inoculum, the site of the implantation, and the host's immune response are all factors of importance.

We have seen cancer of the oral cavity, thyroid gland, breast, stomach, ampulla, pancreas, kidney, large bowel, endometrium, and bladder implanted in various tissues during surgical procedures. The number of times that we have seen this, however, have been relatively few (Ackerman and Wheat[4]). Rarely, this cancerous implantation has been the only tumor that remains after the primary surgery. This implanted cancer has then been surgically excised and the patient cured. We have seen this occur in cancer of the thyroid gland, lung, large bowel, larynx, and endometrium.

Apparently, highly undifferentiated carcinomas with a large inoculum can be implanted fairly readily on a traumatized surface such as the peritoneum. It is not rare to find large numbers of tumor cells in the washings from surgical incisions such as in the neck (Smith and Hilberg[90]), the pleural cavity (Spjut et al.[91]), and the peritoneum. However, the presence of tumor cells in the washings from such wounds does not necessarily mean that the patient will develop local recrudescence. For instance, in patients with pulmonary cancer who had incisional biopsy and frozen section, tumor cells were frequently found in the pleural cavity. In those patients who did not have incisional biopsy, tumor cells were not found in the pleural cavity. There was no difference, however, in the cure rate of those who had tumor cells and those who did not.

Harris and Smith[36] reported that tumor cells were present in the washings from approximately one out of four patients who had surgery for cancer in the head and neck area. Follow-up of these patients demonstrated no correlation in the frequency of local recrudescence in the patients with cancer cells in the washings as compared to the patients with no cancer cells in the washings.

It has been shown experimentally in rats that if there are circulating tumor cells and there is trauma to an organ such as a limb, tumor cells will lodge there and grow (Fisher et al.[24]). The same phenomenon may occur in man (Jewell and Romsdahl[40]). There is no doubt that some of the local recrudescences of tumor are not due to implantation but rather to circulating tumor cells lodging at a site of trauma (Fisher et al.[24]).

There has been an increase in literature on the presence of tumor cells within the bloodstream of a patient with cancer. There are several techniques for their identification (Roberts et al.[73]; Malmgren et al.[52]). If the vein draining a cancer is sampled, cancer cells will often be found. Some of the same patients will also have cancer cells in the peripheral blood. Cancer cells are found in the peripheral blood usually only in patients with advanced disease (Sellwood et al.[87]).

It would seem reasonable to believe that manipulation of a tumor would increase the number of tumor cells in the bloodstream. This could occur through physical examination, rough handling of the tumor at the time of surgery, preparation of the skin prior to operation for cancer of the breast, and dilatation and curettage of the cervix and endometrium. Roberts et al.[73] and Moore et al.[57] demonstrated such an increase in cancer cells in the blood after various types of manipulation. It would also seem reasonable to believe that incurable patients would more often have cancer cells in the blood than curable patients (Fig. 31). Romsdahl et al.[74] showed in malignant melanoma that the presence of

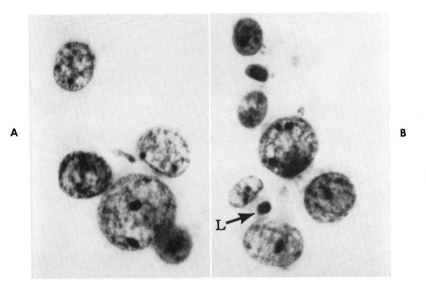

A

B

L→

Fig. 31. Carcinoma of breast. **A,** Direct smear of resected tumor. **B,** Group of cancer cells isolated from peripheral blood (antecubital vein) during skin preparation prior to radical mastectomy. **L,** Lymphocyte. Patient seemed well one year postoperatively with no evidence of disease but died with widespread hematogenous metastases three months later. (Papanicolaou stain; ×1100; from Cole, W. H., et al.: The dissemination of cancer cells, Bull. N. Y. Acad. Med. 34:163-183, 1958.)

tumor cells in the circulating blood after a definitive operative procedure indicated a poor prognosis.

Roberts et al.[72] reported that 7% of 767 patients with cancer who were studied more than five and as many as ten years ago had positive blood samples. The survival rate for curable patients with positive blood samples was no different from that of those with negative blood samples. However, in twenty-three patients with showers of cancer cells demonstrated during operation, only two were alive and well five to ten years postoperatively.

There is an urgent need for reevaluation of the accuracy of statements regarding the presence or absence of tumor cells found in the peripheral blood. Raker et al.[66] studied a series of blood samples from 144 patients. Only two patients were found to have definitely positive samples. Sixty patients were thought to have tumor cells, but reevaluation showed that the cells were, in reality, megakaryocytes. Another patient, who had a fractured rib, had megakaryocytes in the peripheral blood. Spriggs and Alexander[95] also indicated that megakaryocytes can be mistaken for cancer cells. As the quality of preparations improved, the number of patients

with circulating cancer cells diminished (Christopherson[13]). In 255 patients reported by Romsdahl et al.,[75] only thirteen had detectable tumor cells in the blood, and eleven of these patients had disseminated cancer.

We believe that some of the discrepancies cited are due to the incorrect identification of megakaryocytes, lymphocytes, or other cells as malignant cells.

There must be three stages of cancer. In the first stage, cancer will be present in an organ without tumor cells in the peripheral blood. In the second stage, tumor cells will be present in the peripheral blood and all will be destroyed. In the third stage, cancer cells will be present in the peripheral blood, and probably a small percentage will establish themselves in distant organs, grow, and cause the death of the patient. It appears certain that an extremely high percentage of tumor cells released in the bloodstream die without establishment of metastases. Experimentally, fewer than 1% survive (Baserga et al.[8]). The initiation of metastases occurs when tumor emboli are entrapped and attached to the endothelium by fibrous thrombi (Lee[45]).

During or before surgery, is there anything we can do to reduce the numbers of tumor cells that are released in the peripheral blood, and are there any chemotherapeutic substances that should be given to destroy circulating tumor cells? Certainly, the skilled surgeon should manipulate tumors as little as possible and preferably should ligate veins draining the tumor before he proceeds with surgery.

There is in progress a great deal of experimental and clinical work in the use of various substances to prevent the growth of tumor cells liberated within the bloodstream during surgery for cancer. These adjuvant agents have not been proved to be of value in patients with cancer of the lung, large bowel, and stomach. In those with cancer of the breast, their use has been associated with some diminution of local recurrences in the group that received Thio-TEPA. Needless to say, these agents are associated with appreciable complications and can increase the risk of surgery (Veterans Administration Cooperative Study[102]).

Biologic factors

Although metastases may be conditioned somewhat by the anatomic location of a tumor and the pathways available for its spread, there are unknown biologic factors that exist and cloud the picture of tumor dissemination. For instance, carcinoma of the prostate, breast, thyroid gland, and kidney grow luxuriantly and commonly within bone. Skeletal and heart muscles, are seldom the sites of metastases and to only a slightly greater extent are the spleen, pancreas, and kidney. Some tumors nevertheless apparently can grow in any organ. The best example of this is the melanocarcinoma, which in 50% of the cases metastasizes to the heart muscle and is frequently seen in other rare locations. It is known that certain tumors such as the osteosarcoma and the chondrosarcoma rarely grow within lymph nodes.

Anderson and Green[5] believe that there are two or more immune responses in neoplasia: a host immune response against the tumor and a tumor versus host response. The latter process, they believe, is responsible for the peculiar malignancy of a given neoplasm. From this statement it is apparent that lymph nodes in themselves may be responsible for the local destruction of tumor cells. Tumor cells finally grow in a lymph node when the volume, virulence, and lack of immune response combine to allow tumor cells to survive within a given node.

Multiple tumors and multiple foci of origin

There is no doubt that in certain organs multiple tumors occur with greater frequency than on the basis of chance alone. The skin is very frequently the site of multiple carcinomas. This is particularly true in the male exposed to sunlight who develops the so-called tomato skin. Multiple carcinomas appear more quickly in this atrophic skin than it is possible at times to treat them.

In the oral cavity, carcinomas may be multiple. If a patient develops one carcinoma in this region on the basis of leukoplakia and it is cured, then his chance of developing another is fairly high. Sarasin[80] studied slightly over 1000 cases of carcinoma of the oral cavity and found fifty instances in which more than one carcinoma had occurred. The gastrointestinal tract is another site often affected with multiple tumors, as shown by the figures of Slaughter,[89] being particularly common in the large bowel.

A tendency to multiple tumors seems to exist in endocrine organs. When carcinoma occurs in one of two paired organs, the chance that carcinoma will develop in the second organ is greater than average and greater than the likelihood of occurrence of the first tumor.

Spratt and Hoag[94] reviewed the prevalence and sites of simultaneous and the incidence and sites of nonsimultaneous cancers in 1130 patients with colorectal cancer, 710 with mammary cancer, 1853 with cancers of the cervix uteri, 167 with chronic leukemia, and 458 with lymphoma. An additional 1000 consecutive persons with no neoplasm on first examination were also selected. All patients were from the Ellis Fischel State Cancer Hospital, and follow-up was reported up to twenty years. The incidence of new cancers per man-year of risk in the five groups with prior cancers compared to the incidence in the control population with no prior cancers and to the age-specific incidence of cancers in Connecticut for the same period showed that the prior cancer at these sites neither increased nor decreased the risk for developing additional neoplasms. Based entirely on the observed age-specific incidence of cancers, persons living to extreme age could expect to have multiple cancers with great frequency.

However, Cook[18] demonstrated that certain cancers may be followed by another cancer in another organ much more frequently than can be explained by chance. For instance, the esophageal cancer may be followed by a cancer of the pharynx, tongue, or oral cavity, and a lung cancer may be followed by a cancer of the larynx. Einhorn and Jakobsson[21] demonstrated that in younger age groups with carcinoma of the lip, the incidence of new primary malignant tumors in other organs is considerably higher than can be ascribed solely to chance.

These studies have indicated that with increased curability of cancer and with an aging population, many new cancers occur purely on the basis of chance with certain exceptions.

REFERENCES

1 Abbott, K. H., and Adson, A. W.: Primary intracranial lymphosarcoma, Arch. Surg. (Chicago) 47:147-159, 1943.
2 Ackerman, L. V.: Is it cancer? Will it become cancer? In Proceedings of Fourth National Cancer Conference (1960), Philadelphia, 1961, J. B. Lippincott Co., pp. 97-112.
3 Ackerman, L. V., and Ramirez, G. A.: The indications for and limitations of frozen section diagnosis; a review of 1269 consecutive frozen section diagnoses, Brit. J. Surg. 46: 336-350, 1959.
4 Ackerman, L. V., and Wheat, M. W., Jr.: The implantation of cancer—an avoidable surgical risk? Surgery 37:341-355, 1955.
5 Anderson, M. R., and Green, H. N.: Tumour host relationships, Brit. J. Cancer 21:27-32, 1967.
6 Ariel, I. M., and Resnick, M. I.: Altered lymphatic dynamics caused by cancer metastases, Arch. Surg. (Chicago) 94:117-128, 1967.
7 Ashworth, C. T., and Stembridge, V. A.: Utility of formalin-fixed surgical and autopsy specimens for electron microscopy, Amer. J. Clin. Path. 42:466-480, 1964.
8 Baserga, R., Kisieleski, W. E., and Halvorsen, K.: A study on the establishment and growth of tumor metastases with tritiated thymidine, Cancer Res. 20:910-917, 1960.
9 Batson, O. V.: The function of the vertebral veins and their role in the spread of metastases, Ann. Surg. 112:138-149, 1940.
10 Blalock, A., Robinson, C. S., Cunningham, R. S., and Gray, M. E.: Experimental studies on lymphatic blockage, Arch. Surg. (Chicago) 34:1049-1071, 1937.
11 Broders, A. C.: The microscopic grading of cancer. In Pack, G. T., and Livingston, E. M.: Treatment of cancer and allied diseases, vol. 1, New York, 1940, Paul B. Hoeber, Inc., pp. 19-41.
12 Brown, C. E., and Warren, S.: Visceral metastasis from rectal carcinoma, Surg. Gynec. Obstet. 66:611-621, 1938.
13 Christopherson, W. M.: A re-evaluation of the significance of circulating cancer cells in the peripheral blood. In Recent advances in the diagnosis of cancer, Ninth Clinical Conference on Cancer, Anderson Hospital and Tumor Institute; Houston, 1964, Chicago, 1966, Year Book Medical Publishers, Inc.
14 Cole, W. H., Roberts, S., Watne, A., McDonald, G., and McGrew, E.: The dissemination of cancer cells, Bull. N. Y. Acad. Med. 34:163-183, 1958.
15 Coller, F. A., Key, E. B., and MacIntyre, R. S.: Regional lymphatic metastases of carcinoma of the stomach, Arch. Surg. (Chicago) 43:748-761, 1941.
16 Collins, V. P., Loeffler, R. K., and Tivey, H.: Observations on growth rates of human tumors, Amer. J. Roentgen. 76:988-1000, 1956.
17 Coman, D. R.: Mechanisms responsible for the origin and distribution of blood borne tumor metastases; a review, Cancer Res. 13:307-404, 1953.
18 Cook, G. B.: A comparison of single and multiple primary cancers, Cancer 19:959-966, 1966.
19 Croft, P. B., Urich, H., and Wilkinson, M.: Peripheral neuropathy of sensory motor type associated with malignant disease, Brain 90: 31-66, 1967.
20 Dockerty, M. B., and Priestley, J. T.: Lymphosarcoma of the testis, J. Urol. 48:514-523, 1942.
21 Einhorn, J., and Jakobsson, P.: Multiple primary malignant tumors, Cancer 17:1437-1444, 1964.
22 Erickson, C. C., Everett, B. E., Jr., Graves, L. M., Kaiser, R. F., Malmgren, R. A., Rube, I., Schreier, P. C., Cutler, S. J., and Sprunt, D. H.: Population screening for uterine cancer by vaginal cytology; preliminary summary of results of first examination of 108,000 women and second testing of 33,000 women, J.A.M.A. 162:167-173, 1957.
23 Everson, T. C.: Spontaneous regression of cancer, Ann. N. Y. Acad. Sci. 114:721-735, 1964.
24 Fisher, B., Fisher, E. R., and Feduska, N.: Trauma and the localization of tumor cells, Cancer 20:23-30, 1967.
25 Foster, E. A., and Levine, A. J.: Mucin production in metastatic carcinoma, Cancer 16: 506-509, 1963.
26 Gillman, T., and Gillman, J.: Modified liver aspiration biopsy apparatus and technique, with special reference to its clinical applica-

tions as assessed by 500 biopsies, S. Afr. J. Med. Sci. **10**:53-66, 1945.

27 Godwin, J. T.: Aspiration biopsy; technique and application, Ann. N. Y. Acad. Sci. **63**: 1348-1373, 1956 (extensive bibliography).

28 Goldstein, M. N., Burdman, J. A., and Journey, L. J.: Long-term tissue culture of neuroblastoma, J. Nat. Cancer Inst. **32**:165-199, 1964.

29 Grant, L. J., and Trivedi, S. A.: Open lung biopsy for diffuse pulmonary lesions, Brit. Med. J. **1**:17-21, 1960.

30 Greenberg, E., Divertie, M. B., and Woolner, L. B.: A review of unusual systemic manifestations associated with carcinoma, Amer. J. Med. **36**:106-120, 1964.

31 Greenough, R. B.: Early diagnosis of cancer of breast, Ann. Surg. **102**:233-238, 1935.

32 Grinnell, R. S.: The lymphatic and venous spread of carcinoma of the rectum, Ann. Surg. **116**:200-216, 1942.

33 Haagensen, C. D.: Surgical biopsy. In Pack, G. T., and Livingston, E. M.: Treatment of cancer and allied diseases, vol. 1, New York, 1940, Hoeber Medical Division, Harper & Row, Publishers, pp. 42-63.

34 von Hansemann, D.: Ueber asymmetrische Zelltheilung in Epithelkrebsen und deren biologische Bedeutung, Virchow Arch. Path. Anat. **119**:299-326, 1890.

35 Harrington, S. W., and Miller, J. M.: Lymphosarcoma of the mammary gland, Amer. J. Surg. **48**:346-352, 1940.

36 Harris, A. H., and Smith, R. R.: Operative wound seeding with tumor cells; its role in recurrences of head and neck cancer, Ann. Surg. **151**:330-334, 1960.

37 Harvey, H. D., and Auchincloss, H.: Metastases to lymph nodes from carcinoma that were arrested, Cancer **21**:684-691, 1968.

38 Harvey, W. F., and Hamilton, T. D.: Carcino-sarcoma; a study of the microscopic anatomy and meaning of a peculiar cancer, Edinburgh Med. J. **42**:337-373, 1935.

39 Hultborn, K. A., and Törnberg, B.: The biologic character of mammary carcinoma studied in 517 cases by a new form of malignancy grading, Acta Radiol. (Stockholm) (suppl. 196), pp. 1-143, 1960.

40 Jewell, W. R., and Romsdahl, M. M.: Recurrent malignant disease in operative wounds not due to surgical implantation from the resected tumor, Surgery **58**:806-809, 1965.

41 Konikov, N., Bleisch, V., and Piskie, V.: Prognostic significance of cytologic diagnoses of effusions, Acta Cytol. (Balt.) **10**:335-339, 1966.

42 Kósa, M. T.: Chondroblastom in der venösen Blutbahn, Virchow Arch. Path. Anat. **272**: 166-204, 1929.

43 Koss, L. G.: Diagnostic cytology and its histopathologic vases, ed. 2, Philadelphia, 1968, J. B. Lippincott Co.

44 Larson, D. L., Rodin, A. E., Roberts, D. K., O'Steen, W. K., Rapperport, A. S., and Lewsi, S. R.: Perineural lymphatics; myth or fact? Amer. J. Surg. **112**:488-492, 1966.

45 Lee, Y. T.: Experimental studies of metastases; a review, Missouri Med. **65**:36-39, 123-128, 205-210, 1968.

46 Lipsett, M. B.: Humoral syndromes associated with cancer, Cancer Res. **25**:1068-1073, 1965 (extensive bibliography).

47 Lockhart, C., and Ackerman, L. V.: The implications of local excision or simple mastectomy prior to radical mastectomy for carcinoma of the breast, Surgery **26**:577-583, 1949.

48 Loquvam, G. S., and Russell, W. O.: Accessory pancreatic ducts of the major duodenal papilla, Amer. J. Clin. Path. **20**:305-313, 1950.

49 Lynn, J. A., Martin, J. H., and Kingsley, W. B.: Recent developments in the application of electron microscopy to routine diagnostic surgical pathology, Amer. J. Clin. Path. **47**: 373-374, 1967.

50 McGavran, M. H., Bauer, W. C., and Ogura, J. H.: The incidence of cervical lymph node metastases from epidermoid carcinoma of the larynx and their relationship to certain characteristics of the primary tumor; a study based on the clinical and pathological findings for 96 patients treated by primary en bloc laryngectomy and radical neck dissection, Cancer **14**:55-66, 1961.

51 McGavran, M. H., Unger, R. H., Recant, L., Polk, H. C., Kilo, C., and Levine, M. E.: A glucagon secreting Alpha cell carcinoma of the pancreas, New Eng. J. Med. **274**:1408-1414, 1966.

52 Malmgren, R. A., Pruitt, J. C., Del Vecchio, P. R., and Potter, J. F.: A method for the cytologic detection of tumor cells in whole blood, J. Nat. Cancer Inst. **20**:1203-1213, 1958.

53 Marcuse, P. M.: Cytology of short-term tissue cultures; analysis of 600 in vitro preparations from surgical specimens, Lab. Invest. **4**: 293-303, 1955.

54 Meatheringham, R. E., and Ackerman, L. V.: Aspiration biopsy of lymph nodes; a critical review of the results of 300 aspirations, Surg. Gynec. Obstet. **84**:1071-1076, 1947.

55 Miller, R. W.: Relation between cancer and congenital defects in man, New Eng. J. Med. **275**:87-93, 1966 (extensive bibliography).

56 Moloney, G. E.: Lymphosarcoma of the bladder, Brit. J. Surg. **35**:91-94, 1947.

57 Moore, G. E., Sanberg, A. A., and Watne, A. L.: Spread of cancer cells and its relationship to chemotherapy, J.A.M.A. **172**:1729-1733, 1960.

58 Murray, M. R., and Stout, A. P.: The classification and diagnosis of human tumors by tissue culture methods, Texas Rep. Biol. Med. **12**:898-915, 1954.

59 Murray, M. R., Stout, A. P., and Pogogeff, I. A.: Synovial sarcoma and normal synovial tissue cultivated in vitro, Ann. Surg. **12**:843-851, 1944.

60 Nakazawa, H., Rosen, P., Lane, N., and Lattes, R.: Frozen section experience in 3000 cases, Amer. J. Clin. Path. **49**:41-51, 1968.

61 Oberling, C.: Les reticulosarcomes et les réticulo-endothéliol-endothélial de la moelle osseuse, Bull. Assoc. Franc. Cancer **17**:259-296, 1928.

62 O'Brien, P. H., Sherman, J. O., and Beal, J. M.: Lymphatics and malignant disease, Med. Clin. N. Amer. **51**:249-261, 1967.

63 Perera, C. A.: Lymphosarcoma of the lacrimal gland, Arch. Ophthal. (Chicago) **28**:522-529, 1942.

64 Plimpton, C. H., and Gellhorn, A.: Hypercalcemia in malignant disease without evidence of bone destruction, Amer. J. Med. **21**:750-759, 1956.

65 Pressman, J. J., Simon, M. B., Hand, K., and Miller, J.: Passage of fluids, cells and bacteria via direct communications between lymph nodes and veins, Surg. Gynec. Obstet. **115**:207-214, 1962.

66 Raker, J. W., Taft, P. D., and Edmonds, E. E.: Significance of megakaryocytes in the search for tumor cells in the peripheral blood, New Eng. J. Med. **263**:993-996, 1960.

67 Rappaport, H., Winter, W. J., and Hicks, E. B.: Follicular lymphoma; a re-evaluation of its position in the scheme of malignant lymphoma, based on a survey of 253 cases, Cancer **9**:792-821, 1956.

68 Raskin, H. F., Kirnsner, J. B., and Palmer, W. L.: Role of exfoliative cytology in diagnosis of cancer of the digestive tract, J.A.M.A. **169**:789-791, 1959.

69 del Regato, J. A.: Roentgentherapy of lymphosarcomas of the tonsil, radiation therapy, Tumor Institute, Seattle (no. 2), pp. 67-76, 1941.

70 del Regato, J. A.: Discussion of Stout, A. P.: Tumor Seminar, J. Missouri Med. Ass. **46**:259-291, 1949.

71 Renstrup, G.: Leukoplakia of the oral cavity, Acta Odont. Scand. **16**:99-111, 1958.

72 Roberts, S. S., Hengesh, J. W., McGrath, R. G., Valaitis, J., McGrew, E. A., and Cole, W. H.: Prognostic significance of cancer cells in the circulating blood, Amer. J. Surg. **113**:757-762, 1967.

73 Roberts, S., Watne, A., McGrath, B., McGrew, E., and Cole, W. H.: Technique and results of isolation of cancer cells from the circulating blood, Arch. Surg. (Chicago) **76**:334-346, 1958.

74 Romsdahl, M. M., Potter, J. F., Malmgren, R. A., Chu, E. W., Brindley, C. O., and Smith, R. R.: A clinical study of circulating tumor cells in malignant melanoma, Surg. Gynec. Obstet. **111**:675-681, 1960.

75 Romsdahl, M. M., Valaitis, J., McGrath, R. G., and McGrew, E. A.: Circulating tumor cells in patients with carcinoma, J.A.M.A. **193**:1087-1090, 1965.

76 Rosai, J., and Rodriguez, H. A.: Application of electron microscopy to the differential diagnosis of tumors, Amer. J. Clin. Path. **50**:555-562, 1968.

77 Rusznyak, I., Foldi, M., and Szabo, G.: Lymphatic system (translated by M. J. Tobias), Ann Arbor, Mich., 1938, Edwards Brothers, Inc., p. 318.

78 Saltzstein, S. L.: Histologic diagnosis of breast carcinoma with Silverman needle biopsy, Surgery **48**:366-374, 1960.

79 Saltzstein, S. L.: Pulmonary malignant lymphomas and pseudolymphomas, Cancer **16**:928-955, 1963.

80 Sarasin, R.: Les manifestations successives des épithéliomas des muqueuses de la cavité buccale: sont-elles des récidives vraies ou resultent-elles de nouvelles cancérisations? Radiophys. Radiother. **3**:33-76, 1933.

81 Saxton, J.: Personal communication.

82 Schade, R. O. K.: Gastric cytology; principles, methods and results, London, 1960, Edward Arnold (Publishers), Ltd.

83 Schajowicz, F.: Aspiration biopsy in bone lesions, J. Bone Joint Surg. **37-A**:465-471, 1955.

84 Schajowicz, F., and Derqui, J. C.: Puncture biopsy in lesions of the locomotor systems, Cancer **21**:531-548, 1968.

85 Schweitzer, F. C., and Barnfield, W. F.: Ameloblastoma of mandible with metastasis to lungs; report of case, J. Oral Surg. **1**:287-295, 1943.

86 Seefeld, P. H., and Bargen, J. A.: The spread of carcinoma of the rectum; invasion of lymphatics, veins and nerves, Ann. Surg. **118**:76-90, 1943.

87 Sellwood, R. A., Kuper, W. A., Payne, P. M., and Ian Burn, J.: Factors affecting the finding of cancer cells in the blood, Brit. J. Surg. **56**:649-652, 1969.

88 Shafer, W. G., and Waldron, C. A.: A clinical and histopathologic study of oral leukoplakia, Surg. Gynec. Obstet. **112**:411-420, 1961.

89 Slaughter, D. P.: The multiplicity of origin of malignant tumors, Int. Abst. Surg. **79**:89-98, 1944.

90 Smith, R. R., and Hilber, A. W.: Cancer-cell seeding of operative wounds, J. Nat. Cancer Inst. **16**:645-657, 1955.

91 Spjut, H. J., Hendrix, V. J., Ramirez, G. A., and Roper, C. L.: Carcinoma cells in pleural cavity washings, Cancer **11**:1222-1225, 1958.

92 Spjut, H. J., Roper, C. L., and Butcher, H. R., Jr.: Pulmonary cancer and its prognosis; a study of the relationship of certain factors to survival of patients treated by pulmonary resection, Cancer **14**:1251-1258, 1961.

93 Spratt, J. S., Jr., and Ackerman, L. V.: The growth of a colonic adenocarcinoma, Amer. Surg. **27**:23-28, 1961.

94 Spratt, J. S., and Hoag, M. G.: Incidence of multiple primary cancers per man-year of follow-up; twenty-year review from the Ellis Fischel State Cancer Hospital, Ann. Surg. **164**:775-784, 1966.

95 Spriggs, A. I., and Alexander, R. F.: The circulating cancer cell, Lancet **2**:654, 1960.

96 Stewart, F. W.: The diagnosis of tumors by aspiration, Amer. J. Path. **9** (suppl.):801-812, 1933.

97 Stout, A. P.: Is lymphosarcoma curable? J.A.M.A. **118**:968-970, 1942.

98 Takagi, F.: Studies on tumor cells in serous effusion, Amer. J. Clin. Path. **24:**663-675, 1954.

99 Törnberg, B.: See Hultborn and Törnberg.[39]

100 Ultmann, J. E., Koprowski, I., and Engle, R. L., Jr.: A cytological study of lymph node imprints, Cancer **11:**507-524, 1958.

101 Urban, C. H., and McNeer, G.: Relation of morphology of gastric carcinoma to long and short term survival, Cancer **12:**1158-1162, 1959.

102 Veterans Administration Adjuvant Cancer Chemotherapy Cooperative Group: Status of adjuvant cancer chemotherapy, Arch. Surg. (Chicago) **82:**466-473, 1961.

103 Wandall, H. H.: Demonstration of neoplastic cells in the sputum, Acta Path. Microbiol. Scand. **20:**485, 1943.

104 Warren, S.: Chondrosarcoma with intravascular growth and tumor emboli to the lungs, Amer. J. Path. **7:**161-168, 1931.

105 Warren, S., and Meyer, R. W.: Lymph node metastasis of sarcoma, Amer. J. Path. **14:**605-620, 1938.

106 Willis, R. A.: The spread of tumours in the human body, St. Louis, 1961, The C. V. Mosby Co.

107 Wood, S., Jr., Holyoke, E. D., and Yardley, J. H.: Mechanisms of metastasis production by blood-borne cancer cells, Canad. Cancer Conf. **4:**167-223, 1961 (extensive bibliography).

108 Young, J. M.: The thoracic duct in malignant disease, Amer. J. Path. **32:**253-269, 1956.

109 Zeidman, I., and Buss, J. M.: Experimental studies on the spread of cancer in the lymphatic system. I. Effectiveness of the lymph node as a barrier to the passage of embolic tumor cells, Cancer Res. **14:**403-405, 1954.

110 Zeidman, I., Copeland, B. E., and Warren, S.: Experimental studies on the spread of cancer in the lymphatic system. II. Absence of a lymphatic supply in carcinoma, Cancer **8:**123-127, 1955.

Chapter 4

Surgery of cancer

Harvey R. Butcher, Jr., M.D.*

Surgery is the only curative treatment of a variety of malignant tumors. A cancer surgeon requires *technical skill* but, in addition, he must possess a *knowledge of tumor pathology*—the behavior of tumors and the ways of direct extension and of regional and distant metastases that characterize the various malignant tumors. Since all surgical interventions have their limitations and their risk, which the surgeon has to assess, he also must exercise *judgment* (Kennedy et al.[5]). Further, since hazards must not deter a surgeon from rendering a service that can only be obtained through him, he also requires *fortitude*. The prospect of risk and possible impairment must be frankly presented to the patients and relatives. It is not realistic to expect patients to make a difficult choice between possible courses under the emotions of their plight. The surgeon must present the patient with the implications, alternatives, and advisable course, avoiding his own bias: this requires *integrity*.

Surgery and radiotherapy are not competitive, although surgeons and radiotherapists may, at times, appear to be. The surgeon must have an understanding of the indications and limitations of radiotherapy of cancer as well as of effects of irradiation. In some instances in which both surgery and radiotherapy can be carried out with the same measure of success, the choice must be made on the basis of secondary considerations of relative importance (age, expeditiousness, avoidable impairment). In a few instances of the treatment of cancer, a well-planned association of surgery and radiotherapy is indicated, but one-half of each procedure does not necessarily amount to one whole treatment (Moss and Brand[10]).

The manner of surgical treatment for a malignant tumor is dictated by its pathologic nature, its location, its extent, and its previous treatment; past experience with the results of surgery and radiotherapy are helpful in making this decision. Thus, surgery is not justified in the treatment of most manifestations of malignant lymphoma, multiple myeloma, Ewing's sarcoma, cancer of the nasopharynx, in the presence of invasion of unresectable vital structures, etc.

Radical surgical procedures are seldom justified in the presence of signs of incurability due to distant metastases. The preliminary examination of patients before operation should reveal any obvious metastatic manifestations. Radiographic and laboratory examinations, such as roentgenograms of the chest and acid phosphatase determinations, may prove decisive. Others, such as roentgenologic examination of bones, are also imperative in the presence of suggestive symptoms. But extensive bone or gastrointestinal surveys are more often onerous than useful and should not be carried out for routine purposes.

Surgery of primary lesion

In order to be successful, a surgical intervention must be devised and performed for the complete removal of the tumor without breaking its continuity. Such complete extirpation must be possible without undue morbidity and mortality. Surgical procedures, which previously presented a prohibitive morbidity and mortality, have now become possible because of a better knowledge of anesthesia and better preoperative and postoperative care, as well as because of the utilization of antibiotics (Moyer[11]). Whatever the risk, it is the surgeon's duty to assess it and minimize it. All curative surgery is based on the rationale of total extirpation. As is the case in

*Professor of Surgery, Washington University School of Medicine, St. Louis, Mo.

cancer of the breast, clinical signs may be present that reveal *incurability:* this may be translated as *inoperability* of the given case. More often, inoperability results from obvious inability to remove the tumor *in toto* or from a pathologic tally which implies excessive risk to the patient. At best, a surgeon can never be certain that a malignant tumor has been completely removed or that subclinical distant metastases are not present. Evidence of the effectiveness of the separation of the tumor from its human host is obtained only when the operation is not followed by the development of recurrence or metastases.

The risk and possible impairment resulting from a surgical intervention cannot be imposed lightly. A preoperative diagnosis should be reasonably established. Naked-eye gross diagnostic impressions are not sufficient. A preliminary microscopic verification of the nature of the suspected tumor should be carried out. This may imply biopsy during the course of the intervention. *Frozen section* histopathologic diagnosis is a valuable asset in the operating room, but one should not expect it to solve all problems. The surgeon should be prepared to proceed on his own judgment. An understanding of the possibilities of frozen section, of the morphologic diagnosis of various lesions, and of the limitations of the pathologist are required. Frozen section of lesions of the breast may obviate unwarranted mastectomies for sclerosing adenosis, duct ectasia, and fat necrosis. Verification of the suspected diagnosis of adenocarcinoma should also be sought before proceeding with a radical gastrectomy for an ulceration of the lesser curvature. Contrarily, a surgeon must accept the possibility of an occasional right colectomy, for what may prove to be an appendiceal abscess, rather than to subject his patient to the dangers of implantations which will be risked by a colotomy for the purpose of biopsy. Similarly, the involvement of contiguous organs by proved malignant neoplasms may have to be assumed on the basis of inspection and palpation alone, in spite of possible errors, for biopsy may disrupt the "margin of resection" and increase the likelihood of local recurrence (Butcher and Spjut[2]).

Surgery of lymph node metastases

Surgical treatment of metastatic nodes, independent of the treatment of the primary lesion, is indicated in many instances but any sort of removal of nodes is not necessarily justified. In general, what is required is the complete removal of the nodes in a well-conceived resection of the regional lymphatics that will encompass all of the potentially metastatic nodes without cutting through the invaded lymphatic channels. The removal of regional lymph node metastases in continuity with the primary lesion *(en bloc)* is an important principle in the conduct of surgery of certain malignant neoplasms.

A well-indicated radical resection of metastatic nodes for curative purposes may be termed a *therapeutic* dissection. In many instances of the treatment of cancer, a dissection of the regional lymphatics may be advisable in the absence of any clinically ostensible metastatic manifestations—this dissection has been called *prophylactic* by some and *elective* by others.* The obvious purpose of such an action is the early extirpation of metastases that may already be present in a subclinical stage. A radical neck dissection is often advised, in the absence of palpable nodes, for a patient with carcinoma of the lateral border of the tongue (p. 209). In other instances, the prophylactic dissection may be carried out in continuity with the primary lesion. Such is the principle applied in radical mastectomy for cancer of the breast in continuity with the lymph nodes of the axilla or in the removal of part of the lower jaw *en bloc* with the lymphatics of the neck for carcinoma of the lower gingiva.

The usefulness of the prophylactic ("elective") neck dissection in a given set of circumstances may be estimated from an analysis of the following data:

1 % failure of control of primary lesion (A)
2 % occurrence of nodal metastases (B)
3 % operative mortality of dissection (C)
4 % failure of prophylactic dissection on positive nodes (D)

---

*The word elective is unsatisfactory because it only implies choice irrespective of timing. One cannot fathom a systematic "elective" dissection.

$$100\text{-}A = \% \text{ of patients not dying of the primary cancer}$$

$$(100\text{-}A) \times \left(\frac{B \times F}{100}\right) = \% \text{ dying because of nodal metastases if not treated}$$

$$\left((100\text{-}C\text{-}A) \times \frac{B}{100}\right) \times \left(\frac{F - D}{100}\right) = \% \text{ of patients helped by prophylactic neck dissection}$$

$$\left((100\text{-}A) \times \frac{B}{100} \times \frac{100\text{-}C}{100}\right) \times \left(\frac{F - E}{100}\right) = \% \text{ of patients helped by therapeutic neck dissection}$$

5 % failure of *therapeutic* dissections done after metastases become evident (E)

6 Rate of decimation ("rate of dying") of patients with *untreated* metastases (F)

Using these data, the percentage of patients that may be salvaged by prophylactic ("elective") nodal dissection for various forms of cancer may be estimated from the formula in the accompanying box.

Obviously, patients whose primary lesion is not controlled cannot be salvaged by prophylactic or therapeutic dissection of the metastases. Also not helped by "elective" dissections are those patients who prove to have no evidence of metastases. The salvage of prophylactic dissections, among those patients eligible for benefit, must substantially exceed that of therapeutic dissections in order to justify the morbidity and mortality of those who prove to have been subjected needlessly to the prophylactic operation (Table 6). In general, a prophylactic regional dissection is also justified when the dissection in continuity facilitates the adequate removal of the primary lesion (carcinoma of the lower gingiva) or when the nodal metastases along accessible pathways have proven to be frequent (carcinoma of the colon).

At operation, the surgeon may find himself obligated to decide on *abstention* as a wiser course to follow. This may be the case in the presence of widespread peritoneal implants, para-aortic lymph node metastases, liver metastases, or involvement

Table 6. Method of evaluating merits of prophylactic ("elective") versus therapeutic nodal dissection in treatment of cancer

Type of cancer*	Failure to control primary cancer (%)	Occult nodal metastases at time of treatment (%)	Operative mortality (%)	Survival among patients with metastases found in prophylactic nodal dissection specimen (%)	Survival after therapeutic dissection for nodal metastases appearing after primary treatment (%)	Net improvement in survival expected from prophylactic nodal dissection (%)
Epidermoid cancer* of mobile portion of tongue	45	40	2	27	11	+ 2
Epidermoid carcinoma* of lip	5	10	2	42	40	− 1.6
Melanocarcinoma†	60	30	1	30	30	− 0.6
Carcinoma of vulva*	40	48	5	50	30	+ 8
Cancer of breast‡	20	35	1	70‡	40‡	+10

*All data are approximate. See respective chapters.

†See Johnson, R. E.: Occult lymphatic metastases in malignant melanoma of the skin, Ann. Surg. 146:931-936, 1957.

‡Forty-nine of seventy women (70%) survived five years or longer after mastectomy for mammary cancer associated with occult or unsuspected axillary nodal metastases (Barnes Hospital, 1950-1955). Forty-one of 102 women (40%) survived five years or longer after radical mastectomy for mammary cancer associated with palpable axillary metastases. (Stage C mammary cancer is excluded.)

of unresectable structures. A suspicion reached through gross inspection or palpation is seldom justified. Errors may be committed in the presence of omental necrosis, sclerosing hemangiomas, granulomas, etc. Gross impressions of inoperability should be verified by biopsy which, in some instances, may require frozen section techniques. For these purposes, the surgeon would be wise to limit his demands on his surgical pathologist to a bare minimum.

Radical interventions

Most curative surgical procedures applied to the treatment of cancer can be said to be radical. However, the expression is more often applied to those which imply some deformity, dysfunction, or mutilation. The infliction of such impairment is justified in the treatment of many patients with cancer who are not eligible for cure by any other means. Not infrequently, the most mutilating procedures must be offered to those who, by virtue of their youth, may stand to survive for many years. One of the most painful experiences that the surgeon has to face is that often these extreme resections and impairments may prove to be fruitless sacrifices.

A *hemipelvectomy* may be the only recourse in the treatment of various malignant tumors of the pelvic structures or head of the femur. It is justified in the treatment of chondrosarcoma of the head of the femur, or of the acetabulum, in which there is little likelihood of distant metastases. However, such an operation would not be justified for the treatment of Ewing's sarcoma or for metastatic melanoma.

A pelvic *exenteration*, or the removal of pelvic organs in the tissue planes medial to the sciatic nerve roots, is a well-conceived operation capable of salvaging otherwise incurable patients. The principal neoplasms that might be treated by an exenteration of the pelvic organs are extensive carcinomas of the rectum, endometrium, and vagina. The operation yields its best results in the treatment of patients with recurrences or massive necrosis following radiotherapy for cancer of the cervix (Bricker et al.[1]). The results of pelvic exenterations for extensive well-differentiated adenocarcinomas of the rectum, which frequently do not present lymph node metastases (Butcher and Spjut[2]), are better than those of the abdominoperineal resection of all other carcinomas of the rectum (Fig. 32). But the extent of the spread within the pelvis and the character of the tumor are definite limitations in the application of pelvic exenterations.

Palliative surgical interventions

We recognize as palliative procedures those which are intended to relieve symp-

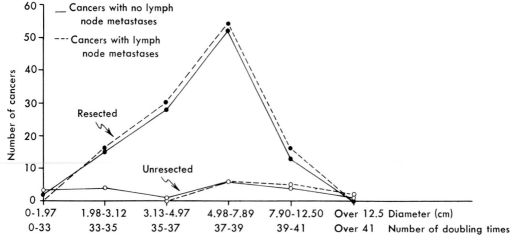

Fig. 32. Distribution of 226 resected and thirty-two unresected colonic carcinomas examined at necropsy with and without lymph node metastases according to seriated diameters of primary carcinomas.

toms or to reduce the severity of a patient's illness without attempt to cure. Surgical interventions that remove "most" of the tumor are not necessarily palliative. Of necessity, the extent of the expected relief must be considered in relation to the morbidity and mortality of the contemplated procedure. Modlin and Walker[7] showed the value of palliative resections for cancer of the colon. Resections for relief of pain, obstructions, infected ulcerations, hemorrhaging, etc., which can be performed without great risk to the patient, are truly palliative, for they relieve the incurable patients of some of his burdens. Prolongation of life may indirectly result, although it is not a requisite. Chordotomies, for example, are well justified for the palliation of pain in definite instances, although they may not extend the life of the patient. Amputations for painful neoplasms of the extremities are justified in some cases, as are gastrectomies for advanced obstructing carcinomas, pneumonectomies for suppurating pulmonary carcinomas, and cystectomies for large infected or hemorrhaging lesions of the bladder, in patients that are not eligible for cure. However, the efficiency of palliative pneumonectomies, gastrectomies, esophagectomies, and cystectomies in the absence of sepsis, obstruction, and hemorrhaging has not been definitely established. The surgeon must avoid rendering a disservice in the name of palliation—he must be able to resist the pressures of those who unwittingly ask that the patient's agony be prolonged.

REFERENCES

1 Bricker, E. M., Butcher, H. R., Jr., Lawler, W. H., Jr., and McAfee, C. A.: Surgical treatment of advanced and recurrent cancer of the pelvic viscera: an evaluation of ten years' experience, Ann. Surg. **152:**388-402, 1960.

2 Butcher, H. R., Jr., and Spjut, H. J.: An evaluation of pelvic exenteration for advanced carcinoma of the lower colon, Cancer **12:**681-687, 1959.

3 Butcher, H. R., Jr.: The utility of ureteroileal urinary diversion in the treatment of irreparable ureteral obstructions, Surg. Gynec. Obstet. **109:**521-525, 1959.

4 Johnson, R. E.: Occult lymphatic metastases in malignant melanoma of the skin, Ann. Surg. **146:**931-936, 1957.

5 Kennedy, C. S., Miller, E. B., McLean, D. C., Perlis, M. D., Dion, R. M., and Horvitz, V. S.: Lumbar amputation of hemicorporectomy for advanced malignancy of the lower half of the body, Ann. Surg. **48:**357-365, 1960.

6 Kiselow, M., Butcher, H. R., Jr., and Bricker, E. M.: Results of the radical surgical treatment of advanced pelvic cancer: a fifteen-year study, Ann. Surg. **166:**428-436, 1967.

7 Modlin, J., and Walker, H. S. J.: Palliative resections in cancer of the colon and rectum, Cancer **2:**767-776, 1949.

8 Moore, G. E.: A plea for valid assessment of surgical therapy; the value of controlled, cooperative clinical trials, Surgery **48:**481-484, 1960.

9 Moore, G. E.: The spread of tumor cells, Proceedings of the Fourth National Cancer Conference, Sept. 13-15, 1960, Philadelphia, 1961, J. B. Lippincott Co., pp. 91-95.

10 Moss, W. T., and Brand, W. N.: Therapeutic radiology, ed. 3, St. Louis, 1969, The C. V. Mosby Co.

11 Moyer, C. A.: The assessment of operative risk. In Allen, J. G., Harkins, H. N., Moyer, C. A., and Rhoads, J. E., editors: Surgery, principles and practice, Philadelphia, 1957, J. B. Lippincott Co., chap. 11, p. 175.

12 Rhoads, J. E.: Development of preventive surgery in the field of cancer, Ann. Surg. **146:**782-789, 1957.

13 Spratt, J. S., Jr., and Ackerman, L. V.: Relationship of the size of colonic tumors to their cellular composition and biological behavior, Surg. Forum **10:**56-61, 1960.

Chapter 5

Radiotherapy of cancer

Three quarters of a century ago the searching observation of an austere German professor of physics resulted in the discovery of "a new kind of ray" which was named, in his honor, the *roentgen ray*. Shortly afterward, a frail, young, and sentimental Polish woman, Marie Sklodowska, chose the subject of her thesis for a degree of Doctor of Sciences and, without suspecting it, embarked on a most fascinating though trying voyage to an unknown destination. The discovery of a new element, *polonium,* named after her country of birth, was but a landmark in the search of this indefatigable woman—loving wife and tender mother, as well as incomparable investigator. Inspired by the serene love and judgment of her French husband and collaborator, Pierre Curie, she pursued a long investigation that led them to the discovery of *radium.*

These remarkable discoveries became the preface of an interminable volume of interrelated discoveries of imponderable magnitude that were to change the old concept of immutable substances and indivisible atoms, that were to project light on the history of matter and its evolution in the cosmos, and that were to lead man to irruption into the infinitesimal planetary system which is the atom, to grasp its secrets, and to acquire possession of the forces of his own destruction. The pleiad of scientists who wrote these new chapters forms a dissonant list of names: Planck, Einstein, Rutherford, de Broglie, Bohr, Irene Curie, Joliot, Lawrence, Compton, Chadwick, Fermi, Oppenheimer.

In the unfolding of scientific interrelations, the ultimate repercussions of the discovery of ionizing radiations cannot as yet be foreseen, but from the start medicine has continuously benefited from their exploitation in the diagnosis and treatment of disease. The development of diagnostic radiology constitutes in itself a major contribution of incalculable value without which modern medicine would lose a great deal of its present solidity. The early application of ionizing radiations brought forth new hope to the incurables, stimulated the study of histopathology of neoplasia, enlarged the interest of surgeons in the treatment of tumors, and gave a most vigorous impulse to cancer research.

Moreover, the advent of radiotherapy of cancer made evident the necessity of close cooperation between pathologists, surgeons, and radiologists for the successful treatment of many tumors and has resulted in the creation of special institutions for treatment and research, as well as for the training of young specialists in the field of cancer. "Those deeply and seriously interested in cancer as one of our greatest problems in medicine today, should ever be mindful of the fact that therapeutic radiology . . . provided the spark to set off a new era in investigation and treatment of neoplastic diseases."*

A knowledge of the chronologic development of therapeutic radiology is paramount to the understanding of its status in medicine, of its present problems, and of its future.

Early in its development, radiotherapy consisted mostly of *radiumtherapy*. The intracavitary and interstitial applications of radium were often made in the operating room and required surgical precautions, surgical exposure, and surgical skill. Naturally the practice of curietherapy fell into the hands of the gynecologists, dermatologists, surgeons, and those who learned the simple techniques of its application. But these men seldom became students of radiobiology or of other important aspects of the growing field of radiotherapy.

The progress of *roentgentherapy* has been slow and undramatic, but it has become a greater and more important part of

---

*From Quick, D.: Therapeutic radiology, Radiology **50:**283-296, 1948.

therapeutic radiology than radiumtherapy. The development of roentgentherapy paralleled for several decades that of radiodiagnosis, for both depended in great part upon the technical advancement of the apparatus. Radiologists familiar with the equipment, its function and dangers, have been responsible for the practice of roentgentherapy and for its progress in the treatment of cancer. There are certain notable radiologists who have equal interest and competence in the diagnostic as well as in the therapeutic aspect of radiology, but the average "general practitioner of radiology" has had considerably more training and is definitely more skilled in radiodiagnosis than in radiotherapy. The modern radiodiagnostician is often by choice a diagnostic consultant operating on a high plane of relationship with other medical specialists. This function requires vast knowledge of a great number of medical problems, a capacity for reflection, a will to follow new developments in a variety of specialties, and considerable time for individual consultation. Not infrequently, the radiologist finds himself too pressed for time to give the necessary attention to the highly dissimilar disciplines of radiophysics, radiobiology, and tumor pathology and the exacting exigencies of the actual everyday practice of medicine. Proof of the unequal interest in the different aspects of radiology may be found in many of the university hospitals in the United States where the departments of radiology are tendered no hospitalization privileges of their own (Regato[172]).

The advent of *radioactive isotopes* in medicine found many a department of radiology entirely unprepared to accept the responsibility for their use and development. Internists, hematologists, physicists, biochemists, and others have become responsible for their therapeutic application. Therapeutic radiology, the very nature of which requires centralization for protection, intelligent application, and research, has been the subject of a pitiful dispersion that has crippled its development. It would be unjust not to add that there are certain departments of radiology that have centralized the authority and responsibility for all therapeutic radiology and in which radiotherapy is practiced with as high

standards as radiodiagnosis. Radiologists themselves recognize the necessity for such departments to be the rule rather than the exception, for the life of thousands of patients and the prestige of the specialty are at stake. The time is approaching when the last organizational step in the long road toward the realization of radiation therapy in its proper place will have been taken—viz., independent departments of radiation therapy or departments of oncology in medical schools (Buschke[28]).

The benefits to be derived from an actual division of diagnostic and therapeutic radiology have been forcefully presented (Portmann[156]; Quick[162]), and the need for greater numbers of radiotherapists has been discussed. However, the procedure leading to a higher standard of practice of therapeutic radiology is not agreed upon. To stiffen the specialty board examinations would only penalize the young student for a poor quality of training for which he was not responsible. To divide large departments of radiology into a department of radiodiagnosis and another of radiotherapy should require more than the availability of rich equipment. To entrust radiotherapy to self-trained neophytes could prove to be the hardest blow yet given to therapeutic radiology.

The solution to this problem depends primarily on the rapid development of *centers of training* in therapeutic radiology. If, for some time to come, a good deal of radiotherapy will have to be administered by general radiologists, it is of the utmost importance that these men be given commensurate training in both radiodiagnosis and radiotherapy. This aim requires first the thorough training of a good number of therapeutic radiologists with academic inclinations who are capable of directing departments of radiotherapy and of organizing the adequate training of general radiologists in the field of therapeutics. In this manner, a high caliber of radiotherapy will be constantly present to the young trainee, and he will be more desirous to receive adequate training as well as more conscious of the tremendous responsibilities of the practice of radiotherapy. Only after this program has been well established will it be timely to raise the minimum requirements of the specialty board examinations in order to stimulate both the offer and the demand for better training (Regato[173]). And as better results are shown in the life-saving indications of radiotherapy, a greater number of physicians will undoubtedly choose to be trained exclusively in this highly exacting, strictly therapeutic aspect of radiology. In 1939, there were only forty-nine physicians practicing radiotherapy in the United States; by 1969, there were nearly 400. The number of trainees in "straight" therapeutic radiology in the United States was 180 at the beginning of 1970, a greater than sixfold increase in the past decade (Regato[176a]).

Adequate training in radiotherapy implies instruction in the physics of radiations enriched by versatile exercise in its everyday utilization. The aim should be to enlighten the student on the possibilities and limitations of the force at his command. ". . . it is surprising how far it is possible to go in giving the learner a real insight into physical principles without covering the blackboard with a mass of symbols and equations."*

A thorough knowledge of radiobiology is also required. Here, it is pertinent to emphasize that present-day radiobiology is infinitely vast—what is paramount to the therapeutic radiologist is a thorough understanding of *human radiophysiology* and of the variants involved in the radiation effects on human tissues. This may be supplemented by theoretical considerations of the mechanism of cellular effects and of quantitative cell biology and by a first-hand exposure of the trainee to experimental work.

The therapeutic radiologist should also have a knowledge of pathology of tumors, without which his other abilities take a lesser significance. By knowledge of pathology we do not imply expert microscopic recognition of specific morphology but a thorough acquaintance with the natural histology of tumors (rate of growth, modes of spread, radiophysiologic response) and of their dynamic character, which is acquired only by prolonged study of cancer patients. Gross pathology as observed at

autopsy and elements of microscopic diagnosis are a useful complement.

But above these essentials, the radiotherapist must have a wide versatile clinical training (Kerr[98]). "No one with experience of the practice of radiation therapy would deny that fundamentally the radiotherapist is a clinician with all that that implies. His technical training is definitely secondary to his medical competence."* His training must be directed by clinicians who consider radiotherapy their vocation, not their hobby.

Young radiologists cannot be inspired to their study of therapeutics by being compelled to deal only with incurables and failures. Their training should be organized to facilitate constant intercourse with cancer surgeons and tumor pathologists. Adequate facilities for examination of both new and old patients and educational clinical histories should be available. Follow-up examinations of patients should be attended by surgeons, pathologists, and other specialists concerned in order to offer a true opportunity for lively discussion and education. It should be obvious that the necessary instruction and experience cannot be provided or acquired in a few months. Visits of short duration and observation of work of large departments, without actual responsibility in the daily work, can only benefit those who are already thoroughly trained.

Physical foundation of radiotherapy

In the gamut of electromagnetic waves that extends from the electric waves (100,000,000,000 cm maximum wavelength) through the radio waves to the visible light (0.0001 cm maximum wavelength) and ultraviolet rays, the roentgen rays, radium, and cosmic rays occupy the other extreme (to a known 0.000,000,000,001 cm wavelength). Radioactivity is the natural property of certain elements found in nature, and it consists of the spontaneous emission of radiations due to a disintegration of their unstable atoms.

Radium has been the most utilized of the naturally radioactive elements. Arti-

---

*From Stead, G.: The place of physics in the training of the medical radiologist (presidential address), Brit. J. Radiol. **21:**373-379, 1948.

*From Mayneord, W. V.: The organization of teaching and research in medical physics, Acta Radiol. (Stockholm) **29:**435-455, 1948.

ficially radioactivated elements also have been adopted for external irradiation as well as for interstitial applications. Roentgen rays are obtained by applying high-voltage electric currents to the electrodes of a specially designed vacuum tube. Other ionizing radiations such as neutrons, protons, and alpha particles have not yet been widely used for therapeutic purposes. Certain phenomena such as that of diffraction and polarization of radiations are compatible with the theory that they are electromagnetic waves. Others, however, such as the photoelectric and Compton's effect, are only explained if one assumes that they are discontinuous *quanta* of energy acting as corpuscular matter.

The beam of radiations that is produced in a roentgen ray tube is not homogeneous, the wavelength of its constituents varying from a maximum to a minimum. An increase in the *kilovoltage* applied to the tube results in a lowering of the minimum wavelength rays within the beam. Since their ability to penetrate matter is greater as their wavelength decreases, an increase in kilovoltage results in a relative improvement of the penetrating ability of the beam of rays.

The range of utilization of roentgen rays in clinical practice extends from *superficial* roentgentherapy (under 10 kv), through *conventional* roentgentherapy (250 to 300 kv) and *supervoltage* roentgentherapy (up to 1000 kv) and *megavoltage* roentgentherapy (over 2 million volts).

As the roentgen rays travel away from their source, they disperse. At points increasingly distant from the target, the beam is distributed over increasingly large surfaces that vary proportionately with the square of the distance. Consequently, as the distance from the source increases, the amount of radiations received by a given surface decreases with the square of the distance (inverse square law).

Interaction of radiations and matter

Among the various properties of radiations are their ability to produce fluorescence of certain substances (utilized in radioscopy), their photochemical effect (utilized in radiography), and their ability to discharge electrically charged bodies to produce ionization. The absorption of radiations by matter depends primarily on (1) the wavelength of the incident radiations, which is directly related to the voltage applied to the tube, and (2) the coefficient of absorption of the matter itself, which increases rapidly with the atomic number of the element. Thus, a thickness of aluminum absorbs less than the same thickness of copper (utilized for filtration), and both absorb considerably less than the same thickness of lead (utilized in protection).

As radiations pass through matter, there is an interaction of one on the other that results in a complex, progressive transformation of the incident energy. Ionizing radiations are capable, by their high intrinsic energy, of disrupting the atoms of the matter they traverse. Because matter is made mostly of empty spaces, it is perfectly possible for a ray or photon to pass through it without being affected, but when it hits an atom, the collision may have either of two types of effect:

1 The *photoelectric effect*, in which the ray loses its entire energy in the dislodgment of an electron from its orbit, with the dislodged electrons becoming negative ions, each one of which may produce several thousand ion pairs along its zigzag path

2 The *Compton effect*, in which the ray loses only part of its energy in the dislodgment of an electron (recoil electron) and proceeds, deviated from its original path (scattered photon), with a reduced energy but capable of further collision

The photoelectric collisions are most frequent in the interaction of low-voltage radiations and matter, their number decreasing (but the range of the dislodged electron increases) as the voltage is raised. The Compton collisions become predominant (and the range of the recoil electrons becomes longer) as the voltage increases. The atom deprived of one of its electrons becomes a positive ion. When another electron replaces the missing one, a *characteristic ray* is emitted, the wavelength of which depends on the nature of the traversed element and the position of the dislodged electron.

The scattered or secondary radiations (photoelectrons, recoil electrons, scattered photons, and characteristic rays) that result from this interaction of radiations and matter may travel in the same direction as the incident radiations (forward scatter), but a portion of it takes a retrograde path (backscatter). Thus at any depth of matter the radiations absorbed result from the addition of the unaltered part of the incident beam plus the forward scatter and the backscatter. In radiotherapy of 200 kv, the unaltered part of the incident beam that reaches a point decreases rapidly with greater depth and becomes inferior to the amount of forward scatter and even backscatter radiations. With supervoltage equipment, the unaltered part of the incident beam that penetrates remains the largest of the three components for a considerably greater depth; the forward scatter remains important, and the backscatter is minimal.

Biologic effects of ionizing radiations

The administration of excessive amounts of radiations to any living tissue results in damage to its different components, damage that affects indiscriminately all living cells in what has been termed a *diffuse cytocaustic effect*. This effect differs in no way from that which is due to an excessive application of heat, cold, or caustic substances. On the contrary, appropriate amounts of radiations of good quality may have an effect only upon certain cells. This latter phenomenon, the *selective cytolethal effect*, is the one utilized in radiotherapy of malignant tumors.

The lethal effect of radiations on living cells is the final result of the ionization produced in their collisions with the components of living tissues. But while the death of the cell may immediately follow in some instances, the damage done may become ostensible only after the cell undergoes mitosis, and still in other instances it is only appreciable in the cell's descendants. Bergonié and Tribondeau[10] noted no visible changes in the appearance and movements of spermatozoa irradiated in vitro, but Bardeen[6] and Regaud and Dubreuil[181] demonstrated that irradiated spermatozoa were either rendered unsuitable for fecundation or resulted in abortive or monstrous fecundations. Guilleminot[71] irradiated dry grain and found that it kept a latent lesion that

brought about anomalies and death at some stage after its germination. The same was true of grain that was not planted for several months following irradiation.

The expression *lethal dose* has no significance in radiobiology. Cells of the same species, simultaneously irradiated, die after receiving extremely variable amounts of radiations. The introduction in biology (Condon and Terrill[39]) of the idea of the discontinuous absorption of the incident energy furnished Lacassagne[104] and Holweck[84] with a means of interpreting the effects of radiations on the cell. Working with different unicellular organisms, they found that irradiation induced several types of lesions among the cells treated and that the relative proportion of these lesions varied with the dose. Interpreting these facts according to the quantum theory (corpuscular nature of radiations), Lacassagne[104] and Holweck[84] attributed these lesions to different qualitative and quantitative effects of radiations on the individual cells:

1 *Immediate death,* due to simultaneous absorption of a large number of particles in the cell, resulting in destruction of the different cellular constituents

2 *Delayed growth* due to partial disintegration of the protoplasm

3 *Suppression of motility* due to an impact on the motor centers

4 *Suppression of reproduction* due to destruction of the centriole

5 *Abortive anomalies of cellular division* due to the destruction of varying quantities of nuclear chromatin

6 *Hereditary malformations* due to a lesion of a particular segment of chromosomic substance (gene)

Lacassagne[104] pointed out that this dissociation of cellular function, this veritable microdissection produced by ionizing radiations, distinguishes them from other physical agents. Effects so far studied can be attributed to the ionization of molecules in the path of the ionizing particles, but Gray[68] showed that the biologic effect is not uniquely determined by the total number of ions but that it is also conditioned by the spatial distribution of ions.

The effects of radiations on living cells cannot be explained, however, on the basis of physical trauma alone, nor can the complicated organization of normal tissues be considered, for the understanding of radiobiology, as the equivalent of an aggregate of unicellular organisms. The chemical effects of ionization of cellular components, the possible changes in the permeability of the cellular membrane, the ionization of circulating minerals and their effect on the interchange of fluids (Zirkle[234]), and the effects of irradiation on the connective tissue, on the blood supply, etc. contribute, in all probability, in a lesser or greater degree to the final results.

Living tissues react very differently to irradiations. Tissues formed by uniform cells, not usually arranged in layers (nervous system, muscle, bone), generally show very poor radiosensitivity (Borak[20]). Their injuries through irradiation are usually an indirect consequence due to resulting fibrosis or impaired vascularity. Tissues composed of multiform cells in continuous transformation, usually arranged in several layers (epidermis, seminiferous tubules), present marked radiosensitivity. But the individual cells of these complex tissues show a very variable degree of response to irradiations, the germ cells (spermatogonias, basal cells of epidermis, lymphoblasts) being considerably more affected than their somatic descendants. This results in latency of the effects that may not make themselves evident for several weeks.

Perthes[146] first noticed the correlation of reproductivity and radiosensitivity of cells. The basic experimental facts were expressed in the form of a general radiobiologic "law" by Bergonié and Tribondeau[11]: "The effect of radiations on living cells is the more intense: (1) the greater their reproductive activity, (2) the longer their mitotic phase lasts, and (3) the less their morphology and function are differentiated."*

In its general application, this "law" has often been found inaccurate. Its relative value is confined to the explanation of the different radiosensitivity of cells within the same tissue, which may be due to the greater vulnerability of cells with marked mitotic activity, but very radiosensitive cells may not have a great reproductivity. The "law" of Bergonié and Tribondeau is of no help in the theoretic establishment of a scale of radiosensitivity of different tissues. Lacassagne[103] found that the follicular cells of the ovary show different degrees of radiosensitivity that do not decrease with the age of the cell. Bloom and Bloom[18] observed that the reticular stem cells of the blood-forming organs are extremely resistant to radiations, although they are more primitive than the free stem cells (blasts).

The intensity of the effects of irradiation and their permanency or atonement depend upon various intrinsic and extrinsic factors. Jolly[90] demonstrated that the radiosensitivity of one-half of the thymus in the rabbit is greatly affected by unilateral ligation of afferent vessels. Thus he proved the importance of blood supply in radiosensitivity. The quality and quantity of radiations have an obvious bearing on the results: the greater the dose and the lesser the quality of the radiations, the less selective is their action, the more marked and diffuse are their effects, and the less reversible are these effects. Fractionation of the total dose results in exactly the opposite effects.

The immediate reaction and the ultimate effect of radiations on the different tissues and organs greatly depend upon the quantity and character of radiations and the circumstances of their application. In addition, the effects produced upon the same type of tissue may be very different in two different animal species, which may lead to controversial experimental findings.

Experimental methods

Puck and Marcus[160] reported their studies on mammalian cell survival, in vitro, in 1956. Hewitt and Wilson[81] wrote on the survival of leukemic cells, in vivo, in 1959. Also in 1959, Elkind and Sutton[56] published their study of the recovery of irradiated cells. These pioneering pieces of work have motivated, in the past decade, a variety of approaches, countless studies, mathematical models, and theories seeking to make a quantitative assessment of the

---

*Translated from Bergonié, J., and Tribondeau, L.: Interprétation de quelques résultats de la radiothérapie et éssai de fixation d'une téchnique rationnelle, C. R. Acad. Sci. (Paris) **143**:983-985, 1906.

effects of ionizing radiations (Conference on Radiobiology and Radiotherapy[40]). The goal would be, of course, the finding of a biologic basis to clinical dosimetry, but the bridge between theory and application is yet to be established (Mendelsohn[128]). A detailed account of the different facets of this work is not in the scope of this chapter. The interested reader is referred to the specific publications of the various workers in this field or monographs on the related fields (Andrews[1]).

Lacassagne[105] irradiated mice while under a state of temporary asphyxia, with cessation of circulation and consequent anoxia of the tissues. He proved that they survived after irradiation, whereas the controls, irradiated to the same dose, died within days. This experiment demonstrated the important role of oxygen in radiobiology and initiated a new chapter of research. Subsequent pieces of work by Loiseleur[117] and by Lacassagne and Latarjet[107] demonstrated the oxidizing effects of irradiations resulting from radioactivation of the molecular oxygen. Their work showed opposite effects depending on molecular mass: *desmolysis* of complex molecules and condensation and *synthesis* of simple ones. This new avenue of radiobiologic research has absorbed the attention of dozens of experimental workers and innumerable laboratory efforts (Lea[114]; Gray[69]). The goal of practical and fruitful *hybaroxic* radiotherapy has yet to be justified (Regato[175]).

On the theory that cell radiosensitivity may not be the same in different phases of the cell reproductive "cycle", considerable experimental work has been produced in an effort to find a rational way toward a better utilization of dose and its optimum relationship to time of delivery (Whitmore and Till[230]; Sinclair[205]; Kallman[93]; Tolmach et al.[218]).

Experimental evidence has been advanced suggesting that DNA is the critical target element for cell killing by ionizing radiations (Epstein[58]). Cells are killed by the beta rays of tritiated thymidine selectively incorporated into nuclear DNA (Painter et al.[141]). As the ingenious researchers have pushed their efforts, the frontiers of radiobiologic research have been expanded.

Human radiophysiology
Effects of irradiation of skin

The effects of irradiation of the skin are a singular example of radiophysiology. The knowledge of these effects is of great importance, since reactions of the skin may become an indicative and limiting factor in radiotherapy. The effects of irradiation on the skin vary greatly with the *dose absorbed*, the quality of radiations, the region of the body, and the individual idiosyncrasy. The quality of radiations and the size of the field have an important bearing on the *dose absorbed* by the skin. The intensity of the immediate reaction is greater, all other conditions being the same, the shorter the time in which the total dose is delivered. The late effects vary according to the fractionation of the total dose and individual idiosyncrasy.

The administration of radiations to the skin may result in an immediate rubicundity or flushness that usually disappears after

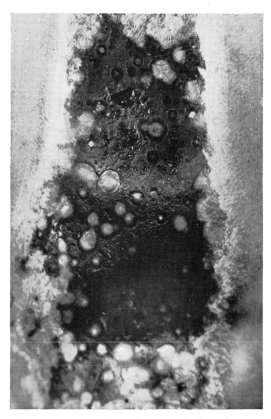

Fig. 33. Moist radioepidermitis of skin showing multiple areas of epidermal repair at borders and center.

a few hours. With a moderate dose, the hair falls or is easily drawn after ten to fourteen days. A larger dose results toward the third week in the development of an erythema that becomes brighter and later may turn to brown. The elimination of large scaly fragments of epidermis, underneath which there is a new thin skin, known as a *dry epidermitis*, may occur between four and five weeks following a single irradiation. With the administration of a somewhat larger dose (or with a larger field or inferior quality of radiations), the erythema ends at three to four weeks in a denudation of the dermis, with or without previous formation of vesicles, in what is known as a *moist epidermitis* (Regaud and Nogier[183]). This denuded area weeps constantly and is subject to easy secondary infection. It is rapidly covered within a few days by the development of confluent, circular islands of new epidermis arising from both the center and borders of the area (Fig. 33). A more intense radioepidermitis takes a considerably longer period to repair, since the epidermis may only grow from the borders of the area. A larger

dose may result in bleeding from the dermis followed by secondary infection and loss of substance, which is known as *acute radiodermitis*, a true radionecrosis of the dermis that is not spontaneously reparable unless it is very limited.

The *permanent sequelae* resulting from irradiation of the skin are also varied. With a small dose the epilation produced is only transistory, but when a radioepidermitis has been produced, the epilation is usually permanent. Except for epilation, there may be little visible sequelae even after a radioepidermitis, but achromia, fibrosis, atrophy, and telangiectasis may gradually develop in very variable degrees (Fig. 34), depending on intensity, region, idiosyncrasy, etc. An intense radioepidermitis with a long period of repair may give place to a discolored atrophic skin that becomes dryer and less pliable (Fig. 35) and may easily

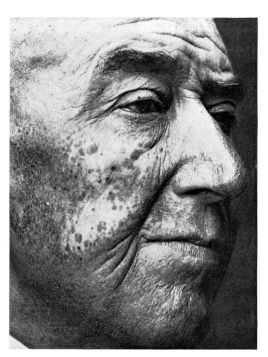

Fig. 34. Slight achromia and atrophy of skin of face several years after roentgentherapy for carcinoma of superior maxilla.

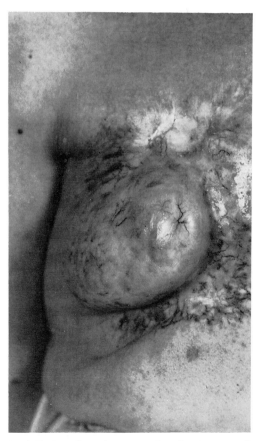

Fig. 35. Atrophic changes with telangiectases of skin of breast following intensive radiotherapy for inoperable carcinoma.

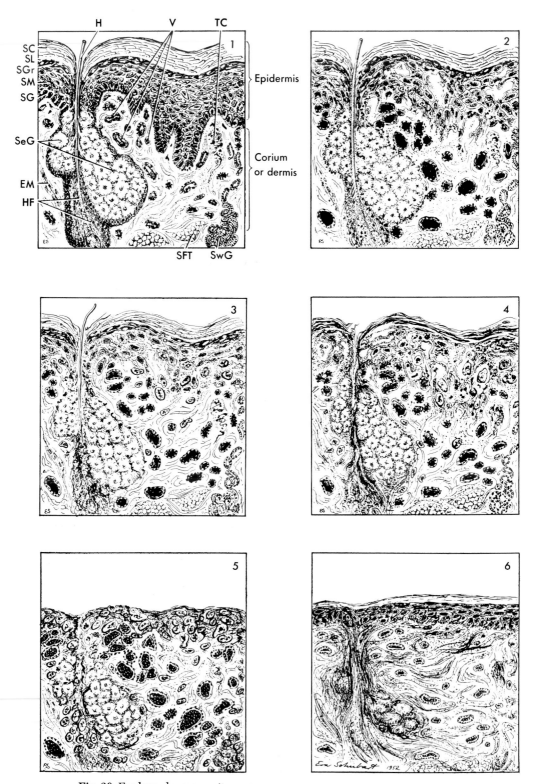

Fig. 36. For legend see opposite page.

break down years later (spontaneously or following trauma and secondary infection). The result is a necrotic ulceration, a *late radiodermitis,* the development of which may be due as much to a lack of local vitality as it is to trauma and infection.

The *radiobiologic mechanism* of skin reactions is one of the best examples of selective cytolethal effect of radiations (Fig. 36). Beyond a certain minimum dose, the administration of a single dose of radiations may destroy the life of the cells of the germinal layer of the epidermis and hair follicles, all or most of which die immediately or shortly afterward in abortive mitoses. The irradiation has very little, if any, effect on the more superficial cells of the epidermis. The hair stops growing and shortly afterward becomes detached from the matrix. Thus, while the normal desquamation of superficial epidermic cells proceeds, the constant supply of cells from the basal layer is stopped and consequently the epidermis becomes thinner, the intercellular spaces become enlarged (edema), and large amounts of polymorphonuclear leukocytes give the area a character of inflammation that justifies the name of epidermitis. Finally, the epidermis entirely disappears in about twenty-six to twenty-eight days. When this occurs, there may have been some reformation of new epidermis, so the dermis is not actually denuded (dry epidermitis). But if the germinal cells have not yet started to repopu-

late the area, the papillae of the dermis lose their normal covering (moist epidermitis) until epidermal growth from around the hair follicles and sweat glands or from the nonirradiated borders of the area finally covers anew the dermis.

Histologically, the late effects of irradiation are characterized by atrophic epidermis, increased pigmentation of the basal layer, and hyalinized dermis with telangiectases and complete absence of skin appendages. Usually there is no thrombosis of blood vessels. These effects are similar to those observed on the scar of burns, but in the latter there is no increase in melanin pigmentation and no telangiectases, and the collagen has a different staining reaction. The experimental irradiation of the skin of mice has shown that the vascular effect was of secondary importance. In cases of acute or late radiodermitis, there is loss of substance and infection of the dermis. The endarteritis that may then be observed is probably a consequence rather than the cause of this untoward effect. The external sheath is the most sensitive part of the hair follicle. The sebaceous glands and the sweat glands are less radiosensitive.

The effects of irradiation of the oral and pharyngeal *mucous membranes* are very similar to those observed on the skin except that, as was pointed out by Coutard,[43] the denudation of the dermis occurs in half the time, thirteen to fourteen days,

Fig. 36. Effects of irradiation of skin. 1, *Normal skin.* Schematic separation of strata showing hair, sebaceous gland, sweat gland, and dermic blood vessels. 2, *Four days after irradiation.* Extensive cytolysis of basal layers and hair bed, resulting in occasional lacunar spaces. All other strata of epidermis remain unchanged except for some edema in stratum malpighii. Papillae are less deep, and there are polymorphonuclear lymphocytes near germinal layer. Dermal vessels are congested with red cells. 3, *Eight days after irradiation.* Stratum malpighii is now reduced to few layers. Other strata are unchanged. Hair is loose from its walls below epidermis but remains attached above. There is less dilatation of vessels, and giant cells have replaced lacunae. 4, *Fifteen days after irradiation.* There are practically no malpighian cells left, and hair has fallen. Stratum granulosum and lucidum are unchanged. Stratum corneum is thinner. 5, *Twenty-six days after irradiation.* All epidermis is gone. Surface of dermis is wavy. Dermic vessels are congested with cells. There are numerous polymorphonuclear leukocytes around hair bed and sweat glands. 6, *Sixty days after irradiation.* New very thin epidermis has formed. Hair follicle and sweat gland duct have become fibrosed. There are fewer vessels in dermis, separated by fibrous tissue. **H,** Hair. **V,** Vessels. **TC,** Tactile corpuscle (Meissner). **SC,** Stratum corneum. **SL,** Stratum lucidum. **SGr,** Stratum granulosum. **SM,** Stratum mucosum. **SG,** Stratum germinativum. **SeG,** Sebaceous glands. **EM,** Erector muscle. **HF,** Hair follicle. **SFT,** Subcutaneous fatty tissue. **SwG,** Sweat gland.

and the dermis is rapidly covered with a diphtheroid membrane. This mucous membrane reaction is known as a *radioepithelitis* (Coutard[43]). Repair is rapid or delayed, depending on the intensity of the irradiation. The columnar epithelium of the nasal fossae and trachea is considerably less radiosensitive and may not be apparently affected by relatively large doses.

Effects of irradiation of gastrointestinal tract

The squamous epithelium of the *esophagus* presents the same radiosensitivity and reactions observed on the mucosa of the oral cavity or pharynx. Clinically, odynophagia is frequently noted in patients receiving irradiation to the mediastinum who may not offer any other signs of irradiation effects. The radioepithelitis of the esophageal mucosa may subside but, depending on the intensity of irradiation and total dose absorbed, the acute reaction may lead to stenosis and necrosis.

Experimental studies in laboratory animals and in human beings have repeatedly established that the irradiation of the *stomach* results in a temporary but often marked diminution of the mucus and acid content of the gastric secretion, even when the dose is not sufficient to produce histologically recognizable lesions (Szegö and Rother[215]; Ivy et al.[86]). This gastric depression has been verified by testing the nocturnal secretion and the response to histamine (Levin et al.[116]). Uropepsin excretion has been found to be increased concomitantly with the decrease in acidity (Rider et al.[187]). This has been attributed to a shift in the direction of pepsinogen diffusion in favor of the bloodstream. Intense irradiation may result in gastritis characterized gastroscopically by hyperemia, edema, hemorrhage, and adherent exudate.

Clinically, ulceration (Palmer[142]) and perforation have been observed months after excessive irradiation of normal stomachs (Brick[24]). Pierce[148a] found the most sensitive cells to be those at the base of the gastric foveola which are responsible for regeneration. Intense irradiation results in degenerative change in the epithelial cells and eventual atrophy of the gastric mucosa (Ricketts et al.[186]).

The mucosa of the *small intestine* shows considerably greater radiosensitivity than the stomach or large bowel. Within a few minutes of the irradiation, early changes in the basal cells of the crypts of Lieberkühn (Tsuzuki[219]), in the villi, and in the lymph follicles may be evident. There is overproduction of mucus, hyperemia, and edema. Later, there may be infection and inflammation. Loose connective tissue appears in the submucosa, and progressive obstruction, extensive ulceration (Fig. 37), and perforation may result (Halls[74]). Moss[132] demonstrated that irradiation of the exteriorized small bowel of rats resulted in a striking decrease of glucose absorption. Malabsorption of various substances of vital importance has been demonstrated experimentally (Dalla Palma[49a]). Permanent injury with malnutrition, diarrhea, and cachexia may result (Martin and Rogers[125]).

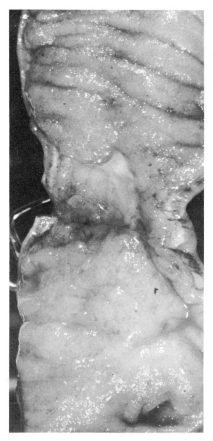

Fig. 37. Effects of irradiation on mucosa of ileum following radiotherapy for carcinoma of cervix. (PCH 64-591.)

Absorption of the muscular layers results in shortening of the irradiated segment. Eddy and Casarett[54a] observed frequent swelling or hypertrophy of endothelial nuclei or cells and increased numbers of endothelial cells in the small arteries.

Clinically, similar changes occur in patients receiving abdominal irradiation for cancer of the cervix, para-aortic metastases, etc. The most marked changes may take place in the ileum: reduction of the intestinal caliber and elasticity may result in ulceration that becomes aggravated by the passage of fecal stream and bacterial infection (Friedman[64]). The frequency of this complication is definitely related to dosage and intensity of irradiation (Brick[24]). Also, laparotomies performed before irradiation seem to increase the chance. Death may occur because of extensive gangrene and perforation. It may be rather simply averted by early suspicion of this complication and surgical intervention (Wiley and Sugarbaker[232]; Mason et al.[126a]; DeCosse et al.[51b]; Ketcham et al.[98a]). Wiernik[231] studied the effects of irradiation on the *jejunal mucosa,* observing a reduction followed by a rise in mitotic activity after a single large dose. With increasing damage of the crypts and villous structures, a change in architecture and epithelial cell population was noted.

The *large bowel* is considerably less vulnerable than the rest of the gastrointestinal tract, but intensive irradiation from uterine and vaginal radium sources or supervoltage roentgentherapy may result in ulceration (Fig. 38) and rarely in perforation (Quan[161]). Following irradiation and in the presence of recurrent or metastatic tumor, the sequence of events may be difficult to interpret, but cases of stenosis have been reported and studied. Histologically, subserosal and submucosal fibrosis, as well as subintimal foam cells in the small arteries, are observed (Perkins and Spjut[145b]).

The irradiation of the *salivary glands* results in rapid thickening of the saliva with qualitative changes together with a diminution of the total amount secreted. Other than this functional effect, seldom is any effect on the salivary glands noted in the course of fractionated therapeutic irradia-

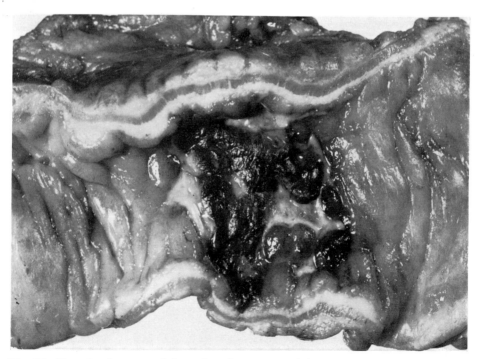

Fig. 38. Necrotic ulceration of large bowel accompanied by extensive submucosal fibrosis. Patient had received dose in excess of 6000 R in six weeks over large bowel. (WU neg. 59-2497.)

tions. *Acute sialadenitis* has been reported in a few cases of accidental intensive irradiation (Kashima et al.[97]). Rarely, an acute swelling of the submaxillary glands is observed at the beginning of treatment. These acute effects are similar, clinically, to the results of chronic inflammatory obstruction of the salivary ducts. Besides being related to intensive irradiation, they may be associated with immunologic deficiencies of the patient. Evans and Ackerman[59] reported patchy destruction of glands and vascular alterations on irradiated submaxillary glands.

The irradiation of salivary glands of rats revealed that the acini, the secretory tubules, and the excretory ducts show decreasing effects (Cherry and Glucksmann[34]). There were changes in the type, amount, and direction of the salivary secretion. Regenerative activity followed the administration of low doses of radiations.

The growth of *teeth* may be retarded by irradiation. Experimental work in animals shows evidence of damage to the odontoblasts of the dentin following irradiation (Kimeldorf et al.[99]). Several years after irradiation of tumors of the oral cavity and pharynx, peculiar, usually painless caries appear in the teeth (Fig. 39), finally

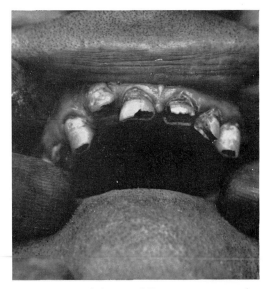

Fig. 39. Dental lesions following treatment for carcinoma of subglottis. (From del Regato, J. A.: Dental lesions observed after roentgentherapy in cancer of the buccal cavity, pharynx and larynx, Amer. J. Roentgen. **42**:404-410, 1939.)

resulting in complete amputation at the neck (Regato[169]). It is most probable that the lesions of teeth observed in man are due to the qualitative and quantitative changes of the saliva (xerostomia), for they occur in the absence of direct irradiation of the teeth or of the jaw.

Experimental evidence (Pohle and Bunting[151]) and clinical experience (Phillips et al.[147]) have long given assurances that the *liver* is not a radiosensitive organ, within therapeutic dose ranges, although liver damage had repeatedly been observed in cases of intensive irradiation (Case and Warthin[32]; Ariel[2]). Supervoltage roentgentherapy has made it possible to irradiate the entire liver with relatively large doses in a relatively short time. As a consequence, there have been reports of "radiation hepatitis" resulting supposedly from these irradiations (Ingold et al.[85]). It is reported that the age of the patients seems to make little difference insofar as the observed parameters are concerned except perhaps in subjects under 1 year of age (Tefft et al.[216a]). The clinical symptoms adduced occur after a few weeks and within six months of the irradiation: gain in weight, abdominal pain, enlarged liver, ascites, and, in some cases, jaundice. In addition the SGOT level may be elevated, and the radiogold liver scan reveals depressed Kupffer cell uptake. The histopathologic evidence, obtained primarily through needle biopsy, is said to be severe sinusoidal congestion or hemorrhage and atrophy of the central hepatic cells (Reed and Cox[166]). The difficulty with this evidence is that the symptoms of liver enlargement and ascites could as well be due to the metastatic disease for which the patients were irradiated. The needle biopsy specimens could possibly reveal the appearance of liver just vacated by the neoplasm. Unquestionably also, acute necrosis may be produced by the irradiation of normal and, perhaps more easily, of diseasesd liver under circumstances of *intense* daily irradiation which need not prevail in clinical radiotherapy. The facts should be susceptible of verification by well-controlled experiments in lower animals and in patients not suffering from metastases in the liver. Radiation injury of the *gallbladder* (Brams and Darnbacher[22]) and of the *biliary tree*

(Case and Warthin[32]) have long been produced experimentally with relatively greater ease.

The *pancreas* is not noticeably affected by irradiations in the therapeutic range, although damage to the gland can be caused by excessive irradiation with interstitial sources. Using rather large doses in single application on exteriorized postoperative pancreatic remnants, Volk et al.[225] were able to study acinar cell damage. Islet cell damage reveals itself after a longer interval.

Effects of irradiation of urinary tract

There is evidence that the *kidney* may be damaged by irradiation within the range of therapeutic dosage (Luxton and Kunkler[19]). Kunkler et al.[102] reported twenty-two patients presenting renal damage in a series of fifty-five men irradiated for metastatic seminoma. Seven of these patients died of renal insufficiency. "Acute" cases occur within six to twelve months after irradiation, with gradual proteinuria, anemia, and hypertension. "Chronic" cases develop insidiously, with proteinuria, anemia, azotemia, and hypertension. Those patients who survive the acute stage do acquire the chronic condition and live for many years. Hypertension with few other symptoms may develop early or late after irradiation. It responds favorably to hypotensive drugs and, when due to unilateral damage, may regress after removal of the damaged kidney.

The reported dose of radiations capable of causing damage is relatively low. It is possible that the required dosage is smaller in the case of children (Sagerman[195]). Fractionation of treatments over a long period of many weeks may be the only safeguard when shielding of the kidneys is not practicable.

Experimental studies have shown that the lesions produced are interstitial and vascular chronic nephritis with degeneration of the tubules, sclerosis of the vessels, and atrophy and hyalinization of the glomeruli (Hartman et al.[75]; Domagk[53]; Redd[165]). Mostofi et al.[134] produced experimentally peritubular congestion and hemorrhage followed by atrophy, interstitial fibrosis, and scarring. Madrazo et al.[121] observed degenerative changes of the epithelial cells, marked tortuosity of glomerular basement membranes plus rarefaction and increase in the mesangial matrix, extensive tubular basement membranes, and increase in the subcellular spaces. The interstitial capillaries showed no significant changes. It must be understood that the experimental evidence gathered by the different workers in dogs and rats has been obtained after the administration of doses of radiations far above those utilized clinically, usually in a single massive application and on previously exteriorized kidneys. Gup et al.[72] showed that irradiation of the kidneys could decrease the glomerular filtration rate and the renal plasma flow. There is no evidence that the *ureters* are affected by radiations within the limits of therapeutic irradiation of the abdomen or pelvis.

The effect of irradiation of the *bladder* can be observed in patients receiving or having received treatment for carcinoma of the cervix. Rarely, a slight dysuria develops during treatment, but cystoscopic examination seldom reveals more than congestion and edema of the mucosa. The bladder mucosa may be entirely covered with false membranes following a course of external pelvic roentgentherapy, but this is inconstant. In heavily irradiated patients, the mucosa may become telangiectatic and atrophic; a late necrotic ulceration may develop which is covered by mineral concretions and is long in healing. Extensive fibrosis between muscle bundles may occur. Sporadic episodes of hematuria are not infrequently observed. Adequate care with antibiotics, cleaning of the bladder, and medical palliation of symptoms frequently result in symptomatic improvement and healing of lesions, except in extreme cases (Pool[154]).

Effects of irradiation of gonads and of embryo

Irradiation of the *testes* results in progressive diminution of their size without loss of sexual appetite and with continued, although diminishing, presence of spermatozoa. The spermatozoa may completely disappear between three and eight weeks after irradiation, the sterilization being temporary or permanent, depending on the character of the therapy. There are no

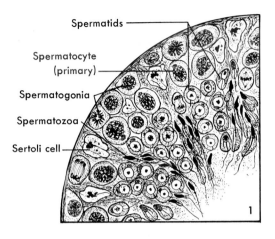

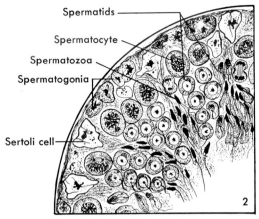

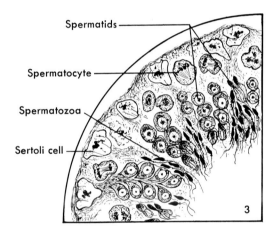

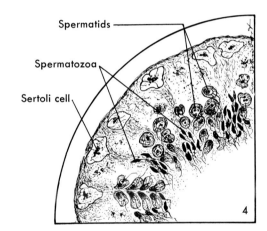

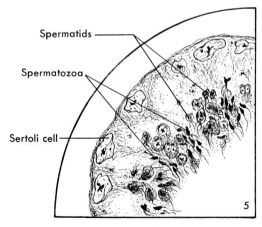

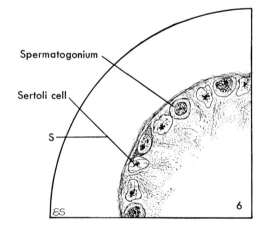

Fig. 40. For legend see opposite page.

changes in the secondary sexual characteristics.

Histologically, there is immediate damage to the spermatogonias, which disappear within a few days, and lesser damage to the more differentiated spermatocytes and spermatids. The destruction of the spermatogonias results in eventual disappearance of spermatocytes, spermatids, and spermatozoa once the maturation of the remaining cells has been completed. Finally, the tubule loses all its germinal epithelium, and only the Sertoli cells remain (Fig. 40). The interstitial cells remain intact, and thus the sterility without impotence is explained. Birke et al.[13] reported no major depression of androsterone or of etiocholanolone in the urine of patients whose testes received daily irradiations. Depending on the dose administered and other factors, spermatogonias may reappear among the Sertoli cells (Regaud and Blanc[180]), and spermatogenesis may eventually be reestablished. Permanent sterilization may also result.

Irradiation of the *ovaries* of young women results in a permanent or temporary arrest of menstruation and development of hot flushes, anxiety, nervousness, etc. characteristic of the menopause although perhaps in a more marked degree. The sexual ardor is quite variably influenced or may not be affected at all. In the experimental animal, the artificial menopause may be accompanied by frigidity (Lacassagne[103]). Irradiation of the ovary may result in the destruction of all follicles contained in the ovary, but these are very differently affected, depending on their degree of maturity at the time of irradiation. The larger, nearly mature follicles are most affected and disappear rapidly. The small primary follicles are very radiosensitive but, because of their large number and small size, may escape a small dose, and they are responsible for the eventual restoration of menstruation. Toward the end of the fourth week, a thoroughly irradiated ovary becomes smooth and decreases in weight. The interstitial glands show very poor radiosensitivity, but the atrophy that follows the disappearance of the follicles results in secondary diminution in the number and in physiologic senescence of these glands (Lacassagne[103]).

Irradiation of the *embryo* in utero during the first half of pregnancy results almost constantly in abortion. Irradiation during the second half may not stop the development of the pregnancy nor produce any visible damage to the fetus (Ronderos[190]), but a large number of malformations of the fetus have resulted, of which microcephaly is the most common (Murphy[136]; Goldstein and Murphy[67]). Important as the experimental work in lower animals is (Brill and Forgotson[25]), it is not justifiable to extrapolate its findings to man (Yamazaki[223]), particularly in respect to dosage. It should be obvious, in spite of alarming lay publicity, that the use of medical radiations for decades has not produced a fraction of the tragic consequences of the ephemeral use of thalidomide.

Effects of irradiation of hemopoietic tissues

Total body irradiation of patients or experimental animals results in an immediate but transient lymphopenia. Following a period of latency, there are also leukopenia, anemia, and thrombocytopenia. Re-

Fig. 40. Effects of irradiation of testis. **1,** *Normal seminal tubule* showing all of different cells and stages of spermatogenesis. **2,** *Two hours after irradiation.* Many spermatogonias are missing. Others are undergoing abnormal mitosis. **3,** *Four days after irradiation.* No spermatogonias are left. Sertoli cells have closed ranks at the base. All other cells have continued their development so that there are fewer primary spermatocytes, some of them showing abnormal mitosis. More mature cells are unchanged. **4,** *Eight days after irradiation.* All primary spermatocytes have disappeared. Cellular column has diminished in height. Some secondary spermatocytes show abnormal mitosis. **5,** *Twenty-one days after irradiation.* No spermatocytes are left. Cellular column is reduced to layer of Sertoli cells. There remain few spermatids, some of which show abnormally shaped heads. **6,** *Thirty-four days after irradiation.* No spermatids are left. Tube has shrunk further. Only Sertoli cells and new spermatogonias are seen.

covery or progressive aggravation and death depend on the intensity and fractionation of the total dose of radiations.

In the circulating blood of rats receiving a single total body irradiation, there is an immediate diminution of lymphocytes, attaining its maximum within twenty-four hours, followed by a reduction in neutrophils, reaching a maximum in seventy-two hours. The diminution of circulating platelets is slower and reaches its maximum toward the eighteenth day (Fig. 41), when all other cells are in frank recovery (Suter[214]).

In man, the reduction in lymphocytes is frequently observed within hours or days. Changes in circulating platelets and anemia may take weeks or months or may become masked by regeneration. Patients exposed to ionizing radiations may show an increase in the number of refractive neutral red bodies in the cytoplasm of circulating lymphocytes (Dickie and Hempelmann[52]), but these and other morphologic changes observed in the circulating blood are not specific (Jacobson et al.[87]). Hemorrhagic

tendencies are thought to be independent of the reduction of megakaryocytes. The changes observed in the circulating blood are a consequence of the irradiation of the hemopoietic organs. The adult circulating blood cells are not radiosensitive.

Irradiation of the *lymphoid tissue* of lymph nodes results in rapid destruction of the lymphoblasts of the germinal centers, but the lymphocytes disappear rapidly also (Heineke[77]). Within a few days repopulation starts and may be complete after several weeks, depending on the intensity of the exposure. Irradiation of the intestinal lymphoid tissue gives the same result but whereas the lymphocytes of Peyer's patches are wiped out, those in the lamina propria of the intestinal villi may remain intact (DeBruyn[51a]).

The *thymus* is also a very radiosensitive organ. Within five days of irradiation, its weight may be reduced by four-fifths (Rudberg[193]). Histologically, the loss results from death of the cortical lymphocytes (thymocytes) and, to a lesser degree, from destruction of the lymphocytes of the

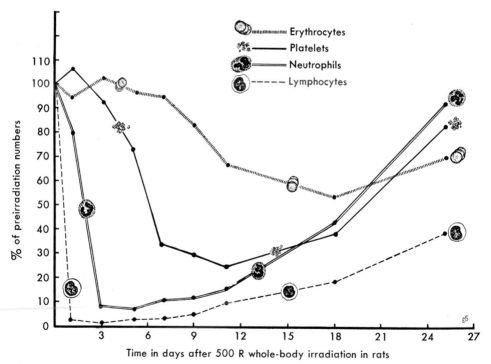

Fig. 41. Graphic demonstration of effects of total body irradiation on circulating blood elements. (Data of Suter et al.; cited in Lawrence, J. S., et al.: Effects of radiation on hemopoiesis, Radiology **51**:400-413, 1948.)

medulla. Hassall's bodies are reported increased (Aubertin and Bordet[4]), and within hours the cortex is reduced to stromal cells. Complete recovery, cellular repopulation, and reestablishment of the thymic structure can be observed after twenty-one to thirty days (Schrek[200]).

Irradiation of the *spleen* follows the same pattern of early destruction of lymphocytes following the lightest irradiation (one to three hours). According to Bloom and Bloom,[18] the medium-sized lymphocytes that predominate in the spleen are entirely destroyed in this first phase, although a few large and small lymphocytes may remain. A second phase of phagocytosis and elimination of debris with consequent shrinkage (three to seventeen hours) is followed by a third phase of relative inactivity (one to nine days) and by eventual proliferation (ten days to four weeks) of lymphocytes (Heineke[77]; Pohle and Bunting[152]; Murray[137]).

Sherman and O'Brien[203] concluded that ionizing radiations seem to have little or no effect on *lymphatic vessels*.

Irradiation of the *bone marrow* results in severe depression of hemopoiesis through changes affecting the megakaryocytes, myelocytes, and erythrocytes. In swine exposed to an atomic explosion, mitotic arrest of hematopoietic cells of the bone marrow appeared after eight hours and progressed to almost complete disappearance of the marrow cells four days after irradiation (Tullis et al.[220]). Lehar et al.[115] noted the persistence of lymphocytes in the irradiated marrow. Heineke[77] considered the cells of the red series to be radioresistant, but other investigators thought their destruction possible (Krause and Ziegler[101]). In general, the difference in radiosensitivity of red and white cells is considered negligible (Lacassagne and Gricouroff[106]). Bloom and Bloom[18] found that, on the contrary, erythrocytes are more radiosensitive than myelocytes and these more so than the megakaryocytes, whereas macrophages, reticular cells, and fat cells were found to be radioresistant. These findings were verified in chickens, in which the recognition of red cells is easy because of the intra-

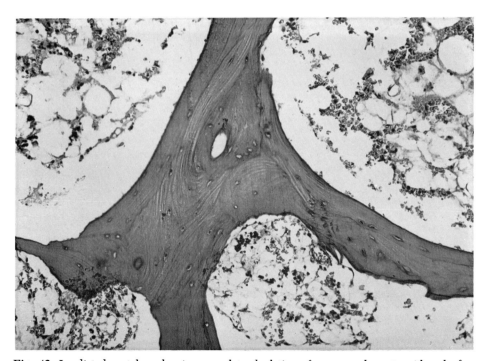

Fig. 42. Irradiated vertebra showing complete depletion of marrow elements with only few persistent reticulum and plasma cells. Cancellous bone is thickened and shows irregular cement lines.

vascular situation of erythropoiesis. Bloom and Bloom[18] found also that the marrow at the growing end of the long bones was more radiosensitive and that regeneration started in the shaft and extended later to the epiphysis and metaphysis. They found no evidence of initial stimulation preceding destruction of blood-forming cells (Fig. 42).

Little evidence has been gathered as to the effect of radiations on the *reticuloendothelial elements* (Brecher et al.[23]). Bloom and Bloom[18] found the reticular stem cell extremely resistant.

Effects of irradiation of cartilage and bone

Growing *cartilage* and *bone* are markedly affected by irradiation, the effects being more remarkable the greater the rate of growth of the irradiated subject and of the irradiated bone. Moreover, the stunting is greater the younger the subject and the greater the intensity of the irradiation. The effects are most striking in the development of symmetrical long bones due to the arrest or retardation of epiphyseal growth (Bisgard and Hunt[14]), where most of the postnatal growth occurs (Hinkel[82]), but flat bones are also affected. The development of bone is affected in width as well as in length (Fig. 43).

Heller[78] observed the first degenerative process in the form of abnormally swollen cartilage cells in the zone of ossification three days after irradiation of rats by means of roentgen rays. Six days later the interdigitation between the cartilage and the metaphyseal bony spongiosa was fully lost. Osteoblasts, the most sensitive of bone cells, disappeared. Dead osteocytes were observed in the lamellae of the spongiosa but not in the cortical bone, and there was only a moderate increase in osteoclasts. From fourteen to thirty-one days after irradiation new primary spongiosa was being laid down against the cartilage plate while the old spongiosa was undergoing gradual resorption. After seventy days the normal pattern of growth was reestablished. The separation of cartilage and bone was not complete until after forty-two to 150 days

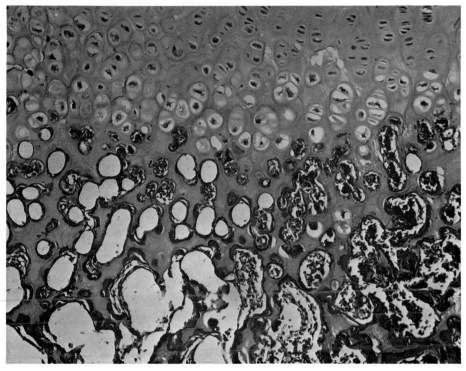

Fig. 43. Epiphysis of irradiated ulna showing irregular epiphyseal junction with swollen cartilage cells.

in mice irradiated internally by means of radioactive strontium.

Retardation of the growth of long bones and scoliotic deformities due to asymmetric development have been observed in children after irradiation for malignant tumors. These changes are directly dependent on the size of the fields, the dose, and the intensity of the irradiation (Whitehouse and Lampe[229]).

Adult cartilage shows little radiosensitivity. Bloom[17] rarely saw any evidence of destruction in the adult epiphyseal cartilage of experimental animals and found the cells of articular cartilages completely resistant. Irradiated cartilage may show changes in staining character and a greater density and fragility and minor cellular changes. Adult bone has long been considered to be radioresistant. However, bony cells have been thought to be more radiosensitive than the interstitial substance of bone lamellae (Heller[78]).

Necrosis of the mandible following irradiation for cancer of the oral cavity is due in great part to the secondary radiations resulting from the high mineral content of the bone and to secondary infection of the irradiated bone. There are clinical examples of necrosis of bones in the absence of infection: the fractures of the neck of the femur following irradiation for carcinoma of the cervix (p. 797) and the fractures of the clavicle and ribs (Pohle and Frank[155]) following irradiation for cancer of the breast. In these cases the irradiation has usually been intense, and there is a long period of latency between the irradiation and the fracture. It is possible that there are cases of necrosis indirectly due to diminished vascularity and persistent or increased strain. Whereas these injuries are avoidable by proper conduct of treatment (fractionation, filtration, small fields), the role of radiations in their production cannot be denied.

Effects of irradiation of lung

Within certain circumstances of intensity of irradiation, total dosage, size of field, etc., the irradiation of *the lung* may result in more or less consequential fibrosis (Freid and Goldberg[63]; Bate and Guttman[8]). In clinical practice this may occur in instances in which irradiation of the lung is an unavoidable risk, but it may also result from incidental irradiation of the lung which could be avoided or minimized. It is not often understood that the immediate consequence of the irradiation of the lung is a *pneumonitis* and that the resulting fibrosis of substitution is greatly dependent on the adequacy and promptness of the medical attention given to the patient subject to this factitial pneumonitis (Warren and Gates[226]) (Fig. 44).

Engelstad[57] reproduced the pulmonary effects of radiations experimentally and noted hyperemia, hypersecretion of mucus, leukocyte infiltration and later degeneration of bronchial epithelium, marked signs of inflammation, and progressive sclerosis. Stetson and Boland[210] irradiated the lungs of dogs under circumstances of dose and fractionation similar to those of clinical delivery. There was correlation between the radiographic and the pathologic findings and, except for those excessively irradiated, there was good recovery. Bennett et al.[9] studied the lungs of patients irradiated for bronchial carcinoma. They found that acute radiation pneumonitis has no single pathognomonic morphologic feature and consists of a combination of alveolar septal thickening, proliferation and desquamation of atypical septal cells, hyaline membrane formation, and pulmonary vascular changes. They believe that the observed alveolar septal changes and foam cell plaques may be considered as highly suspicious of radiation effects. By contrast, Stetson and Boland,[210] working with noncancerous lungs, found no hyaline membrane formation and only slight damage of the larger arteries, in spite of the rather large doses of radiations administered.

The occurrence of pneumonitis should be anticipated in patients undergoing irradiation of the lung and the patients given adequate medical attention before the radiographic opacity, malaise, chills, cough, or fever appears. The best approach is bed rest, administration of antibiotics, and supportive measures. Such attention shortens the duration of the pneumonitis and the resulting fibrosis of substitution.

Effects of irradiation of vascular system

The frequent irradiation of the *myocardium* in clinical radiotherapy has stim-

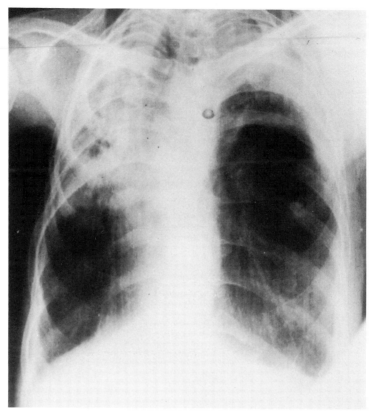

Fig. 44. Resulting pulmonary fibrosis of right upper lobe of lung with retractions of trachea toward right in patient given postoperative roentgentherapy directed to axilla. (PCH 57-566.)

ulated careful study of possible injury to it (Hartman et al.[76]), but the organ has great tolerance (Warthin and Pohle[227]). Whitfield and Kunkler[228] reported transitory asymptomatic changes in the electrocardiograms of irradiated patients. Vaeth et al.[222] studied twenty patients and found no clinical or electrocardiographic changes. Serum glutamic oxalacetic transaminase determinations were also negative. Fajardo et al.[60] studied the morphologic changes induced by clinical irradiation of the heart and found fibrosis to be the hallmark of late effects, with diffuse myocardial fibrosis commonly present but often missed. Experimentally produced changes of the heart were qualitatively identical.

The irradiation of *small vessels* may result in vasodilatation, increased diapedesis, and exudation. Damage to blood vessels has frequently been attributed to changes in the endothelium. Some think that endothelial proliferation is the cause of obliteration of capillaries and even of large veins and arteries, whereas others have found the endothelial cells of large vessels rather radioresistant (Efskind[55]).

It appears that most investigators have exaggerated the importance of vascular findings and have considered them as primary causes of further damage rather than as secondary effects. Rhoades[185] pointed out that the alterations observed in blood vessels of irradiated animals may be secondary to the inflammation in the surrounding connective tissue and that the endothelial swelling observed morphologically might be only an illusion created by the loss of collagen and muscle of the vessels.

Effects of irradiation of eye

In clinical radiotherapy, irradiation of the eye often results in conjunctivitis that is usually mild if uncomplicated. The *cor-*

nea is definitely less sensitive than the conjunctiva and may show no effect, but transient dullness, permanent opacity, and ulceration may occur, depending on the intensity of the irradiation. Thinning of the epithelium, vacuolization of the cytoplasm and degeneration of the nuclei in the cornea follow intense irradiation. Blodi[16] reported that the epithelial damage heals rapidly and that the late effects manifested themselves by a thinning of the corneal fibers, edema, loss of metachromasia, and necrosis. Interstitial keratitis has also been observed clinically and experimentally following intense irradiation. The great regenerative ability of the cornea has also been noted (Poppe[155]). The *iris* has been found to be even less radiosensitive than the cornea.

The *lens* is affected by radiations; indiscriminate irradiation of the orbit and eye may result in cataract and progressive blindness after a period of latency. The use of radium in the treatment of hemangiomas in infants often causes visual impairment and cataracts. However, judicious irradiation of parts of the orbit and of the eye itself may be carried out with proper precautions, avoiding the production of cataracts (Regato[168]). Merriam and Focht[129] did a careful retrospective physical study of doses administered in 100 patients with radiation cataracts and in seventy-three others who were irradiated without resulting cataracts. They found a 50% incidence of progressive loss of vision with doses of 750 R to 1000 R delivered in three weeks to three months. They estimated that 80% of the cataracts could have been avoided by adequate techniques. Histologically, the effects are a complete inhibition of mitoses and eventual cell damage in the germinative epithelial cell (von Sallmann et al.[197]). Nearly all of these must be destroyed before cataract develops. It is possible that partial protection of the lens helps considerably in the recovery (Pirie and Flanders[150]).

Cataracts have been observed in atomic workers exposed to neutrons. The dose necessary to produce damage is apparently less than with roentgen rays, and the latent period is apparently shorter (Krause and Bond[100]). Irradiation cataracts may be successfully operated upon (Reese[167]).

Effects of irradiation of other organs and structures

The *central* and *peripheral nervous systems* have long been considered to be radioresistant. However, heavy irradiation of the spines of monkeys has been shown to result in degeneration of nerve cells and in paralysis (Davidoff et al.[51]). Newborn rats exhibit a greater radiosensitivity of the brain the earlier after birth they are exposed to irradiation. Radiation effects are most commonly found in the subcortical white matter, basal ganglia, cerebellum, hypothalamus, and medulla (Clemente et al.[36]). Using highly penetrating radiations, Arnold et al.[3] studied the effects on the brains of monkeys and concluded that they are not secondary to vascular effects. They consist of a demyelinating process that progressed to actual necrosis of the constituents of the white matter: myelin, glial cells, and axons. Using *tantalum[182]* wire for spotted irradiation of the brain of monkeys, the lesions observed were distributed far more widely than the vascular changes (Bering et al.[12]).

Lampe[111] reported his observation of seven patients who survived seven to fifteen years following intensive radiotherapy for medulloblastoma of the cerebellum. Four of the patients developed epileptic seizures, convulsions, progressive mental deterioration, and, in two, visual impairment. Cases of delayed necrosis of the brain have been reported (Crompton and Layton[46]). Boden[19] observed ten patients with cervical myelitis resulting from irradiation for tumors of the brain stem. Lhermitte's sign of electrical paresthesia may be observed (Jones[91]); paresthesia of the upper and lower extremities may be transient. These symptoms are sometimes followed by muscle weakness, paralysis, and bladder and bowel dysfunction. The severity of the injury is directly related to the intensity of the irradiation.

In 166 patients who survived over sixteen months following irradiation of the spinal cord, Vaeth[221] found three who developed myelitis. He concluded that a single factor, extension of the length of the entire treatment, may be utilized to prevent these untoward effects. Phillips and Buschke[148] related the occurrence of myelitis of the dorsal spine to the intensity of the daily dose administered. In a study reported by Maier et al.,[121a] fifteen of 343 patients surviving three years after radiotherapy developed myelitis of the dorsolumbar cord. Reagan et al.[164] reported ten patients with chronic progressive radiation myelitis following irradiation for cancer of the upper air passages. Four of the patients presented a Brown-Sequard syndrome and six an incomplete transverse myelitis.

Using special staining techniques, Bozzetti and Janovski[21] observed lipid and mucoid degeneration of irradiated pelvic *ganglia*.

Changes observed in irradiated *thyroid glands* suggest that they are due to over-stimulation and exhaustion rather than to the direct effect of radiations: bizarre epithelial cells, suggestion of Hashimoto's disease, follicular atrophy, and widespread fibrosis. Similarly, irradiation of the *suprarenal* glands has no appreciable morphologic effects short of the necrosis produced by massive doses. A lessening of the rise of blood corticosterone level after stimulation by ACTH has been reported as resulting from irradiation of the adrenal glands in rats (Griffith et al.[70]).

Irradiation of *muscles*, smooth as well as striated, does not cause appreciable changes unless the dose is excessive. Under such conditions, the muscle cells may show peculiar or multiple nuclei which may be mistaken for tumor. The effects of radiations on the *connective tissue* everywhere in the body are little known although most significant. There may be alterations of the fibroblasts with edema and hyalinization of the collagen and elastic fibers. These inflammatory effects may be replaced by fibrosis with consequent atresia of the vessels and devitalization of tissues. The final changes depend, of course, on a variety of factors.

Genetic effects of irradiation

Muller[135] demonstrated that irradiation could increase the natural rate of mutations observed in the fruit fly. Stadler,[208] working with barley, demonstrated independently the genetic effect of radiations. Nonsterilizing doses of radiations on the gonads may not cause any deleterious effect on the health of the irradiated individual but may cause important changes in the chromosomes of the spermatozoa or ova, resulting in various types of disability in subsequent generations.

The genetic effects of radiations have been well substantiated in lower animals. Radiation-induced chromosomal anomalies have been observed on euploid human cells in vitro (Puck[159]). Most mutations can be expected to result in an *increase* in the types of abnormalities already occurring in the human population rather than in conspicuous *new* ones. Tangible defects such as malformations, muscular dystrophies, blindness, deafness, hemophilia, epilepsy, etc. occur annually in about 4% of all births in the United States, and half of these defects are estimated to have a genetic origin. In addition, however, gene alterations, once produced, would be transmitted to subsequent generations and would be the cause of "shortened life." They may be eliminated through reverse mutations, which are rare, or through death or failure to reproduce.

The evaluation of genetic effects in man is fraught with uncertainties due to the paucity of data and to the difficult evaluation of what constitutes unequivocal damage. Based on the experimental data obtained in lower animals, it has been concluded that gene mutations in man are *arithmetically* (linearly) proportionate to the dose received by the gonads and *independent of the intensity* or rate of accumulation of the dose received during a lifetime. Thus doubling of the dose received from any source should double the number of mutations. These facts are not completely agreed upon (Russell et al.[194]). *Dose rate* rather than *total dose* may be the most important single factor. An effective threshold dose rate may exist for each biologic species. Whereas a single point mutation may be independent of dose rate, the repair mechanisms may be, on the contrary, very sensitive to dose rate. Unfortunately, world public opinion has been exposed to a great deal of inferences, unwarranted extrapolations, and opinions as to the genetic effects of radiations.

Studies done on the progeny of radiologists (Crow[47]), of radiologic technicians (Tanaka and Ohkura[216]), and on the survivors of the atomic bombardments of Hiroshima and Nagasaki (Neel and

Schull[138]) have failed to demonstrate conclusively any increase in congenital malformations. Kaplan[96] followed and reported on 644 women (18 to 42 years of age) whose ovaries were irradiated to produce transient amenorrhea as treatment for sterility: 351 of these women subsequently conceived a total of 688 times and delivered 566 children (282 boys and 284 girls). Twenty of these children were born dead or died soon afterward. Three had hydrocephalus, one was mentally retarded, one had missing fingers, and one had an extra finger. There were 123 miscarriages among ninety-one women, sixty-eight of whom later safely conceived. At the time of Kaplan's report, there were forty-five grandchildren in the series (twenty-five boys and twenty girls). There was no cancer or leukemia among the children or grandchildren. A reduction in the normal proportion of boys would be expected from sex-linked dominant lethals. Neither the sex ratio (Schull and Neel[202]) nor the occurrence of abnormalities showed a *statistically significant* deviation from the general population, even though all of these women were treated for sterility, in itself a possible genetic abnormality.

Theoretically, there is no "threshold dose" or "permissible dose." The "weighted gonadal dose" received by an individual between conception and 30 years of age in the United States has been estimated to be between 1.5 R and 4.5 R. It is estimated that 60% of this amount is due to natural background radiation (cosmic rays, natural radioactivity, etc.), 27% from radiodiagnostic procedures, 10% from radiotherapeutic procedures and use of radioactive isotopes, 2% from fallout of atomic explosions, and 1% from industrial sources. Geographical differences may be notable. Life in certain areas of India would make the foregoing total gonadal dose ten times greater (Schull[201]).

The extent of fallout radiation will depend on the number of open atomic explosions that may take place in the world atmosphere. A good possibility of important reduction lies in the utilization of perfected radiologic equipment and techniques and discrimination in the use of radiodiagnostic and radiotherapeutic procedures, particularly in children and young individuals. A dispassionate appraisal of this world problem should take into consideration the widespread use of numerous and varied potential mutagenic substances in industry as well as in medicine. In fact, medical progress of many sorts has greatly contributed to keeping alive innumerable individuals with inherited abnormalities who would have been naturally eliminated in yesteryears but who now are capable of transmitting their conspicuous or inconspicuous hereditary abnormalities to their descendants.

Injurious effects of irradiation

In the practice of clinical radiotherapy, injurious effects to organs or structures may result from the treatments or as a consequence of poor planning or neglect. The physician is morally, if not legally, bound to explain the hazards to the patient before treatment and, of course, to conduct the treatment in such a manner as to minimize or avoid injury.

Among all sequelae of radiotherapy, those that show to greatest disadvantage are produced by treatment of benign conditions. Extensive facial changes produced by epilating applications, plantar necrosis following treatment of warts, asymmetrical development of bone following irradiation for hemangioma, etc. are errors of judgment that cannot be justified in most instances. On the other hand, necrosis of the skin and of bone or fibrosis of the lung in patients treated for cancer can well be excused as calculated hazards in view of the gravity of the alternative. In any instance, however, the radiologist should keep his patient informed of the hazards and should obtain a written permit in order to protect his reputation and interests. Irradiation in children may bring about unavoidable interference with the bone development (Rubin et al.[192]; Vaeth et al.[223]). Such potential impairment of growth must be made clear to the parents and acknowledged by them, in writing, before treatments are instituted. Acute injuries are often the result of infection (Miller et al.[130]). Dressing care of radiation reactions should be available and should be provided to all patients. This will reduce complications and will eliminate any impression of negligence. Radiologists should familiarize themselves with the liabilities incurred.

Carcinogenic effects of irradiation

Before the discovery of radiations by man, lung tumors were being induced in *uranium miners* by inhaled radioactive dust. This fact is now well documented. The discovery and early utilization of radiations in diagnosis and treatment promptly brought about obvious manifestations of their carcinogenic powers. Repeated exposures of *physicists* and *radiologists* resulted in carcinomas of the skin of the hands and face. Conservative treatment, often followed by recurrence and metastases, took a heavy toll of the heroic pioneers of radiology.[55a] The industrial uses of radioactive materials also brought forth new hazards. The most notable among these was that of bone tumors developed by *clock dial painters* as a result of the ingestion of small amounts of radioactive materials (Martland[126]). The use of *Thoro-*

trast in diagnostic radiology has resulted in cancer of the liver (McMahon et al.[120]; Baserga et al.[7]).

Carcinomas and sarcomas of the *skin* have been observed following repeated diagnostic exposures, repeated irradiations often for benign conditions, or intensive irradiation for deep-seated tumors. In all of these instances, there is use of low-quality radiations, high total doses, high intensity of exposure, or a combination of these factors. A lapse of several years is necessary before the malignant manifestation. Most carcinomas of the skin that occur as a consequence of intensive irradiation are squamous cell carcinomas presenting similarities to those arising after thermal burns. We have observed a few unequivocal cases of multicentric basal cell carcinomas of the skin of the trunk many years after moderate irradiation (Fig. 45).

Some carcinomas of the *oral cavity, pharynx, larynx, esophagus,* and *large intestine* have been attributed to previous

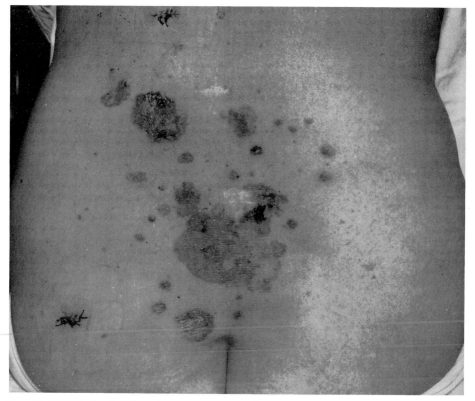

Fig. 45. Multiple basal cell carcinomas arising on skin thirty years after irradiation for ovarian tumor. Similar but fewer lesions were present on front field. (PCH 61-699.)

irradiation. Long follow-up of patients cured of carcinoma of the cervix has revealed rare instances of carcinomas of the *rectum, bladder, ovaries,* and pelvic soft tissues that could be related to radiations (Fernandez-Colmeiro and Chardier[61]). *Soft tissue* sarcomas have been observed in connection with short intensive irradiation to relatively high dose levels. Cases of fibromatosis and fibrosarcoma have been reported (Pettit et al.[146a]). The therapeutic irradiation of *bone,* particularly in children (Cohen and D'Angio[36a]), has resulted in instances of osteosarcoma (Cahan et al.[30]; Castro et al.[33]; Soloway[207]; Sagerman et al.[196]). Cases of chondrosarcoma have also been observed (Perez et al.[145a]). Most of the foregoing instances of cancer of different irradiated tissues suggest direct carcinogenic effect, either chromosomal or cytoplasmic (Kaplan[95]).

There is some evidence that *leukemia* occurs with greater frequency among radiologists than among other physicians (March[122]). A study, in England, of numerous patients given radiotherapy to the spine for ankylosing spondylitis revealed a vastly increased incidence of leukemia (Court-Brown and Doll[41]). Follow-up examination (1946-1964) of the survivors of the atomic bombings of Hiroshima and Nagasaki has revealed a disproportionately higher occurrence of chronic granulocytic leukemia in persons under 29 years of age at the time of exposure and within 1500 meters of the hypocenter (Bizzozero et al.[15]), as compared with the spontaneous occurrence for this age group elsewhere in Japan. Age at the time of the exposure is a covariable to distance. The rate among those 10 to 19 years of age is eighteen times higher and among those under 10 years it is twenty-six times higher than the rate for those not exposed (Miller[131]). The exposure to radiations seems to have increased the incidence of leukemia rather than to have caused it to occur earlier. Studies of children exposed to diagnostic radiations in utero have shown no greater propensity to leukemia than those not exposed (Court-Brown et al.[42]). The data on the survivors of Hiroshima and Nagasaki are not conclusive in reference to any increase in the occurrence of malignant tumors.

For many years, great numbers of new-born infants were routinely irradiated for what was clinically diagnosed as an enlarged thymus. Evidence has been produced that, in some series, a greater-than-expected proportion of *thyroid* and other tumors has subsequently developed (Simpson and Hempelmann[204]; Snegireff[206]). It is possible that the discrepancies observed among these studies are related to differences in age of the children, the size of the field used (Latourette and Hodges[112]), the intensity of the irradiation, and the total dose administered. In a follow-up study of 2878 individuals, Hempelmann et al.[79] reported nineteen carcinomas and twenty-two adenomas of the thyroid gland, whereas the 5006 untreated siblings yielded no carcinomas and only three adenomas. There were, in addition, six cases of leukemia, four salivary gland tumors, one brain tumor, no case of Hodgkin's disease, and fifteen osteochondromas among those irradiated as compared with two, one, two, one, and three, respectively, in their siblings. Another follow-up study of 958 persons irradiated as infants for the same purposes yielded eight thyroid tumors and five osteochondromas, but the total number of malignant tumors was not significantly increased (Pifer et al.[149]).

There is abundant experimental evidence to prove the carcinogenic and leukemogenic effects of local or total body irradiation (Brues[26]). Except for the examples just cited, the human data are far from conclusive. There are suggestions that radiations may, in some instances, act as an indirect agent (Gardner[65]; Kaplan[95]) which, unlike other carcinogens, does require a latent period. Many more facts are required before these theories may eliminate each other (Lamerton[109]). Whether or not there is a human threshold and whether or not hazards can be eliminated or only diminished are problems yet to be solved. It may also have to be acquiesced that man submits of his own free will to considerably greater hazards (Jones[92]).

Radiophysiology of malignant tumors

The irradiation of malignant neoplastic tissue may result in the almost immediate disappearance of all cells in mitosis and, after a short period of time, in an abnormally large number of *degenerative mitoses* followed by death of the cells from accelerated maturation. Whenever this phenomenon can be brought about repeatedly by new irradiations, complete destruction of the tumor can be expected. In a large number of malignant tumors, however, intensive irradiations may not give rise to such a response, and the tumors may continue to grow in spite of irradiations. *This difference in response to irradiation, the different radiosensitivities of malignant tumors, is primarily an attribute of their cell of origin.*

Individual cells within a tumor may present a widely different susceptibility to irradiations. In tumors composed predominantly of radiovulnerable cells (lymphosarcoma, myeloma), the administration of a small dose of radiations results in immediate destruction of a great proportion of these cells and in grossly evident reduction in the size of the tumor, although a recurrence of growth may rapidly follow.

In tumors composed of a variety of cells in different stages of differentiation (epidermoid carcinoma), even a large dose of radiations may not affect the most differentiated cells (horny layer). There may be no grossly ostensible effect for days or even weeks, yet the destruction of the germinal cells eventually results in complete disappearance of the tumor (Fig. 46). In tumors composed mostly of cells that are not radiolabile (osteosarcoma) the most intense irradiation may not produce any immediate or delayed effect.

The foregoing examples illustrate the following:

1 That the *radiosensitivity* of a tumor depends primarily on the radiosensitivity of the cell of origin
2 That the gross reduction in the size of a tumor depends on the proportion of cells that are immediately affected by the irradiation
3 That the lack of immediate ostensible

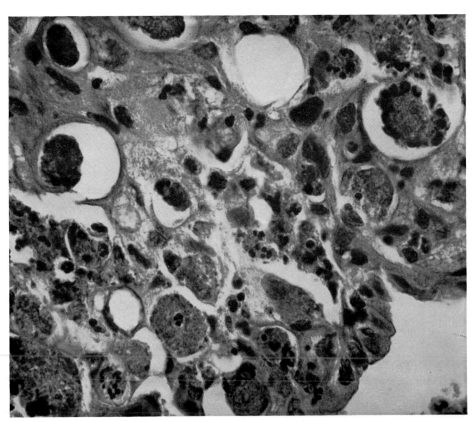

Fig. 46. Marked irradiation effects on epidermoid carcinoma of cervix showing gross aberration of nuclei and cytoplasm.

response does not necessarily indicate radioresistance

4 That radiosensitivity is not synonymous with radiocurability, although the radiocurability of a tumor depends, above all, on its radiosensitivity

Final results in the treatment of radiocurable tumors are considerably more dependent on the feasibility of distributing the necessary dose over the affected area and on skillful handling than on the morphologic variations. A misunderstanding of the radiophysiology of tumors has resulted in a veritable semantic confusion in respect to radiosensitivity. The number of mitotic figures or the proportion of undifferentiated cells may be indicative of the immediate response of a *radiosensitive malignant tumor,* but anaplasia and reproductive activity are not *a priori* signs of radiosensitivity in any or all malignant tumors. A marked degree of differentiation in an epidermoid carcinoma may imply a lesser degree of radiosensitivity, but no epidermoid carcinoma deserves the qualification of *radioresistant.* The qualification is still less fitting to a basal cell carcinoma simply because it may fail to disappear as rapidly as others. The long-standing assumption that *adenocarcinomas* were radioresistant has been widely disproved by the high radiocurability of endometrial adenocarcinomas and others. *Soft tissue* sarcomas and even *malignant melanomas* may show surprising radiosensitivity.

The preliminary condition of radiocurability is radiosensitivity. Radioresistant or faintly radiosensitive malignant tumors are not radiocurable, since their destruction by means of radiations requires a dose so intense that it produces a diffuse cytocaustic effect that implies necrosis of surrounding structures. A relatively small dose of radiations may result in a rapidly noticeable effect in a lymphosarcoma of the tonsil, whereas it may not appreciably affect an epidermoid carcinoma in the same area. Yet, all other conditions being equal, *the total dose required for the sterilization of either tumor does not differ greatly.* Moreover, one type of tumor may be cured by the administration of rather different amounts of radiations, depending on several variable factors, including the period of time over which the treatment is given.

Thus the total dose necessary to sterilize different tumors is certainly not an index of their radiosensitivity.

The establishment of a scale of the radiosensitivity of malignant tumors is the result of clinical observation. In order of decreasing radiosensitivity, we find:

1 Malignant tumors arising from hemopoietic organs (lymphosarcoma, myeloma)
2 Hodgkin's disease
3 Lymphoepitheliomas of the upper air passages
4 Seminomas and dysgerminomas
5 Ewing's sarcoma of the bone
6 Basal cell carcinomas of the skin
7 Epidermoid carcinomas arising by metaplasia from columnar epithelium
8 Epidermoid carcinomas of the mucous membranes, mucocutaneous junctions, and skin
9 Adenocarcinomas of the endometrium, breast, gastrointestinal system, and endocrine glands
10 Soft tissue sarcomas
11 Chondrosarcomas
12 Neurogenic sarcomas
13 Osteosarcomas
14 Malignant melanomas

Some of the latter tumors are truly radioresistant and probably should not be mentioned, but a small proportion of them may present unexpected radiosensitivity (fibrosarcoma and melanoma). One variety of liposarcoma is definitely radiosensitive and is even radiocurable, which is in complete disagreement with the general concept that the radiosensitivity of malignant tumors depends upon the radiosensitivity of their cell of origin. The preceding list is only a scale of average radiosensitivity in each group. Individual tumors may show radiosensitivity in advance of, or following, their place in this rough outline. Rare tumors of varied radiosensitivity are purposely omitted.

It has been demonstrated that interference with the blood supply of a radiosensitive tissue diminishes its radiosensitivity (Jolly[90]). It may be concluded that poor vascular supply is a factor that may conceivably interfere with the radiosensitivity of a tumor. Insufficiently or inadequately irradiated tumors become less responsive to a second series of treatments.

This has been attributed to *radioimmunization* of the tumor cells (Regaud[179]). But whether the radiosensitivity of the tumor cells is actually altered or not, inadequate blood supply (resulting from edema, atrophy, previous surgical interventions, secondary infection, previous burns, previous irradiation) definitely lessens the radiocurability of an otherwise amenable tumor. In reality, this is due to diminished resistance of surrounding tissues that become incapable of tolerating the amount of radiations necessary for the sterilization of the tumor.

The total sterilization of a tumor requires a minimum total dose of radiations capable of destroying all "germinal" cells within a tumor and consequently of discontinuing reproductivity of malignant cells. Radiocurable tumors are those in which the administration of such minimum dose is compatible with sufficient recovery of surrounding normal tissues to assure a *restitutio ad integrum*. This margin between the destruction of the tumor and the untoward effects on neighboring normal tissues decreases as the tumor becomes less radiosensitive. It becomes a negative quantity in nonradiocurable tumors, for the quantity of radiations necessary for the tumor destruction is incompatible with the life of surrounding tissues and implies irreparable injury or death.

If the required amount of radiations is delivered in a single treatment, the margin of safety is very narrow. Regaud[178, 182] established the experimental evidence that it is impossible to sterilize the very radiosensitive tissues of the seminiferous tubules of the testes by the administration of a single large dose of radiations even when the dose is sufficient to produce irremediable damage to the surrounding structures. Conversely, it is very easy to sterilize permanently the testicle of the same animal by the administration of a smaller total dose fractionated and administered at equal intervals. Regaud[178] insisted upon the biologic similarity between permanently growing tissue of the seminiferous tubules and malignant neoplasms. His experiment gave the *coup de grâce* to the then predominant method of single massive doses and effected a turning point in the history of radiotherapy (Regato[176]). Regaud concluded, however, that a protraction beyond twelve days constituted a definite error capable of producing radioimmunization of the tumor.

Coutard[44] noted the possibility and advisability of protraction to several weeks in the treatment of epidermoid carcinomas of the upper air passages and established the basis of the *protracted-fractional method* of treatment, now almost universally accepted. But while the elongation of the treatment does increase the margin of safety, it also enhances the necessity for strict clinical control of the patients. When treatments are administered at a continuous equal daily rate, the *daily dose* is of no apparent consequence when the *total dose* is expressed in the total time of delivery. But when the treatments are discontinued, the relative importance of the daily dose is emphasized. Coutard[45a] experimented with discontinuous intensive irradiations over a period of six weeks on the working hypothesis that epidermoid carcinomas exhibited heights of radiosensitivity at periodic intervals. This approach has been retried in recent years without these basic assumptions or principles (Scanlon[199]; Sambrook[198]; Holsti[83]; Marcial and Frias[123]).

Indications for radiotherapy in treatment of cancer

Radiotherapy has definite primary indications in the treatment of cancer in preference to, or to the exclusion of, other forms of therapy. *Curative radiotherapy* as applied to cancer is a formidable procedure charged with definite risks. It is an all-or-none undertaking which well deserves being called *radical radiotherapy* at par in seriousness with the drastic performances of surgery (Buschke[27]) but differing in results by its conservative character.

The choice of patients with localized lesions to be submitted to radiotherapy requires serious appraisal of the radiosensitivity of the tumor in question, of the material possibility of distributing throughout the tumor area the minimum total amount of radiations capable of sterilizing the tumor, and of the existence of a *margin of safety* assuring the continued viability of the surrounding tissues and serious estimation of whether other forms of treatment offer the same or a better result more expeditiously or with less risk (Moss and Brand[133]).

In *highly radiosensitive tumors* such as lymphosarcoma, lymphoepithelioma, and transitional cell carcinoma of the upper air passages, in seminoma, and in localized myeloma, the opportune and adequate administration of radiations is the undisputed form of curative treatment.

In the *moderately radiosensitive tumors* such as carcinomas of the skin and epidermoid carcinomas of the mucous membranes and mucocutaneous junctions, radiotherapy may be most effective, but the choice of treatment should take into consideration other concomitant circumstances besides favorable radiosensitivity. A small basal cell carcinoma of the skin may promptly and effectively be treated by wide excision. Epidermoid carcinoma arising on a burn scar cannot be given a sufficient amount of radiations without danger of necrosis of the atrophic tissues of the burned area, so that a wide excision and skin graft are often more effective. Surgical excision of an otherwise radiocurable carcinoma of the lower lip facilitates immediate surgical removal of metastases. Epidermoid carcinoma that invades bone does not become radioresistant or even less radiosensitive. In fact, epidermoid carcinomas of the maxillary antrum are curable by roentgentherapy in spite of extensive bone invasion and destruction (Regato[168]). But the invasion of bone diminishes the *margin of safety* between destruction of the tumor and damage to the surrounding tissues, particularly since invasion carries the implication of secondary infection. Since in these cases the sterilization of the tumor by means of radiations may imply long and painful elimination of sequestra, surgical removal of the diseased structures when possible may be less mutilating and more easily tolerated.

Lymph node metastases from squamous cell carcinomas of the oral cavity, pharynx, cervix, etc. are no less radiosensitive than their primary lesion. Evidence of sterilization of lymph node metastases by roentgentherapy and curietherapy has been long available. However, as a matter of practical approach, a lymph node dissection may be the treatment of choice of metastatic lymph nodes, particularly in the neck.

Another group of moderately radiosensitive tumors, the adenocarcinomas, may or may not be radiocurable, depending on the site of origin. Adenocarcinoma of the cervix is as easily sterilized by radiations as epidermoid carcinoma in the same area. Adenocarcinoma of the endometrium can be cured by radiotherapy alone, but it is generally admitted that hysterectomy should follow irradiation whenever possible to assure a greater chance of permanent control. Adenocarcinoma of the breast can sometimes be controlled by radiations but always at the expense of extensive damage to the neighboring tissues; radiotherapy is not justified unless the lesion is inoperable. Adenocarcinomas of the gastrointestinal tract may present variable degrees of radiosensitivity. They are more logically treated by radical surgery, which assures simultaneous treatment of the primary lesion and of the potential, often extensive, metastatic area. Adenocarcinomas of endocrine glands may be radiocurable, and occasional long remissions are effected by the use of radiations.

Poorly radiosensitive or *radioresistant tumors,* such as the soft tissue sarcomas, sarcomas of bone, and malignant melanomas, are rarely radiocurable. Unexpected palliation and occasional sterilization may be obtained in the irradiation of tumors conventionally considered to be radioresistant (Guttmann[73]; Flatman[62]; Buschke[27]).

In addition to the indications of radiotherapy as a curative form of treatment, there are definite indications of *palliative radiotherapy* in advanced or incurable forms of cancer. To conclude that a given tumor is inoperable, however, is not to imply automatically that radiotherapy is indicated, nor are advanced lesions necessarily benefited by radiation therapy. Those who appear most incredulous at the possibilities of curative radiotherapy often demand from it true miracles when other forms of treatment appear impotent or have failed. A great deal of discredit has fallen upon radiotherapy by its systematic association with the hopeless. The use of radiations for psychotherapy results in an adverse psychologic effect deterring other patients who could benefit by, but may refuse, radiotherapy (Lampe[110]).

Palliative radiotherapy may require serious advanced planning. An incomplete treatment or a few sporadic irradiations do not necessarily give relief (Paterson[144]). A variety of incurable conditions, recurrences or metastases of otherwise radiocurable tumors, and recurrences or metastases of tumors that are tributaries of surgery may justify the use of radiotherapy as a palliative measure. In Hodgkin's disease and leukemia adequate radiotherapy results in unquestionable comfort and lengthening of life. In other instances, radiotherapy is applied locally to avert ulceration of a recurrent tumor and to avoid secondary infection or hemorrhage. Radiotherapy of metastatic lesions of the bone, particularly of the head of the femur and of the vertebrae, may avert fractures or paraplegias and may contribute a transitory but definite analgesic effect. Apart from these and a few other instances, radiotherapy is not justified in the patient whose condition is simply hopeless (Parker[143]).

Preoperative and postoperative irradiation

The qualities that characterize the effectiveness of surgery and radiotherapy in the treatment of cancer can seldom be combined to produce an advantageous complementary effect. *"Once inoperable, always inoperable"* is a fairly current dogma among cancer surgeons that seems justified by the majority of facts. In some particular instances, however, such as in the treatment of adenocarcinoma of the endometrium, the administration of preoperative radiotherapy brings about unquestionable improvement of the final results of surgery. In borderline inoperable lesions of the breast and gastrointestinal tract, the administration of radiations results in diminution of secondary infection and inflammation and in a reduction of the size of the tumor that may thus become technically operable.

A true trial of preoperative radiotherapy of *operable* carcinomas of the breast and of the rectum may prove effective in improving results. A randomized experiment would be desirable. Buschke and Galante[29] treated inoperable advanced carcinomas of the oral cavity with supervoltage roentgentherapy and submitted them to subsequent radical surgery with encouraging results. A similar association of successful irradiation with cobalt[60] followed by surgical excision of cervical metastases was reported by Romieu et al.[189]

A controlled experiment in which patients received a "low dose" irradiation preceding neck dissection for metastatic carcinoma resulted in unquestionable reduction in the proportion of recurrences as compared with the nonirradiated controls. The proportion of recurrences on the other side of the neck was the same in both groups (Henschke et al.[80]). Based on their experience with cancer of the upper air passages, breast, and bladder, Nickson and Glicksman[139] advocate "full dose" preoperative radiotherapy followed by radical surgery. In special instances, they would advocate "moderate dose" irradiation immediately followed by surgery. Dutreix et al.[54] experimented with a preoperative plan consisting of a short intensive application of two days, an interval of three weeks, a fractionated course of three weeks, followed by surgery after a few days. The technique seems appropriate especially in advanced cases. Controlled trials of preoperative irradiation in bronchial carcinoma have not confirmed the initial enthusiasm. In general, however, the experimental evidence seems to show that preoperative radiotherapy is the best available surgical adjuvant.

Following surgical intervention, it may be that microscopic fragments of tumor have been left in the operative area or in the region of possible metastases. The *postoperative* administration of an amount of radiations sufficient to sterilize the tumor is seldom possible over such wide areas, and anything short of this dosage is a futile attempt to remedy the irremediable. In some instances of incomplete removal, the cooperation of the surgeon and the pathologist may sufficiently delineate the area of localized residual to make postoperative radiotherapy a worthwhile attempt, if not necessarily a successful one. Careful biopsies of the suspected area and minute examination of surgical specimens are a considerable help. In addition, the surgeon may place metal clips, recognizable in the roentgenograms, in the periphery of the suspected area of involvement. These procedures may facilitate the administration of radiotherapy at the necessary high doses over a restricted area. Too frequently radiotherapy is called upon to follow an operation in which "most" of the tumor has been removed. Those who naïvely cooperate in such travesty gain only the blame for the inevitable failure of such augmentation, and they also contribute to the discredit of radiotherapy.

Technical aspects of radiotherapy of cancer

Roentgentherapy

In the treatment of superficial lesions, the distribution of the necessary dose throughout the tumor offers little difficulty. In order to avoid undesirable penetration of deep tissues, *low voltage*, a *short target-skin distance*, and *no filter* or *weak filtration* are generally employed. In this manner, the differential between the dose absorbed in the surface and that absorbed at any depth is greatly increased. Such treatments are generally of *short duration*. But if the lesion spreads over a large area, or if it invades in depth, or if it is near the eye, cartilaginous areas, or bony surfaces, then it is better to increase the quality of the beam and the margin of safety by increasing the kilovoltage and filtration and further protracting the time of therapy. The principle of practical reproduction of the collimated beam of radiations by a beam of light has now been adopted for cobalt and megavoltage units (Fig. 47).

The qualitative composition of a beam of rays, the relative proportion of radiations of shorter or longer wavelength, is obviously of importance in the appreciation of its physical possibilities. To obtain this information, spectroscopic analysis or other complicated studies are necessary. For practical purposes, the quality of a beam may be appreciated by a study of the absorption curve when it passes through increasing thicknesses of a given material. Since what is generally required is an idea of the penetrating ability of the beam, it has been agreed that this is simply expressed in a figure by the *half-value-layer*— the thickness of material that reduces the incident dose in half. The half-value-layer is usually expressed in millimeter thicknesses of aluminum or copper. It must be remembered, however, that in working

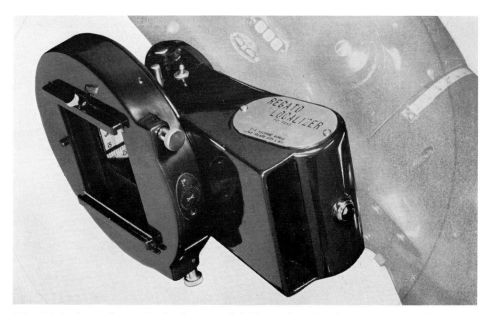

Fig. 47. Lighting device for localization of fields in clinical radiotherapy. Principle of practical reproduction of collimated beam of radiations by beam of light has now been adopted for cobalt and megavoltage units.

with beams of different sources, one may reach an expression of the same half-value-layer for beams of very different qualitative composition.

In the treatment of deep-seated tumors, higher kilovoltage and a *maximum practical target-skin distance* are chosen to assure less diffusion and consequently a larger transmission in depth, and the beam is *heavily filtered*. This results in an improvement of the relative proportion of short-wavelength radiations and in greater ability to penetrate while reducing the proportion of long-wavelength radiations and the undesirable effects of excessive backscatter. The amount and the quality of radiations received by a deep-seated tumor, however, still depend greatly upon the secondary radiations created within the tissues (forwardscatter and backscatter), but an improvement in the *quality* of the incident beam does not result always in an increase of the *quantity* received in depth (Quimby[163]). A problem not yet solved in dosimetry is the appreciation of *quality of radiations absorbed* at different depths in terms of the quality of the incident beam. An improvement in quality results in an increase in the margin of safety, and consequently better quality may be desirable even when at the expense of the quantity. In the irradiation of different areas of the body, the density of the tissues and the quality of radiations used enter into the consideration of energy absorbed.

For several decades, roentgentherapy was limited to levels under 300 kv (*conventional* roentgentherapy), and the radiotherapist was forced to seek a sufficient depth dose by the artifice of cross fire and rotation therapy. The development of *supervoltage* and *megavoltage* roengentherapy has eliminated the previous limitations. Intensive and extensive reactions of the skin are no longer necessary in order to bring to a deeply seated tumor a rather large amount of radiations. Besides greater penetration, the irradiation with these high-voltage beams of radiations results in considerably less backscatter, a reduction of volume dose, and less potential injury or sequelae to the irradiated normal tissues. The advent of high-energy radiations has deceived those who expected that their use would make tumors more radiosensitive and radiotherapy easier to practice.

Multimillion-volt *betatrons* and *linear accelerators* have become part of the armamentarium of special institutions. Provided their use is accompanied by skill and experience, better results may be obtained than with lower voltages. Moreover, these high-energy radiations allow the approach of tumors heretofore incurable by conventional sources of roentgen rays.

Curietherapy

In the treatment of malignant tumors, radium is applied in different fashions that are important to distinguish.

Interstitial curietherapy is the insertion of needles containing radium or other radioactive substances into the tumor. The value of this form of treatment depends on its ability to irradiate the tumor area intensely and yet without considerable effect on the surrounding structures. With some exceptions in which the placement of the sources of radiations can be accurately controlled, interstitial curietherapy often fails to administer a homogeneous irradiation to the tumor area.

Intracavitary curietherapy is the introduction of radium into natural cavities, the best example being in the treatment of carcinoma of the cervix.

Surface curietherapy is the application of radium on a molded apparatus with the purpose of increasing depth dose. In general, the radioactive sources are only 1 cm or 2 cm away from the surface of the tumor.

Finally, *telecurietherapy* is the use of relatively large amounts of radium at a greater distance from the tumor in the treatment of deep-seated malignant neoplasms.

Cobalt[60] teletherapy

The hopes once placed in telecurietherapy have now been revived by artificially radioactivated cobalt. The advantages are the much lower cost, an almost monochromatic beam of radiations, easier protection, and greater possibility of field limitation and of long-range irradiation. Cobalt[60] has the minor disadvantage of a short half-life that forces frequent replacement of the source.

The practical advantages of cobalt[60] tele-

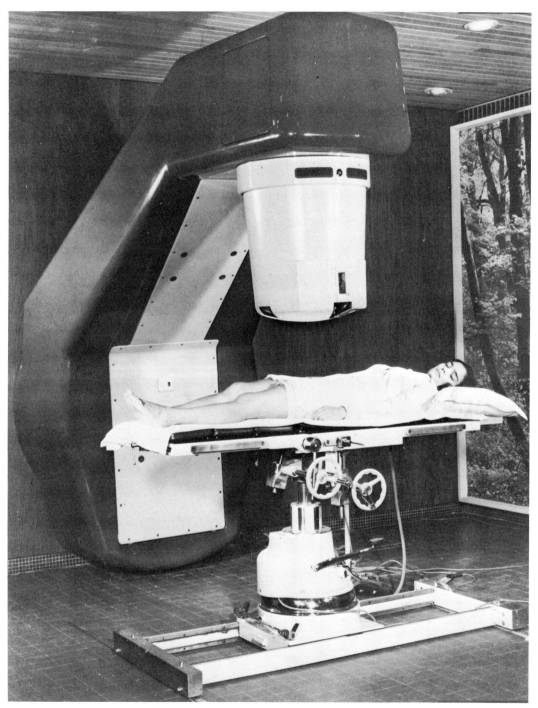

Fig. 48. Sample of 32 million volt (MEV) Linear Accelerator manufactured by Raytheon/Thomson—C. S. F.

therapy have been rapidly absorbed in clinical practice. It is possible by this means to administer larger doses to greater depth with greater impunity. This modality is useful also in the treatment of relatively superficial tumors of the oral cavity, pharynx, and larynx and in the irradiation of radiosensitive but widespread tumors, for there is less systemic effect than with conventional roengentherapy when large fields are used. Cobalt[60] teletherapy has made it possible to cure tumors that were not curable by conventional roentgentherapy, and the curability of some radiocurable tumors has been improved by skilled utilization of cobalt[60] teletherapy. Cesium[137] units have also been developed. Their advantage is primarily the longer half-life and consequent relative economy. Cobalt and cesium are progressively replacing the indications and uses of conventional roentgentherapy.

Dosimetry

The ability of roentgen rays to ionize gases has been utilized for measuring quantity, since the ionization produced is proportional to the quantity absorbed by the gas. An international unit, convenient because of its reproducibility, has been agreed upon: the *roentgen* (R). Ionization chambers or dosimeters that report the amounts of radiations in roentgens are currently used. Because the range of dislodged electrons varies with the voltage, the ionization chambers must be constructed differently for radiations of different quality. Thus the ordinary ionization chamber cannot be used to measure radiations emanating from radium, for instance, in order to express them in roentgens. In expressing doses of radiations in roentgens, it is pertinent to remember that *dose delivered* (measured in air) is not the same as *dose absorbed* (measured in the tissues), that the ionization of air is not equivalent to the ionization of tissues, and that the same amount of radiations absorbed may result in varied effects in different tissues. A biologic unit of dosage is desirable but has never been practical.

The estimation of adequate doses is rather simple in the treatment of superficial lesions, since the optimum amount of radiations accomplishing the required aims is easily found by experience. In the treatment of deep-seated tumors, the estimation of depth dose requires evaluation from depth dose charts and curves of isodose. The appreciation of dose received by a tumor at any depth is at best a rough estimate. It is subject to error in evaluation of the tumor topography, since the actual extension of the tumor may not be known. It is subject to error in appreciation of the depth of the tumor from every point of attack, since human anatomy is variable. It is subject to the errors of the depth dose tables themselves. It is also subject to error in the adaptation of charts based on "average" absorption of living tissues that do not apply to evaluation of depth dose in predominantly bony areas or air-filled organs.

An accurate dosimetry is not possible with the use of radium. The dose expressed in *milligram hours* or *millicuries destroyed* is dose-emitted, whereas the doses actually absorbed vary considerably, depending on the manner of application. Curves of absorption for individual sources and for sets of applicators, with a definite relative arrangement of the sources, have been the subject of a very laudable study by Paterson and Parker.[145] The advent of the *roentgen* as a unit of quantity of radiations has naturally made evident the desirability of expressing radium energy in the same units, but this presents great technical difficulties. A *gamma roentgen* has been defined to which milligram hours can be translated under certain specified circumstances, but the mistake should not be made of adding roentgens and gamma roentgens to express the accurate tumor dose—nothing could be so inaccurate. The present practice is to express depth dose in the form of *absorbed rads* rather than of *administered roentgens*.

The *rad* has been proposed as the unit of absorbed dose (100 ergs/gm). A conversion of roentgens to rads requires that the density of the tissues be known, the conversion factor being different for bone, fat, air, etc. To choose a given average conversion factor, in order to make up for the fact that the treated region may be composed of various tissues, is simply to accept a convenient inaccurate generalization for the sake of intended accuracy.

In other words, such an expression *rads* is often pseudoaccurate.

We do not know, with any degree of accuracy, the optimal dose that should be administered under defined circumstances to assure the sterilization of radiocurable malignant tumors. The expressions *lethal dose* and *cancer dose* have no basis in fact. We have learned through clinical observation that the proportion of tumors of the same variety that are destroyed by radiations increases with the dose. The aim of radiotherapy is to administer as homogeneously as possible throughout the entire potential area of tumor involvement the largest quantity of radiations compatible with the life of irradiated normal tissues. From the point of view of effect on the tumor, it is the minimum dose received at any point of the tumor that is important. From the point of view of untoward effects, it is the maximum dose absorbed at any point that is important (Regato[171]).

Obviously, the expression of the dose at the portals of entry is of no biologic significance. It has become evident that dosage should be expressed at the level of the tumor—hence the expression *tumor dose*. In reality, however, it matters little that most of a tumor may have received a large dose if any part of it has received an insufficient one. It would be better to speak of *minimum tumor dose* (Regato[171]). To calculate the dose at a given point of the anatomy (the midpoint of the nasopharynx or of the pelvis) and to express such dosage as tumor dose is a grotesque misrepresentation. Pragmatic adoption of such expressions as median, average, and modal dose (Sundbom and Asard[213]) cannot be reconciled with the biologic facts. Only the highest dose that has been found safe under the circumstances, delivered as homogeneously as possible throughout the potential tumor area, seems a justifiable goal.

The rate of delivery of any dose plus the length of time in which it was administered are important data for the biologic appraisal of its effects. Ellis[56a] has proposed a theoretical formula which relates total dose, number of fractions, and overall duration of treatments to a quantity named Nominal Standard Dose (NSD). His formula would permit comparison of effects of the different treatment schedules. Obviously, it is meaningless to express a tumor dose without qualifying it by giving the length of time in which it was administered. Moreover, to add a calculated dose of roentgentherapy delivered to a fictional point of the pelvis (A or B) at the slow rate of a few roentgens per day (in several weeks) together with the calculated dose delivered by radium (converted to gamma roentgens) at a tremendously faster rate (in a few hours) and to express the whole as a meaningful didactic panacea is senseless. Obviously, no one should undertake radiotherapy of cancer who has not had a proper background of training and experience. In the present status of our knowledge of therapeutic radiology, the neophyte is more of a menace as he attempts to reproduce a given "tumor dose" in the face of numerous possibilities of error than when he proceeds according to more detailed information.

Clinical roentgentherapy suffers from a profound intoxication with the idea of dose and also from haste in the administration of that dose. In this obsession it is easy to lose sight of many factors in the management of successful radiotherapy. *Elongation* (fractionation) facilitates the task of the radiotherapist by enlarging the *margin of safety*. Elongation of treatments remains the most unexploited and ignored asset of modern radiotherapy.

Radioactive isotopes

The introduction of suspensions or solutions of radioactive materials into the bloodstream was recognized long ago as a possible approach to the treatment of generalized neoplasms. The experimental injection of radium and polonium, however, revealed their concentration in, and injury to, vital structures and disclosed the impossibility of using them to therapeutic advantage. The discovery of artificial radioactivity made it possible to render radioactive many elements such as phosphorus and iodine. However, when they are introduced into the circulation, they accumulate in certain organs or tissues in preference to others, not necessarily those desired. The amount of radiations necessary for the sterilization of a malignant tumor, however radiosensitive, is considerably greater than the amount that can be withstood by the hemopoietic organs and kidneys. Thus this method of treatment fails when applied to cancer.

The development of radioactive isotopes has opened new doors in scientific research, particularly in investigation of metabolism and organ fuction, but in radiotherapy of cancer their contribution at present may well be considered as nil, except in the form of sources for interstitial implantation or external irradiation. Moreover, their use in treatment of benign conditions may prove dangerous because of the risk of later carcinogenesis and is certainly unwarranted when other therapeutic means are effective. Radioactive gold and chromic phosphate have been used for the palliative treatment of metastatic implants and effusion of the pleural and peritoneal cavities. These procedures, even when temporarily successful, do not justify the cost to the patient and the exposure of personnel, particularly when other procedures such as injection of nitrogen mustards and external irradiation may be as effective.

Radiosensitizers

Since the dawn of radiotherapy, efforts have been made to augment the effects of radiations by various means. *Potentiation* of the beam of radiations by simultaneous irradiation from different directions and by implantation of metals within the tumor were among the earliest trials. More recently, attempts have centered on *sensitization* of the irradiated tissues, hoping for a favorable differential between the normal and malignant structures (Bane et al.[5]). Oxygen has been used for this purpose with some experimental support but no clinical success. The laboratory experiments (Gray[69]; Thoday and Read[217]) inevitably led to clinical trials of hybaroxic radiotherapy (Churchill-Davidson et al.[35]; van den Brenk[224]). The better results reported by the early advocates have not been generally substantiated. Hybaroxic radiotherapy does not render radiosensitive hitherto nonresponsive tumors. The door remains open to a controlled clinical experiment (Regato[175]).

Mitchell studied the possible advantages of *synkavit* (Marrian[124]). *Actinomycin D* (D'Angio et al.[50]) and other drugs have been

tried. Unfortunately, many of these drugs are highly toxic, and some have antineoplastic effects of their own that cloud an understanding of their effects. Nevertheless, this is fruitful research. Combinations of radiotherapy with chemotherapy seek *additivity* that may in some instances be favorable. A favorable additivity is obtained in the use of hormones combined with radiotherapy in such tumors as cancer of the breast. True *synergism* does not exist except with the use of combined roentgentherapy and radium if we accept the word as meaning combined effects through the same mechanism of action.

Clinical control of radiotherapy of cancer

The development of our knowledge of the physics of radiations, of radiobiology, and of pathology of tumors has resulted in slow but definite progress in the field of therapeutic radiology. But our limited scientific knowledge of radiations and their effects has not yet rendered simple or routine the daily practice of radiotherapy. Medical observation remains the basis on which important decisions as to its use must be made. The mistake is often made of believing that better equipment means better results. A variety of devices have been developed to help in the actual application of radiations in clinical practice. Bolus and especially shaped cones, measuring calipers, collimators, localizers, dose finders, etc. are intelligent adjuncts but are of limited advantage when evaluated in terms of clinical results. "It has sometimes been urged that cancer is not a disease of spherical masses and point sources, cylinders, rings, discs and line elements; therefore the mathematical and physical solutions to the problem are ridiculously inadequate."* Indeed, medical knowledge remains the dominant asset in radiotherapy of cancer.

Working with radiations at limits of tolerance of normal tissues, it becomes important and delicate to calculate, as precisely as possible, the distribution of dose throughout the irradiated area with the different physical schemes adapted to the topography of the region (Cohen[37]) and

*From Mayneord, W. V.: The organization of teaching and research in medical physics, Acta Radiol. (Stockholm) **29:**435-455, 1948.

to the potential area of tumor involvement (Moss and Brand[133]; Stewart[211]). The use of computers for the purpose of estimating dosimetry has become sufficiently practical for everyday radiotherapy (Kalnaes[94]; Powers et al.[158]), but such pragmatic assistance as a timesaving device does not authorize the belief that it eliminates the need for skill or other important considerations in treatment planning.

The strictly physical planning of radiotherapy leads, beyond certain limits, to frequent failures and accidents. The radiotherapist who plans his treatments on physical charts and mathematical calculations to the exclusion of all other considerations is as dangerous as the most daring empiricist. It is Coutard's greatest contribution to radiotherapy that he demonstrated the primary importance of clinical observation and judgment in the conduct of treatments. Thus the radiotherapist has ceased being a technician whose knowledge and ability are confined to the use of his apparatus. Without underestimating the basic importance of a thorough knowledge of the physics of radiations, the radiotherapist must also be thoroughly acquainted with the character of the disease he is attempting to treat. He must be capable of observing the significant general and local reactions that occur in the course of treatments and of evaluating their importance. Above all, the radiotherapist must be capable of reshaping his plans according to the individual clinical circumstances rather than follow preconceived formulas.

The clinical control of radiotherapy requires full evaluation of the case by the radiotherapist before treatments are started. Secondhand information contributed or recorded is seldom satisfactory, for the information important to radiotherapy is not usually noted by other workers. In his preliminary acquaintance with any lesion, the radiotherapist should evaluate the general condition of the patient, make a record of the symptoms and their intensity, and appreciate the consistency and physical dimensions of the tumor, as well as its topographic spread and depth. Other factors such as secondary infection, inflammation, edema, collateral circulation, etc. must also be carefully recorded. In the course of treatments, the improvement or further deterioration of the general condition, loss or gain in weight, and the persistence or disappearance of symptoms or the onset of new ones, in addition to the changes of the tumor itself, become the factors on which the proper evaluation of the therapy is based. Further, the systemic and local reactions due to the administration of radiations require daily evaluation. It is on the basis of these considerations that the final character of the treatment is shaped.

Systemic effects of irradiations

The indiscriminate administration of radiations results frequently in untoward systemic effects known as *irradiation sickness*, which are only rarely observed when treatments are intelligently conducted. These effects consist of anorexia, nausea, vomiting, lassitude, pallor, lividity, profuse perspiration, and even chills in extreme cases (Jenkinson and Brown[89]). They are most often observed in women and are definitely associated, although the mechanism is not understood, with the irradiation of excessively large fields or with the use of excessive doses for moderate-sized fields. A number of medications have been advocated in the treatment of irradiation sickness, *but the best way to deal with irradiation sickness is to avoid it entirely.* Also, it is important not to assume that any nausea or vomiting that patients may experience during *and after* radiotherapy is necessarily due to irradiation.

In certain very radiosensitive tumors, the *daily dose* is unimportant. Only the administration of a minimum total amount of radiations is necessary to assure local sterilization. In such cases, the required fields are usually large, but since a high daily dose is not necessary, the treatments need only be sufficiently elongated to accumulate the required total dose without general untoward effects or excessive local reactions. In tumors with a moderate radiosensitivity, however, the administration of radiations below a certain daily minimum never results in control of the tumor, even when the total amount administered may be brought to a maximum of tolerance. When tumors of this type are very limited in extent, the daily dose may be raised at least during part of the treatments to achieve their destruction. But when they are extensive, the battle is lost from the start, since a high dosage is not compatible with the use of large fields.

Local effects of irradiations

The daily observation of patients in the course of radiotherapy may reveal signs that require immediate change in the character of the treatment (the daily dose, the size of the field, etc.) lest the too forceful application of radiations results in an early interference with the natural radiosensitivity of the tumor. Such a sign is the edema that may be observed in the very few days of treatment for a carcinoma of the larynx. The necessity for close control and repeated examinations is thereby explained. The regression of a tumor may reveal that its actual extension is greater than had been estimated, requiring a revision of the size or position of portals.

Coutard[45] developed the theory that in the treatment of carcinomas of the upper air passages the sterilization of the tumor could not be expected unless an "epidermicidal" effect was noted on the normal mucous membranes. This meant that in the treatment of these carcinomas the development of a radioepithelitis of the mucosa around the tumor area could be taken for a good sign of sufficient dosage. However, with the rise of cobalt[60] and supervoltage roentgentherapy, the reactions of the mucosa are greatly minimized, particularly with the use of small fields. False membranes are usually limited and of short duration. Adequacy of irradiation of the tumor area requires careful radiographic control.

The *total dose* necessary for the sterilization of a tumor is established by experience. The same total dose rarely produces comparable effects not only because the physical factors of its administration may vary, but also because in the adaptation of the daily delivery to the requirements of the case, the treatments end in different fractionations. The total amount of radiations that may be given to a tissue or region varies with the multiplicity of physical factors and also with the rate of delivery and individual sus-

ceptibility. Only the experience of the radiotherapist can be of value in estimating the proper limits of dosage compatible with viability of normal tissues.

In the conduct of therapeutic radiology, clinical observation and experience may play a great role, but the radiotherapist cannot rely on clinical observation alone any more than he can conduct his treatments on the basis of physical knowledge alone. "To study the phenomena of disease without books is to sail an uncharted sea, while to study books without patients is not to go to sea at all."*

---

*From Osler, Sir W.: Aequanimitas (books and men), Philadelphia, 1904, The Blakiston Co.

REFERENCES

1 Andrews, J. R.: The radiobiology of human cancer radiotherapy, Philadelphia, 1968, W. B. Saunders Co.
2 Ariel, I. M.: Effect of single massive doses of roentgen radiation upon liver; experimental study, Radiology 57:561-575, 1951.
3 Arnold, A., Bailey, P., Harvey, R. A., Laughlin, J. S., and Haas, L. L.: Changes in the central nervous system following irradiation with 23 mev. x-rays from the betatron, Radiology 62:37-46, 1954.
4 Aubertin, C., and Bordet, E.: Action des rayons X sur le thymus, C. R. Soc. Biol. (Paris) 66:1091-1093, 1909.
5 Bane, H. N., Conrad, J. T., and Tarnowski, G. S.: Combination therapy of malignant tumors with ionizing radiations and chemicals; a review, Cancer Res. 17:551-566, 1957.
6 Bardeen, C. R.: Abnormal development of toad ova fertilized by spermatozoa exposed to the roentgen rays, J. Exper. Zool. 4:1-44, 1907.
7 Baserga, R., Yokoo, H., and Henegar, G. C.: Thorotrast-induced cancer in man, Cancer 13: 1021-1031, 1960 (extensive bibliography).
8 Bate, D., and Guttman, R. J.: Changes in lung and pleura following two-million-volt therapy for carcinoma of the breast, Radiology 69:372-383, 1957.
9 Bennett, D. E., Million, R. R., and Ackerman, L. V.: Bilateral radiation pneumonitis, a complication of the radiotherapy of bronchogenic carcinoma, Cancer 23:1001-1018, 1969.
10 Bergonié, J., and Tribondeau, L.: Action des rayons X sur les spermatozoïds de l'homme, C. R. Soc. Biol. (Paris) 57:595, 1904.
11 Bergonié, J., and Tribondeau, L.: Interprétation de quelques résultats de la radiothérapie et éssai de fixation d'une technique rationnelle, C. R. Acad. Sci. (Paris) 143:983-985, 1906.
12 Bering, E. A., Jr., Bailey, O. T., Fowler, F. D., Dillard, P. H., and Ingraham, F. D.: The

effect of gamma radiation on the central nervous system. II. The effects of localized irradiation from tantalum 182 implants, Amer. J. Roentgen. 74:686-700, 1955.

13 Birke, G., Franksson, C., Hultborn, K. A., and Plantin, L.-O.: The effect of roentgen irradiation on the steroid production of the testicles, Acta Chir. Scand. 110:469-474, 1955.

14 Bisgard, J. D., and Hunt, H. B.: Influence of roentgen rays and radium on epiphyseal growth of long bones, Radiology 26:56-64, 1936.

15 Bizzozero, O. J., Johnson, K. G., and Ciocco, A.: Radiation-related leukemia in Hiroshima and Nagasaki, 1946-1964, New Eng. J. Med. 274:1095-1101, 1966.

16 Blodi, F. C.: The effects of experimental x-radiation on the cornea, Arch. Ophthal. (Chicago) 63:20-29, 1960.

17 Bloom, W., editor: Histopathology of irradiation from external and internal sources, National Nuclear Energy Series, Division IV, vol. 22 I, New York, 1948, McGraw-Hill Book Co.

18 Bloom, M. A., and Bloom, W.: The radiosensitivity of erythroblasts, J. Lab. Clin. Med. 32:654-659, 1947.

19 Boden, G.: Radiation myelitis of the cervical spinal cord, Brit. J. Radiol. 21:464-469, 1948.

20 Borak, J.: The biologic basis of the fractionated method of irradiation of malignant tumors, Radiology 30:439-450, 1938.

21 Bozzetti, L. P., and Janovski, N. A.: Degenerative changes in the pelvic ganglia following betatron irradiation, Neurology (Minneap.) 13:788-792, 1963.

22 Brams, J., and Darnbacher, L.: The effect of x-rays on the gallbladder; experimental production of an x-ray cholecystitis, Radiology 13:103-108, 1929.

23 Brecher, G., Endicott, K. M., Gump, H., and Brawner, H. P.: Effects of x-ray on lymphoid and hemopoietic tissues of albino mice, Blood 3:1259-1274, 1948.

24 Brick, I. B.: Effects of million volt irradiation on the gastrointestinal tract, Arch. Intern. Med. (Chicago) 96:26-31, 1955.

25 Brill, A. B., and Forgotson, E. H.: Radiation and congenital malformations, Amer. J. Obstet. Gynec. 90:1149-1168, 1964.

26 Brues, A.: Radiation as a carcinogenic agent, Radiat. Res. 3:272-280, 1955.

27 Buschke, F.: Common misconceptions in radiation therapy, Amer. J. Surg. 101:164-170, 1961.

28 Buschke, F.: Radiation therapy: the past, the present, the future; Janeway lecture, 1969, Amer. J. Roentgen. 108:236-246, 1970.

29 Buschke, F., and Galante, M.: Radical preoperative roentgen therapy in primarily inoperable advanced cancers of the head and neck, Radiology 73:845-848, 1959.

30 Cahan, W. G., Woodard, H. Q., Higinbotham, N. L., Stewart, F. W., and Coley, B. L.: Sarcoma arising in irradiated bone, Cancer 1:3-29, 1948.

31 Cantril, S. T., and Buschke, F.: The clinical usefulness and limitations of supervoltage roentgen therapy, Radiology 53:313-328, 1949.

32 Case, J. T., and Warthin, A. S.: The occurrence of hepatic lesions in patients treated by intensive deep roentgen irradiation, Amer. J. Roentgen. 12:27-46, 1924.

33 Castro, L., Choi, S. H., and Sheehan, F. R.: Radiation induced bone sarcomas; report of five cases, Amer. J. Roentgen. 100:924-930, 1967.

34 Cherry, C. P., and Glucksmann, A.: Injury and repair following irradiation of salivary glands in male rats, Brit. J. Radiol. 32:596-608, 1959.

35 Churchill-Davidson, I., Sanger, C., and Thomlinson, R. H.: High-pressure oxygen and radiotherapy, Lancet 1:1091-1095, 1955.

36 Clemente, C. D., Yamazaki, J. N., Bennett, L. R., and McFall, R. A.: Brain radiation in newborn rats and differential effects of increased age, Neurology (Minneap.) 10:669-675, 1960.

36a Cohen, J., and D'Angio, G. J.: Unusual bone tumors after roentgen therapy of children, Amer. J. Roentgen. 86:502-512, 1961.

37 Cohen, M.: The organization of clinical dosimetry. I. The four stages of clinical dosimetry, Acta Radiol. [Ther.] (Stockholm) 4:233-256, 1966.

38 Comas, F., and Brucer, M.: Irradiation of the ovaries from the urinary excretion of iodine 131, Amer. J. Roentgen. 83:501-506, 1960.

39 Condon, E. U., and Terrill, H. N.: Quantum phenomena in the biological action of x-rays, J. Cancer Res. 11:324-333, 1927.

40 Conference on radiobiology and radiotherapy, Colorado Springs, Colo., Nov. 1-3, 1965 (J. A. del Regato, chairman and editor), Nat. Cancer Inst. Monogr. 24:1-289, Feb., 1967.

41 Court-Brown, W. M., and Doll, R.: Leukemic and aplastic anemia in patients irradiated for ankylosing spondylitis, London, 1957, Medical Research Council, Special Reports Series, no. 295.

42 Court-Brown, W. M., Doll, R., and Hill, A. B.: Incidence of leukemia after exposure to diagnostic irradiation in utero, Brit. Med. J. 2:1539-1545, 1960.

43 Coutard, H.: Sur les delais d'apparition et d'évolution des réactions de la peau, et des muqueuses de la bouche et du pharynx, provoquées par les rayons X, C. R. Soc. Biol. (Paris) 86:1140-1141, 1922.

44 Coutard, H.: Die Röntgenbehandlung der epithelialen Krebse der Tonsillengegend, Strahlentherapie 33:249-252, 1929.

45 Coutard, H.: Principles of x-ray therapy of malignant diseases, Lancet 2:1-12, 1934.

45a Coutard, H.: The conception of periodicity as a possible directing factor in roentgenotherapy of cancer, Proc. Inst. Med. Chicago 10:1-14, 1935.

46 Crompton, M. R., and Layton, D. D.: Delayed radionecrosis of the brain following therapeutic x-radiation of the pituitary, Brain 84:85-91, 1961.

47 Crow, J. F.: Comparison of fetal and infant death rates in progeny of radiologists and pathologists, Amer. J. Roentgen. **73**:467-471, 1955.

48 Crow, J. F.: The estimation of spontaneous and radiation induced mutation rates in man, Eugen. Quart. **3**:201-208, 1956.

49 Curie, P., and Curie, M. P.: Sur la radioactivité provoquée par les rayons de Bécquerel, C. R. Acad. Sci. (Paris) **129**:714-716, 1899.

49a Dalla Palma, L.: Intestinal malabsorption in patients undergoing abdominal radiation therapy. In Gastrointestinal radiation injury: Report of a symposium held at Richland, Wash., U.S.A., Sept. 25-28, 1966 (M. R. Sullivan, editor), Amsterdam, 1968, Excerpta Medica Foundation.

50 D'Angio, G. J., Farber, S., and Maddock, C. L.: Potentiation of x-ray effects by actinomycin D, Radiology **73**:175-177, 1959.

51 Davidoff, L. M., Dyke, C. G., Elsberg, C. A., and Tarlov, I. M.: The effect of radiation applied directly to the brain and spinal cord; experimental investigation on macacus rhesus monkeys, Radiology **31**:451-463, 1938.

51a DeBruyn, P. P. H.: Lymph node and intestinal lymphatic tissue. In Bloom, W., editor: Histopathology of irradiation from external and internal sources, National Nuclear Energy Series, Division IV, vol. 22 I, New York, 1948, McGraw-Hill Book Co.

51b DeCosse, J. J., Rhodes, R. S., Wentz, W. B., Reagan, J. W., Dworken, H. J., and Holden, W. D.: The natural history and management of radiation induced injury of the gastrointestinal tract, Ann. Surg. **170**:369-384, 1969.

52 Dickie, A., and Hempelmann, L. H.: Morphologic changes in the lymphocytes of persons exposed to ionizing radiation, J. Lab. Clin. Med. **32**:1045-1059, 1947.

53 Domagk, G.: Die Röntgenstrahlenwirkung auf das Gewebe, im besonderen befrachtet an den Nieren, Morphologische und funktionelle Veränderungen, Beitr. Path. Anat. **77**:525-575, 1927.

54 Dutreix, J., Schlienger, M., and le Peigneux, M.: Irradiation en deux séries et irradiation préopératoire en deux jours (Résultats préliminaires de 140 observations), J. Radiol. Electr. **48**:167-172, 1967.

54a Eddy, H. A., and Casarett, G. W.: Intestinal vascular changes in the acute radiation intestinal syndrome. In Gastrointestinal radiation injury: Report of a symposium held at Richland, Wash., U.S.A., Sept. 25-28, 1966 (M. R. Sullivan, editor), Amsterdam, 1968, Excerpta Medica Foundation.

55 Efskind, L.: Vaskuläre Veränderungen nach intravenöser Injektion von Thoriumdioxyd (Thorotrast), Acta Chir. Scand. **84**:177-186, 1940.

55a Ehrenbuch der Röntgenologen und Radiologen aller Nationen, Berlin, 1959, Urban & Schwarzenberg.

56 Elkind, M. M., and Sutton, H.: X-ray damage and recovery in mammalian cells in culture, Nature (London) **184**:1293-1295, 1959.

56a Ellis, F.: Dose, time and fractionation: a clinical hypothesis, Clin. Radiol. **20**:1-7, 1969.

57 Engelstad, R. B.: Ueber die Wirkungen der Röntgenstrahlen auf die Lungen, Acta radiol. (Stockholm) (suppl. 19), pp. 1-94, 1934.

58 Epstein, H. T.: Identification of radiosensitive volume with nucleic acid volume, Nature (London) **171**:394-395, 1953.

59 Evans, J. C., and Ackerman, L. V.: Irradiated and obstructed submaxillary salivary glands simulating cervical node metastasis, Radiology **62**:550-555, 1954.

60 Fajardo, L. F., Stewart, J. R., and Cohn, K. E.: Morphology of radiation-induced heart disease, Arch. Path. (Chicago) **86**:512-519, 1968.

61 Fernandez-Colmeiro, J. M., and Chardier, P.: Radio-épithéliomas et radiosarcomes pelviens survenus aprés radiothérapie d'un premier cancer. Étude de 15 observations, Mem. Acad. Chir. (Paris) **82**:981-985, 1956.

62 Flatman, G. E.: Some observations on the treatment of certain radio-resistant tumours, J. Fac. Radiol. **10**:21-26, 1959.

63 Freid, J. R., and Goldberg, H.: Post-irradiation changes in lungs and thorax; clinical, roentgenological and pathological study, with emphasis on late and terminal stages, Amer. J. Roentgen. **43**:877-895, 1940.

64 Friedman, N. B.: Pathogenesis of intestinal ulcers following irradiation, Arch. Path. (Chicago) **59**:2-4, 1955.

65 Gardner, W. U.: Hormonal imbalance in tumorigenesis, Cancer Res. **8**:397-411, 1952.

66 Gastrointestinal radiation injury: Report of a symposium held at Richland, Wash., U.S.A., Sept. 25-28, 1966 (M. R. Sullivan, editor), Amsterdam, 1968, Excerpta Medica Foundation.

67 Goldstein, L., and Murphy, D. P.: Etiology of ill health in children born after maternal pelvic irradiation; defective children born after post-conception pelvic irradiation, Amer. J. Roentgen. **22**:322-331, 1929.

68 Gray, L. H.: Comparative studies of the biological effects of x-rays, neutrons and other ionizing radiations, Brit. Med. Bull. (Special issue on Radiobiology) **4**:11-18, 1946.

69 Gray, L. H.: Radiobiologic basis of oxygen as a modifying factor in radiation therapy, Amer. J. Roentgen. **85**:803-815, 1961.

70 Griffith, M. G., Griffith, J. Q., Jr., Hermel, M. B., and Gershon-Cohen, J.: Effect of irradiation to adrenal upon circulating adrenal cortical hormone in the rat, Radiology **76**:110-112, 1961.

71 Guilleminot, H.: Action comparée des doses massives et des doses fractionées des rayons X sur la cellule végétale à l'état de vie latente, C. R. Soc. Biol. (Paris) **64**:951, 1908.

72 Gup, A. K., Schlegel, J. U., Caldwell, T., and Schlosser, J.: Effect of irradiation on renal function, J. Urol. **97**:36-39, 1967.

73 Guttmann, R. J.: Effect of 2 million volt

roentgen therapy on various malignant lesions of the upper abdomen, Amer. J. Roentgen. **74**:204-212, 1955.

74 Halls, J. M.: Radiation damage of the small intestine, Clin. Radiol. **16**:173-176, 1965.

75 Hartman, F. W., Bolliger, A., and Doub, H. P.: Experimental nephritis produced by irradiation, Amer. J. Med. Sci. **172**:487-500, 1926.

76 Hartman, F. W., Bolliger, A., Doub, H. P., and Smith, F. J.: Heart lesions produced by the deep x-rays; an experimental and clinical study, Bull. Hopkins Hosp. **41**:36-61, 1927.

77 Heineke, H.: Experimentelle Untersuchungen über die Einwirkung der Roentgenstrahlen auf innere Organe, Mitt. Grenzgeb. Med. Chir. **14**:21-94, 1905.

78 Heller, M.: Bone. In Bloom, W., editor: Histopathology of irradiation from external and internal sources, National Nuclear Energy Series, Division IV, vol. 22 I, New York, 1948, McGraw-Hill Book Co.

79 Hempelmann, L. H., Pifer, J. W., Burke, G. J., Terry, R., and Ames, W. R.: Neoplasms in persons treated with x-rays in infancy for thymic enlargement; a report of the third follow-up survey, J. Nat. Cancer Inst. **38**:317-341, 1967.

80 Henschke, U. K., Frazell, E. L., Hilaris, B. S., Nickson, J. J., Tollefsen, H. R., and Strong, E. W.: Value of preoperative x-ray therapy as an adjunct to radical neck dissection, Radiology **86**:450-453, 1966.

81 Hewitt, H. B., and Wilson, C. W.: A survival curve for mammalian leukemia cells irradiated in vivo (implications for the treatment of mouse leukemia by whole-body irradiation), Brit. J. Cancer **13**:69-75, 1959.

82 Hinkel, C. L.: The effect of roentgen rays upon the growing long bones of albino rats. I. Quantitative studies of the growth limitation following irradiation. II. Histopathological changes involving endochondral growth centers, Amer. J. Roentgen. **47**:439-457, 1942; **49**:321-348, 1943.

83 Holsti, L. R.: Split-course radiotherapy of cancer, Acta Radiol. [Ther.] (Stockholm) **6**:313-322, 1967.

84 Holweck, F.: Le problème des quanta en radiobiologie (point de vue physique), Radiophys. Radiother. **3**:235-250, 1934.

85 Ingold, J. A., Reed, G. B., Kaplan, H. S., and Bagshaw, M. A.: Radiation hepatitis, Amer. J. Roentgen. **93**:200-208, 1965.

86 Ivy, A. C., Orndorff, B. H., Jacoby, A., and Whitlow, J. F.: Studies of the effect of x-rays on glandular activity, J. Radiol. **4**:189-199, 1923.

87 Jacobson, L. O., Marks, E. K., and Lorenz, E.: The hematological effects of ionizing radiation, Radiology **52**:371-395, 1949.

88 Jacoby, J.: Experimentelle Untersuchungen über die Schadigungen des Auges durch Röntgenstrahlen, Strahlentherapie **16**:492-498, 1923.

89 Jenkinson, E. L., and Brown, W. H.: Irradiation sickness; a hypothesis concerning the basic mechanism and a study of the therapeutic effect of amphetamine and dextrodesoxyephedrine, Amer. J. Roentgen. **51**:496-503, 1944.

90 Jolly, J.: Action des rayons X sur les cellules. Diminution de la réaction d'un organe sensible par la ligature des artères afferentes, C. R. Soc. Biol. (Paris) **91**:532-534, 1924.

91 Jones, A.: Transient radiation myelopathy (with reference to Lhermitte's sign of electrical paraesthesia), Brit. J. Radiol. **37**:727-744, 1964.

92 Jones, H.: Evaluation and reduction of risks; a concept of lifetime tolerance to radiation, Pediatrics **41**:271-277, 1968.

93 Kallman, R. F.: Evidence for cyclic fluctuations in radiosensitivity and their implications, Conference on radiobiology and radiotherapy, Colorado Springs, Nov. 1-3, 1965 (J. A. del Regato, chairman and editor), Nat. Cancer Inst. Monogr. **24**:205-223, 1967.

94 Kalnaes, O.: Computer program for dose planning with analytical representation of radiation fields, Acta Radiol. [Ther.] (Stockholm) **4**:449-458, 1966.

95 Kaplan, H. S.: Some implications of indirect induction mechanisms in carcinogenesis; a review, Cancer Res. **19**:791-803, 1959.

96 Kaplan, I. I.: Genetic effects in children and grandchildren, of women treated for infertility and sterility by roentgen therapy; report of a study of thirty-three years, Radiology **72**:518-521, 1959.

97 Kashima, H. K., Kirkham, W. R., and Andrews, J. R.: Post-irradiation sialadenitis; a study of the clinical features, histopathologic changes and serum enzyme variations following irradiation of human salivary glands, Amer. J. Roentgen. **94**:271-291, 1965.

98 Kerr, H. D.: Some thoughts on the training of a radiation therapist, Amer. J. Roentgen. **66**:873-879, 1951.

98a Ketcham, A. S., Hoye, R. C., Pilch, Y. H., and Morton, D. L.: Delayed intestinal obstruction following treatment for cancer, Cancer **25**:406-410, 1970.

99 Kimeldorf, D. J., Jones, D. C., and Castanera, T. J.: The radiobiology of teeth, Radiat. Res. **20**:518-540, 1963.

100 Krause, A. C., and Bond, J. O.: Neutron cataracts, Amer. J. Ophthal. **34**:25-35, 1951.

101 Krause, P., and Ziegler, K.: Experimentelle Untersuchungen über die Einwirkung der Roentgenstrahlen auf tierisches Gewebe, Fortschr. Roentgenstr. **10**:126-182, 1906.

102 Kunkler, P. B., Farr, R. F., and Luxton, R. W.: The limit of renal tolerance to x-rays. An investigation of the renal damage occurring following the treatment of tumors of the testis by abdominal baths, Brit. J. Radiol. **25**:190-201, 1952.

103 Lacassagne, A.: Étude histologique et physiologique des éffects produits sur l'ovaire par les rayons X, Thesis, Faculty of Medicine of Lyon, 1913.

104 Lacassagne, A.: Le problème des quanta en

radiobiologie (Point de vue biologique), Radiophys. Radiother. 3:215-234, 1934.

105 Lacassagne, A.: Chute de la radiosensibilité aux rayons X chez la souris nouveau-née en état d'asphixie, C. R. Acad. Sci. (Paris) 215: 231, 1942.

106 Lacassagne, A., and Gricouroff, G.: Action des radiations sur les tissus, Paris, 1941, Masson et Cie.

107 Lacassagne, A., and Latarjet, R.: Diverses actions produites par les rayons ultraviolets sur la souris nonveau-née. Influence de l'asphyxie, C. R. Soc. Biol. (Paris) 137:413-414, 1943.

108 Lacassagne, A., and Loiseleur, J.: Synthèses chimiques consecutives à l'action des rayons X, C. R. Acad. Sci. (Paris) 237:417-419, 1953.

109 Lamerton, L. F.: Radiation carcinogenesis, Brit. Med. Bull. 20:134-138, 1964.

110 Lampe, I.: The radiation therapist in contemporary medicine, Radiology 43:181-183, 1944.

111 Lampe, I.: Radiation tolerance of the central nervous system. In Buschke, F., editor: Progress in radiation therapy, vol. 1, New York, 1958, Grune & Stratton, Inc.

112 Latourette, H. B., and Hodges, F. J.: Incidence of neoplasia after irradiation of thymic region, Amer. J. Roentgen. 82:667-677, 1959.

113 Lawrence, J. S., Dowdy, A. H., and Valentine, W. N.: Effects of radiation on hemopoiesis, Radiology 51:400-413, 1948.

114 Lea, D.: Actions of radiations on living cells, New York, 1947, The Macmillan Co.

115 Lehar, T. J., Kiely, J. M., Pease, G. L., and Scanlon, P. W.: Effect of focal irradiation on human bone marrow, Amer. J. Roentgen. 96: 183-190, 1966.

116 Levin, E., Hamann, A., and Palmer, W. L.: The effect of radiation therapy on the nocturnal gastric secretion in patients with duodenal ulcer, Gastroenterology 8:565-574, 1947.

117 Loiseleur, J.: L'intervention de l'oxygène en radiobiologie, Ann. Inst. Pasteur (Paris) 84: 1001-1009, 1953.

118 Luxton, R. W.: Radiation nephritis, Quart. J. Med. 22:215-242, 1953.

119 Luxton, R. W., and Kunkler, P. B.: Radiation nephritis, Acta Radiol. [Ther.] (Stockholm), 2:169-178, 1964.

120 McMahon, H. E., Murphy, A. S., and Bates, M. I.: Endothelial-cell sarcomas in liver following thorotrast injections, Amer. J. Path. 23:585-611, 1947.

121 Madrazo, A., Suzuki, Y., and Churg, J.: Radiation nephritis; acute changes following high dose of radiation, Amer. J. Path. 54: 507-527, 1969.

121a Maier, J. G., Perry, R. H., Saylor, W., and Sulak, M. H.: Radiation myelitis of the dorsolumbar spinal cord, Radiology 93:153-160, 1969.

122 March, H. C.: Leukemia in radiologists in a 20 year period, Amer. J. Med. Sci. 200:282-286, 1950.

123 Marcial, V. A., and Frias, Z.: Dose fractionation in carcinoma of the base of the tongue; uninterrupted versus split-course irradiation—a prospective study, Amer. J. Roentgen. 108: 30-36, 1970.

124 Marrian, D. H.: Studies of potential radiosensitizing agents: an effect of tetrasodium 2-methyl-1:4-naphthodydroquinone diphosphate (synkavit) on the Ehrlich mouse ascites tumour, Brit. J. Cancer 13:461-468, 1959.

125 Martin, C. L., and Rogers, F. T.: Intestinal reactions to erythema dose, Amer. J. Roentgen. 10:11-19, 1923.

126 Martland, H. S.: The occurrence of malignancy in radioactive persons; a general review of the data gathered in the study of radium dial painters with special reference to the occurrence of osteogenic sarcoma and interrelationship of certain blood diseases, Amer. J. Cancer 15:2435-2516, 1931.

126a Mason, G. R., Guernsey, J. M., Hanks, G. E., and Nelsen, T. S.: Surgical therapy for radiation enteritis, Oncology 22:241-257, 1968.

127 Mayneord, W. V.: The organization of teaching and research in medical physics, Acta Radiol. (Stockholm) 29:435-455, 1948.

128 Mendelsohn, M. L.: Cell-cloning experiments as models for radiotherapy; a critical appraisal, Conference on radiobiology and radiotherapy, Colorado Springs, Colo., Nov. 1-3, 1965 (J. A. del Regato, chairman and editor), Nat. Cancer Inst. Monogr. 24:157-167, 1967.

129 Merriam, G. R., Jr., and Focht, E. F.: A clinical study of radiation cataracts and the relationship to dose, Amer. J. Roentgen. 77: 759-785, 1957.

130 Miller, C. P., Hammond, C. W., and Tompkins, M.: The role of infection in radiation injury, J. Lab. Clin. Med. 38:331-343, 1951.

131 Miller, R. W.: Effects of ionizing radiation from the atomic bomb on Japanese children, Pediatrics 41:257-270, 1968.

132 Moss, W. T.: The effect of irradiating the exteriorized small bowel on sugar absorption, Amer. J. Roentgen. 78:850-854, 1957.

133 Moss, W. T., and Brand, W. N.: Therapeutic radiology, ed. 3, St. Louis, 1969, The C. V. Mosby Co.

134 Mostofi, F. K., Pani, K. C., and Ericsson, J.: Effects of irradiation on canine kidney, Amer. J. Path. 44:707-725, 1964.

135 Muller, H. J.: Artificial transmutation of the gene, Science 66:84-87, 1927.

136 Murphy, D. P.: Ovarian irradiation and health of subsequent child; review of more than two hundred previously unreported pregnancies in women subjected to pelvic irradiation, Surg. Gynec. Obstet. 48:766-779, 1929.

137 Murray, R. G.. The spleen. In Bloom, W., editor: Histopathology of irradiation from external and internal sources, National Nuclear Energy Series, Division IV, vol. 22 I, New York, 1948, McGraw-Hill Book Co.

138 Neel, J. V., and Schull, W. J.: The effect of exposure to the atomic bombs on pregnancy termination in Hiroshima and Nagasaki, National Research Council, National Academy of

Sciences, pub. no. 461, Washington, D. C., 1956.

139 Nickson, J. J., and Glicksman, A. S.: Preoperative radiotherapy in cancer, J.A.M.A. **195:**138-142, 1966.

140 Osler, Sir W.: Aequanimitas (books and men), Philadelphia, 1904, The Blakiston Co.

141 Painter, R. B., Drew, R. M., and Hughes, W. L.: Inhibition of HeLa growth by intranuclear tritium, Science **127:**1244-1245, 1958.

142 Palmer, E. D.: The gastroscopic picture of post-irradiation gastritis, Amer. J. Roentgen. **60:**360-367, 1948.

143 Parker, R. G.: Palliative radiation therapy, J.A.M.A. **190:**1000-1002, 1964.

144 Paterson, R.: The use and abuse of palliative radiotherapy, J. Fac. Radiol. **8:**235-238, 1957.

145 Paterson, R., and Parker, H. M.: A dosage system for gamma ray therapy, Brit. J. Radiol. **7:**592-632, 1934.

145a Perez, C. A., Vietti, T., Ackerman, L. V., Egelton, M. D., and Powers, W. E.: Tumors of the sympathetic nervous system in children; an appraisal of treatment and results, Radiology **88:**750-760, 1967.

145b Perkins, D. E., and Spjut, H. J.: Intestinal stenosis following radiation therapy, Amer. J. Roentgen. **88:**953-966, 1962.

146 Perthes, G.: Ueber den Einfluss der Röntgenstrahlen auf epitheliale Gewebe, inbesondere auf das Carcinom, Arch. Klin. Chir. **71:** 955-1000, 1903.

146a Pettit, V. D., Chamness, J. T., and Ackerman, L. V.: Fibromatosis and fibrosarcoma following irradiation therapy, Cancer **7:**149-158, 1954.

147 Phillips, R., Karnofsky, D. A., Hamilton, L. D., and Nickson, J. J.: Roentgen therapy of hepatic metastases, Amer. J. Roentgen. **71:** 826-834, 1954.

148 Phillips, T. L., and Buschke, F.: Radiation tolerance of the thoracic spinal cord, Amer. J. Roentgen. **105:**659-664, 1969.

148a Pierce, M.: The gastrointestinal tract. In Bloom, W., editor: Histopathology of irradiation from external and internal sources, National Nuclear Energy Series, Division IV, vol. 22 I, New York, 1948, McGraw-Hill Book Co.

149 Pifer, J. W., Hempelmann, L. H., Dodge, H. J., and Hodges, F. J.: Neoplasms in the Ann Arbor series of thymus-irradiated children; a second survey, Amer. J. Roentgen. **103:**13-18, 1968.

150 Pirie, A., and Flanders, P. H.: Effect of x-rays on partially shielded lens of the rabbit, Arch. Ophthal. (Chicago) **57:**849-854, 1957.

151 Pohle, E. A., and Bunting, C. H.: Studies of effect of roentgen rays on liver; histological changes in liver of rats following exposure to single graded doses of filtered roentgen rays, Acta Radiol. (Stockholm) **13:**117-124, 1932.

152 Pohle, E. A., and Bunting, C. H.: Histologische Untersuchungen an der Rattenmilz nach abgestuften Roentgenstrahlendosen, Strahlentherapie **57:**121-131, 1936.

153 Pohle, E. A., and Frank, R. C.: Radiation osteitis of the ribs, J. Bone Joint Surg. **31-A:** 654-657, 1949.

154 Pool, T. L.: Irradiation cystitis, J.A.M.A. **168:** 854-856, 1958.

155 Poppe, E.: Experimental investigations on the effect of roentgen rays on the epithelium of the crystallin lens, Acta Radiol. (Stockholm) **23:**354-367, 1942.

156 Portmann, U. V.: Therapeutic radiology as a specialty, Amer. J. Roentgen. **63:**1-5, 1950.

157 Portmann, U. V.: Clinical therapeutic radiology, New York, 1950, Thos. Nelson & Sons.

158 Powers, W. E., Bogardus, C. R., White, W., and Gallagher, T.: Computer estimation of dosage of interstitial and intracavitary implants, Radiology **85:**135-142, 1965.

159 Puck, T. T.: Action of radiation on mammalian cells. III. Relationship between reproductive death and induction of chromosome anomalies by x-irradiation of euploid human cells in vitro, Proc. Nat. Acad. Sci. **44:**772-780, 1958.

160 Puck, T. T., and Marcus, P. I.: Action of x-rays on mammalian cells, J. Exp. Med. **103:** 653-666, 1956.

161 Quan, S. H.: Factitial proctitis due to irradiation for cancer of the cervix uteri, Surg. Gynec. Obstet. **126:**70-74, 1968.

162 Quick, D.: Therapeutic radiology, Radiology **50:**283-296, 1948.

163 Quimby, E. H.: The history of dosimetry in roentgen therapy, Amer. J. Roentgen. **54:**688-703, 1945.

164 Reagan, T. J., Thomas, J. E., and Colby, M. Y.: Chronic progressive radiation myelopathy, J.A.M.A. **203:**106-110, 1968.

165 Redd, B. L., Jr.: Radiation nephritis; review, case report and animal study, Amer. J. Roentgen. **83:**88-106, 1960.

166 Reed, G. B., and Cox, A. J., Jr.: The human liver after radiation injury, Amer. J. Path. **48:** 597-611, 1966.

167 Reese, A. B.: Operative treatment of radiation cataract, Arch. Ophthal. (Chicago) **21:**476-485, 1939.

168 del Regato, J. A.: Roentgentherapy of epitheliomas of the maxillary sinus, Surg. Gynec. Obstet. **65:**657-665, 1937.

169 del Regato, J. A.: Dental lesions observed after roentgentherapy in cancer of the buccal cavity, pharynx and larynx, Amer. J. Roentgen. **42:**404-410, 1939.

170 del Regato, J. A.: Discussion of paper on roentgentherapy of carcinoma of the lower lip, Radiology **51:**717, 1948.

171 del Regato, J. A.: Cancer of the nasopharynx. In Portmann, U. V.: Clinical therapeutic radiology, New York, 1950, Thos. Nelson & Sons.

172 del Regato, J. A.: Roentgentherapy of carcinoma of the endolarynx, Laryngoscope **61:** 511-516, 1951.

173 del Regato, J. A.: Centers of training in therapeutic radiology (editorial), Postgrad. Med. **14:**161-162, 1953.

174 del Regato, J. A.: Report to the clinical studies panel: suggestions for incorporating stud-

ies using radiotherapy into the clinical studies of the Cancer Chemotherapy National Service Center, Cancer Chemother. Rep. no. 7, pp. 47-49, 1960.

175 del Regato, J. A.: Hybaroxic radiotherapy, Postgrad. Med. 39:87-89, 1966.

176 del Regato, J. A.: Historical changes in time-dose relationship in therapeutic radiology. In Frontiers of radiation therapy and oncology, vol. 3—Relationship of time and dose in the radiation therapy of cancer (San Francisco Cancer Symposium), White Plains, N. Y., 1968, Albert J. Phiebig, pp. 1-5.

176a del Regato, J. A.: The training of therapeutic radiologists (editorial), Radiology 95:703-704, 1970.

177 Regaud, C.: Sur l'erreur du tractionnement, de l'espacement et de la répétition exagérée des doses dans la radiothérapie des cancers, Paris Med. 43:102-106, 1922.

178 Regaud, C.: Influence de la durée d'irradiation sur les éffects déterminées dans le testicule par le radium, C. R. Soc. Biol. (Paris) 86:787-790, 1922.

179 Regaud, C.: Sur la radio-immunisation des tissus cancereux et sur le mechanism de l'action des rayons X et des rayons du radium sur les cellules et sur les tissus vivants en général, Bull. Acad. Med. (Paris) 91:604-607, 1924.

180 Regaud, C., and Blanc, J.: Action des rayons X sur les diverses générations de la lignée spermatique; extrême sensibilité des spermatogonies à ces rayons, C. R. Soc. Biol. (Paris) 61:163-165, 1906.

181 Regaud, C., and Dubreuil, G.: Perturbations dans le developement des oeufs fecondés par des spermatozoïdes roentgénisés chez le lapin, C. R. Soc. Biol. (Paris) 64:1014-1016, 1908.

182 Regaud, C., and Ferroux, R.: Discordances des effects des rayons X, d'une part dans la peau, d'autre part dans le testicule, par le fractionnement de la dose: diminution de la efficacité dans la peau, maintien de l'efficacité dans le testicule, C. R. Soc. Biol. (Paris) 97:431-434, 1927.

183 Regaud, C., and Nogier, T.: Les éffets produits sur la peau par les hautes doses de rayons X sélectionnés par la filtration à travers 3 à 4 millimètres d'aluminium. Applications à la röentgenthérapie, Arch. Electr. Med. 21:49, 97, 1913.

184 Rhoades, R. P.: The lung. In Bloom, W., editor: Histopathology of irradiation from external and internal sources, National Nuclear Energy Series, Division IV, vol. 22 I, New York, 1948, McGraw-Hill Book Co., Inc.

185 Rhoades, R. P.: The vascular system. In Bloom, W., editor: Histopathology of irradiation from external and internal sources, National Nuclear Energy Series, Division IV, vol. 22 I, New York, 1948, McGraw-Hill Book Co., Inc.

186 Ricketts, W. E., Kirsner, J. B., Humphreys, E. M., and Palmer, W. L.: Effect of roentgen irradiation on the gastric mucosa, Gastroenterology 11:818-832, 1949.

187 Rider, J. A., Moeller, H. C., Althausen, T. L., and Sheline, G. E.: The effect of x-ray therapy on gastric acidity and on 17-hydroxycorticoid and uropepsin excretion, Ann. Intern. Med. 47:651-664, 1957.

188 Roentgen, W. C.: On a new kind of rays, Science 3:227-231, 1896.

189 Romieu, C. L., Pourquier, H., Leehardt, P., Gary-Bobo, J., Pages, A., and Pujol, H.: La télécobalthérapie des metastases ganglionnaires cervicales, son apport dans l'association radiochirurgicale: (à propos de 15 cas controlés histologiquement), J. Radiol. Electr. 39:369-377, 1958.

190 Ronderos, A.: Fetal tolerance to radiation, Radiology 76:454-456, 1961.

191 Rubin, P., and Casarett, G. W.. Clinical radiation pathology, Philadelphia, 1968, W. B. Saunders Co.

192 Rubin, P., Duthie, R. B., and Young, L. W.: The significance of scoliosis in postirradiated Wilms's tumor and neuroblastoma, Radiology 79:539-559, 1962.

193 Rudberg, H.: Studien über die Thymus-involution. I. Die Involution nach Röntgenbestrahlung, Arch. Anat. Physiol. (suppl.), pp. 123-124, 1907.

194 Russell, W. L., Russell, L. B., and Kelly, E. M.: Radiation dose rate and mutation frequency, Science 128:1546-1550, 1958.

195 Sagerman, R. H.: Radiation nephritis, J. Urol. 91:332-336, 1964.

196 Sagerman, R. H., Cassady, J. R., Tretter, P., and Ellsworth, R. M.: Radiation induced neoplasia following external beam therapy for children with retinoblastoma, Amer. J. Roentgen. 105:529-535, 1969.

197 von Sallmann, L., Caravaggio, L., Munoz, C. M., and Brungis, A.: Species differences in the radiosensitivity of the lens, Amer. J. Ophthal. 43:693-703, 1957.

198 Sambrook, D. K.: Split-course radiation therapy in malignant tumors, Amer. J. Roentgen. 91:37-45, 1964.

199 Scanlon, P. W.: Radiotherapeutic problems best handled with split-dose therapy, Amer. J. Roentgen. 93:639-650, 1965.

200 Schrek, R.: Cytologic changes in thymic glands exposed in vivo to x-rays, Amer. J. Path. 24:1055-1065, 1948.

201 Schull, W. J.: A geneticist looks at the radiation hazard, Radiology 72:522-528, 1959.

202 Schull, W. J., and Neel, J. V.: Radiation and the sex ratio in man, Science 128:343-348, 1958.

203 Sherman, J. O., and O'Brien, P. H.: Effect of ionizing irradiation on normal lymphatic vessels and lymph nodes, Cancer 20:1851-1858, 1967.

204 Simpson, C. L., and Hempelmann, L. H.. The association of tumors and roentgen-ray treatment of the thorax in infancy, Cancer 10:42-56, 1957.

205 Sinclair, W. K.: X-ray induced heritable damage (small colony formation) in cultured mammalian cells, Radiat. Res. 21:584-611, 1964.

206 Snegireff, L. S.: The elusiveness of neoplasia following roentgen therapy for thymic enlargement in childhood, Radiology **72:**508-517, 1959.

207 Soloway, H. B.: Radiation-induced neoplasms following curative therapy for retinoblastoma, Cancer **19:**1984-1988, 1966.

208 Stadler, L. J.: Mutations in barley induced by x-rays and radium, Science **68:**186-187, 1928.

209 Stead, G.: The place of physics in the training of the medical radiologist (presidential address), Brit. J. Radiol. **21:**373-379, 1948.

210 Stetson, C. G., and Boland, J.: Experimental radiation pneumonitis; radiographic and pathologic correlation, Cancer **20:**2170-2183, 1967.

211 Stewart, J. G.: Dose distribution problems in megavoltage therapy. III. The clinical significance of dose distribution problems, Brit. J. Radiol. **35:**743-749, 1962.

212 Strandqvist, M.: Studien über die Kumulative Wirkung der Rontgenstrahlen bei Fraktionierung, Acta Radiol. (Stockholm) (suppl. 55), pp. 1-293, 1944.

213 Sundbom, L., and Asard, P. E.: Tumour dose concept, Acta Radiol. [Ther.] **3:**135-142, 1965.

214 Suter et al.; cited in Lawrence, J. S., Dowdy, A. H., and Valentine, W. N.: Effects of radiation on hemopoiesis, Radiology **51:**400-413, 1948.

215 Szegö, E., and Rother, J.. Ueber den Einfluss der Röntgenstrahlen auf die Magensaftsekretion, Z. Ges. Exp. Med. **24:**270-288, 1921.

216 Tanaka, K., and Ohkura, K.: Evidence for genetic effects of radiations in offspring of radiological technicians, Proc. 10th Int. Cong. Genet. **2:**287, 1958 (abst.).

216a Tefft, M., Mitus, A., Das, L., Vawter, G. F., and Filler, R. M.: Irradiation of the liver in children: review of experience in the acute and chronic phases, and in the intact normal and partially resected, Amer. J. Roentgen. **108:**365-385, 1970.

217 Thoday, J. M., and Read, J.: Effect of oxygen on frequency of chromosome aberrations produced by x-rays, Nature (London) **160:**608, 1947.

218 Tolmach, L. J., Terasima, T., and Phillips, R. A.: X-ray sensitivity change during the division cycle of HeLa S3 cells and anomalous survival kinetics of developing microcolonies. In Cellular radiation biology, Baltimore, 1965, The Williams & Wilkins Co.

219 Tsuzuki, M.: Experimental studies on the biological action of hard roentgen rays, Amer. J. Roentgen. **16:**134-150, 1926.

220 Tullis, J. L., Lamson, B. G., and Madden,

S. C.: Pathology of swine exposed to total body gamma radiation from an atomic source, Amer. J. Path. **31:**41-71, 1955.

221 Vaeth, J. M.: Radiation-induced myelitis. In Buschke, F., editor: Progress in radiation therapy, vol. III, New York, 1965, Grune & Stratton, Inc.

222 Vaeth, J. M., Feigenbaum, L. Z., and Merrill, M. D.: Effects of intensive radiation on the human heart, Radiology **76:**755-762, 1961.

223 Vaeth, J. M., Levitt, S. H., Jones, M. D., and Holtfreter, C.: Effects of radiation therapy in survivors of Wilms's tumor, Radiology **79:**560-567, 1962.

224 van den Brenk, H. A.: An oxygen barotherapy apparatus for use with 4 MeV accelerator, J. Coll. Radiol. Aust. **5:**113-122, 1961.

225 Volk, B. W., Wellmann, K. F., and Lewitan, A.. The effect of irradiation on the fine structure and enzymes of the dog pancreas. I. Short-term studies, Amer. J. Path. **48:**721-753, 1966.

226 Warren, S., and Gates, O.: Radiation pneumonitis; experimental and pathologic observations, Arch. Path. (Chicago) **30:**440-460, 1940.

227 Warthin, A. S., and Pohle, E. A.: The effect of roentgen rays on the heart, the toleration dose for the myocardium of rats, Amer. J. Roentgen. **25:**635-643, 1931.

228 Whitfield, A. G. W., and Kunkler, P. B.: Radiation reactions in the heart, Brit. Heart J. **19:**53-58, 1957.

229 Whitehouse, M., and Lampe. I.: Osseous damage in irradiation of renal tumors in infancy and childhood, Amer. J. Roentgen. **70:**721-729, 1953.

230 Whitmore, G. F., and Till, J. E.: Quantitation of cellular radiobiological responses. In Annual review of nuclear medicine, vol. 14 (E. Serge, G. Friedlander, and H. P. Noyes, editors), Palo Alto, Calif., 1966, Annual Reviews, Inc.

231 Wiernik, G.: Radiation damage and repair in the human jejunal mucosa, J. Path. Bact. **91:**389-393, 1966.

232 Wiley, H. M., and Sugarbaker, E. D.: Roentgenotherapeutic changes in the small intestine, Cancer **3:**629-640, 1950.

233 Yamazaki, J. N.: A review of the literature on the radiation dosage required to cause manifest central nervous system disturbances from in utero and postnatal exposure, Pediatrics **37**(suppl.):877-903, 1966.

234 Zirkle, R. E.: Relationships between chemical and biological effects of ionizing radiations, Radiology **52:**846-855, 1949.

Chapter 6

Cancer of the skin

Carcinoma
Malignant melanomas

Anatomy

The skin is formed by several layers of epithelium, the *epidermis,* and by a dense underlying layer of connective tissue, the *derma* or *corium.* The basal layer of the epidermis consists of a palisade of somewhat columnar cells. Above the basal layer lie the stratum malpighii, the stratum granulosum, the stratum lucidum, and, finally, the stratum corneum, which consists of desquamating, cornified cells. The sweat and sebaceous glands, hair follicles, vessels, and nerves are found in the corium, which forms papillary projections into the epidermis.

Lymphatics. The skin of the forehead, the temporal and malar regions, the lateral half of the eyelids and outer canthus, and anterior aspect of the ear is drained by the preauricular lymph nodes. The skin of the midline of the forehead, the medial half of the eyelids and inner canthus, and the nose, lips, and cheeks is drained by the submaxillary and cervical lymph nodes. The parietal and occipital regions of the scalp and the skin of the posterior aspect of the ear are drained by the upper cervical nodes (Fig. 49).

The skin of the hand is drained by lymphatics that follow a long course to the epitrochlear and axillary lymph nodes. Many of these lymphatics go directly to the axilla (Fig. 49).

The skin of the anterior and posterior chest walls is drained by the axillary and supraclavicular lymph nodes. The lymphatics of the lumbar region and anterior abdominal wall empty into the inguinal nodes. The lower extremities are almost entirely drained by lymphatics that empty into the inguinal lymph nodes. Only a small area of the skin of the heel is drained by popliteal nodes (Fig. 49).

Carcinoma

Epidemiology

Carcinoma of the skin is one of the most frequent forms of cancer, accounting for 19% of all cancer in men and 11% of all cancer in women. The number of cases of skin cancer observed in different clinics and hospitals depends on the proportion of outdoor workers seen in such institutions.

Chronic exposure to *solar rays* over a period of several decades frequently results in the production of carcinoma of the exposed areas of the skin. This is most often observed in individuals occupied in outdoor work, such as farmers and sailors (Unna[92]) (Fig. 50). The greater amount of sunshine that prevails in the tropics and subtropics may be responsible for a greater incidence of cancer of the skin among the inhabitants of these areas. Blum[5] pointed out that ultraviolet rays of shorter wavelength than 3,200 Å, capable of carcinogenesis in experimental animals, compose only a small fraction of sunlight and that this fraction changes greatly with latitude. The chronicity of the exposure seems to be the most important factor, but the intensity of the exposure also probably plays an important role. Sailors, as a whole, de-

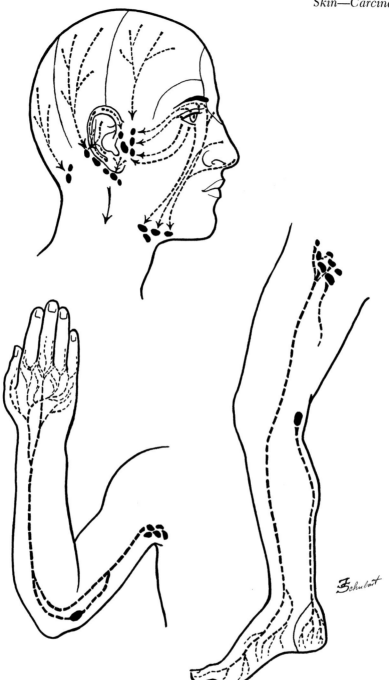

Fig. 49. Lymphatics of skin of face, upper extremity, and lower extremity.

velop carcinomas at an earlier age than farmers.

Blum's experimental studies have led to the simple theory that the proliferation of a few cells is progressively accelerated by successive doses and that they outstrip their fellows to constitute a tumor. How-

ever, neoplastic cells differ from their fellows not only in their faster proliferation, but also in their inability to undergo normal maturation, which implies deep character changes. That there is always a relatively long period of latency and that carcinomas of the skin also arise on the

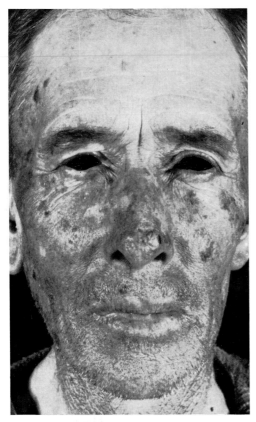

Fig. 50. Typical appearance of farmer's face showing almost normal skin of forehead and multiple dyskeratotic changes of skin of nose, cheeks, and nasolabial folds.

basis of long-standing thermal burns or scars suggest that ultraviolet rays may only produce an underlying atrophy on the basis of which cancer eventually develops. It has been suggested that chronic solar exposure of inadequately pigmented skin leads to collagen degeneration of the dermis and nutritional deficiency of the epidermis that would predispose to cancer (Mackie and McGovern[58]). There seems to be a direct relationship between sebaceous gland density of exposed skin and frequency of basal cell carcinomas (Graham and McGavran[32]).

There are definite racial differences in respect to the susceptibility to the development of carcinoma of the skin, but these differences seem to be related simply to the texture of the skin and its pigment content. In general, persons with a ruddy complexion, such as average Scandinavians

and North Germans, seem to develop carcinomas of the skin after chronic exposure to solar rays much more frequently than persons with coarser or darker skin. It is well known that Arabs, South American Indians (Roffo[76]), and blacks are only slightly susceptible to the development of carcinoma of the skin. In South Africa, cancer of the skin is much more common in whites and albinos than in the deeply pigmented Bantu (Oettlé[68]). Schrek[79] collected twenty cases of carcinoma of the skin in blacks and found a comparable number in exposed and unexposed areas and an equal distribution in both sexes. He concluded that chronic inflammatory lesions were more important than exposure to solar rays as a causative factor of carcinoma of the skin in blacks. The great majority of cutaneous carcinomas observed in the black population of Tanganyika were squamous cell carcinomas arising from scars and chronic ulcerations of the skin of the extremities (Sequeira and Vint[80]).

A rare hypersensitivity of the skin to solar rays leads to a condition known as *xeroderma pigmentosum* and to the development of multiple carcinomas of the skin in children (Fig. 51) (Rouvière[78]). The condition is hereditary and is supposedly due to an incompletely sex-linked gene (Haldane[33]) or to an independent autosomal gene (Koller[42]). Thus it becomes important to investigate the family history in order to discover additional early cases and to institute measures to prevent the development of carcinoma (Lynch et al.[55]).

Another important physical agent capable of producing carcinoma of the skin is the *roentgen ray*. Exposure to the primary beam of radiations or, more frequently, to scattered radiations reflected from objects hit by the primary beam causes the development of a complex properly called *xeroderma pigmentosum roentgenologicum*. The lesions frequently end in carcinomatous changes. Many worthy pioneers in the field of radiology paid with their lives for the knowledge that resulted in the present methods of protection.[20a]

In addition to the occupational form of cancer due to roentgen rays, carcinomas of the skin may also rarely develop upon medically irradiated areas. In general,

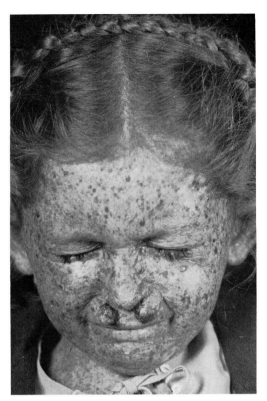

Fig. 51. Child suffering from xeroderma pigmentosum. Such a patient inevitably dies of multiple skin carcinomas.

these carcinomas develop many years after an accidental overexposure, or following excessive unfiltered irradiation, or after large areas or areas close to bone have been irradiated. The intensity of the exposure, the low quality of the primary beam used, and the excessive scattered radiation with the use of large fields are usually responsible for the ultimate development of carcinoma (Mitchell and Haybittle[62]).

Carcinomas may arise also as a late effect of irradiations that left little or no visible sequelae, such as treatment of acne. Totten et al.[89] reported on twenty patients with cancer of the skin who had had previous radiotherapy for benign conditions. The carcinomas developed fourteen to forty-five years after the administration of radiotherapy. The long interval between the radiation exposure and the development of carcinoma deserves emphasis. A conclusion of cause to effect with a relatively short interval should be considered

spurious. In general, the relationship of carcinoma of the skin to previous medical exposure to radiations requires close scrutiny.

Many supposed carcinomas arising in the borders of an area of radioepidermitis in a recently irradiated region are of questionable identity (Larsson[45]). In excessively irradiated areas, a late radiodermatitis may result, and after many years a carcinoma may develop on this indolent ulcer. But here carcinoma develops on atrophic, poorly vascularized tissue on a basis similar to that on which it occurs in burn scars and probably without relationship to the cause of these changes. Finally, carcinoma of the skin arising after irradiation of lupus vulgaris is only questionably due to the irradiation, since carcinoma may arise from a lupus that has not been irradiated.

Carcinomas of the skin may develop in relationship with certain chemical agents, the most frequently incriminated being *arsenic*. The occurrence of a keratosis of the skin in individuals exposed to arsenicals in their work or as a consequence of medicinal applications has been widely observed, but the incidence of arsenical carcinomas is rather small in comparison with the widespread industrial and medicinal exposure to this agent. Characteristic of the carcinomas of the skin developing in patients who have received arsenical treatment is their frequent location in the palm of the hand, on the plantar region of the foot, and in the inguinal region. In a limited area of the southwest coast of Taiwan, cancer of the skin is often attributed to arsenic because of its high concentration in the drinking water (Yeh[98]; Tseng et al.[91]).

Prunés,[71] of Chile, first observed in 1918 and later reported carcinoma of the skin in *nitrate* workers. Most of the lesions developed on the hands and feet, probably because of a carcinogenic agent contained in saltpeter plus added trauma (Fig. 52).

Tar and *pitch* have also been recognized as causative agents of carcinoma of the skin, but in many of the reported cases the concomitant exposure to solar rays may have played an important role.

Carcinomas developing on the skin of workers in oil refineries, machinists, metal lathe workers, etc. have been attributed to

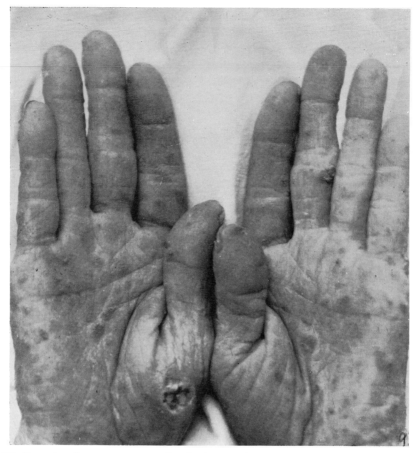

Fig. 52. Extensive dermatitis associated with obvious ulcerated epidermoid carcinoma in nitrate worker. (Courtesy Prof. L. Prunés, Santiago, Chile.)

the carcinogenic activity of *oils* and *paraffins* (Hueper[36]). The classical example of carcinoma of the scrotum of chimney sweepers, due to soot, is rarely seen today, but it is now observed among workers exposed to oils (Cruickshank and Squire[14]).

In 511 cases of cancer of the extremities reported by Browne et al.,[8] 347 were located on the upper extremities (67.9%) and 167 on the lower extremities (32.1%). In almost three-fourths, the carcinomas arose in areas of altered skin. In 110 there was a history of previous irradiation, in forty-two there were burn scars, and in twenty-four the lesions developed on the basis of an arsenical keratosis.

The occurrence of carcinoma on burn scars is frequently observed (Treves and Pack[90]). As a general rule, carcinomas developing on scars of severe burns occur twenty to forty years after the accident and arise usually from long-standing ulcerations (Giblin et al.[27]). Lawrence[48] reported ninety-three cases of cancer of the skin which developed, for the most part, on severe and penetrating burns. This study revealed that the older the patient at the time of the burn, the shorter the interval before the development of cancer. Thus it may be concluded that alterations due to age make the skin more susceptible to the development of cancer. A peculiar form of carcinoma of the skin of the abdomen and thighs is frequently observed in India among indigent Kashmiris. The carcinomas arise on the scars of burns caused by an earthenware bowl (kangri) that is filled with smoldering wood charcoal and worn under the garments as a portable calefactor (Neve[66]).

Epidermoid carcinoma can arise in the

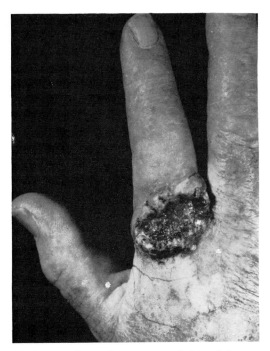

Fig. 53. Epidermoid carcinoma of skin of dorsum of index finger. With exception of face, dorsum of hand is most frequent location of carcinoma arising on basis of long-standing dyskeratotic changes.

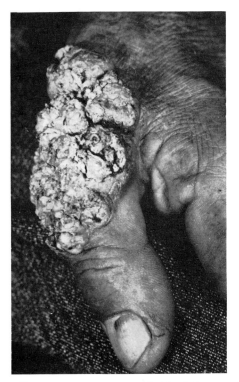

Fig. 54. Verrucous carcinoma of skin of dorsum of thumb.

sinus tracts of chronic osteomyelitis; the histologic diagnosis of such occurrences may be difficult (Johnson and Kempson[38]; Cruickshank et al.[13]). Carcinomas also arise from pilonidal sinuses presenting special problems of treatment (Milch et al.[61]). Epidermoid carcinoma also develops rarely from chronic draining sinuses produced by infection following war wounds. Gillis and Lee[28] reported thirty-four epidermoid carcinomas developing in such wounds and occurring after a time interval of no less than eighteen years.

Men are more frequently subject to carcinoma of the skin, perhaps because a greater number of them do outside work and because of differences in the chronicity of exposure. In carcinomas of the skin of unexposed areas (trunk and extremities), the proportion of males and females is usually comparable. Although the age of affected patients is variable, carcinoma of the skin, except for xeroderma pigmentosum, is very seldom observed in young individuals.

Pathology
Gross pathology

Carcinomas of the skin are divided into two main types: basal cell and epidermoid. The early basal cell carcinoma usually has a gray, somewhat translucent appearance and may be present as a small nodule beneath the thinned-out overlying epithelium. If it contains large amounts of mucin, it may have a cystic appearance and may even shell out of its bed. Large basal cell carcinomas frequently contain areas of yellowish necrosis. The epidermoid carcinoma, often keratinizing, may show yellowish gray areas on cross section. The large epidermoid carcinoma with an ulcerated surface is heavily infected. The infrequently observed carcinomas of the sweat glands are usually deeply invasive and at times cystic.

Carcinoma of the skin varies in its manner of growth. It may develop outward, producing a burgeoning tumor, it may develop inward, infiltrating and ulcerating the underlying tissues, or it may spread

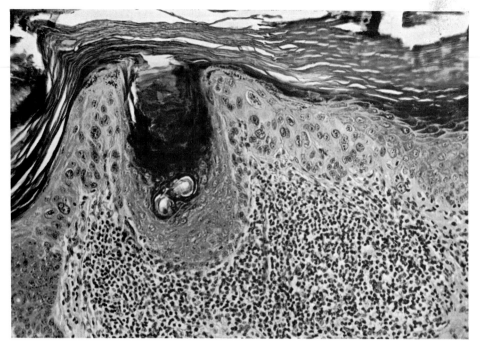

Fig. 55. Senile keratosis showing focal atypical changes in overlying epidermis. (Moderate enlargement.)

parallel to the surface of the skin, involving the epidermis alone or including the papillary layers. Both basal cell and epidermoid carcinomas may involve a wide zone with little infiltration in depth. As epidermoid carcinomas grow deeper, they often become fixed to underlying structures either because of inflammation or because of actual invasion. Epidermoid carcinoma of the dorsal surface of the hand is particularly prone to become fixed to underlying fascia, and it is impossible to determine grossly whether such fixation is inflammatory or neoplastic. The indolent, slowly growing basal cell carcinoma may, over a period of years, destroy the entire side of the face, eat away the cartilage of the nose, destroy the bone of the antrum, and cause death through hemorrhage.

If treated inadequately, both epidermoid carcinoma and basal cell carcinoma may heal over their surface and begin to spread in the deeper structures. This deep encroachment with spreading growth with many fine tendrils of tumor is often unappreciated by the surgeon, and exploration of a small previously treated basal cell carcinoma may reveal a tumor with unexpected deep ramifications. The carcinomas of the sweat gland often recur locally and may invade underlying bone.

Microscopic pathology

The earliest microscopic changes of carcinoma of the skin are difficult to evaluate. These changes can occur in a single focus or in multiple areas. The earliest changes observed in an area of senile keratosis resemble mere hyperplasia and thickening of the epidermis, but disorganization begins to show particularly in the basal layers in the form of increased mitotic activity and the presence of vacuolated and monster cells with several nuclei (Fig. 55). These changes are designated as *carcinoma in situ* because the basal layer remains intact. However, progress may lead to invasion of the corium and to definitely invasive epidermoid carcinoma. *Seborrheic keratosis* does not undergo carcinomatous changes.

The *basal cell carcinoma* arising from the basal layer of the epithelium has many different patterns, one variety of which often merges into the other. These tumors can form solid masses and lacy strands,

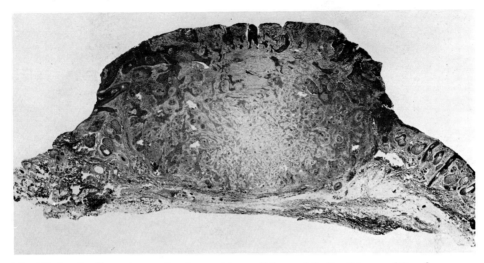

Fig. 56. Basal cell carcinoma showing excision well beyond limits of tumor. (Very low-power enlargement.)

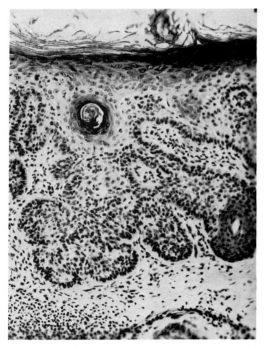

Fig. 57. Early typical basal cell carcinoma of skin. (Moderate enlargement.)

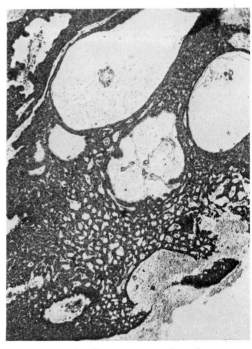

Fig. 58. Basal cell carcinoma, adenoides cystica, with typical cystic zones. (Low-power enlargement.)

show foci of keratinization, or suggest hair follicle origin. Rather infrequently, they are cystic with areas of mucin (Figs. 57 and 58). Lennox and Wells[50] concluded that it is impossible and impractical clinically and, in particular, pathologically to differentiate the different types of basal cell carcinoma. The designation basosquamous carcinoma has little significance, for these tumors do not mestastasize.

Multiple foci of origin of basal cell carcinomas often appear, particularly in the superficial spreading variety. The peripheral cells of the tumor masses frequently have a palisade arrangement. Inflammation may accompany these tumors (plasma cells, lymphocytes, mononuclears), but usually this inflammatory exudate does not infiltrate the tumor proper. The individual cell of the basal cell carcinoma is characteristically polygonal, with oval nuclei, fine

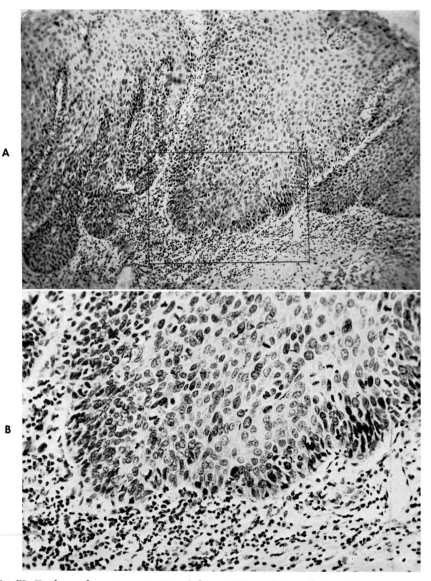

Fig. 59. Epidermoid carcinoma in situ of skin. **A,** Hyperplasia and intact basement membrane. **B,** Disorganization of architecture, numerous mitotic figures, and vacuolated cells. (**A,** Low-power enlargement; **B,** high-power enlargement.)

chromatin, and poorly defined cytoplasmic outlines. Mitoses are usually few in number.

Melanin pigment may be found within basal cell carcinomas in relatively small amounts. Infrequently, however, tumors with excessive melanin pigment may be observed. The microscopic pattern of these basal cell carcinomas is no different from the rest. This pigment may be in dendritic cells, both in the basal cells of the epidermis and in the tumor. In sixty-six cases reported by Birrell,[4] 77% were on the face or neck.

The *epidermoid carcinomas* of the skin, often well differentiated, do not differ microscopically from squamous carcinomas arising in other locations. In some instances, the carcinomatous changes may be confined to the epidermis, and there is no infiltration in depth. The rare type of spindle cell epidermoid carcinoma has a rapid evolution and can be classified as highly malignant (Martin and Stewart[59]).

Carcinomas of sweat glands occur relatively infrequently. They arise from specialized ciliary, apocrine (axillary, inguinal region), and ceruminous glands. Sweat gland tumors closely caricature the normal sweat glands, may be deeply invasive, are slow growing, and can, at times, show evidence of nerve sheath invasion. The tumor may have a papillary cystic character.

Benign tumors of the skin arising from sweat glands of the head or neck may resemble mixed tumors of salivary gland origin. They may produce mucin (Lennox et al.[49]). Stout and Gorman[83] reported 134 cases. None were malignant. Hirsch and Helwig[34] described this tumor under the name of chondroid syringoma.

Sebaceous gland carcinomas are rare. Microscopically, they suggest origin from sebaceous glands, contain fat, and grow relatively slowly. Welton and Helwig[94] reported thirty-three sebaceous carcinomas (in thirty-one patients). The average age of the patients was 55 years, and 88% of the tumors were located on the head. Six patients developed local recrudescence, but none showed metastases. This group of relatively rare carcinomas is usually cured by local excision.

Epidermoid carcinomas have been reported arising from sebaceous cysts, but we have never seen such a case. Invariably the "sebaceous cyst" contains well-differentiated, keratinized squamous epithelium. Sebaceous cyst is an incorrect designation because these cysts do not contain sebum. They contain keratin and are more properly designated as keratinous cysts (McGavran and Binnington[57]). We have never seen such a lesion metastasize or recur after removal (Fig. 72).

Metastatic spread

The basal cell carcinomas, although stubbornly and deeply invasive, practically never metastasize. Dahlgren and Martensson[16] were able to collect thirty-six instances of basal cell carcinomas that metastasized. The sweat gland carcinomas have a tendency to local recurrence and metastasize only rarely (Smith[82]) (Fig. 60).

Epidermoid carcinomas of the exposed areas of the skin metastasize infrequently. In a series of 444 patients with squamous cell carcinomas of the skin treated at the Ellis Fischel State Cancer Hospital, fifty-two (11%) presented metastases. Large size of the primary lesion and history of recurrences were the principal factors associated with metastases (Modlin[63]). In another series of 413 cases studied at the Roswell Park Memorial Institute, twenty

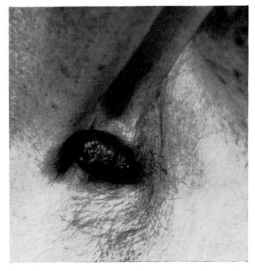

Fig. 60. Raised nonulcerated carcinoma of apocrine axillary sweat glands in male patient. Lesion was excised, recurred three years later, and patient finally died with distant metastases.

patients presented metastases on admission and fifteen developed them later, for a total of 8% (Katz et al.[39]). The proportion of metastases varies according to anatomic region: those of the dorsum of the hand in 1 out of 5 and those of the lower extremities in about 1 out of 3.

The regions of the exposed areas of the body where epidermoid carcinoma shows the greatest tendency to metastasize are the ear and the dorsum of the hand (Regato[74]). Johnson and Ackerman,[37] in a microscopic study of carcinomas of the hand, found that the lesions did not show metastases in any case in which the infiltration remained superficial to the level of sweat glands. A study of 335 cases of epidermoid carcinomas of the extremities showed sixty-six (20%) metastases (Taylor et al.[85]). In general, the large size, long duration, histologic undifferentiation, deep infiltration, and previous inadequate treatments usually result in a relatively greater incidence of metastases (Lavedan et al.[47]).

Clinical evolution

The typical patient with carcinoma of the skin is an elderly man showing signs of chronic exposure to solar rays. Such chronic exposure results in variable changes, depending on the racial character of the person. In favored subjects, a permanent suntan takes place with slight thickening of the skin and no deep changes. In others, the corium is affected, with resulting vasodilatation and permanent hyperemia of the exposed areas. In still others, the changes are uneven with alternate patches of pigmentation and discoloration, the vasodilatation becomes pronounced with telangiectatic, somtimes angiomatous, spots, and the skin becomes dry and atrophic with a tendency to hyperplasia and abnormal keratinization. The tendency to develop carcinoma is least with the first and greatest with the last of these three types of response to chronic exposure.

In farmers, the chronic changes are most marked on the nose, cheeks, ears, upper cervical regions, and dorsum of hands. The skin of the forehead is usually protected by a hat or cap, and the contrast between the skin of the neck and that of the chest is marked at the neckline. Hyperkeratotic lesions that develop predominantly in these regions eventually give place to the development of carcinoma. Seborrheic keratosis of the nonexposed areas of the skin is said to give rise to basal cell carcinomas, but we have never seen a case. Carcinomas may also arise from areas of the skin which, although chronically exposed to solar rays, have not been visibly altered.

The distribution of carcinomas of different types is not the same. Basal cell carcinomas predominate on the nose, eyelids, skin of the upper and lower lips, and chin, whereas epidermoid carcinomas predominantly occur on the dorsum of the hands, ears, and temples (Lacassagne[43]). More carcinomas of the forehead are found in women (57%), whereas a much smaller proportion (15%) of carcinomas of the ear is found in women. The explanation for these facts lies, of course, in the characteristic headgear worn by men and women and the natural protection afforded by the hair of women (Regato[74]).

Basal cell carcinomas may or may not develop from a preexisting area of hyperkeratosis, and they occur most frequently on the skin of the scalp, nose, nasolabial fold, eyelids, skin of upper and lower lips, chin, and forehead. They are rarely found on the anterior aspects of the ears, preauricular, temporal, and cervical regions, or dorsum of the hands.

Typically, these lesions have a pearly appearance and are usually well circumscribed. In the larger ulcerated lesions, the pearly appearance is observed only in the rolled borders of the tumor. Their growth is slow, and not infrequently lesions have been present for years before medical consultation is sought.

Basal cell carcinomas may be predominantly exophytic, but a variety known as *rodent ulcer* is characterized by its destructive capacity, and advanced lesions may destroy cartilage and bone extensively in their slow but tenacious growth (Fig. 79). Still another variety may present a serpiginous, superficial development, forming arcs of a circle around areas of normal skin. These lesions have been described as *flat cicatricial epitheliomas* because of their apparent spontaneous tendency to heal in one area while developing further in other

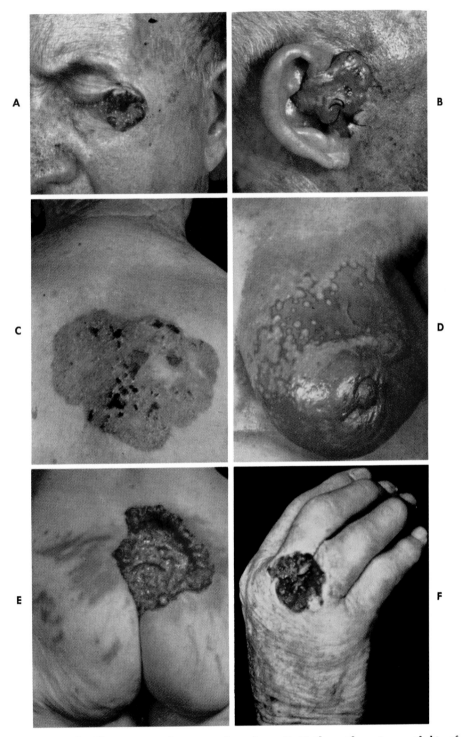

Plate 1. **A,** Basal cell carcinoma of outer canthus of eye. **B,** Epidermoid carcinoma of skin of preauricular region. **C,** Typical slowly growing, extensive, nonulcerated lesion of skin of posterior chest wall (Bowen's disease). **D,** Area of moist radioepidermitis showing peripheral and central regeneration of epithelium following palliative roentgentherapy for advanced carcinoma of breast. **E,** Basal cell carcinoma of skin of intergluteal space. **F,** Epidermoid carcinoma of skin of dorsum of hand.

areas. They are also designated as *field-fire type* of carcinoma.

Basal cell carcinomas arising on unexposed areas of the skin are frequently multiple, nonulcerated, scaly lesions that rarely are darkly pigmented.

Epidermoid carcinomas arise most often from preexisting patches of hyperkeratosis and occur predominantly on the skin of the cheeks, ears, and preauricular, temporal, and malar regions, as well as on the dorsum of the hands. They are rarely found on the forehead, eyelids, nose, nasolabial folds, chin, or skin of the lips.

The typical epidermoid carcinoma begins as a warty area. The keratotic surface may be removed, and the bleeding base rapidly covers itself with a crust that acquires larger proportions each time. Finally, an ulceration develops which may be superficial but usually has indurated borders and a more or less marked secondary infection. The growth of an epidermoid carcinoma is more rapid than that of a basal cell carcinoma, but the long history of preexisting keratoses seldom permits a proper evaluation of the time of development.

Epidermoid carcinomas are not necessarily excavating. Some present an extensive outgrowth and only superficial ulceration, but more often there is some degree of infiltration and fixation to deep structures. Still others have a superficial spread or may present multicentric growths arising from neighboring areas of hyperkeratinization that finally become confluent. Invasion of fascia, muscles, cartilage, and bone may take place. Local and referred pain is not infrequent due to secondary infection and the infiltrating properties of the tumor. Bleeding is not frequent, but at times very severe hemorrhage occurs from exophytic as well as from ulcerating lesions.

Epidermoid carcinomas of the unexposed areas of the skin usually arise from burn scars or other scars or on chronic inflammatory lesions but a few arise from apparently normal skin.

Bowen,[6] in 1912, described an atypical and proliferative "precancerous" lesion of the skin which later, at the suggestion of Darier, was called *Bowen's disease*. This lesion is pale red and slightly raised and

may acquire large dimensions. It usually appears on the unexposed areas of the skin but has been observed also on the skin of the face. The growth is very slow (five to thirty-five years). It seldom becomes ulcerated. Two or more such lesions may be observed simultaneously, although most patients present with a single plaque. This characteristic clinical entity has been identified with certain histologic changes that are thought by many investigators to be diagnostic.

Unfortunately, when a histologic criterion is chosen for the diagnosis, many other lesions of the skin and even of the mucous membrane which do not present a comparable clinical character become assimilated in this disease. The result is rather confusing. Metastases are seldom observed from these lesions. To add to the confusion, basal cell carcinomas arising often simultaneously from the skin of the chest develop over periods of years and may present a comparable clinical ap-

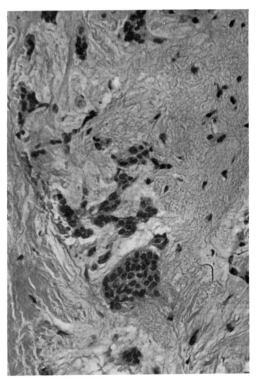

Fig. 61. Malignant sweat gland tumor that recurred in 55-year-old woman and was located in retroauricular area of neck. (×260; WU neg. 59-77.)

pearance, although their histopathology is quite different. In summary, Bowen's disease is undoubtedly a pathologic entity with a characteristic clinical appearance that can be, however, mimicked by other pathologic processes. It should not be confused microscopically with epidermoid carcinoma in situ.

Graham and Helwig[31] found frequent association of Bowen's disease of the skin with internal malignant tumors, suggesting that it is a manifestation of systemic carcinogenesis. In thirty-five cases studied, they found one or more internal primary malignant tumors present in twenty-eight (80%).

Carcinomas of the sweat glands are rare. They may originate from specialized sweat glands (apocrine, ciliary, and ceruminous) and are consequently observed around the anus, eyelids, and ears. They are also observed, however, on the skin of the axilla and scrotum. Their growth is slow. They tend to remain localized but may recur locally (Fig. 61). Regional nodes are seldom implicated. Teloh[86] collected twenty-three cases of sweat gland carcinoma. Keasby and Hadley[40] had eight sweat gland carcinomas with metastases in their group of 235 sweat gland tumors and also reported three carcinomas of sweat glands under the title of "clear-cell hidradenoma." Most tumors of ceruminous glands are benign (Cankar and Crowley[9]).

Carcinomas of the sebaceous glands are rare and develop slowly. They occur most often on the upper eyelids but may also be found on the scalp, ear, forehead, nose, chin, chest, and scrotum.

Diagnosis

The diagnosis of carcinomas of the skin can be made clinically in the majority of cases, but a biopsy should always be taken for confirmation, for "the final diagnosis of skin cancer lies under the pathologist's microscope, not in the clinician's eye."*
In a series of over 2000 carcinomas of the skin, 90% were accurately diagnosed clinically, whereas in over 1000 lesions that were diagnosed clinically as benign, 15%

---

*From O'Donnell, W. E., et al.: Early detection and diagnosis of cancer, St. Louis, 1962, The C. V. Mosby Co.

were found to be carcinoma on histologic examination (Torrey and Levin[88]). The histologic variety of carcinoma can be suspected with a high percentage of accuracy on the basis of the gross appearance of the lesion and its location. In a thorough study of a large number of cases, the clinical diagnosis of basal cell carcinoma was only 75% accurate (Lightstone et al.[53]).

Carcinomas developing in areas of pre-existing keratoses are often epidermoid, although this is not always true. A knowledge of the time of development and the history of previous treatments is of help in avoiding errors of diagnosis. Biopsy specimens should be removed from the clean borders of the ulcerated areas, should be deep, and should include some normal skin.

Differential diagnosis

The existence of definite *precancerous dermatoses* is unquestionable. Hyperkeratoses of the skin of the face and hands, resulting from chronic exposure to solar rays, often become carcinomatous. The same is true of senile keratoses of the skin of the unexposed areas of the body and of arsenical keratoses. Arsenical keratoses often appear in the palms and plantas and present clavuslike elevations. Their malignant potentialities should be considered rather than their benign appearance. Of ninety-three lesions diagnosed clinically as keratotic, 37% were actually found to be carcinoma (Torrey and Levin[88]). A biopsy,

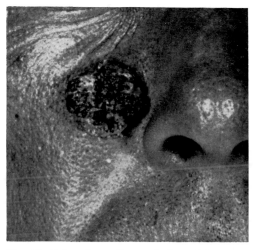

Fig. 62. Infected papilloma of skin of face suggesting carcinoma.

and often repeated biopsies, will be necessary to establish an accurate diagnosis.

Cornu cutaneum is a keratotic malformation that needs to be treated with care since 5% to 10% of these lesions present epidermoid carcinoma at their base. *Seborrheic keratoses* should be differentiated from senile keratoses. The seborrheic keratoses usually arise on the unexposed areas of the skin, particularly of the interscapular region and about the waistline, are often covered with greasy scales, have a granular surface, and occur in a relatively young age group (Eller and Ryan[21]). They practically never become carcinoma but may become ulcerated or pigmented and be mistaken clinically for melanoma.

The lesion often designated as *keratoacanthoma* (molluscum sebaceum) is frequently mistaken both clinically and histologically for carcinoma. The lesion may be single or multiple, it occurs predominately on the face and hands (Linell and Mansson[52]) of adolescents or young adults (Epstein et al.[22]), and it has a definite tendency to spontaneous regression (De Mora-gas et al.[19]; Witten and Kopf[97]) (Fig. 64). This lesion may be familial (Currie and Smith[15]). Keratoacanthomas may show rapid growth and are usually circular in shape with a central crater. Micro-

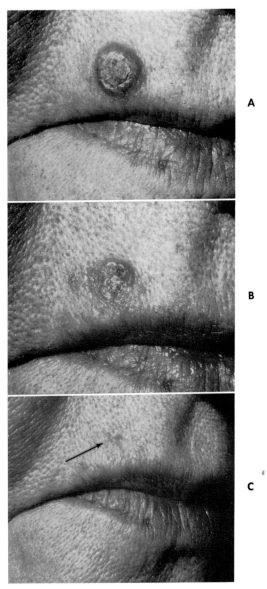

Fig. 64. Classic example of keratoacanthoma. **A,** Original lesion of two months' duration. **B,** Appearance of lesion one month after biopsy (no therapy was given). **C,** End result of spontaneous involution six months after original photograph taken. Arrow indicates all that can be seen of lesion. (From Witten, V. H., and Kopf, A. W.: Some common misconceptions regarding nevi and skin cancers, Med. Clin. N. Amer. 43:731-752, 1959.)

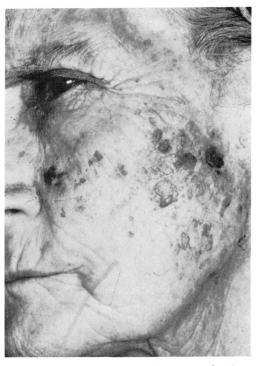

Fig. 63. Numerous pigmented, greasy, seborrheic keratoses. Such lesions only rarely undergo change to basal cell carcinoma.

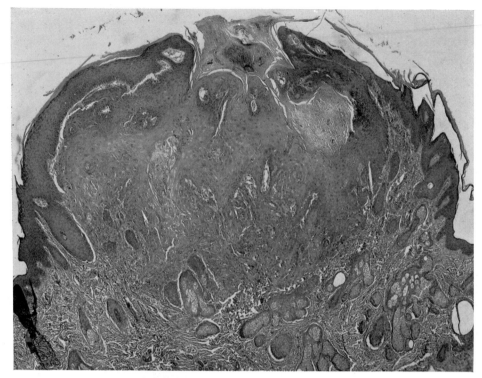

Fig. 65. Well-delimited keratoacanthoma of short duration on skin of face. Note central keratinized core and cup-shaped pattern. (Low power; WU neg. 60-2315.)

scopically, they are well delineated and easily identifiable (Fig. 65).

Frequently mistaken for recurrent carcinoma are the verrucoid lesions or exuberant granulations that occur after radiotherapy of cancer of the skin (Gartmann[25]).

Lesions of *psoriasis* may be confused with multiple basal cell carcinomas of the skin of the chest. The typical occurrence of psoriasis on the skin of the elbows and knees may suffice to make the diagnosis, but biopsy may be necessary.

The serpiginous type of *tertiary syphilis* of the skin may reproduce the appearance of a superficially spreading basal cell carcinoma. The inflammatory type of syphilitic lesion of the skin of the nose may also be confused with carcinoma. The biopsy easily solves these problems of diagnosis.

Forty-three cases of *reticulohistiocytic granuloma* of the skin were reported by Purvis and Helwig.[72] The lesions measured 1.5 mm to 2 cm and were usually single, rarely multiple. They occurred as a nodular lesion in the dermis and consisted of typical giant cells and histiocytes.

They are considered to be a reactive process of the reticuloendothelial elements. They are often mistaken microscopically for a malignant skin tumor.

Nonpigmented nevi may be confused clinically with basal cell carcinomas. This is also true of the *nonpigmented malignant melanoma,* which may, in addition, be misdiagnosed histologically as a basal cell carcinoma. The lack of radiosensitivity of the lesion should betray the error in diagnosis.

Pigmented papillary nevi may become ulcerated and infected and appear clinically as a malignant tumor. A *sebaceous adenoma* may resemble a basal cell carcinoma because of its pearly appearance, but it is usually softer. Benign, verrucous, chronic inflammatory lesions of the skin may spread over large areas and appear as an extensive carcinoma.

Pseudoepitheliomatous hyperplasia is often confused microscopically with epidermoid carcinoma because of the deep penetration of the rete ridges and the apparent isolated nests of epidermal cells found deep in the biopsy. In this condition, poly-morphonuclear leukocytes are often seen infiltrating the isolated islands of squamous epithelium. This does not usually occur in epidermoid carcinoma. The individual squamous cells are also well differentiated and, if serial sections are made, the deeply penetrating fingers of epithelium are seen to be continuous. This condition occurs in many chronic inflammatory lesions such as tuberculosis, syphilis, and varicose ulcers. The changes are particularly prominent in blastomycosis (Winer[96]).

Kempson and McGavran[41] reported twenty-one instances of *atypical fibroxan-thomas* of the skin. This tumor occurs in sun-damaged skin of elderly patients. It forms an ulcerated nodular mass and mimics highly malignant tumors histo-logically.

Lesions of *neurofibromatosis* (Reckling-hausen's disease) appear as multiple, non-ulcerated, subcutaneous tumors of various dimensions. Pigmentary disturbances (café-au-lait spots) may precede or accompany these nodular lesions. They have an easily recognizable histologic appearance.

A rare lesion of the skin of the forehead and scalp, variously referred to as endo-thelioma, cylindroma, or "*turban tumor*," may be confused clinically and histologi-cally with basal cell carcinoma. The "tur-ban tumor" is a benign epithelial lesion characterized by multicentric development and slow growth. The individual lesions have a translucent grayish appearance (Ronchese[77]), at times appear pearly, and may attain large dimensions (Fig. 66). Crain and Helwig[12] studied seventy-nine of these tumors and concluded that they arose from eccrine sweat apparatus. In their series, the lesions were often solitary and almost always located in the head and neck area.

Glomus tumors are rare, generally aris-ing near the nail bed of the fingers and toes, but may also be found on the fore-arm and other parts of the body. They are characteristically exquisitely painful and do not become ulcerated. The original description of these tumors was made by Masson.[60] The glomus is a normal vascular anastomosis without intervening capillaries and includes a special arrangement of muscle and nerve tissue. Murray and

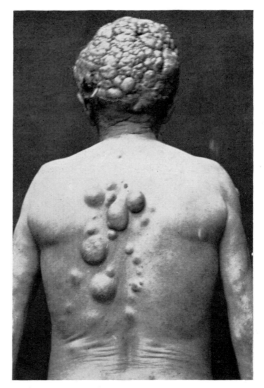

Fig. 66. Typical nodular turban tumor of long duration with innumerable lesions of scalp and posterior chest wall. This condition appeared in several members of same family.

Stout[65] identified the epitheloid cell of the glomus tumor as the pericyte of Zimmer-mann, thus offering an explanation for the occurrence of these tumors in parts of the body where glomus is not normally present.

Kaposi's sarcoma is a malignant lesion often of slow evolution. It used to be re-ported as commonest in Italian and Jewish men 50 to 70 years of age. We know now that it is extremely common in certain parts of Africa, where it occurs not only in adults, but also in children. In equatorial Africa, it makes up 10% of all malignant neoplasms.

The first lesions usually begin on an extremity as a slightly raised nodule. In some instances, it can simulate pyogenic granuloma. As the disease becomes more advanced with increasing numbers of nodules, edema appears (Figs. 67 and 68). This edema is a sign of advanced disease and is not in any way related to etiology. At this stage, arteriography and soft tissue roentgenograms invariably show numerous

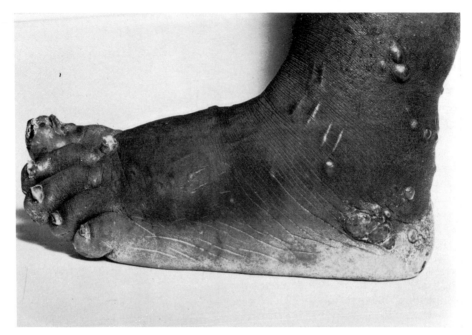

Fig. 67. Kaposi's sarcoma of foot of black man in Uganda demonstrating nodules and edema. Edema is sign of advanced disease. Note linear marks of witch doctor. (Courtesy Dr. J. N. P. Davies, Albany, N. Y.)

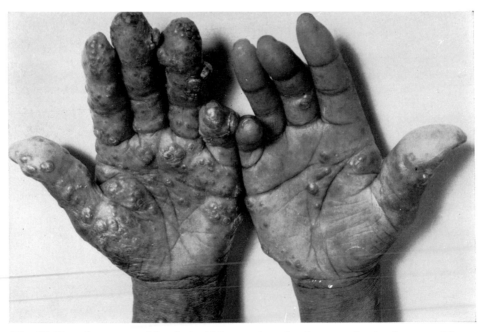

Fig. 68. Kaposi's sarcoma of hands in African patient showing extensive involvement. (Courtesy Dr. J. N. P. Davies, Albany, N. Y.)

deep-seated nodules (Palmer[69]). It undoubtedly has multiple foci of origin. At autopsy, involvement of the gastrointestinal tract, lymph nodes, liver, and bone often is noted. The cell of origin is in doubt. Microscopically, the pattern is typical, composed of a vascular element and a sarcomatous-like stroma.

Kaposi's sarcoma is best treated by radiotherapy (Cohen et al.[10]). Arterial perfusion with nitrogen mustard in advanced cases may give excellent palliation (Cook[11]).

Dermatofibrosarcoma protuberans, an unusual fibromatous tumor of the skin (Darier and Ferrand[18]; Hoffmann[35]), is often observed on the skin of the trunk but may occur in other areas such as on the forehead. This tumor is very slow growing and is usually adherent to the skin although movable over the underlying tissues. It has been observed in individuals of all ages. Dermatofibrosarcoma seldom produces any symptoms or affects the general health of the patient. If inadequately excised, it will recur locally. It practically never metastasizes. We have seen a patient with dermatofibrosarcoma protuberans of the skin of the abdomen. This lesion recurred after inadequate excision, disseminated widely, and caused the death of the patient (Adams and Saltzstein[1]). Adequate, well-conceived surgery of the primary lesion is usually curative.

Mycosis fungoides is a malignant skin condition with the microscopic appearance of a lymphoma. It is easily confused with the skin manifestations of leukemia and Hodgkin's disease, and for this reason its identity has been contested. Mycosis fungoides develops in the form of raised skin plaques which pass through several periods of development over many years, extend over large areas of the body, and may become bright red or brown in color (Fig. 69).

Gall[24] reviewed the natural life history of mycosis fungoides. In some instances, the chronic pruritic dermatitis becomes stationary, and in others it may regress or progress to a plaque stage, nodular stage, and systemic stage. It is impossible to predict the course of a given case. According to Reed and Cummings,[73] hyperplastic reticulosis may undergo transformation to *malignant reticulosis in situ* which, in turn, may become invasive and systemic, with a much shorter clinical course than its predecessor.

Mycosis fungoides is very radiosensitive and locally radiocurable. Survivals of fifteen to twenty years are common. This superficial and multicentric lesions is ideally suited for irradiation by means of electron beams of limited penetration. Repeated treatments, ulceration, infection, and systemic course often lead to eventual death.

The rare *calcifying epithelioma of Malherbe* is often located in the region of the head (about 50%), occurs frequently in young individuals, is covered by intact skin, and is usually small. Microscopically, it is made up of globular masses or bands of epithelial cells surrounded by a vascular connective tissue capsule (Setala[81]). The epidermis is not involved. Hyalinization, cornification, and a patchy calcification occur in the medullary portion.

Metastatic carcinoma of the skin may

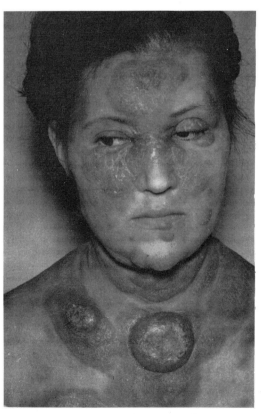

Fig. 69. Mycosis fungoides extensively involving skin. Lesions in all stages of development.

occasionally be mistaken for a primary lesion, particularly when a solitary metastasis becomes ulcerated, but this error occurs infrequently. Gates[26] reported a collected series of 231 cases of metastatic carcinoma of the skin from lesions in the breast, stomach, ovary, uterus, kidney, etc. There was a solitary skin metastasis in only nine instances. Although the metastatic lesion usually appears near the source of origin, it may be found very distant from the primary tumor.

Hemangiomas of the skin seldom are confused with cancer. They may be present at birth or may appear in the first months of life. Their rapid growth or unesthetic appearance may lead to hasty or unwarranted therapeutic decisions. Hemangiomas that exhibit no growth, or which are seen after their growth has stopped, may be best managed by *abstention,* for four out of five will disappear, leaving little or no sequelae by the time the child is 5 to 7 years of age (Lister[54]; Lampe and Latourette[44]; Modlin[64]; Walter[93]). Those that would not disappear entirely may leave the child less disfigured than if he is vigorously treated by any of the various means. Some may be excised later. To avoid being led into unwarranted treatment, the medical attention should turn to the usually alarmed, uninformed, ashamed, and insecure young mother of the infant, without whose concourse the child may eventually end in unscrupulous or inexperienced hands. Lesions that are seen in their period of growth may be irradiated *lightly* (200 R to 300 R at the most) in order to stop their development. Aggressive irradiation, particularly interstitial irradiation by means of radon seeds, is to be proscribed, for it only leads to unsightly overeffects that will require long and costly plastic surgery. Port-wine stains that persist are best handled by cosmetic makeup.

Treatment

Carcinomas of the skin are theoretically curable by a variety of therapeutic means, such as the application of escharotics, cryotherapy, electrocoagulation, cautery excisions, scalpel excisions, curietherapy, and roentgentherapy. In practice, however, the *injudicious* application of any of these methods is responsible for frequent failures that render incurable what originally was a rather innocent lesion. Following are the most common causes of failure in the treatment of carcinoma of the skin:

1 The administration of treatment by unskilled personnel without supervision
2 The systematic use of a single method or technique of treatment to cover all eventualities
3 The lack of histopathologic confirmation of clinical diagnoses and, in the case of surgical excisions, lack of microscopic verification of the adequacy of the treatment
4 The concept of primary healing as a criterion of cure
5 The self-satisfaction emanating from lack of adequate follow-up of patients

In carcinoma of the skin, as in other forms of cancer, the skill with which therapy is applied may be more important than the choice of method, but there is no special advantage attached to many of the methods that are used except that they do not require great skill. *The treatment of carcinoma of the skin may be reduced to the choice between its destruction by means of radiations or its eradication by means of surgical excision.* The choice of therapy depends mostly on the location of the tumor, on its extension, and on the history of previous treatment. When the control of the disease can be accomplished with equal certainty by either radiotherapy or surgery, preference may be given to the type of treatment that assures a better esthetic result or to the one that can be accomplished with greater ease, but no such practical consideration should be entertained when the chances of control of the disease are hampered by the choice of method.

Surgery will be chosen in some instances because its radical intervention offers the patient the best chances of permanent control of a carcinoma. In other instances, surgery will be favored only because of its expeditious character. Radiotherapy will be indicated because of its ability, when adequately applied, to destroy the carcinomatous tissue selectively without mutilation or dysfunction and with little or no visible sequelae. In other cases, radiotherapy will be indicated because the extension of the lesion and its infiltration of deep structures make its treatment by surgery entirely impossible. In other instances, radiotherapy will be chosen only because it will accomplish with less difficulty what would require repeated surgical interventions and/or cosmetic repair. But whether surgery or radiotherapy is employed, it must be applied by experienced physicians who have a definite knowledge of the pathology of cancer.

Surgery

A wide surgical excision is a very satisfactory form of treatment for carcinomas of the skin whenever the excision can be carried out without subsequent dysfunction or esthetic impairment. This applies to small lesions of the cheeks and cervical regions, where a surgical excision can accomplish without difficulty and in a single act the complete eradication of the tumor. Cautery excisions have no particular advantage and, in fact, modify the specimen, rendering its histologic study unsatisfactory.

The adequacy of a surgical excision should always be verified by microscopic study of properly selected sections of the specimen (Figs. 56 and 70). If tumor extends to the limits of the excision, the probability of recurrence is present, and a wider excision of the diseased area or the administration of radiotherapy should be contemplated. In epidermoid carcinomas of the skin, histologic signs of incomplete removal imply a 50% chance of clinical recurrence according to Glass et al.[30]

Three-fourths of these recurrences appear within six months, and there is a 25% mortality rate associated with such instances. Recurrences are more frequent after excision of large lesions. In general, a margin of 1 cm beyond the apparent limits of the tumor is sufficiently safe for the excision of well-delimited tumors. Although making their incision well around the surface of the lesion, unskilled surgeons may cut through the tumor in the deeper areas (Fig. 70). Even in the case of an early, apparently harmless, basal cell carcinoma, such an error may lead to a diffusely infiltrating and deep recurrence with a lessened chance of cure.

When the limits of the lesion are not well outlined or when its extension is such that the resulting wound cannot be closed without deformity, treatment by surgery should be wide excision followed by skin graft. However, treatment by radiotherapy is probably preferable to surgery, particularly if the lesions occur near the eye, ear, or nose. Mastery of surgery and distrust of other methods sometimes lead to unnecessarily elaborate surgical treatment (pedicle graft from forehead for carcinoma of the tip of the nose) or to biased inexpeditious procedures (surgery for carcinoma of the eyelids) that do not offer better chances of control and often result in unnecessary deformity or dysfunction.

When a small carcinoma is surrounded by multiple hyperkeratotic lesions, a wide excision, including these potentially malignant lesions, followed by a skin graft may

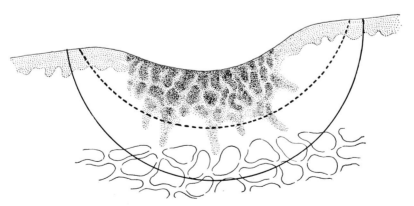

Fig. 70. Small carcinomas of skin are very often excised wide enough but not deep enough (dotted line). Pathologic examination should be directed to ascertaining complete removal of tumor.

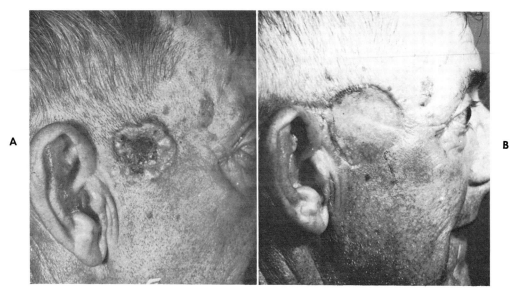

Fig. 71. A, Carcinoma of skin of temporal region. **B,** Following excision and graft.

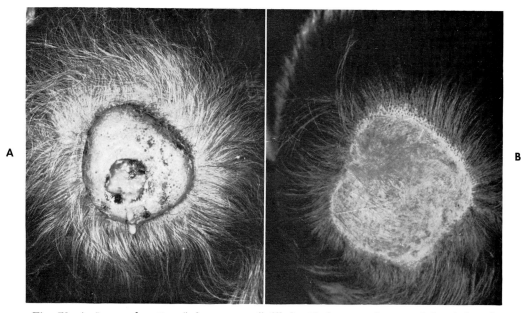

Fig. 72. A, Large ulcerating "sebaceous cyst" filled with keratinized material first believed clinically and microscopically to be carcinoma. Subsequent study demonstrated that lesion was perfectly benign. This type of lesion has often been designated as epidermoid carcinoma arising within sebaceous cyst. **B,** Following excision and graft.

be the most satisfactory means of avoiding repeated treatments to neighboring areas. Superficial carcinomas of the skin of the scalp are adequately treated by excision and skin graft (Figs. 71 and 72). Lesions of the dorsum of the hand that have not invaded in depth can also be very satisfac-torily controlled by an excision and graft (Fig. 73). The expeditious character of the procedure is an important factor here, but carcinomas of the dorsum of the hands may be adherent to tendons, and their surgical treatment may imply mutilation or impair-ment of function. In such cases, prefer-

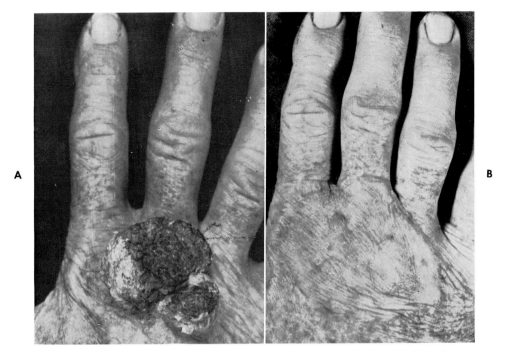

Fig. 73. A, Epidermoid carcinoma of dorsum of hand. B, Following excision and skin graft. Patient has remained without evidence of disease over five years.

ence should be given to roentgentherapy. This will, of necessity, be a laborious, protracted course of treatment that may achieve the conservative control of the disease and that does not interfere with a radical intervention in case of failure. Obviously, in extremely advanced cases of carcinoma of the skin of the hands, nothing but an amputation is logically indicated.

Surgery is also the treatment of choice for carcinomas of the skin of unexposed areas of the body. Often in these areas a large amount of tissue can be excised without inconvenience. Simple excisions, excisions followed by skin grafts, or amputations should be considered in cases of carcinoma of the lower extremities. In all tumors arising from scars or from lupus vulgaris, the surgical treatment is the method of choice. Whenever a carcinoma of the sweat glands is suspected, preference should be given to its surgical removal. In carcinomas in which inadequate irradiation has resulted in marked changes and in recurrence, a radical surgical excision, no matter how laborious or extensive, is usually the only hope of cure. In carcinomas arising on irradiated skin, the intensity

of the irradiation has usually caused marked changes, and excision followed by skin graft is the treatment of choice (Brown et al.[7]). It is important that burn scars be excised and grafted when this is feasible, for carcinoma only rarely develops in a primary grafted burn (Arons et al.[2]).

In the treatment of metastatic carcinoma from primary lesions of skin, the radical dissection of the lymph nodes of the neck, axilla, or inguinal regions is the logical therapeutic approach. A prophylactic dissection of the regional lymph nodes is seldom indicated in any location after control of the primary carcinoma of the skin (Johnson and Ackerman[37]; Lavedan et al.[47]; Dargent[17]).

Radiotherapy

Curietherapy. Radium has been used successfully in the treatment of carcinoma of the skin, both in surface application and in interstitial implantation. The surface application of radium requires the time-consuming preparation of special molds and very careful planning of the treatment, but at best its results are not so satisfactory as

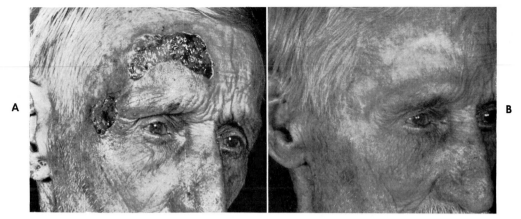

Fig. 74. A, Basal cell carcinoma of skin of forehead and frontotemporal region. **B,** Following roentgentherapy.

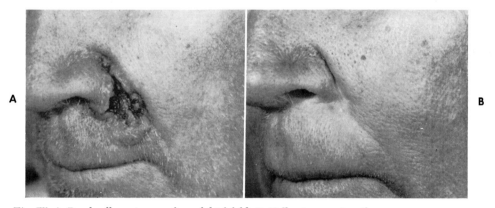

Fig. 75. A, Basal cell carcinoma of nasolabial fold. **B,** Following roentgentherapy.

those of adequate roentgentherapy in regard to the control of the disease and the esthetic result. Interstitial curietherapy is an expeditious method of treatment which is justified only in small lesions. In these, however, a surgical excision is often more convenient. The interstitial application of radium carries the unquestionable danger of nonsterilization of the tumor due to uneven distribution of radiations and also the high possibility of late radionecrosis of the treated area.

Roentgentherapy. Of all the forms of treatment of carcinoma of the skin, roentgentherapy is the one that has the widest range of indications and the greatest adaptability to the peculiarities of the given cases, but it also requires application with the greatest skill. Roentgentherapy is actually contraindicated in very few instances, such as in carcinomas arising from

scars. In most other instances where surgery is preferable, the choice is purely a practical one.

The success of roentgentherapy depends on its ability to achieve as nearly as possible the homogeneous distribution of a minimum amount of radiations throughout the entire tumor area that will assure complete destruction of the tumor. Failures may result from insufficient irradiation or uneven distribution of radiations. In carcinomas arising in certain areas of the face, the aim of sterilization of the tumor is closely followed by the important consideration of preserving the normal structures and of avoiding disfigurement. In the treatment of carcinomas of the eyelids, the inner and outer canthi, the skin of the ears, the preauricular and retroauricular regions, and the skin of the nose and of extensive or diffusely infiltrating

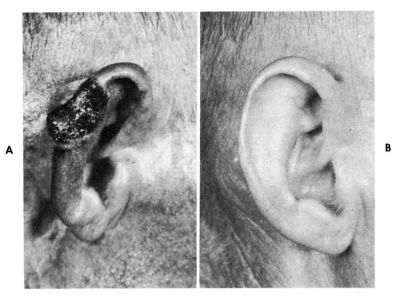

Fig. 76. A, Basal cell carcinoma of ear. B, Following roentgentherapy. Note excellent cosmetic result. (From del Regato, J. A., and Vuksanovic, M.: Radiotherapy of carcinomas of the skin overlying the cartilages of the nose and ear, Radiology **79**:203-208, 1962.)

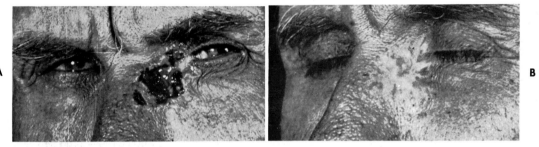

Fig. 77. A, Basal cell carcinoma of inner canthus of left eye. B, Following roentgentherapy. Patient has remained without recurrence over five years.

lesions elsewhere, the suppleness of roentgentherapy and its adaptability to the peculiar requirements of the lesion or of the region cannot be excelled by any other method (Regato[74]).

The invasion, or the proximity, of a tumor to cartilaginous or bony structures is not a contraindication to roentgentherapy but simply a circumstance requiring special adaptation of techniques. Single treatments using unfiltered radiations can be applied with impunity in the treatment of small lesions or of those so situated that the resulting atrophy can be easily dissimulated. But the systematic irradiation with low filtration results in a relative high proportion of primary recurrences. Late radionecroses are frequent when such massive treatment is applied to skin lesions overlying bone, such as the preauricular and retroauricular regions. Painful chondronecrosis often follows the application of unfiltered radiations to lesions of the nose and ears.

On the contrary, well-filtered radiations applied with convenient fractionation eliminate these untoward effects while assuring the success of this conservative treatment (Levi[51]). When the cartilage is involved by tumor, loss of substance will result (Tori[87]), but the defect may be limited to a minimum by the administration of antibiotics and by adequate dressing care. The size of the lesion and its location will determine the quality of radiations needed, the maximum daily dose administered, and the required elongation. The minimum total dose that is necessary to sterilize the tumor will vary with the size of the field, the quality of the radiations, and the average daily dose (Regato[74]). The esthetic result depends greatly upon the proper balance of these factors. This implies, unquestionably, a diversity of techniques to be applied to the circumstances of the case, and it forbids the utilization of a convenient but irrational standard technique.

Proper adaptation of treatment may entirely do away with complications and sequelae. Cataracts, which develop in patients with carcinoma of the eyelids treated with radium, need not occur if a properly adapted technique of roentgentherapy is used. Regato[74] reported 117 consecutive basal cell carcinomas of the eyelid successfully treated without a single occurrence of cataract (Fig. 78).

The treatment of carcinomas of the skin with special low-voltage equipment of the Chaoul type (contact therapy) offers no special advantage except for the rapid delivery of large amounts of low-quality radiations. Such practical aspect is far from compensating for the unequal distribution of radiations or excessive sequelae. The method accomplishes nothing that cannot be excelled with the adequate administration of conventional roentgentherapy. Under certain circumstances, the defect resulting from adequate irradiation of an extensive carcinoma may best be repaired by immediate cosmetic surgery. Contrary to usual belief, the freshly irradiated area, provided it is clean, is readily amenable to pinch grafts, split-thickness grafts, or pedicle grafts.

Basal cell and epidermoid carcinomas of the skin show a different radiosensitivity but are equally radiocurable. No differences in dosage of radiations are warranted, and there is no greater chance of recurrence in either case provided the treatments are adequate. Recurrences following roentgentherapy can be ascribed and often traced back to a definite defect in the technique of treatment. No carcinoma of the skin can be called radioresistant. The reputed radioresistance of the adenoides cystica type of basal cell carcinoma is a myth.

In general, metastatic adenopathies from epidermoid carcinomas are more satisfactorily managed by radical surgical treatment. In the case of isolated preauricular metastases, thorough roentgentherapy may succeed in sterilizing the node without causing a facial paralysis. Because of this, its use may be considered.

Prognosis

Carcinomas of the skin have the best prognosis of all malignant tumors that affect man. But, as has been pointed out, this relative advantage is frequently wasted by the administration of inadequate treatment leading to incurability. Consequently, the greatest efforts should be made to

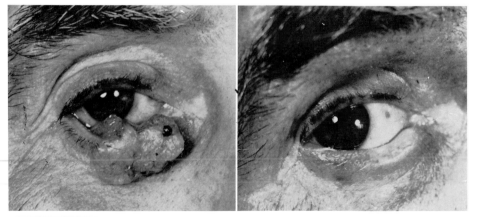

Fig. 78. A, Basal cell carcinoma of skin of lower eyelid with invasion of conjunctiva. **B,** Following roentgentherapy.

assure adequate treatment even in the most incipient lesions.

Under ideal circumstances, failures of treatment can be reduced to a negligible minimum, and few untreated cases are seen that may be considered incurable. For a large group of patients with carcinoma of the skin, the period of control may be reasonably limited to three years, since recurrences are rare after that period. In presenting statistics of results, most authors have been confronted with the problem of a large number of deaths due to intercurrent disease in groups of patients who, as a rule, are advanced in age. Patients who die of intercurrent disease within this period cannot be entirely eliminated in the computation of results, for some could have developed recurrence of carcinoma. If these cases are included in the statistics and considered as failures, the result is equally inaccurate.

In a series of 825 basal cell carcinomas treated by roentgentherapy at the Ellis Fischel State Cancer Hospital, there were sixty recurrences, but fifty-seven of these

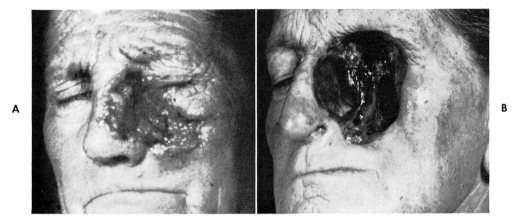

Fig. 79. **A,** Advanced basal cell carcinoma of skin of cheek that invaded nasal fossa, maxillary antrum, and orbit. **B,** Following administration of roentgentherapy over seven-week period. Patient remained well for years in spite of destruction produced by tumor. Notice almost complete absence of sequelae due to treatment.

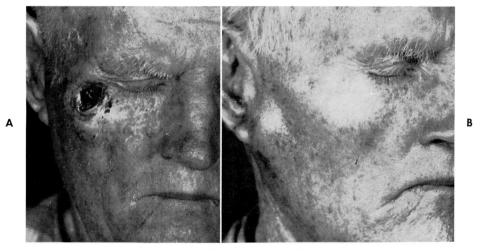

Fig. 80. **A,** Epidermoid carcinoma of malar region. **B,** Following roentgentherapy for primary lesion. Later, preauricular metastasis developed, proved by biopsy. Patient was well and without facial paralysis three years after roentgentherapy to lymphadenopathy.

were controlled by subsequent treatment. The remaining three cases were advanced lesions in aged patients. There were 149 deaths from intercurrent diseases and twenty-two patients lost to follow-up; 655 patients survived three years or more, or an absolute three-year survival rate of 79% (Regato [74a]). Of 117 consecutive basal cell carcinomas of the eyelid treated by roengentherapy, there were nine recurrences, all of which were controlled by subsequent treatment, and a three-year absolute survival rate of 86%. There were no recurrences in the group followed from three to eight years (Regato[74]).

Regato and Vuksanovic[75] reported on a series of fifty-six consecutive cases of carcinoma of the skin overlying the cartilages of the nose and ear. There were only three recurrences after roentgentherapy, all subsequently controlled, and not a single case of chondronecrosis.

Lauritzen et al.[46] reported a series of 2900 basal cell carcinomas treated by surgery or radiotherapy. There was a total recurrence rate of 3.4%, with 70% of the postoperative recurrences appearing within the first two years after surgery, and 98% of all the recurrences were controlled by subsequent surgery or radiotherapy.

Baclesse and Dolfus[3] reported 414 cases of carcinoma of the eyelids treated at the Fondation Curie by contact roentgentherapy or low-voltage roentgentherapy. There were ninety-six recurrences, sixty-one of which were controlled by subsequent treatment. Wildermuth and Evans[95] reported on a group of seventy-one determinate patients with carcinoma of the eyelids irradiated at the Tumor Institute of Seattle. There were four recurrences, two of which were subsequently controlled.

Statistics on smaller numbers of selected cases may show a still better proportion of good results. The site and the size of the lesion have a definite bearing on the prognosis, but very advanced basal cell carcinomas that have received no previous therapy may still be controlled (Fig. 79). The presence of a metastatic adenopathy darkens the prognosis of epidermoid carcinomas. Recurrences following inadequate excision or irradiation have the worst prognosis.

REFERENCES

1 Adams, J. T., and Saltzstein, S. L.: Metastasizing dermatofibrosarcoma protuberans, Amer. Surg. **29**:879-886, 1963.

2 Arons, M. S., Lynch, J. B., Lewis, S. R., and Blocker, T. G., Jr.: Scar tissue carcinoma. Part I. A clinical study with special reference to burn scar carcinoma, Ann. Surg. **161**:170-188, 1965.

3 Baclesse, F., and Dolfus, M. A.: Le traitement roentgenthérapique des cancers palpebraux. Étude de 414 cas ayant un recul minimum de cinq ans (1), J. Radiol. Electr. **39**:832-840, 1958.

4 Birrell, J. H. W.: Pigmented basal cell tumours of the skin, Aust. New Zeal. J. Surg. **22**:47-59, 1952.

5 Blum, H. F.: On the mechanism of cancer induction by ultraviolet radiation, J. Nat. Cancer Inst. **11**:463-495, 1950.

6 Bowen, J. T.: Precancerous dermatoses, J. Cutan. Dis. **30**:241-255, 1912.

7 Brown, J. B., McDowell, F., and Fryer, M. P.: Surgical repair of radiation lesions, Surg. Gynec. Obstet. **88**:609-622, 1949.

8 Browne, H. J., Coventry, M. B., and McDonald, J. R.: Squamous carcinoma of the extremities, Proc. Staff Meet. Mayo Clin. **28**:590-598, 1953.

9 Cankar, V., and Crowley, H.: Tumors of ceruminous glands; a clinicopathological study of 7 cases, Cancer **7**:67-75, 1964.

10 Cohen, L., Palmer, P. E., and Nickson, J. J.: Treatment of Kaposi's sarcoma by radiation, Acta Un. Int. Cancr. **18**:502-509, 1962.

11 Cook, J.: Kaposi's sarcoma treated with nitrogen mustard, Lancet **1**:25-26, 1959.

12 Crain, R. C., and Helwig, E. B.: Dermal cylindroma (dermal eccrine cylindroma), Amer. J. Clin. Path. **35**:504-515, 1961.

13 Cruickshank, A. H., McConnell, E. M., and Miller, D. G.: Malignancy in scars, chronic ulcers and sinuses, J. Clin. Path. **16**:573-580, 1963.

14 Cruickshank, C. N. D., and Squire, J. R.: Skin cancer in the engineering industry from the use of mineral oil, Brit. J. Indust. Med. **7**:1-11, 1950.

15 Currie, A. R., and Smith, J. F.: Multiple primary spontaneous-healing squamous cell carcinomata of the skin, J. Path. Bact. **64**:827-839, 1952.

16 Dahlgren, S., and Martensson, B.: Metastasizing basal-cell carcinoma, Acta Path. Microbiol. Scand. **59**:335-340, 1963.

17 Dargent, M.: Le problème ganglionnaire dans les épitheliomas cutanés, J. Med. Lyon **34**:301-802, 1953.

18 Darier, J., and Ferrand, M.: Dermatofibromes progressifs et recidivants ou fibrosarcomes de la peau, Ann. Derm. Syph. (Paris) **5**:545-570, 1924.

19 De Moragas, J. M., Montgomery, J., and McDonald, J. R.: Keratoacanthoma versus squamous-cell carcinoma, Arch. Derm. (Chicago) **77**:390-395, 1958.

20 Dillon, J. S., and Spjut, H. J.: Epidermoid

carcinoma occurring in acne conglobata, Ann. Surg. **159**:451-455, 1963.

20a Ehrenbuch der Roentgenologen und Radiologen aller Nationen, Berlin, 1959, Urban & Schwarzenberg.

21 Eller, J. J., and Ryan, V. J.: Senile keratosis and seborrhic keratosis, Arch. Derm. Syph. **22**:1043-1060, 1930.

22 Epstein, N. N., Biskind, G. R., and Pollack, R. S.: Multiple primary self-healing squamous cell "epitheliomas" of the skin, Arch. Derm. (Chicago) **75**:210-223, 1957.

23 Forbis, R., Jr., and Helwig, E. B.: Pilomatrixoma (calcifying epithelioma), Arch. Derm. (Chicago) **83**:608-618, 1961.

24 Gall, E. A.: Enigmas in lymphoma; reticulum cell sarcoma and mycosis fungoides, Minn. Med. **38**:674-681; 705, 1955.

25 Gartmann, H.: Pseudorezidive nach Ro-Nahbestrahlung von Hautkarzinomen, Derm. Wschr. **126**:710-718, 1952.

26 Gates, O.: Cutaneous metastases of malignant diseases, Amer. J. Cancer **30**:718-730, 1937.

27 Giblin, T., Pickrell, K., Pitts, W., and Armstrong, D.: Malignant degeneration in burn scar; Marjolin's ulcer, Ann. Surg. **162**:291-297, 1965.

28 Gillis, L., and Lee, E. S.: Cancer as a sequel to war wounds, J. Bone Joint Surg. **33-B**:167-179, 1951.

29 Glass, R. L., Spratt, J. S., Jr., and Perez-Mesa, C.: Epidermoid carcinoma of lower extremities; an analysis of 35 cases, Arch. Surg. (Chicago) **89**:955-960, 1964.

30 Glass, R. L., Spratt, J. S., Jr., and Perez-Mesa, C.: The fate of inadequately excised epidermoid carcinoma of the skin, Surg. Gynec. Obstet. **122**:245-248, 1966.

31 Graham, J. G., and Helwig, E. B.: Bowen's disease and its relationship to systemic cancer, Arch. Derm. (Chicago) **80**:133-159, 1959.

32 Graham, P. G., and McGavran, M. H.: Basal-cell carcinomas and sebaceous glands, Cancer **17**:803-806, 1964.

33 Haldane, J. B. S.: Search for incomplete sex-linkage in man, Ann. Eugenics **7**:28-57, 1936.

34 Hirsch, P., and Helwig, E. B.: Chondroid syringoma; mixed tumor of skin, salivary gland type, Arch. Derm. (Chicago) **84**:835-847, 1961.

35 Hoffman, E.: Ueber das knollentreibende Fibrosarkom der Haut (Dermatofibrosarkoma protuberans), Derm. Z. **43**:1-28, 1925.

36 Hueper, W. C.: Occupational tumors and allied diseases, Springfield, Ill., 1942, Charles C Thomas, Publisher.

37 Johnson, R. E., and Ackerman, L. V.: Epidermoid carcinoma of the hand, Cancer **3**:657-666, 1950.

38 Johnson, L. L., and Kempson, R. L.: Epidermoid carcinoma in chronic osteomyelitis: diagnostic problems and management; report of ten cases, J. Bone Joint Surg. **47-A**:133-145, 1965.

39 Katz, A. D., Nrbach, F., and Lilienfeld, A. M.: The frequency and risk of metastases in

40 Keasbey, L. E., and Hadley, G. G.: Clear-cell hidradenoma, Cancer **7**:934-952, 1954.

41 Kempson, R. L., and McGavran, M. H.: Atypical fibroxanthomas of the skin, Cancer **17**:1463-1471, 1964.

42 Koller, P. C.: Inheritance of xeroderma and its chromosome mechanism, Brit. J. Cancer **2**:149-155, 1948.

43 Lacassagne, A.: Repartition des differentes varietés histologiques d'épithéliomas de la peau (plus particulzerment ceux de la tête) suivant les regions anatomiques, le sexe et l'âge, Ann. Derm. Syph. (Paris) **4**:497-514, 613-640, 722-754, 1933.

44 Lampe, I., and Latourette, H. B.: The management of cavernous hemangioma in infants, Postgrad. Med. **19**:262-270, 1956.

45 Larsson, L.: Tubercle-like structures in late irradiation injuries of the skin, Acta Radiol. (Stockholm) **31**:17-27, 1949.

46 Lauritzen, R. E., Johnson, R. E., and Spratt, J. S., Jr.: Pattern of recurrences in basal cell carcinoma, Surgery **57**:813-816, 1965.

47 Lavedan, J., Ennuyer, A., and Soenen, A.: Fréquence de adenopathie secondaires aux cancer cutanés de la tête et du cou, en fonction de la localisation, de l'extension en surface et du degré d'infiltration, Rev. Med. Liege **5**:415-418, 1950.

48 Lawrence, E. A.: Carcinoma arising in the scars of thermal burns, Surg. Gynec. Obstet. **95**:579-588, 1952.

49 Lennox, B., Pearse, A. G. E., and Richards, H. G. H.: Mucin secreting tumors of the skin with special reference to the so-called salivary tumor of the skin and its relation to hidradenoma, J. Path. Bact. **64**:865-880, 1952.

50 Lennox, B., and Wells, A. L.: Differentiation in the rodent ulcer group of tumours, Brit. J. Cancer **5**:195-212, 1951.

51 Levi, L. M.: The roentgen treatment of cutaneous carcinoma involving cartilage, Amer. J. Roentgen. **61**:380-386, 1949.

52 Linell, F., and Mansson, B.: Molluscum pseudocarcinomatosum, Acta Radiol. (Stockholm) **48**:123-140, 1957.

53 Lightstone, A. C., Kopf, A. W., and Garfinkel, L.: Diagnostic accuracy—a new approach to its evaluation; results in basal cell epitheliomas, Arch. Derm. (Chicago) **91**:497-502, 1965.

54 Lister, W. A.: Natural history of strawberry nevi, Lancet **1**:1429-1434, 1938.

55 Lynch, H. T., Anderson, D. E., Krush, A. J., and Mukerjee, K.: Cancer; heredity and genetic counseling, Cancer **20**:1796-1801, 1967.

56 McGavran, M. H.: Ultrastructure of pilomatrixoma (calcifying epithelioma), Cancer **18**:1445-1456, 1965.

57 McGavran, M. H., and Binnington, B.: Keratinous cysts of the skin, Arch. Derm. (Chicago) **94**:499-508, 1966.

58 Mackie, B. S., and McGovern, V. J.: The mechanism of solar carcinogenesis, Arch. Derm. (Chicago) **78**:218-244, 1958.

59 Martin, H. E., and Stewart, F. W.: Spindle-cell epidermoid carcinoma, Amer. J. Cancer **24**:273-298, 1935.

60 Masson, P.: Les glomus cutanés de l'homme, Bull. Soc. Franc. Derm. Syph. **42**:1174-1245, 1935.

61 Milch, E., Berman, L., and McGregor, J. K.: Carcinoma complicating a pilonidal sinus; review of the literature and report of a case, Dis. Colon Rectum **6**:225-231, 1963.

62 Mitchell, J. S., and Haybittle, J. L.: Carcinoma of the skin appearing 49 years after a single diagnostic roentgen exposure, Acta Radiol. (Stockholm) **44**:345-350, 1955.

63 Modlin, J. J.: Cancer of the skin; surgical treatment, Missouri Med. **51**:364-367, 1954.

64 Modlin, J. J.: Capillary hemangiomas of the skin, Surgery **38**:169-180, 1955.

65 Murray, M. R., and Stout, A. P.: The glomus tumor; investigation of its distribution and behavior and the identity of its "epithelial" cell, Amer. J. Path. **18**:183-203, 1942.

66 Neve, E. F.: Kangri-burn cancer, Brit. Med. J. **2**:1255-1256, 1923.

67 O'Donnell, W. E., Day, E., and Venet, L.: Early detection and diagnosis of cancer, St. Louis, 1962, The C. V. Mosby Co.

68 Oettlé, A. G.: Skin cancer in Africa; presented at the Conference on Biology of Cutaneous Cancer, Philadelphia, Pa., April 6-11, 1962.

69 Palmer, P. E. S.: Radiological changes of Kaposi's sarcoma, Acta Un. Int. Cancr. **18**:400-412, 1962.

70 Piers, F.: Sunlight and skin cancer in Kenya, Brit. J. Derm. **60**:319-332, 1948.

71 Prunés, L. R.: Cancer de los salitreros (o enfermedad del salitre). Personal communication, 1956.

72 Purvis, E., and Helwig, E. B.: Reticulo-histiocytic granuloma of the skin, Amer. J. Clin. Path. **24**:1005-1015, 1954.

73 Reed, R. J., and Cummings, C. E.: Malignant reticulosis and related conditions of the skin, Cancer **19**:1231-1247, 1966.

74 del Regato, J. A.: Roentgen therapy of carcinoma of the skin of the eyelids, Radiology **52**:564-573, 1949.

74a del Regato, J. A.: Unpublished data, 1947.

75 del Regato, J. A., and Vuksanovic, M.: Radiotherapy of carcinomas of the skin overlying the cartilages of the nose and ear, Radiology **79**:203-208, 1962.

76 Roffo, A. H.: Cancer y sol, Bol. Inst. Med. Exp. Estud. Trat. Cancer **10**:417-439, 1933.

77 Ronchese, F.: Multiple benign epithelioma of scalp (turban tumors), Amer. J. Cancer **18**:875-887, 1933.

78 Rouvière, G.: Le xeroderma pigmentosum, Thesis, Faculty of Medicine of Toulouse, 1910.

79 Schrek, R.: Cutaneous carcinoma. IV. Analysis of 20 cases in Negroes, Cancer **4**:119-127, 1944.

80 Sequeira, J. H., and Vint, F. W.: Malignant melanoma in Africans, Brit. J. Derm. **46**:561-567, 1934.

81 Setala, K.: Calcifying epitheliomata of the skin (type malherbe); a new growth probably derived from the pilous tissue, Ann. Chir. Gynaec. Fenn. **37**:6-34, 1948.

82 Smith, C. C. K.: Metastasizing carcinoma of the sweat-glands, Brit. J. Surg. **43**:80-84, 1955.

83 Stout, A. P., and Gorman, J. G.: Mixed tumors of the skin of the salivary gland type, Cancer **12**:537-543, 1959.

84 Taylor, H. B., and Helwig, E. B.: Dermatofibrosarcoma protuberans; a study of 115 cases, Cancer **15**:717-725, 1962.

85 Taylor, G. W., Nathanson, I. T., and Shaw, D. T.: Epidermoid carcinoma of the extremities with reference to lymph node involvement, Ann. Surg. **113**:268-275, 1941.

86 Teloh, H.: Sweat-gland carcinoma, Cancer **8**:1003-1008, 1955.

87 Tori, G.: Studio clinico statisco sulla fisioterapie del cancro del padiglione auriculare, Radioterap. Radiobiol. Fis. Med. **8**:184-208, 1952.

88 Torrey, F. A., and Levin, E. A.: Comparison of clinical and pathologic diagnoses of malignant conditions of the skin, Arch. Derm. Syph. (Chicago) **43**:532-535, 1941.

89 Totten, R. S., Antypas, P. G., Dupertuis, S. M., Gaisford, J. C., and White, W. L.: Pre-existing roentgen-ray dermatitis in patients with skin cancer, Cancer **10**:1024-1030, 1957.

90 Treves, N., and Pack, G. T.: The development of cancer in burn scars; an analysis and report of 34 cases, Surg. Gynec. Obstet. **51**:749-782, 1930.

91 Tseng, W. P., Chu, H. M., How, S. W., Fong, J. M., Lin, C. S., and Yeh, S.: Prevalence of skin cancer in an endemic area of chronic arsenicism in Taiwan, J. Nat. Cancer Inst. **40**:453-463, 1968.

92 Unna, P. G.: Carcinom der Seemanshaut. In Die Histopathologie der Hautkrankheiten, Berlin, 1894, A. Hirschwald.

93 Walter, J.: On the treatment of cavernous haemangioma with special reference to spontaneous regression, J. Fac. Radiol. **5**:134-140, 1953.

94 Welton, W. A., and Helwig, E. G.: Adenomas and carcinomas of the sebaceous glands (to be published).

95 Wildermuth, O., and Evans, J. C.: The special problem of cancer of the eyelid, Cancer **9**:837-841, 1956.

96 Winer, L. H.: Pseudoepitheliomatous hyperplasia, Arch. Derm. Syph. (Chicago) **42**:856-867, 1942.

97 Witten, V. H., and Kopf, A. W.: Some common misconceptions regarding nevi and skin cancers, Med. Clin. N. Amer. **43**:731-752, 1959.

98 Yeh, S.: Relative incidence of skin cancer in Chinese in Taiwan; with special reference to arsenical cancer, Nat. Cancer Inst. Monogr. **10**:81-102, 1962.

99 Yeh, S., How, S. W., and Lin, C. S.: Arsenical cancer of skin; histologic study with special reference to Bowen's disease, Cancer **21**:312-339, 1968.

Malignant melanomas

This section is devoted exclusively to malignant melanomas of the skin. Malignant melanomas of the nasal fossa, oral cavity, bronchus, vagina, etc. are discussed in the corresponding sections or chapters.

Epidemiology

Malignant melanomas of the skin occur with equal frequency in individuals of both sexes, most often between 40 and 70 years of age. They are a rarity in children, but about forty-five such cases have been reported (Skov-Jensen et al.[66]; Lerman et al.[39]). These tumors also occur on the skin of black people (Morris and Horn[48]). At the Charity Hospital of New Orleans, where about half of the patients are black, Muelling[49] collected eighty cases of malignant melanomas of the skin, 25 of them in blacks. A greater incidence of melanomas of the skin is reported among South African Bantus than among American blacks (Shapiro et al.[65]). In Uganda Africans, malignant melanomas appear to be related to black discrete pigment spots on the soles of the feet (Lewis[40]; Kiryabwire et al.[33]). In India, the most common site of origin is the lower extremities, with a high percentage occurring on the sole of the foot (Sampat and Sirsat[61]). This is also true of the Bantu (Oettlé[53]) (Fig. 81). Hewer[25] reported forty-seven cases in black people of the Sudan, three-fourths of which developed in the lower extremity. There is an apparent relatively greater incidence of these tumors in Australia than in other countries (McGovern and Mackie[42]).

Malignant melanomas frequently arise from preexisting benign nevi. Trauma and chronic irritation may play a role in this transformation (Lea[36]). McGovern and Mackie[42] believe that dermic changes subsequent to chronic solar exposure may influence the development of these tumors in elderly persons. They rarely arise on the basis of xeroderma pigmentosum (Van Patter and Drummond[76]). They can be multiple (Kahn and Donaldson[31a]).

Pathology
Gross pathology

The benign nevus may have many diverse forms, ranging from flat to sessile to papillary (Fig. 82). Sometimes it is hairy,

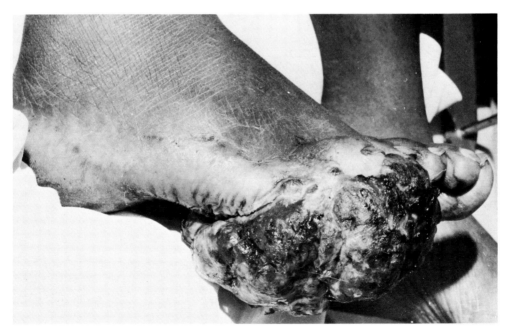

Fig. 81. Typical ulcerating melanoma occurring in commonest site in Bantu. (Courtesy Mr. J. A. Hunt, Johannesburg, South Africa; WU neg. 69-13 3823.)

and its color may vary from the normal shade of skin to coal black. The junctional nevus is flat, usually fawn-colored, and hairless and is most likely to undergo malignant change (Traub and Keil[73]).

The malignant melanoma has indefinite margins and is usually deeply pigmented, superficially ulcerated, and firm (Fig. 83). It is unusual to find it totally nonpigmented. Fingers of brownish black pigment may extend from the tumor and, as it grows, well-delineated, slightly elevated satellite nodules may be observed. The cut section of the tumor shows the extension to be much deeper and broader than its surface area might indicate.

The *freckle-type melanoma* of the skin tends to be superficial, spreading through the outer layers of the skin. The *subungual melanoma* is usually well demarcated beneath the nail bed limited by the fascial planes of the distal phalanx. This limitation of spread is similar to that in infection, hence the designation by Hutchinson[28] as "melanotic whitlow." Gibson et al.[23] reported thirty-eight cases of subungual melanoma, most of which developed under the fingernails. Two-thirds were found in a thumb or great toe.

Microscopic pathology

The microscopic appearance of the nevus may have several variants. Nevi are congenital malformations whose development is dependent on two components: the in-traepidermal melanoblasts and the nerves of the dermis (Masson[46]). The neval cells have different locations, and from their distribution various names have been given (Fig. 84).

The type of nevus that undergoes malignant change is called the junctional nevus (Fig. 85). In this type, the neval cells are both in the dermis and seemingly within the epidermis. There is excessive activity at the dermoepidermal junction. If the neval cells lie entirely within the dermis, it is called an intradermal nevus, a type that almost never undergoes malignant change. In a certain number of instances, both types appear in combination. In children, excessive activity is often seen at the dermoepidermal junction. For instance, in a review of 156 moles occurring in children, there were 100 (70%) that showed junctional change (Ackerman[1]).

The blue nevus is made up of interlacing strands of fibrous tissue associated with ribbonlike, melanin-containing cells in the dermis. Invariably an area of nonpigmented corium is present between the tumor and the epidermis. These lesions are usually small (about 1 cm) and may occur in the region of the sacrum, buttock, dorsum of the feet, ankles, toes, wrist, hands, and fingers.

The microscopic appearance of the melanocarcinoma is exceedingly variable. It

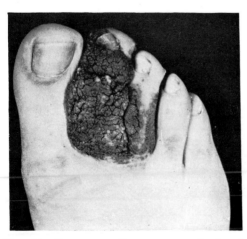

Fig. 82. Benign, papillary, pigmented, sharply demarcated nevus of toe.

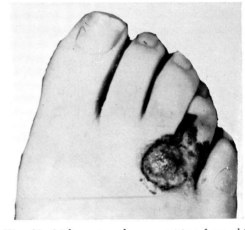

Fig. 83. Malignant melanoma arising from skin of toe with ulceration and typical sooty halo about periphery. Leg was amputated and radical inguinal dissection done. Patient died four months later with extensive metastases.

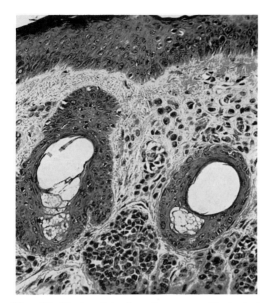

Fig. 84. Benign intradermal nevus with typical arrangement of neval cells in small clusters entirely in dermis. This type practically never undergoes malignant transformation.

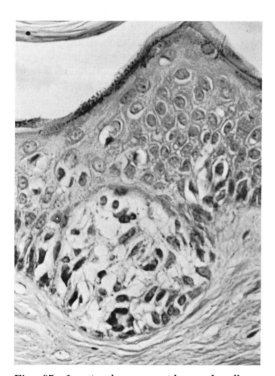

Fig. 85. Junctional nevus with neval cells at dermoepidermal junction. Great proportion of malignant melanomas arise from this type of nevus. (High power.)

may suggest a basal cell carcinoma, a fibrosarcoma, an epidermoid carcinoma, or a tumor of nerve origin (Fig. 86). If it is nonpigmented, it may be particularly difficult to diagnose. The amount of melanin varies but, when present, it is both within and outside the cells. In contrast to hemosiderin, which is golden yellow and forms large granules, melanin is rather finely granular and has a brown color. It is not unusual to find very large cells that bear a superficial resemblance to ganglion cells.

The greatest difficulty in microscopic diagnosis lies in certain early borderline lesions in which junctional changes are ob-

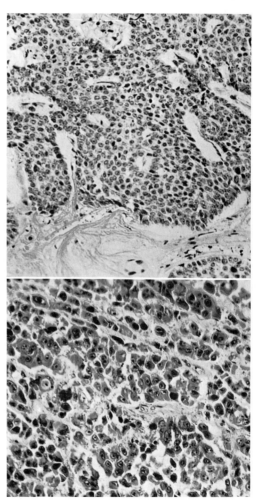

Fig. 86. Two different malignant melanomas with moderate but equal enlargement. Note dissimilar size of cells and histologic pattern, one superficially resembling basal cell carcinoma and other resembling tumor of nerve origin.

served (Ackerman[1]). The first changes suggesting malignancy include increase in size of the cells, prominence of the nucleus as related to the size of the cytoplasm, prominence of nucleoli, and, at times, the presence of mitotic figures. Invasion of the dermis by malignant-appearing cells is important evidence of malignant change in a junctional nevus. This change may be focal. In the presence of considerable pleomorphism, many abnormal mitotic figures, and invasion of lymphatics or blood vessels, the diagnosis is obvious.

Metastatic spread

In malignant melanoma of the skin, the regional lymph nodes are frequently involved. In addition, the tumor may metastasize widely to the lungs, liver, spleen, and practically any organ. In about half of all cases examined at autopsy, metastases

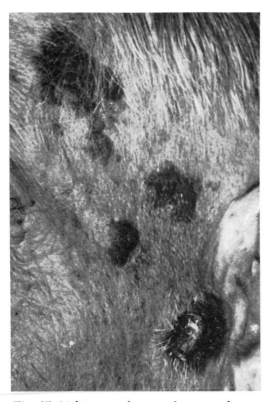

Fig. 87. Malignant melanoma of preauricular region arising from one of multiple benign nevi of skin of face. Lesion was excised and radical neck dissection done. Nodes were negative. Patient was living and well eight years after intervention.

are found in the heart. Bone metastases may pass clinically unnoticed, but routine investigation may reveal their occurrence (Wilner and Breckenridge[83]). Cases of transplacental metastases from mother to fetus have been reported (Reynolds[59]). Metastatic lesions vary in color from light pigmentation to sooty black.

Clinical evolution

About two-thirds of malignant melanomas of the skin arise from preexisting benign nevi (Webster et al.[80]). Many years may elapse before, explosively or insidiously, the benign nevus becomes malignant (Figs. 87 and 88). In some cases, there is a clear history of trauma or irritation (by belt, collar band, brassiere) preceding the malignant change. The most significant symptoms of malignant transformation are *sudden increase in rate of growth, darkening of pigmentation,* and *bleeding.*

The moles most likely to undergo malignant changes are those microscopically diagnosed as *junctional nevi.* They are usually flat, soft, dark brown, and hairless (Ackerman[1]). The black, hairless mole, however, is also dangerous. In children, moles only rarely become malignant. Large, hairy, black, congenital verrucous moles, the bathing trunk nevus (Conway[9]), the naevus unius lateris (Pack and Sunderland[56]), and the blue nevus (Allen and Spitz[2]) only very rarely undergo malignant transformation.

Malignant melanomas may develop from apparently normal skin. They are observed

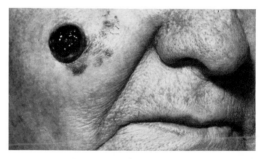

Fig. 88. Malignant melanoma of skin of cheek arising from pigmented melanotic freckle of Hutchinson that had been present for thirty years. (PCH 61-087.)

in fair-skinned persons who freckle easily and in "sandy-haired" individuals whose skin does not tan easily. In blacks, a history of previous mole is infrequent, and the melanomas usually develop in relatively nonpigmented areas such as the plantar surface of the foot (Pack et al.[55]).

Malignant melanomas are found most frequently on the lower extremities (Table 7) and on the face (Sylven and Hamberger[72]) and neck. *A persistent tumor on the plantar region of the foot, pigmented or nonpigmented, should be considered a malignant melanoma until proved otherwise.* This tumor often presents a history of previous inadequate treatment and is commonly diagnosed as a plantar wart or some inflammatory process before the true diagnosis is established.

The *melanotic freckle* is a superficial lesion usually of long duration (Hutchinson[27]; Dubreuilh[16]). It is usually found on the skin of the face of elderly persons as a series of confluent, variously pigmented, not well-defined giant freckles (Fig. 89). It may also be found on nonexposed areas of the skin (Jackson et al.[29]). Wayte and Helwig[79] reported eighty-five cases of melanotic freckle. Forty-five presented focal invasion, but metastases occurred in only four.

Table 7. History of preexisting mole in malignant melanoma*

Location of lesion	Lesions	% total lesions	Previous mole
Lower extremities	68	37	31
Head	62	33	30
Chest	25	14	15
Upper extremities	24	13	13
Trunk	6	3	3
Total	185	100	92

*From Ackerman, L. V.: Malignant melanoma of the skin, Texas J. Med. **45:**735-744, 1949.

Diagnosis

The strictly clinical diagnosis of pigmented lesions of the skin is associated with a high percentage of error. In a series of 151 malignant melanomas diagnosed microscopically (Becker[3]), the clinical diagnosis had been correct in only seventy-two (48%), whereas in 161 lesions diagnosed clinically as malignant melanomas, the diagnosis was microscopically confirmed in only seventy-two (43%). When the malignant melanoma is not pigmented, the proportion of errors is even greater. In the presence of a suspected lesion, a biopsy should be resorted to. There is no evidence that an incisional biopsy causes spread of malignant melanoma (Epstein et al.[19]). However, it is preferable to perform a wide excision when such an excision does not imply deformity or dysfunction.

Regional lymph node metastases may appear early. Das Gupta and McNeer[12] studied the distribution of regional lymph node metastases in reference to location of the primary lesion: from primary lesions of the scapular region, metastases occurred in the ipsilateral axilla and rarely in the cervical region, and from lesions below the eighth rib, the metastases occurred in the ipsilateral groin. Metastases seldom are found in the epitrochlear and popliteal nodes.

A thorough examination should include palpation of the liver, which is often the site of voluminous metastases. Radio-

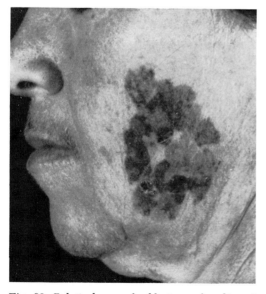

Fig. 89. Relatively rare freckle type of malignant melanoma with superficial character. Lesion was excised and radical neck dissection done. Nodes were negative. Patient was living and well eight years after operation. This type of malignant melanoma does not require prophylactic regional node dissection.

graphic examination of the lungs should be routine. The radiographic diagnosis of the presence or absence of lymph node metastases by means of lymphangiography is notably unreliable (Cox et al.[10]). Metastatic melanoma from unsuspected primary lesions may cause symptoms capable of suggesting a host of conditions of the respiratory, gastrointestinal, nervous, and other systems. There is some evidence (Smith and Stehlin[67]) that a certain proportion of malignant melanomas of all sites of origin may undergo spontaneous regression and disappearance so as to be unidentifiable even at autopsy. Such possibility should be kept in mind. The taking of an adequate history is the best safeguard against important errors in diagnosis. Because several cases of malignant melanoma have been known to develop in several members of the same family, it is a good measure to examine the close relatives of the patient (Turkington[75]).

Differential diagnosis

Malignant melanomas may be confused with many other pigmented lesions of the skin. Pigmentation may be due either to melanin or to some other pigment such as hemosiderin.

Infected, ulcerating *hemangiomas* may exactly simulate melanoma. *Seborrheic keratoses*, particularly when infected and heavily impregnated with melanin pigment, may be difficult to distinguish from melanoma except on pathologic examination. This is also true of the *pigmented basal cell carcinoma*. The lesion variously known as sclerosing hemangioma (Gross and Wolbach[24]; Dawson[13]) or *dermatofibroma lenticulare*, or *histiocytoma* but best designated as *subepidermal nodular fibrosis* (Rentiers and Montgomery[58]) may be misinterpreted as a melanoma both grossly and microscopically (Black et al.[55]). Pigmented *epidermoid carcinomas* of the skin (Stewart and Bonser[70]; Lennox[38]), *Kaposi's sarcoma*, and various pigmented lesions may also be clinically confused with malignant melanomas.

The *spindle cell nevus* in a child is often confused with malignant melanoma (Spitz[68]). The lesion is usually elevated, highly vascularized, and under 1 cm in diameter (Figs. 90 to 92). Echevarria and Ackerman[18] have observed over thirty such cases. They have been called *juvenile melanoma*, but this is a poor term, for it suggests a malignant lesion to clinicians. A preferable designation would be spindle cell and epithelioid cell nevus. In a review of 2600 nevi, there were 430 malignant melanomas and twenty-seven spindle cell and epithelioid cell nevi (Kernen and Ackerman[32]). These nevi can occur rarely in adults.

Blue nevi may be confused clinically with malignant melanomas. Rodriguez and Ackerman[60] studied forty-five large, cellular, blue nevi (Fig. 93). The majority of the patients were in their twenties, and thirty-one were females. More than half of the lesions were located in the buttocks, and none was malignant. Blue nevi also occur on the skin near the hairline of the scalp.

Treatment
Prevention

It is impractical and unwarranted to remove all benign nevi of the skin to prevent their malignant transformation. The average adult has fifteen to twenty such lesions. But it is fruitful to excise certain nevi on the basis of location and other considerations. Any nevus should be removed that is subject to chronic irritation by collar, belt, or shoe or to infection. Junctional nevi of the genitals are better removed. Junctional nevi of the palm of the hand and sole of the foot (Allen and Spitz[2])

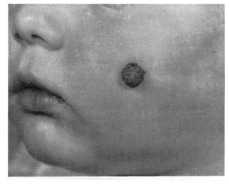

Fig. 90. Spindle cell nevus in young child. It was red and elevated and measured 1 cm × 1 cm. (From Kernen, J. A., and Ackerman, L. V.: Spindle cell nevi and epithelioid cell nevi [so-called juvenile melanomas] in children and adults, Cancer 13:612-625, 1960; WU neg. 61-988).

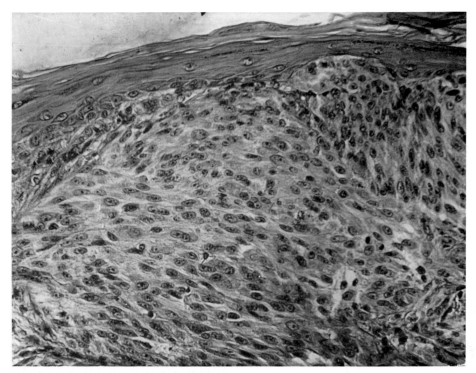

Fig. 91. Spindle cell nevus in 1½-year-old child. Note elongated fusiform cells with uniform nuclei. (×300; WU neg. 58-125.)

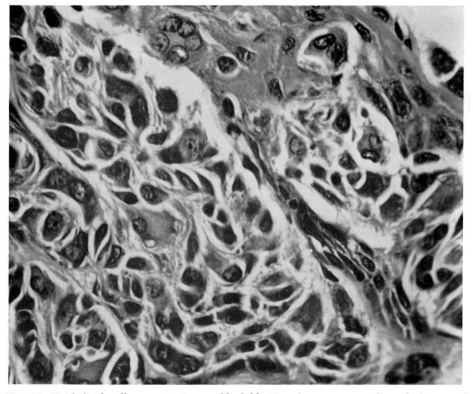

Fig. 92. Epithelioid cell nevus in 9-year-old child. Note bizarre giant cells and absence of mitotic figures. (×600; WU neg. 52-4082.)

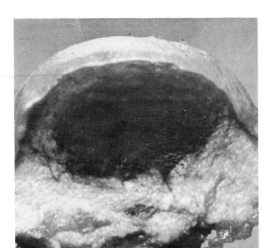

Fig. 93. Large, cellular, blue nevus occurring in buttock of young girl. (WU neg. 55-3892.)

show a very low rate of malignant transformation (Wilson and Anderson[84]), and thus their removal is not advisable (Van Scott et al.[77]) on a prophylactic basis.

Incomplete removal of a junctional nevus may be followed by a regrowth of the pigmented cells around the scar. Such recurrences do not imply malignant change (Schoenfeld and Pinkus[64]). Although spindle cell and epithelioid cell nevi, of children or adults, do not undergo malignant transformation, they should be removed by conservative surgical excision (Kopf[34]).

Surgery

In the treatment of malignant melanomas of the skin, a wide surgical excision is the treatment of choice. A radical excision, in surface and in depth, often requires a skin graft to fill the defect. A careful examination before surgery should look for the possibility of satellite nodules that should be included in the excision. Cautery excisions offer no advantage and spoil the possibility of an adequate histopathologic study of the specimen. An inadequate excision may be revealed by careful microscopic study. Local recurrences may occur even after radical excisions (Fig. 94).

In extensive lesions, particularly of the

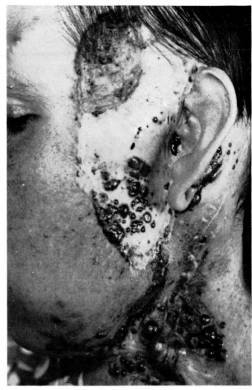

Fig. 94. Innumerable skin recurrences and cervical lymph node metastases following wide excision and neck dissection for malignant melanoma of skin of face. Tumor can be seen growing through grafted skin.

lower extremity, where a wide excision is compromised at some point, an amputation is indicated and preferable. Whenever a wide excision of a melanoma of the skin of the foot would result in impairment of pedal function, a midleg amputation should be preferred. Similarly, amputations of fingers or toes is the approach of choice in subungual melanomas.

Because of their occasional dissemination through the lymphatics of the skin, it has been recommended that these tumors be excised en bloc with the overlying skin and the regional lymphatic nodes. When the primary lesion and the draining nodes are in close proximity, an en bloc dissection is indicated (Raven[57]). When the primary lesion is located at a considerable distance from its corresponding lymph nodes, as lesions of the foot are from the inguinal region, we feel that such dissection cannot be of any particular value in-as much as metastases also occur through deep lymphatics.

Therapeutic lymphatic dissection. An excision of the involved nodes, when they are located in an area of immediate lymphatic drainage, is definitely indicated provided, of course, there are no distant metastases. This dissection is most successful in tumors of the skin of the head, which metastasize to the cervical lymph nodes. The therapeutic dissection of the inguinal nodes is seldom successful because deep inguinal and often iliac node metastases are almost invariably present. Even a hemipelvectomy is unwarranted, for invariably there is involvement beyond the lymph nodes encompassed by the operation.

Prophylactic* lymphatic dissection. When the tumor is located in an area from which the lymphatic drainage is predictable, a radical dissection of the anticipated metastatic node areas used to be considered mandatory in spite of the fact that the nodes did not appear clinically involved. It is granted that if a patient develops a malignant melanoma in the midline of the anterior or posterior chest, it would be impossible to predict the node-draining areas, and prophylactic node dissection would not be indicated. The number of times that a prophylactic dissection turns out to be a therapeutic dissection is not well established in the literature.

Palpation of the axilla in search of metastatic nodes is notoriously inaccurate. It would appear that there is greater justification for prophylactic dissection of the axillary nodes than nodes in other areas. Nicolle et al.[51] studied the relationship of the depth of infiltration of the malignant melanoma of the skin and the occurrence of regional lymph node metastases. In lesions that had been only widely excised and had no clinically detectable adenop-

athy, half of the patients developed metastases when the primary tumor was found infiltrating beyond the superficial sweat glands. This apparently logical concept remains to be verified.

Sandeman[62] has presented convincing evidence that prophylactic lymph node dissection does not increase the cure rate in patients with malignant melanoma. His five-year survival rate in those with lymph node dissection is 28%, and in the patients who were only observed, the rate was 57%. Olsen[54] also follows this principle and does not advocate prophylactic dissection. Her experience is based on more than 900 cases. Sandeman[62] believes that there is no disadvantage in waiting until the metastatic nodes become clinically ostensible to institute surgical treatment.

Radiotherapy

Malignant melanomas of the skin have long been categorized as "radioresistant" tumors. We have been surprised to observe that not only are they often responsive to irradiation, but also may be remarkably radiosensitive and locally radiocurable. Some have advocated radiotherapy for the treatment of metastases (Hilaris et al.[26]; Sandeman[63]) (Fig. 95) or as a postoperative adjuvant (Dickson[15]; Nitter[52]). If this latter course were substantiated, it is likely that radiotherapy might prove to be of greater value as a preoperative measure. Jørgsholm and Engdahl[31] have proposed that radiotherapy be used as a palliative measure whenever surgery cannot be carried out by virtue of location, extent, or age of the patient. We have irradiated with an aim to cure one unquestionable malignant melanoma of the skin of the temporal region involving the outer canthus, with dark pigmentation and raised indurated areas. The lesion has entirely disappeared, and more than five years later there are no residual pigmentation, sequelae, or metastases.

Chemotherapy

Systemic administration of drugs has brought very poor response from these tumors. Notable cases of regression and unquestionable palliation have been brought about by regional perfusion of drugs in concentrations that would not be permis-

---

*The word prophylactic as used here does not, of course, mean preventive, but simply treatment administered early when the metastases, if present, are still in a subclinical stage and not clinically apparent. The word elective is neither a good substitute nor any more accurate. It only means that one might or might not *choose* to do the procedure. When the prophylactic dissection is not carried out *systematically*, it may be proper to say that a patient received an elective prophylactic dissection.

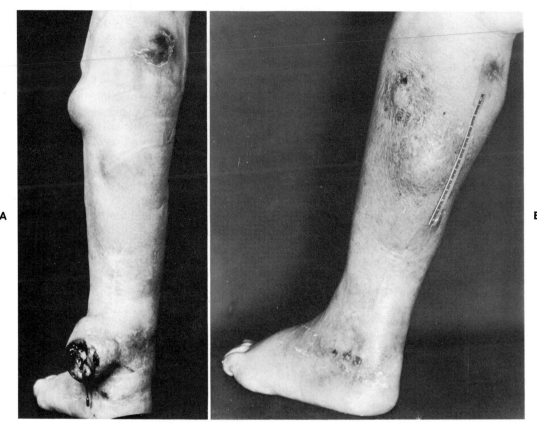

Fig. 95. A, Skin metastases from malignant melanoma before treatment with interstitial irradiation. **B,** One year after completion of interstitial irradiation. (From Hilaris, B. S., et al.: Value of radiation therapy for distant metastases from malignant melanoma, Cancer 16:765-773, 1963.)

sible in systemic administration (Stehlin and Clark[69]; Creech and Krementz[11]). Favorable results have also been observed by combination of the effects of chemotherapy and radiotherapy (Falkson et al.[20]) and of chemotherapy and surgery (Stehlin and Clark[69]).

Prognosis

The undisturbed clinical course of malignant melanoma of the skin is usually swift and fatal, but unpredictable exceptions have been observed. Cases of long survival in spite of visceral metastases defy rationalization. More baffling yet are the cases of spontaneous regression and even of spontaneous healing of the primary lesion (Smith and Stehlin[67]). Treatment of advanced cases has occasionally been accompanied by unexpected results that the

uninformed or unsuspecting may attribute to the particular features of the treatment employed.

Lewis et al.[40a] demonstrated autoantibodies in patients with malignant melanoma. For the most part, these autoantibodies were confined to those in whom the disease was well localized. In a limited number of patients who had been followed, autoantibodies disappeared as the disease became widely disseminated.

In the evaluation of results of treatment of malignant melanomas of the skin, it is important first to eliminate from any group of cases the benign pigmented lesions which may have been histologically mistaken for malignant melanomas (Truax et al.[74]): atypical nevi, cellular and giant blue nevi, spindle cell and epithelioid cell nevi (so-called juvenile melanoma), and superficial malignant melanoma without invasion of the dermis.

Patients with malignant melanomas of the skin may be divided into four groups in regard to prognosis:

1 Those with distant metastases when first seen are hopeless and live between one and one-half to three years.

2 Those with clinically obvious regional metastatic adenopathy have a prognosis of less than 10% for a five-year survival.

3 Those without clinically ostensible adenopathy whose nodes are proved to contain microscopic evidence of metastases have a fair prognosis of 15% to 25%.

4 Those with microscopically negative lymph nodes have an excellent prognosis of 50% to 60% for a five-year survival.

The foregoing considerations presuppose adequate radical surgical treatment.

In a series of 341 patients reported upon by Sylven,[71] only 291 of which were eligible for curative treatment, ninety-one (35%) were living and well after five years. Kragh and Erich[35] reported on a series of eighty-five patients with malignant melanomas of the skin of the head and cervical regions, with a five-year survival of 49% after surgical treatment of primary and secondary manifestations. Fortner et al.[22] had a five-year survival of 35% in a series of 194 patients with *operable* malignant melanomas of the skin. The rate was 19% for those who were found to have involved nodes (109) and 55% for those without metastatic adenopathy (eighty-five).

The usefulness of prophylactic dissections is difficult to ascertain (Johnson[30]; Block and Hartwell[6]). Retrospective studies may yield paradoxical results (Sandeman[62]). It is obvious that this question can only be resolved by a properly controlled prospective clinical trial. In 243 patients with malignant melanoma of the skin treated with an aim to cure at the Massachussetts General Hospital, the five-year and ten-year survival rates for patients undergoing prophylactic node dissections were 77% and 64%, respectively, for patients with negative nodes and 59% and 38% for those with positive nodes.

McPeak and Constantinides[44] reported on the results of amputation of the lower extremity in patients who were not eligible for any other approach. A preoperative exploration established whether or not there was involvement beyond the scope of amputation. Of forty-six patients so carefully chosen, there were fifteen free of disease (30%) five years after operation. The results of groin dissection on patients with positive nodes vary considerably. Fortner et al.[21] had a five-year survival rate of over 20%. It appears that radiotherapy judiciously applied may be successful in the treatment of metastases. Sandeman[63] reported ten patients surviving five years in a series of thirty-seven cases irradiated.

Shingleton[65a] reported on thirty-five patients with malignant melanoma of the skin and subcutaneous tissues, a majority of whom presented lymph node metastases. Following treatment with perfusion of phenylalanine mustard, fourteen patients survived two years and four were apparently disease free after five years.

Certain factors automatically confer an unfavorable prognosis to malignant melanoma of the skin, such as the site of origin, mostly because of the variety or gravity of lymphatic drainage. The outlook of melanomas of the skin of the lower extremities is worse than that of those of the upper extremity. The rare case of malignant melanoma of the skin of children has a very poor prognosis. Previous inadequate treatment followed by recurrence, and consequent delay, result in unfavorable prognosis. Lymph node metastases of the inguinal region have a very poor prognosis (Booher and Pack[7]) even when very radical procedures are instituted (McPeak et al.[45]).

Conversely, melanomas of the skin of the face, which are diagnosed earlier, and their cervical lymph node metastases have a relatively favorable prognosis. Lesions that prove to have very superficial infiltration (Lund and Ihnen[41]; Nicolle et al.[51]; Decosse and McNeer[14]) are cured in greater proportions. Women with these tumors have a better prognosis (Lehman et al.[37]; Watson[78]), and they seem to suffer no deleterious effects from pregnancy (White et al.[82]).

Subungual melanoma of the skin have a

more fortunate outlook. The so-called freckle type of malignant melanoma must be separated from superficial melanoma, because the freckle type has a much better prognosis (Clark and Mihm[8]).

REFERENCES

1 Ackerman, L. V.: Malignant melanoma of the skin, Amer. J. Clin. Path. **18**:602-604, 1948.
2 Allen, A. C., and Spitz, S.: Malignant melanoma; a clinico-pathologic analysis of the criteria for diagnosis and prognosis, Cancer **6**:1-45, 1953.
3 Becker, S. W.: Pitfalls in the diagnosis and treatment of 151 malignant melanomas, Arch. Derm. Syph. (Chicago) **69**:11-30, 1954.
4 Biology of melanomas—Special publication of New York Academy of Sciences, 1948.
5 Black, W. C., McGavran, M. H., and Graham, P.: Nodular subepidermal fibrosis, Arch. Surg. (Chicago) **98**:296-300, 1969.
6 Block, G. E., and Hartwell, S. W.: Malignant melanoma, Ann. Surg. **154**:88-101, 1962.
7 Booher, R. J., and Pack, G. T.: Malignant melanoma of the feet and hands, Surgery **42**:1084-1121, 1957.
8 Clark, W. H., Jr., and Mihm, M. C., Jr.: Lentigo maligna and lentigo-maligna melanoma, Amer. J. Path. **51**:39-67, 1969.
9 Conway, Herbert: Bathing trunk nevus, Surgery **6**:585-597, 1939.
10 Cox, K. R., Hare, W. S. C., and Bruce, P. T.: Lymphography in melanoma; correlation of radiology with pathology, Cancer **19**:637-647, 1966.
11 Creech, O., and Krementz, E. T.: Regional perfusion in melanoma of limbs, J.A.M.A. **188**:855-858, 1964.
12 Das Gupta, T., and McNeer, G.: The incidence of metastasis to accessible lymph nodes from melanoma of the trunk and extremities—its therapeutic significance, Cancer **17**:897-911, 1964.
13 Dawson, E. K.: Sclerosing angioma; a non-melanotic pigment tumor of the skin, Edinburgh Med. J. **55**:655-674, 1948.
14 DeCosse, J. J., and McNeer, G.: Superficial melanoma, Arch. Surg. (Chicago) **99**:531-534, 1969.
15 Dickson, R. J.: Malignant melanoma; a combined surgical and radiotherapeutic approach, Amer. J. Roentgen. **79**:1063-1070, 1958.
16 Dubreuilh, W.: De la melanose circonscrite precancereuse, Ann. Derm. Syph. (Paris) 3 (5th ser.):129-204, 1912.
17 Dubreuilh, W.: De la melanose circonscrite precancereuse. I. Melanose conjonctivale et palpebrale, Ann. Derm. Syph. (Paris) 3(5th ser.):205-230, 1912.
18 Echevarria, R., and Ackerman, L. V.: Spindle and epithelioid cell nevi in the adult; clinico-pathologic report of 26 cases, Cancer **20**:175-189, 1967.
19 Epstein, E., Bragg, K., and Linden, G.: Biopsy and prognosis of malignant melanoma, J.A.M.A. **208**:1369-1371, 1969.
20 Falkson, G., deVilliers, P. C., Falkson, H. C., and Fichardt, T.: Natulan (Procarbazine) combined with radiotherapy in management of inoperable malignant melanoma, Brit. Med. J. **2**:1473-1474, 1965.
21 Fortner, J. G., Booher, R. J., and Pack, G. T.: Results of groin dissection for malignant melanoma in 220 patients, Surgery **55**:485-494, 1964.
22 Fortner, J. G., Das Gupta, T., and McNeer, G.: Primary malignant melanoma on the trunk; an analysis of 194 cases, Ann. Surg. **161**:161-169, 1965.
23 Gibson, S. H., Montgomery, H., Woolner, L. B., and Brunsting, L. A.: Melanotic whitlow (subungual melanoma), J. Invest. Derm. **29**:119-129, 1957.
24 Gross, R. E., and Wolbach, S. B.: Sclerosing hemangiomas; their relationship to dermatofibroma, histiocytoma, xanthoma and to certain pigmented lesions of the skin, Amer. J. Path. **19**:533-551, 1943.
25 Hewer, T. F.: Malignant melanoma in coloured races; the role of trauma in its causation, J. Path. Bact. **41**:473-477, 1935.
26 Hilaris, B. S., Raben, M., Calabrese, A. S., Phillips, R. F., and Henschke, U. K.: Value of radiation therapy for distant metastases from malignant melanoma, Cancer **16**:765-773, 1963.
27 Hutchinson, J.: Lentigo-melanosis; a further report, Arch. Surg. (London) **5**:253-256, 1894.
28 Hutchinson, J.: Melanosis often not black; melanotic whitlow, Brit. Med. J. **1**:491, 1886.
29 Jackson, R., Williamson, G. S., and Beattie, W. G.: Lentigo meligna and malignant melanoma, Canad. Med. Ass. J. **95**:846-851, 1966.
30 Johnson, R. E.: Occult lymphatic metastases in malignant melanoma of the skin, Ann. Surg. **146**:931-936, 1957.
31 Jørgsholm, B., and Engdahl, I.: Malignant melanoma, Acta Radiol. (Stockholm) **44**:417-433, 1955.
31a Kahn, L. B., and Donaldson, R. C.: Multiple primary melanoma; case report and study of tumor growth in vitro, Cancer **25**:1162-1169, 1970.
32 Kernen, J. A., and Ackerman, L. V.: Spindle cell nevi and epithelioid cell nevi (so-called juvenile melanomas) in children and adults; a clinicopathologic study of 27 cases, Cancer **13**:612-625, 1960.
33 Kiryabwire, J. W. M., Lewis, M. G., Ziegler, J. L., and Loefler, I.: Malignant melanoma in Uganda, E. Afr. Med. J. **45**:498-507, 1968.
34 Kopf, A. W., and Andrade, R.: Benign juvenile melanoma. In The year book of dermatology 1965-1966 (Kopf, A. W., and Andrade, R., editors), Chicago, 1966, Year Book Medical Publishers, Inc.
35 Kragh, L. V., and Erich, J. B.: Malignant melanomas of the head and neck, Ann. Surg. **151**:91-96, 1960.
36 Lea, A. J.: Malignant melanoma of the skin; the relationship to trauma, Ann. Roy. Coll. Surg. Eng. **37**:169-176, 1965.
37 Lehman, J. A., Jr., Cross, F. S., and Richey,

W. G.: Clinical study of forty-nine patients with malignant melanoma, Cancer 19:611-619, 1966.

38 Lennox, B.: Pigment patterns in epithelial tumors of the skin, J. Path. Bact. 61:587-598, 1949.

39 Lerman, R. I., Murray, D., O'Hara, J. M., Booher, R. J., and Foote, F. W.: Malignant melanoma of childhood; a clinicopathologic study and a report of 12 cases, Cancer 25: 436-449, 1970.

40 Lewis, M. G.: Malignant melanoma in Uganda (the relationship between pigmentation and malignant melanoma on the soles of the feet), Brit. J. Cancer 21:483-495, 1967.

40a Lewis, M. G., Ikonopisov, R. L., Nairn, R. C., Philips, T. M., Fairley, G. H., Bodenham, D. C., and Alexander, P.: Tumour-specific antibodies in human malignant melanoma and their relationship to the extent of the disease, Brit. Med. J. 3:547-552, 1969.

41 Lund, R. H., and Ihnen, M.: Malignant melanoma, Surgery 38:652-659, 1955.

42 McGovern, V. J., and Mackie, B. S.: The relationship of solar radiation to melanoblastoma, Aust. New Zeal. J. Surg. 28:257-262, 1959.

43 McNeer, G., and Das Gupta, T.: Life history of melanoma, Amer. J. Roentgen. 93:686-694, 1965.

44 McPeak, C. J., and Constantinides, S. G.: Lymphangiography in malignant melanoma, Cancer 17:1586-1594, 1964.

45 McPeak, C. J., McNeer, G. P., Whiteley, H. W., and Booher, R. J.: Amputation for melanoma of the extremity, Surgery 54:426-431, 1963.

46 Masson, P.: Les naevi pigmentaires; tumeurs nerveuses, Ann. Anat. Path. (Paris) 3:417-453, 657-696, 1926.

47 Masson, P.: My concept of cellular nevi, Cancer 4:9-38, 1951.

48 Morris, G. C., and Horn, R. C.: Malignant melanoma in the Negro, Surgery 29:223-230, 1951.

49 Muelling, R. J.: Malignant melanoma, a comparative study of the incidence in the Negro race, Milit. Surg. 103:359-364, 1948.

50 Mundth, E. D., Guralnick, E. A., and Raker, J. W.: Malignant melanoma; a clinical study of 427 cases, Ann. Surg. 162:15-28, 1965.

51 Nicolle, F. V., Mathews, W. H., and Palmer, J. D.: Treatment of malignant melanomas of the skin, Arch. Surg. (Chicago) 93:209-214, 1966.

52 Nitter, L.: The treatment of malignant melanoma with special reference to the possible effect of radiotherapy, Acta Radiol. (Stockholm) 46:547-562, 1956.

53 Oettlé, A. G.: Epidemiology of melanomas in South Africa. Symposium on Structure and control of the melanocyte, Sixth International Pigment Cell Conference; Berlin/Heidelberg/New York, 1966, Springer-Verlag, pp. 292-308.

54 Olsen, G.: The malignant melanoma of the skin; new theories based on a study of 500 cases, Danish Med. Bull. 14:229-238, 1967.

55 Pack, G. T., Davis, J., and Oppenheim, A.: The relation of race and complexion to the incidence of moles and melanomas, Ann. N. Y. Acad. Sci. 100:719-742, 1963.

56 Pack, G. T., and Sunderland, D. A.: Naevus unius lateris, Arch. Surg. (Chicago) 43:341-375, 1941.

57 Raven, R. W.: The properties and surgical problems of malignant melanoma, Ann. Roy. Coll. Surg. Eng. 6:28-55, 1950.

57a del Regato, J. A.: The training of therapeutic radiologists (editorial), Radiology 95:703-704, 1970.

58 Rentiers, P. L., and Montgomery, H.: Nodular subepidermal fibrosis (dermatofibroma versus histiocytoma), Arch. Derm. Syph. (Chicago) 59:568-583, 1949.

59 Reynolds, A. G.: Placental metastases from malignant melanoma, Obstet. Gynec. 6:205-209, 1955.

60 Rodriguez, H. A., and Ackerman, L. V.: Cellular blue nevus; a clinicopathologic study of 45 cases, Cancer 21:393-405, 1968.

61 Sampat, M. B., and Sirsat, M. V.: Malignant melanoma of the skin and mucous membranes in Indians, Indian J. Cancer 3:228-254, 1966.

62 Sandeman, T. F.: Treat or watch? An evaluation of elective treatments of clinically uninvolved nodes in malignant melanoma, Med. J. Aust. 1:42-46, 1965.

63 Sandeman, T. F.: The radical treatment of enlarged lymph nodes in malignant melanoma, Amer. J. Roentgen. 97:967-979, 1966.

64 Schoenfeld, R. J., and Pinkus, H.: The recurrence of nevi after incomplete removal, Arch. Derm. (Chicago) 78:30-35, 1958.

65 Shapiro, M. P., Keen, P., Cohen, L., and Murray, J. F.: Skin cancer in the African Bantu, Brit. J. Cancer 7:45-47, 1953.

65a Shingleton, W. W.: Perfusion chemotherapy for recurrent melanoma of extremity; a progress report, Ann. Surg. 169:969-973, 1969.

66 Skov-Jensen, T., Hastrup, J., and Lambrethsen, E.: Malignant melanomas in children, Cancer 19:620-626, 1966.

67 Smith, J. L., Jr., and Stehlin, J. S., Jr.: Spontaneous regression of primary malignant melanomas with regional metastases, Cancer 18: 1399-1415, 1965.

68 Spitz, S.: Melanomas of childhood, Amer. J. Path. 24:591-619, 1948.

69 Stehlin, J. S., Jr., and Clark, R. L.: Melanoma of the extremities; experiences with conventional treatment and perfusion in 339 cases, Amer. J. Surg. 110:366-383, 1965.

70 Stewart, M. J., and Bonser, G. M.: Melanin-forming epidermal tumours of the skin; a study of 57 personally observed cases, J. Path. Bact. 60:21-33, 1948.

71 Sylven, B.: Malignant melanoma of the skin; report of 341 cases treated during the years 1929-1943, Acta Radiol. (Stockholm) 32:33-59, 1949.

72 Sylven, B., and Hamberger, C. A.: Malignant melanoma of the external ear, Ann. Otol. 59: 631-647, 1950.

73 Traub, E. F., and Keil, H.: "Common mole";

its clinico-pathologic relations and question malignant degeneration, Arch. Derm. Syph. (Chicago) 41:214-252, 1940.

74 Truax, H., Barnett, R. N., Hukill, P. B., Campbell, P. C., and Eisenberg, H.: Effect of inaccurate pathological diagnosis on survival statistics for melanoma, Cancer 19:1543-1547, 1966.

75 Turkington, R. W.: Familial factor in malignant melanoma, J.A.M.A. 192:77-82, 1965.

76 Van Patter, H. T., and Drummond, J. A.: Malignant melanoma occurring in xeroderma pigmentosum; report of a case, Cancer 6:942-947, 1953.

77 Van Scott, E. J., Reinertson, R. P., and McCall, C. B.: Prevalence, histological types, and significance of palmar and plantar nevi, Cancer 10:363-367, 1953.

78 Watson, E. C.: Melanoma; a ten-year retrospective survey in New Zealand, Aust. New Zeal. J. Surg. 33:31-46, 1963.

79 Wayte, D. M., and Helwig, E. B.: Melanotic freckle of Hutchinson, Cancer 21:893-911, 1968.

80 Webster, J. P., Stevenson, T. W., and Stout, A. P.: Symposium on reparative surgery; the surgical treatment of malignant melanomas of the skin, Surg. Clin. N. Amer. 24:319-339, 1944.

81 White, L. P.: Studies on melanoma. II. Sex and survival in human melanoma, New Eng. J. Med. 260:789-797, 1959.

82 White, L. P., Linden, G., Breslow, L., and Harzfeld, L.: Studies on melanoma; the effect of pregnancy on survival in human melanoma, J.A.M.A. 177:235-238, 1961.

83 Wilner, D., and Breckenridge, R. L.: Bone metastasis in malignant melanoma, Amer. J. Roentgen. 62:388-394, 1949.

84 Wilson, F. C., Jr., and Anderson, P. C.: A dissenting view on the prophylactic removal of plantar and palmar nevi, Cancer 14:102-104, 1961.

Chapter 7

Cancer of the respiratory system and upper digestive tract

Nasal fossae
Maxillary sinus
Oral cavity
Nasopharynx

Oropharynx
Laryngopharynx (hypopharynx)
Endolarynx
Lung

Nasal fossae

Anatomy

The nasal fossae are roughly pyramidal spaces, one on each side of the nasal septum, opening externally through the anterior nares and communicating posteriorly with the nasopharynx through the choanae, laterally with the maxillary sinuses, and superiorly with the sphenoid sinus, the ethmoid cells, and the frontal sinuses (Fig. 96).

Physiologically and clinically, the nasal fossa is divided into a lower or respiratory portion comprising the inferior meatus, middle meatus, inferior turbinate, and free border of the middle turbinate and an upper or olfactory portion above these structures.

The lower or *respiratory* portion of the nasal fossa, which is richly vascularized and through which air circulates, is covered by a cylindrical cell ciliated epithelium, the so-called respiratory epithelium. The cells have a distinct basement membrane, goblet cells that secrete mucus are interspersed, and lymphoid tissue is found, but its density is not very marked except near the posterior choanae. Sparse pigmented cells are found in the submucosa. Metaplasia of the cylindrical epithelium toward squamous epithelium is very commonly found.

The upper or *olfactory* portion of the nasal fossa lies above a hypothetical horizontal line passing at the level of the free border of the middle turbinate. This is a narrow space through which air does not circulate. It is not as well vascularized and is rich in yellow pigment, the locus luteus. The olfactory nerve distributes its fine fibrils over this area.

Lymphatics. The *anterior* lymphatics follow a forward direction, pass between the cartilages to reach the teguments of the face, and become continuous with the superficial lymphatics of the skin of the nose and cheek. The *posterior* lymphatics gather into three main trunks:

1 An upper group, which drains the superior turbinates and leads to the retropharyngeal lymph nodes
2 A middle group, which drains the lower turbinate and lower meatus and passes under the eustachian tube to end in the deep nodes of the internal jugular chain
3 A lower group, which includes most of the lymphatic drainage of the floor of the nasal fossae and septum, that follows the direction of the soft palate and joins the lymphatics of the tonsil to terminate in the lymphatics of the anterior jugular chain (Fig. 97)

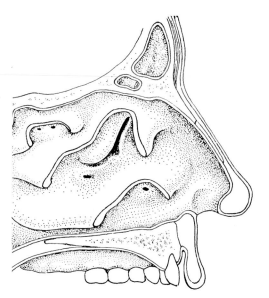

Fig. 96. Lateral view of nasal fossa. Parts of turbinates have been removed to demonstrate openings that establish communication with maxillary sinus and frontal sinus.

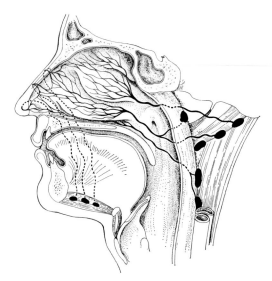

Fig. 97. Lymphatics of nasal fossa. Anterior lymphatics lead to submaxillary lymph nodes. Posterior lymphatics are drained by retropharyngeal and anterior jugular nodes.

Epidemiology

Benign and malignant tumors of the nasal fossae are rare, and even an approximate incidence cannot be computed since the cases have been so very sporadically reported.

Malignant tumors of the nasal fossa are found in men as well as in women, but the proportion in women seems to be slightly larger than that generally found for cancer of the upper air passages. Only 113 cases of malignant tumors of the nasal fossae were seen at the Memorial Hospital for Cancer and Allied Diseases in New York during a period of twenty years (Frazell and Lewis[14]). The number of these tumors seen in hospitals in certain areas of Africa seems unquestionably higher (Clifford[10]). In particular, there seems to be a high occurrence of melanomas (Lewis and Martin[26]).

Pathology

Gross and microscopic pathology

Although tumors of the nasal fossae are relatively rare, this region is the site of origin for a variety of benign and malignant tumors, the histogenesis of which may be quite difficult to establish.

The most common growths are *polyps.*

These are usually associated with inflammatory lesions but may accompany malignant tumors of the nasal fossae and accessory sinuses. Nasal polyps are usually fibroepithelial tumors arising from the lower turbinate. They are characteristically pedunculated, and about half are ulcerated. The bulk of the tumor is formed by loose edematous connective tissue, but sometimes it may present cystic dilatations, which may lead to an erroneous diagnosis of cystadenoma. Pyogenic granuloma and squamous papillomas occur most frequently just within the nasal fossa. They are usually inflammatory and are found most often in men in the fourth decade of life. *Hemangiomas* arise from the septum and the lower turbinate. They have the shiny, bluish appearance of hemangiomas developing under mucous membrane.

Extramedullary *plasmacytomas* are rare tumors. Hellwig[19] found only 127 cases reported between 1905 and 1942. The majority of these tumors seem to arise in the nasal fossae and accessory sinuses and to occur in men 40 to 70 years of age. Stout and Kenny[38] collected a total of 104 cases, of which eighty-six had a known single site of origin, forty-eight arising in the nasal cavity, nasopharynx, and nasal sinuses.

Astacio et al.[3] reported the presence of plasma cell myeloma following rhinoscleroma. Chronic inflammatory lesions may contain large numbers of plasma cells and may be erroneously diagnosed as plasmacytomas. In the benign processes, however, there is usually an intermingling of plasma cells with other inflammatory cells, and the presence of Russell bodies in the cytoplasm of plasma cells (eosinophilic hyaline droplets) is more often seen in benign than in malignant lesions. Lesions in which there is no actual replacement of tissue by plasma cells are unlikely to be malignant (Rawson et al.[31]). When the lesion presents broad sheets of normal-appearing plasma cells, the differentiation between benign and malignant lesions may be difficult, but when the plasma cells are atypical with great variation in size and form of cells and nuclei with mitotic figures and accompanying tumor giant cells, the lesion is invariably malignant (Ringertz[33]).

Extramedullary plasmacytomas may remain localized for a long time. They can be locally sterilized by irradiation. Their relationship to the subsequent development of multiple myeloma may not be suspected, particularly in view of the long time interval that may elapse between the occurrence of the primary lesion and its dissemination.

Myxomas may arise from the ethmoid region. They are characteristically soft, slowly growing tumors that microscopically show a typical syncytium. *Chondromas* and *chondrosarcomas* may arise from the cartilage of the nasal septum and in the ethmoid. *Enchondromas* have been reported arising from the ethmoid region or at the junction of the septum and the floor of the nasal fossa. *Fibro-osteomas* may arise from the ethmoid (Billing and Ringertz[7]). *Neurilemomas* have also been reported to arise in the nasal fossa in the form of a firm, reddish, nonulcerated mass (Bogdasarian and Stout[8]). Most of these tumors are pathologic rarities.

An important group of tumors arising from the nasal fossa and also from the accessory sinuses are the *mucous and salivary gland tumors*. They arise from the floor of the nasal fossa and from the ethmoid region. The true incidence of this type of tumor has been underestimated.

In general, these neoplasms are benign. The malignant variant cannot always be diagnosed with biopsy.

The majority of these tumors are well encapsulated and destroy surrounding tissue by unrelenting expansion. Their histologic character is varied, and for this reason they have been reported under a large number of labels: adenocarcinomas, chondrosarcomas, endotheliomas, myxochondromas, etc. (p. 535). Some of them may be confused with carcinomas. They are of epithelial origin and present great microscopic variation. Although they are identical in nature with tumors of the major salivary glands, they also develop in the oral cavity (p. 241), oropharynx, and trachea and from lacrimal and salivary glands. Increased knowledge of these tumors has resulted in their grouping under the heading of mucous and salivary gland tumors (Ahlbom[1]).

Badib et al.[4a] reported a series of fifty-seven cases of malignant tumors of the nasal fossa: thirty-two squamous cell carcinomas, eleven adenocarcinomas, five salivary gland tumors, four anaplastic carcinomas, three lymphoepitheliomas, and two melanomas.

The most common malignant tumors of the nasal fossae are the *epidermoid carcinomas*. Eighty-eight of the 113 cases reported by Frazell and Lewis[14] fell in this group. They usually arise from the middle and inferior turbinates and rarely from the ethmoid region and septum. The majority of these tumors are polypoid or papillary, at times becoming superficially necrotic. They invade the thin wall that separates the nasal fossa from the maxillary sinus and penetrate the antrum. They may produce obstruction of the lacrimal duct and also may be accompanied by frontal sinusitis.

Adenocarcinomas most often arise from the glands in the olfactory mucous membrane. These tumors diffusely invade the thin bone of the area and extend to one or both orbits, with consequent displacement of the eye. They also extend to the nasopharynx and to the base of the skull, resulting in early invasion of the cranium. Histologically, adenocarcinomas may present a pseudopapillary arrangement covered by a single layer of epithelium greatly resembling that of an adenocarcinoma of the large bowel (Ringertz[33]). These tumors, however, may present themselves as mucin-producing adenocarcinomas. They are formed by cylindrical or prismatic cells similar to those seen on the olfactory mucosa. Mucus is secreted more or less abundantly, giving the tumors a peculiar soft consistency which is responsible for their being called colloid carcinomas. Sometimes the mucus is not abundant and bone formation is found. These bone fragments may be a distinctive feature of the tumor or may be due to the presence of invaded bone. Rarely are the frontal and sphenoid sinuses invaded by these tumors, but they may be filled with polypoid masses (Hautant et al.[18]).

Tumors having a neurogenous origin have been observed in the nasal cavity. Among these are *neurofibromas, ganglioneuromas,* and *meningiomas. Gliomas* supposedly arising from embryonal detachments of the central nervous system have also been reported in this area. They may be veritable encephaloceles communicating with the ventricles or, more often, may be composed of a solid mass of autonomous glial tissue (Black and Smith[6]). They are usually seen in newborn infants and only rarely in adults. *Pituitary chromophobe tumors* of the nasal cavity, not directly related to the pituitary gland, have been reported (Kay et al.[23]).

Olfactory neuroepithelial tumors, first described by Berger et al.[5] as "esthésioneuroépithélioma olfactif," arise from the upper part of the nasal fossa (Grahne[17]). They are often mistaken for undifferentiated carcinomas and lymphosarcomas (Gerard-Marchant and Micheau[15]).

Malignant melanomas of the nasal fossa have been observed. Ravid and Esteves[30] collected 117 recorded instances. These tumors arise from the nasal vestibule, the septum, and also from the turbinates. They have been found in white as well as in black patients, mostly past 40 years of age. These neoplasms often protrude from the nares and have a bloody, black discharge.

Lymphosarcomas are the second most frequent malignant tumor of the nasal fossa. They develop from lymphoid tissue that is particularly dense around the choanae. More often, lymphosarcomas found

in this area have originated in the nasopharynx and have invaded the nasal fossa secondarily. They are soft and rapid growing and produce a deformity of the nose. They invade the maxillary sinus and the orbit. So-called *lymphoepitheliomas* are rare in the nasal fossae. They may develop near the choanae.

Metastatic spread

Metastases to the retropharyngeal lymph nodes from tumors arising in the olfactory area are rare, but they occur more frequently than is suspected from malignant tumors of the respiratory area of the nasal fossae. Metastases to the submaxillary region are occasionally seen, and distant blood-borne metastases to the lungs, liver, brain, and bones have also been observed. However, most authors have been struck by the relatively lesser metastasizing ability of some of these tumors, particularly the salivary gland type and adenocarcinomas.

Ringertz[30] found only two cases of distant metastases in twenty-seven reported cylindrical cell carcinomas. Lymphosarcomas may present cervical or mediastinal metastases early in their development. Hellwig[19] collected nine cases of plasmacytomas that also involved bone, in four of which there were also lymph node metastases. In seven of the cases, the primary lesion presented in the nasal fossa. Neuroepithelial tumors metastasize (Fisher[13]) and sometimes may disseminate through the spinal fluid (Riemenschnieder and Prior[32]).

Clinical evolution

Whether a tumor of the nasal fossa is benign or malignant, the most common presenting symptoms are nasal obstruction, nasal discharge, and epistaxis. Tumors that develop in the respiratory portion of the nasal fossa may rapidly produce obstruction and, later, deformity of the nose (Fig. 98), deviation of the nasal septum, and partial obstruction of the opposite fossa. Tumors of the olfactory region, on the other hand, usually produce a partial bilateral obstruction which only becomes complete in very advanced cases. When tumors of the ethmoid region develop posteriorly, they may invade the nasopharynx. When they develop anteriorly, they flatten the bridge of the nose, may invade the skin, and ul-

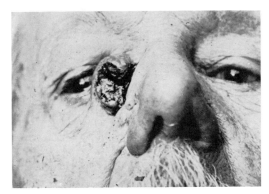

Fig. 99. Carcinoma of ethmoid that has invaded anteriorly through soft tissues and has ulcerated skin of naso-orbital region.

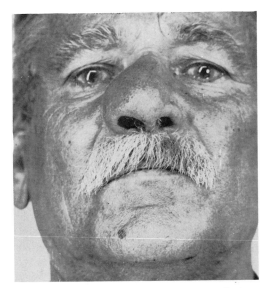

Fig. 98. Epidermoid carcinoma of nasal fossa producing deformity of nose and enlargement of anterior naris.

cerate at the inner canthus of the eye (Fig. 99). Sometimes there is simple lateral displacement of the eye with some exophthalmos and chemosis. As the tumor increases and invades both orbits, the eyes become widely separated (Fig. 100), but generally the movements and the vision of the eye are preserved. Nasal discharge and epistaxis may or may not be present, but no conclusions can be drawn from the intensity of the bleeding, for benign tumors frequently bleed more than malignant tumors. Pain is an important sign, for it is rarely present in benign tumors unless caused by concomitant sinusitis. In malignant tumors, the pain is progressive and severe.

Some of the malignant tumors of the nasal fossa develop relatively fast, facilitating the clinical diagnosis, but others, such as the cylindrical cell carcinomas of the ethmoid and the malignant variety of the mucous and salivary gland tumors, may develop slowly over a period of years without evidence of metastases. Some of plasma cell myelomas present a fast evolution, but others develop slowly and may recur years after treatment.

A variety of secondary symptoms may appear, such as lacrimation and dacrocystitis due to compression of the lacrimal duct. These signs are particularly common

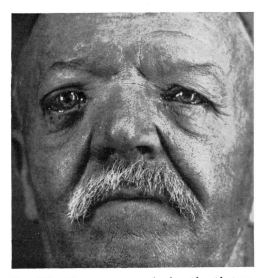

Fig. 100. Adenocarcinoma of ethmoid with invasion of both orbits and wide separation of eyes.

with ethmoid tumors (Öhngren[28]). Symptoms of frontal and maxillary sinusitis may also be present.

Early metastases do not occur in most malignant tumors of the nasal fossa with the exception of the lymphosarcoma, which may metastasize to the submaxillary region and the mediastinum and cause symptoms before the primary lesion is suspected. In these cases, the discovery of the primary lesion in the nasal fossa is only a consequence of the perspicacity of the examiner. Epidermoid carcinomas may metastasize to the retropharyngeal and submaxillary regions. Other malignant tumors of the nasal fossa metastasize predominantly to distant organs through the bloodstream. Plasma cell tumors also involve bones, and in some cases the development of an osseous involvement marks the clinical onset (Ringertz[33]).

Diagnosis

The diagnosis of tumors of the nasal fossa requires a careful evaluation of the history, a thorough anterior and posterior rhinoscopy, multiple roentgenographic studies, and a skilled appraisal of the histologic character of the tumor.

Anterior rhinoscopy often reveals only evidence of turbinate edema, and profuse bleeding may interfere with proper visualization. Only repeated examinations can overcome these difficulties. Posterior rhinoscopy is particularly helpful in tumors of the ethmoid. This examination may be done best with a rubber catheter as a soft palate retractor (Fig. 186). Profuse bleeding after removal of benign polyps in an aged patient should be carefully investigated (Hautant et al.[18]). Benign polyps are often due to, and found together with, malignant tumors of the nasal fossa and the maxillary sinus. The removal of a polyp under these circumstances may provide some relief but may delay the proper diagnosis.

Little of value can be said about the aspect of these lesions for their clinical differentiation. Papillary bleeding tumors may be either benign or malignant, and a smooth, nonulcerated mass may sometimes hide a malignant tumor. Melanomas are easily recognized because of their grayish black color. Hemangiomas have a typical shiny bluish appearance, but this may be obscured by excessive bleeding. Plasmacytomas are often pedunculated and, at times, ulcerated. They rarely occur in patients under 40 years of age.

Roentgenologic examination

Radiographic examination of the skull may be extremely valuable. In benign tumors that produce obstruction, there may be edema and opacity of the nasal fossa and accessory sinuses. When displacement occurs, there is seldom actual bone destruction. The same elements are present in malignant tumors but, in addition, there is an obvious break in the continuity of the bones (Figs. 101 and 102) with decalcification. Lesions of the ethmoid may invade the sphenoid, and extensive destruction of the base of the skull may be seen. Opacity of the accessory sinuses cannot always be regarded as evidence of extension of a malignant tumor, but may simply be due to block.

Biopsy

The removal of a specimen of tumor for pathologic examination may be quite dif-

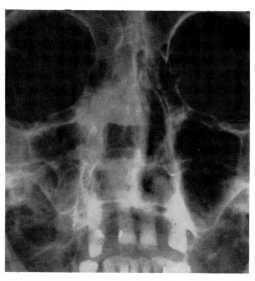

Fig. 101. Carcinoma of ethmoid with bone destruction and opacity of anterior ethmoid cells.

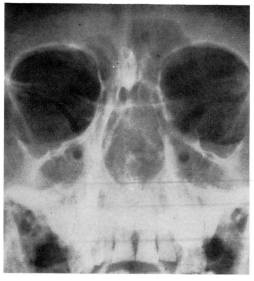

Fig. 102. Carcinoma of ethmoid with extensive destruction of septum.

ficult because of edema of the turbinates, and repeated trials may be necessary. When the tumor is not accessible through anterior or posterior rhinoscopy, a needle biopsy may be the next best means of obtaining a specimen.

Differential diagnosis

Fibromas that are reported to be found in the nasal fossa are generally nasopharyngeal fibromas that extend into the nasal fossa and even protrude through the nostrils (Fig. 194). These tumors may regress spontaneously after puberty.

Rhinoscleromas have been confused with carcinoma of the nasal fossa. These granulomatous lesions are frequently observed in Central Europe and Central and South America. A few have been seen in patients of Mexican extraction in southern California. The hypertrophic and ulcerating types of rhinoscleroma may dilate the nasal fossae and produce all the symptoms of a malignant tumor. Histologically, the lesion appears as a granuloma with plasma cell infiltration and abundant collagen fibers. Giant cells very similar to the Sternberg-Reed cells in Hodgkin's disease may be present.

Cases of so-called *lethal midline granuloma* may originate in the nasal fossae (Singh et al.[35]) and, by virtue of their overwhelming necrosis and systemic progression, may be confused with malignant tumors in this area. *Wegener's granulomatosis* is another condition of unknown etiology and serious clinical course that may be confused with malignant tumors of the nasal fossa or other areas of the upper air passages. Opinions are divided as to the identity of these last two conditions (Spear and Walker[37]; Brown and Woolner[9]). Tumors of the ethmoid may be confused with the very rare primary tumors of the frontal sinus. The tumors of the frontal sinus, however, are strictly unilateral and displace the eye laterally and downward (Fig. 103.) A roentgenologic examination is helpful in establishing the diagnosis.

Some forms of tertiary syphilis of the nasal fossa may be histologically confused with lymphosarcoma. Others that are ulcerated may be taken for carcinomas. On histologic examination, the syphilitic lesions present a protean appearance, but their nature is usually suspected by their granulomatous character and a positive serologic test.

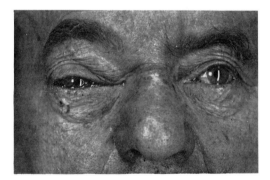

Fig. 103. Carcinoma of right frontal sinus with lateral and downward deviation of eye.

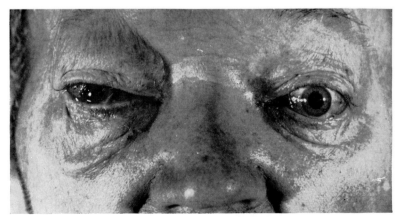

Fig. 104. Local invasion of ethmoid region by meningioma. Note chemosis and lateral deviation of right eye.

Rarely, meningiomas of uncertain origin (optic nerve, cerebral or meningeal tissues, or a congenital fault in the region of the Schneiderian membrane) can develop in the orbit and be confused with malignant neoplasms of the ethmoid (Fig. 104).

Treatment

Surgery

The treatment of the different tumors of the nasal fossae varies considerably, depending on the nature of the lesion at hand. An accurate diagnosis is consequently necessary before therapy is chosen.

Most of the benign tumors can be adequately excised through the anterior naris. By this process the tumor very often has to be morseled, and some of the lesions may eventually recur because obviously the excisions may be incomplete. Some benign tumors, however, may be encapsulated and so large that a major surgical procedure is required to remove them in toto. A lateral rhinotomy followed by curettement is sometimes necessary for advanced benign tumors. Denker and Kahler[11] proposed a resection of the superior maxilla, including the ethmoid. Holmgren[20] performed a similar operation but preferred the use of electrosurgery, also advocated by New and Devine[27] and others. Hautant et al.[18] perfected a technique for the removal of ethmoid tumors that consisted of a block resection of the ethmoid, including part of the floor of the orbit and the upper and middle turbinates. The operation was followed by intracavitary curietherapy, and in his hands this technique gave interesting results. It was attended, however, by serious complications, such as meningitis, hemorrhages, radionecrosis, loss of the eye, etc.

Tumors of the nasal septum may be widely excised without much difficulty, but often they require removal of parts of the ethmoid.

Radiotherapy

Epidermoid carcinomas, lymphoepitheliomas, lymphosarcomas, plasmacytomas, and neuroepithelial tumors of the nasal fossae are best treated by irradiation. Intracavitary applications of radium are handicapped by inability to appraise the true extent of these tumors. Lymphosarcomas, olfactory neural tumors, and epidermoid carcinomas should be treated by roentgentherapy alone. The external radiotherapy must be administered so that the tumor is homogeneously irradiated with a sufficient dose for its sterilization. With cobalt[60] and supervoltage units, adequate irradiation presents some practical difficulties. Complex radiotherapeutic approaches, such as the use of wedge filters and protectors, may be introduced to avoid overirradiation of the eyes, brainstem, or cervical spine. In this process, it is important that no part of the tumor fails to receive the desirable amount of radiations. In lymphosarcomas, the commonest error is the administration of an insufficient dose.

Adenocarcinomas of the ethmoid are seldom sterilized by external irradiation and should preferably be treated by surgery when possible.

Prognosis

Benign tumors of the nasal fossae have a tendency to hemorrhage or to become infected, and for this reason the prognosis is not always good. When they are advanced and treated surgically, the risk of hemorrhage is great. Short-term follow-up of slow-growing malignant tumors is meaningless, for recurrences may not be manitest for years (Baclesse[14]).

Frazell and Lewis[14] reported on a total of sixty-eight cases of epidermoid and adenocarcinomas treated by radical surgery with thirty-eight (56%) five-year survivals. Ethmoid tumors (adenocarcinomas, salivary gland type, etc.) have been treated successfully by surgical extirpation. Hautant et al.[18] reported that nine of twenty-one patients operated upon were living after four to twelve years. Öhngren[28] reported on fifty-seven patients treated with electrosurgery, with a 42% three-year survival. Plasmocytomas have been temporarily controlled by irradiation (Andersen[2]). Melanomas have a poor prognosis (Ringertz[33]). Only four patients (13%) were alive at five years in a series of thirty-one cases of melanoma, with adequate follow-up, filed with the Armed Forces Institute of Pathology (Holdcraft and Gallagher[19a]).

In a series of fourteen cases of cancer, presumably all carcinomas, of the nasal septum treated at the M. D. Anderson

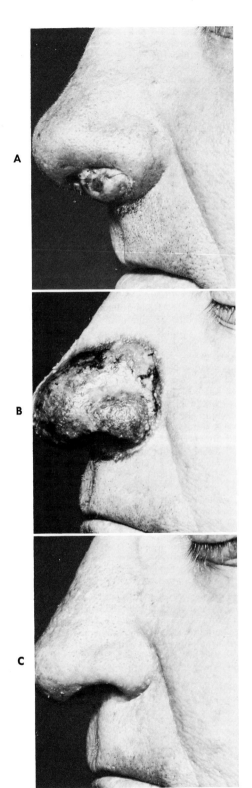

A

B

C

Fig. 105. **A**, Moderately well-differentiated squamous cell carcinoma probably arising from lower septum and filling nasal fossa anteriorly. **B**, Height of most severe skin reaction following 4350 R (skin) in eighteen days with 200 kv roentgentherapy. **C**, Appearance of skin one month later. (From Parker, R. G.: Carcinoma of the nasal fossa, Amer. J. Roentgen. **80**:766-774, 1958.)

Hospital in Houston, twelve patients were living and well after four years. Seven were treated solely by surgery, six received radiotherapy, and one was treated by both measures (Jesse et al.[22]). In a series of fifty-seven patients with malignant tumors of the nasal fossa treated at the Roswell Park Memorial Institute in Buffalo, N. Y., thirty by radiotherapy, thirteen by surgery, and fourteen by a combination of surgery and radiotherapy, 56% survived five years (Badib et al.[4a]).

The prognosis of adenocarcinomas is poor. Ringertz[33] reported that eight of eighteen patients with cylindrical cell carcinoma remained well five years after treatment. Parker[29] reported survivals of three and one-half to ten years in seven of ten patients treated by external roentgentherapy for carcinoma of the nasal fossa at the Tumor Institute of Seattle (Fig. 105). Esthesioneuroepithelioma has been treated successfully by irradiation (Hutter et al.[21])

REFERENCES

1 Ahlbom, H. E.: Mucous- and salivary-gland tumours, Acta Radiol. (Stockholm) (suppl. 23), pp. 1-452, 1935.
2 Andersen, P. E.: Extramedullary plasmocytomas, Acta Radiol. (Stockholm) **32**:365-374, 1949.
3 Astacio, J. N., Noubleau, V. M., Alfaro, D. A., and Vilanova, C. S.: Plasmocitomas extramedulares de los tractos respiratorio superior y gastro-intestinal. Relacion escleroma-plasmocitoma, Arch. Col. Med. El Salvador **18**:213-248, 1965.
4 Baclesse, F.: Les cancer du sinus maxillaire d'ethmoide et des fosses nasales, Ann. Otolaryng. (Paris) **69**:465-485, 1952.
4a Badib, A. O., Kurohara, S. S., Webster, J. H., and Shedd, D. P.: Treatment of cancer of the nasal cavity, Amer. J. Roentgen. **106**:824-830, 1969.
5 Berger, L., Luc, and Richard: L'esthésioneuroépithéliome olfactif, Bull. Ass. Franc. Cancer **13**:410-421, 1924.
6 Black, B. K., and Smith, D. E.: Nasal glioma, Arch. Neurol. Psychiat. **64**:614-630, 1950.

7 Billing, L., and Ringertz, N.: Fibro-osteoma; a pathologico-anatomical and roentgenological study, Acta Radiol. (Stockholm) 27:129-152, 1946.

8 Bogdasarian, R. M., and Stout, A. P.: Neurilemoma of the nasal septum, Arch. Otolaryng. (Chicago) 38:62-64, 1943.

9 Brown, H. A., and Woolner, L. B.: Findings referable to the upper part of the respiratory tract in Wegener's granulomatosis, Ann. Otol. 69:810-829, 1960.

10 Clifford, P.: Malignant disease of the nose and nasal sinuses in East Africa, Brit. J. Surg. 48: 15-25, 1960.

11 Denker, A., and Kahler, O.. Handbuch der Hals-, Nasen-, Ohrenheilkunde, vol. 5, Berlin, 1929, Julius Springer.

12 Dodd, G. T., Collins, L. C., Egan, R. L., and Herrera, J. R.: The systematic use of tomography in the diagnosis of carcinoma of the paranasal sinuses, Radiology 72:379-393, 1959.

13 Fisher, E. R.: Neuroblastomas of the nasal fossa, Arch. Path. (Chicago) 60:435-439, 1955.

14 Frazell, E. L., and Lewis, J. S.: Cancer of the nasal cavity and accessory sinuses; a report of the management of 416 patients, Cancer 16: 1293-1301, 1963.

15 Gerard-Marchant, R., and Micheau, C.: Microscopical diagnosis of olfactory esthesioneuromas; general review and report of 5 cases, J. Nat. Cancer Inst. 35:75-82, 1965.

16 Grace, C. C.: Malignant melanoma of the nasal mucosa, Arch. Otolaryng. (Chicago) 46: 195-210, 1947.

17 Grahne, B.: Olfactory neuroblastoma, Acta Otolaryng. (Stockholm) 59:55-64, 1965.

18 Hautant, A., Monod, O., and Klotz, A.: Les épithéliomas ethmoido-orbitaires. Leur traitement par l'association chirurgie-radium; résultats éloignés, Ann. Otolaryng. (Paris), pp. 385-421, 1933.

19 Hellwig, C. A.: Extramedullary plasma cell tumors as observed in various locations, Arch. Path. (Chicago) 36:95-111, 1943.

19a Holdcraft, J., and Gallagher, J. C.: Malignant melanomas of the nasal and paranasal sinus mucosa, Ann. Otol. 78:5-20, 1969.

20 Holmgren, G.: Die Diathermiebehandlung der bosartigen Tumoren der Nasennebenholen, des Naso-und Mesopharynx, Acta Otolaryng. (Stockholm) (suppl. 7), pp. 301-335, 1928.

21 Hutter, R. V. P., Lewis, J. S., Foote, F. W., Jr., and Tollefsen, H. R.: Esthesioneuroblastoma; a clinical and pathological study, Amer. J. Surg. 106:748-753, 1963.

22 Jesse, R. H., Butler, J. J., Healey, J. E., Jr., Fletcher, G. H., and Chau, P. M.: Paranasal sinuses and nasal cavity. In McComb, W. S., and Fletcher, G. H.: Cancer of the head and neck, Baltimore, 1967, The Williams & Wilkins Co., chap. 10.

23 Kay, S., Lees, J. K., and Stout, A. P., Pituitary chromophobe tumors of the nasal cavity, Cancer 3:695-704, 1950.

24 Largiader, F.: A rare nasal tumor; aesthesioneuroepithelioma of the olfactory nerve, Pract. Otorhinolaryng. (Basel) 23:373-383, 1961.

25 Lewis, J. S., Hutter, R. V. P., Tollefsen, H. R., and Foote, F. W.: Nasal tumors of olfactory origin, Arch. Otolaryng. (Chicago) 81:169-174, 1965.

26 Lewis, M. G., and Martin, J. A. M.: Malignant melanoma of the nasal cavity in Uganda Africans, Cancer 20:135-141, 1967.

27 New, G. B., and Devine, K. D.: Neurogenic tumors of nose and throat, Arch. Otolaryng. (Chicago) 46:163-179, 1947.

28 Öhngren, L. G.: Malignant tumors of the maxillo-ethmoidal region; a clinical study with special reference to the treatment with electrosurgery and irradiation, Acta Otolaryng. (Stockholm) (suppl. 19), pp. 1-476, 1933.

29 Parker, R. G.: Carcinoma of the nasal fossa, Amer. J. Roentgen. 80:766-774, 1958.

30 Ravid, J. M., and Esteves, J. A.: Malignant melanoma of the nose and paranasal sinuses and juvenile melanoma of the nose, Arch. Otolaryng. (Chicago) 72:431-444, 1960.

31 Rawson, A. J., Eyler, P. W., and Horn, R. C.: Plasma cell tumors of the upper respiratory tract, Amer. J. Path. 26:445-461, 1950.

32 Riemenschneider, P. A., and Prior, J. T.: Neuroblastoma originating from olfactory epithelium (esthesioneuroblastoma), Amer. J. Roentgen. 80:759-765, 1958.

33 Ringertz, Nils: Pathology of malignant tumors arising in the nasal and paranasal cavities and maxilla, Acta Otolaryng. (Stockholm) (suppl. 27), pp. 1-405, 1938.

34 Sekulic, B.: Naso-pharyngeal fibromata enclosed in the pharyngo-maxillary fossa, Rev. Laryng. (Bordeaux) 80:978-985, 1959.

35 Singh, M. M., Stokes, J. F., Drury, R. A. B., and Walshe, J. M.: The natural history of malignant granuloma of the nose, Lancet 1: 401-403, 1958

36 Smith, K. R., Jr., Schwartz, H. G., Luse, S. A., and Ogura, J. H.: Nasal gliomas; a report of five cases with electron microscopy of one, J. Neurosurg. 20:968-982, 1963.

37 Spear, G. S., and Walker, W. G.: Lethal midline granuloma (granuloma gangraenescens) at autopsy, Bull. Hopkins Hosp. 99:313-332, 1956.

38 Stout, A. P., and Kenny, F. R.: Primary plasma-cell tumors of the upper air passages and oral cavity, Cancer 2:261-278, 1949.

39 Tauxe, W. N., McDonald, J. R., and Devine, K. D.: A century of cylindromas; short review and report of 27 adenoid cystic carcinomas arising in the upper respiratory passages, Arch. Otolaryng. (Chicago) 75:364-376, 1962.

Maxillary sinus

Anatomy

The maxillary sinus occupies the center of the superior maxillary bone. Roughly, it forms a triangular pyramid with its base toward the nasal fossa and its summit toward the malar region. The anterior wall corresponds to the cheek and the canine fossa and extends up to the border of the floor of the orbit. The roof or upper wall corresponds to the floor of the orbit and the posterior wall is related to the pterygomaxillary fossa (Fig. 106). The base is formed by a thin wall divided in two by the insertion of the inferior turbinate. The orifice of communication between the maxillary sinus and the nasal fossa is found in the upper half of this wall. The maxillary sinus is lined by a columnar ciliated epithelium.

Lymphatics. The lymphatics of the maxillary sinus communicate with those of the nasal fossa and consequently end in the retropharyngeal, submaxillary, and anterior jugular lymph nodes.

Epidemiology

Malignant epithelial tumors of the maxillary antrum constitute the majority of malignant tumors in this region. They are found more frequently in men than in women and occur predominantly in patients 40 to 70 years of age. A greater proportion of women has been found in some series (Markowitz[20]).

Carcinomas of the antrum have been reported in patients who had been given Thorotrast (Markowitz[20]; Buda et al.[7]). These and other tumors of the upper jaw seem to be peculiarly frequent in Africa (Clifford[8]; Dodge[12]). There is increased frequency of carcinoma of the nasal cavity and sinuses in woodworkers (Acheson et al.[1]).

Pathology

Gross pathology

The majority of carcinomas of the maxillary sinus originate in the *infrastructure* (or lower half) in close contact with the dental roots and their nerves. They expand the anterolateral wall of the sinus and distend the soft tissues (Fig. 107), very rarely invading and ulcerating them. In

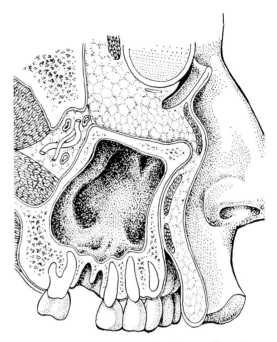

Fig. 106. Sagittal section of right maxillary sinus showing its close relationship with dental roots, floor of orbit, and pterygomaxillary fossa.

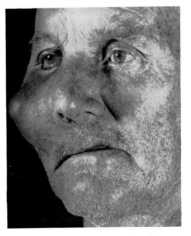

Fig. 107. Advanced carcinoma of infrastructure of maxillary sinus with typical deformity of anterolateral wall and filling of nasolabial region.

their downward extension, they produce a filling of the upper gingivobuccal gutter, causing enlargement of the upper gingiva, loosening the anterior molars and premolars, ulcerating the gingiva, and finally extending submucosally to involve the entire half of the hard palate. They displace the nasal turbinates medially and produce nasal obstruction but rarely ulcerate the tissues of the nasal fossa.

Tumors of the infrastructure very seldom develop posteriorly. Such rare posterior tumors rapidly invade the pterygomaxillary fossa and the posterior ethmoid cells. Further extension to the hard palate is sometimes accomplished at the level of the last gross molar.

Carcinomas of the antrum originate less often in the *suprastructure* than in the infrastructure, usually laterally at the summit of the sinusal pyramid. They rapidly invade the malar bone and the outer half of the floor of the orbit and later extend to the temporal fossa. At first the skin is only distended but may later be invaded.

Less frequently, tumors of the suprastructure develop medially, rapidly invading the ethmoid and the inner half of the floor of the orbit, extending anteriorly at the level of the naso-orbital region. Invasion of the orbit is rarely followed by invasion of the eye. Usually the eye is only displaced.

Whether carcinomas of the maxillary sinus arise in the infrastructure or the suprastructure, they may extend throughout the antrum and to surrounding structures in every direction. In advanced lesions, invasion of the floor of the orbit and the malar bone occur frequently, and there may be some extensive destruction of the alveolar process. Extension to the pterygomaxillary structures is almost a constant finding in terminal disease. Ulceration of the markedly distended soft tissues of the cheek occurs only in the late stage. With secondary infection, an accompanying pansinusitis often results.

Microscopic pathology

The overwhelming majority of tumors of the antrum are moderately differentiated epidermoid carcinomas developing by metaplasia from the mucosa. Large, clear cells presenting nuclear monstrosities are often observed, resembling those seen in recently irradiated carcinomas (Fig. 108). Takashi[32] described in detail some of the microscopic variance of carcinomas of this area.

Although they constitute a minority, adenocarcinomas also develop from the lining of the antrum (Batsakis et al.[3]). In

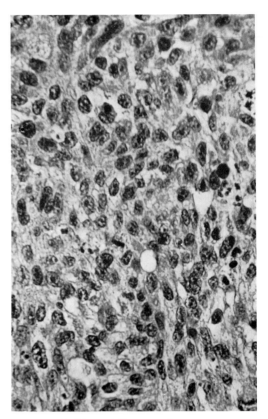

Fig. 108. Highly undifferentiated squamous cancer of maxillary sinus in 72-year-old man. (×370; WU neg. 61-75.)

a series of 261 cases, there were forty-three adenocarcinomas (Frazell and Lewis[16]). Depending on concepts, institutions, and authors, the term adenocarcinoma may or may not include other antral tumors (cylindromas, salivary gland tumors, etc.).

Metastatic spread

Metastases from carcinomas of the maxillary antrum are observed only in late stages. They usually appear in the submaxillary and cervical lymph nodes but rarely may be found in the retropharyngeal lymph nodes. Tumors of the suprastructure that develop laterally may invade the subcutaneous tissues and metastasize to the preauricular lymph nodes. Distant metastases are uncommon.

Clinical evolution

The majority of patients with carcinomas of the maxillary antrum first complain of a toothache, loosening of teeth, inability to apply a dental plate, or a superior maxillary tumefaction suggesting a dental abscess. An anterolateral tumefaction is typical of most tumors of the infrastructure and may appear without giving any symptoms. This tumefaction distends the soft tissues, which become reddened, and may finally ulcerate. Oral extension of the tumor appears as a smooth, nonulcerated tumefaction of the upper gingiva and hard palate. An ulceration may occur in the upper gingiva, around the teeth, or through a tooth socket. The tumor may extend beneath the mucosa to involve half of the hard palate. The rare tumors of the infrastructure that develop posteriorly show no external tumefaction. They are attended by diffuse pain and trismus.

Nasal discharge and epistaxis may be the first symptom in carcinomas of the suprastructure, followed by an external tumefaction in the malar region or the naso-orbital area. Lacrimation and dacryocystitis may also occur. Trismus is seldom an early symptom except in the few tumors that develop near the posterior wall and invade the pterygomaxillary fossa. In general, there is little or no initial pain, but as the tumor develops, and particularly as it invades the floor of the orbit, pain in the infraorbital region may become intense. There may be a burning sensation and other paresthesias along the distribution of the superior maxillary nerve. Waltner and Fritton[34] found numbness of the cheek in four patients, in three of whom there was no radiographic evidence of bone involvement.

In tumors of the suprastructure developing medially, the ethmoid region and the floor of the orbit are invaded early. There is an external tumefaction in the naso-orbital region, and the eye is displaced laterally. The movements of the eye are seldom affected, and chemosis is not frequently observed, but dacryocystitis frequently complicates the picture. In tumors of the suprastructure developing laterally, an external tumefaction appears first in the malar region, later extending to the temporal fossa. The eye is displaced medially. There is frequently marked chemosis but no impairment of the movements of the eye (Fig. 112). Invasion of the skin with secondary infection occurs in late stages.

Carcinomas of the maxillary antrum do not metastasize early. Those that ulcerate into the oral cavity most frequently present a submaxillary and upper cervical metastasis. A preauricular adenopathy may accompany tumors of the suprastructure that develop in the malar region when the subcutaneous tissues have been invaded (Regato[24]). Distant metastases occur infrequently.

The majority of patients in whom carcinoma of the maxillary antrum is not controlled by treatment die from local spread, hemorrhage, bronchopneumonia, undernourishment, and cachexia.

Diagnosis

The early diagnosis of carcinomas of the maxillary sinus is, unfortunately, seldom made. Because of the frequency of dental symptoms, members of the dental profession are largely responsible for their early detection. Unfortunately, the symptoms are usually interpreted to be due to other more common benign conditions, and, in general, tooth extractions and curettements or even minor surgical interventions are attempted before the true diagnosis is established.

The clinical examination should include palpation of the tumor area, including the floor of the orbit, the hard palate, and the upper gingivobuccal gutter. Anterior rhinoscopy may reveal narrowing of the nasal fossa or the presence of concomitant polyps. Rarely is the tumor directly accessible through the nasal fossa. Posterior rhinoscopy should be carried out to eliminate the possibility that the tumor originated in the nasopharynx and invaded the antrum secondarily.

Roentgenologic examination

The radiographic examination of the maxillary sinus requires good technique and roentgenograms taken in several positions. Usually, one or two anterior views and a lateral view are taken. In addition, tomograms and a roentgenogram of the base of the skull may be useful.

The radiographic examination is not diagnostic in early cases, for the only abnormality usually observed is a clouding of the sinus (Pfahler and Vastine[23]) (Fig. 109). As the tumor progresses, evidence of its destroying character may be found in

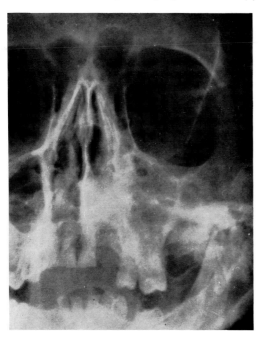

Fig. 109. Early carcinoma of left maxillary antrum showing cloudiness of sinus and lower half of nasal fossa.

the decalcification of the malar bone, floor of the orbit, or anterior wall. Evidence of asymmetry of the posterior wall may be observed in the roentgenogram of the base of the skull. Opacity of the ethmoid cells, the frontal sinuses, or even the opposite maxillary sinus is sometimes observed in carcinomas of the maxillary antrum. When found in the immediate vicinity of the tumor, these changes may correspond to neoplastic invasion. More often they represent inflammatory complications accompanying the tumor.

Biopsy

When the tumor has ulcerated into the oral cavity, a biopsy specimen can usually be removed with ease. It is very seldom possible to obtain a biopsy from the nasal fossa. In general, the tumor is entirely enclosed, and a specimen can be obtained only through an incision. It is often satisfactory to withdraw a fragment of the tumor through a large needle. The fragment should be fixed and processed as any other biopsy specimen to permit sectioning and staining. Biopsy of a lesion through a Caldwell-Luc fenestration is often done.

Differential diagnosis

A variety of conditions have to be considered in the differential diagnosis of tumors of the maxillary antrum.

Maxillary sinusitis seldom produces a tumefaction, and its clinical evolution and marked inflammatory elements often facilitate its diagnosis.

Papillary squamous metaplasia may form a tumorlike mass within the antrum and cause smooth erosion of bone. On biopsy of this lesion, the complexity of the pattern and the layering of squamous cells may lead a pathologist unfamiliar with this microscopic pattern to make a diagnosis of papillary carcinoma. These lesions may also involve the nasal fossa, may recur after removal and, under extremely rare circumstances, may undergo transition to carcinoma. A variety of rare benign and malignant tumors of the superior maxillary region may offer difficulties in clinical differential diagnosis, but most of them are easily differentiated when a biopsy is available.

Dentigerous cysts usually occur in young adults. They cause no symptoms but may grow to considerable size. When they contain a tooth, their diagnosis is easily made by roentgenographic examination.

Odontomas are tumors in which two or more tissues of the tooth germ are present (enamel, dentin, cementum). They occur in young individuals, are directly caused by faulty tooth formation, and may be solid or cystic. Radiographic examination reveals the presence of one or more teeth, and the enamel may have a radial arrangement.

Nonsecreting cysts and *retention cysts* arising from the mucosa of the sinus are usually the result of chronic inflammation. *Mucoceles* may cause facial deformity and bone erosion. They commonly arise from the frontal and ethmoid sinuses (Schuknecht and Lindsay[28]).

Ameloblastomas occur in the superior maxilla much less frequently than in the mandible. In a review of 379 cases, Robinson[27] found only 16% in the upper jaw. There was an almost equal distribution in both sexes, and the average duration of the tumor was eight and one-half years. Although ameloblastomas have been found in a 4-month-old infant and in older persons, they are most frequently diagnosed in patients 25 to 35 years of age. There may be a history of an unerupted tooth or of trauma. The tumors develop very slowly without pain and become ulcerated and secondarily infected in the oral cavity only after teeth have been extracted. They are surrounded by a thick shell of bone. Some of them are cystic, and others are solid. In the cystic variety, the cavities are lined with a smooth membrane. The cysts contain a clear, yellowish, fibrinous fluid and are separated by thin bony walls. Their histologic appearance is characteristic (p. 247). The polycystic type is easily recognized on radiographic examination, but this examination alone is not diagnostic because confusion with so-called giant cell reparative granuloma is very possible. A monocystic ameloblastoma is difficult to differentiate from an odontogenic cyst or from a fibro-osteoma. The contour of the ameloblastoma is somewhat lobulated. The dentigerous cyst contains the crown of a tooth pressed away from the alveolar process, whereas the ameloblastoma may contain a tooth

completely surrounded by tumor. Ameloblastomas are treated surgically, but radiotherapy may bring about desirable conservative results (Baclesse et al.[2]). Radiotherapy, however, has not been widely tried.

Fibro-osteoma (or ossifying fibroma) is

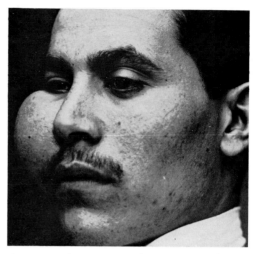

Fig. 110. Fibro-osteoma of superior maxillary region developing from infraorbital region.

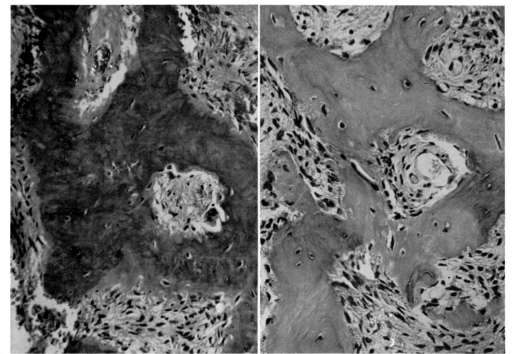

Fig. 111. Fibro-osteoma of maxilla at two different time periods showing practically no change. **A,** Biopsy taken at 25 years of age. **B,** Biopsy taken at 36 years of age. If anything, stroma is more cellular. (×250; **A,** WU neg. 59-80; **B,** WU neg. 59-81.)

a tumorlike lesion observed in patients 10 to 30 years of age. Fibro-osteomas are not related to osteitis fibrosa cystica of hyperparathyroidism. In the superior maxilla, fibro-osteomas occurring in the infraorbital region usually have the appearance of a small button or mushroom (Billing and Ringertz[5]), but they become broad-based as they grow (Fig. 110). They may invade the entire surface of the maxillary bone and obliterate the sinus. Radiographic examination, however, can show the sinus wall to be displaced without evidence of bone rupture or mucosal swelling. The most common of these neoplasms is an entirely eburnified tumor usually called fibroosteoma, but another variety may present more fibrous tissue than bone and for this reason they are called ossifying fibromas. Radiographic examination of these lesions may consequently show varying degrees of bone density, but the age of the patient and the painless, slow development greatly facilitate the differential diagnosis.

True *giant cell tumors* of the maxilla are rare, but they do exist. *Giant cell reparative granulomas* are nonneoplastic giant cell lesions (Jaffe[18]). There are also lesions of the maxilla that are secondary to hyperparathyroidism.

The *mucous* and *salivary gland types* of tumor arise from the mucosa of the maxillary sinus, just as they do from the mucosa of the nasal fossa and oral cavity. Ringertz[26] reported six of his own cases together with nine collected from the literature. The majority occurred in patients 40 to 59 years of age. These tumors develop very slowly and, although the majority are benign, some may be malignant and capable of metastasizing (p. 542).

Mucous and salivary gland tumors are well circumscribed, generally encapsulated, and in their expansion destroy, but seldom infiltrate, the surrounding tissues. They have varied histologic appearances. Surgical excision usually results in permanent cure with the exception of the malignant varieties, which may recur repeatedly following excision. Radiotherapy has been found to be successful in some cases.

Lymphosarcomas of the maxillary antrum have been reported in young patients (Dargent et al.[10]). Not infrequently, they arise in the nasal fossa and nasopharynx, invading the antrum secondarily. However, the possibility of their arising in the maxillary sinus cannot be denied. Lymphosarcomas are radiosensitive, and about half of the patients can be cured by adequate irradiation. Massive tumors of the Burkitt type are common in Africa.

Extramedullary plasmacytomas originate frequently in the antrum (Stout and Kenney[31]). The primary tumor may remain unnoticed even in the presence of extensive bone involvement. *Neurilemomas* and *malignant melanomas* have also been found to originate within the sinus cavity. The rare *melanotic neuroectodermal tumor* (so-called retinal anlage tumor) occurs in children, and it is benign. It is undoubtedly a tumor of neural crest origin (Borello and Gorlin[6]).

Ewing's tumors have been reported arising in the superior maxillary region of young persons. A histopathologic diagnosis of Ewing's tumor requires elimination of the possibility that the lesion may actually represent a metastasis from an unsuspected neuroblastoma of the adrenal gland (p. 701). In the adult, metastatic lesions of the superior maxilla from carcinomas of the kidney, breast, thyroid gland, etc. have been observed (Bernstein et al.[4]).

Chondromas and *myxomas* are rare tumors. They are observed in young persons and grow slowly and painlessly, sometimes undergoing calcification. They usually develop from the canine fossa or the molar and palatal processes and are contained in a capsule of connective tissue.

Chondromas are made up of hyaline cartilage, with occasional transition to osteoid or even bony areas, and a greater or lesser amount of mucinous material. When formed by a syncytium of cells in abundant mucoid tissue, they are usually diagnosed as pure myxomas. Radiographically, they are transparent and may present spotted calcifications. Treatment by surgical excision is most often successful.

Sarcomas of the superior maxilla are very rare and may be observed in the young child as well as in the adult. They may develop rapidly to attain huge dimensions. Pain is often an early symptom, and the rapidity of growth, although variable, is greater than that of benign tumors. The teeth become loose and may fall spontaneously. Paresthesias of the skin and mucous membrane of the mouth may also be present.

Innumerable varieties of sarcomas have been described, depending on their tissue content, but most of these varieties do not necessarily have a different histogenesis. The osteosarcoma, the chondrosarcoma, and the fibrosarcoma are the most common of the maxillary sarcomas. Osteosarcoma may be associated with Paget's disease of the bone, and it has been seen to follow therapeutic irradiation (Hora and Weller[17]).

Radiographic examination may reveal osteolytic or osteosclerotic changes (osteosarcoma), irregular, blotchy calcification (chondrosarcoma), or soft, transparent tissues entirely (fibrosarcoma). The histologic examination determines the diagnosis of these three varieties. The development of these tumors usually results in pulmonary metastases and death within a period of two years. A wide surgical excision should be attempted when possible. A few fibrosarcomas are radiosensitive but have not proved radiocurable in this area. The prognosis is very poor.

Epidermoid carcinomas of the upper gingiva may rapidly invade the antrum and reproduce the clinical appearance of an antral carcinoma that has ulcerated the gingiva. In surgical statistics, the former cases are usually grouped with carcinomas of the antrum. The differential diagnosis can be made here on the basis of the chronology of the developments. Moreover, carcinomas of the upper gingiva are usually more differentiated, keratinizing carcinomas.

In summary, the differential diagnosis of carcinomas of the maxillary sinus offers little difficulty in the majority of cases. Most benign tumors develop in young individuals, in whom carcinomas of the antrum are the exception. The same is true of many of the noncarcinomatous malignant tumors of this area (Ewing's sarcoma, osteosarcoma). The remaining few cases that might be confused are easily diagnosed on biopsy.

Treatment
Surgery

The surgical extirpation of maxillary tumors often requires excision of an important part of the facial structures along the anatomic lines first established by Gensoul (Dechaume[11]). Less radical excisions are only suitable for limited lesions of the floor of the antrum. In carcinomas that have invaded the orbit, the ethmoid, or pterygoid fossa, even the most radical procedure will be insufficient. Contraindications to surgery are as follows:

1 Invasion of the pterygomaxillary fossa
2 Invasion of the orbit or of the temporal fossa
3 Invasion of the skin
4 Invasion of the ethmoid
5 Distant metastases (presence of cervical metastases not necessarily a contraindication to surgery)

Radical excisions may require subsequent cosmetic surgery or prosthetic appliances (Schuknecht and Lindsay[28]).

Electrocautery and electrosurgery have been favored by some surgeons for the extirpation of maxillary tumors (Öhngren[21]). However, the success of the procedure seems to depend more on its thoroughness than on any particular virtues of surgical diathermy.

Radiotherapy

Curietherapy. Radium has been used in the treatment of maxillary tumors, mostly as a complementary procedure to the opening of the antrum and removal of the grossly visible tumor. But radium alone has also been applied successfully. Tod[33] described a technique in which the radium was placed within the antrum, under anesthesia, through an artificial opening. Treatment by means of intracavitary curietherapy requires that either the entire tumor or the postoperative residual be within the range of effectiveness of the source of radiations. It is not possible to estimate whether or not such is the case in most instances.

Roentgentherapy. External irradiation was thought, for a long time, to be incapable of controlling maxillary tumors and thus was called upon only as a means of palliation. It was also assumed that a therapeutic dosage would inevitably result in radionecrosis of the bone. A group of ten patients with inoperable carcinomas of the maxillary antrum receiving external roentgentherapy as the only form of treatment

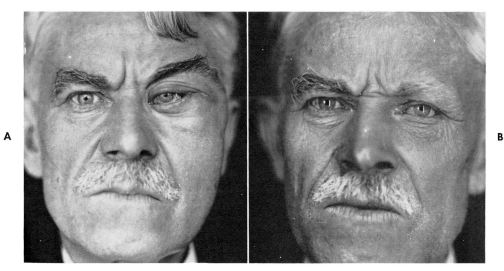

Fig. 112. **A,** Carcinoma of maxillary antrum developing in suprastructure with early invasion of floor of orbit and temporal fossa. **B,** Five years after administration of roentgentherapy. Treatments were protracted over a period of six weeks, and eye was protected during part of treatment. Vision was perfect five years after treatment. (From del Regato, J. A.: Roentgentherapy in epitheliomas of the maxillary sinus, Surg. Gynec. Obstet. **65**:657-665, 1937; by permission of Surgery, Gynecology & Obstetrics.)

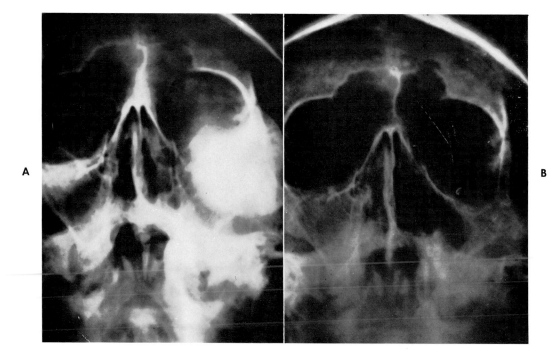

Fig. 113. **A,** Complete destruction of floor of orbit and invasion of temporal fossa. **B,** Seven years after administration of roentgentherapy. Note reformation of floor of orbit at lower than normal level and postirradiation cloudiness of opposite maxillary sinus.

was first reported in 1937 (Regato[24, 25]). This study revealed that patients could be cured, with preservation of vision, even when the orbit had been widely invaded by the tumor (Fig. 112). The necessity of fractionating the treatment and protecting the lens during part of the treatment was emphasized. These tumors have great radiosensitivity and metastasize late, two qualities that are advantageous for roentgentherapy. Invaded bone recalcifies following irradiation (Fig. 113), although in some instances the elimination of sequestra may result. The fractionated administration of roentgentherapy over a period of five to six weeks appears most satisfactory for avoiding untoward effects. Short treatments with a high daily dose may also be successful, but the danger of radionecrotic complications of the bone when higher doses are used does not justify this procedure, and the results are not improved.

Successful roentgentherapy of carcinomas of the maxillary antrum requires detailed care and minute evaluation. A detailed study of the physical distribution of radiations throughout the region is of great help in the evaluation of the usefulness of different fields (Ennuyer et al.[13]). Supervoltage roentgentherapy and cobalt[60] teletherapy permit a more homogeneous distribution of good quality radiations, thus minimizing the hazards and permitting the administration of a larger dose. Irradiation by these means requires special procedures to protect the eyes. The use of wedge filters has its ideal indication in the irradiation of these tumors. Bataini and Ennuyer[2a] found the use of electron therapy particularly encouraging in preliminary trials in carcinomas of this area.

Radiotherapy is often associated with surgery in the treatment of maxillary tumors. Administered postoperatively, it is usually called upon to remedy what has proved to be an inoperable condition. If the extent of the residual disease is limited, roentgentherapy may prove fruitful in some instances. Preoperative irradiation has been preferred in some institutions. Dalley[9] reported on a series of patients treated by external roentgentherapy followed by surgery. In at least ten of these no residual evidence of tumor was found in the surgical specimen. In spite of this, such combined treatment continues to be advocated (Spratt et al.[29, 30]; Lederman[19a]).

Prognosis

Carcinomas of the maxillary antrum that develop in the infrastructure have the best prognosis, but whatever the form of treatment applied, it must be radical. Öhngren[21] reported on forty-five patients with carcinomas of the antrum, fifteen (33%) of whom were living five years or more after treatment. The treatment consisted of electrothermic excisions, electrocoagulation, and curietherapy. In a series of 162 cases of carcinomas of the superior maxilla treated at the Mayo Clinic by a combination of diathermic surgery and irradiation, the relative five-year survival rate was 39.4% (Erich and Kragh[14]).

Windeyer[35] reported 21% five-year survivals among a group of eighty-two patients treated by combined methods from 1925 to 1937. Tod[33] reported forty-six patients living and well (25%) in a series of 222 patients treated. Dalley[9] reported the results of preoperative radiotherapy and surgery in sixty-seven patients treated at the Royal Marsden Hospital, with eighteen patients (26%) surviving five years.

Regato[24] reported on ten patients treated with roentgentherapy alone, of whom four remained well five years or longer. None of the patients treated could have been cured by the widest surgical excision. In a series of thirty-three patients treated by supervoltage roentgentherapy at the Tumor Institute of Seattle (Parker[22]), twelve remained well from three to ten years.

REFERENCES

1 Acheson, E. D., Cowdell, R. H., Hadfield, E., and Macbeth, R. G.: Nasal cancer in woodworkers in the furniture industry, Brit. Med. J. 2:587-596, 1968.

2 Baclesse, F., Dechaume, M., and Calle, R.: Les améloblastomes (ou adamantinomes) et les épithéliomas adamantins (Les résultats obtenus à longue échéance par les radiations), J. Radiol. Electr. 46:113-122, 1965.

2a Bataini, J. P., and Ennuyer, A.: Electronthérapie des épithéliomas des sinus de la face. Résultats a trois ans, Bull. Cancer (Paris) 56:61-66, 1969.

3 Batsakis, J. G., Holtz, F., and Sueper, R. H.: Adenocarcinoma of nasal and paranasal cavities, Arch. Otolaryng. (Chicago) 77:625-633, 1963.

4 Bernstein, J. M., Montogomery, W. W., and Balogh, K., Jr.: Metastatic tumors to the

maxilla, nose, and paranasal sinuses, Laryngoscope 76:621-650, 1966.

5 Billing, L., and Ringertz, N.: Fibro-osteoma; pathologico-anatomical and roentgenological study, Acta Radiol. (Stockholm) 27:129-152, 1946.

6 Borello, E. D., and Gorlin, R. J.: Melanotic neuroectodermal tumor of infancy—a neoplasm of neural crest origin, Cancer 19:196-206, 1966.

7 Buda, J. A., Conley, J. J., and Rankow, R.: Carcinoma of the maxillary sinus following thorotrast instillation; a further report, Amer. J. Surg. 106:868-871, 1963.

8 Clifford, P.: Malignant disease of the nose and nasal sinuses in East Africa, Brit. J. Surg. 48:15-25, 1960.

9 Dalley, V. M.: Malignant disease of the antrum, Brit. J. Radiol. 32:378-385, 1959.

10 Dargent, M., Gignoux, M., and Gaillard, J.: Le traitement des tumeurs malignes primitives du maxillaire superieur, Paris, 1948, Masson et Cie.

11 Dechaume, M.: De la résection totale du maxillaire supérieur dans le traitement des tumeurs malignes (operation de Gensoul), Thesis, Faculty of Medicine of Lyon, 1927.

12 Dodge, O. G.: Tumors of the jaw, odontogenic tissues and maxillary antrum (excluding Burkitt lymphoma) in Uganda Africans, Cancer 18:205-215, 1965.

13 Ennuyer, A., Folichon, A., Bertoluzzi, M., and Calle, R.: À propos des techniques roentgenthérapiques des tumeurs du sinus maxillaire et du sinus ethmoidal, J. Radiol. Electr. 32:476-491, 1951.

14 Erich, J. B., and Kragh, L. V.: Results of treatment of squamous cell carcinoma of the upper jaw and antrum, Amer. J. Surg. 100:401-416, 1960.

15 Ewing, J.: Review and classification of bone sarcomas, Arch. Surg. (Chicago) 4:485-533, 1922.

16 Frazell, E. L., and Lewis, J. S.: Cancer of the nasal cavity and accessory sinuses: a report of the management of 416 patients, Cancer 16:1293-1301, 1963.

17 Hora, J. F., and Weller, W. A.: Postradiation osteogenic sarcoma of the maxilla, Ann. Otol. 71:321-329, 1962.

18 Jaffe, H. L.: Giant-cell reparative granuloma, traumatic bone cyst, and fibrous (fibro-osseous) dysplasia of the jawbones, Oral Surg. Oral Med. Oral Path. 6:159-175, 1953.

19 Lacharité, H.: Radiothérapie des tumeurs des os à cellules géantes, Un. Med. Canada 57:587-651, 1928; also J. Radiol. Electr. 12:521-535, 1928.

19a Lederman, M.: Tumours of the upper jaw; natural history and treatment, J. Laryng. 84:369-401, 1970.

20 Markowitz, A. M.: Malignant tumors of the upper jaw, Surgery 47:443-452, 1960.

21 Öhngren, L. G.: Malignant tumors of the maxillo-ethmoidal region, Acta Otolaryng. (Stockholm) (suppl. 19), pp. 1-476, 1933.

22 Parker, R. G.: Personal communication, 1961.

23 Pfahler, G. E., and Vastine, J. H.: Roentgen diagnosis of cancer of the accessory sinuses, Arch. Otolaryng. (Chicago) 31:561-587, 1940.

24 del Regato, J. A.: Roentgentherapy in epitheliomas of the maxillary sinus, Surg. Gynec. Obstet. 65:657-665, 1937.

25 del Regato, J. A.: Sur la roentgenthérapie des épithéliomas du sinus maxillaire, Paris, 1937, Arnette.

26 Ringertz, N.: Pathology of malignant tumors arising in the nasal and paranasal cavities and maxilla, Acta Otolaryng. (Stockholm) (suppl. 27), pp. 1-405, 1938.

27 Robinson, H. B. G.: Histologic study of the ameloblastoma, Arch. Path. (Chicago) 23:644-673, 1937.

28 Schuknecht, H. F., and Lindsay, J. R.: Benign cysts of the paranasal sinuses, Arch. Otolaryng. (Chicago) 49:609-630, 1949.

29 Spratt, J. S., Jr., and Mercado, R., Jr.: Therapy and staging in advanced cancer of the maxillary antrum, Amer. J. Surg. 110:502-509, 1965.

30 Spratt, J. S., Jr., Mercado, R., Jr., Perez-Mesa, C., and Haun, C. L.: Carcinoma of the maxillary antrum; coordinated roentgen-surgical therapy, Missouri Med. 61:1003-1010, 1964.

31 Stout, A. P., and Kenney, F. R.: Primary plasma-cell tumors of the upper air passages and oral cavity, Cancer 2:261-278, 1949.

32 Takashi, M.: Carcinoma of paranasal sinuses, Amer. J. Path. 32:501-519, 1956.

33 Tod, M. C.: The treatment of cancer of the maxillary antrum by radium, Brit. J. Radiol. 21:270-275, 1948.

34 Waltner, J. G., and Fritton, R. H., Jr.: Anesthesia of the cheek; an early sign of carcinoma of the maxillary sinus, Ann. Otol. 65:955-959, 1956.

35 Windeyer, B. W.: Malignant tumors of the upper jaw, Brit. J. Radiol. 16:362-366, 1943; 17:18-24, 1944.

Oral cavity

Lower lip

Upper lip

Mobile portion of
tongue

Floor of mouth

Buccal mucosa

Lower gingiva

Upper gingiva

Hard palate

Lower jaw

Malignant tumors of the oral cavity make up about 5% of all forms of cancer occurring in the human body. Tumors that develop within the oral cavity present a distinct character and clinical course, are treated differently, and have a widely different prognosis, depending on their points of origin. It is regrettable that the medical literature abounds in the therapeutic discussions in which various carcinomas of the oral cavity are considered together as "cancer of the mouth," for it is neither possible nor rational to treat all of these tumors as a single unit.

There has been an increasing number of articles concerning the etiology of cancer of the oral cavity, for the most part dealing with smoking and the use of alcohol. Multicentric carcinomas of the oral cavity often are found in patients in whom heavy smoking is associated with alcoholism (Keller[1]). Trauma and dental irritation are of lesser importance. Carcinoma of the lower lip is undoubtedly related to chronic exposure to sunlight. A marked difference in the frequency of various types of cancer of the oral cavity is found in India as compared with western countries (Paymaster[2]; Shanta and Krishnamurthi[3]). In a series of 1130 cases of oral carcinomas reported from Ceylon, 743 arose from the buccal mucosa and only 168 from the tongue (Tennekoon and Bartlett[6]). This high occurrence seems to be related to the habit of betel nut chewing.

There is evidence that alcohol is of some importance, particularly if the intake is at a high level, 7 oz or more per day (Wynder et al.[8]). There is also a high frequency of the use of tobacco, either through chewing or pipe, cigar, or cigarette smoking, in patients with cancer of the oral cavity. In cancer of the buccal mucosa there is the most evidence for the relation between tobacco chewing and cancer. Trieger et al.[7] pointed out that there is a high incidence of some degree of liver dysfunction in postmenopausal women who have epidermoid carcinoma of the oral cavity and that patients with cancer of the oral cavity have a high frequency of cirrhosis. Undoubtedly, there are multiple factors concerning the development of this type of cancer.

The value of cytodiagnosis as a screening procedure for normal individuals remains in doubt. It is certainly not indicated in patients with visible lesions that can be biopsied. Cytodiagnosis may be helpful when done repeatedly in debatable lesions. (Shapiro and Gorlin[4]) or in the follow-up of carcinomas treated by radiotherapy (Silverman et al.[5]).

In order to understand the behavior of different tumors of the oral cavity and to formulate indications of treatment of the primary lesions and their metastatic adenopathy, this discussion of cancer of the oral cavity will be divided into the following sections: (1) lower lip, (2) upper lip, (3) mobile portion of tongue (anterior two-thirds), (4) floor of mouth, (5) buccal mucosa, (6) lower gingiva, (7) upper gingiva, (8) hard palate, and (9) lower jaw.

REFERENCES

1 Keller, A. Z.: Cirrhosis of the liver, alcoholism and heavy smoking associated with cancer of the mouth and pharynx, Cancer **20**:1015-1022, 1967.

2 Paymaster, J. C.. The problem of oral, oropharyngeal, and hypopharyngeal carcinoma in India, Brit. J. Surg. **44**:467-471, 1957.

3 Shanta, V., and Krishnamurthi, S.: Further study in aetiology of carcinomas of the upper alimentary tract, Brit. J. Cancer **17**:8-23, 1963.

4 Shapiro, B. L., and Gorlin, R. J.: An analysis of oral cytodiagnosis, Cancer **17**:1477-1479, 1964.

5 Silverman, S., Jr., Sheline, G. E., and Gillooly, C. J., Jr.: Radiation therapy and oral carcinoma;

radiation response and exfoliative cytology, Cancer **20**:1297-1300, 1967.

6 Tennekoon, G. E., and Bartlett, G. C.: Effect of betel chewing on the oral mucosa, Brit. J. Radiol. **23**:39-43, 1969.

7 Trieger, N., Taylor, G. W., and Weisberger, D.: The significance of liver dysfunction in mouth cancer, Surg. Gynec. Obstet. **108**:230-234, 1959.

8 Wynder, E. L., Bross, I. J., and Feldman, R. M.: A study of the etiological factors in cancer of the mouth, Cancer **10**:1300-1323, 1957.

Lower lip

Anatomy

The lower lip is a muscular and cutaneous fold that forms the lower half of the anterior wall of the oral cavity and its external opening. It varies considerably in thickness, shape, and size according to the race and age.

Transversely it extends between the buccal commissures and vertically from its free border to a horizontal depression that separates the lip from the chin. The same mucous membrane that covers the lower gingiva reflects upon itself to form the gingivolabial gutter and the posterior aspect of the lower lip. As it extends to the free border, it passes through a gradual transition into the vermilion area of the lower lip. The vermilion area is remarkable for its red or pink color. It presents thin anteroposterior irregularities on its surface, with a moderate depression in the midline. It ends brusquely in a regular curved distinctive line called the vermilion border that separates it neatly from the skin.

Lymphatics. The lymphatics of the *mucous membrane* of the lip and vermilion border gather in three trunks, one medial and two lateral. The medial trunk descends directly to the chin and ends in one of the submental nodes. The lateral trunks follow an oblique direction, cross the lower border of the mandible with the facial vessels, and usually end in one of the prevascular submaxillary nodes (Fig. 114). These lymphatics very rarely cross the midline to end in the nodes of the opposite side.

The lymphatics of the *skin* of the lower lip also end in the submental and submaxillary lymph nodes, but the medial lymphatics are richer and often cross the midline to end in the submental and submax-

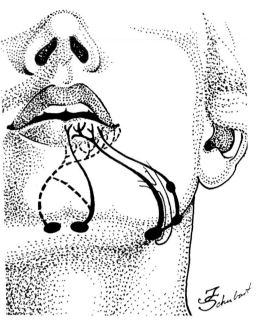

Fig. 114. Lymphatics of lower lip which end in submental and prevascular submaxillary lymph nodes but sometimes stop in facial nodes. Lymphatics of skin of lower lip (dotted line) may cross midline to end in submental and submaxillary nodes of opposite side.

illary lymph nodes of the opposite side (Fig. 114).

In addition to this classical termination of the lymphatics of the lower lip, it must be noted that in some cases these lymphatics may end in one of the mandibular nodes of the facial group (Rouvière[25]). These nodes are situated just below the subcutaneous tissues of the face, generally along the trajectory of the facial vessels and lateral to the horizontal branch of the mandible. They are not constant.

Epidemiology

Carcinoma of the lower lip includes lesions that develop on either the mucous membrane or the vermilion area. Carcinomas that develop on the cutaneous aspect of the lower lip, usually basal cell carcinomas, should be labeled carcinomas of the skin of the lower lip and should be considered with other lesions of the skin of the face.

In the United States, cancer of the lower lip constitutes only 0.6% of all cancer in man. In the 1947 cancer survey, the sex-

Table 8. Age incidence of patients with carcinoma of lower lip

Age (yr)	Judd and Beahrs[12]	Burkell[3]	Widmann[34]	Total	%
10-19	1	0	0	1	—
20-29	12	10	3	25	1.5
30-39	73	53	15	141	8.7
40-49	150	92	35	277	17.1
50-59	235	165	78	478	29.5
60-69	179	133	79	391	24.1
70-79	101	67	77	245	15.1
80-89	23	14	21	58	3.6
90+	0	0	2	2	—
	774	534	310	1618	99.6

age adjusted incidence rates were 5.3 for males and 0.7 for females per 100,000. Carcinomas of the lower lip constitute 25% to 30% of all carcinomas of the oral cavity and occur predominantly in men in the later decades of life. Seldom seen in young individuals (Ledlie and Harmer[15]; Gárciga[9]), this form of cancer is also rare in women except in countries where it follows the Plummer-Vinson syndrome (Ahlbom[1]). Carcinoma of the lower lip is rare in blacks. Leffall and White[16] reported two black patients with carcinoma of the lower lip in a series of seventy-five cases of carcinomas of the oral cavity registered at the Freedmen's Hospital of Washington, D. C. from 1948 to 1963.

Tobacco, and in particular the habit of pipe smoking, has been considered responsible for the development of carcinoma of the lower lip, which is often referred to as "cancer of pipe smokers." The assumption that the heat of the pipestem habitually applied to the same side of the lower lip over a period of years may end in the production of carcinoma is as well established in the mind of the medical profession as in that of the lay public. It is also argued that the porous clay pipes and the wooden stems permit seepage of tarry products that come in direct contact with the lower lip on the dependent side of the pipestem.

However, the infrequent occurrence of carcinomas of the upper lip, which is equally affected by the heat of the pipestem, the not infrequent occurrence of carcinoma of the lower lip toward the midline and its rather infrequent occurrence at the buccal commissure, where most pipe smokers hold the stem, and the rarity of carci-

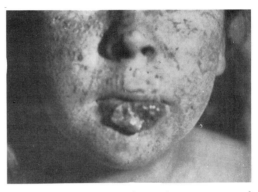

Fig. 115. Carcinoma of lower lip in young girl with xeroderma pigmentosum. (Courtesy Dr. Leonardo Guzmán, Santiago, Chile.)

noma of the lower lip in blacks who smoke pipes should be sufficient evidence to eliminate this argument. In addition, among patients with carcinoma of the lower lip, pipe smokers constitute a minority.

Long-standing exposure to sunshine, wind, and frost (farmers, sailors, etc.) is by far the most frequent cause of carcinoma of the lower lip. Chronic exposure to sunshine over a period of fifteen to thirty years results in dryness and hyperkeratosis of the exposed aspect of the lower lip. This hyperkeratosis may gradually develop into a superficial area of ulceration which later becomes indurated and is found to be carcinomatous. The effects of solar rays are variable and may require different length of exposure or intensity, depending on individual susceptibility. Blond-skinned persons are easily affected. Carcinoma of the lower lip is observed rarely in children suffering from xeroderma pigmentosum (Fig. 115).

Pathology

Gross pathology

Most carcinomas of the lower lip develop on the portion of the vermilion border that lies outside of the line of contact with the upper lip at a point equally distant from the midline and buccal commissure (Figs. 116 to 118). They may develop in the middle third of the lower lip and less frequently may start at the buccal commissure. In general, carcinoma develops on a long-standing hyperkeratotic lesion. In certain instances there may be pathologic alteration of the entire vermilion surface of the lower lip. Under these circumstances, multiple foci of origin may occur, and the patient may develop several independent carcinomas of the lower lip.

There are three distinct types of carcinoma of the lower lip: exophytic, ulcerating, and verrucous. The majority of lesions are of the exophytic type (Fig. 116). The lip becomes thickened, and induration may involve an entire half of the lower lip, whereas the ulceration is limited to the vermilion border and is comparatively small. These lesions may become bulky and in later stages may present spontaneous necrosis with loss of substance.

The ulcerating form of carcinoma of the lower lip usually starts with an ulceration of the vermilion border which immediately creates a defect (Fig. 118), whereas the tumefaction itself is limited to the area immediately surrounding it. These lesions are slower in their development but usually infiltrate the entire depth of the lip.

The verrucous type usually extends toward the cutaneous side of the lower lip. It has a very irregular surface and appears to be ulcerated only in the crevices. It develops very slowly, may involve the entire width of the lip, and may even extend to the chin. This type, however, has little tendency to extend to the mucous membrane aspect of the lower lip or to infiltrate in depth.

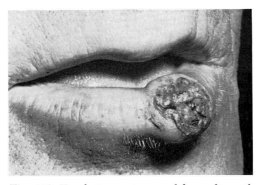

Fig. 116. Exophytic carcinoma of lower lip with central ulceration and raised, rolled borders.

Microscopic pathology

The overwhelming majority of malignant tumors of the lower lip are epidermoid carcinomas. More than two-thirds of all carcinomas of the lower lip are well differentiated. The proportion of anaplastic carcinomas is small. The microscopic diagnosis of epidermoid carcinoma should be relatively simple. The general tendency, however, is to overdiagnose and to include some benign lesions. Keratoacanthomas and extreme hyperplasias accompanied by chronic inflammation are often diagnosed as carcinomas. Reported series of carcino-

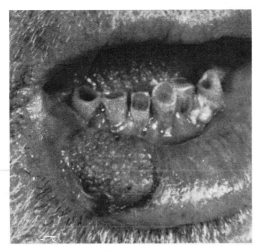

Fig. 117. Superficially ulcerating epidermoid carcinoma of lower lip, usually preceded by "blister."

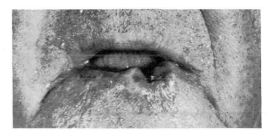

Fig. 118. Ulcerating carcinoma of lower lip with diffuse infiltration.

mas of the lower lip are likely to contain variable percentages of these benign lesions incapable of metastasizing.

The well-differentiated carcinomas (Grade I) usually include a group of papillary lesions that we call verrucous carcinomas and that arise also from other areas of the oral cavity. These tumors have been variously referred to by different authors, but no effort has been made to individualize them as a clinicopathologic entity.

Basal cell carcinomas do not arise on the mucous membrane or vermilion area of the lip. However, having arisen on the skin of the lower lip, they may invade these areas secondarily. Such cases should be considered as carcinomas of the skin.

Metastatic spread

Lymph node metastases are neither early nor frequent. The most frequently invaded nodes are the prevascular submaxillary nodes on the same side as the lesion. Carcinomas of the middle third of the lower lip may metastasize to the submental nodes but do so infrequently. Lesions of or near the buccal commissure may metastasize, also rarely, to the buccal nodes within the substance of the cheek, and the nodes may adhere to the lateral aspect of the mandible and erode the bone before they are recognized. Contralateral metastases are infrequent unless the lesion has invaded the midline. Distant metastases are rarely observed even at autopsy.

Clinical evolution

The most important single detail in the history of patients with carcinoma of the lower lip is the description of the onset on the basis of a "blister." This blister evidently precedes the development of a superficial ulceration (Fig. 117). In many other cases, there is a history of recurrent scabs that finally leave a superficial bleeding ulceration. This process may last many years, which explains the unusually long duration in some patients. Rarely does a carcinoma develop from an entirely normal lower lip. In general, the development of a carcinoma of the lower lip is rather slow and produces no symptoms until it has reached a rather advanced stage. Not infrequently, these lesions are ignored for years before advice is sought.

The reported incidence of metastases from carcinoma of the lower lip varies with the institutions. As many as 20% of patients registered may present a metastatic adenopathy (Modlin[20]), but the proportion of metastases is lower in the group who have received no previous treatment (Regato[23]). The proportion of metastases that develop after treatment of the primary lesions varies, of course, with the effectiveness of the treatment. In general, the reported incidence of metastases in that group varies from 6% to 12%. In a series of 179 patients presenting no clinical evidence of metastases at the time of treatment, only eleven subsequently developed metastases (Regato[23]). Most metastases present within two years following the discovery of the primary lesion. The likelihood of their occurrence increases with the duration of the primary lesion and the increase in its size. However, some very large lesions are observed which never metastasize. The risk also increases with unsuccessful treatment of the primary lesion and repeated recurrences. The proportion of metastases increases with the undifferentiated character of the tumor (Cross et al.[4]).

Table 9. Histologic differentiation of carcinomas of lower lip (comparison of figures from four sources reveals great discrepancy)

Grade	*Judd and Baehrs*[12]	*Ward and Hendrick*[32]	*Widman*[34]	*Ackerman and del Regato*
I	328	107	119	142
II	305	114	51	36
III	94	32	25	4
IV	14	16	3	—
Not graded	33	—	61	13
Totals	774	269	259	195

Diagnosis

Although most carcinomas of the lower lip can be easily recognized clinically, some of the early lesions arising from an area of hyperkeratosis and presenting only superficial ulceration may not be clinically evident and can be diagnosed only by biopsy. The same applies to a carcinoma with the gross appearance of so-called leukoplakia which may be taken for a benign or only "precancerous" lesion.

The biopsy specimen of lesions of the lower lip should be obtained with a scalpel, should be sufficiently deep, and should include a part of the surrounding normal skin. In the case of verrucous carcinoma particularly, superficial biopsies may show nothing but hyperkeratinization and chronic inflammation. If the clinical impression suggests malignant disease, additional biopsies should be taken sufficiently deep from the borders of the lesion.

The presence of palpable lymph nodes in the submental or submaxillary regions of patients with carcinomas of the lower lip is inconclusive if the nodes are less than 2 cm in diameter, for they are often a consequence of bad oral hygiene or secondary infection of the tumor. Nodes more than 2 cm in diameter are most often metastatic. Their metastatic nature can easily be proved by needle biopsy, thus expediting adequate treatment. In general, the clinical appraisal of metastases is surprisingly inaccurate. Only approximately two-thirds of cases considered clinically as having metastases are actually proved on microscopic examination (Judd and Beahrs[12]).

Differential diagnosis

Few other lesions of the lower lip may be clinically confused with carcinoma. Secondarily *infected hyperkeratoses* may become ulcerated and bulky, bleed easily, and reproduce the gross appearance of carcinoma, but biopsy will easily solve the problem of diagnosis. The appearance of a white patch on the lower lip, usually diagnosed clinically as *leukoplakia*, may be due to carcinoma or to hyperkeratosis. The true nature of such a lesion can only be decided on biopsy.

Deficiency *cheilitis* is never accompanied by induration and is usually present at the commissures on both sides. Syphilitic *chancres* of the lower lip are rare. They never grow over 1.5 cm in diameter. They may become indurated, but the base is clear and regular. *Hemangiomas* of the lower lip have a characteristic bluish appearance and are not indurated or ulcerated unless traumatized.

Treatment

The medical literature abounds in controversial statements regarding treatment of carcinoma of the lower lip and its metastases.

Treatment of primary lesion

It is generally admitted that skillful surgical excision, roentgentherapy, or curietherapy may contribute a high percentage of local cures in carcinoma of the lower lip. But whereas some authors readily acknowledge that radiotherapy offers a better esthetic result, others assert that surgery is the method of choice in this respect. These differences of opinion are not explained on the basis of varied surgical techniques but rather on the basis of a very unequal variety of radiotherapeutic skills and experiences.

Radiotherapy

Interstitial or surface applications of radium, once the standard radiotherapeutic approach, have given way to the more supple, adaptable, and effective techniques of roentgentherapy.

External roentgentherapy is a considerably more satisfactory means of treatment than surface curietherapy. Whether the lesions are small or extensive or exophytic or excavating, roentgentherapy can definitely cure the overwhelming majority of carcinomas of the lower lip and contributes the best esthetic results. Good results are not possible, however, by routine application of roentgentherapy with fixed factors of quality of radiations as well as of daily and total dosage and total duration of treatment. Intelligent variations of the quality of radiations used (100 to 200 kv, 3 mm of aluminum to 2 mm of copper filtration), depending on the extension and infiltrating quality of the tumor, will determine the outcome. There is also need for an intelligent elongation of the treatments

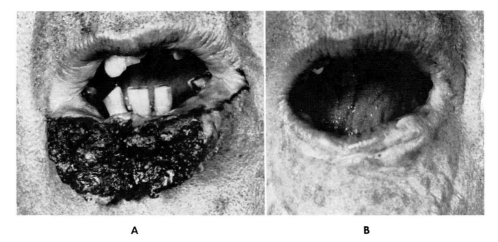

A   **B**

Fig. 119. A, Carcinoma of lower lip extending over two-thirds of its length. B, Three years following roentgentherapy, with only defect that due to destruction by tumor. Treatments were fractionated over five weeks.

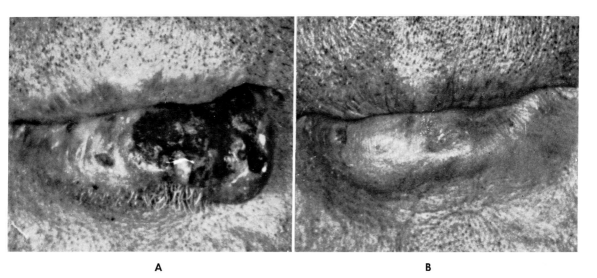

A   **B**

Fig. 120. A, Carcinoma of entire half of lower lip. B, Five years after roentgentherapy. Note absence of atrophy of telangiectasia.

(one to six weeks) and of the total dose of radiations, depending on the character and extension of the tumor (Mitchell and Mitchell[19]). In the proper evaluation of all these factors and their wise application, there is no room for amateur radiotherapists. Because of unquestionable possibilities of error, conservative treatment should not be undertaken without previous biopsy. External roentgentherapy is capable of sterilizing with greater certainty small and large tumors of the lower lip. In addition, the proficiency of its adaptation to the particular circumstances of the case

contributes to the best esthetic results (Figs. 119 and 120).

Surgery

Blond persons with a redundant lower lip who are chronically exposed to sunshine may develop multicentric areas of dyskeratosis and carcinoma in situ of the vermilion area of the lower lip. In the absence of frank infiltrating carcinoma, these patients benefit greatly by a cheiloplasty which removes the vermilion area and slides the oral mucosa of the lower lip to meet the skin. This cosmetic surgery,

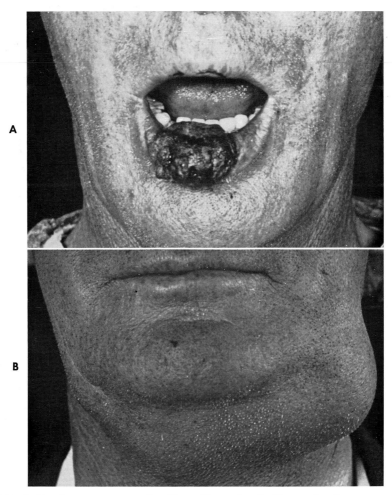

Fig. 121. A, Exophytic carcinoma of midline of lower lip. B, Six months after roentgentherapy. Bilateral submaxillary metastases had developed rapidly.

vulgarly referred to as a "lip shave," is very efficient in eliminating the chance of subsequent infiltrating carcinoma and often improves the patient's appearance. When a small area of infiltrating carcinoma is present, the operation may be combined with a V-shaped excision at its site (Jesse[11]; Paletta et al.[22]).

A V-shaped excision is the simplest form of surgical treatment. It is a minor procedure that can be done under local anesthesia and does not require hospitalization. A wedge-shaped section of the entire thickness of the lower lip is removed, allowing a margin of at least 0.5 cm beyond the recognized limits of the tumor. This operation implies only a diminution in the length of the lower lip with consequent decrease in the size of the oral opening.

The excision of small lesions from rather large mouths produces a satisfactory esthetic result if care is exercised in the approximation of the margins after removal. With small mouths and thin lower lips, however, the most limited excision results in constricted oral openings that may interfere with speech or the introduction of a dental appliance. For this reason, a V-shaped excision should be done only in patients with large mouths and thick lower lips. Other forms of local excision leaving an elliptic defect give an undesirable esthetic result and offer no additional advantage. For lesions requiring excision of more than one-fourth of the entire length of the lower lip, a V excision is not satisfactory, and some form of cheiloplasty has to be considered.

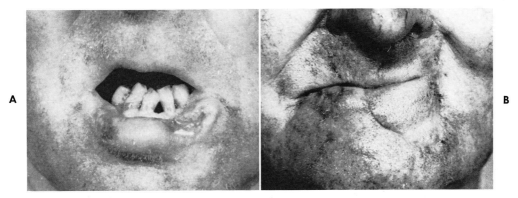

Fig. 122. **A,** Large ulcerated carcinoma of the lower lip. **B,** Following Estlander operation.

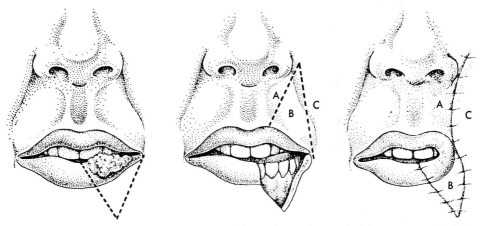

Fig. 123. Estlander operation for carcinoma of lower lip. Defect created by V excision filled by flap from upper lip.

Defects caused by surgical excisions of lesions of the lower lip may be filled by sliding the soft tissues of the cheek toward the midline. These tissues provide a shield for the teeth but lack mobility and may not be sufficient to contain food in the oral cavity. The Estlander[8] procedure consists in the repair of a defect caused by a V-shaped excision of the lip by a flap of the same shape rotated from the opposite lip to form a new buccal commissure (Figs. 122 and 123). The asymmetry resulting from this type of cheiloplasty may be corrected by subsequent cosmetic surgical steps. Schewe[26] reported a technique for reconstruction of the lower lip following extensive excision of deeply infiltrating carcinomas of 2.5 cm or more in diameter. The procedure is a one-stage operation.

In the surgical treatment of extensive lesions of the lower lip, particularly those that may extend to the cheek, a wide excision of the affected tissues and repair of the defect by a graft may be preferable. Most of these cases require additional surgical management of a submaxillary adenopathy, but the long surgical procedures, tedious as they may be, are well justified.

Treatment of lymph node metastases
Surgery

The treatment of choice of metastatic adenopathies from carcinomas of the lower lip is a radical neck dissection. Such treatment should not be undertaken, however, unless the primary lesion has been or is assumed to be controlled. Because the metastases from carcinoma of the lower lip may often be confined to nodes in the submaxillary region and upper cervical region, a compromise procedure has been

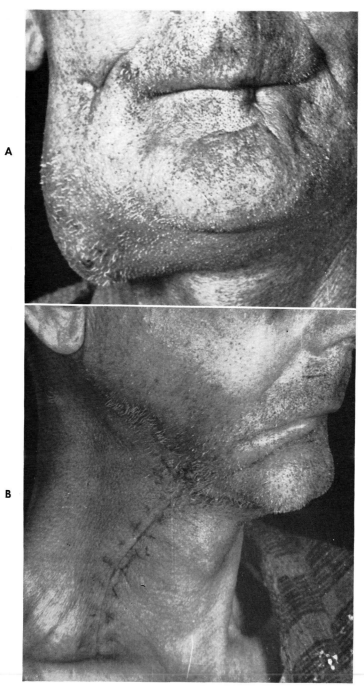

Fig. 124. **A,** Metastatic carcinoma of submaxillary region from surgically excised primary lesion of lower lip. Metastatic nodes were adherent to mandible. **B,** Following combined jaw resection and neck dissection. Patient remained free of disease three years following treatment. (From Sugarbaker, E. D., and Gilford, J.: Combined jaw resection neck dissection for metastatic carcinoma of cervical lymph nodes secondarily involving the mandible, Surg. Gynec. Obstet. **83:**767-777, 1946; by permission of Surgery, Gynecology & Obstetrics.)

advocated and practiced. But, even though a supraomohyoid dissection may be satisfactory in many cases, the limited operation is not anatomically sound and leads to more frequent recurrences (Modlin[20]; Klippel and Eckert[13]).

When the primary lesion invades or approaches the midline, the therapeutic neck dissection on the affected side may be extended to include the prophylactic dissection of the contralateral submental and submaxillary nodes. Not infrequently, metastatic nodes adhere to or invade the mandible. In such cases, an enlarged procedure is indicated and, when necessary, removal of the mandible in continuity is justified (Fig. 124). The presence of metastases on both sides of the neck is not a contraindication to surgical treatment. Bilateral neck dissections have been performed successfully (Leclerc and Roy[14]; Tailhefer[29]).

Radiotherapy

External irradiation is capable, under certain circumstances, of destroying metastatic adenopathies. However, this form of treatment requires extensive irradiation of the oral cavity and mandible and would not be justified when a neck dissection is practicable. It should be considered as a second choice when surgery is not possible.

Prophylactic* treatment of lymph node metastases

Prophylactic treatment of submaxillary metastases means the administration of treatment to the nodes before metastatic disease has become clinically evident. The decision for such a treatment is made upon the basis that early metastases may thus receive early treatment.

Prophylactic treatment of the submaxillary region by means of external roentgentherapy is not justified unless the total

---

*The word prophylactic as used here does not, of course, mean preventive, but simply treatment administered early when the metastases, if present, are still in a subclinical stage and not clinically apparent. The word elective is neither a good substitute nor any more accurate. It only means that one might or might not *choose* to do the procedure. When the prophylactic dissection is not carried out *systematically*, it may be proper to say that a patient received an elective prophylactic dissection.

amount of radiations administered is sufficient to sterilize an epidermoid carcinoma if it were present. This amount of radiations implies an extensive irradiation of the oral cavity and mandible which is not justified as a routine procedure.

Prophylactic neck dissection in patients with carcinoma of the lower lip is also unwarranted as a routine procedure. Its relative merits should be judged on the basis of the following factors (Regato[22a]):

1 *Percentage of patients who do not have a metastasis at the time of treatment of the primary lesion but will develop one later.* In a series of 146 patients without metastases on admission, only nine developed them subsequently (Backus and DeFelice[2]). This implies that if the operation is systematically done, it will serve no purpose in 84% to 94% of all the patients operated on.

2 *Chances of a permanent local sterilization of the primary lesion after adequate treatment.* Whether the treatment applied is surgical (Eckert and Petry[6]) or radiotherapeutic (Schreiner and Christy[27]), the cure rate of the primary lesion is about 95%.

3 *Comparison of the cure rate of prophylactic neck dissections with the cure rate of therapeutic neck dissections.* In a series of fifty-seven patients with microscopically proved metastases following prophylactic neck dissection, twenty-four (42%) survived five years (Eckert and Petry[6]). On the other hand, the curability of the submaxillary metastases is not much lower when the treatment is applied after the metastases have become clinically evident (Backus and DeFelice[2]). In a series of fifteen patients with metastases occurring after treatment of the primary lesion, Modlin[20] reported eight living and well after five years (53%).

4 *Proportion of patients who will be lost through inoperability when the metastases are allowed to become clinically evident before they are treated.* Because metastases are usually limited to the submaxillary region and, in most instances, remain localized there, the patients are seldom inoperable when first seen.

5 *Operative mortality of neck dissec-*

tions. The neck dissection practiced for prophylactic purposes usually yields a very low operative mortality. However, the risk will have to be sustained by a majority of patients who would not stand to benefit by the operation.

In general, the merits of a prophylactic neck dissection are overbalanced by the fact that there is a greater risk. The small group that will eventually develop metastases have a fair chance of survival with adequate radical treatment after the metastases have become clinically evident. It may be wise, however, to electively apply the prophylactic procedure to the small group in which, because of the greater chances of subsequent metastases, the balance is in favor of the operation. When the lesions grow rapidly to large dimensions, when the pathologic examination reveals a rather undifferentiated carcinoma, when the tumor has invaded the buccal commissure and the upper lip, or when there has been previously unsuccessful treatment, an "elective" prophylactic neck dissection is justified. In most instances, however, the assurance of a close follow-up is sufficient safeguard.

Prognosis

In 1965, 149 males and 23 females died in the United States from cancer of the lower lip, a mortality rate of 0.1 per 100,000. Indeed, the prognosis of carcinoma of the lower lip is excellent—the few deaths from it are due to inadequate treatment. Of 299 carcinomas small enough to be treated by a V excision, 94% showed no evidence of recurrence (Eckert and Petry[6]). In a series of 287 patients treated by superficial roentgentherapy, there was a crude five-year survival rate of 81.4% and a corrected survival rate of 95% (Dick[5]).

Regato and Sala[24] reported on a series of 498 consecutive patients with carcinoma of the lower lip without ostensible metastases on admission to the Ellis Fischel State Cancer Hospital. Only twenty-three of these patients died with cancer, including five with advanced lesions who received only palliative treatment. In 306 patients with lesions less than 2 cm in diameter treated mostly by surgery, there were seven local recurrences, seventeen subsequent metastases, and only five deaths from cancer. In 192 patients with lesions 2 cm to 12 cm in diameter treated mostly by radiotherapy, there were eighteen local recurrences, twenty-two subsequent metastases, and eighteen deaths from cancer (Table 10).

Watson and Burkell[33] reported on 1205 consecutive patients treated at the Saskatchewan Cancer Clinics, mostly by means of radium implantation, with a five-year survival in 1011 (83%). There were sixty-four recurrences and twenty-nine deaths from cancer. The prognosis of patients with recurrent lesions from any kind of treatment is less favorable, probably because

Table 10. Carcinoma of lower lip in patients without previous treatment and without metastases on admission: choice of treatment and results related to size of lesion, 1940-1953*

Size	Form of treatment	Patients	Dead without cancer within 3 yr	Total local recurrences†	Subsequent metastases‡	Dead from cancer	Well 3 yr or more	Absolute 3-yr survival
Less than 2 cm	Surgery	210	35	7	14 (2)	4	171	
	Curietherapy	34	4	—	3	1	29	82%
	Roentgentherapy	62	11	—	—	—	51	
2 cm to 12 cm	Surgery	45	10	5 (2)	1	2	33	
	Curietherapy	13	2	1	2 (1)	2	9	73%
	Roentgentherapy	129	21	12	19 (4)	9	99	
	Total	493	83	25	39 (7)	18	392	78%

*From del Regato, J. A., and Sala, J. M.: The treatment of carcinoma of the lower lip, Radiology **73**:839-844, 1959.
†Local recurrences without metastases. All subsequently controlled except the two noted in parentheses.
‡Figures in parentheses indicate concomitant recurrences.

of a combination of factors, including greater malignancy, size, and duration of lesions and greater proportion of metastases (Regato and Sala[24]).

Although the size of the lesion is an important factor in the prognosis, even lesions that involve the entire lower lip and extend beyond it are curable. Several authors have pointed out that the radio-curability of these lesions does decrease with the increase in the size of the lesions (Gladstone and Kerr[10]; von Essen[7]). The apparent lesser radiocurability of the larger as well as of the recurrent lesions may be due also to greater degree of malignancy requiring larger dosage, to less intensive irradiation of larger lesions, or to inadequate appraisal of the actual limits of the tumor. There is definite evidence that the curability decreases as the carcinomas are less differentiated (Cross et al.[4]; Ward and Hendrick[32]).

When a metastasis is present on initial examination, the chance of survival after treatment of the primary lesion and the metastatic nodes is lower than just mentioned (but better than that of other lesions of the oral cavity presenting metastases). Modlin[20] reported thirteen five-year survivals (53%) in a series of twenty-five patients with histologically verified metastases who had therapeutic neck dissections. In fifty-four patients who had therapeutic neck dissections for metastatic nodes from cancer of the lower lip, thirty (55%) remained well (Regato and Sala[24]).

The presence of bilateral metastases further diminishes the percentage of cures, but it is still rather good. In a series of twenty-six cases of bilateral metastases collected by Taylor and Nathanson,[30] there were five cures (20%) after surgical treatment.

Attempts to remove submaxillary lymph nodes, even when they have become adherent to the skin or to the mandible, will yield a good percentage of satisfactory results although at the expense of some permanent deformity and a higher operative mortality (Sugarbaker and Gilford[28]).

REFERENCES

1 Ahlbom, H. E.: Simple achlorhydric anaemia, Plummer-Vinson syndrome, and carcinoma of the mouth, pharynx, and esophagus in women, Brit. Med. J. 2:331-339, 1936.

2 Backus, L. H., and DeFelice, C. A.: Five-year end results in epidermoid carcinoma of the lip with indications for neck dissection, Plast. Reconstr. Surg. 17:58-63, 1956.

3 Burkell, C. C.: Cancer of the lip, Canad. Med. Ass. J. 62:28-33, 1950.

4 Cross, J. E., Guralnick, E., and Daland, E. M.: Carcinoma of the lip, a review of 563 case records of carcinoma of the lip at the Pondville Hospital, Surg. Gynec. Obstet. 87:153-162, 1948.

5 Dick, D. A. L.: Clinical and cosmetic results in squamous cancer of the lip treated by 140 kV. radiation therapy, Clin. Radiol. 13:304-312, 1962.

6 Eckert, C. T., and Petry, J. L.: Carcinoma of the lip, Surg. Clin. N. Amer. 24:1064-1076, 1944.

7 von Essen, C. F.: Roentgen therapy of skin and lip carcinoma: factors influencing success and failure, Amer. J. Roentgen. 83:556-570, 1960.

8 Estlander, J. A.: Méthode d'autoplastie de la joue ou d'une lèvre par un lambeau emprunté a l'autre lèvre, Rev. Int. Med. Chir. 1:344-356, 1877.

9 Gárciga, C. E.: Cancer de los labios, Havana, Cuba, 1948, Seoane, Fernandez y Cia.

10 Gladstone, W. S., and Kerr, H. D.: Epidermoid carcinoma of the lower lip; results of radiation therapy of the local lesion, Amer. J. Roentgen. 79:101-113, 1958.

11 Jesse, R. H.: Extensive cancer of the lip, Arch. Surg. (Chicago) 94:509-516, 1967.

12 Judd, E. S., and Beahrs, O. H.: Epithelioma of the lower lip, Arch. Surg. (Chicago) 59:422-432, 1949.

13 Klippel, A., and Eckert, C.: Suprahyoid neck dissection for epidermoid carcinoma of the lower lip: an appraisal of its use in one hundred and thirty patients, Amer. Surg. 24:107-111, 1958.

14 Leclerc, Georges, and Roy, Jean: La résection successive des deux jugulaires internes au cours des évidements ganglionnaires bilatéraux du cou, Presse Med. 40:1382-1383, 1932.

15 Ledlie, E. M., and Harmer, M. H.: Cancer of the mouth; a report on 800 cases, Brit. J. Cancer 4:6-19, 1950.

16 Leffall, L. D., Jr., and White, J. E.: Cancer of the oral cavity in Negroes, Surg. Gynec. Obstet. 120:70-72, 1965.

17 Martin, H.: The treatment of cervical metastatic cancer, Ann. Surg. 114:972-985, 1941.

18 Martin, H., MacComb, W. S., and Blady, J. V.: Cancer of the lip, Ann. Surg. 114:226-242, 341-368, 1941.

19 Mitchell, J. S., and Mitchell, M.: Fractionation in radiotherapy of cancer of the lip, Acta Radiol. [Ther.] (Stockholm) 6:299-312, 1967.

20 Modlin, J.: Neck dissections in cancer of the lower lip, Surgery 28:404-412, 1950.

21 Newell, E. T., Jr.: Carcinoma of the lip, Arch. Surg. (Chicago) 38:1014-1029, 1939.

22 Paletta, F. X., Coldwater, K., and Booth, F.: The treatment of leukoplakia and carcinoma-

in-situ of the lower lip, Ann. Surg. **145**:74-80, 1957.

22a del Regato, J. A.: Tratamiento de las adenopatías metastásicas del cuello, Arch. Cubanos Cancerol. **6**:311-316, 1947.

23 del Regato, J. A.: Roentgen therapy of carcinoma of the lower lip, Radiology **51**:499-508, 1948.

24 del Regato J. A., and Sala, J. M.: The treatment of carcinoma of the lower lip, Radiology **73**:839-844, 1959.

25 Rouvière, H.: Anatomy of the human lymphatic system, Ann Arbor, Mich., 1938, Edwards Brothers, Inc.

26 Schewe, E. J.: A technic for reconstruction of the lower lip following extensive excision for cancer, Ann. Surg. **146**:285-290, 1957.

27 Schreiner, B. F., and Christy, C. J.: Results of irradiation treatment of cancer of the lip; analysis of 636 cases from 1926-1936, Radiology **39**:293-297, 1942.

28 Sugarbaker, E. D., and Gilford, J.: Combined jaw resection neck dissection for metastatic carcinoma of cervical lymph nodes secondarily involving the mandible, Surg. Gynec. Obstet. **83**:767-777, 1946.

29 Tailhefer, A.: Traitement chirurgical des adénopathies du cancer de la langue. Resultats éloignés, Mem. Acad. Chir. (Paris) **62**:977-983, 1936.

30 Taylor, G. W., and Nathanson, I. T.: Lymph node metastases, New York, 1942, Oxford University Press.

31 Walker, A. W., and Schewe, J. E., Jr.: Nasolabial flap reconstruction for carcinoma of the lower lip; an eleven-year follow-up study, Amer. J. Surg. **113**:783-786, 1967.

32 Ward, C. F., and Hendrick, J. W.: Results of treatment of carcinoma of the lip, Surgery **27**:321-342, 1950.

33 Watson, T. A., and Burkell, C. C.: Cancer of the lip, J. Canad. Ass. Radiol. **6**:41-46, 1955.

34 Widmann, B. P.: Cancer of the lip, Amer. J. Roentgen. **63**:13-24, 1950.

Upper lip

Anatomy

The upper lip is a muscular and cutaneous fold that forms the upper half of the anterior wall of the oral cavity and its external opening. It varies considerably in shape according to race and age. Transversely it extends from the buccal commissures and vertically from the free border to the base of the nose in the center and to the nasolabial folds on each side. The mucous membrane that covers the upper gingiva reflects upon itself to form the gingivolabial gutter and the posterior aspect of the upper lip. As it extends to the free border, it passes through a gradual transition into the vermilion area of the upper lip. The vermilion area is remarkable for its red or pink color. It ends brusquely in a regular curved line which separates it neatly from the skin. The substance of the upper lip is formed by numerous thin muscles, the most important of which is the orbicularis oris.

Lymphatics. The lymphatics of the upper lip are more numerous than those of the lower lip. Those of the mucous membrane may gather into five trunks that end in the preauricular nodes of the parotid gland, in the upper cervical nodes just below the parotid gland, in the prevascular and retrovascular submaxillary nodes, and in the submental nodes. Occasionally, a small number of these lymphatic trunks end in the buccinator group of facial nodes, which are always found outside of the buccinator muscle and its fascia and above a line extending from the buccal commissure to the lobule of the ear.

The lymphatics of the skin of the upper lip follow a similar course to those of the mucous membrane, but some may cross the midline to end in the submental and submaxillary lymph nodes of the opposite side (Fig. 125).

Epidemiology

Carcinomas of the upper lip occur considerably less often than those of the lower lip. In 555 cases of cancer of the lip reported by Saggioro,[8] 473 were in the lower lip, thirty-five in the commissures, and only forty-seven in the upper lip. There seems to be a greater proportion of women with carcinoma of the upper lip than with carcinoma of the lower lip.

Perhaps the low incidence of carcinoma of the upper lip is the best argument against the possible causative effect of tobacco, and particularly pipe smoking, in the production of these tumors. The upper lip is, however, better protected against the action of actinic rays.

Pathology
Gross and microscopic pathology

Carcinoma of the upper lip may appear in the form of an exophytic growth rather frequently near the midline. In some cases,

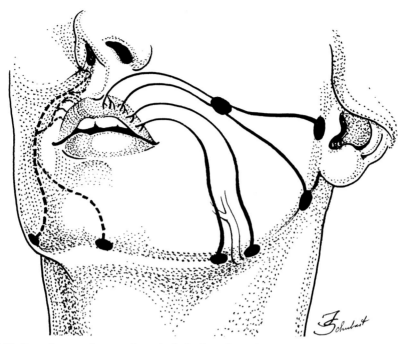

Fig. 125. Lymphatics of upper lip which lead to buccal, parotid, and upper cervical nodes as well as to prevascular and retrovascular submaxillary lymph nodes. Lymphatics of skin of upper lip (dotted line) may cross midline to terminate in submental and submaxillary nodes of opposite side.

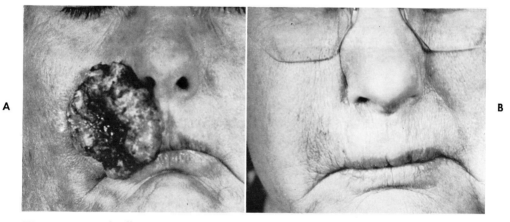

Fig. 126. A, Basal cell carcinoma arising from skin of upper lip. **B,** Following roentgentherapy.

the tumor is barely or not at all ulcerated, and it infiltrates the entire thickness of the lip. Some lesions are verrucous and rather superficial.

The majority of tumors of the upper lip are epidermoid carcinomas, but it should be borne in mind that these may sometimes appear as spindle cell carcinomas that may be confused with other tumors.

Tumors of the mucous and salivary gland type may also develop in the upper lip. These lesions are usually benign but present a variety of appearances that may make the pathologic diagnosis difficult, particularly since this type of lesion is not common. Salivary gland tumors are more frequently found (9 to 1) in the upper than in the lower lip (Eggers[3]).

Basal cell carcinomas in this area originate in the skin of the upper lip (Fig. 126).

Metastatic spread

Metastases from a carcinoma of the upper lip may go directly to the upper cervical region and to the preauricular nodes of the parotid gland as well as to the submaxillary region. The metastases are usually widespread in these areas. Martin et al.[5] reported twenty-one cases, ten of which (48%) eventually metastasized.

Clinical evolution and diagnosis

As a general rule, a carcinoma of the upper lip grows more rapidly than its counterpart on the lower lip. It is generally exophytic and superficially ulcerated. The differential diagnosis with salivary gland tumors is easily made on the basis of the great difference in their speed of development and time of evolution and on the fact that salivary gland tumors are not ulcerated. Their histology is characteristic (p. 535).

The spindle type of epidermoid carcinoma also has little tendency to ulcerate. Carcinomas of the upper lip metastasize earlier and more frequently than those of the lower lip. Hemangiomas occur in the upper lip (Fig. 127) but offer no difficulty in diagnosis.

Treatment

Carcinomas of the upper lip may be treated successfully by radiotherapy (Fig. 128). However, tumors of the spindle cell type and salivary gland tumors are best treated by surgical excision. In such instances, an Estlander operation is indicated. This consists of a triangular-shaped exci-

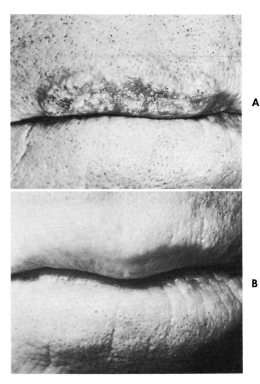

Fig. 128. **A,** Squamous cell carcinoma of mucocutaneous junction of upper lip treated by radiotherapy with total dose of 5000 R in thirty-one days. **B,** Twelve years after radiotherapy, only sequela being epilation of moustache near border of upper lip. (PCH 54-1053.)

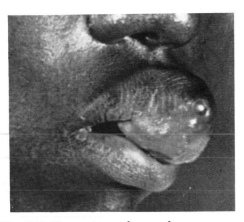

Fig. 127. Hemangioma of upper lip.

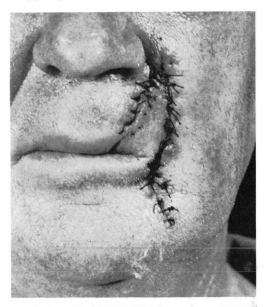

Fig. 129. Estlander operation for malignant tumor of upper lip. Defect created by excision filled by triangular flap from lower lip.

sion to be filled with an identical flap from the corresponding part of the lower lip that is turned around a thin pedicle to form a new buccal commissure (Fig. 129).

Prognosis

Prognosis in carcinomas of the upper lip is not so good as that in carcinomas of the lower lip. Eckert and Petry[2] reported twelve patients treated surgically with six surviving five years and six treated by curietherapy with three surviving five years.

REFERENCES

1 Backus, L. H., and DeFelice, C. A.: Five-year end results in epidermoid carcinoma of the lip with indications for neck dissection, Plast. Reconstr. Surg. **17**:58-63, 1956.
2 Eckert, C. T., and Petry, J. L.: Carcinoma of the lip, Surg. Clin. N. Amer. **24**:1064-1076, 1944.
3 Eggers, H. E.: Mixed tumors of lip, Arch. Path. (Chicago) **26**:348-353, 1938.
4 von Essen, C. F.: Roentgen therapy of skin and lip carcinoma; factors influencing success and failure, Amer. J. Roentgen. **83**:556-570, 1960.
5 Martin, H. E., MacComb, W. S., and Blady, J. V.: Cancer of the lip, Ann. Surg. **114**:226-368, 1941.
6 Martin, H. E., and Stewart, F. W.: Spindle-cell epidermoid carcinoma, Amer. J. Cancer **24**:273-298, 1935.
7 Rouvière, H.: Anatomy of the human lymphatic system, Ann Arbor, Mich., 1938, Edwards Brothers, Inc.
8 Saggioro, C.: Osservazioni statiche su 555 casi di epitheliomi del labbro nel centro tumori di padova, Radiol. Clin. (Basel) **23**:166-181, 1954.
9 Stout, A. P.: Tumor seminar, Texas J. Med. **41**:564, 1946.
10 Watson, T. A., and Burkell, C. C.: Cancer of the lip, J. Canad. Ass. Radiol. **6**:41-46, 1955.

Mobile portion of tongue

Anatomy

The tongue is a muscular organ which lies over the floor of the mouth and has the form of a flattened cone extending anteroposteriorly. The mobile portion (its anterior two-thirds) is that part which extends anteriorly to the lingual V formed by the vallate papillae. It is this portion that belongs in the oral cavity proper. The base of the tongue, situated behind the lingual V, is anatomically situated in the oropharynx.

The superior surface of the tongue is slightly convex. Its inferior surface is attached to the floor of the mouth except for its anterior third. The lateral borders of the tongue are rounded and correspond to the dental arches.

The muscles of the tongue have their strongest attachment on the hyoid bone and are divided in the midline by a fibrous septum. The tongue is covered by a stratified squamous epithelium, beneath which abundant mucous and serous glands are located. The irregular appearance of the dorsal surface is due to the presence of numerous and varied papillae. The mucous membrane is firmly adherent to the underlying muscle.

Lymphatics. The network of lymphatics of the anterior two-thirds of the tongue is almost entirely independent from that of the base or pharyngeal aspect. The network of lymphatics of the mucous membrane is rich and intercommunicates with the equally rich muscular network. These lymphatics gather into several collecting trunks: apical lymphatics, marginal lymphatics, and central lymphatics.

The lymphatics of *the tip* of the tongue gather into two main collecting trunks that run along the direction of the frenulum on each side of the midline. They take a posterior and downward direction, pass under the digastric muscle and inside the hyoid bone, and terminate in the supraomohyoid node of the internal jugular chain in the midcervical region. A second collecting trunk of lymphatics of the tip of the tongue ends in the submental nodes, but this is seldom observed in the adult and consequently has no clinical significance.

The collecting trunks of the *lateral border and inferior surface* of the tongue may follow one of two directions: (1) run medially to the submaxillary gland toward the nodes on the anterior jugular chain; the more anteriorly these lymphatics originate in the tongue, the lower the node in the neck in which they will end (Fig. 130); (2) run laterally to the submaxillary gland, ending in the submaxillary group of nodes. The greater number of trunks take the first direction.

The *central lymphatics* drain the medial two-thirds of the dorsal surface of the

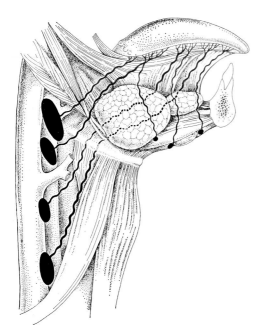

Fig. 130. Lymphatics of tongue illustrating that more anteriorly they originate in tongue, lower may be their draining lymph nodes.

tongue, anterior to the vallate papillae. They may run medially to the submaxillary gland, ending in the jugular chain of nodes, or laterally to the submaxillary gland, ending in the submaxillary nodes (Fig. 131). These trunks often cross the midline to end in the submaxillary and jugular nodes of the opposite side of the neck.

Epidemiology

In the 1947 cancer survey in the United States, the age-adjusted incidence rates for cancer of the tongue were 4.2 and 1.2 per 100,000 for male and female whites and 2.7 and 1.1 per 100,000 for male and female nonwhites. For white males 40 to 44 years old, the rate is approximately 0.7 but rises thereafter to around 40 per 100,000 in those 80 to 84 years of age. Venables and Craft[67] reported on thirteen patients under 30 years of age.

Excluding the lower lip, carcinomas of the tongue constitute the greatest single group of malignant tumors of the oral cavity. Wookey et al.[71] found 342 lingual

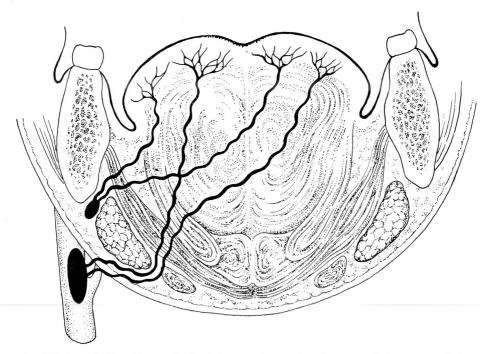

Fig. 131. Lymphatics of tongue in frontal section illustrating that areas of dorsum are drained by trunks that may cross midline to end in submaxillary or cervical lymph nodes on opposite side. (After Rouvière, H.: Anatomie des lymphatiques de l'homme, Paris, 1933, Masson et Cie.)

carcinomas among 839 cases of cancer of the oral cavity, whereas Cade and Lee[10] found 380 in a series of 550 cases. A greater relative occurrence of cancer of the oral cavity in Sweden has been associated with preexisting Plummer-Vinson syndrome. The latter deficiency disease is reportedly diminishing.

A high coincidence of syphilis and carcinoma of the tongue was reported in the past. Trieger et al.[65] found evidence of syphilis in 18% of his patients.

Poor oral hygiene is often associated with carcinoma of the tongue. It is not unusual to find a carcinoma of the lateral border of the tongue next to a jagged, carious tooth. As in other forms of cancer of the upper air passages, the use of tobacco, cigar and pipe smoking and particularly the chewing of snuff (Peacock et al.[45]) and other forms of tobacco, has been incriminated as a causative factor. An association of the use of tobacco and alcohol has been invoked (Wynder et al.[72]). Three out of four of the patients reported by Trieger et al.[65] were heavy drinkers, almost 50% had unequivocal evidence of hepatic cirrhosis, and 90% smoked excessively.

In India there is a disproportionate occurrence of cancer of the tongue (Khanolkar[30]). In a total of 30,000 cases of cancer recorded at the Tata Memorial Hospital of Bombay from 1941 to 1955, there were 4200 carcinomas of the tongue. However,

the base of the tongue was affected three times more frequently than the anterior two-thirds (Paymaster and Shroff[44]). Among Gujaratis, lesions of the base of the tongue predominate, whereas the opposite is true among Deccanis. This high occurrence has been attributed to the habit of chewing betel nut mixed with slaked lime and tobacco.

Leukoplakia is often discussed as a precancerous lesion of the oral cavity (Robinson[50]). It is dangerous to presume a diagnosis of "leukoplakia" on any visible white patch on the oral mucosa, for often the appearance is the same in the presence of frank carcinoma.

Pathology
Gross pathology

Carcinomas of the mobile portion of the tongue arise most frequently on the lateral border (Fig. 132). Jacobsson[27] studied 174 cases of carcinoma of the anterior two-thirds of the tongue, of which 82% arose in the lateral border, 11% on the dorsum, and 6% on the tip.

Of the 149 patients surviving for five or more years reported by Sturdy,[62] twelve (8%) developed a second primary lesion. It is not uncommon to see areas of neighboring carcinoma in situ in specimens of surgical excisions of carcinomas of the oral cavity. Thus, as more lesions are controlled by adequate treatment, surgical or radiotherapeutic, a larger proportion of second lesions may be expected (Ackerman and Johnson[1]).

Some lesions of the tongue are predominantly infiltrating and may show extensive involvement without much ulceration. Others present wide and superficial ulceration with some, but not very deep, infiltration. Still others may present wide ulceration with extensive infiltration of the underlying muscle.

Lesions that develop on the lateral border of the tongue usually extend submucously toward the anterior pillar of the soft palate, which they may secondarily invade and ulcerate. They also may extend toward the floor of the mouth but may not reach it until the tumor is far advanced. Lesions of the ventral surface of the tongue extend directly toward the floor of the mouth, and in many instances it is dif-

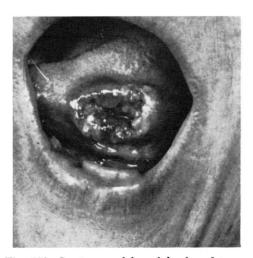

Fig. 132. Carcinoma of lateral border of tongue showing raised borders and ulcerating center.

ficult or impossible to establish whether the lesion arose on the tongue or on the floor of the mouth. The ulceration is usually in the form of an elongated, fissurelike loss of substance with submucous and muscular infiltration which rapidly becomes attached to the mandible. As a general rule, the attachment to the mandible does not imply invasion of the bone, which is safeguarded by its periosteum. Lesions that develop on the tip of the tongue are usually ulcerating with little infiltration, but cases of extensive involvement and even spontaneous amputation have been reported. Deeply infiltrating carcinomas of the tongue that spread toward its posterior third may invade and perforate the large lingual vessels.

Microscopic pathology

The overwhelming majority of tumors developing in the tongue are epidermoid carcinomas, and most of these are rather undifferentiated. A few, however, may show a little tendency to keratinization. It is fairly common to see areas of carcinoma in situ in direct association with invasive cancer. This finding has therapeutic implications whether surgery or radiotherapy is used. Polypoid squamous carcinoma of the tongue with pseudosarcoma has been reported by Sherwin et al.[56]

Metastatic spread

Approximately two-thirds of all patients with carcinoma of the tongue present a metastatic adenopathy during the course of the disease. The nodes of the jugular chain, particularly the high subdigastric nodes, are most frequently invaded. Submaxillary adenopathies are also observed but less frequently. Bilateral metastases are not uncommon, particularly when the primary lesion crosses or approaches the midline. Distant metastases are seldom observed during the early course of the disease, but the proportion of cases with visceral involvement, found at autopsy, may be surprisingly high.

Clinical evolution

The most common presenting symptom of carcinoma of the tongue is a growth or very slight local pain. Usually there is coexistent poor oral hygiene, and not infrequently the growth is lying against a carious tooth. Later, when the tumor becomes ulcerated and secondarily infected, *otalgia* on the same side as the lesion, a certain degree of *hypersalivation,* and *dysphagia* may occur. *Pain* is an important symptom except in the early stages of disease. In a great number of patients it may become excruciating and radiate to the entire side of the face and head.

Very early carcinoma may show only a slight thickening of a patch of mucous membrane, with or without superficial erosion and without subjective symptoms (Jacobsson[27]). Later, the lesion may appear as a slightly raised and indurated area with eventual development of spontaneously bleeding crevices. As the area of induration extends, the center of the tumor becomes ulcerated and secondarily infected. At times, there is accompanying glossitis or stomatitis. With infiltrating lesions, the movements of the tongue become more and more limited.

About 40% of all patients with carcinoma of the tongue are first examined after a metastatic adenopathy has already developed, and about 40% of those without node involvement when first seen develop an adenopathy later. Although a metastatic adenopathy may develop early in the evolution of the disease, the chances of its appearance become greater the longer the tumor has been present, and these chances are also greater as the primary lesion increases in size. Taylor and Nathanson[64] reported that 40% of the patients whose primary lesion had been present for three months presented a coexisting metastasis and that 90% of those whose lesions had been present for a year had already developed metastases. They also found that only 22% of the primary lesions measuring 1 cm in diameter presented a metastatic node, whereas 92% of those measuring 4 cm were accompanied by a metastasis. In a study of 763 cases of carcinoma of the tongue, Ash[2] found that 256 of the patients (33%) had metastases on admission and that 225 of the remainder (29%) presented metastases later (i.e., nearly two-thirds of all cases).

Metastatic nodes from a primary lesion of the tongue are most commonly found in the upper cervical region just below the angle of the mandible at the level of the carotid bulb area. Less frequently, nodes will be found in the submaxillary region or lower in the neck. Involved submental nodes are rare. Individual nodes rarely grow to large dimensions.

Bilateral metastases are not infrequent, particularly in those with the more advanced lesions and with lesions that develop in the midline. In 306 cases of carcinoma of the anterior two-thirds of the tongue in which the lesion was strictly unilateral, Roux-Berger[53] found only 6% bilateral metastases, whereas in 188 cases in which the lesion was close to or beyond the midline, he found 32% bilateral metastases. On the opposite side of the neck, the metastases are more often found in the submaxillary and upper cervical region. Seldom are supraclavicular nodes involved.

Without treatment, patients with carcinoma of the tongue usually die within a short period of time because of hemorrhage, aspiration pneumonia, or some other complication. The danger of hemorrhage, which may be fatal, is always present in spite of preventive ligation of the external carotid artery (Diamant and Hamberger[16]). In addition, when intense pain is present, the administration of sedatives and hypnotics contributes to the further deterioration of the general condition. Distant metastases from primary carcinoma of the tongue used to be considered a rather rare occurrence, but with the improved results in the treatment of the primary lesion and the regional lymph node metastases, a greater percentage of distant metastases has been observed (Braund and Martin[6]).

Diagnosis

When a carcinoma of the tongue is suspected, an effort should always be made to establish the approximate duration of both the symptoms and the lesion, for this information may have a bearing on the therapeutic decisions. The intensity of any pain should also be recorded, because it may give a clinical idea of the differentiation of the tumor and its infiltrating ability.

It should be remembered that early diagnosis of carcinoma of the tongue is often missed not because the patient delays consultation but because of the apparent innocence of very early lesions. The dentist in particular is in the unique position of observing early lesions and of obtaining the pertinent clinical history. He also has the unparalleled opportunity to biopsy areas of leukoplakia and to follow their development: His diagnostic and therapeutic knowledge are of utmost importance (Burford[7]; Buschke and Cantril[8]). A greater instruction and training in the early diagnosis of oral tumors is desirable in the dental schools for this reason (Martin et al.[39]).

Clinical examination

Examination of the tongue should never be limited to the visual findings. There should be a thorough palpation of the tumor area, for this often results in doubling the visual appreciation of the actual volume of the tumor.

Palpation of the neck in search of metastatic nodes should be thorough. An inflammatory enlargement of the submaxillary gland is often confused with a metastatic node, but the inflammatory enlargement is usually discoid in shape, and there is no neoplastic induration. Bimanual palpation of the submaxillary region with a finger placed in the floor of the mouth may help to eliminate errors. The cervical region proper should also be investigated, particularly at the level of the carotid bulb. When both sides of the neck are palpated at the same time, the examiner may unconsciously push the hyoid bone toward one side and have the impression of palpating a node with the other hand. This may be obviated by palpating only with one hand, and there may be some advantage in palpating the neck while standing behind the seated patient. It is much more difficult to palpate lymph nodes in a patient with a thick, short, muscular neck than in a patient with a thin neck.

Frequently, because the primary lesion is secondarily infected, enlarged nodes may be merely inflammatory, and it is impossible to decide clinically whether or not they are metastatic. The chance of their being metastatic, however, increases with their size. Taylor and Nathanson[64] found that only 20% of the nodes less than 1 cm in diameter were shown to be metastatic, whereas 99% of those reaching a diameter of 3 cm showed evidence of carcinomatous involvement.

Staging

Under the designation of TNM (for tumor, regional nodes, and distant metastases) a clinical classification has been proposed by the International Union Against Cancer. Such staging has usefulness for purposes of comparisons. (Deckers and Maisin[14]). MacComb and Fletcher[35] have adopted the following definitions for the various stages of the primary lesion:

T₁ Carcinoma less than 2 cm in greatest diameter

T₂ Carcinoma 2 cm to 4 cm in diameter with minimal infiltration

T₃ Carcinoma more than 4 cm in diameter confined to one side of tongue with or without extension to floor of mouth

T₄ Carcinoma involving more than half of tongue, or massive extension to floor of mouth, or involvement of mandible

In a series of 74 patients with carcinoma of the tongue treated at the M. D. Anderson Hospital of Houston, the distribution was as follows: T₁, fifty-three; T₂, fifty; T₃, thirty; T₄, forty-one. Since these figures do not include fifty-nine patients who were not treated and thirty-seven whose lesions were too advanced for treatment, the distribution in the four stages was about equal.

Biopsy

Biopsy specimens from an ulcerated lesion of the tongue should be taken with a scalpel, for specimens taken with a grasping or even a cutting forceps are usually insufficient and limited to the more superficial layers of the lesion. A wedge-shaped specimen, including some of the surrounding normal mucous membrane, should be taken from the borders of the ulceration. One or two sutures may be necessary to avoid excessive bleeding.

In the majority of instances, a needle biopsy of the nodes has only an academic interest inasmuch as, if the results are negative, the possibility of a metastasis somewhere in the neck is not necessarily eliminated, and consequently it does not preclude the indication for a radical neck dissection.

Differential diagnosis

White patches on the surface of the mucous membranes, frequently diagnosed clinically as *"leukoplakia,"* may prove, on histopathologic examination, to be due to typical or atypical hyperplasia, to carcinoma in situ, or to actual invasive carcinoma (Waldron and Schafer[68]). Some pathologists would only make a histopathologic diagnosis of leukoplakia when such areas show evidence of dyskeratosis. Renstrup[48] studied eighty cases of clinical leukoplakia, only two of which presented dyskeratosis.

Tuberculous lesions of the tongue are usually painful circinated, nonindurated ulcerations without deep infiltration of the muscle and are secondary to pulmonary tuberculosis. A *primary syphilitic chancre,* usually found toward the tip of the tongue, may sometimes give the impression of an early carcinoma. Differential diagnosis should be done both by dark-field examination of the exudate and by biopsy in view of the possibility of the coexistence of the two conditions.

Median rhomboid glossitis may be mistaken clinically for carcinoma of the tongue. Rhomboid glossitis is a developmental anomaly in which the tuberculum impar persists in the median line of the posterior portion of the dorsum of the tongue, a rare location for carcinoma. Microscopically, there is considerable acanthosis, hyperplasia of the epithelium, and chronic inflammation (Fig. 133).

Inflammatory conditions of the tongue are easily eliminated on the basis of their rapid development, extensive areas of tenderness, and lack of definite ulceration or induration. *Pyogenic granulomas* are common (Fig. 134). Localized areas of inflammation caused by injury, particularly on the lateral borders, might be more difficult to differentiate and might require a microscopic examination. Lacassagne[32] called attention to the frequent error in diagnosis connected with the development of a *lingual tonsillitis.* This consists of a hypertrophy of the organ folliatum situated on the tongue at the insertion of the anterior pillar of the soft palate.

Other tumors of the tongue are rare. They include *chondroma, osteoma* (Jahnke and Daly[28]), *salivary gland tumors, malig-*

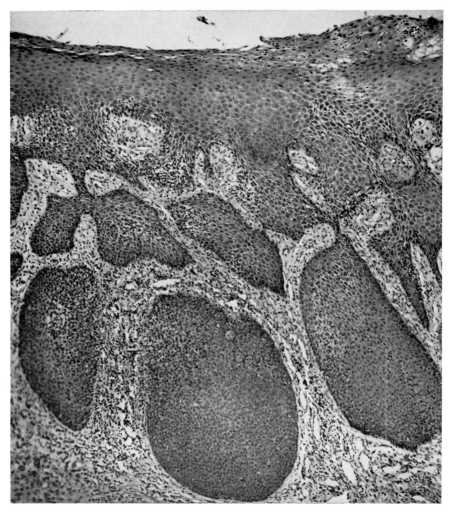

Fig. 133. Median rhomboid glossitis in 40-year-old man with reddish flat growth on posterior midsurface of tongue. Clinical diagnosis of cancer was made, and area was excised rather than incised. (x83; WU neg. 61-74.)

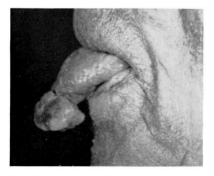

Fig. 134. Pyogenic granuloma of tip of tongue.

nant melanoma (Principato et al.[46]), and *neurofibroma* (Flicinski[22]). We have seen seven *malignant lymphomas,* nine *granular cell myoblastomas,* four *neurofibromas,* and five *neurilemomas. Fibrosarcomas* of the tongue following radiation therapy for previous carcinoma have been reported (Castigliano[11]).

Treatment

Although there is wide agreement on certain phases of the treatment of carcinoma of the tongue and its cervical metastases, there is still some diversity of opinion about the methods of approach and the techniques to be used.

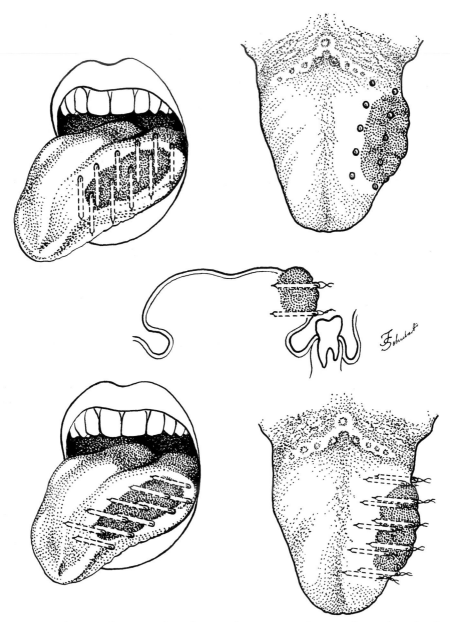

Fig. 135. Technique of interstitial irradiation of carcinoma of tongue by means of radium element needles. Needles are first implanted as shown in top diagrams. After half of dosage has been given, they are placed in perpendicular direction (bottom diagrams). Thus, homogeneous irradiation is assured.

Radiotherapy

The most effective treatment in the majority of carcinomas of the tongue is the *interstitial irradiation* by means of radium element needles or other radioactive materials. The procedure requires skill and proper evaluation of the dimensions of the potentially involved area. The calculation of dosage is comparatively simple. It is preferable to utilize needles containing 1 mg of radium per centimeter of length and needles 15 mm to 40 mm in length with 0.5 mm of wall thickness. We have found advantage in delivering half of the precalculated dose with the needles placed in one direction and the other half through

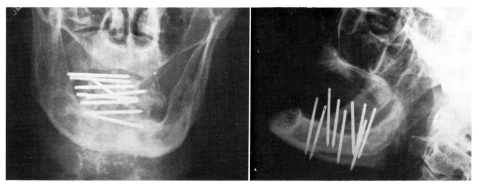

Fig. 136. Roentgenograms showing successive implants of radium needles perpendicular to each other to equalize dosage.

a new implant of needles in a plane or planes perpendicular to the first (Figs. 135 and 136). The entire procedure is usually achieved within ten days. The patients must be hospitalized and kept comfortable through necessary nasal feeding and medications.

The interstitial implantation of *radon seeds* has long been abandoned as inaccurate. The use of cobalt pellets spaced in nylon threads or cobalt needles is very satisfactory (Morton et al.[42]). This approach yields a large proportion of local sterilization of the tumor (Fletcher and Stovall[21]). A method gaining approval is that which places plastic tubings ("gutters") well threaded through the tumor area, with radiologic control when necessary, for subsequent loading with cobalt[60], iridium[192], gold[198], or other radioisotopic materials (Pierquin[45a]). The procedure is safer for the personnel and allows for very adequate dosimetry.

Peroral roentgentherapy has limited indications which are confined to small lesions of the anterior third of the tongue. It requires considerable care and cooperation from the patient. *External irradiation* has been used, more and more, as a preliminary procedure before the interstitial implant. Alone, it seldom succeeds in the complete destruction of infiltrating carcinomas of the tongue. Moreover, the rather large dose that is required is, per force, spread over a wider area which has to be irradiated. With cobalt[60] and supervoltage roentgentherapy, a preliminary external irradiation can be carried out without producing important reactions of the skin or mucous membranes. The resulting regression of tumor volume and secondary infection facilitate the subsequent and definitive interstitial implant. If a combination of external and interstitial irradiation is planned, it is important that the time lapse between the two procedures be commensurate with the daily dose received—too long a lapse implies that the implant may be done on an already recurrent tumor.

Except in rare circumstances, radiotherapy, in any form, has little place in the treatment of lymph node metastases from carcinoma of the tongue. Irradiation of metastatic nodes may be done as a preoperative or as a palliative procedure.

Surgery

The indications for surgery in the treatment of carcinoma of the tongue are limited to very small lesions that can be widely excised without resulting dysfunction and also carcinomas in a syphilitic tongue. In a series of 174 consecutive patients treated by MacComb and Fletcher,[37] twenty-eight were treated surgically (nineteen of the lesions were stages T_1 or T_2) and 146 received radiotherapy. The advocates of surgery have continued to use primarily the surgical approach, utilizing several different procedures ranging from wide excision (Kremen and Arhelger[31]) to total glossectomy (Donaldson et al.[17]) to wide excision with removal of the mandible (Slaughter et al.[57]), usually combined with a radical neck dissection. The frequent presence of cervical metastases and the haste to deal with them are usually the basis on which the decision to operate is made.

The accepted treatment of a metastatic

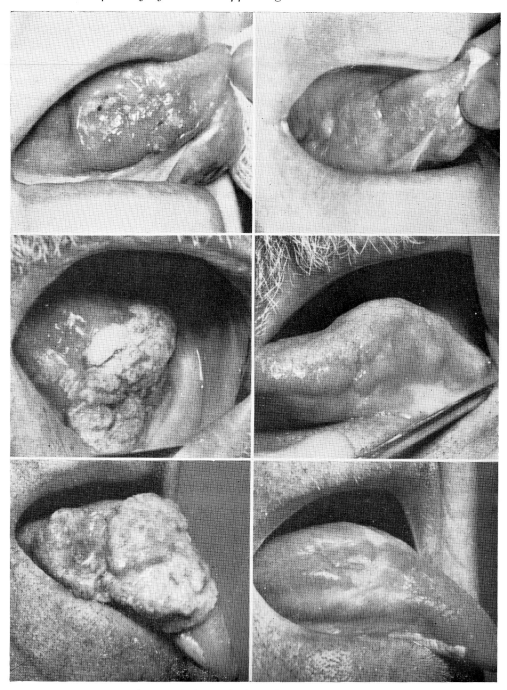

Fig. 137. Carcinomas of tongue before and after radiotherapy. Treatment consisted of external roentgentherapy followed by interstitial curietherapy. (Courtesy Toronto Institute of Radiotherapy, Toronto General Hospital, Toronto, Canada.)

cervical adenopathy from a primary carcinoma of the tongue is a *radical neck dissection*. There can be no compromise in this choice. Local excisions of nodes or even partial neck dissections should not be done. They are worse than abstention.

A radical dissection implies the block excision of the submaxillary contents, sternocleidomastoid muscle, and internal jugular vein and of the nodes, fat, and connective tissue that surround these structures from the midline to the anterior border of the trapezius muscle and from the mandible to the clavicle. This classic operation, the technique of which was perfected by Maitland[36] and Crile,[12] is sometimes handicapped by the fact that the most commonly invaded nodes (the subdigastric group) are very close to, or partially hidden below, the upper limit of the dissection. Roux-Berger[53] suggested the extension of the operation by dividing the posterior belly of the digastric muscle at its insertion on the hyoid bone. This appears to be the most useful means of gaining several centimeters in order to perform a higher ligature of the internal jugular vein after the subdigastric group of nodes has been largely exposed.

With the use of antibiotics, it is no longer necessary to waste time, for a radical neck dissection may be satisfactorily performed immediately after completion of the radiotherapy of the primary lesion. It would not be reasonable today to await satisfactory healing of the primary lesion and radiation reactions. Large or fixed adenopathies may be considered inoperable particularly when adherent to the carotid artery. Under very special circumstances, the ligation of the carotid artery may be justified (Moore and Baker[1]).

A clinically evident metastasis on the opposite side of the neck obviously darkens the prognosis, but bilateral neck dissections have been performed successfully in such cases. The problem here is that of resecting both internal jugular veins and handling the unquestionable disturbances that result in some instances, but consecutive ligation of both internal jugular veins is possible and may be warranted in certain instances (Tailhefer[63]). The ligation of the internal jugular vein seems to result in a definite increase in intracranial pressure, which is more marked when the operation is bilateral (Jones[29]; Gius and Grier[24]). This complication is not a very serious one, however, and one-stage bilateral neck dissections have been carried out successfully (Staley and Scanlon[61]).

A radical dissection may result in partial facial paralysis or paralysis of the trapezius muscle, with a corresponding drop of the shoulder, often accompanied by pain. At times, there are also sensory problems such as hyperesthesias of the neck and shoulder. The possibility of these sequelae should be presented to the patient before the operation so that he may accept them more readily if they occur.

Prophylactic treatment of cervical metastases

The prophylactic treatment of cervical metastases means *the administration of treatment before the metastatic lymph nodes have become clinically evident.* By this treatment it is hoped that in a sizable number of instances the procedure will be therapeutic for early, undetected metastases in the subclinical stage.

A *prophylactic neck dissection* in patients with carcinoma of the tongue has unquestionable merits. In the discussion of this controversial issue, arguments that are valid against the prophylactic neck dissection in carcinoma of the lower lip do not apply when carcinoma of the tongue is considered. The relative merits of a prophylactic neck dissection may be best judged on the basis of the following factors (Regato[47]):

1 *Proportion of cases that do not present ostensible metastases at the time of the treatment of the primary lesion but will present metastases later.* In carcinoma of the tongue, the proportion is high, of the order of 35% to 40%. Kremen and Arhelger[31] found twelve cases of microscopic metastases (46%) in a series of twenty-six patients with clinically negative nodes (Table 11).

2 *Chances of permanent local sterilization of the primary lesion.* This depends, of course, on the proportion of early and advanced cases and on the adequacy of the treatment. In a total of 390 consecutive cases, Ash[2] reported 218 (56%) locally controlled by radiotherapy.

3 *Greater cure rate of prophylactic neck dissections (in which nodes are histologically positive) over that of therapeutic neck dissections (on proved metastatic nodes).* Roux-Berger[53] showed a five-year survival rate of 27% as compared with one of 11% (Table 13). Others have been impressed by the same facts (Guiss and MacDon-

ald[25]; Kremen and Arhelger[31]). It remains impossible to show the merits of an early intervention as compared with a later one (Hayem et al.[26]) unless a properly randomized study is undertaken.

4 *Number of patients lost through inoperability when the operation is deferred.* It is true that this factor may be minimized by close follow-up. By waiting, one may eliminate the more malignant group which may also show local recurrence and distant metastases. It is no less true that by operating on the remainder, one may have an illusion of a better relative result. But any institution bears witness to the cases of cervical metastases that have become inoperable in a short time and that were theoretically curable by early intervention.

5 *Operative mortality of neck dissections.* A mortality of under 2% has been the rule for years, particularly due to advances in anesthesia and the advent of antibiotics.

Arguments in reference to prophylactic neck dissections tend to confuse the issues. Fayos and Lampe[19] maintain their position against it on the basis of an *a posteriori* analysis of their own material. This

Table 11. Histologic findings in carcinoma of tongue treated by prophylactic or therapeutic dissection; lymph node involvement*

	Cases	Positive	Negative	% involvement
Clinically negative nodes	26	12	14	46
Clinically palpable nodes	12	7	5	59
Total	38	19	19	50

*From Kremen, A. J., and Arhelger, S. W.: Early cancer of the oral cavity with special reference to cancer of the tongue, Postgrad. Med. **27:**422-427, 1960.

Table 12. Results of interstitial irradiation of carcinoma of tongue systematically followed by prophylactic neck dissection in patients without clinically ostensible metastases (1919-1942)*

Size of lesion	With negative lymph nodes	Well 5 yr	With positive lymph nodes	Well 5 yr
I. Primary lesion less than 2 cm	23	18	12	8
II. Primary lesion 2 cm to 3 cm localized to border	37	15	36	11
III. Primary lesion 3 cm to 4 cm, or extending across midline, or diminishing protraction of tongue	19	5	19	2
IV. Primary lesion more than 4 cm, or involvement of neighboring area, or almost complete fixation	9	2	11	0
Total	88	40	78	21

Data on seven patients with unclassified lesions, two of whom survived, are not included.
*Data from Roux-Berger, J. L., et al.: Cancer de la partie mobile de la langue. Le curage ganglionnaire prophylactique est-il justifié? Statistique de la Fondation Curie, Mem. Acad. Chir. (Paris) **75:**120-126, 1949.

Table 13. Comparative results of prophylactic and therapeutic neck dissections on patients with positive and negative lymph nodes*

	Patients	Well 5 yr	5-yr cure rate (%)
Prophylactic neck dissections	173	63	36
Lymph nodes not involved	92	41	45
Lymph nodes found involved	81	22	27
Therapeutic neck dissections	154	29	19
Lymph nodes not involved	49	18	37
Lymph nodes found involved	105	11	11

*From Roux-Berger, J. L., et al.: Cancer de la partie mobile de la langue. Le curage ganglionnaire prophylactique est-il justifié? Statistique de la Fondation Curie, Mem. Acad. Chir. (Paris) **75:**120-126, 1949.

retrospective approach eliminates cases in which subsequent developments (local recurrence, distant metastases) have shown the procedure useless or "unjustified" (Van Slooten and Buwalda[66]). Others, objecting to the word prophylactic and substituting "elective," contribute only to the confusion (Southwick et al.[59]). The word elective carries no implication of timing or of intent but simply of choice. Some carry out an occasional *elective* prophylactic neck dissection. What we advocate, until a randomized study is done, is a *systematic* prophylactic neck dissection in all patients.

Prognosis

In 1965, there were 1611 deaths from cancer of the tongue in the United States, or a crude death rate of 0.8 per 100,000. The overall results of treatment are better in women than in men, but they have remained about the same from 1949 to 1964 (Cutler et al.[13]).

Adequate local treatment will succeed in healing a rather large proportion of carcinomas of the tongue. Of 390 patients treated at the Ontario Institute of Radiotherapy from 1929 to 1947, 219 (56.2%) appeared to have been locally controlled (Table 14). Wasserburger[69] reported on a larger series treated by electrosurgery plus

interstitial curietherapy. All but one of the 162 patients with Stage I lesions were controlled.

In a symposium arranged by the American Radium Society in 1949, the overall result of the treatment of 1636 cases reported by four different European authors (Table 15) was 23% absolute five-year survivals. A series of 235 patients treated at the Radiumhemmet of Stockholm showed a five-year cure rate of 30% (Jacobsson[27]). A series of 465 patients treated at the Holt Radium Institute of Manchester was reported to show a five-year survival rate of 28% (Paterson[43]). Of 342 patients treated at the Ontario Institute of Radiotherapy and the Department of Surgery of the University of Toronto, 115 patients (33.6%) were living at the end of five years (Wookey et al.[71]).

Lyall and Schetlin[34] treated seventy-six unselected patients by surgical excision and neck dissection with twenty-nine (38%) five-year survivals. In a series of 269 patients treated surgically at the Mayo Clinic by Erich and Kragh,[18] the five-year survival rate was 46%. MacComb and Fletcher[35] selected twenty-eight patients for surgical excision of the primary lesion, nineteen of whom had stage T_1 or T_2 lesions, and eighteen patients (64%) survived five years. They treated the remaining 146 patients not eligible for surgical excision of the primary lesion by irradiation and neck dissection with forty-eight (33%) five-year survivals. Thus sixty-six (37%) of the total of 174 patients treated survived.

It is obvious in the analysis of papers on this subject that excellent treatment of metastases is no help when the proportion of local recurrences is too high and, on the other hand, that excellent radiotherapy of the primary lesion cannot compensate for

Table 14. Results of radiumtherapy of primary carcinoma of tongue*

Stage	No.	Controlled	% controlled
Early	195	150	76.4
Late	195	69	35.4
Total	390	219	56.2

*From Ash, C. L., and Millar, O. B.: Radiotherapy of cancer of the tongue and floor of the mouth, Amer. J. Roentgen. 73:611-619, 1955.

Table 15. Results of treatment of carcinoma of anterior two-thirds of the tongue

	Baud[4] (Paris) 1919-1941	Berven[5] (Stockholm) 1921-1942	Cade[9] (London) 1924-1939	Windeyer[70] (London) 1931-1942	Total 1919-1942
Patients treated	724	403	365	144	1,636
Dead of intercurrent diseases	100	34	?	9	143
Dead or living with cancer	462	267	234	93	1,056
Lost to view	14	0	32	2	48
Well five years or more	148	102	99	40	389
Five years symptomless rate	20%	25%	24%	28%	23%

the loss due to inadequate surgical management of metastases. This malignant tumor requires the best in both the radiotherapist and the surgeon.

The prognosis depends primarily on whether or not a metastasis develops. Jacobsson[27] reported on 103 patients who did not develop metastases, with a 52% five-year survival. Som[58] reported on sixty-one patients treated by interstitial irradiation and neck dissection. Two-thirds of those without metastases, or with only microscopically detected metastases, were cured, whereas only one-fourth of the patients with clinically ostensible metastases survived.

The combination of a small lesion and microscopic metastases treated early yields good results. There is a direct correlation between the size of the lesion and the possibility of metastasis (Monaco et al.[40]). In MacComb and Fletcher's series[35] at the M. D. Anderson Hospital in Houston, fifty-two (50%) of a total of 103 patients with primary lesions T_1 and T_2 survived following treatment, whereas only fifteen (20%) of seventy-three patients with primary lesions T_3 and T_4 survived. The relatively recent use of cobalt[60] and supervoltage roentgentherapy seems to have brought some improvement in results (Fayos and Lampe[19]).

It is clear that the important point in the prognosis of carcinomas of the tongue is the presence or absence of actual node involvement and the early or delayed treatment of such metastasis. For this reason, lesions that have been present for a short time or that have not become very large have a fair prognosis, but the metastasizing ability of the tumor partly reflected in its microscopic features should also be taken into consideration. Lesions that develop near the midline or that have invaded beyond it will have a worse prognosis because of their potential ability to metastasize to the opposite side of the neck. Carcinomas invading the anterior pillar of the soft palate or that have actually invaded the mandible have a very bad prognosis because of frequent failure to be locally sterilized. Aged patients can seldom tolerate the necessary treatments and are subject to greater possibilities of complications.

Cade and Lee[10] reported a greater curability of women with carcinoma of the tongue. Thirty-six of 103 women were reported well (35%) as compared with eighty-eight men well in a series of 415 (21%). Although carcinoma of the tongue seems to occur at an older age in women, the prognosis is relatively better even in the presence of metastases (Spitalier et al.[60]; Shedd et al.[55]).

Gibbel et al.[23] reported on forty-eight cases of carcinoma of the tongue with associated syphilis with only three patients (6.2%) surviving at the end of five years.

Patients with postirradiation recurrences or nonsterilization in the tongue are not necessarily hopeless. Roux-Berger[52] reported on 103 cases of nonsterilization or recurrences following radiumtherapy that were surgically excised, with ten patients remaining well after five years. Thirty-four other such cases were retreated by radiotherapy, with five patients surviving 5 years after the second treatment.

REFERENCES

1 Ackerman, L. V., and Johnson, R.: Present-day concepts of intra-oral histopathology, Proc. Nat. Cancer Conf. 1:403-414, 1954.

2 Ash, C. L.: Oral cancer; a twenty-five year study, Amer. J. Roentgen. 87:417-430, 1962.

3 Ash, C. L., and Millar, O. B.: Radiotherapy of cancer of the tongue and floor of the mouth, Amer. J. Roentgen. 73:611-619, 1955.

4 Baud, J.: End results of radiotherapy of cancer of the tongue, Amer. J. Roentgen. 63:701-711, 1950.

5 Berven, E.: End results of treatment of cancer of the tongue, Amer. J. Roentgen. 63:712-715, 1950.

6 Braund, R. R., and Martin, H. E.: Distant metastasis in cancer of the upper respiratory and alimentary tracts, Surg. Gynec. Obstet. 73:63-71, 1941.

7 Burford, W. N.: The dentist's responsibility in oral tumors, Amer. J. Orthodont. Oral Surg. (Oral Surg. Sect.) 29:612-622, 1943.

8 Buschke, Franz, and Cantril, S. T.: Dentist and cancer, Radiation Therapy, Tumor Inst., Seattle (no. 1), pp. 48-64, 1940.

9 Cade, S.: Treatment of cancer of the tongue, Amer. J. Roentgen. 63:716-718, 1950.

10 Cade, S., and Lee, E. S.: Cancer of the tongue; a study based on 653 patients, Brit. J. Surg. 44:433-446, 1957.

11 Castigliano, S. G.: Fibrosarcoma of the tongue after x-irradiation therapy for squamous cell carcinoma of the tongue; report of cases, J. Oral Surg. 26:197-200, 1968.

12 Crile, G.: Excision of cancer of the head and neck with special reference to plan of dissec-

tion based on 132 operations, J.A.M.A. **47:** 1780-1786, 1906.

13 Cutler, S. J., et al.: End results in cancer, report no. 3, Washington, D. C., 1968, National Cancer Institute.

14 Deckers, P. C., and Maisin, J.: Le cancer de la langue, J. Radiol. Electr. **42:**655-662, 1961.

15 Denoix, P.-F., and Hayem, G.: A propos de l'indication du curage cervical dans les cancers de la portion mobile de la langue sans adénopathie clinique, Mem. Acad. Chir. (Paris) **84:**592-597, 1958.

16 Diamant, H., and Hamberger, C. A.: The risks of haemorrhage in carcinoma of the tongue, Acta Otolaryng. (Stockholm) **75:**20-35, 1949.

17 Donaldson, R. C., Skelly, M., and Paletta, F. X.: Total glossectomy for cancer, Amer. J. Surg. **116:**585-590, 1968.

18 Erich, J. B., and Kragh, L. V.: Results of treatment of squamous cell carcinoma of the anterior part of the tongue, Amer. J. Surg. **98:**677-682, 1959.

19 Fayos, J. V., and Lampe, I.: Radiotherapy of squamous cell carcinoma of the oral portion of the tongue, Arch. Surg. (Chicago) **94:**316-321, 1967.

20 Fletcher, G. H., MacComb, W. S., and Braun, E. J.: Analysis of sites and causes of treatment failures in squamous cell carcinomas of the oral cavity, Amer. J. Roentgen. **83:**405-411, 1960.

21 Fletcher, G. H., and Stovall, M.: A study of the explicit distribution of radiation in interstitial implantations. II. Correlation with clinical results in squamous cell carcinomas of the anterior two-thirds of the tongue and floor of the mouth, Radiology **78:**766-782, 1962.

22 Flicinski, E.: Neurofibromatosis of the tongue in von Recklinhausen's disease, Otolaryng. Pol. **18:**153-155, 1964.

23 Gibbel, M. I., Cross, J. H., and Ariel, I. M.: Cancer of the tongue, Cancer **2:**411-423, 1949.

24 Gius, J. A., and Grier, D. H.: Venous adaptation following bilateral radical neck dissection with excision of the jugular veins, Surgery **28:** 305-321, 1950.

25 Guiss, L. W., and MacDonald, I.: End results and causes of failure in treatment of intraoral carcinoma, Amer. J. Roentgen. **83:**412-420, 1960.

26 Hayem, M., Flamant, R., Schwartz, D., and Denoix, P.: Should lymph nodes be removed as a matter of principle or not? The surgical treatment of the lymph nodes of the neck in cases of cancer of the mobile portion of the tongue, J. Chir. (Paris) **85:**189-198, 1963.

27 Jacobsson, F.: Carcinoma of the tongue, Acta Radiol. (Stockholm) (suppl. 68), pp. 1-184, 1948.

28 Jahnke, V., and Daly, J. F.: Osteoma of the tongue, J. Laryng. **82:**273-275, 1968.

29 Jones, R. K.: Increased intracranial pressure following radical neck surgery, Arch. Surg. (Chicago) **63:**599-603, 1951.

30 Khanolkar, V. R.: Oral cancer in Bombay, India; a review of 1,000 consecutive cases, Cancer Res. **4:**313-319, 1944.

31 Kremen, A. J., and Arhelger, S. W.: Early cancer of the oral cavity with special reference to cancer of the tongue, Postgrad. Med. **27:**422-427, 1960.

32 Lacassagne, A.: L'organe folié de la langue, cause possible d'un diagnostic erroné de cancer, Radiophys. Radiother. **2:**587-594, 1930.

33 Lampe, I.: Personal communication, 1955.

34 Lyall, D., and Schetlin, C. F.: Cancer of the tongue, Ann. Surg. **135:**489-496, 1952.

35 MacComb, W. S., and Fletcher, G. H.: Cancer of the head and neck, Baltimore, 1967, The Williams & Wilkins Co.

36 Maitland, H. L.: Radical method of extirpating malignant growths in the neck, secondary to mouth carcinoma, Aust. Med. Gaz. (Sydney) **25:**497-503, 1906 (discussion, p. 530).

37 Marchetta, F. C., and Mattick, W. L.: Carcinoma of the tongue, Surgery **40:**378-386, 1956.

38 Martin, H. E.: The treatment of cervical metastatic cancer, Ann. Surg. **114:**972-985, 1941.

39 Martin, H. E., Munster, H. and Sugarbaker, E. D.: Cancer of the tongue, Arch. Surg. (Chicago) **41:**888-936, 1940.

40 Monaco, A. P., Buckley, M., and Raker, J. W.: Carcinoma of the oral cavity. I. Carcinoma of anterior two-thirds of the tongue—results of surgical treatment, New Eng. J. Med. **266:** 575-579, 1962.

41 Moore, O., and Baker, H. W.: Carotid-artery ligation in surgery of the head and neck, Cancer **8:**712-726, 1955.

42 Morton, J. L., Callendine, G. W., Jr., and Myers, W. G.: Radioactive cobalt[60] in plastic tubing for interstitial radiation therapy, Radiology **56:**553-557, 1951.

43 Paterson, R.: Discussion of the treatment of cancer of the tongue, Proc. Roy. Soc. Med. **40:** 412-415, 1947.

44 Paymaster, J. C., and Shroff, P. D.: The problem of carcinoma of the tongue in India, Amer. J. Surg. **94:**450-454, 1957.

45 Peacock, E. E., Jr., Greenberg, B. G., and Brawley, B. W.: The effect of snuff and tobacco on the production of oral carcinoma: an experimental and epidemiological study, Ann. Surg. **151:**542-550, 1960.

45a Pierquin, B.: Précis de curiethérapie. Endocuriethérapie, plesiocuriethérapie, Paris, 1964, Masson et Cie.

46 Principato, J. J., Sika, J. V., and Sander, H. C.: Primary malignant melanoma of the tongue; a case report and review of the literature, Cancer **18:**1641-1645, 1965.

47 del Regato, J. A.: Tratamiento de las adenopatías metastásicas del cuello, Arch. Cubanos Cancerol. **6:**311-316, 1947.

48 Renstrup, G.: Leukoplakia of the oral cavity, Acta Odont. Scand. **16:**99-111, 1958.

49 Richards, G. E.: The treatment of cancer of the tongue, Amer. J. Roentgen. **47:**191-206, 1942.

50 Robinson, H. B. G.: Practical application of

experimental cancer research, J. Amer. Dent. Ass. **54**:524-529, 1957.

51 Roux-Berger, J. L.: Le curage des ganglions du cou dans le cancer de la langue, Radiophys. Radiother. **1**:257-264, 1927; also Presse Med. **35**:881, 1927.

52 Roux-Berger, J. L., and Baud, J.: Traitement des récidives linguales du cancer de la partie mobile de la langue, Mem. Acad. Chir. (Paris) **75**:446-453, 1949.

53 Roux-Berger, J. L., Baud, J., and Courtial, J.: Cancer de la partie mobile de la langue. Le curage ganglionnaire prophylactique est-il justifié? Statistique de la Fondation Curie, Mem. Acad. Chir. (Paris) **75**:120-126, 1949.

54 Sachs, M. D.: Metastases from carcinoma of the tongue, Amer. J. Roentgen. **42**:833-842, 1939.

55 Shedd, D. P., von Essen, C. F., Ferraro, R. H., Connelly, R. R., and Eisenberg, H.: Cancer of tongue in Connecticut, 1935-1959, Cancer **21**:89-96, 1968.

56 Sherwin, R. P., Strong, M. S., and Vaughn, C. W., Jr.: Polypoid and junctional squamous cell carcinoma of the tongue and larynx with spindle cell carcinoma ("pseudosarcoma"), Cancer **16**:51-60, 1963.

57 Slaughter, D. P., Roeser, E. H., and Smejkal, W. F.: Excision of the mandible for neoplastic diseases, indications and techniques, Surgery **26**:507-522, 1949.

58 Som, M. L.: Carcinoma of the mobile portion of the tongue; follow-up of previous study, Arch. Otolaryng. (Chicago) **87**:511-514, 1968.

59 Southwick, H. W., Slaughter, D. P., and Trevino, E. T.: Elective neck dissection for intraoral cancer, Arch. Surg. (Chicago) **80**:905-909, 1960.

60 Spitalier, J. M., Colonna D'Istria, J., and Colonna D'Istria, P. P.: A propos des carcinomes épidermoïdes de la langue mobile chez la femme, Bull. Ass. Franc. Cancer **51**:225-234, 1964.

61 Staley, C. J., and Scanlon, E. F.: Bilateral radical neck dissection, Amer. J. Surg. **98**:851-857, 1959.

62 Sturdy, D. E.: Cancer of the mouth; 11-year follow-up of 800 cases, Brit. J. Cancer **13**:13-19, 1959.

63 Tailhefer, A.: Traitement chirurgical des adénopathies du cancer de la langue; résultats éloignés, Radiophys. Radiother. **3**:419-428, 1936; also Mem. Acad. Chir. (Paris) **62**:977-983, 1936.

64 Taylor, G. W., and Nathanson, I. T.: Lymph node metastases, New York, 1942, Oxford University Press.

65 Trieger, N., Ship, I. I., Taylor, G. W., and Weisberger, D.: Cirrhosis and other predisposing factors in carcinoma of the tongue, Cancer **11**:357-362, 1958.

66 Van Slooten, E. A., and Buwalda, G.: Indications for radical neck dissection in cancer of the tongue, Nederl. T. Geneesk. **107**:1625-1629, 1963.

67 Venables, C. W., and Craft, I. L.: Carcinoma of the tongue in early adult life, Brit. J. Cancer **21**:645-650, 1967.

68 Waldron, C. A., and Schafer, W. G.: Current concepts of leukoplakia, Int. Dent. J. **10**:350-367, 1960 (extensive bibliography).

69 Wasserburger, K.: Das Zungenkarzinom, Strahlentherapie **107**:161-182, 1958.

70 Windeyer, B. W.: End results and treatment of cancer of the tongue, Amer. J. Roentgen. **63**:719-726, 1950.

71 Wookey, H., Ash, C., Welsh, W. K., and Mustard, R. A.: The treatment of oral cancer by a combinaton of radiotherapy and surgery, Ann. Surg. **134**:529-540, 1951.

72 Wynder, E. L., Bross, I. J., and Feldman, R. J.: A study of the etiological factors in cancer of the mouth, Cancer **10**:1300-1321, 1957.

Floor of mouth

Anatomy

The floor of the mouth or inferior wall of the oral cavity is a semilunar area circumscribed anteriorly by the lower dental arch and posteriorly by the inferior surface of the tongue (Fig. 138). In depth, it extends to the mylohyoid muscle, which separates it from the suprahyoid region. It

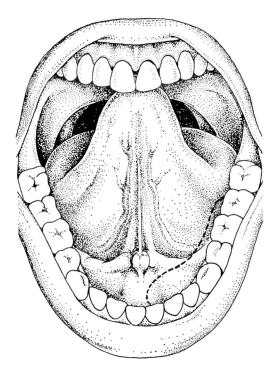

Fig. 138. Floor of mouth showing projection of sublingual gland (dotted line).

is divided in the midline by a mucous fold, the frenulum, on each side of which a small nodule with a central orifice (the openings of the canal of Wharton) can be seen. Lateral to these there are two smaller orifices corresponding to the canals of the sublingual glands.

The floor of the mouth is covered by the same squamous epithelium that covers the rest of the oral cavity. Below the mucous membrane are found the sublingual glands, the anterior pole of the submaxillary gland with its canal, and numerous vessels and nerves.

Lymphatics. The lymphatics of the floor of the mouth are continuous with those of the tongue and sublingual gland. They empty into the submaxillary nodes and the nodes of the anterior jugular chain. Laterally, they are continuous with those of the lower alveolar ridge (Rouvière[15]).

Epidemiology

Carcinomas of the floor of the mouth constitute approximately 15% of all carcinomas of the oral cavity. They are primarily observed in elderly men. The reported proportion of women varies widely from country to country: 4% in Chile (Rahausen and Sayago[13]), 22% in Puerto Rico (Correa et al.[5]), 33% in Norway (Alsos[2]). Tobacco smoking, particularly in the form of cigars, has been incriminated as a causative factor (Wynder et al.[18]). Heavy consumption of alcohol (Alford and Klopp[1]) and bad oral hygiene are also found to be associated with these tumors.

Pathology
Gross pathology

Carcinomas of the floor of the mouth arise most often on one or the other side of the midline. In most instances, they present only a deep fissurelike ulceration, the bulk of the tumor having developed submucously (Fig. 139). In other instances, the tumor is superficially ulcerated throughout, without apparently invading in depth (Fig. 140).

These tumors rapidly extend beyond the midline and become adherent to the inner aspect of the mandible. Their extension into the tongue is less frequent. However, there are instances in which it is difficult to establish whether the tumor had a lingual origin or whether the tongue was invaded secondarily. Direct extension of the tumor to the submaxillary and sublingual glands is sometimes observed, or extension may occur through the muscular layer to the submaxillary region.

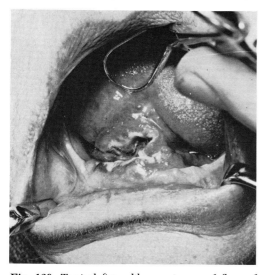

Fig. 139. Typical fissurelike carcinoma of floor of mouth extending to anterior midline.

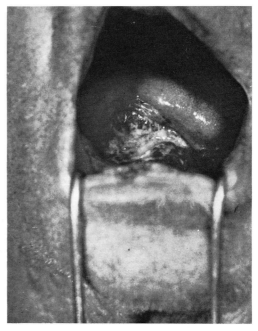

Fig. 140. Exophytic carcinoma of floor of mouth extending beyond midline and over lingual mucosa.

Microscopic pathology

Most carcinomas of the floor of the mouth are moderately differentiated epidermoid carcinomas.

Metastatic spread

Metastases from carcinomas of the floor of the mouth are found more often in the submaxillary region than are metastases from carcinoma of the tongue, and they are also more often bilateral. Metastatic implants in the anterior jugular chain of lymph nodes also take place, but this seldom occurs until after the tumor has metastasized to the submaxillary region.

Most patients with carcinoma of the floor of the mouth develop an adenopathy sometime during the course of the disease (Correa et al.[5]). Bilateral metastases are frequent even when the primary lesions appear to be confined to one side (Dargent and Papillon[6]; Laborde and Taillard[8]). Distant metastases are exceptional.

Clinical evolution

The most common presenting symptom of carcinoma of the floor of the mouth is an indurated growth felt by the tip of the tongue. Later, when the tumor becomes ulcerated, there may be *otalgia, hypersalivation,* and progressive *difficulties in speech. Bleeding* may occur, but hemorrhage is infrequent. About one-fourth of all the patients present a submaxillary adenopathy when first seen. This is often bilateral and adherent to the mandible. In many instances, the submaxillary tumefaction is actually a direct extension of the tumor. A few carcinomas of the floor of the mouth may be inconspicuous, and their clinical onset is characterized by development of a submaxillary adenopathy. The primary lesion may be found in an apparently innocent patch of sublingual leukoplakia.

Left to themselves, most carcinomas of the floor of the mouth produce complications directly related to secondary infection and malnutrition.

Diagnosis

As a rule, there is very little difficulty in establishing a diagnosis of carcinoma of the floor of the mouth. Examination should always be accompanied by a thorough digital palpation. In most instances, a biopsy is easily obtainable. When there is no large ulceration, the specimen may have to be taken with a scalpel on the indurated borders of the fissure. A needle biopsy of suspected metastatic lymph nodes may establish a definite diagnosis. This should always be done, particularly when the patient is to be treated entirely by radiotherapy.

Differential diagnosis

Few benign conditions of the floor of the mouth offer a problem of differential diagnosis. So-called *leukoplakia* of the floor of the mouth presents as a whitish patch of the mucous membrane. There is no certainty as to the neoplastic or nonneoplastic nature of such a clinical finding until it is verified by biopsy (Waldron and Schafer[17]). There is little evidence that a great number of these lesions when proved to be benign actually undergo malignant transformation, but many carcinomas of the oral cavity, which are often multicentric, present a whitish appearance.

A *chronic inflammatory obstruction* of the submaxillary or sublingual ducts produces a tumefaction of the floor of the mouth that may become indurated and displace the tongue upward. In some instances, this produces considerable pain and dysphagia and is accompanied by a hard bilateral tumefaction of the submaxillary regions which may appear as a metastatic adenopathy. In these cases, however, the absence of ulceration, the relatively rapid progression of the condition, and periods of spontaneous improvement militate against the diagnosis of carcinoma. This obstruction of the submaxillary and sublingual ducts is most often due to mucous plugs.

A *ranula* is more often a unilateral and cystic retention of saliva in the sublingual or submaxillary glands due to salivary calculus. There is no ulceration in a ranula, the tumefaction is fluctuant, and the roentgenogram may show a calcified calculus.

Sublingual salivary gland tumors are rare (Stuteville and Corley[16]). They are slow growing, nonulcerated, and rubbery in consistency and have a typical histologic appearance (p. 535).

Treatment
Surgery

A few small carcinomas of the floor of the mouth may be easily and widely excised. Many others do not allow for a sufficient margin of uninvolved tissues. In very few instances is a wide excision practicable in this area without resulting dysfunction. The mandible presents a definite impediment to an adequate excision even when it has not been reached by tumor. Often, in order to achieve an adequate excision, either the mandible or a good part of the tongue, or both, may have to be removed.

In the presence of clinically ostensible metastases, a *therapeutic* radical neck dissection is the treatment of choice. Patients with carcinoma of the floor of the mouth and metastatic adenopathy are not always eligible for a standard neck dissection. Adherence of metastasis to the mandible and bilaterality of the adenopathy may force the choice of a more radical procedure. Direct extension of the primary lesion to the mandible and into the submaxillary region often dictates the logic of a surgical *en bloc* resection of all the involved structures. When this procedure is indicated, preoperative irradiation of the primary lesion and of the metastatic nodes may favor better results.

Independently of the treatment chosen for the primary lesion, a *prophylactic* radical neck dissection is advocated by some because of the frequent occurrence of metastases (MacFee[10]) and the relative advantage of instituting treatment before the metastatic nodes become clinically ostensible. A prophylactic neck dissection is sometimes carried out in continuity with the surgical excision of the primary lesion but so-called "pull through" operations, intended to bypass the mandible, have been found wanting. Following irradiation of the primary lesion, a prophylactic neck dissection can and should be carried out in most instances.

Radiotherapy

Peroral roentgentherapy can be used successfully in the treatment of very few superficial carcinomas in this area. Radium has long been utilized in the treatment of primary carcinomas of the floor of the mouth (Reverdy and Courtial[14]). *Surface* applications requiring specially made molds have given reasonable results in skillful hands. Melville[12] combined a surface intraoral application with a submaxillary one. These procedures have given way to the greater reliability and more homogeneous external irradiation by means of cobalt[60] or supervoltage units.

Interstitial implantation of radium element or cobalt needles remains a very adequate means for the intensive irradiation of carcinomas limited to the floor of the mouth (Figs. 141 and 142). Specially

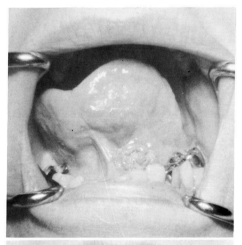

A

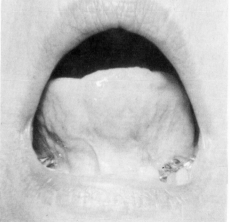

B

Fig. 141. **A,** Exophytic carcinoma of left side of floor of mouth next to frenulum in 60-year-old woman. Patient treated by radium needle implantation in double plane. Dose rate was 40 R per hour, and total dose of 7000 R was delivered in seven days. **B,** Following radiotherapy. (Courtesy Dr. Robert Lindberg, Houston, Texas.)

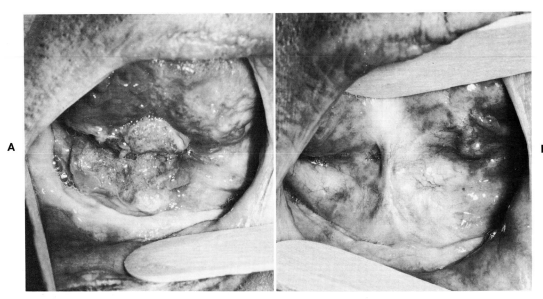

Fig. 142. A, Carcinoma of floor of mouth extending under surface of tongue. Patient treated with single plane tantalum wire implant, receiving 5000 R in 126 hours. This was followed by external irradiation to a dose of 1500 R to midline in eight days. B, Atrophy and slight telangiectases resulting from interstitial irradiation seven years later. (Courtesy Staff, Department of Radiotherapy, Princess Margaret Hospital, Toronto, Canada.)

contrived implantations make dose calculations less accurate and dose distribution less homogeneous than with similar procedures elsewhere. Irradiation of the mandible is unavoidable, and bone necrosis often occurs.

External irradiation by means of conventional roentgentherapy was often rejected because of the intense and uncomfortable oral reactions that resulted. The advent of cobalt[60] and supervoltage roentgentherapy has made more acceptable a rational course of external irradiation as a preliminary procedure before interstitial curietherapy or surgical excision (Buschke and Galante[4]). In advanced cases with submaxillary and midcervical metastases, the preliminary irradiation has already given better results (MacComb and Fletcher[9]).

Prognosis

The prognosis of carcinomas of the floor of the mouth is relatively better than that of carcinomas of the tongue. Failure of treatment of cancer of the floor of the mouth is only rarely related to distant metastases. Extensive local lesions with invasion of the bone even in the absence of

lymph node involvement are practically never cured.

In a series of 273 consecutive patients, Reverdy and Courtial[14] reported sixty (22%) well five years after curietherapy and surgery. Eight of thirty-nine with proved metastases remained well. The five-year net survival rate in a series of 427 patients treated at the Holt Radium Institute was found to be 32% (Dobbie[7]).

Ash[3] reported on 184 patients treated by radiotherapy at the Ontario Cancer Institute of Toronto, with a crude five-year survival of 40.2% (Table 16). MacComb and Fletcher[9] reported their results at the M. D. Anderson Hospital in Houston: in a series of 108 patients treated mostly by radiotherapy, but also by surgery alone (one out of five) or a combination of both treatments, forty-six patients (42%) survived five years.

In a selected series of eleven patients treated surgically, Alford and Klopp[1] reported seven living five years (65%). In a series of sixty-two unselected patients treated by radiotherapy exclusively, for both the primary and metastatic lesions, twenty-nine (46.8%) were reported well after five years (Martin and Martin[11]). In

Table 16. Carcinoma of floor of mouth; five-year survival rates by stages (1929-1955)*

	Crude 5-yr survival rate† (%)	Net 5-yr survival rate‡ (%)	Adjusted 5-yr survival rate§ (%)
Stage I (less than 1.5 cm)	59.4	73.1	70.7
Stage II (less than 3 cm)	47.0	57.4	61.0
Stage III (less than one-half tongue)	28.8	31.9	41.1
Stage IV (more than one-half tongue)	20.7	21.4	27.6
All stages (184 cases)	40.2	46.5	54.3

*Data from Ash, C. L.: Oral cancer; a twenty-five year study, Amer. J. Roentgen. 87:417-430, 1962.
†Precentage of traced patients alive and well.
‡Excluding death from intercurrent diseases.
§Percentage of expected number of survivors.

Ash's series,[3] the crude five-year survival for patients with carcinomas of the floor of the mouth measuring less than 1.5 cm was 59.4%.

REFERENCES

1 Alford, T. C., and Klopp, C. T.: The surgical treatment of cancer of the floor of the mouth, Cancer 11:1-3, 1958.

2 Alsos, T.: Cancer of the oral cavity treated at the Norwegian Radium Hospital, Cancer 13:925-931, 1960.

3 Ash, C. L.: Oral cancer; a twenty-five year study, Amer. J. Roentgen. 87:417-430, 1962.

4 Buschke, F., and Galante, M.: Radical pre-operative roentgen therapy in primarily inoperable advanced cancers of the head and neck, Radiology 73:845-949, 1959.

5 Correa, J. N., Bosch, A., and Marcial, V. A.: Carcinoma of the floor of the mouth; review of clinical factors and results of treatment, Amer. J. Roentgen. 99:302-312, 1967.

6 Dargent, M., and Papillon, J.: Le cancer du plancher de la bouche, Paris, 1955, Masson et Cie.

7 Dobbie, J. L.: Carcinoma of the floor of the mouth, Brit. J. Surg. 41:250-253, 1953.

8 Laborde, S., and Taillard, P.: Les cancers du plancher buccal, Bull. Ass. Franc. Cancer 34:153-161, 1947.

9 MacComb, W. S., and Fletcher, G. H.: Cancer of the head and neck, Baltimore, 1967, The Williams & Wilkins Co.

10 MacFee, W. F.: Carcinoma of the floor of the mouth; clinical observations and surgical treatment, Ann. Surg. 149:172-187, 1959.

11 Martin, C. L., and Martin, J. A.: Treatment of cancer of the floor of the mouth and its cervical metastases by irradiation, Southern Med. J. 51:1017-1025, 1958.

12 Melville, A. G. G.: The double radium mould treatment of carcinoma of the floor of the mouth and lower alveolus, Brit. J. Radiol. 13:337-344, 1940.

13 Rahausen, A., and Sayago, C.: Cancer of the floor of the mouth, Amer. J. Roentgen. 75:515-518, 1958.

14 Reverdy, J., and Courtial, J.: Le traitement des cancers du plancher de le bouche à la Fondation Curie de 1924 à 1941, Bull. Ass. Franc. Cancer 34:162-176, 1947.

15 Rouvière, H.: Anatomie des lymphatiques de l'homme, Paris, 1933, Masson et Cie.

16 Stuteville, O. H., and Corley, R. D.: Surgical management of tumors of intraoral minor salivary glands, Cancer 20:1578-1586, 1967.

17 Waldron, C. A., and Schafer, W. G.: Current concepts of leukoplakia, Int. Dent. J. 10:350-367, 1960.

18 Wynder, E. L., Navarette, A., Aróstegui, G. E., and Llambés, J. L.: Study of environmental factors in cancer of the respiratory tract in Cuba, J. Nat. Cancer Inst. 20:665-673, 1958.

Buccal mucosa

Anatomy

The cheeks, which form the lateral walls of the oral cavity, are formed by the buccinator muscle which is covered on its outer surface by a fairly thick layer of fat tissue and skin. Internally it is covered by a smooth squamous epithelium, which has considerably less surface than the cutaneous aspect of the cheek (Fig. 143). The term buccal mucosa is now generally applied to that part of the oral mucous membrane that is connected with the cheek or bucca. It extends from the upper to the lower gingivobuccal gutters, where the mucous membrane reflects itself to cover the upper and lower alveolar ridges, and from the commissure of the lips to the ascending ramus of the mandible. The parotid duct opens at the level of the posterosuperior quadrant of this surface at about the level of the second superior gross molar.

Lymphatics. The lymphatics of the buccal aspect of the cheek form collecting trunks that pierce the buccinator muscle and follow the direction of the facial vein, ending in the submaxillary and upper cervical lymph nodes. Any involved cervical lymph nodes are usually situated in

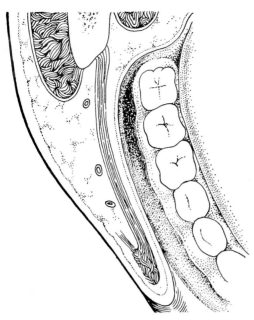

Fig. 143. Buccal mucosa showing close relationship of mucous membrane and muscle.

the prevascular group of the submaxillary region.

The lymphatics of the buccal mucosa may end in the buccinator group of the superficial facial nodes that are sometimes found over the outer surface of the buccinator muscle above a horizontal line extending from the buccal commissure to the lobule of the ear (Fig. 125). Rarely, some of them may end in the lower parotid nodes.

Epidemiology

The incidence of carcinoma of the buccal mucosa appears to be quite variable according to regions and countries. In general, it occurs only one-third or one-fourth as often as carcinoma of the tongue and, on an average, is found predominantly in patients of a more advanced age, than those who present other forms of oral carcinomas. The ratio of males to females has been reported as high as 10 to 1 by Richards,[20] who found an average age of 64 years.

The use of tobacco, particularly for chewing, appears to have an important role in the etiology of these tumors. It is our impression that in some rural areas of the United States carcinoma of the

buccal mucosa may occur even more frequently than carcinoma of the tongue, and admittedly tobacco chewing may play a role in this difference (Friedell and Rosenthal[9]).

In southern India, the incidence of carcinoma of the oral cavity is high. The tumors occur in younger male individuals, the peak age incidence being at least one decade below that found in the United States. Among 576 cases of carcinoma of the oral cavity reported by Khanolkar,[12] 315 (55%) arose from the buccal mucosa. He found the incidence of this carcinoma four times greater in Decanni Hindus than in Gujaratis. In northern India, the buccal mucosa was the most frequent site of carcinoma in patients who chewed and/or smoked tobacco (Wahi et al.[26, 27]).

Davis[7] observed that carcinoma of the buccal mucosa is also common in the Philippine Islands but is more frequently found in women. These curious phenomena have been attributed to the widespread habit of chewing betel nut (or buyo). This habit is prevalent among the natives of India, Ceylon, Malaysia, Thailand, Indochina, and the Philippine Islands, but the incidence of carcinoma of the oral cavity is not the same in all places where betel nut chewing is common. These variations have been explained in terms of changes in the ingredients or in the fashion of chewing (Orr[17]). It is possible that the betel chewing only supplements bad oral hygiene and that dietary factors may be overwhelmingly more important (Khanolkar[12]).

The cud consists of finely cut Areca nuts (betel palm), slaked lime, spices (cardamom, nutmeg, and others), and buyo leaves from the Piper betel plants (Hueper[10]). Tobacco may or may not be added to the composition. The betel nut is rich in tannic acid. The lime sweetens the bitter taste of the leaves which contain essential oils. The chewing of these ingredients results in the formation of a bright red dye. The cud is usually carried between the lower teeth or gums and the buccal mucosa, often all day and even during the night (Veliath[24]).

Sirsat and Doctor[22] studied the buccal mucosa of three groups of Indians: (1) those who chewed betel nut with tobacco with evidence of oral carcinoma, (2) those who chewed betel nut with tobacco without clinical evidence of cancer, and (3) nonchewers and nonsmokers without oral lesions. They found evidence of dyskeratosis in the first two groups, evidence of unsuspected carcinoma in two persons in the second group, and no evidence of dyskeratosis in the control group. These findings are objective evidence that tobacco plays a role in the causation of carcinoma of the oral cavity.

Pathology
Gross pathology

Carcinomas that arise on the buccal aspect of the cheeks develop rather frequently in association with an area of leukoplakia. In fact, except for carcinomas of the tongue, there is no other lesion of the oral cavity that is so frequently associated with a leukoplakic patch. The lesions most commonly arise on that part of the buccal mucosa that lies against the lower third molar, but they also may arise from the middle of the buccal area against the occlusal line of the teeth and from the neighborhood of the commissure of the lips.

Grossly, there are three distinct types of carcinomas of the buccal mucosa: the exophytic, the ulcerating, and the verrucous.

The *exophytic* papillary growths are usually soft and whitish in appearance. They are commonly associated with, and preceded by, leukoplakia, and they usually become thick but not necessarily extensive. They are more commonly found at the level of the buccal commissure.

The *ulcerating* lesions are not so common but often present a deep excavation with diffuse surrounding infiltration. They invade the buccinator muscle rather early in their development and also extend to the anterior pillar of the soft palate and to the lower alveolar ridge. Actual invasion of the bone is not infrequent. Extension to the pharyngomaxillary fossa occurs easily from posteriorly situated lesions. The ulceration may extend through the entire thickness of the cheek to ulcerate the skin. When the buccal commissure is involved, the lesion may enlarge the opening of the mouth.

The *verrucous* type of carcinoma of the buccal mucosa is a built-up lesion with a pebbly, mammillated surface. The tumor may be relatively soft but, with coexisting infection, induration becomes prominent. These lesions spread considerably on the surface but also may extend to involve the soft tissues and the underlying bone (Ackerman[1]). Kraus and Perez-Mesa[13] studied 105 cases of verrucous carcinoma, seventy-seven of which were located in the oral cavity, with fifty occurring on the buccal mucosa.

Microscopic pathology

Carcinoma in situ may precede the development of invasive carcinoma of the buccal mucosa as well as carcinoma elsewhere in the oral cavity (Slaughter[23]; Byars and Anderson[6]) (Fig. 144). It may be observed on the periphery of an infiltrating carcinoma but also may be found removed from the area of infiltration or as a first manifestation of the disease. There appears to be little doubt that eventually carcinomas in situ become invasive and even capable of destroying bone, but the time lapse is variable (Ackerman and Johnson[2]). Most carcinomas of the buccal mucosa are well differentiated.

It is worthy of special note that in the verrucous type of carcinoma repeated biopsies may reveal only hyperkeratinization, hyperplasia, and chronic inflammation. The time lost in taking multiple biopsies for establishing a diagnosis means delay in treatment.

Microscopically, long fingers of well-differentiated squamous epithelium dip deeply into the tissues but maintain their basement membrane. As the process becomes more advanced, considerable inflammation is present just beneath this basement membrane. The tumor insinuates itself into the soft tissues of the cheek and can extend to the surface, where it may ulcerate (Fig. 145). No matter how extensive or how deeply invasive, it maintains its extremely well-differentiated pattern.

Metastatic spread

Only about half of all carcinomas of the buccal mucosa present a metastasis during their development. Actually, the percentage of metastases found in any series will depend considerably on the number of

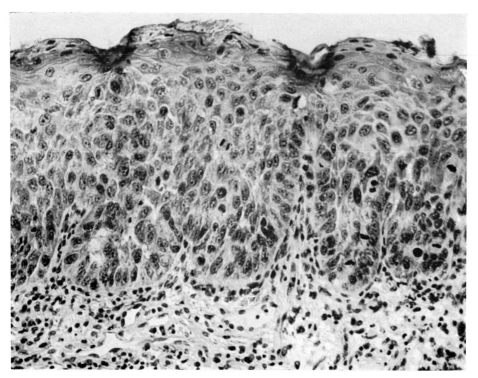

Fig. 144. Carcinoma in situ. Disorganization of all layers of epidermis with innumerable mitotic figures. Basement membrane intact. (Moderate enlargement.)

verrucous type of carcinomas included, for these very seldom metastasize. The ulcerating and exophytic types metastasize with the usual frequency of all carcinomas of the oral cavity. Metastases more often appear in the submaxillary region but rarely in the parotid gland group of lymph nodes.

Distant metastases infrequently occur, as in other carcinomas of the oral cavity. In ten cases of carcinoma of the buccal mucosa seen at autopsy, Braund and Martin[4] reported four with distant metastases.

Clinical evolution

The onset of carcinomas of the buccal mucosa is usually insidious. Frequently, the lesion has infiltrated sufficiently to produce *trismus* by the time the first examination is made. A submaxillary *adenopathy* is sometimes the first clinical symptom, and *bleeding* may be present in variable degrees. *Pain* is very intense in the ulcerating forms but may not appear at all in extensive stages of the verrucous type of carcinoma.

Exophytic lesions grow to be considerably bulky and may interfere with mastication. Ulcerating lesions can involve the entire surface of the buccal mucous membrane and be surrounded by indurated, edematous tissues. In these cases, there is usually a marked amount of secondary infection. Left to themselves, the exophytic and ulcerating lesions of the buccal mucosa invade and destroy the entire cheek and present metastases to the submaxillary and upper cervical regions. The general condition of the patient is affected because of the secondary infection and inability to masticate.

The verrucous type of carcinoma produces practically no functional defect and is accompanied by very little induration. In a rapid examination, the extension of the lesion to the adjacent structures may not be evident. The advanced verrucous carcinoma may produce considerable destruction of the upper alveolar ridge and mandibular bone, terminating fatally without even metastasizing to the submaxillary region.

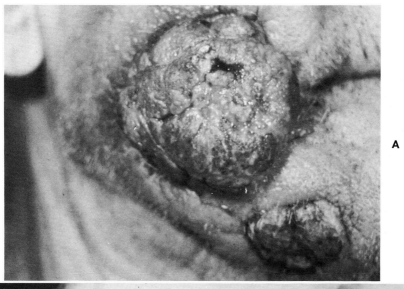

A

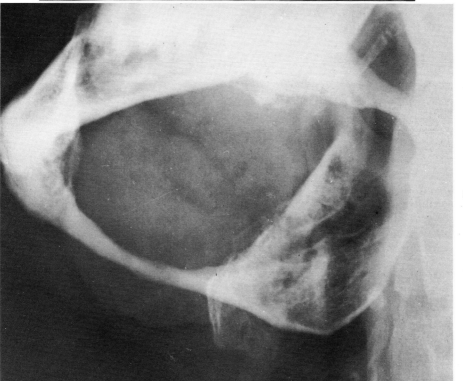

B

Fig. 145. A, Verrucous carcinoma of buccal mucosa that has invaded through skin of cheek and floor of mouth. **B,** Mandible has been invaded and eroded extensively. (**A,** WU neg. 65-1680; **B,** from Kraus, F. T., and Perez-Mesa, C.: Verrucous carcinoma, Cancer **19:**26-38, 1966; WU neg. 64-5814.)

Diagnosis

There are a few benign conditions of the buccal mucosa, and they offer little difficulty in the differential diagnosis. Mucous cysts are usually multiple, small, and separated by areas of normal mucous membrane. Leukoplakia is frequently found, particularly around the commissure of the lips, usually in the form of an isolated patch of raised whitish mucous membrane. Although these areas of leukoplakia may disappear upon improvement in oral hygiene, they should be biopsied or excised because areas of leukoplakia that appear benign may show evidence of carcinoma on microscopic examination.

The verrucous type of carcinoma of the buccal mucosa appears clinically as a benign condition because of its lack of ulceration, secondary infection, and symptomatology. In addition, repeated biopsies may show nothing but hyperkeratinization, hyperplasia, and chronic inflammation. It is important to remember that, in spite of this, the lesions will behave with a rather malignant local character although they seldom metastasize. After several local excisions and recurrences, the diagnosis of well-differentiated epidermoid carcinoma is invariably finally established.

Salivary and mucous gland tumors are found around the orifice of the parotid duct and are generally well defined, nonulcerating, slowly growing tumors. In a collected series of 760 benign minor salivary gland tumors (Fine et al.[8]), forty-four arose from the buccal mucosa. The majority of these oral salivary tumors are pleomorphic adenomas (mixed tumors) (Vellios and Shafer[25]). Next in frequency are the mucoepidermoid carcinomas. Usually they can be adequately excised.

Treatment

Good results may be obtained in the treatment of early carcinomas of the buccal mucosa by both surgical excision and radiotherapy. The cure of tumors that have already invaded adjacent structures will depend greatly on the method of approach.

Radiotherapy

Roentgentherapy. External roentgentherapy has been used as a preparatory measure before interstitial curietherapy or surgical excision. As such, roentgentherapy seems to be of unquestionable value. Used alone as a curative measure, however, it gives inconstant and not sufficiently good results to justify its systematic and exclusive use. Peroral roentgentherapy is practical only in limited lesions of the posterior half of the buccal mucosa and in particular in those that have already invaded the anterior pillar of the soft palate. In these cases, a combination of external and peroral irradiation may be, but is not often, sufficient to control the lesion.

Curietherapy. The best results in the treatment of carcinoma of the buccal mucosa appear to have been obtained by interstitial curietherapy with radium element needles. Richards[20] used this form of treatment in conjunction with external and peroral roentgentherapy with good results. The insertion of radium element needles allows a concentrated but sufficiently homogeneous irradiation to eradicate a limited carcinoma without damage to the adjacent structures. This type of irradiation cannot be applied to lesions that have already invaded the upper or lower alveolar ridge or the anterior pillar of the soft palate. It may be very successful in all lesions that are sufficiently sepa-

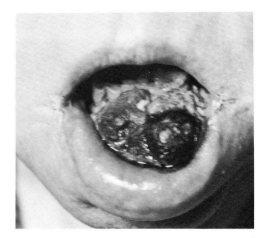

Fig. 146. Large verrucous carcinoma of buccal mucosa, lower gingiva, and floor of mouth. Patient had habitually placed snuff in this area for more than fifty years. Lesion regressed completely after midline radiation dose of 5500 R (betatron) in forty-three days. One month later, larger tumor mass had regrown. (From Kraus, F. T., and Perez-Mesa, C.: Verrucous carcinoma, Cancer **19:** 26-38, 1966; WU neg. 57-5361.)

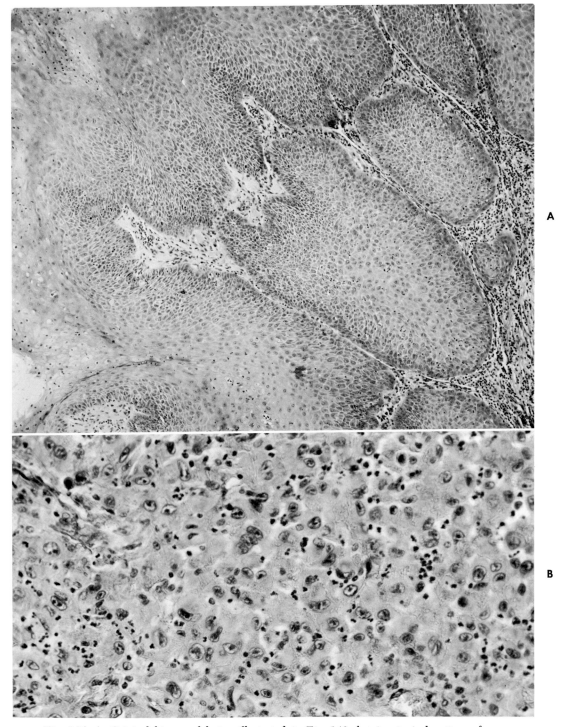

Fig. 147. A, Original biopsy of lesion illustrated in Fig. 146 showing typical pattern of verrucous carcinoma. **B,** Tumor appearing after radiation therapy was poorly differentiated epidermoid carcinoma. Surgical excision with neck dissection failed to control undifferentiated
carcinoma. Patient died of disseminated carcinoma and local infection in neck nine months
after initial radiation therapy. (**A,** ×85; WU neg. 65-393; **B,** ×300; WU neg. 62-4544; **A** and **B**
from Kraus, F. T., and Perez-Mesa, C.: Verrucous carcinoma, Cancer **19:**26-38, 1966.)

rated from those structures to avoid untoward effect.

The exophytic type of lesion is particularly suitable for interstitial curietherapy. Seldom, however, are the ulcerating lesions sufficiently well delimited to justify its use.

Interstitial irradiation of the buccal mucosa has the added advantage that its failure does not necessarily imply the failure to cure the disease, for as soon as a recurrence is detected, a radical excision can be carried out just as well and perhaps better than if it had been done in the first place. Recurrences not being the rule, this sequence is well justified. Perez et al.[19] reported on three cases of verrucous carcinoma of the oral cavity which regressed promptly under irradiation. The postirradiation recurrences revealed a highly undifferentiated carcinoma (Figs. 146 and 147).

Surgery

Early accessible lesions of the buccal mucosa may be successfully excised. In some instances, a wide excision of the buccal mucosa may be followed by a skin graft. These limited excisions, however, are justified only in the very early lesions and are still often followed by a recurrence.

For moderately advanced ulcerating lesions of the buccal mucosa and for all such lesions that have already invaded the lower alveolar ridge or that have metastasized to the submaxillary region, the wisest and most successful procedure is a radical en bloc excision of the primary lesion and its adenopathy. An atypical form of radical neck dissection which includes resection of part of the mandible and some other oral structures is usually done with appreciable success for radical treatment of carcinomas of the buccal mucosa or of the lower alveolar ridge. When the tumor has invaded the soft palate, the upper alveolar ridge, or the pterygoid fossa, even the most radical operation is bound to result in failure. Verrucous carcinomas that have invaded and destroyed the mandible, however, may be successfully treated by this type of surgery. Lengthy and tedious plastic repair is sometimes necessary following this radical excision, and the cosmetic result, although not perfect, may eventually be satisfactory (Fig. 148). In spite of any disadvantages, however, this operation is

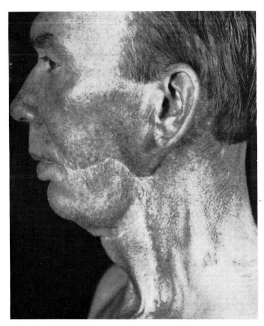

Fig. 148. Satisfactory cosmetic result in patient treated for carcinoma of buccal mucosa by radical surgical excision.

well justified when applied to the aforementioned lesions that are not curable by any other means.

Prognosis

The prognosis of ulcerating lesions of the buccal mucosa is rather poor, but that of verrucous carcinomas is excellent (Kraus and Perez-Mesa[13]). The prognosis of exophytic lesions depends on the stage of their development. Lampe[14] reported on the treatment of thirty consecutive cases of carcinoma of the buccal mucosa by roentgentherapy with fifteen patients well at the end of five years. Jackson and New[11] reported on 107 cases, of which only ninety-three were followed, with forty-eight patients surviving five years after surgical treatment. Modlin and Johnson[15] reported eleven patients (47%) surviving five years in a series of twenty-seven with carcinoma of the buccal mucosa and lower gingiva treated by combined jaw resection and neck dissection. He had an operative mortality of 6%.

Paymaster[18] reported the results of the treatment of 467 patients with carcinoma of the buccal mucosa by different methods with 43% five-year survivals. There were

Table 17. Cancer of buccal mucosa; results of treatment in 467 patients*

Mode of treatment	Cases	No evidence of disease at end of 5 yr	
		Cases	%
Radiotherapy and surgery	170	92	54
Surgery	75	36	48
Radiotherapy	222	72	32
Total	467	200	43

*From Paymaster, J. C.: Cancer of the buccal mucosa; a clinical study of 650 cases in Indian patients, Cancer 9:431-435, 1956.

no details of the proportion of patients with metastases and the results of treatment when metastases were present (Table 17). In a series of 374 patients treated at the Ontario Cancer Institute, mostly by curietherapy, 132 (35.3%) were reported well after five years (Ash[3]). O'Brien and Catlin[16] reported on 248 patients with carcinoma of the buccal mucosa treated by surgery with a 42% five-year survival rate.

REFERENCES

1 Ackerman, L. V.: Verrucous carcinoma of the oral cavity, Surgery 23:670-678, 1948.
2 Ackerman, L. V., and Johnson, R.: Present-day concepts of intraoral histopathology. In Proceedings of the Second National Cancer Conference, vol. 1, New York, 1952, American Cancer Society, Inc., pp. 403-414.
3 Ash, C. L.: Oral cancer; a twenty-five year study, Amer. J. Roentgen. 87:417-430, 1962.
4 Braund, R. R., and Martin, H. E.. Cancer of the upper respiratory and alimentary tracts, Surg. Gynec. Obstet. 73:63-71, 1941.
5 Buschke, Franz, and Cantril, S. T.: The dentist and cancer, Radiation Therapy, Tumor Inst., Seattle (no. 1), pp. 48-64, 1940.
6 Byars, L. T., and Anderson, R.: Multiple cancer of the oral cavity, Amer. Surg. 18:386-391, 1952.
7 Davis, G. G.: Buyo cheek cancer, J.A.M.A. 64:711-718, 1915.
8 Fine, G., Marshall, R. B., and Horn, R. C., Jr.: Tumors of the minor salivary glands, Cancer 13:653-669, 1960.
9 Friedell, H. L., and Rosenthal, L. M.: The etiologic role of chewing tobacco in cancer of the mouth, J.A.M.A. 116:2130-2135, 1941.
10 Hueper, W. C.: Occupational tumors and allied diseases, Springfield, Ill., 1942, Charles C Thomas, Publisher.
11 Jackson, H. S., and New, G. B.: Carcinoma of the buccal mucosa; treatment and end results, Surg. Gynec. Obstet. 91:232-241, 1950.
12 Khanolkar, V. R.: Oral cancer in India, Acta Un. Int. Cancr. 15:67-77, 1959.
13 Kraus, F. T., and Perez-Mesa, C.: Verrucous carcinoma, Cancer 19:26-38, 1966.
14 Lampe, I.: Radiation therapy of cancer of the buccal mucosa and lower gingiva, Amer. J. Roentgen. 73:628-635, 1955.
15 Modlin, J., and Johnson, R. E.: The surgical treatment of cancer of the buccal mucosa and lower gingiva, Amer. J. Roentgen. 73:620-627, 1955.
16 O'Brien, P. H., and Catlin, D.: Cancer of the cheek (mucosa), Cancer 18:1392-1398, 1965.
17 Orr, Ian M.. Oral cancer in betel nut chewers in Travancore, Lancet 2:575-580, 1933.
18 Paymaster, J. C.: Cancer of the buccal mucosa; a clinical study of 650 cases in Indian patients, Cancer 9:431-435, 1956.
19 Perez, C. A., Kraus, F. T., Evans, J. C., and Powers, W. E.: Anaplastic transformation in verrucous carcinoma of the oral cavity after radiation therapy, Radiology 86:108-115, 1966.
20 Richard, G. E.: Radiation therapy of carcinoma of the buccal mucosa (cheek). In Pack, G. T., and Livingston, E. M.: Treatment of cancer and allied diseases, vol. 1, New York, 1940, Hoeber Medical Division, Harper & Row, Publishers, pp. 327-344.
21 Rouvière, H.: Anatomie des lymphatiques de l'homme, Paris, 1933, Masson et Cie.
22 Sirsat, M. V., and Doctor, V. D.: A histopathologic study on the effect of tobacco chewing on the buccal mucosa in Indians and its relationships to cancer, Brit. J. Cancer 21:277-284, 1967.
23 Slaughter, D. P.: Multicentric orgin of intraoral carcinoma, Surgery 20:133-146, 1946.
24 Veliath, D. G.: The problem of cancer in India, J. Indian Med. Ass. 19:397-399, 1950.
25 Vellios, F., and Shafer, W. G.: Tumors of the intraoral accessory salivary glands, Surg. Gynec. Obstet. 108:450-456, 1959.
26 Wahi, P. N., Lahiri, B., Kehar, U., and Arora, S.: Oral and oropharyngeal cancers in North India, Brit. J. Cancer 19:627-641, 1965.
27 Wahi, P. N., Kehar, U., and Lahiri, B.: Factors influening oral and oropharyngeal cancers in India, Brit. J. Cancer 19:642-660, 1962.

Lower gingiva

Anatomy

The lower gingiva is formed by the soft tissues that cover the alveolar ridge of the mandible. The mucous membrane of the floor of the mouth extends laterally and forward to cover the inner aspect of the alveolar process, where it becomes continuous with the periosteum of the alveoli. The mucous membrane joins between the teeth with that which covers the outer aspect of the alveolar ridge, and when teeth are not present, the mucous membrane entirely covers the free border of the mandible. Laterally, the mucous membrane

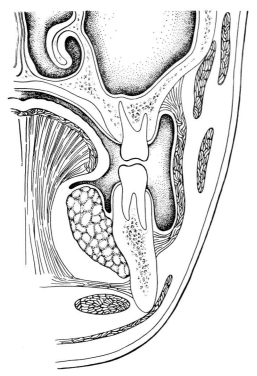

Fig. 149. Frontal section of upper and lower jaws illustrating medial and lateral contours of lower gingiva and its close relationship to floor of mouth and sublingual gland as well as to buccal mucosa and buccinator muscle.

extends over the outer surface and reflects upon itself in the gingivobuccal and gingivolabial gutters, where it joins with the buccal and labial mucous membrane (Fig. 149). At the level of the alveolar ridge, the mucous membrane is rather thick with underlying rich connective tissue and, unlike the mucous membrane of the rest of the oral cavity, is not provided with glands.

Lymphatics. Rouvière[20] divided the lymphatics of the lower gingiva into a lateral and a medial network. The lymphatics of the lateral aspect gather into several trunks that pass through the insertions of the buccinator muscle and follow the facial vein to end in the submaxillary lymph nodes. The lymphatics of the region of the incisors may end in the submental lymph nodes. The medial lymphatics pass through the mylohyoid muscle and end predominantly in the submaxillary nodes, which are found in front of the submaxillary gland. Others follow an opposite direction, passing outside of the styloglossus muscle and inside of the digastric muscle, and end for the most part in the subdigastric group of lymph nodes (Fig. 150).

Epidemiology

In a group of 8828 patients with cancer seen at Emory University during a period of twenty years, there were 512 malignant tumors of the oral cavity. Of these, seventy-

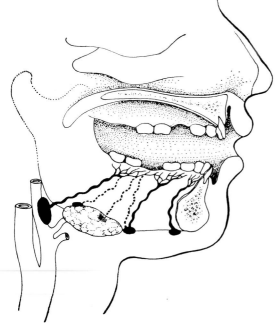

Fig. 150. Medial and lateral lymphatics of lower gingiva leading to submental, submaxillary, and subdigastric lymph nodes.

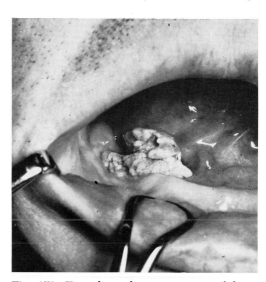

Fig. 151. Typical exophytic carcinoma of lower gingiva.

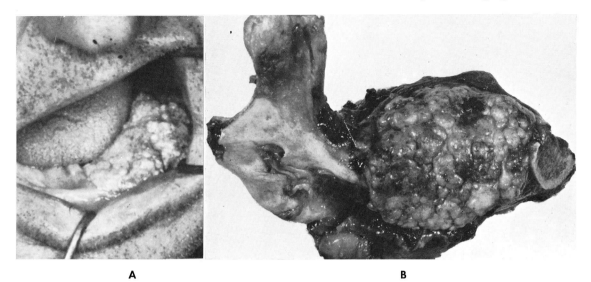

A B

Fig. 152. A, Typical verrucous carcinoma of lower gingiva showing granulating surface and extensive development. B, Surgical specimen after block resection of mandible from midline to condyle. Specimen includes submaxillary contents.

nine or about 1% of the total were carcinomas of the gingivae. Sixty-three of the lesions were located in the lower gingiva, and more than half of the patients were female (Wilkins and Vogler[24]).

Carcinomas of the lower gingiva are predominantly found at an older age than is usual for other forms of cancer of the oral cavity and are very rarely found in individuals under 40 years of age.

Pathology
Gross pathology

Carcinomas of the lower gingiva usually arise in the molar area or posterior third of the dental arch. They are sometimes found in the premolar or middle third area but are very rarely seen to arise in the anterior third or midline area.

Grossly, the most common forms of carcinoma of the lower gingiva can be divided into three types: exophytic, ulcerating, and verrucous.

The *exophytic* type of lesion is a cauliflower-like outgrowth which is seldom confined to the gingiva. This lesion bleeds easily and has a tendency to spontaneous necrosis (Fig. 151).

The *ulcerating* type of growth is usually accompanied by extensive invasion of the mandible with exposure of the bone.

The *verrucous* type of carcinoma is char-

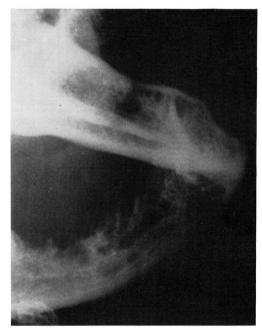

Fig. 153. Same lesion illustrated in Fig. 152 showing diffuse involvement of bone.

acterized by a granular, noninfected, superficial growth which may spread to the buccal mucosa, lower lip, and floor of the mouth and, in advanced cases, may invade the bone (Fig. 152).

Laterally, tumors of the lower gingiva easily spread to the subcutaneous fat and

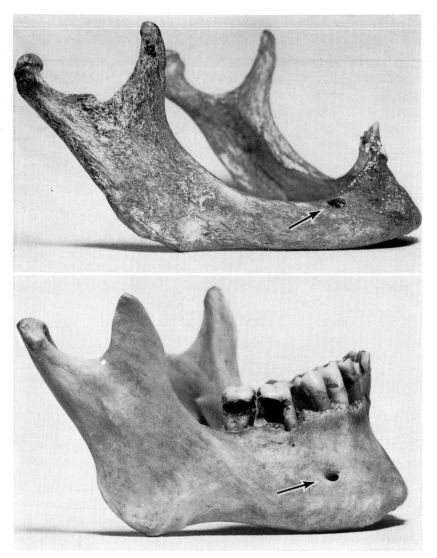

Fig. 154. Graphic demonstration of great difference in distance of mental foramen from gingival mucosa in edentulous and dentulous mandibles. This has important practical significance in patients with cancer of gingiva. (Specimens courtesy Dr. L. T. Byars, St. Louis, Mo.; WU negs. 60-8619 and 60-8618.)

skin of the cheek, producing an outside tumefaction that is continuous with the primary growth, and then they may rapidly break through the skin. Medially, these tumors often extend to the floor of the mouth, where they invade the sublingual tissues, but only exceptionally do they succeed in spreading directly to the submaxillary fossa. Posteriorly, the spread of these tumors to the retromolar area puts them in the region of the anterior pillar of the soft palate, from which they can extend to the

pterygomaxillary fossa. In depth, they extend through the alveoli to the center of the mandible, at times producing wide areas of bone destruction (Fig. 153). They can also extend along the periosteum for a considerable distance, unsuspected clinically and radiographically.

Byars[8] emphasized that invasion of the mental foramen may occur with carcinoma. This invasion is facilitated by atrophy so that the distance the tumor has to travel to invade the nerve foramen is a relatively short one in comparison with the distance between the alveolar margin and the foramen in a normal mandible (Fig. 154). With invasion of the mental foramen, the necessity of doing a hemisection of the mandible increases. If partial resection is done, the gap can be breeched by a prosthesis.

Microscopic pathology

The great majority of carcinomas of the lower gingiva are epidermoid and, as a rule, are rather differentiated. Melanocarcinomas and adenocarcinomas have been observed rarely.

It is worthy of note that in the verrucous type of carcinoma a single biopsy may show only hyperkeratinization, hyperplasia, and chronic inflammation and that only on repeated biopsies or on examination of a surgical specimen can a definite diagnosis of epidermoid carcinoma be made. Microscopically, the tumor is characterized by long fingers of squamous epithelium extending deep into the tissues but maintaining its basement membrane (Fig. 155). It maintains a well-differentiated pattern throughout.

Metastatic spread

In a series of 275 cases of carcinoma of the lower gingiva studied by Taylor and Nathanson,[23] metastases were present in 178 (65%). The first metastatic node is usually in the submaxillary region. It usually becomes attached to the mandible, forming a single block with the primary lesion. Rarely is there subdigastric node involvement without a previous submaxillary metastasis. Jugular chain nodes are often secondarily involved. Distant metastases are found in about one-third of carcinomas of the lower gingiva that come to autopsy.

Clinical evolution

Generally, carcinomas of the lower gingiva are first noticed because they interfere with the proper fitting of a denture or because of bleeding on mastication. The dentist is most often consulted about these difficulties, and consequently he holds a great part of the responsibility for the early diagnosis. There is often a history of extraction of teeth and of surgical incisions for a suspected alveolar abscess before a

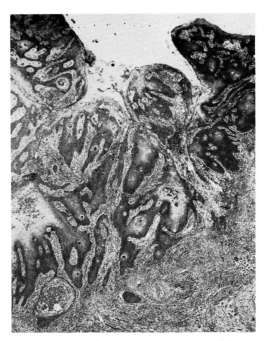

Fig. 155. Typical verrucous carcinoma of lower gingiva showing long fingers of deeply invading, well-differentiated squamous epithelium. Basement membrane intact.

correct diagnosis is established. There may be a spontaneous *bleeding*, but this is usually associated with exophytic tumors. *Otalgia* on the same side as the lesion often accompanies secondary infection. *Trismus* is sometimes observed, particularly when the tumor develops posteriorly. Severe pain often accompanies the ulcerating type of lesion that has developed extensive invasion of the bone. In verrucous carcinomas, there may be a remarkable absence of all symptoms in spite of the extension of the tumor.

On examination of the gingiva, the most common lesion is an exophytic, rubbery growth extending to the floor of the mouth and to the gingivobuccal gutter. Less commonly, the lesion is ulcerated, exposing the mandible and accompanied by considerable induration and infiltration of the surrounding tissues. Superficial nonulcerated and nonsecondarily infected lesions of the verrucous type usually extend to adjacent structures. They have a typical granular appearance, and their exact limits may be difficult to establish (Fig. 152). Not infrequently, carcinomas of the lower gingiva may present a superficial whitish appearance which is often diagnosed, clinically, as "leukoplakia."

An outside tumefaction of the lower portion of the cheek with adherence to, and ulceration of, the skin is not uncommonly found. Enlargement of the submaxillary lymph nodes is present in more than half of the cases, and, although not always, they are most often metastatic. The submaxillary tumefaction may represent direct extension of the tumor but, because of ulceration and secondary infection, there may be inflammatory enlargement of the lymph nodes and of the submaxillary gland.

Death usually occurs in unsuccessfully treated cases or in posttreatment recurrences and is usually caused by complications such as hemorrhage and bronchopneumonia. Distant metastases, although sometimes found, are seldom directly responsible for the death.

Diagnosis
Clinical examination

Examination of a carcinoma of the lower gingiva should not be limited to mere inspection but should always be completed by careful palpation of the floor of the mouth, gingivobuccal gutter, soft palate, and soft tissues of the cheek. In general, the diagnosis of the primary lesion will offer no difficulties, but the clinical impression should always be substantiated by a biopsy. The careful inspection and palpation should establish as far as possible the extent of the tumor and consequently will be of capital importance in the therapeutic decisions.

Roentgenologic examination

A roentgenogram of the mandible is an absolute requisite in all cases of carcinoma of the gingiva, for it may reveal evidence of bone invasion even when this is not clinically suspected (Fig. 153). On the other hand, lack of radiographic evidence of bone invasion is not an absolute proof of its absence. Also, it is frequent that in surgical specimens the carcinomatous infiltration is found to extend far beyond the radiographic evidence of such extension. Swearingen et al.[22] studied 100 cases of carcinoma of the lower gingiva, fifty-six of which "invaded or eroded the mandible." They apply the term invasion for actual

infiltration of the medullary bone and erosion to the roentgenographic evidence of extension into the bone. In their series, there were thirteen false-positive interpretations of erosion. At times, invasion of the mental foramen by carcinoma can be demonstrated.

Differential diagnosis

Chronic inflammatory ulcerations of the gingiva, which are sometimes observed in the area of defective teeth, may be taken for early carcinomatous lesions. Such inflammatory ulcerations will disappear rapidly after extraction of carious teeth and improvement of the oral hygiene. If there is outgrowth in addition to the ulceration, a biopsy should be done at the time of extraction.

Chronic inflammatory outgrowths of the gingival mucous membrane are smooth tonguelike projections found between the teeth. They are usually small but are sometimes large enough to cover two or three teeth (Bernick[4]). They may bleed easily when traumatized, and they give the impression of a neoplasm.

Inflammatory masses of the gingiva may show irregular epithelial proliferation, and these changes may be so prominent that secondary destruction of the mandible will take place. This may be interpreted by the radiologist as invasion of the mandible by cancer. *Pseudoepitheliomatous hyperplasia* may also be misinterpreted by the pathologist as epidermoid carcinoma (Ackerman and McGavran[2]) (Fig. 156).

Peripheral giant cell tumors are commonly observed on the gingiva, more often in the premolar area but also in the area of the molars. They are smooth, shiny tumefactions with some areas of induration and others of considerable softness. Their clinical appearance is typical, and biopsy will rapidly substantiate the clinical impression. In children, the clinical diagnosis will have the added support of the fact that carcinomas of the lower gingiva are practically never seen in juveniles. When these lesions have received an injury such as incision or extraction of teeth, they may become ulcerated and secondarily infected. When secondary infection takes place, central necrosis, pain, and even trismus may contribute to give them the appearance of

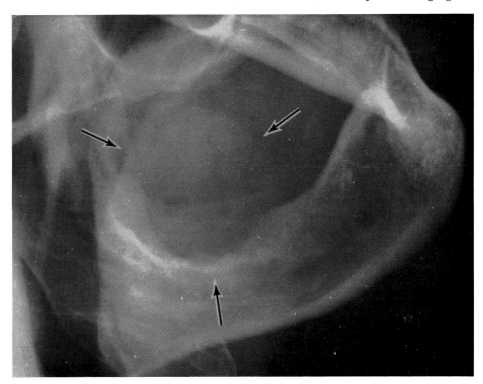

Fig. 156. Local destruction of mandible in presence of soft tissue inflammatory mass (arrows). This lesion was misinterpreted by both pathologist and radiologist as epidermoid cancer. Mandibular resection was done, and mass was entirely inflammatory. (WU neg. 57-4722.)

a malignant tumor. These giant cell tumors develop slowly and recur following incomplete excisions.

Some rare inflammatory lesions of the mandible may show a fibrous structure and appear pedunculated, becoming ulcerated only after trauma. Simple *fibromas* arising from the periodontal membrane are usually well encapsulated, their vascularity decreasing with age (Bernier[5]). *Leukemia* may present a rather characteristic swelling of the gums, which is sometimes an early manifestation of the disease (Moloney[17]).

The whitish appearance of the mucous membrane usually referred to as *leukoplakia* may be due to incipient infiltrating carcinoma, to carcinoma in situ, or to areas of hyperkeratosis which may or may not be associated with cancer.

Primary benign and malignant *tumors of the mandible,* as well as *metastatic lesions* to this bone, may become ulcerated in the mouth and suggest rarely a primary carcinoma of the lower gingiva. When this takes place, the biopsy will make the dif-

ferential diagnosis, for it usually will reveal evidence of a type of tumor (adenocarcinoma, ameloblastoma, etc.) very different from the epidermoid carcinomas that are usually found in this region.

Treatment
Radiotherapy

Surface and interstitial radiumtherapy, once the main approach to the treatment of these carcinomas, have given way to the applications of peroral roentgentherapy and external irradiation by means of cobalt[60] or supervoltage roentgentherapy. Cases of carcinoma of the lower gingiva are curable by means of radiations even when the mandible has been eroded. (Lampe[12]). The use of external irradiation and the highly penetrating radiations of cobalt[60] and supervoltage units is justified by the relatively lesser absorption of these radiations by the mandible and the frequent association with an adjacent metastatic node. Verrucous carcinomas do regress under irradiation. Perez et al.[18] reported instances of apparent postirradiation transformation into undifferentiated carcinoma.

Preoperative radiotherapy has come into greater use as its advocates have shown that adequate utilization of high-quality radiations not only do not interfere with subsequent surgery, but also yield improved results. Krishnamurthi and Shanta[11] reported practically no morbidity with the use of cobalt[60] preoperatively. As pointed out by Bacq,[3] the tendency has been toward an association of cobalt[60] teletherapy and surgery and away from radium applications or surgery alone in the treatment of these tumors.

Surgery

A local excision of a carcinoma of the gingiva through the mouth aims to conserve part of the horizontal branch of the mandible and to maintain continuity of the mandibular arch. Such an operation is justified only in early cases in which the tumor is limited to the alveolar ridge of the mandible. Under these circumstances, however, roentgentherapy is just as successful. Resections of a good part of the horizontal branch of the mandible and immediate substitution by bone graft have been successfully carried out (Finochietto et al.[10]; Conley and Pack[9]).

In the treatment of lesions that have already invaded the surrounding structures, which present bone invasion or lymph node metastases, the only curative form of treatment is a radical resection of the mandible and the submaxillary and cervical lymph nodes. This radical operation includes not only a resection of the entire half of the mandible, but also a neck dissection. This operation proves successful in a very small proportion of patients in whom the nodes are found invaded, but these few patients could seldom be saved by any other procedure.

A complete resection of one-half of the bone is preferable to its division at the level of the angle of the mandible. If the mandible is divided close to, but not beyond, the midline, there is seldom a deviation of its normal position, and patients are able to masticate without difficulty. If the operation does not require excision of large portions of skin, the facial defect is not marked.

Prophylactic neck dissection

When a radical resection of the mandible is done, it should always be accompanied by neck dissection, whether nodes are palpable or not. On the other hand, when a conservative form of treatment is decided upon for early lesions in which no metastatic nodes are palpable, there is the question of treating possible metastatic lymph nodes. In general, the patients chosen for a conservative form of treatment have early, usually differentiated tumors with a small chance of developing metastases, and for this reason a prophylactic neck dissection may not be justified. In addition, if there is a recurrence of the primary lesion after such conservative treatment, with or without an adenopathy, the proper means of approach will be a radical surgical excision with neck dissection.

Prognosis

With an adequate therapeutic approach, the prognosis of carcinoma of the lower gingiva is rather good. In MacComb and Fletcher's series[13] of 108 patients at the M. D. Anderson Hospital in Houston (1947 to 1960), two-thirds of whom were treated by surgery alone, there were thirty-seven (34%) living and well at five years, forty-three verified failures, one lost to follow-up, and twenty-seven presumably dead of intercurrent disease.

Lampe[12] treated thirty-three patients with carcinoma of the lower gingiva with radiotherapy from 1940 to 1950. Of these, eleven lived from three to ten years without evidence of recurrence, five of whom had shown roentgenographic evidence of bone invasion before treatments. Of the twenty-two patients who were not cured, ten had shown bone invasion. The five-year survival rate in a series of fifty-six patients treated at the Roswell Memorial Institute was 19%. No patient with metastases on admission or who developed metastases later was cured (Mattick and Meehan[14]).

Modlin and Johnson[16] performed a combined jaw resection and neck dissection on twenty-seven patients with carcinoma of the lower gingiva or buccal mucosa. They had an operative mortality of 6%, and eleven patients (47%) survived five years without recurrence or metastases. The five-year survival rate in a group of twenty-one patients with carcinoma of the lower gingiva treated by various methods at the Ellis Fischel State Cancer Hospital was 49% (Schwarz et al.[21]).

Krishnamurthi and Shanta[11] studied a series of 188 patients with carcinoma of the lower gingiva, 130 (69%) of whom showed evidence of bone erosion and 166 (88%) of whom had lymph node metastases. These patients were irradiated and some of them subsequently submitted to resection. Thirty-seven were offered and accepted the combined procedure and of fourteen at risk, ten lived three years. Twenty-three required no surgery and of eleven at risk, seven were well three years.

REFERENCES

1 Aboulker, Paul: Les épithéliomas du maxillaire inférieur; variétés anatomocliniques et traitement, Ann. Otolaryng. (Paris) 58:121-149, 1939.
2 Ackerman, L. V., and McGavran, M. H.: Proliferating benign and malignant epithelial lesions of the oral cavity, J. Oral Surg. 16:400-413, 1958.
3 Bacq, J.: Les épithéliomas de la muqueuse de recouvrement du maxillaire inférieur, J. Belg. Radiol. 46:515-543, 1963.
4 Bernick, S.: Growths of the gingiva and palate. I. Chronic inflammatory lesions, Oral Surg. Oral Med. Oral Path. 1:1029-1041, 1948.
5 Bernier, J. L.: Differential diagnosis of oral lesions, Oral Surg. Oral Med. Oral Path. 2:617-627, 690-703, 1949.
6 Blair, V. P., Moore, S., and Byars, L. T.: Cancer of the face and mouth, St. Louis, 1941, The C. V. Mosby Co.
7 Burford, W. N., Ackerman, L. V., and Robinson, H. B. G.: Symposium on twenty cases of benign and malignant lesions of the oral cavity, from the Ellis Fischel State Cancer Hospital, Columbia, Missouri, Amer. J. Orthodont. Oral Surg. (Oral Surg. Sect.) 30:353-398, 1944.
8 Byars, L. T.: Extent of mandibular resection required for treatment of oral cancer, Arch. Surg. (Chicago) 70:914-922, 1955.
9 Conley, J. J., and Pack, G. T.: Surgical treatment of malignant tumors of the inferior alveolus and mandible, Arch. Otolaryng. (Chicago) 50:513-540, 1949.
10 Finochietto, R., Turco, N. B., and Canale, A.: Hemiresección de maxilar inferior, prótesis inmediata, injerto de hueso ilíaco, Semana Med. 50:65-71, 1944.
11 Krishnamurthi, S., and Shanta, V.: Evaluation of treatment of advanced primary and secondary gingival carcinoma, Brit. Med. J. 5340:1261-1263, 1963.
12 Lampe, I.: Radiation therapy of cancer of the buccal mucosa and lower gingiva, Amer. J. Roentgen. 73:628-635, 1955.
13 MacComb, W. S., and Fletcher, G. H.: Cancer of the head and neck, Baltimore, 1967, The Williams & Wilkins Co.
14 Mattick, W. L., and Meehan, D. J.: Carcinoma of the gum, Surgery 29:249-254, 1951.
15 Melville, A. G. G.: The double radium mould treatment of carcinoma of the floor of the mouth and lower alveolus, Brit. J. Radiol. 13:337-344, 1940.
16 Modlin, J., and Johnson, R. E.: The surgical treatment of cancer of the buccal mucosa and lower gingiva, Amer. J. Roentgen. 73:620-627, 1955.
17 Moloney, W. C.: Clinical significance of oral lesions in acute leukemia, New Eng. J. Med. 222:577-579, 1940.
18 Perez, C. A., Kraus, F. T., Evans, J. C., and Powers, W. E.: Anaplastic transformation in verrucous carcinoma of the oral cavity after radiation therapy, Radiology 86:108-115, 1966.
19 Quick, D.: Carcinoma of the lower jaw, Amer. J. Surg. (new series) 1:360-364, 1926.
20 Rouvière, H.: Anatomie des lymphatiques de l'homme, Paris, 1933, Masson et Cie.
21 Schwarz, H., Lesser, J. H., and Sammons, V. E.: The treatment of cancer of the lower gingiva, Acta Un. Int. Cancr. 10:262-270, 1954.
22 Swearingen, A. G., McGrew, J. P., and Palumbo, V. D.: Roentgenographic pathologic correlation of carcinoma of the gingiva involving the mandible, Amer. J. Roentgen. 96:15-18, 1966.
23 Taylor, G. W., and Nathanson, I. T.: Lymph node metastases, New York, 1942, Oxford University Press.
24 Wilkins, S. A., and Vogler, W. R.: Cancer of the gingiva, Surg. Gynec. Obstet. 105:145-152, 1957.

Upper gingiva

Anatomy

The upper gingiva is formed by the tissues that cover the alveolar ridge of the upper maxilla. It is formed by fibrous tissue that is continuous with the periosteum of the bone and by a stratified squamous epithelium similar to that of the rest of the oral cavity. This mucous membrane is rather thick and does not contain glands. Around the neck of the teeth the gingiva forms an overlapping collar. The upper gingiva extends only a few millimeters medial to the neck of the teeth. Laterally, it is considerably more extensive. The epithelium that covers it is reflected upon itself deep in the gingivobuccal and gingivolabial gutters to become the buccal mucosa and the mucous membrane of the upper lip.

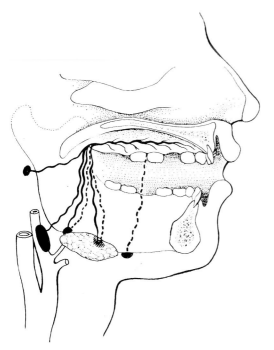

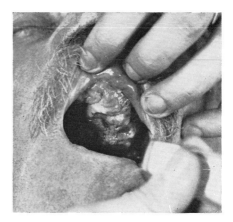

Fig. 158. Typical papillary carcinoma of upper gingiva.

Fig. 157. Lymphatics of upper gingiva, which end in submaxillary or jugular lymph nodes and rarely in retropharyngeal nodes.

Lymphatics. Rouvière[7] divides the lymphatics of the upper gingiva into a lateral and a medial network. The lateral group of lymphatics pierces through the upper insertions of the buccinator muscle, follows the facial vein to the submaxillary region, and ends in submaxillary lymph nodes. The medial group follows an anteroposterior direction and joins the lymphatics of the hard and soft palates behind the dental arch. From there on they form part of the same group but often end in lymph nodes of the anterior jugular chain. More rarely, they will end in the submaxillary and retropharyngeal lymph nodes (Fig. 157).

Epidemiology

Carcinomas of the upper gingiva are not so common as those of the lower gingiva. The usual proportion is 1 to 4 (Wilkins and Vogler[8]). They are usually reported together with carcinomas of the maxillary antrum under the heading of cancer of the upper jaw, and for this reason it is difficult to estimate the approximate incidence. They occur predominantly in men in the fifth and sixth decades of life.

Ill-fitting dentures, carious teeth, and

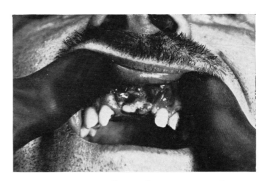

Fig. 159. Rare epidermoid carcinoma of upper gingiva at midline.

syphilis have been incriminated as causative factors in carcinoma of the upper gingiva as in other carcinomas of the oral cavity. A large proportion of the patients are found to be users of tobacco, particularly chewers of regular tobacco (Wilkins and Vogler[8]) or of snuff (pulverized tobacco).

Pathology
Gross pathology

Carcinomas of the upper gingiva are usually papillary, presenting deep crevices and a keratinized surface (Fig. 158). They usually develop over the molar and premolar areas and very rarely on the anterior midline (Fig. 159). Extension toward the hard palate is often submucous, giving an adjacent smooth tumefaction that seldom extends beyond the midline. Lateral spread to the upper gingivobuccal gutter by extension of the ulceration is much more common. Extension into the floor of the

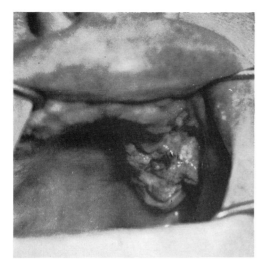

Fig. 160. Verrucous type of carcinoma of upper gingiva.

maxillary antrum through the alveoli usually occurs earlier in those patients who still have their teeth, inasmuch as disease loosens the teeth, and the tumor can easily spread through the alveolar canal. Invasion of the soft structures of the cheek and upper lip is only seen in very advanced cases. In general, the soft structures are merely displaced.

Microscopic pathology

Almost all carcinomas of the upper jaw are well differentiated. Verrucous carcinomas, which are more frequently found on the buccal mucosa and the lower jaw, are also observed on the upper gingiva (Fig. 160). Mucous and salivary gland tumors, which occur more often on the hard palate, may arise near the medial limits of the upper gingiva or on its lateral aspect. These tumors may present variable microscopic patterns (p. 535).

Metastatic spread

Carcinomas of the upper gingiva metastasize most frequently to the submaxillary lymph nodes. Seldom do they reach the upper jugular nodes without first metastasizing to the submaxillary region. The chances of metastatic spread increase with the invasion of the gingivo-buccal gutter and buccal mucosa, with the undifferentiation of the tumor, and with the overall size of the primary lesion. Bilateral metas-

tases are seldom seen. Verrucous carcinoma seldom metastasizes.

Clinical evolution

Carcinomas of the upper gingiva are usually first noticed because of their interference with the fitting of a denture or because of ulceration around teeth. For these reasons, the dentists are often first consulted. In general, there is a friable papillary outgrowth extending over the middle or posterior third of the upper gingiva (Fig. 158). As a rule, there are few other symptoms except otalgia when there is coexistent secondary infection. Spontaneous bleeding may also be observed. Trismus is found only in very advanced cases.

A submaxillary adenopathy is usually found in patients with moderately advanced lesions, particularly when disease has invaded laterally. Upper cervical metastases are sometimes observed, but distant metastases are very uncommon. Death often occurs from complications such as hemorrhage and bronchopneumonia.

Diagnosis

Carcinomas of the maxillary antrum that develop on the infrastructure of the superior maxilla may extend to the upper gingiva and become ulcerated therein. It may be impossible in some cases to establish with certainty the gingival or the antral point of departure of an epidermoid carcinoma. In the majority of cases, however, the carefully recorded details of the history and the physical findings will speak eloquently enough for one or the other point of origin.

Primary carcinomas of the maxillary antrum usually produce a smooth, nonulcerated tumefaction in the upper gingivo-buccal gutter, and loosening of the teeth usually precedes the development of a gingival ulceration. In addition, nasal discharge, bleeding, or nasal obstruction may have preceded the appearance of a tumefaction or ulceration of the upper gingiva.

In carcinomas of the upper gingiva, on the other hand, the loosening of the teeth occurs after the growth has eroded around them. The ulceration is present from the beginning and is usually wider, and the extension to the antrum occurs late. In addition, the microscopic examination of a biopsy specimen from the antrum will reveal a rather undifferentiated carcinoma whereas, as a general rule, those arising on the gingiva are rather differentiated keratinizing carcinomas. The point of origin, however, cannot be determined on a microscopic basis.

Roentgenologic examination

Roentgenologic examination of the superior maxilla will be helpful in establishing the extent of bone destruction as well as that of the invasion of the maxillary antrum. In primary tumors of the upper gingiva, the maxillary antrum may be cloudy due to neighboring edema, but the bone destruction is limited to the alveolar border. In carcinomas of the antrum, the bone destruction is in general more extensive.

Differential diagnosis

Several benign growths occur in the upper gingiva which can be easily differentiated from malignant tumors. Peripheral giant cell tumors (epulis) are usually shiny, grow around the teeth with a varied consistency, and have no ulceration (Fig. 161). Ulceration and secondary infection occur when teeth have been extracted from the diseased gum. Fibrous epulis is usually a pedunculated, nonulcerated, rubbery growth (Fig. 161). These benign growths may be present in both young and aged people. In children, the differential diagnosis of benign lesions will be simplified because of the age. Other conditions of the upper gingiva, such as hypertrophic gingivitis, are easily recognized.

The commonest location of malignant melanoma of the oral cavity is in the upper gingiva (Fig. 162). Seventy-five of ninety-three cases of malignant melanoma of the oral cavity reported by Chaudhry et al.[3] originated on the upper jaw. These lesions are easily identified by their dark color (Baxter[2]). Primary central tumors of the upper jaw, such as ameloblastomas, dentigerous cysts, primary tumors of the antrum or nasal fossa, sarcomas of the bone, and metastatic carcinomas of the upper maxilla may produce a tumefaction of the upper gingiva and a loosening of the teeth. In later stages, they result in a wide ulceration of the oral cavity. The differential diagnosis of the point of origin is not always possible in these cases, but the history, physical findings, clinical sequence of events, and biopsy should help.

Treatment

Radiotherapy

As has been stated, the majority of the carcinomas of the upper gingiva are well-differentiated tumors that metastasize late or are carcinomas of the verrucous type that only rarely metastasize. Although external irradiation can sterilize these lesions, a skillful surgical excision of these tumors is usually successful also. Peroral roentgentherapy is feasible in limited growths that can be included in a circular field of

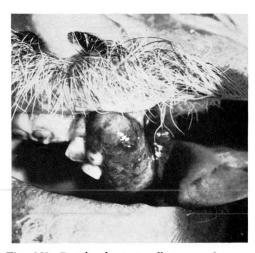

Fig. 161. Peripheral giant cell tumor of upper gingiva.

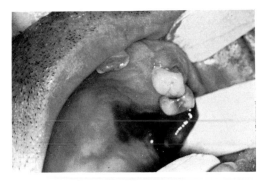

Fig. 162. Malignant melanoma of upper gingiva extending onto hard palate. Lesion was surgically resected.

irradiation. If peroral roentgentherapy is to be used, its role should be only a complementary one after external irradiation.

Radiotherapy finds its best indications in early lesions (not more than 3 cm in diameter) that are exophytic in type and that have a moderate degree of histologic differentiation. In these cases, a wide surgical excision is still possible if a recurrence manifests itself.

Surgery

A wide surgical excision of tumors of the upper gingiva that have invaded the lower structure of the maxilla is often successful. This treatment usually implies a resection of parts of the hard palate and maxillary bone, but the extent of the resection will depend, of course, on the extent of the disease.

As a general rule, the operation can be done through the opening of the mouth. In patients with more advanced lesions, however, it may be necessary to enlarge the opening by an incision around the ala nasi and midline of the upper lip. These resections do not need to extend to the floor of the orbit and consequently change the symmetry of the face very little. The resections often result in a large perforation of the hard palate into the nasal fossa and maxillary antrum, which must be occluded by specially fitted prosthetic appliances.

In those tumors of the upper gingiva that have invaded beyond the midline or those that have already infiltrated the buccal mucosa, the chances of success by a surgical resection are considerably diminished. Now and then, however, a heroic approach by excision of large areas of the cheek and bone may be successful.

It has been the custom in the past to follow this atypical resection of the maxilla by an intracavitary application of curietherapy. The success of this form of treatment, however, depends on the wide excision of the tumor. A combination of supervoltage roentgentherapy or cobalt[60] teletherapy with radical surgery may prove more fruitful (MacComb and Fletcher[4]).

When a cervical adenopathy is present, a radical neck dissection is indicated. In the absence of a palpable cervical adenopathy, an excellent attitude is justified, for only a small percentage of the patients will develop a metastasis after the primary lesion has been controlled.

Prognosis

An adequate therapeutic approach will contribute a rather good percentage of results. In a series of forty-seven patients treated at the Memorial Hospital for Cancer and Allied Diseases in New York, Martin[5] reported twelve five-year survivals (25%). A report on forty-five patients treated at the Roswell Park Memorial Institute showed eight patients (18%) well five years (Mattick and Meehan[6]).

REFERENCES

1 Ackerman, A. J.: Prosthetic reconstruction of the face and mouth following cancer therapy. In Pack, G. T., and Livingston, E. M.: Treatment of cancer and allied diseases, vol. 1, New York, 1940, Paul B. Hoeber, Inc., pp. 508-518.
2 Baxter, H.: A review of malignant malanoma of the mouth, Amer. J. Surg. **51**:379-386, 1941.
3 Chaudhry, A. P., Hampel, A., and Gorlin, R. J.: Primary malignant melanoma of the oral cavity; a review of 105 cases, Cancer **11**:923-928, 1958.
4 MacComb, W. S., and Fletcher, G. H.: Planned combination of surgery and radiation in treatment of advanced primary head and neck cancers, Amer. J. Roentgen. **77**:397-414, 1957.
5 Martin, H. E.: Cancer of the gums (gingivae), Amer. J. Surg. **54**:765-806, 1941.
6 Mattick, W. L., and Meehan, D. J.: Carcinoma of the gum, Surgery **29**:249-254, 1951.
7 Rouvière, H.: Anatomie des lymphatiques de l'homme, Paris, 1933, Masson et Cie.
8 Wilkins, S. A., Jr., and Vogler, W. R.: Cancer of the gingiva, Surg. Gynec. Obstet. **105**:145-152, 1957.

Hard palate

Anatomy

The hard palate is a U-shaped area limited anteriorly and laterally by the upper dental arch which forms the roof of the mouth. Its anterior two-thirds are formed by the palatine process of the superior maxilla. Its posterior third is formed by the horizontal portion of the palatine bone. In the midline of the hard palate there is a linear raphe. The mucous membrane is a stratified squamous epithelium that appears corrugated and pale on the anterior third of the roof of the mouth but is smooth and darker on the posterior two-thirds.

The bone is covered by dense tissues

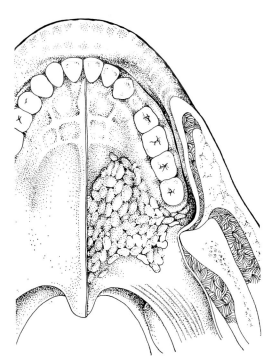

Fig. 163. Inferior view of hard palate showing mucosal rugae on anterior half and racemose glands lying beneath epithelium on posterior half.

formed by the periosteum and mucous membrane that are intimately adherent on the anterior half. The palatine glands, a group of some 250 independent though closely packed glandular aggregates, lie between the mucous membrane and the periosteum (Fig. 163) on the posterior half of the hard palate. These racemose glands, producing mostly mucus, are continuous with those found near the anterior surface of the soft palate (about 100) and those found in the uvula (about twelve).

Lymphatics. According to Rouvière,[18] the network of lymphatics of the hard palate runs posteriorly to a point behind the dental arch, from which it diverges in three directions: (1) to the deep lymph nodes of the neck, (2) to the lymph nodes of the submaxillary region, and (3) to the retropharyngeal lymph nodes.

Of these, only the first is constantly present. The lymphatic vessels traveling to the deep nodes of the neck pass under the mucous membrane of the retromolar space, descend along the anterior border of the vertical branch of the mandible, pass inside of the submaxillary gland, and end in the deep nodes of the subdigastric group on the anterior jugular chain. The lymphatics of the roof of the mouth may cross the midline and end on the corresponding nodes of the opposite side.

Epidemiology

A large proportion of the tumors that develop on the hard palate are of the mucous and salivary gland type. They arise from the mucous and minor salivary glands, and although they may be found elsewhere in the oral cavity, they are most frequently found on the hard palate (Reynolds et al.[17]). These tumors have a similarity to others that arise from the main salivary glands.

In a collected series of 760 benign minor salivary gland tumors (Fine), fifty-eight arose from the hard palate and fifty-three from the soft palate. These locations were second only to the upper lip in the distribution of these tumors. The benign variety seems to predominate in women (Vellios and Shafer[21]).

Epidermoid carcinomas of the hard palate are very rare. In a series of about 5000 cases of cancer of the oral cavity observed from 1907 to 1938 by New and Hallberg,[12] there were only twenty-five epidermoid carcinomas of the hard palate. There is only one epidermoid carcinoma for every three or four mucous and salivary gland tumors of the hard palate, and, unlike these, the carcinomas are seldom observed in female patients.

In Vizagapatam, India, Kini and Subba-Rao[8] found fifty-two carcinomas of the palate among 335 cases of carcinoma of the oral cavity. This high occurrence has been considered to be due to irritation from the habit of smoking a local type of cigar, *chutta*, a poor substitute for tobacco. The lighted end repeatedly goes out, and the smokers resort to Adda Poga, or reverse smoking, putting the lighted end inside the mouth. Large areas of leukoplakia usually precede the development of carcinoma (Khanolkar and Suryabai[7]) (Fig. 164). This style of reverse smoking is also favored by laundresses and cooks in Panama and Venezuela. Carcinomas of the hard palate also develop in these individuals. The changes brought about by heat chronically applied to the mucosa of the

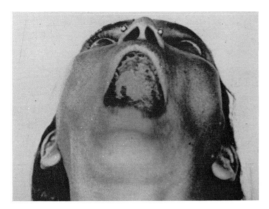

Fig. 164. Chutta cancer in Hindu. (Courtesy Dr. V. R. Khanolkar, Bombay, India.)

hard palate may be as important as (Reddy et al.[14]), or perhaps more important than, the fact that this results from smoking tobacco.

Pathology

Gross pathology

Mucous and salivary gland tumors develop on the posterior half of the hard palate on one side of the midline (Fig. 168). In general, they are well encapsulated and have a polylobated surface. They may extend to the adjacent area of the soft palate and grow through it to the nasopharynx. Without showing any tendency to ulceration of the mucous membrane, they may erode into the maxillary bone and erupt into the floor of the nasal fossa or the maxillary antrum. On section, they contain hyalinized connective tissue that forms septa. Cartilage may also be present.

Epidermoid carcinomas of the hard palate are usually superficially ulcerated and rarely localized. The ulceration may extend beyond the midline and invade secondarily the upper gingiva or the soft palate, and later the bone.

Microscopic pathology

In the hard palate, the majority of the mucous and salivary gland tumors are of the mixed tumor type. Renstrup and Pindborg[15] reported twenty-seven tumors of the palate, of which fifteen were mixed tumors, nine were adenoid cystic carcinomas, and three were mucoepidermoid carcinomas. The distribution was similar in the series reported by Kohn et al.[9]

Epidermoid carcinomas of the mucous membrane of the hard palate are the same as other oral carcinomas. A whitish appearance of the mucous membranes usually referred to as "leukoplakia" is often observed. These thickened areas of the mucosa may represent carcinoma in situ or simple hyperkeratosis, but in some instances it may be found to show early infiltrating carcinoma. At times, epidermoid carcinomas of the hard palate may be of the same verrucous type that has been described in other areas of the oral cavity.

Metastatic spread

Malignant salivary gland tumors have a tendency to distant blood-borne spread, but they may also metastasize through the lymphatics to the submaxillary lymph nodes. Squamous cell carcinomas, on the contrary, seldom metastasize at a distance, although relatively infrequently they metastasize to the submaxillary group of nodes.

Clinical evolution

Salivary gland tumors of the hard palate are characterized by a slow growth, sometimes developing over a period of twenty years or even longer. In general, the benign tumors present no symptoms except in patients with advanced lesions, in whom their presence may give rise to difficulties in speech and deglutition. Malignant tumors may cause pain and oral and nasal hemorrhages, as well as secondary infection and necrosis. They are usually first noticed because they interfere with the use of dental plates, but several years may elapse before advice is sought.

There is little difference in the rate of growth of the benign and the malignant tumors. Some lesions develop faster after they have been present for many years, but this is not necessarily a sign of malignant transformation. Only rarely do benign tumors become malignant. Even the malignant group of mucous and salivary gland tumors present a rather low grade of malignancy. They develop very slowly in most cases and metastasize only in the late stages.

The benign tumors, whether treated or not, seldom cause death. The malignant tumors may finally ulcerate the mucous membranes and develop distant metastases, often causing death by hemorrhage, bronchopneumonia, or cachexia.

Epidermoid carcinomas of the hard palate may arise in the midline or on one or the other side of the hard palate close to the upper gingiva. They are usually superficially ulcerated and metastasize in only one-fourth or one-third of the cases. Distant metastases are rare. Death occurs as a consequence of local spread, infection, and pulmonary complications.

Diagnosis

A thorough palpation of mucous and salivary gland types of tumors of the hard palate will reveal that they are hemispherical in shape (Fig. 168) and well delimited, with a polylobated surface and a rubbery consistency. The limits of the malignant tumors are hard to establish. Although there is little difference in the rate of growth of the benign and the malignant tumor and although slow growth is not of diagnostic significance, rapid growth does favor the diagnosis of malignant tumor. In general, the malignant tumors occur in older patients. Pain often accompanies the malignant tumor, but, of course, the presence of metastases is, in the final analysis, the only definite criterion of malignancy of these tumors.

Epidermoid carcinomas offer little difficulty in recognition. They are widely ulcerated, and biopsy is possible without difficulty. In the verrucous type of carcinoma, repeated biopsies may show only hyperkeratinization and chronic inflammation before a positive diagnosis of carcinoma is made.

Roentgenologic examination

Radiographic examination of the hard palate and the maxilla is always of value in the differential diagnosis with other tumors of this region. Perforation of the palatine bone by tumor may be present in both benign and malignant tumors. In the benign tumor, however, the perforation is sharply outlined, whereas in the malignant group the perforation through the bone may be quite diffuse.

Biopsy

Ulcerative lesions are biopsied without difficulty. In nonulcerated lesions that are

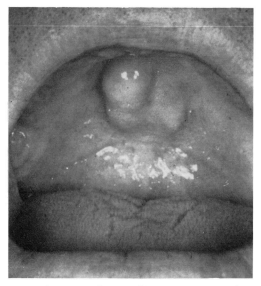

Fig. 165. Torus palatinus. (Courtesy Dr. Hamilton B. G. Robinson, Columbus, Ohio.)

frequently salivary gland neoplasms, the surgeon must be careful that he carries his biopsy into the lesion. Superficial biopsies do not demonstrate the tumor.

Differential diagnosis

In general, the clinical examination may establish a strong presumptive diagnosis of salivary gland tumor. It can be differentiated with ease from the exostoses of the bones of the palate, called *torus palatinus*, which occurs usually at the midline of the anterior third of the palate (Fig. 165). *Papillomas* of the mucosa of the hard palate could be taken for early carcinomas. They are characteristically papillary and well outlined and may be pedunculated or may be attached by a broad base (Bernick[2]). Their histology is characteristic.

Syphilitic gumma of the hard palate is rare. In the presence of ulceration and secondary infection, it may be difficult to differentiate this syphilitic lesion from an epidermoid carcinoma. The biopsy, however, will show only chronic inflammation, and the lesion will disappear rapidly under antisyphilitic treatment.

Dentigerous cysts and *ameloblastomas* of the upper jaw may grow slowly in the form of a nonulcerated, smooth tumefaction that may be confused with salivary and mucous gland tumors. These tumors of the jaw, however, usually arise in the

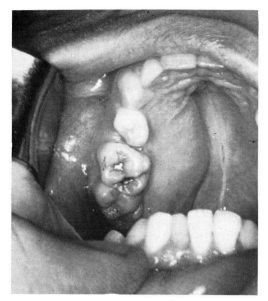

Fig. 166. Hypertrophy and hyperplasia of palatine glands suggesting tumor. (Courtesy Dr. Hamilton B. G. Robinson, Columbus, Ohio.)

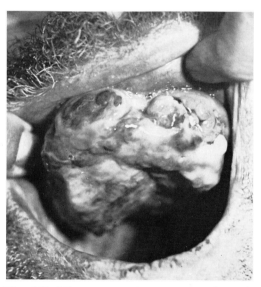

Fig. 167. Fibrosarcoma of superior maxilla with invasion and ulceration of hard palate.

region of the upper alveolar ridge. The same may be true of a carcinoma of the antrum. It should be noted that the same type of mucous and salivary gland tumors may arise from the maxilloethmoidal region and that in their development they may secondarily extend to the palate.

A differential diagnosis with the rare sarcomas of the maxilla (Fig. 167) may be difficult upon inspection, but the presence of pain and ulceration and the rapidity of growth may help to distinguish them. The biopsy will be conclusive in most instances.

Malignant melanomas of the oral cavity arise most often from the area of the hard palate and the maxilla (Chaudhry et al.[3]). A blue nevus of the hard palate was reported by Harper and Waldron.[5]

Treatment
Surgery

Salivary and mucous gland tumors, whether benign or malignant, require surgical excision in the young patient. In early benign lesions the excision will be rather simple because of the usual encapsulation of the tumor. In the more advanced lesions with bone perforation, the difficulties in excision, extent of the defect, and chances of local recurrence are considerably greater.

Sometimes a subperiosteal excision of a benign tumor can be performed without touching the integrity of the bone. Very often, however, the salivary gland tumor is not detachable from the bone without breaking its capsule, and the excision implies the necessity of extirpation of part of the hard palate. This results in a permanent opening into the antrum and nasal fossa. (Fig. 168). The resulting defect will be well worth the elimination of the chance of recurrence. This defect may be easily alleviated by the use of a prosthesis. In very extensive tumors that have involved the infrastructure of the superior maxilla and the nasal fossa, a radical excision implies a major defect (Öhngren[13]). In general, the success of any type of technique depends greatly on skillful performance (Stuteville and Corley[20]).

Epidermoid carcinomas of the mucous membrane of the hard palate that are well delimited should also be treated surgically. A radical neck dissection is the treatment of choice for metastatic adenopathy of the neck.

Radiotherapy

Mucous and salivary gland tumors develop slowly as a rule and do not present a large number of cellular mitoses. Theoretically, they should not be radiosensitive

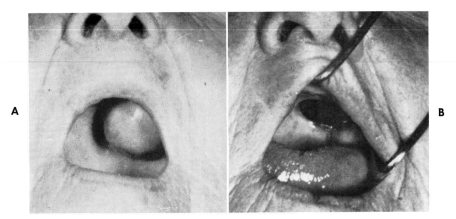

Fig. 168. **A,** Typical smooth unilateral hemispherical mucous and salivary gland type of tumor of hard palate. **B,** After surgical excision. Resulting defect communicating with nasal fossa was easily occluded by prosthesis.

and, in fact, are only slightly so, although the more malignant they are, the more they are affected by radiations. Ahlbom[1] reported that in some cases the tumor shows definite radiosensitivity. However, radiosensitivity does not imply radiocurability. Actually, when these tumors are treated by radiotherapy alone, they do show a slow and delayed response; the value of preoperative and postoperative irradiation is questionable. Some malignant varieties show surprising radiosensitivity (Hobaek[6]), particularly adenocarcinoma of the cylindromatous type.

Radiotherapy in the form of external roentgentherapy as well as specially fitting radium molds may be applied to epidermoid carcinomas of the hard palate that have already extended beyond the midline and are consequently not resectable. Very little experience has been accumulated in the treatment of these uncommon epidermoid carcinomas, but their treatment by radiation therapy when resection is impossible is well justified.

Prognosis

The prognosis of the benign mucous and salivary gland tumors is very good. It is difficult to give an estimate of the prognosis of the malignant tumors because the material reported is not usually comparable. In a series of sixty patients with salivary gland tumors of the hard and soft palates, benign and malignant, surgically treated by New and Hallberg,[12] twenty (33%) were reported living five years or longer after treatment.

The prognosis of epidermoid carcinomas of the hard palate is not so good as that of salivary gland tumors in general. In the verrucous type, however, which seldom metastasizes, a wide excision will often be followed by a definite cure.

The adenoid cystic type of salivary gland tumor has a poor prognosis. Only one of six patients reported by Kohn et al.[9] was cured. Stiebitz[19] reported similar poor results in his five patients.

REFERENCES

1 Ahlbom, H. E.: Mucous- and salivary-gland tumours, Acta Radiol. (Stockholm) (suppl. 23), 1935.
2 Bernick, S.: Growths of the gingiva and palate. III. Epithelial growths, Oral Surg. Oral Med. Oral Path. **2:**217-228, 1949.
3 Chaudhry, A. P., Hampel, A., and Gorlin, R. J.: Primary malignant melanoma of the oral cavity; a review of 105 cases, Cancer **11:**923-928, 1958.
4 Fine, G., Marshall, R. B., and Horn, R. C., Jr.: Tumors of the minor salivary glands, Cancer **13:**653-669, 1960.
5 Harper, J. C., and Waldron, C. A.: Blue nevus of the palate; report of a case, Oral Surg. Oral Med. Oral Path. **20:**145-149, 1965.
6 Hobaek, A.: Intraoral mucous- and salivary-gland mixed tumors, Acta Radiol. (Stockholm) **32:**229-247, 1949.
7 Khanolkar, V. R., and Suryabai, B.: Cancer in relation to usages, Arch. Path. (Chicago) **40:** 351-361, 1945.
8 Kini, M. G., and Subba-Rao, K. V.: Problem of cancer, Indian Med. Gaz. **72:**677-679, 1937.
9 Kohn, E. M., Dahlin, D. C., and Erich, J. B.: Primary neoplasms of the hard and soft palates

and the uvula, Proc. Mayo Clin. **38**:233-241, 1963.

10 Martin, H. E.: Tumors of the palate (benign and malignant), Arch. Surg. (Chicago) **44**: 599-635, 1942.

11 Masson, P., and Peyron, R.: A propos des tumeurs mixtes des glandes salivaires. Spécificité cellulaire et tumeurs mixtes, Bull. Ass. Franc. Cancer **7**:219, 1914.

12 New, G. B., and Hallberg, O. E.: The end-results of the treatment of malignant tumors of the palate, Surg. Gynec. Obstet. **73**:520-524, 1941.

13 Öhngren, L. G.: Malignant tumours of the maxillo-ethmoidal region, Acta Otolaryng. (Stockholm) (suppl. 19), pp. 1-476, 1933.

14 Reddy, D. G., Reddy, D. B., and Rao, P. R.: Experimental production of cancer with tobacco tar and heat, Cancer **13**:263-269, 1960.

15 Renstrup, G., and Pindborg, J. J.: Salivary gland tumors of the palate, Acta Path. Microbiol. Scand. **49**:417-425, 1960.

16 Reuterwall, O.: Cited in Ahlbom, H. E.: Mucous- and salivary-gland tumours, Acta Radiol. (Stockholm) (suppl. 23), 1935.

17 Reynolds, C. T., McAuley, R. L., and Rogers, W. P., Jr.: Experience with tumors of minor salivary glands, Amer. J. Surg. **111**:168-174, 1966.

18 Rouvière, H.: Anatomie des lymphatiques de l'homme, Paris, 1933, Masson et Cie.

19 Stiebitz, R.: Die Tumoren der Gaumenschleimdrüsen, Wien. Med. Wschr. **114**:247-249, 1964.

20 Stuteville, O. H., and Corley, R. D.: Surgical management of tumors of intraoral minor salivary glands—report of 80 cases, Cancer **20**: 1578-1586, 1967.

21 Vellios, F., and Shafer, W. G.: Tumors of the intraoral accessory salivary glands, Surg. Gynec. Obstet. **108**:450-456, 1959.

Lower jaw

Anatomy

In the adult, the lower jaw or mandible is a single bone with a symphysis in the midline. It is usually divided into a *corpus* and two ascending branches. The corpus is horseshoe-shaped and is formed by two lateral branches. The superior borders of these branches form the alveolar ridge and lodge the teeth. The ascending branches of the mandible are roughly rectangular. Their internal surfaces contain the orifice of entrance of the dental nerve and artery. The posterior borders of the ascending branches end in the condyle.

The mandible is formed mostly by spongy bone entirely surrounded by remarkably dense bone. Each half of the mandible contains a long canal running horizontally along the dental roots. This canal is occupied by the dental nerve and vessels.

The teeth and their immediate supporting structures have a complex origin. At about the sixth week of intrauterine life, the oral epithelium proliferates in twenty places to form the anlages for the ten maxillary and ten mandibular deciduous teeth. From these primordia the enamel organs of the deciduous teeth differentiate, and the same epithelial proliferations contribute the anlages for the thirty-two permanent teeth. Each tooth bud undergoes a complex differentiation until enamel organs evolve.

Each enamel organ consists of an outer squamous epithelial layer, an inner columnar epithelial layer (ameloblasts), a central core of stellate reticulum, and a less differentiated stratum intermedium. The enamel organ lays down the enamel and also, by proliferation of its apical end, forms a tube of epithelium, the sheath of Hertwig, which outlines the future tooth root. Within the hollow of the enamel organ, the mesenchymal tissue differentiates into the dental papillae that contribute the dentin and the pulp. The mesodermal tissues surrounding the developing tooth contribute the cementum of the tooth, the periodontal membrane, and the alveolar and supporting bone. During this process, epithelial rests may be left behind from the sheath of Hertwig and from the dental lamina, which connects the oral mucosa to the young enamel organ (Robinson[41]).

Epidemiology

Tumors of the lower jaw are relatively rare in comparison with other oral neoplasms. In general, they are found in relatively young patients. *Fibro-osteomas* and *giant cell reparative granulomas* develop most commonly in adolescents. About 70% of *ameloblastomas* are found in patients 10 to 35 years old, and *Ewing's sarcomas* are found generally in persons under 20 years of age. *Osteosarcomas* of the jaw may be found in persons of all ages.

Tumors of the jaw are relatively common in Africa. In a series of eighty-nine primary bone tumors reported from Ghana, seventy arose from the mandible or maxilla (Kovi and Laing[30]). Slavin and Cameron[44a] collected fifty-six cases of ameloblas-

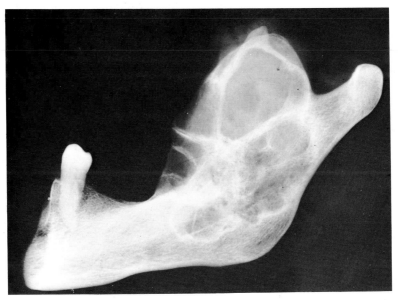

Fig. 169. Roentgenogram of surgical specimen showing ameloblastoma of mandible with typical cystic areas and trabeculations.

tomas in Africans from Tazmania and Uganda over a period of eight years. Forty-eight of these lesions appeared in the mandible. However, the largest single group of tumors is composed of a *malignant lymphoma* first described by Burkitt,[14] in Uganda, in 1958. This tumor seems to originate frequently in the mandible or maxilla of African children generally under 10 years of age. Similar tumors have been reported in New Guinea (Booth et al.[12]) and Singapore (Shanmugaratnam et al.[42]).

Pathology

Gross and microscopic pathology

A few tumors of the lower jaw warrant detailed description.

The *fibro-osteoma* of the mandible is usually multilocular or diffuse, involving the corpus. On section, the tumor shows a variable resistance according to its cellularity. Microscopically, it exhibits a great difference in connective tissue maturation. Connective tissue is interlaced with bone spicules, and the tumor varies from the very cellular to eburnating (Billings and Ringertz[10]).

True giant cell tumors of the bone of the mandible are extremely rare lesions. Most of the tumors of the mandible containing giant cells are not true neoplasms

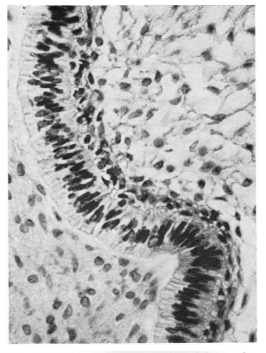

Fig. 170. Solid ameloblastoma. From left to right, mesenchymal cell stroma, ameloblast-like cells, stratum intermedium–like layer, and stellate cells can be seen mimicking normal enamel organ.

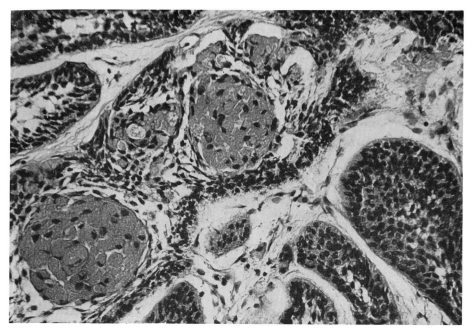

Fig. 171. Adamantinoma showing classic pattern and collections of granular cells as reported by McCallum and Cappell.[34] (×250; WU neg. 59-82.)

and fall into the group described by Jaffe[28] as *giant cell reparative granulomas.* This term is a descriptive one and a poor designation for this entity. The lesion does contain giant cells, but it is not a granuloma and the word reparative does not apply. However, it is impossible to dislodge this name from the literature. The lesion can be peripheral, arises from the interdental papilla, and presents a broad-based smooth surface. It can arise centrally in the mandible and maxilla. The premolar and molar areas of the mandible are the preferred site (Bhaskar et al.[9]). Other lesions containing giant cells are related to hyperparathyroidism, and in such cases the chemical findings, particularly the elevation of the alkaline phosphatase level, may be helpful. We believe it best to separate the various lesions that contain giant cells, for each has a different clinical evolution (Waldron[48]). Tombridge[47] believes that "cherubism," a rare condition in children with bilateral involvement of the mandible, is in reality a giant cell reparative granuloma.

The *ameloblastoma* is an epithelial tumor derived from cells that have a potentiality for enamel formation. This tumor is more commonly found in the mandible (85%) than in the upper jaw. It forms a cystic mass within the body of the mandible and often reveals surface lobulations. On section, the consistency is usually firm, but it may be cystic with fibrous trabeculae or occasional bone spicules. The tumor is sometimes found in some transitional phase between solid and cystic forms. Sonesson[46] pointed out that after separation of the soft part of the ameloblastoma from the capsule, a finely lobulated surface (like the mould of a blackberry) may be observed.

Microscopically, the young or solid ameloblastoma shows epithelial proliferation in a connective tissue stroma of mesenchymal type of cells. The epithelium is arranged in cords, strands, or follicles strikingly similar to the arrangement of the epithelium in dental buds, dental laminae, or enamel organs. The differentiation of these dental anlage-like structures continues up to the point where function (laying down of enamel) begins. The cells of an ameloblastoma do not assume this function. Degeneration begins instead at the expense of the central stellate cells of the enamel organ's homologues. This retrogression leads to the formation of a multicystic tumor. The tall columnar cells of the solid ameloblastoma may be compressed to cuboidal or squamous forms, and the stellate central cells are replaced by mucoid fluid. Any transitional stage between these two extremes, solid or cystic, may be observed, but careful examination reveals the arrangement of cells in the form of odontogenic tissues in some areas. The adamantinoma may have foci of granular cells (McCallum and Cappell[34]) (Fig. 171).

Sonesson[46] believes that all types of odontogenic cysts have a tendency to develop adamantinomas, and he reported ten such cases. Other authors are of the same view (Goldman[22]; Bernier[5]).

Ewing's sarcomas arise from within the marrow cavity and thicken the cortical bone; the tumor cells gradually permeate by way of the haversian canals through the cortex to elevate the periosteum. The cellular appearance is similar to that observed in other bones (p. 899).

Osteosarcomas occur more often in the lower than in the upper jaw (Fig. 172). They may present all the variants characteristic of this form of tumor. They may arise on the basis of a preexisting Paget's disease or, rarely, fibrous dysplasia. In general, they grow rapidly and may become ulcerated within the mouth.

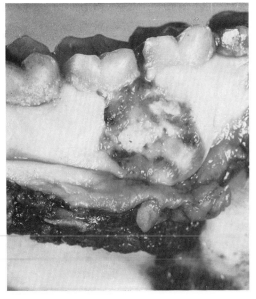

Fig. 172. Osteosarcoma of mandible in 50-year-old man. Segmental resection was done. (WU neg. 60-2968.)

Metastatic spread

Fibro-osteomas and giant cell reparative granuloma do not metastasize. Ameloblastomas are tumors that have a capacity to invade locally, but they have practically no tendency to metastasize (Hoke and Harrelson[27]). Many metastasizing tumors are epidermoid carcinomas, whereas others are the adenoid cystic type of salivary gland carcinoma. Small and Waldron[45] found only twenty-one possibly malignant ameloblastomas in his collected series of 1036 cases. Several of these would have to be rejected for lack of adequate data.

Ewing's sarcoma quite characteristically involves other bones, the regional lymph nodes, and the lungs. Osteosarcomas metastasize with preference to the lungs but not to regional nodes. Burkitt's tumors metastasize widely but to the thyroid gland, liver, pancreas, kidneys, and ovaries in greater proportion than other malignant lymphoid tumors (Wright[49]). The involvement of superficial lymph nodes is less and that of para-aortic nodes usually massive.

Clinical evolution

The *fibro-osteoma* usually appears at the age of puberty. As the tumor gradually increases in size, it causes no pain, and any symptoms that develop are due to the mechanical difficulties induced by deformity and swelling.

Giant cell reparative granulomas develop slowly and may reach a huge size. They usually appear as nonulcerated tumefactions of the outer aspect of the mandible, or they may enlarge the width of the alveolar ridge. The teeth become separated and displaced. When teeth are extracted, a granulating, easily bleeding tissue may appear in the socket. Pain is seldom present unless secondary infection has taken place. The general condition of the patient is affected if the tumor interferes with eating or if there is marked bleeding or infection. This tumor may also develop centrally within the mandible, where it may show a single area of radiolucency or a soap bubblelike lesion.

The slow progress of *ameloblastomas* rarely produces any symptoms. Occasionally, however, these tumors cause numbness in the region of the intramandibular nerve or may cause a toothache. Over a period of years, the tumor may attain a large size (Fig. 173). Fractures of the bone may be a complication of these tumors. At times, secondary infection occurs through the mouth. These tumors distend but do not infiltrate the surrounding soft tissues. They rarely cause death.

Ewing's sarcomas develop faster than the tumors previously discussed. Pain accompanies their growth, becoming progressively intense. The mass may rapidly involve both sides of the mandible. Both

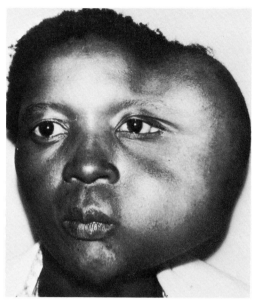

Fig. 173. Huge ameloblastoma in young African girl which was treated successfully by surgery. (Courtesy Dr. Ian Smith, Johannesburg, R.S.A.)

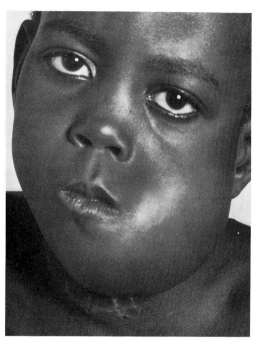

Fig. 174. Extensive lymphoma (Burkitt's tumor) involving mandible and maxilla in young African boy. (Courtesy Dr. J. N. P. Davies, Albany, N. Y.)

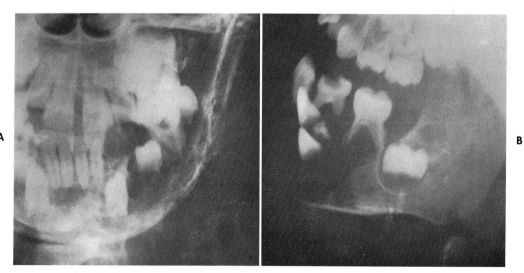

Fig. 175. Burkitt's tumor in African child (Uganda). **A,** Frontal projection demonstrating extensive destruction of mandible with large soft tissue mass that contains parallel radiating calcifications. **B,** Lateral projection showing extensive osteolytic defect in which destruction involves alveolar process around roots of teeth. (Courtesy Dr. J. N. P. Davies, Albany, N. Y.)

local and distant metastases are frequently found.

Osteosarcoma of the mandible is invariably accompanied by severe pain and sometimes fever. A history of loosening of the teeth is usually given. The evolution of the tumor is rapid, with equally rapid deterioration of the general condition. Distant metastases are the rule.

Davies[17] reported the unusual multicentric lymphoma (Burkitt's tumor) of the mandible and maxilla in children (Fig. 174). These tumors occurred between the ages of 2.5 and 14 years. The involvement of the mandible and maxilla and the orbital areas is frequently the presenting sign (Fig. 175). *Burkitt's tumor* is a multicentric malignant lymphoma occurring frequently in the mandible of children (Fig. 175). It may be accompanied by pain (Burkitt and O'Conor[15]). This tumor has been thought to be a specific entity assimilated, on a morphologic basis, to other tumors occurring in other parts of the world in adult individuals and in other organs. There is some question as to the specificity of the histologic pattern (Dorfman[19]). Burkitt and O'Conor[15, 37] reported in detail the findings in 106 children.

Diagnosis

Diagnosis of tumors of the mandible may be very difficult. Slow evolution and lack of symptoms generally designate a fibro-osteoma, giant cell reparative granulomas, or ameloblastoma. Rapidity of growth and pain in a young individual point to a diagnosis of Ewing's sarcoma or osteosarcoma.

The roentgenographic appearance of adamantinomas has been variously described as characteristic. A cystic multiloculated image is typical. Sonesson[46] thinks that different-sized, not completely divided, compartments and irregular sclerosis of the bony wall are additional characteristics that help to establish a radiographic diagnosis of ameloblastoma. Giant cell reparative granulomas, and various other multiloculated lesions may give the same image. Fibromyxomas of the mandible present a thin-laced pseudoloculated appearance (Sonesson[46]). Ewing's tumors may present bone spicules at right angles to the surface of the mandible that may also be seen in osteosarcomas. Sherman and Melamed[43] described the variegated pattern of osteosarcoma of the jaw. Garrington et al.[20] emphasize that a symmetrically widened periodontal membrane space may be a significant early finding.

Differential diagnosis

There is usually no difficulty in the diagnosis of fibro-osteoma, for the clinical history and roentgenographic findings are typical.

The giant cell reparative granulomas have to be differentiated from all other lesions that cause a cystic area within the mandible. The giant cell reparative granuloma occurring in association with hyperparathyroidism cannot be distinguished microscopically from other giant cell reparative granulomas (Black and Ackerman[11]). Patients presenting a giant cell lesion of the mandible should have a roentgenographic study of other bones and alkaline phosphatase determination to be certain that the changes are not due to a functioning parathyroid tumor. In the latter, the alkaline phosphatase level is always elevated. True aneurysmal bone cyst may involve the mandible (Bhaskar et al.[9]). Focal chronic osteomyelitis may be confused roentgenologically and pathologically with a variety of benign lesions (Schmaman et al.[41a]).

A rare tumor designated as a calcifying epithelial odontogenic neoplasm does occur in the mandible and maxilla. It has a rather typical microscopic pattern, is benign, but may recur after surgical excision (Abrams and Howell[1]).

Ameloblastomas may cause considerable difficulty, for they also have to be differentiated from various cystic lesions. We have seen two instances of suspected ameloblastoma in which the mandible was invaded secondarily, first by a mixed tumor of the submaxillary gland and second by a mixed tumor of the alveolar ridge. In each instance, the invaded mandible showed a cystic area.

Two lesions confused microscopically with ameloblastoma are ameloblastic fibroma and adenoameloblastoma. Both lesions are completely benign and do not recur following simple excision (Halperin et al.[26]). Bhaskar[8] believes that the adenoameloblastoma arises from the wall of a follicular cyst.

Odontogenesis	Cysts and neoplasm	Origin of lesions

Proliferation

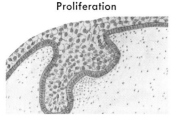

Solid ameloblastoma

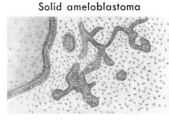

The ameloblastoma is an epithelial neoplasm which resembles dental laminae and enamel organs until the period of amelogenesis. It may be derived from cells of the oral epithelium with a tendency to odontogenesis, from remnants of the sheath of Hertwig or the dental lamina (epithelial rests) or from aberrant tooth buds. It begins as a solid tumor aping the dental anlage and enamel organ but never forms enamel. It degenerates at the expense of the stellate reticulum to become a multicystic tumor.

Differentiation

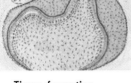

Cystic ameloblastoma

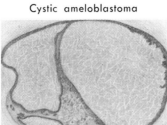

Tissue formation

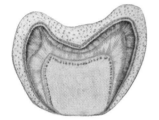

Primordial cyst

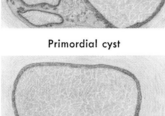
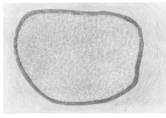

The primordial cyst is a cyst of the jaw derived from the enamel organ in its early stages. Before tissue formation begins, the stellate reticulum breaks down and fluid collects between the inner and outer enamel epithelium. The cyst is formed by internal pressure.

Tissue formation

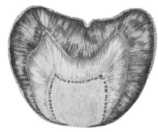

Dentigerous cyst

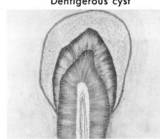

The dentigerous cyst is a cyst of the jaw containing the crown of a tooth. It is usually described as formed by a breakdown of the stellate reticulum during amelogenesis. This would produce hypoplastic enamel. It appears to be formed within the reduced enamel epithelium.

Erupted tooth

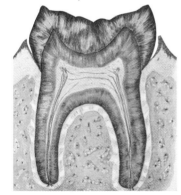

Periodontal cyst

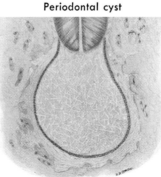
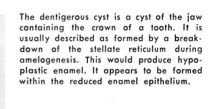

The periodontal cyst is a cyst formed in the periodontal membrane usually at the root end of a pulpless infected tooth. The epithelial lining is derived from the epithelial rests (usually remnants of the sheath of Hertwig). It is commonly the sequel of a dental granuloma, in which either resting or proliferating epithelium is a constant finding.

Plate 2. Classification of cysts of jaws. (From Robinson, H. B. G.: Classification of cysts of jaws, Amer. J. Orthodont. Oral Surg. [Oral Surg. Sect.] **31**:370-375, 1945.)

Rarely, the very cellular fibro-osteoma can be confused microscopically with osteosarcoma. However, neoplastic osteoid will not be present, and the roentgenographic picture and clinical history are sufficient to make the differentiation. The formation of a tumor nodule outside of bone in which roentgenologically there is destruction of the mandible is almost certain evidence of an osteosarcoma. In its undifferentiated state, an osteosarcoma may be difficult to differentiate from Ewing's sarcoma. The response to radiations alone often makes the diagnosis. Ewing's tumors may be confused with osteomyelitis.

Cysts of the jaw often enter into the differential diagnosis of these tumors. The developmental cysts of the oral cavity are derived from ectodermal remnants and can be divided into periodontal, dentigerous, and primordial.

Gorlin et al.[24] carefully reviewed the complex problem of odontogenic tumors and modified the classification of Pindborg. Many of these tumors are rare and poorly understood. Some are confused with the ameloblastoma and are thought to be much more malignant than their true nature. These include ameloblastic adenomas and ameloblastic fibromas.

Periodontal cysts are often symptomless and cause remarkably little bulge in spite of their wide spread. They are usually preceded by a dental granuloma on an infected pulpless tooth. In the lower jaw, they occur three times more frequently in the molar and premolar regions (Sonesson[46]). The cysts are usually closed sacs formed in the periodontal membrane. They are lined by stratified squamous epithelium (rarely columnar) and have a connective tissue capsule. Roentgenographically, they most often give a unilocular, radiolucent image with a distinct outline. Three varieties are recognized:

1 Periapical, in which a root is usually seen projecting to, or into, the radiolucent area
2 Lateral (or paradental), in which the root is seen alongside the cyst
3 Residual (which constitutes as many as half of all cases according to Sonesson[46]), in which the cyst develops in an edentulous region of the jaw at a site previously occupied by a root

Periodontal cysts must be differentiated from primordial cysts, dentigerous cysts, and osteitis fibrosa cystica.

Dentigerous cysts are caused by degenerative changes in the enamel epithelium of unerupted teeth or odontomes and may become very large. They are unilocular, are attached to the neck of the tooth, and are lined by stratified squamous epithelium in a connective tissue capsule. Roentgenographically, the dentigerous cysts are radiolucent and unilocular with a definite cortical margin, showing the crown of the responsible tooth in the part of the cyst that is farthest from the original site, with its long axis pointing toward the center of the cyst (Sonesson[46]). So-called eruption cysts occurring on an erupting third molar are simply late dentigerous cysts. Rarely after removal of the tooth there may be a residual dentigerous cyst. Sonesson[46] believes that in addition to these pericoronal dentigerous cysts there are others (paradental) in which the tooth is placed tangentially to the cyst. Squamous carcinoma rarely arises from the epithelial lining of these cysts (Angelopoulos et al.[2]).

Primordial cysts are formed by retrogression of the stellate reticulum in enamel organs or tooth buds at any time before calcium is deposited, often developing near the angle of the mandible and often becoming infected. Multiple primordial cysts sometimes occur as a familial disease. Roentgenographically, primordial cysts appear as unilocular, multilocular, or multiple cysts in which the various compartments are generally uniform in size (Sonesson[46]) and present, unlike periodontal cysts, a definite cortical margin. Often, several distinct cysts may give a fictitious radiographic impression of multilocularity. Primordial cysts are often confused with ameloblastomas on the roentgenograms.

Bernier[5] divides odontogenic tumors into two types. Those lesions occurring during the first stage of tooth formation do not contain calcified dental tissues and are referred to as "soft." Those occurring in the second stage may contain dentin, enamel, or cementum and are spoken of as "hard." These extremely rare dentinomas are best defined as "an odontogenic tumor composed of dentin, connective tissue, and odontogenic epithelium."[*] A complex syndrome associated with oral anomalies, including primordial cysts or odontogenic keratocysts, has been reported (Gorlin et al.[25]).

Metastatic carcinoma in the mandible is observed. The most common sites of origin are the breast, lung, and kidney (Clausen and Poulsen[16]). The metastases may be accompanied by pain, swelling, and loosening of the teeth. These symptoms and signs may occur before the primary tumor is recognized.

Treatment

Giant cell reparative granulomas often recur after local excisions but can be cured by wide resections. The question is only whether or not radical mutilating treatment is justified for a benign condition in young patients. Curettement may be a satisfactory form of treatment for the central type. Roentgentherapy is the treatment of choice for the peripheral type. The regression of these tumors is slow and a large amount of radiations is not required. Small repeated series of treatments over months may be satisfactory. Cases of *ameloblastomas* may be conservatively and successfully treated by roentgentherapy (Baclesse et al.[3]).

Simple surgical enucleation is not adequate treatment for ameloblastomas. In a series reported by Goldwyn et al.,[23] there were eight recurrences out of fourteen enucleations. Resection with preservation of the mandible is well indicated.

Ewing's sarcomas are very radiosensitive and have been successfully treated by radiations. Surgical excision of these tumors ends invariably in failure. Roentgentherapy need not be very intensive. A fractionated course of treatments is preferable in order to facilitate recalcification without untoward effect on the skin or mucous membranes. When radiotherapy fails, it is most often due to the unsuspected presence of distant metastases. Radiation therapy is indicated for the treatment of the rare reticulum cell sarcomas (Gerry and Williams[21]).

Surgical excision of *osteosarcoma* of the mandible and maxilla is the only recommended treatment. The surgeon must plan the excision so that he will not cut through tumor, and this may make his excisions radical at times (Fig. 172). It is not necessary to dissect lymph nodes because they are practically never involved (Kragh et al.[31]). Primary radiation therapy is not recommended.

Some *Burkitt's tumors* have reacted favorably to administration of methotrexate (Oettgen et al.[38]), increasing considerably the normal life expectancy (Ngu[36]). Cyclophosphamide has been found to be a highly effective form of treatment for Burkitt's lymphoma, and multiple doses are more beneficial than single doses (Ziegler et al.[51]). This is apparently the most effective agent. For obvious reasons, a reasonable trial of skillfully delivered radiotherapy has not been made on a sample of Burkitt's tumors in Africa.

Prognosis

The prognosis of fibro-osteoma is excellent. Giant cell reparative granulomas have an excellent prognosis provided they are adequately treated. Ameloblastomas have a good prognosis with constant good results if the tumor is adequately resected. If ameloblastomas are only enucleated, local recurrences may be expected in a high percentage of instances. Radiation therapy may be successful rarely in the cure of a primary reticulum cell sarcoma of bone. Osteosarcoma of the jaws has an unexpected rather favorable prognosis. In thirty-five patients eligible for five years or more of follow-up, eleven were well in a series reported by Kragh et al.[31] In a series of 245 cases of Burkitt's tumor treated with cytoxan, Burchenal[12a] reported thirty-eight (15%) with remissions of one to seven years.

REFERENCES

1 Abrams, A. M., and Howell, F. V.: Calcifying epithelial odontogenic tumors, J. Amer. Dent. Ass. **74**:1231-1240, 1967.
2 Angelopoulos, A. P., Tilson, H. B., Stewart, F. W., and Jaques, W. E.: Malignant transformation of the epithelial lining of the odontogenic cysts, Oral Surg. Oral Med. Oral Path. **22**:415-428, 1966.
3 Baclesse, F., Dechaume, M., and Calle, R.: Les améloblastomes (ou adamantinomes) et les épithéliomas adamantins, J. Radiol. Electr. **46**:113-122, 1965.
4 Baclesse, F., and Letouze, G.: Considérations radio-cliniques à propos de 14 cas d'adamantinomes, Presse Med. **58**:372-374, 1950.
5 Bernier, J. L.: Tumors of the odontogenic apparatus and jaws. In Atlas of tumor pathology,

---

[*]From Pindborg, J. J.: On dentinomas; with report of a case, Acta Path. Microbiol. Scand. **105** (suppl.):135-144, 1955.

Sec. IV, Fasc. 10a, Washington, D. C., 1960, Armed Forces Institute of Pathology.

6 Bernier, J. L., and Tiecke, R. W.: Compilation of material received by registry of oral pathology, J. Oral Surg. 9:341-348, 1951.

7 Bhaskar, S. N.. Oral tumors of infancy and childhood, Pediatrics 63:195-210, 1963.

8 Bhaskar, S. N.: Adenoameloblastoma; its histogenesis and report of 15 new cases, J. Oral Surg. 22:218-226, 1964.

9 Bhaskar, S. N., Bernier, J. L., and Godby, F.: Aneurysmal bone cyst and other giant cell lesions of the jaws; report of 104 cases, J. Oral Surg. 17:30-41, 1959.

10 Billings, Lars, and Ringertz, Nils: Fibro-osteoma, Acta Radiol. (Stockholm) 27:129-152, 1946.

11 Black, B. K., and Ackerman, L. V.: Tumors of the arathyroid; a review of twenty-three cases, Cancer 3:415-444, 1950.

12 Booth, K., Burkitt, D. P., Bassett, D. J., Cooke, R. A., and Biddulph, J.: Burkitt lymphoma in Papua, New Guinea, Brit. J. Cancer 21:657-664, 1967.

12a Burchenal, J. H.: Long-term survivors in acute leukemia and Burkitt's tumor, Cancer 21:595-599, 1968.

13 Burford, W. N., Ackerman, L. V., and Robinson, H. B. G.: Symposium on twenty cases of benign and malignant lesions of the oral cavity, from Ellis Fischel State Cancer Hospital, Columbia, Missouri, Amer. J. Orthodont. Oral Surg. (Oral Surg. Sect.) 30:353-398, 1944.

14 Burkitt, D.: Sarcoma involving jaws in African children, Brit. J. Surg. 46:218-223, 1958-1959.

15 Burkitt, D., and O'Conor, G. T.: Malignant lymphoma in African children. I. A clinical syndrome, Cancer 14:258-269, 1961.

16 Clausen, F., and Poulsen, H.: Metastatic carcinoma to the jaws, Acta Path. Microbiol. Scand. 57:361-374, 1963.

17 Davies, J. N. P.: Cancer in Africa. In Collins, D. H.: Modern trends in pathology, New York, 1959, Hoeber Medical Division, Harper & Row, Publishers, chap. 8, pp. 132-160.

18 Dorfman, R. F.: Childhood lymphosarcoma in St. Louis, Missouri clinically and histologically resembling Burkitt's tumor, Cancer 18:418-430, 1965.

19 Dorfman, R. J.: Diagnosis of Burkitt's tumor in the United States, Cancer 21:563-574, 1968.

20 Garrington, G. E., Scofield, H. H., Cornyn, J., and Hooker, S. P.: Osteosarcoma of the jaws, Cancer 20:377-391, 1967.

21 Gerry, R. G., and Williams, S. F.: Primary reticulum-cell sarcoma of the mandible, Oral Surg. Oral Med. Oral Path. 8:568-581, 1955.

22 Goldman, H. M.: The value of microscopic examination of lesions of the jaw; case report of ameloblastoma in cystic walls, J. Oral Surg. 3:241-254, 1945.

23 Goldwyn, R., Constable, J., and Murray, J. E.: Ameloblastoma of the jaw, New Eng. J. Med. 269:126-129, 1963.

24 Gorlin, R. J., Chaudhry, A. P., and Pindborg, J. J.: Odontogenic tumors; classification, histopathology, and clinical behavior in man and domesticated animals, Cancer 14:73-101, 1961 (extensive bibliography).

25 Gorlin, R. J., Vickers, R. A., Kellen, E., and Williamson, J. J.: The multiple basal-cell nevi syndrome; an analysis of a syndrome consisting of multiple nevoid basal-cell carcinoma, jaw cysts, skeletal anomalies, medulloblastoma, and hyporesponsiveness to parathormone, Cancer 18:89-104, 1965.

26 Halperin, V., Carr, R. F., and Peltier, J. R.: Follow-up of adenoameloblastomas, Oral Surg. Oral Med. Oral Path. 24:642-647, 1967.

27 Hoke, H. F., Jr., and Harrelson, A. B.: Granular cell ameloblastoma with metastases to the cervical vertebrae; observations on the origin of the granular cells, Cancer 20:991-999, 1967.

28 Jaffe, H. L.: Tumors and tumorous conditions of the bones and joints, Philadelphia, 1958, Lea & Febiger.

29 Jaffe, H. L., Lichtenstein, L., and Portis, R. B.: Giant cell tumor of bone; its pathologic appearance, grading, supposed variants and treatment, Arch. Path. (Chicago) 30:993-1031, 1940.

30 Kovi, J., and Laing, W. N.: Tumors of the mandible and maxilla in Accra, Ghana, Cancer 19:1301-1307, 1966.

31 Kragh, L. V., Dahlin, E. C., and Erich, J. B.: Osteogenic sarcoma of the jaws and facial bones, Amer. J. Surg. 96:496-505, 1958.

32 Lichtenstein, L.: Giant-cell tumor of bone; current status of problems in diagnosis and treatment, J. Bone Joint Surg. 33-A:143-150, 1951.

33 Lucas, R. B., and Thackray, A. C.: The histology of adamantinoma, Brit. J. Cancer 5:289-300, 1951.

34 McCallum, H. M., and Cappell, D. F.: Adamantinoma with granular cells, J. Path. Bact. 74:365-369, 1957.

35 Nielsen, J.: Swei Fälle von Ewing-Sarkom im Uterkiefer, Acta Radiol. (Stockholm) 21:286-291, 1940.

36 Ngu, V. A.: The African lymphoma (Burkitt tumour); survivals two years, Brit. J. Cancer 19:101-107, 1965.

37 O'Conor, G. T.: Malignant lymphoma in African children. II. A pathological entity, Cancer 14:270-283, 1961.

38 Oettgen, H. F., Burkitt, D., and Burchenal, J. H.: Malignant lymphoma involving the jaw in African children; treatment with methotrexate, Cancer 16:616-623, 1963.

39 Phemister, D. B., and Grimson, K. S.: Fibrous osteoma of the jaws, Ann. Surg. 105:564-583, 1937.

40 Pindborg, J. J.: On dentinomas; with report of a case, Acta Path. Microbiol. Scand. 105 (suppl.):135-144, 1955.

41 Robinson, H. B.: Histologic study of the ameloblastoma, Arch. Path. (Chicago) 23:664-673, 1927.

41a Schmaman, A., Smith, I., and Ackerman, L. V.: Benign fibro-osseous lesions of the mandible and maxilla, Cancer 26:303-312, 1970.

42 Shanmugaratnam, K., Tan, K. K., and Lee, K. W.: Lymphoma of the Burkitt type in Singapore, Int. J. Cancer 2:576-580, 1967.

43 Sherman, R. S., and Melamed, M.: Roentgen characteristics of osteogenic sarcoma of the jaw, Radiology 64:519-527, 1955.

44 Slaughter, D. P., Roeser, E. H., and Smejkal, W. F.. Excision of the mandible for neoplastic disease; indications and techniques, Surgery 26:507-522, 1949.

44a Slavin, G., and Cameron, H. M.: Ameloblastomas in Africans from Tazmania and Uganda, Brit. J. Cancer 23:31-38, 1969.

45 Small, I. A., and Waldron, C. A.: Ameloblastoma of the jaws, Oral Surg. Oral Med. Oral Path. 8:281-297, 1955 (extensive bibliography).

46 Sonesson, A.: Odontogenic cysts and cystic tumours of the jaws, Acta Radiol. (Stockholm) (suppl. 81), pp. 1-159, 1950.

47 Tombridge, T. L.: Familial giant cell reparative granuloma of the mandible ("cherubism"), Amer. J. Clin. Path. 37:196-203, 1962.

48 Waldron, C. A.: Fibrous and granulomatous lesions of the jaw bones, Amer. J. Surg. 94:877-881, 1957.

49 Wright, D. H.: Burkitt's tumour; a post-mortem study of 50 cases, Brit. J. Surg. 51:245-251, 1964.

50 Zegarelli, E. V., Napoli, N., and Hoffman, P.: The cementoma, Oral Surg. Oral Med. Oral Path. 17:219-224, 1964.

51 Ziegler, J. L., Morrow, R. H., Jr., Fass, L., Kyalwazi, S. K., and Carbone, P. P.: Treatment of Burkitt's lymphoma with cyclophosphamide (Makerere University, Kampala, Uganda, and National Cancer Institute, National Institutes of Health, U.S.A.); presented at the Tenth International Cancer Congress, Houston, Texas, May, 1970.

Nasopharynx

Anatomy

The nasopharynx or epipharynx is an open chamber situated below the base of the skull and behind the nasal fossa. It has an irregularly cubic form with six walls, two of which, the lateral walls, are symmetric. It is 4 cm in its transverse diameter, 4 cm in height, and 2 cm to 3 cm in anteroposterior diameter. The nasopharynx is the only one of the three portions of the pharynx that does not make up part of the digestive tract and that is incapable of obliteration.

The *anterior wall* is formed by the posterior nares or choanae, oval-shaped openings communicating with the nasal fossa and separated in the midline by the nasal septum. The *posterior wall* lies at the level of the first two cervical vertebrae and is sometimes continuous with the roof of the nasopharynx. Laterally, it extends to form the posterior limits of the fossae of Rosenmüller. The *inferior wall* is a virtual one, formed by the soft palate. It extends from the posterior border of the palatine bones to the free border of the soft palate itself. The *roof* or *upper wall* corresponds to the body of the occipital bone and to the adjacent part of the sphenoid. It is almost entirely made up of the lymphoid tissue that forms the pharyngeal tonsil, or tonsil of Luschka, divided in the midline by a deep fissure that extends anteroposteriorly and ends in a small depression, the pharyngeal bursa. The pharyngeal tonsil is relatively large in children but is atrophied in the adult. The *lateral walls*, the most important of all, contain the pharyngeal orifice of the tubae auditivae (eustachian tubes). These openings are small, triangular, and infundibular in appearance. They are surrounded by a ridge, the torus tubarius, due to the salience of cartilage above and behind the opening but not below or in front of it (Fig. 176). A depression may be formed behind it that is called the recessus pharyngeus (fossa of Rosenmüller).

The mucous membrane that covers the nasopharynx is formed by a stratified cylindrical and ciliated epithelium. This epithelium extends on the posterior wall and becomes squamous at the oropharynx and abruptly at the free border of the soft palate. Beneath the lining epithelium there are numerous closed lymphoid follicles in the corium. These lymphoid structures are particularly abundant on the rim of the eustachian tube (tonsil of Gerlach), but they are present on the lateral and posterior walls as well as on the nasopharyngeal surface of the soft palate, where they contribute to form the upper arch of Waldeyer's ring.

The posterior and lateral walls of the nasopharynx are surrounded by the pharyngeal fascia, which is strongly attached to the base of the skull just in front of the

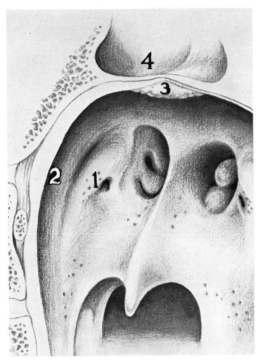

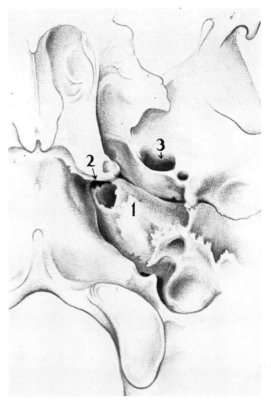

Fig. 176. Posterolateral view of nasopharynx. **1,** Choanae, posterior extremity of second and third turbinates, and eustachian tubes. **2,** Rosenmüller's fossa. **3,** Roof of tonsil of Luschka. **4,** Very close relationship with sphenoidal sinus.

Fig. 177. Bony structures of base of skull, left side. **1,** Position of petrous portion of temporal bone. **2,** Foramen lacerum. **3,** Foramen ovale. This petrosphenoidal portion of base of skull provides easy access into middle cerebral fossa.

foramen magnum posteriorly and to the petrous portion of the temporal bone laterally. At the level of the eustachian tubes this fascia is divided into a sort of gutter which is responsible for the strong attachment of the tubes to the base of the skull. The fascia thus forms a fibrotic chamber entirely closed and very resistant that is continuous with the fibrous tissue occupying the foramen lacerum (Truffert[58]). This anatomic conception is important for understanding the extension of tumors of the nasopharynx toward the middle cerebral fossa. The foramen lacerum and the foramen ovale constitute a zone of little resistance and an easy pathway into the cranium (Fig. 177). This "petrosphenoidal crossway" (Jacod[22]) is in close relationship to two very important anatomic structures: the gasserian ganglion and its branches and the cavernous sinus. The abducens nerve (VI) passes through the areolar

cavity of the cavernous sinus, and the oculomotor nerve (III) and the trochlear nerve (IV) are found in its lateral wall (Fig. 178). The optic nerve (II) lies medial to the cavernous sinus.

The roof of the nasopharynx is in direct relation with the occipital bone and sphenoidal sinus, as well as the cavernous sinus. The posterior wall is in relation to the first two cervical vertebrae through the medium of the pharyngeal fascia and the superior constrictor muscles. In front of the eustachian tube, the lateral wall of the pharynx is in relation with the maxillopharyngeal space, limited externally by the vertical ramus of the mandible. In this space is found the mandibular nerve descending from the foramen ovale. It must be noted that the facial and acoustic nerves (VII and VIII) are situated fairly high and are protected by the strong petrous portion of the temporal bone. Behind the eustachian

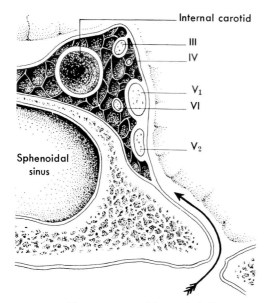

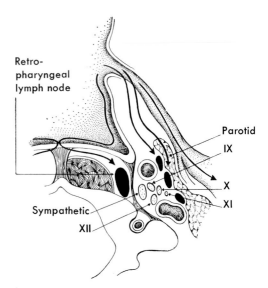

Fig. 178. Oblique section of base of skull passing through sphenoidal sinus and cavernous sinus. Arrow illustrates way in which tumors of nasopharynx come rapidly in contact with third, fourth, fifth, and sixth cranial nerves which are in substance of or in lateral wall of cavernous sinus.

Fig. 179. Lymphatics of nasopharynx which end in retropharyngeal lymph nodes or in Krause group of nodes of anterior jugular chain. Note relationship of these lymph nodes with last four cranial nerves and cervical sympathetic nerve in retroparotidian space.

tube the fossa of Rosenmüller is in close relationship with the retroparotidian space, which is limited anteriorly by the parotid gland and the styloid process and its muscles, posteriorly by the transverse process of the first cervical vertebrae, and laterally by the sternocleidomastoid muscle. This retroparotidian space contains the internal carotid artery, the internal jugular vein, and the glossopharyngeal, vagus, spinal accessory, and hypoglossal nerves (IX, X, XI, and XII), as well as cervical sympathetic nerve, as they emerge from the base of the skull (Fig. 179). Lateral to these structures three or four small lymph nodes may also be found.

Lymphatics. The lymphatics of the roof and of the posterior wall of the nasopharynx run anteroposteriorly and join at the midline. After passing through the pharyngeal fascia, they run to the right or left toward the retropharyngeal nodes. Some of the lymphatics, however, end in the highest nodes in the internal jugular and spinal chains on either side. The lymphatic vessels of the lateral wall of the pharynx are particularly rich at the level of the eustachian tube. They also follow an anteroposterior

direction and may end in the retropharyngeal node or on the highest node of the jugular and spinal chains of the same side (Fig. 179). Some of these deep cervical nodes of the jugular chain are very highly situated, and three or four of them may be found very near the emergence of the last cranial nerves.

Epidemiology

The incidence of cancer of the nasopharynx can only be estimated. In cancer centers, tumors of the nasopharynx are variously reported as making up between 0.5% and 1% of all cases of cancer. Malignant tumors of the nasopharynx are most commonly found in patients 40 to 45 years of age. Epidermoid carcinomas are rarely seen in patients under 25 years of age, but lymphosarcomas are seen both in children and in very aged persons. Approximately two-thirds of all tumors of the nasopharynx occur in males.

The considerably greater relative occurrence of these tumors among Chinese has long been observed (Digby et al.[10]; Yeh[66]; Pang[37]; Clifford[7a]). A variable number of cases diagnosed in coastal American cities

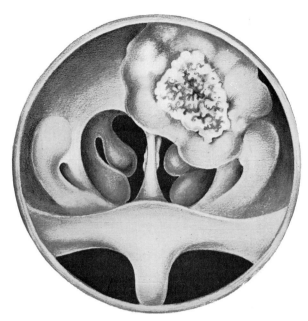

Fig. 180. Carcinoma of roof and left lateral wall of nasopharynx showing extensive ulceration and some surrounding infiltration.

are found in Chinese and frequently, as has been pointed out by Ho,[20] in natives of China. Buell[5] has shown that the incidence among Chinese born in America is considerably reduced, possibly because of selection against a genotype, but the incidence is still twenty times greater among them than among other Americans. The average age of Chinese is lower than that of Caucasians with nasopharyngeal tumors (Teoh[54]). Cancer of the nasopharynx has also been found to be relatively frequent in Malays (Loke[30]) and among Kenya Africans (Clifford and Beecher[8]), with about the same age and sex distribution found in Chinese. On the other hand, it has been pointed out[51] that these tumors are rare among Japanese and Hindus.

Pathology

Gross pathology

Grossly, tumors of the nasopharynx may develop into three distinct categories: ulcerated, lobular, and exophytic.

The *ulcerated* lesions are most frequently found on the posterior wall or deep in Rosenmüller's fossa (Fig. 180). Less frequently, they are situated on the lateral wall in front of the eustachian tube or on the roof of the nasopharynx. These rare

ulcerated lesions are often well-differentiated epidermoid carcinomas. The ulcerations are small and necrotic and progressively infiltrate the neighboring tissues. Those that develop on the lateral wall or on the roof of the nasopharynx are canalized by the pharyngeal fascia toward the petrosphenoidal region of the base of the skull. They tend to enlarge and destroy the foramina and to spread into the middle cerebral fossa. There they may remain subdural or may invade the dura and the bones. Invasion of the petrous portion of the temporal bone is rare. In this area, the tumor comes into contact with several cranial nerves (II, III, IV, V, VI), which are compressed but not necessarily invaded (Fig. 178).

The *lobulated* form of nasopharyngeal tumors arises most commonly from the eustachian tube area, which becomes rapidly obliterated. The tumor has a grapelike, polypoid appearance and may not show ulceration anywhere on its surface. More commonly, however, a small ulceration in great disproportion to the size of the tumor is visible (Fig. 181). This form of development is usually observed in an undifferentiated epidermoid carcinoma. The tumor infiltrates around the eustachian tube, and when it spreads forward, it may extend into the maxillopharyngeal space and compress the mandibular branch of the fifth cranial nerve. In spreading downward, it may interfere with the normal excursion of the soft palate on the side of the lesion. It easily spreads to the petro sphenoidal region of the base of the skull. It does not, however, grow rapidly enough to cause symptoms from compression of

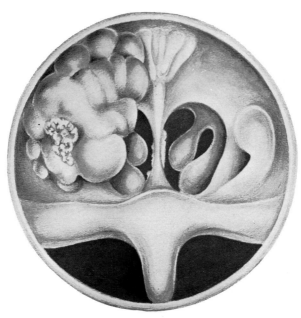

Fig. 181. "Lymphoepithelioma" of right eustachian tube area showing polylobated outgrowth with little ulceration. Undifferentiated carcinomas have similar appearance.

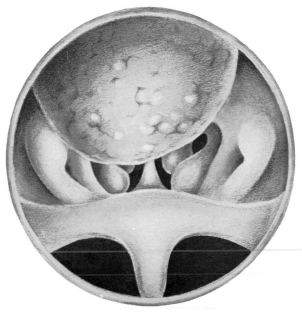

Fig. 182. Lymphosarcoma of roof of nasopharynx showing ulceration and bilateral obstruction of choanae. Lymphosarcomas arising in Rosenmüller's fossa seldom become very large and are usually discovered only after distant metastases are evident.

the nerve, although the nerve may be surrounded by tumor. It is only late in the development, long after tumor has spread into the middle cerebral fossa, that it decalcifies the bones of the base of the skull. In very advanced stages, tumor may invade the orbit through the inferior orbital fissure and may invade the maxillary sinus most commonly through the ethmoid.

The *exophytic* type of growth is usually a hemispheric, nonulcerated, sometimes pedunculated, smooth tumor that may arise from the roof and rapidly fill the nasopharyngeal cavity. It pushes the soft palate downward and spreads toward the choanae and the nasal fossa (Fig. 182). It rapidly reaches the maxillary sinus and the orbit, producing marked unilateral exophthalmos. This exophytic tumor has even been seen protruding through the anterior naris. This form of development is typical of lymphosarcomas of the pharyngeal tonsil. Those lymphosarcomas that develop from the eustachian tube area do not show much tendency to grow toward the nasopharyngeal cavity but spread in the submucosa toward the base of the skull. They do not compress the cranial nerves until they become quite bulky, and even then the nerve paralyses are few and limited. Erosion of the base of the skull is also seldom observed in lymphosarcomas.

Microscopic pathology

Lymphosarcomas are rather infrequent, making up only a small percentage of the primary tumors of the nasopharynx. Keratinizing epidermoid carcinomas of the nasopharynx are rare. The remaining number is represented by a rather large group of tumors, mostly so-called lymphoepitheliomas, which are variously diagnosed as undifferentiated epidermoid carcinomas, transitional cell carcinomas, lymphoepitheliomas, and even incorrectly as lymphosarcomas.

The *differentiated squamous cell carcinomas* of the nasopharynx are clear-cut diagnostic entities. The difficulty in microscopic diagnosis lies with the larger number of anaplastic undifferentiated epidermoid carcinomas.

Regaud[43] and Schmincke,[49] in 1921, simultaneously but independently described a new form of tumor that was called *lym-*

phoepithelioma. Regaud[43] acted upon the necessity of classifying differently a group of cases that clinically, pathologically, and radiotherapeutically were being recognized to behave in a different and characteristic manner. The name lymphoepithelioma was given as a suggestion that they arose from the normal lymphoepithelial structures that are present in the tonsils, base of the tongue, nasopharynx, thymus, and Peyer's patches of the small intestine. No case has yet been reported, however, arising in the latter organ. Histologically, so-called lymphoepitheliomas are formed by cords of clear epithelial cells with indistinct limits, forming a sort of syncytium. The nuclei of these cells are clear, frequently lobated, and contain one or two voluminous nucleoli (Fig. 183). They show frequent mitoses. These cords of probable epithelial cells are homogeneously infiltrated by lym-

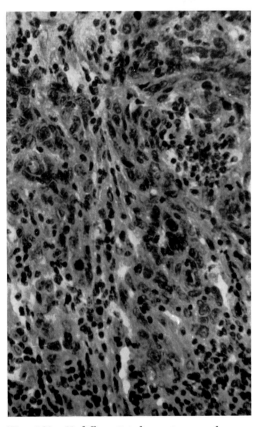

Fig. 183. Undifferentiated carcinoma of nasopharynx within lymph node. Nonkeratinizing masses of tumor cells are intermingled with collections of lymphocytes. This could be designated as "lymphoepithelioma." (×350; WU neg. 61-79.)

phocytes and occasional plasma cells. This constant presence of epithelial cells and lymphocytes is what gives to these tumors their original character.

Teoh[54] studied thirty-one Chinese patients with epidermoid carcinoma of the nasopharynx at autopsy in Hong Kong. He reported that in those with so-called lymphoepitheliomas the lymphoid elements were not found in the metastases. At autopsy he found no difficulty in diagnosing all these cases as carcinomas of the nasopharynx, and lymphocytes appeared to be incidental components of the tumors. It is likely, therefore, that these tumors are, in reality, highly undifferentiated carcinomas. Yeh and Cowdry[67] reviewed 1000 nasopharyngeal lesions, of which 988 were carcinomas. The remainder were of various types. Practically none of them were keratinized. After thorough study, they were of the opinion that the term lymphoepithelioma should be discarded, for it represented only carcinoma infiltrating preexisting lymphoid tissue. It seems certain that most of the undifferentiated tumors of the nasopharynx, including so-called lymphoepitheliomas, are squamous cell carcinomas. Svoboda et al.[53] demonstrated, by electron microscopy, that these tumors form keratin fibrils.

Lymphosarcomas are not frequent primary tumors of the nasopharynx. The variable proportions of these tumors found in the medical literature are due to the fact that in the past many pathologists designated as lymphosarcomas the tumors which others called lymphoepitheliomas. The tendency, at present, is to designate these tumors as undifferentiated carcinomas, leaving a small proportion of genuine lymphosarcomas. The details of microscopic pathology of malignant tumors of the lymphoid structures are given in the chapter on pathology (p. 53).

Tumors of mucous and salivary gland type may occur in the nasopharynx. They usually arise from Rosenmüller's fossa. Among these, *adenoid cystic carcinoma* has been reported occasionally. Extramedullary *plasmacytomas* have been found in the nasopharynx, and they may develop the widespread bone lesions of multiple myeloma. Ennuyer et al.,[12] in an extensive review, point out their slow clinical evolution, their

radiosensitivity, and the rarity of lymph node metastases.

Metastatic spread

A metastatic adenopathy is usually present with every tumor of the nasopharynx. The retropharyngeal nodes are often invaded, particularly in tumors of the roof and posterior and lateral walls of the nasopharynx, but they seldom become very large when involvement is from tumors of the lateral wall. An early metastasis may be found in the Krause group of nodes, which are very highly placed close to the last four cranial nerves and the cervical sympathetic nerve as they emerge from the base of the skull. As these nodes enlarge, compression of the nerves with a resulting paralytic syndrome takes place (Regato[41]). From the Krause group of nodes lymphatic permeation leads to the nodes of the internal jugular chain and not infrequently to the spinal chain of nodes placed just beneath the trapezius muscle behind the jugular chain, which follows a divergent direction.

In lymphosarcomas, the invasion of the lymph nodes of the neck, supraclavicular regions, axillae, mediastinum, etc. seems to progress in an orderly fashion. Lymphoepitheliomas are capable of presenting distant metastases to the bones, lungs, and liver (Ch'in and Szutu[7]). Such metastases are the exception in epidermoid carcinomas and are only rarely observed in lymphosarcomas.

Clinical evolution

The nasopharynx is the most frequent blind spot in the diagnosis of all tumors of the aerodigestive tract. The majority of patients with malignant tumors of the nasopharynx are seen because of a cervical adenopathy without any symptoms referable to a primary lesion in the nasopharynx. The next most common symptoms are hypoacousia, nasal obstruction, cranial nerve paralysis, and pain.

A unilateral painless upper cervical *adenopathy* is often the first sign of the disease, the metastatic nodes usually developing in the submastoid area (Greenberg[18]). Nodes of the internal jugular chain following the course of the sternocleidomastoid muscle may also be invaded. It is not uncommon, however, to have consecutive involvement of nodes of the spinal chain following the anterior border of the trapezius muscle. The lymphadenopathy is most often unilateral, rapidly growing, bulky (6, 8, or 10 cm in diameter), somewhat lobulated, and accompanied by considerably smaller nodes in the corresponding chain. This is the typical lymphadenopathy of very undifferentiated epidermoid carcinomas. The very rare cases of differentiated carcinomas present a small, rounded adenopathy, usually confined to the upper cervical region. In lymphosarcomas, the adenopathy may be unilateral or bilateral, depending on whether the tumor arises from the lateral wall or on the roof and posterior wall of the nasopharynx. Lymphosarcomas also grow rapidly but are considerably softer and quickly extend to other elements of the spinal and internal jugular chains. In some cases of lymphosarcoma, the cervical adenopathy may be small, whereas mediastinal or retroperitoneal metastases may be considerably larger.

A unilateral diminution in the sense of hearing, *hypoacousia*, is very commonly found accompanying tumors of the nasopharynx, but especially in so-called lymphoepitheliomas and lymphosarcomas. This is, of course, due to an obliteration of the internal orifice of the eustachian tube. The hypoacousia may be so insidious that the impairment of hearing may not have been noticed. A certain number of patients will give a history of long-standing unilateral hypoacousia. This is sometimes connected with long-standing chronic inflammatory lesions that may have contributed to the development of the tumor.

A definite *nasal twang* in speech is sometimes noticed, a consequence of the lack of nasopharyngeal resonance, obstruction of the choanae, and mechanical interference with the normal movements of the soft palate. *Nasal obstruction* is not infrequent in lymphosarcomas. *Nasal bleeding* or retropharyngeal bleeding is a rare occurrence. *Pain* results from compression of the trigeminal nerve or its branches and from invasion of the bones of the skull. The character of the pain is usually related to the motor paralyses that also result from the compression of the fifth nerve. They will be described together.

Trotter described a triad of symptoms that he thought were associated with "endotheliomas" of the tubal area: (1) hypoacousia, (2) impaired movements of the soft palate, and (3) neuralgia within the territory of the mandibular nerve. Trotter's clinical description of this triad fits perfectly the development of malignant tumors of the eustachian tube with forward extension, interfering mechanically with the movement of the soft palate and irritating the mandibular branch of the fifth nerve in the maxillopharyngeal space. *Cranial nerve paralyses* are not frequently the first symptoms of tumors of the nasopharynx, except in children, but they are not uncommon later in the development of these tumors. In a large series of patients with cancer of the nasopharynx, Godtfredsen[16] found 38% presenting neurologic symptoms. The percentage is doubled in children. These cranial nerve paralyses appear most often in the form of two syndromes: the petrosphenoidal syndrome of Jacod, produced by direct extension of the neoplasm, and the syndrome of the retroparotidian space of Villaret, due to the development of the metastatic adenopathy (Regato[41]). A unilateral paralysis of all of the cranial nerves has sometimes been observed in patients with advanced cancer of the nasopharynx. In general, however, such extensive paralyses are associated with neoplasms of the base of the skull proper, such as fibrosarcoma and osteosarcoma.

The *petrosphenoidal syndrome* results from the compression of the second, third, fourth, fifth, and sixth cranial nerve and consequently is characterized by unilateral neuralgia of the trigeminal type with total unilateral ophthalmoplegia and amaurosis. As a general rule, this syndrome starts by sudden paralysis of the abducens nerve (VI) and by pain in the supraorbital and superior maxillary regions (V). Unless treatment is administered at this time, the syndrome rapidly progresses with a palpebral ptosis, fixation of the eye, and finally loss of sight (Fig. 184). The sensory disturbances due to compression of the fifth nerve pass through various stages. As a general rule, there is pain first and then hyperesthesia of the cutaneous territory of the ophthalmic and superior maxillary nerves. The pain seems to center around

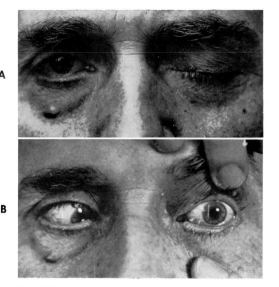

A

B

Fig. 184. Carcinoma of nasopharynx. **A**, Palpebral ptosis produced by compression of third cranial nerve. **B**, Complete fixation of left eye due to compression of third, fourth, and sixth cranial nerves.

the floor of the orbit. In the mouth, there may be a painful anesthesia of one side of the tongue, floor of the mouth, and buccal mucosa. The motor difficulties resulting from compression of the mandibular branch result in paralysis of the temporal, internal pterygoid, and masseter muscles. These muscles become atrophied after the paralysis has been present for some time, and as a consequence there may be a slight asymmetry of the face that could be taken for a facial paresis. Lack of corneal reflex in cases of ophthalmoplegia suggests direct extension along the petrosphenoidal pathways (Lambert et al.[25]).

The *syndrome of the retroparotidian space* results from the compression of the ninth, tenth, eleventh, and twelfth cranial nerves and the cervical sympathetic nerve (Fig. 185). This is usually the consequence of the development of retropharyngeal or retroparotidian metastases that compress these nerves as they emerge from the base of the skull. The compression of these nerves results in difficulties in deglutition because of hemiparesis of the superior constrictor muscle, in perversion of the sense of taste in the posterior third of the tongue (IX), in a hyperesthesia, hypoesthesia, or anesthesia of the mucous membrane of the

soft palate, pharynx, and larynx, and in respiratory and salivary problems (X). In addition, there is a paralysis and atrophy of the trapezius and sternocleidomastoid muscles, as well as a hemiparesis of the soft palate (XI) and a hemiparalysis and atrophy of one side of the tongue (XII). All of this is usually accompanied and sometimes preceded by a narrowing of the palpebral fissure, enophthalmia, and myosis characteristic of Horner's syndrome due to compression of the cervical sympathetic nerve.

There are instances in which the paralysis of the last four cranial nerves and the sympathetic nerve do not coincide, and limited syndromes only may be present. The syndrome of Jackson, as described by him, is a hemiparalysis of the soft palate, larynx, and tongue, which would correspond to a compression of the eleventh and twelfth cranial nerves. Such is also the case when only the ninth, tenth, and eleventh nerves are compressed, resulting in a syndrome of the jugular foramen (Vernet[60]). There may be, in addition to these three nerves, also a paralysis of the hypoglossal nerve without any evidence of compression of the cervical sympathetic nerve.

The natural evolution of malignant tumors of the nasopharynx that are not controlled is mostly toward the generalization of the disease. In epidermoid carcinomas, however, invasion of the meninges, hemorrhage, and secondary infection or severe pain and deterioration of the general condition may be observed at the terminal stages without generalized metastases. In so-called lymphoepitheliomas, lung, bone, and liver metastases are not rare. In lymphosarcomas, the generalization is mostly in the lymphatic system. In infants, lymphosarcoma metastasizes rapidly to the mediastinum.

Diagnosis

It is only in the past fifty years, due to the progress of otolaryngology, that tumors of the nasopharynx have been diagnosed correctly. However, even today many pass undiagnosed. Errors in diagnosis are due primarily to disregard of the pharynx at examination. Actually, this examination does not require special skill or instruments. In addition, it has not been suf-

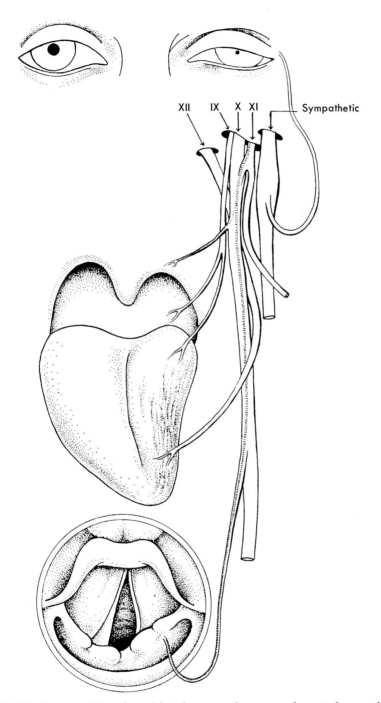

Fig. 185. Distribution of branches of last four cranial nerves and cervical sympathetic nerve in reference to their compression by tumors of nasopharynx. Compression of all these nerves results in Horner's syndrome, hemiparalysis of soft palate and of wall of pharynx, hemiparalysis of tongue, and hemiparalysis of larynx, plus sensory disturbances.

ficiently emphasized that patients with cervical adenopathy, particularly those between 30 and 50 years of age but also younger and older patients, may have a primary tumor of the nasopharynx. A safe approach would be to assume the presence of such a primary nasopharyngeal lesion in all patients with metastatic tumor of the upper cervical region unless otherwise demonstrated. This statement is reinforced by the fact that the clinical onset of more than half of all primary tumors of the nasopharynx is characterized by the development of cervical adenopathy. Simmons and Ariel[50] reported on a series of 150 patients with cancer of the nasopharynx, 125 of whom presented metastases on admission. On an average, patients waited over three months following onset of symptoms before consulting a physician. Seven months elapsed before the correct diagnosis was established, and correct treatment was applied only after a period of ten months.

The final diagnosis of the pathologic entity must be made by biopsy, but clinically the diagnosis may be suggested by the symptoms. Clinical onset by a cervical adenopathy is most often connected with lymphosarcomas and so-called lymphoepitheliomas. An early bilateral adenopathy is most often associated with a primary lymphosarcoma. Nasal obstruction, particularly if bilateral, is also most frequently the result of the forward development of a lymphosarcoma. Rapid invasion of the nasal fossae and orbit may be found in both lymphosarcomas and lymphoepithelioma, but it is most common in the former. The presence of visceral metastases suggests highly undifferentiated carcinoma. Invasion of cervical veins is often responsible (Riggs et al.[45]). Cranial nerve paralyses are almost constantly found in carcinomas and may be observed in some lymphosarcomas (particularly in children). The intensity of pain is usually mild in lymphosarcomas and severe in carcinomas. Bone erosion is most commonly found in carcinomas. Nasal and postnasal bleeding is an almost exclusive sign of carcinomas.

Method of examination

No examination of the nasopharynx should be done without a previous inspection of the oral cavity, oropharynx, hypopharynx, and larynx. This may reveal an impairment of the movements of the soft palate due to the presence of a tumefaction behind it. In addition, it may reveal the presence of a paralysis of the soft palate, pharynx, and larynx due to compression of the cranial nerves.

A very simple method of examination of the nasopharynx is the *digital exploration.* This can be done without anesthesia but is considerably easier if done after spraying the area with an anesthetic solution. Palpation of both sides of the nasopharynx may reveal asymmetry, indurations, or tumefactions. An inspection of the pharynx should always be made following palpation, for some tumors bleed after manipulation.

The examination of the nasopharynx by means of a mirror, the *posterior rhinoscopy,* is sometimes possible in patients with a large retrovelar space and subnormal pharyngeal reflexes. A sensory lack in the soft palate and pharynx should lead to the suspicion that the vagus nerve is being compressed by tumor. A posterior rhinoscopy, however, is best accomplished by means of a soft palate retractor. The general practitioner, nevertheless, can make a very thorough exploration of the nasopharynx without the help of any special instrument.

After a thorough spraying of the posterior wall of the pharynx, the soft palate, and the floor of the nasal fossa with an anesthetic solution, an interval of a few minutes should be allowed to elapse. Then a rubber catheter (urethral catheter, Fr. 12) can be introduced through the nostril on the opposite side of the suspected lesion while the patient breathes deeply with his mouth open. As soon as the tip of the catheter is visible behind the soft palate, it may be grasped with a clamp and brought outside the mouth (Fig. 186). By progressively tightening this elastic catheter, the soft palate will be brought forward and a very satisfactory posterior rhinoscopy will be possible with a large laryngeal mirror (Fig. 187). In general, the introduction of one catheter is sufficient, but a very perfect view can be had by duplicating the procedure on the other side. For this examination, it is more satisfactory for the examiner to use a headlight rather than a reflecting head mirror.

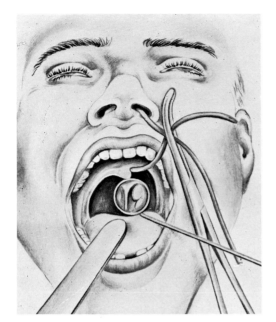

Fig. 186. Easiest way to examine nasopharynx is to insert through nostril a rubber catheter which is retrieved behind soft palate by means of forceps and brought out of mouth, where it is kept tense by means of a clamp. Only light spray anesthesia is necessary.

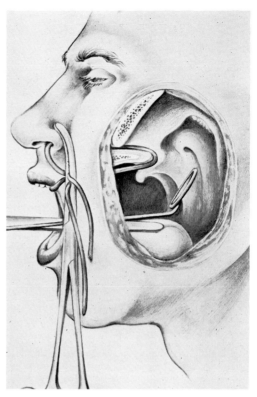

Fig. 187. Progressive retraction of soft palate by rubber catheter permits wide view of nasopharynx without great discomfort to patient.

A posterior rhinoscopy will allow a wide view of the choanae and the posterior extremities of the middle and lower turbinates. Opoline areas of lymphoid tissue may be seen developing in the floor of the nasal fossa or on the sides of the septum in normal individuals and should not be mistaken for tumor. A better view of the lateral walls of the nasopharynx may be obtained by displacing the examining mirror to one or the other side. Outgrowth tumefactions may be seen easily, but submucous nonulcerated infiltrations and deeply ulcerated lesions in Rosenmüller's fossa and the roof of the nasopharynx may require repeated examinations. Because of the numerous anatomic variations of the normal nasopharynx, the symmetry of the two sides should be noted.

The *endoscopic examination* by means of a specially designed instrument has been advocated by some authors. The difficulties of this type of examination are those common to all forms of endoscopic examination. The examiner will have a monocular view and very little sense of distance. This type of examination cannot replace a thorough posterior rhinoscopy, but it has its indications and is a valuable additional means of examination in competent hands.

Cranial nerve paralysis

Cranial nerve paralyses are not, of course, an exclusive feature of nasopharyngeal tumors. In order to be able to make a differential diagnosis, a thorough knowledge of the symptoms produced by the compression of each nerve is necessary.

Olfactory nerve (I). The olfactory nerve is seldom compressed by nasopharyngeal tumors unless the disease has become very extensive. In addition, it is always difficult to ascertain the presence of a unilateral deficiency of the olfactory sense, particularly when there is also nasal obstruction.

Optic nerve (II). Compression of the optic nerve results in complete unilateral amaurosis. The nerve is usually compressed between the chiasm and the optic foramen just medial and anterior to the cavernous sinus.

Oculomotor nerve (III). Compression of the oculomotor nerve results in paralysis of the upper, lower, and inner rectus muscles of the eye and also of the inferior oblique and levator palpebrae muscles. This causes complete fixation of the eye except for its lateral movement, and it also causes palpebral ptosis. The nerve is usually compressed inside the cavernous sinus or on its lateral wall.

Trochlear nerve (IV). Compression of the trochlear nerve results in paralysis of the superior oblique muscle of the eye. Rarely observed alone, it most often accompanies compression of the oculomotor nerve in the cavernous sinus.

Trigeminal nerve (V). The trigeminal nerve is both a motor and sensory nerve which divides into three branches: (1) the ophthalmic, (2) the superior maxillary, and (3) the mandibular. Of these, the first two branches are strictly sensory, but the latter is both sensory and motor. All three branches may be compressed at their origin in the gasserian ganglion. The mandibular branch may be compressed alone in the maxillopharyngeal space.

Compression of sensory fibers of the fifth nerve results in neuralgic pain of the supraorbital and superior maxillary regions. This may be accompanied by hyperesthesia and followed by hypoesthesia and anesthesia. In the mouth, there is most often painful anesthesia of half the tongue, floor of the mouth, buccal mucosa, and hard palate.

The compression of the motor fibers of the mandibular branch results in paralysis of the temporal, internal pterygoid, and masseter muscles. This is evidenced by the inability to protrude the lower jaw so as to bring the lower teeth in front of the upper teeth. The total compression of the fifth nerve is evidenced by the lack of corneal reflex.

Abducens nerve (VI). Compression of this nerve produces paralysis of the external rectus muscle of the eye, which results in diplopia and internal strabismus. The abducens nerve is very vulnerable because of its long subdural trajectory, and it is the most sensitive of all the cranial nerves.

Facial nerve (VII). Compression of the facial nerve causes a typical peripheral facial paralysis. However, this nerve is well

protected by the petrous portion of the temporal bone and is seldom compressed by nasopharyngeal tumors.

Acoustic nerve (VIII). Compression of the acoustic nerve results in loss of hearing and in vertigo. Evidence of its compression requires special verification. This nerve is also rarely reached by nasopharyngeal tumors.

Glossopharyngeal nerve (IX). There is still considerable discussion as to the resulting abnormalities from compression of the glossopharyngeal nerve. According to Vernet,[60] its compression results in a paralysis of the constrictor superior muscle of the pharynx. Paralysis of this muscle may be evidenced by a transversal movement of the posterior wall of the pharynx (curtain movement of Collet) when a pharyngeal reflex occurs. This would be due to a unilateral contraction of the constrictor superior muscle. The sensory disturbances are characterized by a perversion of the sense of taste on the posterior third of the tongue.

Caussé,[6] in reviewing a number of cases with injuries or experimental division of the glossopharyngeal nerve, failed to find the "curtain sign" in any of them. He agreed that the sense of taste of the base of the tongue was probably regulated by this nerve, although the exact area is vari-

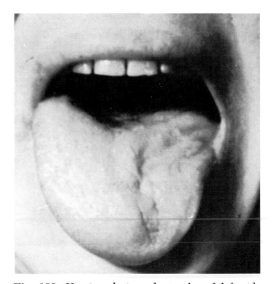

Fig. 188. Hemiparalysis and atrophy of left side of tongue caused by carcinoma of lateral wall of nasopharynx.

able. According to him, the division of the glossopharyngeal nerve results in a lowering of the arch of the soft palate. It is not demonstrated, however, whether these motor fibers originate, as they may, in the spinal accessory nerve.

Vagus nerve (X). There has been confusion as to the physiology of the vagus nerve. The work of Vernet[60] established the fact that it is an entirely sensory nerve and that all of its motor fibers that go to the pharynx, larynx, and heart originate in the spinal accessory nerve and pass to the vagus nerve through an anastomosis in the base of the skull. Compression of the vagus nerve is responsible for the anesthesia of the soft palate, pharynx, and larynx that results in passage of food into the trachea and consequent cough. In addition, there may be cardiorespiratory difficulties such as tachycardia and tachypnea. Congestive lesions of the base of the lung on the same side as the nasopharyngeal lesion have been attributed to vasomotor and trophic disturbances due to compression of the vagus nerve. Further, there may be hypersalivation or hyposalivation, but these are very inconstant.

Hyperesthesia of the tragus is a very good sign of compression of the vagus nerve, the cutaneous fibers of which go to the external auditory canal.

Spinal accessory nerve (XI). The spinal accessory nerve is strictly a motor nerve,

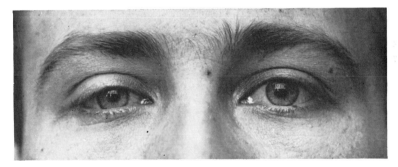

Fig. 189. Horner's syndrome as presenting symptom of tumor of right side of nasopharynx.

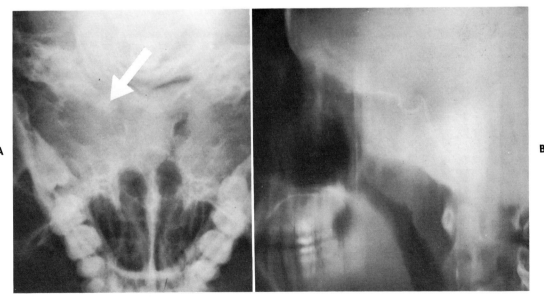

Fig. 190. **A,** Roentgenogram of base of skull showing erosion (arrow) of petrosphenoidal region. **B,** Tomogram showing greater detail of nasopharyngeal tumor. (**A,** Courtesy Dr. Robert Lindberg, M.D. Anderson Hospital, Houston, Texas; **B,** courtesy Dr. Betty Hathaway, National Cancer Institute, Bethesda, Md.)

and it supplies the vagus nerve with its motor fibers. Its compression results in paralysis and atrophy of the trapezius and sternocleidomastoid muscles (external branch) and in a hemiparalysis of the soft palate and larynx of the same side (internal branch). As a result of this compression, there will be atrophy of the cervical muscles, lowering of the arch of the soft palate, and dysphonia.

Hypoglossal nerve (XII). The hypoglossal nerve is a purely motor nerve innervating half of the tongue. Its compression results in rapid atrophy of one side of the tongue, which in protraction will deviate toward the paralyzed side (Fig. 188).

Cervical sympathetic nerve. The cervical sympathetic nerve provides the fibers going to the orbital fascia and those that are responsible for the dilation of the iris. Its compression results in a constriction of the pupil, a retraction of the eye into the orbit, and a consequent narrowing of the palpebral fissure, known as Horner's syndrome (Fig. 189).

Roentgenologic examination

Radiographic examination is a valuable adjunct in the diagnosis of malignant tu-

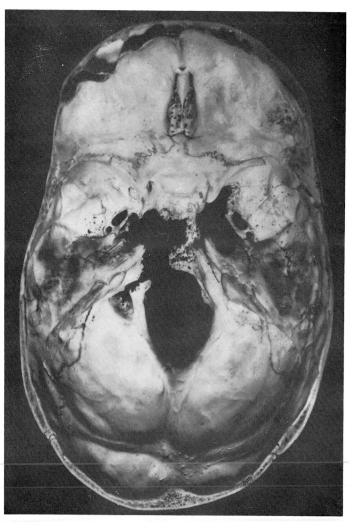

Fig. 191. Erosion of bones of base of skull by malignant tumor of nasopharynx. (Courtesy Prof. A. Fialho; from Pinto Vieira, A.: Radiotherapy of cancer of the nasopharynx, Acta Un. Int. Cancr. **10:**335-344, 1954.)

mors of the nasopharynx. A lateral projection may reveal enlargement of the soft tissues of the posterior wall that had not been suspected on clinical examination. It may also show decalcification of the walls of the sphenoidal sinus that may extend to the clinoid processes. Anteroposterior views of the skull are also useful in establishing evidence of the invasion of ethmoid cells, orbit, nasal fossae, and maxillary sinuses. Roentgenograms of the base of the skull (Fig. 190) are of great importance (Belanger and Dyke[4]), and stereoscopic views may be necessary (Baylin et al.[3]). On careful study of these films, a unilateral decalcification of the bones of the skull (especially of the petrosphenoidal region) betrays the extension of the tumor in the direction of the middle cerebral fossa. Most often the decalcification is found to enlarge the foramen ovale or the foramen lacerum (Fig. 191). Baclesse and Dulac[2] made a most careful study of the radiologic anatomy of the nasopharynx and of the radiographic findings in nasopharyngeal tumors. Lateral roentgenograms may show a typical enlargement or opacity in the region of the tumor (Fig. 192).

Staging

Ho[20a] has proposed the following grouping of his cases for purposes of reporting (letters and figures in parentheses designate elements of the TNM classification):

Stage I
Tumor confined to nasopharyngeal mucosa (T_1)

Stage II
Extension to adjacent areas of soft tissues and compression of nerves below the skull (IX, X, XI, XII, and sympathetic) (T_2) and/or lymph nodes in upper cervical region (N_1)

Stage III
Extension of tumor to base of skull (T_3) and/or to lower cervical lymph nodes (N_2)

Stage IV
Involvement of supraclavicular lymph nodes (N_3) or overlying skin

A

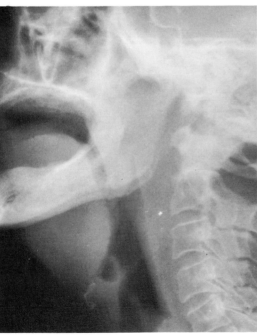

B

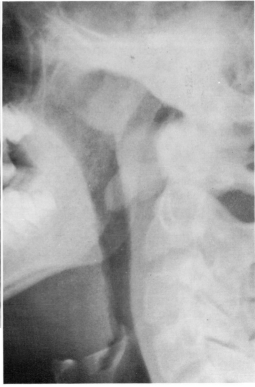

Fig. 192. **A,** Widening of posterior wall and tumor in nasopharynx. **B,** Tumor of nasopharynx. (**A,** Courtesy Dr. Robert Lindberg, M. D. Anderson Hospital, Houston, Texas; **B,** courtesy Dr. Betty Hathaway, National Cancer Institute, Bethesda, Md.)

Stage V

Lymph node or visceral metastases below clavicle

Ho's classification does not take account of differences in unilateral and bilateral adenopathy, only of their level. Presumably Stage III will include compression of one or more cranial nerves in the middle cerebral fossa (III, IV, V, VI).

Biopsy

A biopsy specimen is relatively easy to obtain in the majority of exophytic nasopharyngeal lesions. A curved forceps introduced behind the palate can reach into the lesions of the roof or Rosenmüller's fossae. Smaller lesions of the eustachian tube may need to be biopsied through the nasal fossae with visual control by posterior rhinoscopy. A specimen may be impossible to obtain from infiltrating lesions surrounded by edema. Cytologic study of nasopharyngeal exudate can establish a diagnosis of probability of malignant tumors of the nasopharynx. A needle biopsy of the metastatic nodes is frequently easier to obtain for confirmation of the diagnosis. It should always be done.

Differential diagnosis

A paralysis of the facial nerve (VII) may be present in the course of *acute otitis media,* together with some irritation of the trigeminal nerve (V). In such cases, however, the temporal pain is predominant, and there is an elevation of temperature. The otitis seldom includes compression of other nerves. Facial nerve paralysis is seldom due to a nasopharyngeal tumor unless the tumor is in the last stages of development. When a paralysis of the facial nerve is accompanied by loss of hearing and vertigo, nystagmus, cerebellar symptoms, nausea, choked disk, and symptoms of compression of the fifth, ninth, tenth, or eleventh nerve, the diagnosis should turn toward a possible tumor of the acoustic nerve. In the presence of an ophthalmoplegia without evidence of compression of the fifth nerve, the disturbance will probably be found in the orbit itself and is most often produced by benign bone tumors.

Individual lesions or paralytic syndromes of the last four cranial nerves and the cervical sympathetic nerve have been reported as a result of injuries (particularly war injuries), but paralysis of these nerves may occur in the course of inflammatory conditions of the middle ear with an adenopathy in the retroparotidian space or a possible phlebitis of the jugular vein. Here, again, the cause of the paralysis will be betrayed by the typical acute inflammatory picture of the case. Salivary gland tumors of the parotid gland may come in direct contact with the last four cranial nerves in the retroparotidian space and produce a compression of these nerves, and the same is true of nasopharyngeal chordomas. Both of these tumors, however, present a very slow growth, and this factor will help in the differential diagnosis. The same is true of craniopharyngiomas, which occur predominantly in children (Gordy et al.[17]). In these cases, evidence of focal calcification in the roentgenogram may help in the differential diagnosis (Whittaker[63]).

Cranial nerve paralysis may occur as a consequence of syphilitic meningitis, but in these cases very often the paralyses are bilateral, and they do not follow a particular group, pattern, or syndrome. They seem to attack particularly the ocular muscles and the trigeminal nerve. The specific reactions in the blood and the spinal fluid will be of help in establishing the diagnosis of syphilis. Intracranial tumors may also cause cranial nerve paralysis, but these are constantly accompanied by symptoms of compression of the pyramidal tract and increased intracranial pressure.

There are but few benign conditions of the nasopharynx that may be mistaken for malignant tumors. In children, one should be aware of the often exaggerated pharyngeal tonsil, which may be unusually large (adenoids). The adenopathy that accompanies benign conditions of the nasopharynx is usually discrete, bilateral, multiple, and tender. A retropharyngeal abscess may cause chronic osteomyelitis of the base of the skull and thus result in a suspicion of tumor of the nasopharynx (Eagleton[11]).

Malignant granuloma is a rare progressive disease that may involve the soft tissue of the face, underlying bone, sinuses, hard palate, soft palate, and pharynx. It usually has a prolonged, progressive course terminating in death (Hultberg et al.[21]). It may be confused clinically with a malig-

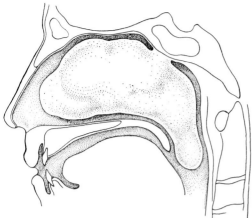

Fig. 193. Nasopharyngeal fibroma illustrating its pedunculated attachment to base of skull and its well-encapsulated extension toward nasal fossa and pharynx.

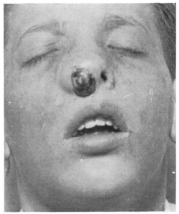

Fig. 194. Nasopharyngeal fibroma protruding through right nostril in 12-year-old boy.

nant neoplasm. Radiotherapy, ACTH, or cortisone may temporarily arrest the course of the disease.

Nasopharyngeal fibromas are predominantly found in boys 10 to 16 years of age (Härkönen and Malmio[19]). These tumors arise at the union of the roof and posterior wall of the nasopharynx (Fig. 193) in the form of a shiny, nonulcerated, rubbery tumor. They may fill the nasopharynx, extend to the nasal fossae, protrude through the naris (Fig. 194), and invade the maxillary sinuses. They may produce extensive deformity of the face ("frog face"). Biopsies and incomplete excisions are often followed by serious hemorrhage and the creation of secondary adhesions and false pedicles. Microscopically, these tumors are made up of myxomatous connective tissue with star-shaped cells and prominent vascularization. The vascular component is thought by Sternberg[52] to be an integral part of the tumor.

Spontaneous regression of these tumors is not so frequent as suggested by the medical literature. Arteriographic studies confirm the vascularity of the lesion (Fig. 195). Such studies may be helpful in determining adequacy of resection (McGavran et al.[30a]). Transnasal resections are done blindly under considerable bleeding and are frequently followed by recurrence. Transmaxillary resections involve considerable mutilation. Rodriguez[46] recommends

the transpalatine approach which gives excellent exposure and permits adequate removal of the entire tumor. Others prefer the transantral approach (Apostol and Frazell[1]). Mild irradiation may result in arrest of development and reduction in size and vascularity, which may obviate surgery or allow it to be done in safety. Since these tumors may be related to an excess of estrogens, they have been treated favorably by administration of androgens —yet they have also responded to the administration of estrogens (Schiff[48]).

Nasopharyngeal *chordomas* are malignant tumors that develop at the expense of vestigial remnants of the notochord. The commonest sites of development are the sacrococcygeal region, nasopharynx, and cervical region. Rarely, these lesions may arise in the lumbar and dorsal spine (Dahlin and MacCarty[9]). Their histologic appearance is characteristic (p. 508). In the nasopharynx, chordomas may extend to destroy the sphenoid and ethmoid sinuses and to cause cranial nerve paralyses. Calcific particles may be detected in the roentgenogram. Encephalography and ventriculography may help to establish the diagnosis (Wood and Himadi[65]). Radiation therapy will frequently give definite palliation for this neoplasm (Windeyer[64]). A rare case of sarcoma botryoides of the nasopharynx has been described (Prior and Stoner[40]).

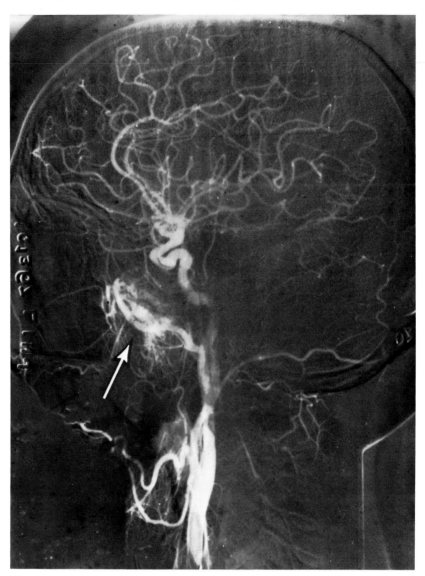

Fig. 195. Lateral projection (subtraction technique) following injection of contrast medium into common carotid artery. Internal maxillary artery is enlarged, indicating increased flow through it. Tumor blush (arrow) in nasopharyngeal area confirms presence of nasopharyngeal angiofibroma. (Courtesy Dr. J. Taveras, St. Louis, Mo.; WU neg. 67-9774.)

In generalized cases of *sarcoidosis*, the nasopharynx may be the site of clinical, roentgenographic, and histologic manifestations of this disease (Larsson[26]). Sarcomas of the bones or soft tissues of the base of the skull are rare.

Treatment

Surgery

The complete surgical extirpation of nasopharyngeal malignant tumors, regard-

less of early diagnosis or small size of the lesion, is an impossibility. Their diffusely infiltrating character and early metastasizing ability put them beyond the scope of this form of treatment. Because the first relay of lymphatic spread is usually an inaccessible lymph node close to the base of the skull, a radical neck dissection cannot be successful in the treatment of their cervical metastases (Perez et al.[38]).

Table 18. Five-year survival at different institutions*

Series	Patients	5-yr survivors
University of California Hospital, San Francisco, Calif.	82	23 (28.2%)
Martin-Blady: Memorial Hospital, New York, N. Y.	87	20 (23.0%)
Kramer: Middlesex, London	54	8 (15.0%)
Lenz: Presbyterian and Montefiore Hospitals, New York, N. Y.	44	13 (29.6%)
Nielsen: Radium Center, Copenhagen, Denmark	77	11 (14.3%)
Smedal-Watson: Lahey Clinic, Boston, Mass.	39	13 (33.3%)

*From Vaeth, J. M.: Nasopharyngeal malignant tumors; 82 consecutive patients treated in a period of twenty-two years, Radiology **74**: 364-372, 1960.

Radiotherapy

Most malignant tumors of the naso-pharynx are radiosensitive and theoretically radiocurable. The difficulty encountered in their radiotherapeutic management has been the administration of a sufficiently high amount of radiations throughout the vast area of primary infiltration and secondary involvement. The task of irradiating, as homogeneously as possible, the deep-seated primary lesion, its possible involvement of the middle cerebral fossa, its prevertebral first relay of node involvement, and the cervical metastases, on one or both sides, require careful planning of approaches and dosimetry (Regato[42]; Kramer[24]; Folichon et al.[14, 15]). The development of supervoltage roentgentherapy and cobalt[60] teletherapy has facilitated the task (Fletcher and Million[13]) but has increased the possibilities of untoward effects on the cervical spine that are observed with the use of excessively large fields and intensive irradiation (Tan and Khor[53a]). But careful treatment planning and fractionation usually permit a sufficient and relatively homogeneous irradiation of the potential areas of tumor involvement.

Intracavitary radiumtherapy was frequently sought, in combination with conventional roentgentherapy, to increase the irradiation of the deeply situated primary lesion. This approach is seldom used now, except perhaps for the irradiation of limited nasopharyngeal recurrences (Vaeth[59]; Wang and Schulz[62]).

A rapid regression of symptoms usually accompanies the first administrations of radiotherapy. The hypoacousia may disappear, but it also may continue to the end of the treatment because of increased edema. Cranial nerve paralysis of the petro-sphenoidal group may also regress and vanish. The same is not true, however, of the paralysis due to compression of the retroparotidian group of nerves, which may persist in spite of the sterilization of the tumor. Pain is usually relieved after a few weeks of treatment, but in some instances, probably because of invasion rather than compression of the gasserian ganglion, intense pain in the trigeminal area will persist and will require continuous administration of narcotics.

During the course of treatment, a radio-epithelitis of the mucous membrane may develop. Because of the treatment of nodes, radioepithelitis of the hypopharynx will cause dysphagia and weight loss. In general, the latter can be managed by a well-balanced high-caloric, high-vitamin liquid diet.

The most common complication in the course of treatment is an otitis media with its characteristic intense pain and rapid elevation of temperature. This will almost always react favorably to the administration of antibiotics.

Prognosis

The prognosis of cancer of the naso-pharynx today is relatively good exclusively to the credit of radiotherapy. Results reported from different institutions are usually based on a relatively small number of patients (Table 18). Gotfredsen[16] collected 266 cases from four different Scandinavian institutions with fifty-nine (22%) of the patients living and well five years after irradiation. In seventy patients with malignant tumors of the nasopharynx reported by Perez et al.,[38] twenty-four survived more than five years free from tumor. However, four of the survivors later developed recrudescence and/or distant metastases. Of 467 patients treated during 1965 at the Institute of Radiology in Hong Kong, Ho[20a] reported 117 (25%) living and well. Using his proposed classification

Table 19. Results of radiotherapy for carcinoma of the nasopharynx (Institute of Radiology, Hong Kong)*

Stage	Cases	Alive and well (4 yr)	%
I	29	19	65
II	37	21	57
III	243	65	27
IV	128	12	10
V	30	0	0
	467	117	25

*From Ho, J. C.: Natural history and treatment of nasopharyngeal cancer (Tenth International Cancer Congress, Houston, Texas, May, 1970), Int. J. Cancer (to be published).

(p. 269), the relative results were as shown in Table 19.

The relative prognosis of the different histologic varieties is most favorable to lymphosarcomas, with a five-year survival rate of 50% (Lenz[28]; Fletcher and Million[13]). It is least favorable for the well-differentiated squamous cell carcinoma (Baclesse and Dulac[2]; Nielsen[36]; Pierquin et al.[38a]). The clinical absence of metastases confers a relatively better prognosis (Vaeth[59]; Scanlon et al.[47]), but proved metastatic nodes are sterilized in a high proportion of cases (Million et al.[33]). Prognosis is relatively better in women than in men (Lederman[27]), whereas the outlook in children is almost consistently fatal. Involvement of the base of the skull implies an ominous prognosis. The presence of cranial nerve paralysis usually compromises the results. Of 113 patients with neurologic manifestations reported by Thomas and Waltz,[55] only nine survived. Distant metastases may also be the cause of failure. Patients living without evidence of recurrence at the end of five years usually remain well. Late recurrences or metastases are rare.

REFERENCES

1 Apostol, J. V., and Frazell, E. L.: Juvenile nasopharyngeal angiofibroma; a clinical study, Cancer 18:869-878, 1965.

2 Baclesse, F., and Dulac, G.: Les tumeurs malignes du rhinopharynx, Bull. Ass. Franc. Cancer 31:160-177, 1943.

3 Baylin, G. J., Reeves, R. J., and Kerman, H. D.: A roentgen and clinical study of nasopharyngeal malignancies, Southern Med. J. 42:467-476, 1949.

4 Belanger, W. G., and Dyke, C. G.: Roentgen diagnosis of malignant nasopharyngeal tumors, Amer. J. Roentgen. 50:9-18, 1943.

5 Buell, P.: Nasopharynx cancer in Chinese of California, Brit. J. Cancer 19:459-470, 1965.

6 Caussé, R.: Les signes de la paralysie du glosso-pharyngien, Ann. Otolaryng. (Paris), pp. 44-58, 1936.

7 Ch'in, K. Y., and Szutu, C.: Lymphoepithelioma; a pathological study of 97 cases, Chin. Med. J. (Peking) (suppl. 3), pp. 94-119, 1940.

7a Clifford, P.: On the epidemiology of nasopharyngeal cancer, Int. J. Cancer 5:287-309, 1970 (excellent review).

8 Clifford, P., and Beecher, J. L.: Nasopharyngeal cancer in Kenya; clinical and environmental aspects, Brit. J. Cancer 18:25-43, 1964.

9 Dahlin, D. C., and MacCarty, C. S.: Chordoma; a study of fifty-nine cases, Cancer 5:1170-1178, 1952.

10 Digby, K. H., Fook, W. L., and Che, Y. T.: Nasopharyngeal carcinoma, Brit. J. Surg. 28:517-537, 1941.

11 Eagleton, W. P.: New classification of bones, forming skull based on their function and embryologic origin as influencing kind, course and frequency of infections of individual bones, with surgical applications, especially as to relation of osseous infections to meningitis, Arch. Otolaryng. (Chicago) 24:158-189, 1936.

12 Ennuyer, A., Bataini, P., Helary, J., and Chavanne, G.: Les plasmocytomes des voies aéro-digestives superieures; a propos de 248 cas dont 19 traités à la Fondation Curie, Bull. Cancer (Paris) 50:53-100, 1963.

13 Fletcher, G. H., and Million, R. R.: Malignant tumors of the nasopharynx, Amer. J. Roentgen. 93:44-55, 1965.

14 Folichon, A., Ennuyer, A., Bertoluzzi, M., and Calle, R.: Mesures directes de doses de rayons a l'hypophyse du cadavre dans les conditions röntgenthérapiques habituelles, J. Radiol. Electr. 31:170-174, 1950.

15 Folichon, A., Ennuyer, A., Bertoluzzi, M., and Calle, R.: Mesures a l'aide de microchambres de Sievert, des doses reçues au niveau du rhinopharynx du cadavre et du malade, dans les conditions techniques röntgenthérapiques habituelles, J. Radiol. Electr. 32:48-55, 1951.

16 Godtfredsen, E.: Ophthalmologic and neurologic symptoms at malignant nasopharyngeal tumours, Acta Psychiat. Neurol. Scand. (suppl. 34), pp. 1-323, 1944.

17 Gordy, P. D., Peet, M. M., and Kahn, E. A.: The surgery of the craniopharyngomas, J. Neurosurg. 6:503-517, 1949.

18 Greenberg, B. E.: Cervical lymph node metastasis from unknown primary sites; an unresolved problem in management, Cancer 19:1091-1095, 1966.

19 Härkönen, M., and Malmio, K.: On the treatment of nasopharyngeal fibroma and its results, Acta Otolaryng. (Stockholm) 67(suppl.):33-40, 1948.

20 Ho, J. C.: Nasopharyngeal carcinoma in Hong Kong. In Cancer of the nasopharynx, UICC Monograph Series I, New York, 1967, Medical Examination Publishing Co., pp. 58-63.

20a Ho, J. C.: Natural history and treatment of nasopharyngeal cancer (Tenth International

Cancer Congress, Houston, Texas, May, 1970), Int. J. Cancer (to be published).

21 Hultberg, S., Koch, H., Moberger, G., and Martensson, G.: Malignant granuloma, Acta Radiol. (Stockholm) 47:229-248, 1957.

22 Jacod, M.: Sur la propagation intracranienne des sarcomes de la trompe d'eustache syndrome durcarrefour petro-sphenoidal paralysie des 2e, 3e, 4e, 5e et 6e paires craniennes, Rev. Neurol. (Paris) 37:33-38, 1921.

23 Kobayashi, H., Suzuki, H., Ishikawa, D., and Miyasaki, T.: Radiological treatment of malignant tumors of the nasopharynx, oropharynx and hypopharynx, Clin. Radiol. 10:249-258, 1965.

24 Kramer, S.: The treatment of malignant tumours of the nasopharynx, Proc. Roy. Soc. Med. 43:867-874, 1950.

25 Lambert, V., Snelling, M., Flatman, G. E., and Lederman, M.: Discussion of treatment of cancer of the nasopharynx, Proc. Roy. Soc. Med. 47:547-560, 1954.

26 Larsson, L. G.: Nasopharyngeal lesions of sarcoidosis, Acta Radiol. (Stockholm) 36:361-373, 1951.

27 Lederman, M.: Cancer of the nasopharynx; its natural history and treatment, Springfield, Ill., 1961, Charles C Thomas, Publisher.

28 Lenz, M.: Roentgen therapy of primary cancer of the nasopharynx, Amer. J. Roentgen. 48:816-832, 1942.

29 Little, J. B., Schulz, M. D., and Wang, C. C.: Radiation therapy for cancer of the nasopharynx, Arch. Otolaryng. (Chicago) 77:621-624, 1963.

30 Loke, Y. W.: Nasopharyngeal cancer in the Malays, Brit. J. Cancer 20:226-230, 1966.

30a McGavran, M. H., Sessions, D. G., Dorfman, R. F., Davis, D. O., and Ogura, J. H.: Nasopharyngeal angiofibroma, Arch. Otolaryng. (Chicago) 90:68-78, 1969.

31 Macomb, W. S.: Juvenile nasopharyngeal fibroma, Amer. J. Surg. 106:754-763, 1963.

32 Martin, H., Ehrlich, H. E., and Abels, J. C.: Juvenile nasopharyngeal angiofibroma, Ann. Surg. 127:513-536, 1948.

33 Million, R. R., Fletcher, G. H., and Jesse, R. H., Jr.: Evaluation of elective irradiation of the neck for squamous-cell carcinoma of the nasopharynx, tonsillar fossa and base of tongue, Radiology 80:973-988, 1963.

34 Muir, C. S.: Cancer of the buccal cavity and nasopharyngeal angiofibroma; a clinical study, Cancer 18:869-878, 1965.

35 New, G. B.: Highly malignant tumors of the nasopharynx and pharynx, Trans. Amer. Acad. Ophthal. 36:39-44, 1931.

36 Nielsen, J.: Roentgen treatment of malignant tumors of the nasopharynx, Acta Radiol. (Stockholm) 26:133-154, 1965.

37 Pang, L. Q.: Carcinoma of the nasopharynx, Arch. Otolaryng. (Chicago) 82:622-628, 1965.

38 Perez, C. A., Ackerman, L. V., Mill, W. B., Ogura, J. H., and Powers, W. E.: Cancer of the nasopharynx; factors influencing prognosis, Cancer 24:1-17, 1969.

38a Pierquin, Y., Cachin, D., Chassagne, R., Lefur, R., and Bigot, R.: Étude de 49 cas de carcinomes épidermoides du cavum traités a l'Institut Gustave-Roussy de 1960 a 1965, Presse Med. 76:1565-1566, 1968.

39 Pinto Vieira, A.: Radiotherapy of cancer of the nasopharynx, Acta Un. Int. Cancr. 10:335-344, 1954.

40 Prior, J. T., and Stoner, L. R.: Sarcoma botryoides of the nasopharynx, Cancer 10:957-963, 1957.

41 del Regato, J. A.: Neurological manifestations of cancer of the nasopharynx, St. Louis Med. Soc. Weekly Bull. 40:331-332, 1946.

42 del Regato, J. A.: Cancer of the nasopharynx. In Portmann, U. V., editor: Clinical therapeutic radiology, New York, 1950, Thos. Nelson & Sons.

43 Regaud, C.; cited in Reverchon, L., and Coutard, H.: Lymph-épithéliome de l'hypopharynx traité par röntgenthérapie, Bull. Mem. Soc. Franc. Otorhinolaryng. Congr., May, 1921.

44 Reverchon, L., and Coutard, H.: Lympho-épithéliome de l'hypopharynx traité par röntgenthérapie, Bull. Mem. Soc. Franc. Otorhinolaryng. Congr., May, 1921.

45 Riggs, H. E., Rupp, C., Ray, H., and Yaskin, J. C.: Cranial nerve syndromes associated with nasopharyngeal malignancy, Arch. Neurol. Psychiat. (Chicago) 77:473-482, 1957.

46 Rodriguez, H.: A new surgical approach to nasopharyngeal angiofibroma, Cancer 19:458-460, 1966.

47 Scanlon, P. W., Rhodes, R. E., Jr., Woolner, L. B., Devine, Kenneth D., and McBean, J. B.: Cancer of the nasopharynx, Amer. J. Roentgen. 99:313-325, 1967.

48 Schiff, M.: Juvenile nasopharyngeal angiofibroma; a theory of pathogenesis, Laryngoscope 69:981-1016, 1959.

49 Schmincke, A.: Ueber lymphoepitheliale Geschwulste, Beitr. Path. Anat. 58:161-170, 1921.

50 Simmons, M. W., and Ariel, I. M.: Carcinoma of the nasopharynx, Surg. Gynec. Obstet. 38:763-775, 1949.

51 Smoke and nasopharyngeal cancer, Lancet 2:833-834, 1965.

52 Sternberg, S. S.: Pathology of juvenile nasopharyngeal angiofibroma—a lesion of adolescent males, Cancer 7:15-28, 1954.

53 Svoboda, D., Kirchner, F., and Shanmugaratnam, K.: Ultrastructure of nasopharyngeal carcinoma in American and Chinese patients; an application of electron microscopy to geographic pathology, Exp. Molec. Path. 4:189-204, 1965.

53a Tan, B. C., and Khor, T. H.: Radiation myelitis in carcinoma of the nasopharynx, Clin. Radiol. 20:329-331, 1969.

54 Teoh, T. B.: Epidermoid carcinoma of the nasopharynx among Chinese; a study of 31 necropsies, J. Path. Bact. 73:451-465, 1957.

55 Thomas, J. E., and Waltz, A. G.: Neurological manifestations of nasopharyngeal malignant tumors, J.A.M.A. 192:103-106, 1965.

56 Todd, I. D. H.: Treatment of solitary plasmacytoma, Clin. Radiol. 16:395-399, 1965.

57 Trotter, W.: Malignant tumours of the nasopharynx, Lancet 1:1277, 1911.

58 Truffert, P.: Les aponevroses de la trompe d'eustache, Ann. Mal. Oreille, Larynx **41**:498-507, 1922.

59 Vaeth, J. M.: Nasopharyngeal malignant tumors; 82 consecutive patients treated in a period of twenty-two years, Radiology **74**: 364-372, 1960.

60 Vernet, Maurice: Le syndrome du trou dechire posterieur. Les paralysies laryngees associees, Thesis, Faculty of Medicine, Lyon, 1916.

61 Villaret, M.: Le syndrome de l'espace retroparotodien posterieur, Paris Med. **21**:430, 1917.

62 Wang, C. C., and Schulz, M. D.: Management of locally recurrent carcinoma of the nasopharynx, Radiology **86**:900-903, 1966.

63 Whittaker, L. R.: Nasopharyngeal cancer in Kenya; radiological appearances, Brit. J. Cancer **18**:44-48, 1964.

64 Windeyer, B. W.: Chordoma, Proc. Roy. Soc. Med. **52**:1088-1100, 1959.

65 Wood, E. H., Jr., and Himadi, G. M.: Chordomas; a roentgenologic study of sixteen cases previously unreported, Radiology **54**:706-716, 1950.

66 Yeh, S.: A histological classification of carcinoma of the nasopharynx with a critical review as to the existence of lymphoepithelioma (University of Taipei, Formosa), Cancer **15**: 895-920, 1962.

67 Yeh, S., and Cowdry, E. V.: Incidence of malignant tumors in Chinese, especially in Formosa, Cancer **7**:425-436, 1954.

Oropharynx

Soft palate
Tonsil

The oropharynx extends between two horizontal planes, one passing through the soft palate when in a horizontal position and the other passing at the level of the hyoid bone (Fig. 196). This region includes the lower surface of the soft palate, the palatine tonsil, the lingual tonsil, the base of the tongue, the free border of the epiglottis, and the part of the pharyngeal walls included between its limits (Fig. 197).

A variety of tumors may develop within the oropharynx, each offering different diagnostic, pathologic, therapeutic, and prognostic problems. They will be discussed on an anatomic basis as follows: (1) soft palate, (2) tonsil, (3) base of the tongue, and (4) periepiglottic area, including glossopharyngeal sulcus, glossoepiglottic fossa, free portion of the epiglottis, pharyngoepiglottic fold, and oropharyngeal wall.

Soft palate

Anatomy

The soft palate or velum is a muscular structure strongly attached to the posterior border of the hard palate. From this point of attachment it extends first horizontally and then downward to form the uvula in the midline. The two anterior pillars of the soft palate originate at the base of the uvula and find their insertion near lateral

Base of tongue
Periepiglottic area

aspects of the base of the tongue. These two pillars form an elongated arcade interrupted only in the midline by the uvula. Also from the base of the uvula spring the posterior pillars, which follow a posterior and downward direction and insert themselves on the lateral wall of the pharynx. Between these two pillars there is on each side an excavation, the tonsillar fossa, which is normally occupied by the palatine tonsil.

The mucous membrane that covers the lower aspects of the soft palate is a continuation of the mucous membrane of the mouth, and it has a stratified squamous character. In the region adjacent to the hard palate there is a group of independent glandular aggregates, about 100 in number, producing mostly mucous. They are found in front of the palatine fascia (Fig. 163). About twelve more of these glands are found in the uvula.

Lymphatics. The soft palate is relatively rich in lymphatics, particularly at the midline. They all converge toward a group of nodes found below the anterior belly of the digastric muscle immediately in front of the jugular chain (Fig. 198).

Epidemiology

Carcinomas of the soft palate are most often observed in men in the sixth and seventh decades of life. In a series of

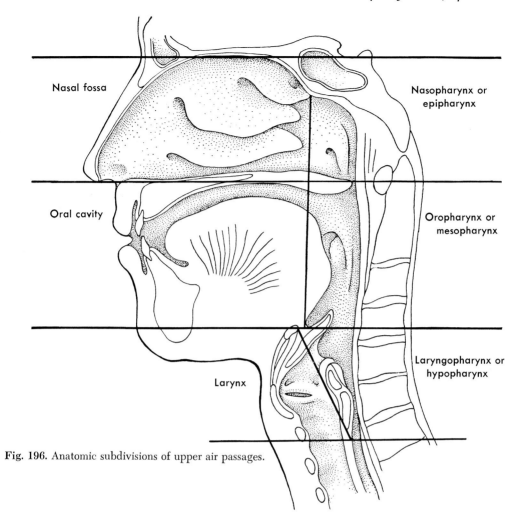

Nasal fossa

Nasopharynx or epipharynx

Oral cavity

Oropharynx or mesopharynx

Laryngopharynx or hypopharynx

Larynx

Fig. 196. Anatomic subdivisions of upper air passages.

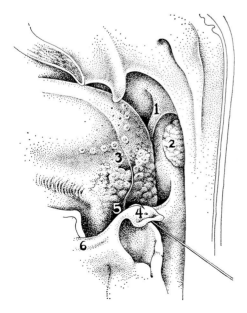

eighty-four patients studied by Perussia,[42] 90% were men, and fifty-two patients (62%) were between 50 and 69 years of age.

Pathology

Gross pathology

Carcinomas of the soft palate are usually found on the anterior pillar or on the supratonsillar fossa. They rarely arise from the posterior pillar. The majority are ulcerated and diffusely infiltrating. A very small number of lesions that usually develop on the anterior pillar may be papillary in character (Fig. 199). Extension

Fig. 197. Posterolateral view of oropharynx. **1,** Anterior pillar of soft palate. **2,** Tonsil. **3,** Base of tongue. **4,** Free portion of epiglottis. **5,** Valleculae. **6,** Pharyngoepiglottic fold.

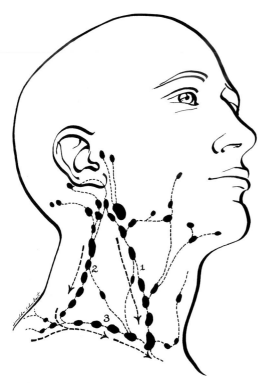

Fig. 198. Lymphatic chains of neck. 1, Anterior or jugular chain. 2, Posterior or spinal chain. 3, Transverse or supraclavicular chain.

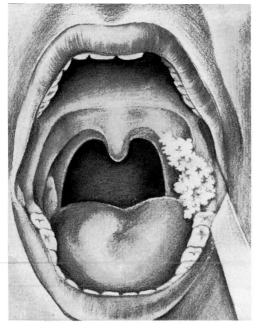

Fig. 199. Papillary epidermoid carcinoma of anterior pillar of soft palate extending over base of tongue and buccal mucosa.

toward the buccal mucosa and toward the hard palate is common. Deep extension into the pterygoid fossa is not infrequent.

Microscopic pathology

Carcinomas of the soft palate are epidermoid in type and usually well differentiated. A few cases, however, will show little tendency to differentiation. Adenocarcinomas, which are described as developing in this region, are invariably tumors of salivary gland origin (Marcial-Rojas and Leon-Antoni[30]).

Metastatic spread

Carcinomas of the soft palate do not metastasize early, but the proportion of metastases increases with their duration and size. The most frequently involved node is one high in the jugular chain.

Clinical evolution

The first symptom of carcinoma of the soft palate is *odynophagia,* rapidly followed by *local pain* that radiates to the entire side of the face and head. *Pain* is an important symptom. *Dysphagia* may become very marked. *Trismus* may be present in apparently early lesions, betraying the deep infiltration that usually accompanies these tumors. *Bleeding* is not frequent but is sometimes present.

An adenopathy will not be found at the time of examination in the majority of patients. When it appears, it is a discrete, barely palpable upper cervical node located just below the angle of the mandible. This is usually a hard node showing a very slow growth. Later, shotty nodes might be felt in other areas of the neck.

Left to itself, carcinoma of the soft palate develops slowly, but the general condition of the patient rapidly deteriorates. The necessity for the administration of strong sedatives and the marked dysphagia contribute to impoverish the general condition further. Most patients with carcinoma of the soft palate, whether treated or untreated, die with the disease confined to the soft palate and cervical region.

Diagnosis

In examining the patients, an effort should always be made to differentiate

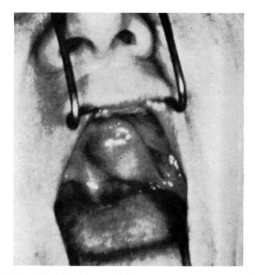

Fig. 200. Benign mixed tumor of mucous and salivary gland type developing on left side of soft palate. Lesion was treated by surgical excision.

those carcinomas arising in the soft palate proper and those arising in the tonsil and extending to the soft palate secondarily. This is not always possible.

Carcinomas of the soft palate will show a superficial necrotic ulceration with retraction and immobility of the surrounding area. Digital palpation will reveal a diffuse induration well beyond the ulceration. A specimen for biopsy can be secured only by means of a cutting instrument.

Next to the hard palate, the soft palate is the most frequent site of development of mucous and salivary gland tumors. These are nonulcerated, slowly growing, submucous tumors, mostly benign but sometimes malignant, which develop near the anterior surface of the palate in front of the palatine aponeurosis and which seldom occur in the midline (Fig. 200). They are usually well encapsulated and can be easily excised. Their histology is characteristic (p. 535).

Treatment

Most carcinomas of the soft palate are, as a rule, markedly differentiated, develop slowly, show little radiosensitivity, and have characteristics that seem appropriate for surgical excision. Surgical excision, however, is usually unsatisfactory. It is difficult to excise the lesion without cutting through tumor whose exact limits are difficult to ascertain. Excision of carcinomas of the soft palate in continuity with a good portion of the lower jaw and the lymphatics of the neck has been advocated.

Roentgentherapy may be applied externally, including the metastatic node when present, and also through the oral opening. It is possible to deliver an adequate dose by these two approaches. Supervoltage roentgentherapy and cobalt[60] permit very satisfactory irradiation of the primary lesion and the cervical metastases. A combined approach of radical radiotherapy and radical surgery is preferred by some (Fletcher et al.[16]) for carcinomas of the palatine arch.

Treatment of the metastatic adenopathy should be surgical. Although usually only upper cervical nodes are invaded, a radical neck dissection should be carried out.

Prognosis

The exact curability of carcinomas of the soft palate is difficult to ascertain from the literature, for these tumors are usually reported in the same group with tumors of the tonsil or of the hard palate. The inclusion in this category of carcinomas arising in the "retromolar trigone" area also vitiates comparisons, for the latter often result from spread of carcinomas of the lower gingiva or buccal mucosa. Perussia[42] reported on a series of fifty-nine patients with histologically proved lesions treated by radiotherapy, from 1928 to 1945, with sixteen (27%) remaining well five years after treatment. This group did not include any patients with lesions of the anterior pillar which are reputedly more difficult to control. In general, carcinomas of the soft palate presenting trismus and deep infiltration are not curable by radiations.

Tonsil

Anatomy

The palatine tonsils are two lymphoid organs situated on each lateral wall of the pharynx between the anterior and posterior pillars of the soft palate. Externally, the tonsils are in relation with the lateral wall of the pharynx and, beyond this, with the maxillopharyngeal space.

Each tonsil is covered by a closely adherent capsule that sends deep prolongations into the lymphoid tissue. The tonsils are lined by a stratified squamous epithelium, a continuation of the surrounding mucous membrane, but at the level of the tonsillar crypts the mucous membrane takes a pseudoreticular aspect and is infiltrated by numerous lymphocytes.

Lymphatics. The rich lymphatics of the tonsil gather in four or six trunks which, after passing through the lateral wall of the pharynx, end in the subdigastric nodes that lie anterior to the jugular chain.

Epidemiology

Cancer of the tonsil is the second most common form of cancer of the upper air passages, superseded only by carcinomas of the laryngopharynx. It accounts for 1.5% to 3% of all forms of cancer.

Carcinomas of the tonsil are most frequently found in men in their sixth and seventh decades of life. Perussia[43] studied a series of 139 patients, of whom ninety-three (67%) were between 50 and 69 years of age and 125 (90%) were men. One-third of lymphosarcomas, however, are found in women. Luzzatti[27, 28] studied a series of 125 lymphosarcomas of the pharynx, sixty-three of which arose in the palatotonsillar region. Lymphosarcomas are found more often than carcinomas during the third and fourth decades of life.

Pathology

Gross pathology

The different tumors developing in the tonsil may present individual gross features that are worthy of note.

Carcinomas of the tonsil usually arise near the upper pole and are commonly exophytic, superficially ulcerated tumors (Fig. 201). Their spread to the soft palate often occurs at the level of the supratonsillar fossa or toward the anterior pillar. Invasion of the posterior pillar is rarely observed, but extension to the glossopharyngeal sulcus is common. Rider[49] emphasizes the frequency of involvement of the base of the tongue.

A rather large group of tumors of the

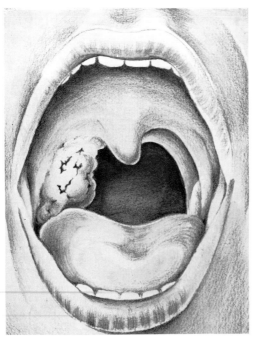

Fig. 201. Epidermoid carcinoma of tonsil with beginning extension to soft palate. These tumors are generally exophytic and show little tendency to infiltrate in depth.

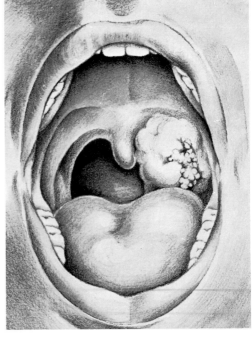

Fig. 202. "Lymphoepithelioma" of tonsil presenting polylobated, polypoid appearance and only limited ulceration.

tonsil variously designated as lymphoepitheliomas, transitional cell carcinomas, or *undifferentiated carcinomas* present as smooth, mostly submucous, somewhat lobulated tumors, with either minimal or no visible ulceration (Fig. 202). They do not infiltrate deeply, and their spread is superficial. In advanced cases, they may become superficially ulcerated throughout. The impression given is a different one.

Lymphosarcomas of the tonsil develop submucosally and may attain large proportions without presenting an ulceration. The surface of the tumor is covered by the same mucous membrane as the soft palate (Fig. 203). Trauma, therapeutic incisions, or biopsy may cause secondary infection which sometimes results in an extensive necrosis of the tumor area. At times, a lymphosarcoma may be superficially ulcerated in its early development and extend superficially beyond the midline in a horseshoe fashion. Some lymphosarcomas of the tonsil are rather small and appear grossly as a purely inflammatory tonsil.

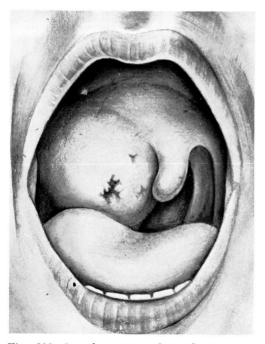

Fig. 203. Lymphosarcoma of tonsil. Tumor is usually smooth, shiny, and almost spherical in shape due to submucous extension. Ulceration occurs only after trauma.

Microscopic pathology

Carcinomas are the most common of tonsillar tumors. Of these, a great proportion are rather undifferentiated squamous cell carcinomas. The great majority of the tumors present a slight differentiation with little or no keratinization. A goodly number will show no keratinization at all and will be included in what is usually called transitional cell carcinomas. This latter designation is not a well-established one. The tumors should probably be considered as *nonkeratinizing carcinomas*.

Lymphosarcomas are usually subdivided into several groups according to the character of their cells and stroma. These groups do not correspond to any clinical entity, and they do not have any therapeutic or prognostic value but are only of interest to the pathologist.

The microscopic diagnosis of lymphosarcoma is not always easy, and this is particularly true when the specimen comes from a lymph node. In cases in which the primary lesion has not been identified in the upper air passages, the pathologist will need the help of the clinician and of further laboratory investigations in order to make a differential diagnosis with other malignant lymphomas.

Metastatic spread

The typical metastatic adenopathy from *carcinomas* of the tonsil is a high jugular node, in the subdigastric group of nodes, immediately lateral to the primary growth (Fig. 204). Subsequent metastases lower in the jugular and supraclavicular chains, axilla, and mediastinum may be observed. Blood-borne metastases are rare in carcinomas.

Undifferentiated carcinomas ("lymphoepitheliomas") metastasize earlier than other carcinomas to nodes in the jugular chain. Their permeation to additional nodes is faster and their volume larger. In patients with advanced lesions, metastases to lungs, liver, and bones are frequently observed.

An early, frequently large, and often bilateral cervical adenopathy is characteristic of lymphosarcomas of the tonsil. However, some lymphosarcomas of the tonsil may grow to obstructive size without significant adenopathy. Unsuccessfully treated

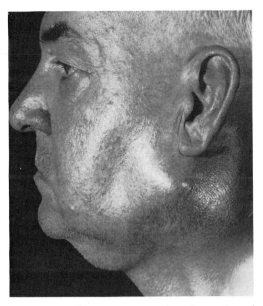

Fig. 204. Voluminous metastatic adenopathy of upper cervical and submaxillary region in carcinoma of tonsil.

lesions advance to present generalized metastases with predominance in the lymphatic system.

Clinical evolution

A mild pharyngeal discomfort or sensation of foreign body accompanied or followed by slight odynophagia is usually the first symptom in *carcinoma* of the tonsil. This symptom is so trivial that the patient may delay considerably his consultation with a physician. Pain is infrequently present except in advanced cases. Otalgia on the same side as the lesion and dysphagia occur in moderately advanced cases. Examination will reveal an enlarged, irregular tonsil usually presenting an ulcerated area in its center. This area may be found indurated but seldom is fixed. When the tumor has spread outside the tonsil, there will be a superficial nodularity of the anterior pillar or supratonsillar fossa, generally not ulcerated. An enlarged lymph node will almost invariably be present in the upper cervical region behind the angle of the mandible. Its appearance may have preceded or accompanied the symptoms caused by the primary lesion. This adenopathy is rapid growing and usually fixed but not adherent to the skin. Subsequent

metastatic nodes in the neck, axilla, and mediastinum appear successively. Scanlon et al.[51] reported that 50% of patients with carcinoma of the tonsil presented metastases.

It is characteristic of *undifferentiated carcinomas* ("lymphoepitheliomas") that the primary lesion may be so discrete as to pass unnoticed. The fact that it is seldom widely ulcerated and that it does not infiltrate in depth accounts for the lack of symptoms caused by the primary lesion. The first symptom is very often the development of a rapidly growing adenopathy. This is found in the upper cervical region behind the angle of the mandible, is usually soft with no tendency to fixation, and is most commonly accompanied by smaller nodes in adjacent areas. In advanced cases, distant metastases to lymph nodes and to the lungs, liver, and bone are not exceptional.

Lymphosarcomas of the tonsil have varied forms of clinical onset worthy of consideration. They may be divided into three clinical groups according to their mode of onset (Regato[46]).

The first group (obstructive) is characterized by the rapid growth of a non-ulcerated, tonsillar tumefaction that may acquire huge dimensions and interfere considerably with deglutition and respiration. There may be no adenopathy or only a rather discrete node palpable in the angulomandibular region.

The second group (inflammatory) is characterized by a history of repeated inflammatory-like attacks of pharyngitis accompanied by fever. An upper cervical adenopathy may appear during this acute stage but will show intermittent spontaneous regression without ever entirely disappearing. The diagnosis can be made only by continued observation of the patient and by biopsy.

The third group (early metastasizing) is considerably more common. The lesion of the tonsil is silent and consequently often overlooked. It may be represented by a small focus of tumor within the tonsil or by a pedunculated tumor hidden in the glossoepiglottic fossa. Metastatic nodes first appear in the cervical region on the same side as the primary lesion and are promptly succeeded by other nodes in the axilla and the mediastinum. The tumor may rapidly become widespread, and for this reason many patients may have an initial examination when the disease has become generalized. In generalized disease, the poor general condition of the patient, the symptoms of mediastinal enlargement, etc. are predominant in the clinical picture, and the primary point of origin in the tonsil may not be established.

Diagnosis

Taking into consideration details of the clinical history and the gross appearance, the pathologic entity of a tumor of the tonsil may be suspected at clinical examination. However, this suspicion should always be confirmed by biopsy. The specimens for microscopic examination are easily removed from this area by means of any grasping forceps.

Biopsy of the metastatic nodes should always be done as a matter of record. Other diagnostic measures such as roentgenograms are seldom of additional value in the diagnosis of extension of the local disease but may be very useful in the diagnosis of distant metastases, particularly of the mediastinum. A routine roentgenogram of the chest should always be taken in all patients suspected of having a lymphosarcoma or "lymphoepithelioma.'"

Differential diagnosis

Tuberculosis of the tonsil and soft palate is usually characterized by a superficial grayish ulceration surrounded by confluent areas of false membrane. Generally, there will also be advanced tuberculosis of the lungs.

Syphilitic gumma of the palatotonsillar region is a rare occurrence. It usually has punched-out borders and is not accompanied by induration. Primary tumors of the parotid gland that develop deeply may sometimes produce a deformity of the lateral wall of the oropharynx and a displacement of the tonsillar region, which may be taken for a tumor of this area. Such tumors present a very slow development and do not become ulcerated.

Treatment
Surgery

Removal of a tumor of the tonsil is seldom possible within basic principles of cancer surgery: the tumors develop in a region where surgical planes are nonexistent; they grow in close relationship to the unresectable vessels of the neck; they are often undifferentiated carcinomas or lymphosarcomas which, as a rule, are least curable by surgery, and they are almost invariably accompanied by a voluminous metastatic adenopathy which, in itself, may make surgery prohibitive.

A radical surgical procedure implies wide removal of the primary lesion and radical neck dissection in continuity. This demands removal of part of the mandible and implies a nonneglible operative mortality (Terz and Farr[56]). This extensive surgical resection requires cosmetic procedures such as chest or forehead flaps that are far from simple, desirable, or satisfactory (Calamel and Hoffmeister[8]; Baker and Weiner[4]). The radiocurability of many of these tumors without mutilation, even in the presence of voluminous metastases, has served as a deterrent to many surgeons. Others, on the contrary, have based their approach on the poor results of radiotherapy at their own institutions. At any rate, in recent years there have been renewed surgical trials in the treatment of tonsillar tumors, some of them in combination with radiotherapy. Within ten days of the administration of a moderate amount of radiations (2000 R to 3000 R in two to three weeks), Staple et al.[55] proceed to a surgical resection of the tonsil, soft palate, pharyngeal wall, base of the tongue, and cervical lymph nodes. The benefits of such an approach remain to be substantiated.

Often, this apparently eclectic attitude is deceiving. A comparison of the results obtained in the treatment of carcinomas of the tonsil (1959-1961) at two different leading institutions of the city of Paris was most rewarding in this respect. At the Fondation Curie, 114 patients received cobalt[60] teletherapy alone, whereas at the Gustave-Roussy Institute 113 patients received combinations of supervoltage roentgentherapy, interstitial curietherapy, and surgery. The four-year survival rate was identical (41% to 42%) at the Fondation Curie for patients with or without a palpable adenopathy (Ennuyer and Bataini[13]). At the Gustave-Roussy Institute the four-year survival for patients without adenopathy was 40% but that of patients with metastatic nodes was only 20% (Pierquin et al.[44]).

Radiotherapy

Skillful administration of radiotherapy is the treatment of choice of most patients with cancer of the tonsil with or without cervical metastases. Since the majority of tumors do not require a high daily dose, it is best to fractionate the treatments over a period of five to six weeks. Bilateral irradiation is often desirable, particularly in lymphosarcomas (Regato[46]). Cobalt[60] teletherapy or supervoltage roentgentherapy permits a rather homogeneous irradiation of the potential area of primary and neighboring metastatic involvement to a desirable high dosage without great intensity of reactions.

Perez et al.[41] reported on 134 patients with carcinomas of the tonsil treated by four different methods: surgical resection of the primary lesion, interstitial implantation of radon, preoperative irradiation, and external irradiation alone. Their results suggested to them that radiotherapy alone is the treatment of choice, but they felt that further trials of preoperative irradiation are necessary.

Peroral roentgentherapy is unsatisfactory, for it irradiates the affected area unevenly and only partially. Interstitial implantation of radioactive sources may be utilized only as a complement or for the management of residual or recurrent foci (Rider[49]).

The use of cobalt[60] teletherapy and supervoltage roentgentherapy in preference to conventional roentgentherapy has reduced the intensity of skin and mucous membrane reactions, and consequent dysphagia, previously observed. Late complications may be, on the contrary, increased. As a consequence of the unavoidable irradiation of both the parotid and submaxillary glands, often on both sides, there is a resulting chronic dryness of the mucous membranes of the mouth and

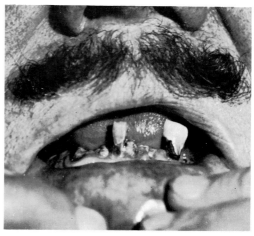

Fig. 205. Typical dental caries occurring after roentgentherapy for tumors of pharynx or oral cavity. (From del Regato, J. A.: Dental lesions observed after roentgen therapy in cancer of the buccal cavity, pharynx and larynx, Amer. J. Roentgen. **42:**404-410, 1939.)

pharynx. Fractionation of the total dose over several weeks is the only possible way of minimizing this irremediable effect.

Caries, regardless of the initial good condition of the teeth (Fig. 205), is a result of the quantitative and qualitative changes of the saliva and not a result of direct irradiation (Regato[45]). Preliminary extraction of teeth in bad condition, and sometimes of others, may prove the only valid precaution (Regato[45]; Grant and Fletcher[18]).

Necrosis of soft tissues of the mouth or pharynx is sometimes observed (Schulz[52]), resulting in pain and possible hemorrhage. Necrosis of the mandible is the most serious complication, usually resulting from intensive irradiation of the bone (Grant and Fletcher[18]), and may be fatal. In general, although a high dose is desirable, it may not have to be delivered in too short a time. Adequate utilization of available sources may permit a homogeneous distribution to avoid overirradiation of any area. Dosage may be kept at optimum levels.

Prognosis

In Fletcher and Lindberg's series[15] of fifty-two patients with *carcinoma* of the tonsil treated with supervoltage roentgentherapy from 1954 to 1963 at the M. D.

Anderson Hospital, nineteen (36.5%) were living at the end of five years. Absence of palpable adenopathy raises the results (Schulz[52]; Rider[49]; Pierquin et al.[44]). Involvement of the base of the tongue may cause a lesser prognosis (Rider[49]). Women seem to have a relatively better prognosis than men.

The excellent results of radiotherapy in *lymphosarcomas* of the tonsil have been long recognized (Regato[46]). Ennuyer et al.[14] reported on 191 patients with tonsillar lymphosarcomas who received radiotherapy, with sixty-seven (35%) five-year survivals. Of 79 patients without palpable adenopathy, forty-one (51%) remained well.

Base of tongue

Anatomy

The base of the tongue is that portion situated behind the sulcus terminalis or lingual ∨ formed by the circumvallate papillae. Laterally, it extends to form the glossopharyngeal sulcus which lies between it and the lateral wall of the pharynx. Posteriorly, it forms the anterior wall of the glossoepiglottic fossae or valleculae. A fold that is situated in the midline and extends from the base of the tongue to the free border of the epiglottis separates the valleculae.

The base of the tongue lacks most of the different papillae that cover the anterior two-thirds, but it is richer in the neurogenic elements of the sense of taste or taste buds. It is lined by a stratified squamous epithelium covering numerous tubercles or encapsulated lymphoid nodules which give an irregular appearance to its surface. This mucous membrane is not so firmly adherent to the underlying muscle at the base of the tongue as it is on the anterior two-thirds.

Lymphatics. The lymphatic network of the base of the tongue is markedly independent from the rest of the lymphatics of the tongue. The collecting trunks pass through the lateral pharyngeal wall just below the palatine tonsil, ending in the subdigastric group of nodes which drain most of the lymphatics of the oropharynx.

Epidemiology

Cancer of the base of the tongue is not so frequent as cancer of the mobile portion. The usual distribution is four to six carcinomas of the anterior two-thirds for every carcinoma of the base of the tongue. In India, the proportions are reversed. Khanolkar[21] found that the proportion of carcinomas of the base is greater in Moslems, Deccani Hindus, and Gujarati Hindus, but in the latter this form of cancer is twice as common as in the others. In Puerto Rico, carcinoma occurs more frequently in the base of the tongue than in all other areas of the pharynx or oral cavity, including the lower lip (Marcial[29]).

In India, as in Puerto Rico, male patients outnumber female patients with this form of cancer. Use of tobacco and alcoholism seem to play an important etiologic role, but it is likely that nutritional factors are also important.

Pathology
Gross pathology

Most of the malignant tumors of the base of the tongue are squamous cell carcinomas. Rarely, other tumors are found such as connective tissue sarcomas and tumors of salivary gland origin (p. 535).

Epidermoid carcinoma of the base of the tongue is one of the most infiltrating types of cancer of the upper air passages. The tumors seldom affect the outside dimensions of the base of the tongue, but they

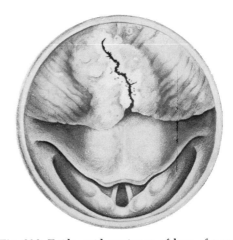

Fig. 206. Epidermoid carcinoma of base of tongue presenting fissurelike ulceration and deep, diffuse infiltration.

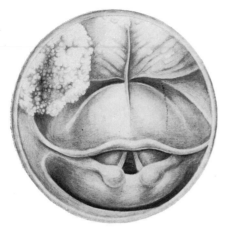

Fig. 207. Carcinoma of glossopharyngeal sulcus.

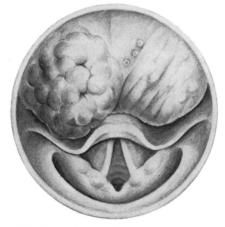

Fig. 208. "Lymphoepithelioma" of base of tongue presenting polypoid appearance and visible ulceration.

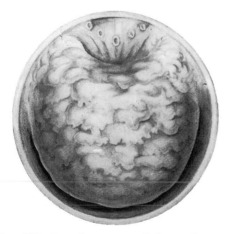

Fig. 209. Lymphosarcoma of base of tongue coming in contact with posterior pharyngeal wall and covering larynx. Usually, there is no ulceration or, rarely, superficial ulceration due to trauma.

infiltrate deep into the muscles. Fissurelike ulcerations may be found on either side of the base of the tongue and are often in the midline (Fig. 206). These ulcerations are surrounded by diffusely disseminated tumor. In 225 cases of carcinoma of the base of the tongue reported by Roux-Berger and Jadlovker,[50] ninety-seven extended on both sides of the midline. Only 128 lesions were strictly unilateral.

Undifferentiated carcinomas ("lymphoepitheliomas") are usually nonulcerated, polypoid, unilateral tumors (Fig. 208).

Lymphosarcomas of the base of the tongue arise from the multiple submucous lymphoid nodules of this organ and are usually bilateral and nonulcerated. They may rapidly fill the entire distance between the base and the posterior wall of the tongue (Fig. 209).

Microscopic pathology

Unlike carcinomas of the tonsil, epidermoid carcinomas that develop in the base of the tongue are usually well differentiated. So-called "lymphoepitheliomas" or transitional cell carcinomas are, in reality, undifferentiated carcinomas. Lymphosarcomas developing from the base of the tongue are similar in character to other such primary tumors of the upper air passages.

Metastatic spread

The metastatic adenopathy from *carcinomas* of the base of the tongue are usually bilateral and are found high in the jugular chain of nodes. Distant metastases are rare. *Undifferentiated carcinomas* ("lymphoepitheliomas") usually present an early bilateral and voluminous upper cervical adenopathy. Spread to other lymphatic areas, lungs, and liver is observed in patients with generalized disease. *Lymphosarcomas* almost invariably present a large cervical adenopathy, often bilateral. Spread to the axilla, mediastinum, and retroperitoneal region occurs early.

Clinical evolution

The onset of *carcinomas* of the base of the tongue is usually accompanied by diffuse *pain* which may become rapidly marked. *Odynophagia* and *dysphagia* customarily accompany this pain and contribute to a rapid deterioration of the general physical condition. Difficulty in protraction of the tongue will interfere with speech, making it unintelligible. Hemorrhages may appear in patients with advanced lesions. An adenopathy is usually found in the upper cervical region. The nodes, however, are often small and non-tender and remain stationary over a long period of time. Metastatic nodes are often bilateral. Uncontrolled carcinomas seldom become generalized. Patients may die from the consequences of hemorrhage, pain, narcotics, and undernourishment.

The onset of *undifferentiated carcinomas* ("lymphoepitheliomas") is characteristically silent. The first manifestation may be the appearance of a metastatic adenopathy in the upper cervical region. The primary lesion seldom produces any symptoms, and its discovery is usually the result of perspicacity on the part of the examiner. Seldom does pain, odynophagia, or dysphagia accompany these tumors. The

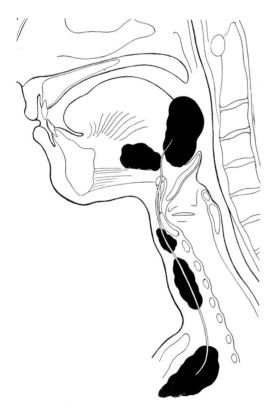

Fig. 210. Thyroglossal cysts may be found at base of tongue or on anterior midline of neck.

adenopathy is usually unilateral, rapid growing, and soft, with little tendency to fixation to the underlying tissues or to the skin. Successive metastases to the lower cervical region, mediastinum, axilla, lungs, and liver are not infrequent in uncontrolled cases.

The clinical evolution of *lymphosarcoma* of the base of the tongue is very much like that of lymphosarcoma of the tonsil. It may develop without causing any symptoms until it has become large enough to hinder deglutition and produce mechanical dysphagia and a nasal twang to the voice. Metastatic nodes, which may or may not be present, are discrete.

On the other hand, lymphosarcoma of the base of the tongue may remain locally unsuspected, presenting a very slow growth, with the clinical onset and course dominated by the development of metastatic adenopathy of the cervical regions or distant lymphatic nodes. When the primary lesion has not been suspected or found, such generalized cases may lead to the diagnosis of primary lymphosarcoma of these nodes. Lumbar pain and rapid loss of weight are indicative of retroperitoneal metastases and generalized disease.

Diagnosis
Differential diagnosis

A condition worthy of mention in the differential diagnosis of tumors of the base of the tongue is a *thyroglossal cyst* in this area. This cyst may develop from remnants of the thyroglossal duct anywhere in the anterior midline of the neck and less often under the base of the tongue (Fig. 210). It is congenital but is usually found in female patients who present a physiologic enlargement of the cyst during puberty or pregnancy. Enlargement of the cyst has also been noticed after oophorectomy or thyroidectomy. Thyroglossal cysts are characterized by nonulcerated, slightly lobulated tumefactions, usually on the midline of the base of the tongue.

The base of the tongue is sometimes the site of origin of *salivary and mucous gland tumors*. These are very slow-growing, nonulcerated, painless tumors which may acquire voluminous dimensions (Fig. 211) and interfere with deglutition and speech. They may be benign or malignant (p. 535)

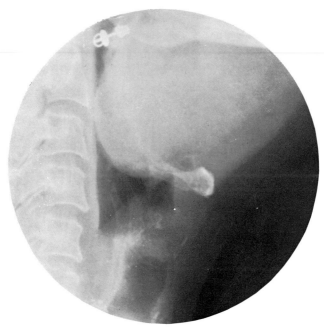

Fig. 211. Salivary gland tumor at base of tongue. Note obliteration of vallecula and bending of free border of epiglottis. (Courtesy Tumor Clinic, National Cancer Institute, Baltimore, Md.)

and generally develop so slowly that abstention may even be justified in the aged patient (Marcial-Rojas and Leon-Antoni[30]).

Hypertrophic lymphoid tissue of the base of the tongue may be injured, become inflamed, and appear as a tumor. *Telangiectatic vessels* of the mucosa may bleed and cause alarm. In all of these instances, a biopsy will solve the problem of diagnosis, but care should be taken in removing the specimen. *Neurofibromas, plasma cell tumors, sarcomas* of all types, and even *metastatic melanomas* have been seen in this location.

Treatment
Surgery

Surgical treatment of tumors of the base of the tongue through an oral approach is well justified in benign lesions such as lingual thyroid lesions or benign salivary tumors but is not satisfactory in malignant tumors. Larger operations such as lateral pharyngotomy or transhyoid pharyngotomy would seem justified in the treatment of epidermoid carcinomas because of the almost constant failure of radiotherapy in such infiltrating tumors. But these radical surgical procedures invariably fail to cure. In the treatment of undifferentiated carcinomas ("lymphoepitheliomas") and lymphosarcomas, highly radiosensitive and radiocurable, such operations are hardly justified.

Neck dissections for the metastatic nodes from epidermoid carcinomas of the base of the tongue are well indicated. However, sterilization of the primary lesion is seldom obtained. In addition, metastatic carcinoma from a primary lesion in the base of the tongue is quite often bilateral, and the undertaking of the double operation with its higher operative mortality will require further assurance that the risk is worth taking. Roux-Berger and Jadlovker[50] reported eight patients well five years after operation in a series of forty-two who had radical neck dissections for metastatic epidermoid carcinoma of the base of the tongue. Four of these eight patients, however, showed no actual metastatic involvement of the nodes.

Radiotherapy

In view of the poor alternative, the treatment of tumors of the base of the tongue is usually entrusted to the therapeutic radiologist. Whereas in the past interstitial implantation of radioactive sources was utilized, it is not really possible to achieve an adequate irradiation in this area by such means. With cobalt[60] and supervoltage, it is now possible to distribute homogeneously a large dose of radiations throughout the base of the tongue and immediately lateral areas of metastatic involvement.

Prognosis

The prognosis of epidermoid carcinomas of the base of the tongue is ominous. Very few cases are locally cured. The majority of patients, however, benefit by considerable transitory palliation when treated by external irradiation.

In a series of 143 patients with squamous cell and anaplastic carcinomas treated from 1945 to 1962 at the Royal Marsden Hospital of London, Dalley[11] reported eighteen surviving five years (12%) and eight (28%) of twenty-eight patients living who had no metastatic adenopathy. Martin and Martin[32] treated a series of forty patients with a combination of external roentgentherapy and interstitial radiumtherapy for both the primary lesion and the cervical metastasis, with a five-year survival rate in fifteen patients (38%).

The curability of lymphosarcomas of the base of the tongue is rather high when the disease is diagnosed before it has spread beyond the limits of the neck. Most treatment failures are due to the presence of unsuspected distant metastases. In an unpublished review of twelve patients with lymphosarcoma of the base of the tongue treated at the Fondation Curie from 1920 to 1932, four appeared well five years after the treatment (Regato[44a]).

Periepiglottic area

Anatomy

The free portion of the epiglottis is that part found above the level of the hyoid bone. It is composed of cartilage surrounded by fibroelastic tissue and is covered by a thin mucous membrane. Laterally, it is attached to the walls of the pharynx by two fibroelastic membranes, the pharyngo-epiglottic folds. Anteriorly, the free portion of the epiglottis and the base of the tongue form the valleculae (or glossoepiglottic fossae) that lie on each side of the glossoepiglottic fold (Fig. 197).

The lateral and posterior walls of the oropharynx extend from the level of a horizontal plane passing by the soft palate to the level of another plane passing through the hyoid bone.

Epidemiology

Carcinomas of the periepiglottic area are seen only half as often as those of the hypopharynx. They are encountered predominantly in men in the fifth and sixth decades of life.

Pathology
Gross pathology

Carcinomas of the *glossopharyngeal sulcus* extend superficially both over the surface of the tongue and over the lateral wall of the pharynx and tonsil. They are superficially necrotic and seldom infiltrate to any depth. They are usually accompanied by a unilateral upper cervical adenopathy (Fig. 207).

Carcinomas of the *glossoepiglottic fossae* or valleculae are noninfiltrating. They grow in the narrow space between the base of the tongue and the epiglottis and usually become deeply excavated (Fig. 212). Retention of particles of food in the excavation causes considerable secondary infection and discomfort. Very rarely, carcinomas of this area will infiltrate the muscles of the tongue and produce a deep excavation into that organ similar to that of carcinomas of the base of the tongue. Most carcinomas of the valleculae are unilateral.

Carcinomas of the *free portion of the epiglottis* are usually bulky, presenting large areas of spontaneous necrosis and abundant secondary infection. Their infiltration does not often extend beyond the free border of the epiglottis itself, even though this border is usually totally destroyed (Fig. 213). The spontaneous necrosis of these tumors creates considerable secondary infection which, in turn, has its repercussions on the general condition of the patient. These tumors arise on the border line of the endolarynx and oro-

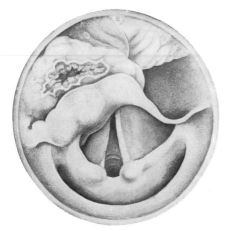

Fig. 212. Carcinoma of right side of glossoepi-glottic fossa (vallecula), with secondary infiltration of epiglottis and pharyngoepiglottic fold. Note edema of right false cord, which may represent tumor extension through cartilage of epiglottis.

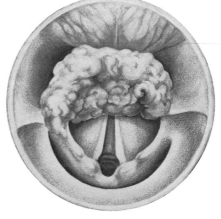

Fig. 213. Carcinoma of free portion of epiglottis. These tumors usually show superficial necrosis and, although extensive, are among most curable of carcinomas of pharynx.

pharynx. They may be classified with carcinomas of the larynx or pharynx. The latter is preferable because of their clinical behavior and frequency of metastases.

Carcinomas of the *pharyngoepiglottic fold* expand between the free portion of the epiglottis and the lateral wall. As a consequence, the epiglottis is distorted and the larynx somewhat displaced (Fig. 214). These tumors seldom infiltrate. They become bulky, presenting superficial ulcerations.

Carcinomas of the *lateral wall* of the oropharynx are seldom confined to the strict anatomic limits of this region. Most of them extend downward to the lateral wall of the hypopharynx and are similar in character to the tumors of the lateral wall of the piriform sinus. They may infiltrate early the lateral wings or superior horns of the thyroid cartilage and sometimes quickly invade the internal carotid artery.

Carcinomas of the *posterior wall* of the oropharynx appear as smooth tumefactions that grow forward, narrowing the antero-posterior diameters of this region. The tumor may come in contact with the soft palate and even the base of the tongue. These rare tumors may finally ulcerate, usually in the midline, because of the trauma of food ingestion.

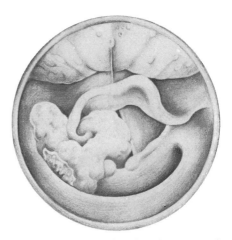

Fig. 214. Carcinoma of right pharyngoepiglottic fold. These rare tumors are usually extensive and consequently difficult to identify as to point of departure. Free portion of epiglottis is curled due to lateral compression.

Microscopic pathology

All of the tumors of this area are epidermoid carcinomas with a lesser degree of differentiation generally than the epidermoid carcinomas of the oral cavity.

Metastatic spread

Carcinomas of the periepiglottic area often metastasize to the nodes in the mid-jugular chain, often bilaterally, with sub-

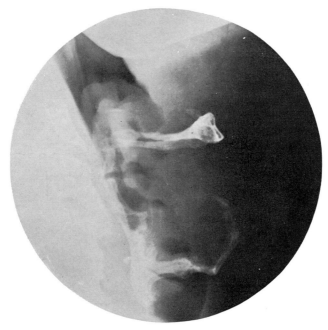

Fig. 215. Extensive exophytic carcinoma of epiglottis occupying almost entire hypopharynx.

sequent extension to other nodes of the same chain. In generalized disease, distant metastases are found, not infrequently, at autopsy.

Clinical evolution

Very frequently, carcinomas of the peri-epiglottic area will manifest themselves by a metastatic cervical adenopathy, whereas the primary lesion has given no symptoms of its presence. In the majority of cases, the only symptom caused by the primary lesion is merely a slight sore throat or mild *odynophagia*. With advancement of the disease, these symptoms become more marked, and *dysphagia* may appear. *Cough*, particularly following ingestion of food, is rather frequent. *Hoarseness* is present only in patients with very advanced tumors with accompanying edema of the false cords. *Pain* is a rare symptom. The general condition of the patient is more rapidly affected than in any other group of tumors of the pharynx, or larynx. Because of the dysphagia and secondary infection, the patients may lose considerable weight and appear cachectic.

A rapid-growing adenopathy of the mid-cervical and upper cervical regions is an almost constant finding and, depending on the location of the primary lesion, is very often bilateral. These adenopathies are usually rapid growing and may acquire large dimensions. They form a bulky mass made up of conglomerate matted nodes and smaller nodes that may be found in the direction of the anterior cervical chain. In the majority of patients with carcinomas of the periepiglottic area, adenopathy may appear before the primary lesion has given any symptoms. Distant metastases to the mediastinum, lungs, and abdominal viscera are not infrequently found at autopsy. The percentage is among the highest for tumors of the upper air passages.

Diagnosis

The diagnosis of carcinomas of the peri-epiglottic area does not offer great difficulties. The lesions are usually of a typical carcinomatous appearance, and the clinical impression may be easily confirmed by biopsy. The removal of specimens for microscopic examination is rather easy in this area.

When a cervical adenopathy is the first symptom, a thorough search for the primary lesion in the epiglottis and other areas of the pharynx and mouth should precede any therapeutic undertaking, for there exists a great number of other conditions, benign and malignant, that may be confused with the metastatic carcinomatous mass of the neck. The diagnosis of these conditions should always be made by exclusion if the search for the primary lesion in the pharynx has been fruitless.

Radiographic examination of the soft tissues of the neck will always be of some additional interest in establishing the limits of extension of a tumor (Fig. 215). This is not always possible on pharyngeal examination.

Differential diagnosis

Tuberculous adenitis may sometimes produce a picture of metastatic carcinoma of the neck. If a thorough examination of the pharynx and oral cavity fails to reveal any suspicious area or point of departure, an aspiration of the cervical mass will most often resolve the problem of diagnosis. Tuberculous adenopathies usually contain thick caseous material, whereas metastatic adenopathies are most often solid. It must be remembered that metastatic epidermoid carcinoma within lymph nodes may undergo almost complete cystic degeneration and contain broken down keratin that may be mistaken for caseous tuberculosis.

An *inflammatory* cervical adenopathy may or may not be bilateral. The nodes, as a rule, are tender and accompany some inflammatory condition of the oral cavity or pharynx. It should not be forgotten, however, that some forms of lymphosarcoma and Hodgkin's disease have a pseudoinflammatory clinical behavior. Inflammatory conditions are considerably more frequent in younger individuals in whom carcinomatous lesions are unusual. No clinical diagnosis of inflammatory adenopathy should be made, however, even in young individuals, without a thorough examination of the nasopharynx, where an early lesion may be hidden.

Branchiogenic cysts of the neck may sometimes be confused with a metastatic adenopathy. They may appear in patients of all ages and are most frequently found just below the angle of the jaw. Aspiration usually brings a transparent mucoid fluid. Although most branchiogenic cysts of the neck are superficial, some may develop beneath the superficial fascia or even near the lateral pharyngeal wall (Bailey[3]; Ward et al.[57]).

Thyroglossal cysts present along the anterior midline of the neck and consequently are seldom confused with a metastatic adenopathy (Marshall and Becker[31]). When the thyroglossal cyst develops at the level of the thyroid cartilage, however, it may be laterally situated (Bailey[3]). Dermoid cysts of the neck are most often found in early life. They contain well-developed structures (hair, teeth) and may show calcification on the roentgenogram (New and Erich[37]).

Carotid body tumors develop in the upper cervical region at the level of the bifurcation of the common carotid artery. Their incidence is the same in male and female patients (MacComb[29]), and they often occur in the third and fourth decades of life. They have been found in several members of the same family and are sometimes bilateral. Tumors similar to these can arise from the aortic body or from the glomus jugulare (Lattes[24]) and from cells associated with the ganglion nodosum of the vagus nerve. These organs consist of nonchromaffin, nonepinephrine-producing bodies with sensory innervation. They must be distinguished from tumors arising from the adrenal medulla. They probably represent chemoreceptors. Of this group the carotid body tumors are the most common.

Neoplasms of the carotid body are usually firmly adherent at the bifurcation of the common carotid artery, and their removal implies great risk (Lahey and Warren[23]; LeCompte[25]) in about half of the cases. Most of these tumors are symptomless and present slow growth, but they may compress the esophagus, larynx, or vagus nerve and cause dysphagia, dysphonia, etc. Angiography may be helpful in establishing a preoperative diagnosis (Idbohrn[20]). The tumors have firm, well-defined capsules, are globular in shape, and usually are not more than 5 cm in diameter. On section, they have a homogenous surface varying from pinkish gray to reddish brown. Prominent vascularization may be observed. Microscopically, they are made up of cell nests with uniform cells without mitotic activity. These nests are surrounded by a vascular stroma, well demonstrated by a reticulin stain. These neoplasms are practically never malignant (Monro[36]; Lahey and Warren[23]). They have been incorrectly diagnosed as malignant because of their intimate relation with carotid vessels and because of cellular variation. The chances of metastases are remote. We have seen only one instance in a regional lymph node.

Excision is the treatment of choice and frequently may necessitate ligation of the internal carotid artery if complete removal is to be obtained. In some instances, incomplete resection may be justified in view of the high operative risk (may reach 30%) and the morbidity, which may be as high as 80% due to injury to the central nervous system. In some patients, particularly in those with tumors of long duration with no symptoms, a diagnostic biopsy is all that is necessary, whereas in others resection is unavoidable due to pressure symptoms or recurrence. Proper precautions (Pemberton and Livermore[40]) and attempts to replace the resected artery may reduce the considerable risk involved. Few of these tumors have been treated by radiotherapy, but a few instances of successful radiotherapy have been recorded (Bevan and McCarthy[7]; Hartmann[19]; Lahey and Warren[23]). Tumors of the glomus jugulare do respond well to irradiation therapy, and it is preferable to treat them by this modality than by surgery.

A *branchiogenic carcinoma* (i.e., carcinoma developing at the expense of the embryonic remnants of the branchial clefts) is no longer believed to constitute a true entity. The overwhelming majority of cases reported as branchiogenic carcinoma are actually metastatic carcinomas from unsuspected primary lesions. In weighing the available evidence, Martin et al.[34] concluded that although the theory is attractive, there is no proof that cancer arises on branchial remnants. Small undifferentiated carcinomas of the pharynx and of the scalp, undetected clinically, have been known to produce large metastatic lesions of the neck. The nasopharynx, base of the tongue, piriform sinuses, etc. are common sites of undetected carcinomas. Irradiation may mask or eradicate an unsuspected primary lesion. Forgotten, unorthodox, or self-applied treatments to carcinomas of the skin may be the cause of confusion. Carcinomas of the lung and thyroid gland do metastasize to the cervical region. Other primary sites, such as the stomach and the breast, may be more readily suspected.

Since the diagnosis of branchiogenic carcinomas is not established histologically, the clinician is responsible for the search for the primary lesion. That one is not found only implies that further search is necessary before the lesion is properly labeled (Dargent and Blanchet[12]).

Cervical adenopathy in cases of unsuspected *lympathic leukemia* may offer confusion with lymphosarcomas. The condition of the spleen, the blood count, or bone marrow biopsy will help in the differential diagnosis. Cases of *Hodgkin's disease* that are not typical on biopsy may also be confused with lymphosarcoma.

To summarize the diagnosis of cervical tumors, careful consideration should be given to the history, length of evolution, consistency and position of the mass, and the presence of symptoms or physical findings elsewhere in the body. Although a needle biopsy may not offer a definite diagnosis, it is of great value. The diagnosis of epidermoid carcinoma, lymphosarcoma, or "lymphoepithelioma" of a metastatic mass of the neck should lead to the suspicion that a primary lesion exists in the upper air passages.

Treatment
Radiotherapy

Because of their location, high degree of radiosensitivity, and the almost constant presence of cervical adenopathy, carcinomas of the periepiglottic area are recognized to be the domain of radiotherapy. External irradiation usually requires moderately large fields because of the frequent presence of metastatic adenopathies. In the presence of bilateral cervical metastases, the problem becomes that of irradiating the primary lesion and its adenopathies at a high dose level.

Supervoltage roentgentherapy and cobalt[60] teletherapy allow a more homogeneous and intensive irradiation than is possible with conventional roentgentherapy. In cases of markedly unilateral involvement, additional anteroposterior and posteroanterior fields may be useful.

Surgery

A limited number of chosen carcinomas, particularly of the free border of the epiglottis, have been treated by surgery with relative success. The procedure most often used is either a radical laryngectomy (del Sel and Agra[53]) or a supraglottic (horizontal) hemilaryngectomy that preserves the vocal function (Leroux-Robert[26]; Ogura[38]). A prophylactic or therapeutic radical neck dissection may be done in continuity with either of these procedures, for if nodes are not clinically ostensible, there is great chance of their presence in a subclinical stage.

Prognosis

The prognosis of carcinomas of the periepiglottic area, as well as that of carcinoma of the glossopharyngeal sulcus and posterior wall of the oropharynx, is relatively good. When these tumors become secondarily infected and there is loss of weight and a foul breath, the clinical impression is unfavorable. Yet a number of these tumors respond well to radiotherapy and patients should always be given a chance of receiving a complete treatment.

In the majority of publications available, tumors of the periepiglottic area are included in reports of carcinomas of the hypopharynx. The good results obtained are largely based on the carcinomas of the periepiglottic area. Although there are no available figures to illustrate the favorable prognosis of this group of tumors, it may be said without hesitancy that they have the most favorable prognosis among carcinomas of the pharynx with the exception only of carcinomas of the palatine tonsil.

The most frequent cause of treatment failure is not the inability to sterilize the primary lesion but the difficulty of sterilizing oversized, secondarily infected metastases. Some of the patients who are cured locally may die within the first three years as a consequence of development of distant metastases. Baclesse[2] reported on 102 patients with epidermoid carcinoma of the vallecula and free portion of the epiglottis treated in Coutard's service from 1920 to 1938, sixteen of whom were living and

well after five years. Dalley[11] reported on a series of sixty-one patients with carcinoma of the vallecula treated mostly by radiotherapy at the Royal Marsden Hospital of London with seven (11%) surviving five years.

REFERENCES

1 Allen, G. W., and Hemenway, W. G.: Carcinoma of the tonsil; surgical treatment, Laryngoscope 70:246-257, 1960.
2 Baclesse, F.: Résultats éloignés du traitement roentgenthérapique des épithéliomas glossoépiglottiques (base linguale, vallecules, épiglotte), J. Radiol. Electr. 25:190-193, 1942-1943.
3 Bailey, H.: Clinical aspects of branchial fistula, Brit. J. Surg. 21:173-182, 1933.
4 Baker, R. R., and Weiner, S.: Clinical management of tonsillar carcinoma. Surg. Gynec. Obstet. 121:1035-1038, 1965.
5 Bardwil, J. M., Reynolds C. T., Ibanez, M. L., and Armando-Luna, M.: Report of one hundred tumors of the minor salivary glands, Amer. J. Surg. 112:493-497, 1966.
6 Baud, J.: L'association de la radiumpuncture aux irradiations externes dans le traitement des épithéliomas de la région amygdalienne, Paris Med. 1:142-151, 1941.
7 Bevan, A. D., and McCarthy, E. R.: Tumors of the carotid body, Surg. Gynec. Obstet. 49:764-779, 1929.
8 Calamel, P. M., and Hoffmeister, F. S.: Carcinoma of the tonsil; comparison of surgical and radiation therapy, Amer. J. Surg. 114:582-586, 1967.
9 Conley, J. J.: The management of carotid body tumors, Surg. Gynec. Obstet. 117:722-732, 1963.
10 Coutard, Henri: Roentgentherapy of epitheliomas of the tonsillar region, hypopharynx and larynx from 1920 to 1926, Amer. J. Roentgen. 28:313-331, 1932.
11 Dalley, V. M.: The place of radiotherapy in the treatment of tumors of the base of the tongue, Amer. J. Roentgen. 93:20-28, 1965.
12 Dargent, M., and Blanchet, H.: Contribution au diagnostic des tumeurs apparemment primitives du cou, Bull. Ass. Franc. Cancer 34:2-18, 1947.
13 Ennuyer, A., and Bataini, P.: Treatment of supra-glottic carcinomas by telecobalt therapy, Brit. J. Radiol. 38:661-666, 1965.
14 Ennuyer, A., Helary, J., and Bataini, P.: Résultats de la radiothérapie des lymphoréticulosarcomes des voies aéro-digestives supérieures; statistique de la Fondation Curie, Bull. Ass. Franc. Cancer 50:413-422, 1961.
15 Fletcher, G. H., and Lindberg, R. D.: Squamous cell carcinomas of the tonsillar area and palatine arch, Amer. J. Roentgen. 96:574-587, 1966.
16 Fletcher, G. H., MacComb, W. S., Chau, P. M., and Farnsley, W. G.: Comparison of medium voltage and supervoltage roentgen ther-

apy in the treatment of oropharynx cancers, Amer. J. Roentgen. 81:375-401, 1959.

17 Gary-Bobo, J., Pourquier, H., and Lamarque, J. L.: Irradiation des cancers de l'amygdale par télécobalt a propos de 74 cas traités au C.A.C. de Montpellier, Rev. Laryng. (Bordeaux) 83: 961-962, 1963.

18 Grant, B. P., and Fletcher, G. H.: Analysis of complications following megavoltage therapy for squamous cell carcinomas of the tonsillar area, Amer. J. Roentgen. 96:28-36, 1966.

19 Hartmann, H.: Tumeur du corpuscule carotidien, ablation, incomplète, Radiothérapie. Guérison, Mem. Acad. Chir. (Paris) 62:1404-1408, 1936.

20 Idbohrn, H.: Angiographical diagnosis of carotid body tumours, Acta Radiol. (Stockholm) 35:115-123, 1951.

21 Khanolkar. V. R.: Cancer in India in relation to race, nutrition and customs. In symposium on geographical pathology and demography of cancer, sponsored by the World Health Organization, July, 1950.

22 Klopp, C. T., and Schurter, M.: The surgical treatment of cancer of the soft palate and tonsil, Cancer 9:1239-1243, 1956.

23 Lahey, F. H., and Warren, K. W.: A long term appraisal of carotid body tumors with remarks on their removal, Surg. Gynec. Obstet. 92:481-491, 1951.

24 Lattes, R.: Nonchromaffin paraganglioma of ganglion nodosum, carotid body, and aortic-arch bodies, Cancer 3:667-694, 1950.

25 LeCompte, P. M.: Tumors of the carotid body and related structures (chemoreceptor system). In Atlas of tumor pathology, Sect. IV, Fasc. 16, Washington, D. C., 1951, Armed Forces Institute of Pathology.

26 Leroux-Robert, J.: La laryngectomie horizontale sus-glottique conservatrice de la fonction vocale, Bull. Acad. Nat. Med. (Paris) 139: 358-364, 1955.

27 Luzzatti, G.: Risultati della radioterapia dei sarcomi della faringe trattati dal 1928-1945 (125 casi). I. Impostazione generale e presentazione della casistica, Tumori 44:87-136, 1958.

28 Luzzatti, G.: Risultati della radioterapia dei sarcomi della faringe trattati dal 1928-1945 (125 casi). II. Analisi della casistica, discussione e conclusioni, Tumori 46:383-410, 1960.

29 MacComb, W. S.: Carotid body tumors, Ann. Surg. 127:269-277, 1948.

29a Marcial, V. A.: Carcinoma of the base of the tongue, Amer. J. Roentgen. 81:420-429, 1959.

29b Marcial, V., and Frías, Z.: Pilot study of dose fractionation in carcinoma of the base of the tongue; uninterrupted vs. split-course irradiation, Amer. J. Roentgen. 108:30-36, 1970.

30 Marcial-Rojas, R. A., and Leon-Antoni, E. de: Adenoid cystic carcinoma of seromucous glands of the head and neck, Ann. Surg. 157:409-418, 1963.

31 Marshall, S. F., and Becker, W. F.: Thyroglossal cysts and sinuses, Ann. Surg. 129:642-651, 1949.

32 Martin, C. L., and Martin, J. A.: Carcinoma

of the posterior tongue treated with radiation, Radiology 66:835-841, 1956.

33 Martin, H. E., and Morfit, H. M.: Cervical lymph node metastasis as the first symptom of cancer, Surg. Gynec. Obstet. 78:133-159, 1944.

34 Martin, H., Morfit, H. M., and Ehrlich, H.: The case for branchiogenic cancer (malignant branchioma), Ann. Surg. 132:867-887, 1950.

35 Mead, P. H.: Surgery or radiotherapy for tonsil cancer? Cancer 16:195-198, 1963.

36 Monro, R. S.: The natural history of carotid body tumours and their diagnosis and treatment, Brit. J. Surg. 37:445-453, 1950.

37 New, G. B., and Erich, J. B.: Dermoid cysts of the head and neck, Surg. Gynec. Obstet. 65:48-55, 1937.

38 Ogura, J. H.: Supraglottic subtotal laryngectomy and radical neck dissection for carcinoma of the epiglottis, Laryngoscope 68:983-1003, 1958.

39 Ogura, J. H., Saltzstein, S. L., and Spjut, H. J.: Experiences with conservation surgery in laryngeal and pharyngeal carcinoma, Laryngoscope 71:258-276, 1961.

40 Pemberton, J. D., and Livermore, G. R.: Surgical treatment of carotid body tumors: value of anticoagulants in carotid ligation, Ann. Surg. 133:837-852, 1951.

41 Perez, C. A., Mill, W. B., Ogura, J. H., and Powers, W. E.: Carcinoma of the tonsil: sequential comparison of four treatment modalities, Radiology 94:649-659, 1970.

42 Perussia, A.: Rendiconto clinico-statistico dei carcinomi della bocca e del faringe trattati dal 1928 al 1945. II. Risultati della radioterapia nei carcinomi del palato molle (84 casi), Radiol. Med. (Torino) 36:378-412, 1950.

43 Perussia, A.: Rendiconto clinico-statistico dei carcinomi della bocca e del faringe trattati dal 1928 al 1945. IV. Risultati della radioterapia nei carcinomi della ragione amigdalo-glosso-palatina e delle pareti del mesofaringe (139 casi), Radiol. Med. (Torino) 36:735-783, 1950.

44 Pierquin, B., Raynal, M., Ennuyer, A., and Bataini, P.: Étude comparative des résultats concernant les épithéliomas de la région amygdalienne traités à l'Institut Gustav-Roussy et à la Fondation Curie, Ann. Radiol. (Paris) 9: 815-824, 1966.

44a del Regato, J. A.: Unpublished data, 1937.

45 del Regato, J. A.: Dental lesions observed after roentgen therapy in cancer of the buccal cavity, pharynx and larynx, Amer. J. Roentgen. 42:404-410, 1939.

46 del Regato, J. A.: Roentgentherapy of lymphosarcomas of the tonsil, Radiation Therapy, Tumor Inst., Seattle (no. 2), pp. 67-76, May, 1941.

47 del Regato, J. A.: La roentgenterapia de los tumores del seno maxilar, de la faringe, y laringe, Rev. Med. Cir. Habana 45:58-65, 1941.

48 Reverchon, L., and Coutard, H.: Lymphoépithéliome de l'hypopharynx traité par röntgenthérapie, Bull. Mem. Soc. Franc. Otorhinolaryng., Congress, May, 1921.

49 Rider, W. D.: Epithelial cancer of the tonsillar area, Radiology 78:760-765, 1962.

50 Roux-Berger, J. L., and Jadlovker, M.: L'en-
vahissement lymphatique dans les cancers de
la base de la langue, Presse Med. **48:**249-250,
1940.
51 Scanlon, P. W., Gee, V. R., Erich, J. B.,
Williams, H. L., and Woolner, L. B.: Carcinoma of the palatine tonsil, Amer. J. Roentgen.
80:781-786, 1958.
52 Schulz, M. D.: Tonsil and palatine arch cancer—treatment by radiotherapy, Laryngoscope
75:958-967, 1965.
53 del Sel, J., and Agra, A.: Cancer de la laringe,
Rev. Argent. Otorinolaryng. **16:**1-30, 1947.
54 Sprong, D. H., and Kirby, F. G.: Familial

carotid body tumors, Ann. West. Med. Surg.
3:241-242, 1949.
55 Staple, T. W., Holtz, S., Ogura, J., and Powers,
W. E.: Carcinoma of the tonsil, results of
radiation therapy and consideration for combined radiation and surgical treatment, Missouri Med. **62:**909-911, 1965.
56 Terz, J. J., and Farr, H. W.: Carcinoma of the
tonsillar fossa, Surg. Gynec. Obstet. **125:**581-
590, 1967.
57 Ward, G. E., Hendrick, J. W., and Chambers,
R. G.: Branchiogenic anomalies, Western J.
Surg. **57:**536-549, 1949.

Laryngopharynx (hypopharynx)

With the exception of tumors arising on the posterior wall of the hypopharynx, most carcinomas of this region sooner or later invade the larynx. For this reason, they have often been erroneously included in the group of laryngeal tumors and called *extrinsic* carcinomas of the larynx together with other tumors that actually arise within the larynx.

The usual points of origin of carcinoma of the laryngopharynx are (1) the *posterior wall,* (2) the *lateral wall of the piriform sinus,* (3) the *medial wall of the piriform sinus,* and (4) the *retrocricoid region.* In this group we are also including the rather common carcinoma of the *arytenoepiglottic fold* that arises from the limiting border of the hypopharynx and endolarynx and anatomically belongs as much in one as in the other of these regions. Not included in this group are those tumors that arise on the free border of the epiglottis or the pharyngoepiglottic fold and that anatomically correspond to the oropharynx. But the reader must become aware of the fact that throughout the literature, particularly the surgical publications in this field, the carcinomas of the aryepiglottic fold and the free border of the epiglottis may be included in the supraglottic group of tumors of the larynx (Ogura et al.[37, 38]; Smith et al.[46]).

Anatomy

The laryngopharynx or hypopharynx surrounds the larynx posteriorly and laterally and extends between two horizontal planes, one of which passes through the hyoid bone and the other through the lower border of the cricoid cartilage. These limits correspond to the levels of the third and sixth cervical vertebrae.

The laryngopharynx is formed by two elongated pear-shaped gutters, the *piriform sinuses,* which extend on both sides of the larynx posteriorly from the pharyngoepiglottic fold to the mouth of the esophagus (Fig. 216). Laterally, the piriform sinus lies against the inner aspect of the thyroid cartilage. Behind the posterior border of the thyroid cartilage, the internal carotid artery runs very near the lateral wall of the hypopharynx (Fig. 217). The medial wall of the piriform sinus is formed by the arytenoepiglottic fold above and by the muscles that form the mouth of the esophagus below. Through this thin layer of muscles the piriform sinus is in very close relationship with the ventricle of the larynx and also with the outer aspect of the cricoid cartilage.

The lining of the hypopharynx is formed by stratified squamous epithelium beneath which are abundant mucous glands.

Lymphatics. The many lymphatics of the laryngopharynx converge toward an orifice in the thyrohyoid membrane which is equidistant from the hyoid bone and the thyroid cartilage (Fig. 218). This orifice also gives passage to the superior laryngeal artery. Through it the lymphatics find their exit and immediately form several diverging trunks that terminate in the anterior and external nodes of the internal jugular chain (Rouvière[43]).

Epidemiology

The proportion of carcinomas of the hypopharynx to carcinomas of the larynx varies from one country to another (Paymaster[31]; Dutta-Chaudhuri et al.[11]). The occurrence of hypopharyngeal tumors seems to follow that of carcinoma of the oral cavity as the occurrence of endolaryngeal tumors follows that of bronchial carcinomas. These tumors are predominantly found in men between 40 and 60 years of age. One exception is notable, that of carcinomas of the retrocricoid region, the great majority of which are found in women. In a series of ninety-eight carcinomas of the retrocricoid region reviewed by Turner,[49] eighty-five were found in women.

Ahlbom[2] pointed out the frequency with which carcinoma of the oral cavity, pharynx, or esophagus in women is accompanied by the Plummer-Vinson syndrome (sideropenia). This syndrome is characterized by

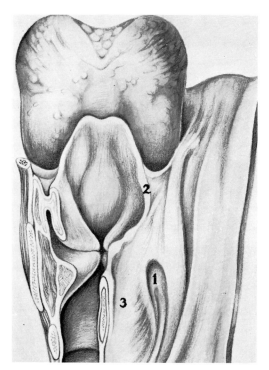

Fig. 216. Posterior view of larynx and laryngopharynx. 1, Piriform sinus. 2, Arytenoepiglottic fold. 3, Postcricoid region. Section on left side allows view into larynx.

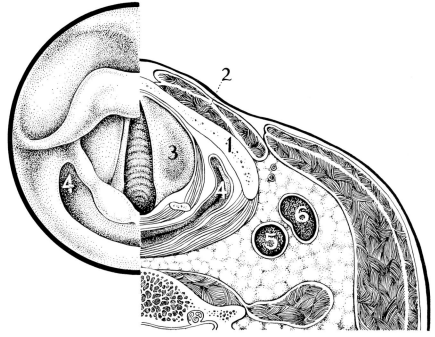

Fig. 217. Mirror view of pharynx and larynx on left and transverse section of neck just above true cord on right. 1, Thyroid cartilage. 2, Prelaryngeal muscles. 3, Laryngeal ventricle. 4, Piriform sinus. 5, Common carotid artery. 6, Internal jugular vein. Note close relationship between artery and lateral wall of piriform sinus and laryngeal ventricle.

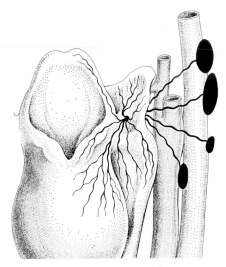

Fig. 218. Lymphatics of laryngopharynx.

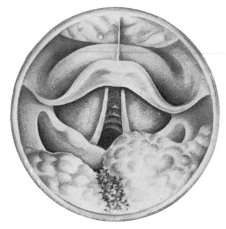

Fig. 219. Laryngeal view of carcinoma of posterior wall of laryngopharynx showing fissurelike ulceration surrounded by nodules.

anemia, achlorhydria, and general signs of atrophy of the mucous membrane, mouth, and pharynx. The disease is due to an alimentary deficiency. There is usually a history of loss of teeth in early life and chronic dysphagia. About 25% of the patients show moderate enlargement of the spleen, and koilonychia (spoon-shaped nails) is also often observed. This syndrome is a true precancerous condition that may be present for many years before any manifestation of cancer is found.

In Jacobsson's series[21] of 322 patients with carcinoma of the hypopharynx treated at the Radium-hemmet of Stockholm, 203 (60%) were women, and 90% gave signs of sideropenia. A large proportion of women among patients with carcinoma of the hypopharynx is also observed in Denmark, England, and Australia (Watts[50]) but not in the United States (Wynder et al.[53]). Changes in diet have resulted in a reduction in the occurrence of these cases (Jacobsson[22]). A high percentage of patients, both male and female, with cancer of the hypopharynx have a history of excessive use of tobacco and alcohol. Hollinger and Rabbitt[19] reported three cases of carcinomas arising in previously irradiated areas of the pharynx and larynx and found nine others in the literature. The irradiation had been for nonneoplastic conditions and had been given at least sixteen years previously.

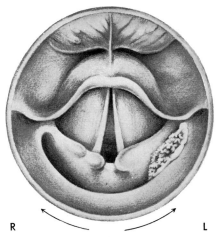

R L

Fig. 220. Carcinoma of lateral wall of piriform sinus without invasion of larynx and showing only slight edema of arytenoid.

Pathology
Gross pathology

Carcinomas of the *posterior wall* of the hypopharynx usually extend diffusely and present a central fissurelike ulceration that rapidly becomes necrotic (Fig. 219). They habitually infiltrate downward toward the esophagus but seldom invade the prevertebral muscles or any important structure. These tumors occur almost exclusively in men.

Carcinomas of the *lateral wall of the piriform sinus* rapidly invade the lateral wing of the thyroid cartilage. Partly be-

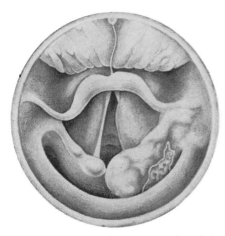

Fig. 221. Mirror view of carcinoma of medial wall of piriform sinus showing considerable edema of arytenoid and arytenoepiglottic fold and tumefaction of left false cord hiding true cord. Because of marked edema, these tumors are easily confused with primary carcinomas of endolarynx and are usually classified as such. Actually, primary lesion is outside of anatomic limits of endolarynx.

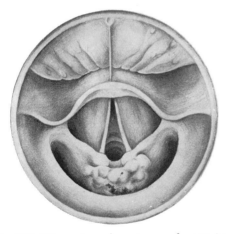

Fig. 222. Mirror view of carcinoma of retrocricoid region. These tumors occur predominantly in women, although carcinomas of laryngopharynx in women are not common.

cause of the trauma of deglutition and also because of the infiltrating nature of these tumors, an extensive area of necrosis develops (Fig. 220). This sometimes dissects on both sides of the thyroid wing and may produce an external tumefaction on the side of the larynx. Tumors of the lateral wall of the hypopharynx may invade the internal carotid artery.

Carcinomas of the *medial wall of the piriform sinus* may invade the larynx

through the laryngeal ventricle, the true cord may be infiltrated, and the false cord becomes edematous (Fig. 221). Invasion of the outer aspect of the cricoid cartilage may occur, but this is not frequent.

Carcinomas of the *retrocricoid region* are usually well-differentiated nodular tumors arising on the mucous membrane of the mouth of the esophagus anteriorly (Fig. 222). They infiltrate insidiously the anterior wall of the esophagus, where they seem to develop rather rapidly. The growth may become annular once it descends into the esophagus proper. As a consequence of the development, the larynx and trachea are displaced forward. Lederman[27] would designate these carcinomas as cricopharyngeal and would make them a subdivision of a group of "epiesophageal" lesions.

Cancer of the *arytenoepiglottic fold* is usually an exophytic, typically "cauliflower" type of growth (Fig. 223). The tumor is friable and extends over both the laryngeal and pharyngeal aspects of the arytenoepiglottic fold (Fig. 224). As a consequence, there is obstruction of the piriform sinus and neighboring edema of the false cord. These carcinomas are frequently included in the surgical series of carcinomas of the larynx (Smith et al.[46]; Ogura et al.[37]).

Due to the considerable secondary infection that usually accompanies these tumors and also because they hinder deglutition, *necrotizing bronchopneumonia* (aspiration pneumonia) may develop. Necrosis of the bronchial walls and suppuration of the lung parenchyma are invariably present. The distribution is lobular and is localized to one or more bronchopulmonary segments. The bronchi are diffusely infected and may contain purulent material. Central softening of the involved areas and often occasional small abscesses may be found (Ackerman et al.[1]).

Microscopic pathology

The overwhelming majority of tumors of the hypopharynx are epidermoid carcinomas, most of which are rather undifferentiated. In general, however, they are less differentiated than carcinomas of the endolarynx. Most of these tumors are undifferentiated with infiltrating borders, but

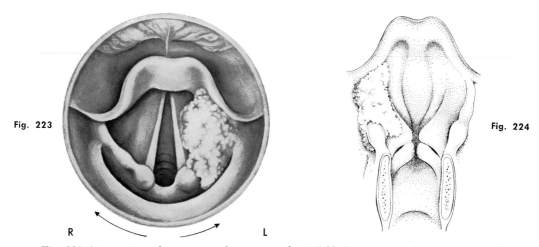

Fig. 223

Fig. 224

R   L

Fig. 223. Mirror view of carcinoma of arytenoepiglottic fold showing typical exophytic growth extending over laryngeal wall of epiglottis and over false cord, with some diminution of movements of larynx due to mechanical obstruction.

Fig. 224. Posterior view of carcinoma of arytenoepiglottic fold illustrated in Fig. 223 showing superficial extension to epiglottis, arytenoid, piriform sinus, and false cord.

a small percentage have sharply delimited pushing borders (Figs. 225 and 226).

Polypoid carcinomas of the piriform sinus are rare. They often have a distinctive histology and may be associated with sarcomatous or pseudosarcomatous stroma (Cornes and Lewis[8]).

Metastatic spread

Carcinomas of the hypopharynx are almost constantly accompanied by a metastatic node, usually large, in the middle portion of the jugular chain. Sometimes the metastatic nodes may be found in the supraclavicular region. Lymphatic permeation may produce mediastinal adenopathy in advanced cases.

Invasion of the jugular vein may result in thrombosis and distant blood-borne metastases. In autopsies on sixty-two patients with metastatic carcinoma of the neck, Willis[51] found twenty-nine invasion of the jugular vein, and of these twenty-four had visceral metastases.

Clinical evolution

The most common first symptom of carcinomas of the hypopharynx is the appearance of *odynophagia*, which is sometimes unilateral. Progressive *dysphagia* will also be present and will contribute to rapid loss of weight and asthenia. *Otalgia* on the

same side as the lesion often follows closely the appearance of the first symptom. *Hoarseness* is present only when the tumor has invaded the larynx or has displaced it sufficiently to interfere with phonation. *Cough*, particularly after ingestion of food, may be present and in some patients is almost constant. *Dyspnea* is rare, being present sometimes when tumors of the piriform sinus have invaded the larynx and obstructed the glottis. In general, respiratory difficulty, when present, is not very marked. Local *pain* in either side of the neck may occur and will be particularly intense when the tumors have invaded the cartilaginous structures of the larynx. *Hemoptysis* is very rarely observed but, when present, is serious, betraying in most instances invasion of the carotid artery. Most tumors of the hypopharynx are secondarily infected and necrotic, causing *maladorous breath*. Occasionally there may be *expectoration* of necrotic material, fragments of the tumor, or cartilage.

Metastatic nodes in the cervical region are most often unilateral. They follow closely the appearance of the first symptoms, but in some instances the *adenopathy may be the first clinical sign of disease*. The metastatic nodes usually grow rapidly and become voluminous. They are soft and movable and may be found anywhere

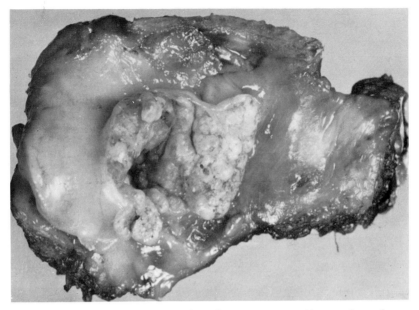

Fig. 225. Large, ulcerating cancer of piriform fossa measuring 2.5 cm × 3 cm that occurred in 46-year-old man who was exceedingly heavy drinker and smoker. Total duration of symptoms was three months. Supraglottic resection was done (sparing larynx), including neck dissection. Seventy-one lymph nodes were negative. Patient continued to drink, developed carcinoma of midesophagus seven years later, and died the following year. There was no recurrence of piriform fossa cancer. (WU neg. 60-7515.)

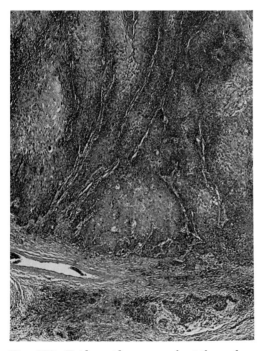

Fig. 226. Epidermoid cancer of piriform fossa shown in Fig. 225. Note pushing margins. Detailed study showed isolated areas of carcinoma in situ present. (WU neg. 60-7821A.)

along the sternocleidomastoid muscle but are present most commonly in the mid-cervical region. However, submaxillary and supraclavicular nodes may also be observed. In forty-five cases of carcinomas of the piriform sinus reported by Pietrantoni et al.,[41] thirty-five showed clinical evidence of metastasis.

Some tumors of the lateral wall of the pharynx present a tumefaction in the mid-cervical region at the level of the posterior border of the thyroid cartilage. This tumefaction is usually due to direct extension of the tumor and secondary infection and should not be confused with an adenopathy. Carcinomas of the mouth of the esophagus may displace the larynx and trachea forward and give a clinical impression of goiter.

Distant metastases are seldom found in the early stages of the disease, but they usually develop sometime during its course. Coutard[8a] reported on eighty-nine patients with carcinoma of the hypopharynx, nineteen of whom (21%) remained locally cured. Ten of these nineteen patients died from pulmonary, hepatic, and osseous me-

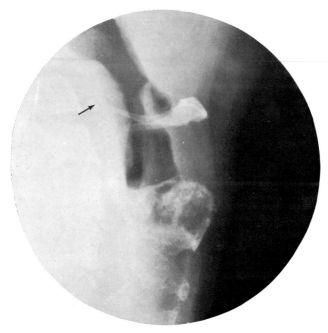

Fig. 227. Carcinoma of posterior wall of pharynx. Note thickness and irregularities of wall. (PCH 58-239.)

tastases three to seven years after the treatment, whereas the primary lesion remained apparently controlled. It is obvious that distant metastases from carcinoma of the pharynx are not often seen, but this is because so few lesions are locally sterilized that the patients do not live long enough for the development of such metastases.

Because of dysphagia and accompanying malnutrition and because of frequent secondary infection and necrosis, aspiration pneumonia may develop. This may occur before, during, or after treatment. It is usually accompanied by only slight fever but a rapid pulse. Because of these factors (loss of weight, absence of fever, poor general condition) the patient may appear to have generalized metastatic spread.

Diagnosis

The diagnosis of tumors of the laryngopharynx by indirect pharyngoscopy offers little difficulty. Even when the cooperation of the patient cannot be immediately secured, repeated examinations through the mirror will contribute more information than will be obtained by direct pharyngoscopy.

Roentgenologic examination

Lateral roentgenograms of the soft tissues of the neck will contribute additional details of the topography of the tumor. Enlargement of soft tissue spaces and displacement and decalcification of cartilages are often observed. In tumors of the retrocricoid area and in some tumors of the piriform sinus, the lateral projection may be complemented by another taken while maintaining air under pressure in the pharynx (Valsalva's maneuver). This procedure allows a certain amount of air to enter the upper portion of the esophagus, permitting a better outline of the mouth of the esophagus.

In some instances, contrast media may add to the simple soft tissue roentgenogram; planigraphy is also utilized, preferably coronal tomograms, which may be of additional value (Fletcher and Jing[13]). Roentgenograms of the chest should be routinely taken in these patients. Mediastinal adenopathy and pulmonary metastases may be observed. Often the lungs may show signs of bronchopneumonia because of aspiration of food or necrotic material.

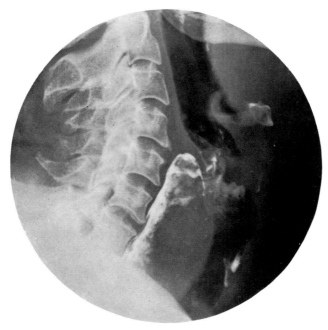

Fig. 228. Carcinoma of retrocricoid area showing compression of trachea and infiltration of mouth of esophagus. Contrast barium permits visualization of most of tumor on anterior wall of esophagus. (Courtesy Radium Institute, University of Paris, Paris, France.)

Biopsy

A biopsy can always be easily obtained from tumors of the hypopharynx through indirect pharyngoscopy. The only difficulty is that very often only necrotic material is obtained at the first trial, and the biopsy has to be repeated. Biopsy may have to be obtained by direct pharyngoscopy which has the advantages of better exposure and of an opportunity to observe the lower limits of the ulceration. A needle biopsy of metastatic lymph nodes should always be done as a matter of record.

Differential diagnosis

A roentgenogram of the chest may give the false impression of pulmonary metastases. The changes found in *aspiration pneumonia* have a lobular distribution and are present mostly in the lower lobes (Fig. 229). These changes are characterized by a patchy cloudiness, but areas of rarefaction may appear in the center of the opaque areas as the disease progresses.

Retropharyngeal abscesses may offer a problem of differential diagnosis. They are soft, fluctuant, and nonulcerated, and digital palpation is usually sufficient to estab-

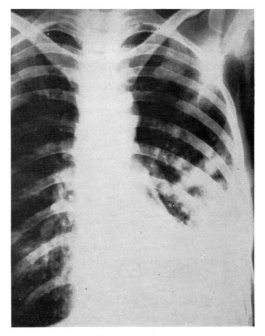

Fig. 229. Typical necrotizing pneumonia characterized by patchy areas of increased density which could be confused with metastatic carcinoma. (From Ackerman, L. V., et al.: Necrotizing bronchopneumonia; its relation to radiation therapy of cancer of the oral cavity, Amer. J. Roentgen. **53**:281-289, 1945.)

lish the diagnosis. *Neurilemomas* arising from the deep cervical nerves, protruding in the pharynx, and causing dysphagia have been rarely observed (Koop et al.[26]). They often pulsate and, when arising from the vagus nerve, may be accompanied by paralysis of a vocal cord (Slaughter and dePeyster[45]).

The problem of cervical *metastases from unknown primary lesions* is an important one, for although the primary lesion is often found in the pharynx, this is not always the case. In many instances, a radical neck dissection has been done with relatively favorable results (Jesse and Neff[24]). In others, irradiation of the metastatic adenopathy and of the underlying unsuspected primary lesion may lead to permanent control. In general, however, the prognosis is poor (France and Lucas[14]).

Treatment
Surgery

Interventions aiming at the extirpation of hypopharyngeal carcinomas, without simultaneous removal of the larynx, are infrequently possible or successful. In a few selected patients, they have been carried out with some measure of success (McGavran et al.[35]). The excision of a carcinoma of the medial wall of the piriform sinus, in continuity with the larynx and a neck dissection, is a more rational though mutilating procedure (Fig. 230).

Sylvestre Begnis[48] performed thirty-seven pharyngolaryngectomies, fourteen of these with simultaneous neck dissections, five of them bilateral. This procedure has been adopted by an increasing number of adepts (Alonso[3]; Leroux-Robert and Ennuyer[31]; Ogura et al.[37]; Letton and Wilson[33]). The practice of pharyngolaryngectomy, with or without neck dissection, followed by postoperative radiotherapy has been advocated by Leroux-Robert and Ennuyer[31].

For the treatment of retrocricoid carcinomas, as well as for those of the mouth of the esophagus, Wookey[52] perfected a surgical technique for a laryngoesophagectomy followed by an ingenious reconstruction of the pharynx in several stages. Extensive surgery is indicated and at times fruitful in cases of postirradiation residual or recurrent carcinoma in spite of consid-

erable mutilation and deformity (Coleman[7]).

Radiotherapy

It was the challenge of carcinoma of the pharynx, incurable by surgery, that opened the opportunities of early clinical research in radiotherapy of cancer. But whereas these tumors and their metastases are highly radiosensitive, the rapidity of their growth, the volume that they attain, the important structures they invade, and the difficulties in healing the necrotized areas frequently interfere with a successful result. Short, intensive treatments are seldom fruitful. It is primarily in an attempt to obtain better results in this area that Coutard[9] first devised a method of discontinued irradiations which has subsequently been readvocated for the same purposes. Cobalt[60] teletherapy and supervoltage roentgentherapy have brought the relative advantage of better quality radiations which permit a more homogeneous irradiation of the primary and metastatic lesions and fewer chances of necrosis. In a comparison of eighty patients treated with cobalt[60] and another series of eighty treated by conventional roentgentherapy, Gary-Bobo et al.[17] found that, at the end of four years, eleven patients from the former series were alive while none from the latter survived.

Leroux-Robert and Ennuyer[32] have practiced and advocated a combination of surgical treatment and *postoperative* radiotherapy. The practice of *preoperative* radiotherapy has been less exploited and is perhaps more fruitful (Bryce[5]; Strong et al.[47]).

Chemotherapy

Various drugs have been tried in the treatment of laryngopharyngeal tumors, for the most part without much effect or success. *Methotrexate* produces a definite regression that occasionally may appear complete, only to be followed by a strikingly fast recurrence. Associations of chemotherapy and radiotherapy have appeared promising (Friedman and Daly[15]; Perez-Tamayo and Soberon[40]). The drug, however, is not a radiosensitizer. Any success may be attributed to an additivity of effects.

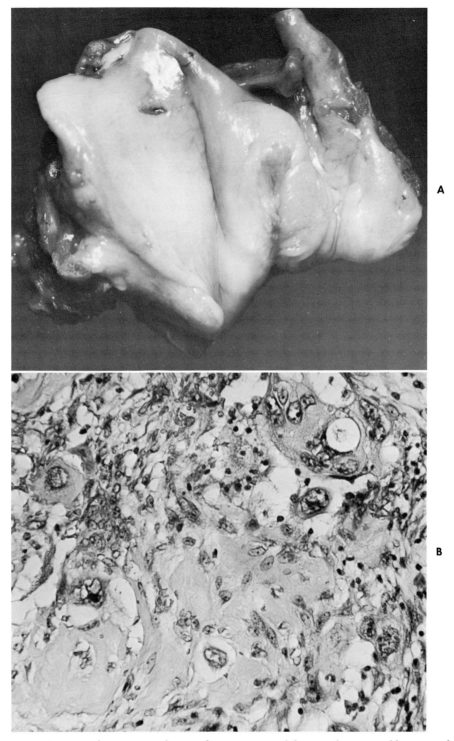

Fig. 230. A, Surgical specimen of supraglottic portion of larynx of 64-year-old man with carcinoma of right anterior medial piriform fossa. Patient received radiotherapy preoperatively (3000 R). Operation also included right radical neck dissection. No definite tumor could be found in region of piriform fossa. **B,** One lymph node in neck showing keratinized squamous carcinoma with profound irradiation effect. Patient living and well two years later. (**A,** WU neg. 68-6988; **B,** ×300; WU neg. 68-7298.)

Prognosis

Jacobsson[21] reported on 242 patients treated at the Radiumhemmet of Stockholm, with twenty-three (9.5%) five-year survivors. MacComb and Fletcher[34] reported on 182 patients treated for carcinoma of the piriform sinus (sixty-two by surgery, fifty-one by radiations alone, and sixty-nine by a combination of both), with thirty-nine patients (21%) living and well at the end of three years. Of 146 patients at risk, twenty-three (15%) were well five years.

McGavran et al.[35] reported fifty-two selected patients with carcinoma of the piriform sinus treated by partial pharyngectomy and supraglottic laryngectomy with radical neck dissection in continuity, with forty-three showing histologic evidence of metastases. Of thirty-four at risk, thirteen (38%) survived five years. Letton and Wilson[33] reported on eighteen patients who had a radical surgical procedure without operative mortality, six of whom lived twelve years. Chardot et al.[6] had eighteen patients at risk following pharyngolaryngectomy and neck dissection, with five living five years. In forty-four favorable cases treated surgically, Bryce[5] reported 23% of the patients surviving five years. The results were half as good in lesions of the piriform sinus as for those elsewhere in the hypopharynx.

Radiotherapy obtains its best results in carcinomas of the posterior wall, arytenoepiglottic fold, and medial wall of the piriform sinus. Retrocricoid carcinomas are seldom cured by radiotherapy. However, Hultberg[20] reported a survival rate of 17% in a small series of patients irradiated for carcinomas of the *lower half* of the piriform sinus, mostly retrocricoid lesions. The results of radiotherapy for carcinomas of the *upper half* of the piriform sinus are relatively better. Lederman[30] reported that results in a series of 673 patients were poor, particularly in the presence of metastases.

A series of thirty-six patients treated by Leroux-Robert and Ennuyer[32] with surgery and postoperative radiotherapy yielded ten five-year survivors.

REFERENCES

1 Ackerman, L. V., Wiley, H. M., and LeMone, D. V.: Necrotizing bronchopneumonia; its relation to radiation therapy of cancer of the oral cavity, Amer. J. Roentgen. **53:**281-289, 1945.

2 Ahlbom, H. E.: Simple achlorhydric anaemia, Plummer-Vinson syndrome, and carcinoma of the mouth, pharynx, and oesophagus in women, Brit. Med. J. **2:**331-333, 1936.

3 Alonso, J. M.: Conservative surgery in cancer of the larynx, Trans. Amer. Acad. Ophthal. **51:**633-642, 1947.

4 Baclesse, F.: Tumeurs malignes du pharynx et du larynx; étude anatomotopographique et radiographique, Paris, 1960, Masson et Cie.

5 Bryce, D. P.: Preoperative irradiation in the treatment of carcinoma of the hypopharynx, Canad. Med. Ass. J. **93:**1147-1151, 1965.

6 Chardot, C., Pigache, R., Carolus, J.-M., and Landes, P.: 100 pharyngo-laryngectomies "monobloc" avec conservation de la continuité digestive; résultats chirurgicaux et cancerologiques, Ann. Chir. **18:**1308-1316, 1964.

7 Coleman, C. C., Jr.: Surgical treatment of extensive cancers of the mouth and pharynx, Ann. Surg. **161:**634-644, 1965.

8 Cornes, J. S., and Lewis, M. S.: Polypoid carcinomas of the pharynx with sarcomatous or pseudosarcomatous stroma, Brit. J. Surg. **53:**340-344, 1966.

8a Coutard, H.: De la roentgenthérapie des cancers du pharynx, Radiophys. Radiother. **3:**203-212, 1934.

9 Coutard, H.: Conception of periodicity as possible directing factor in roentgenotherapy of cancer (Lewis Linn McArthur Lecture), Proc. Inst. Med. Chicago **10:**310-323, 1935.

10 Coutard, Henri: Roentgentherapy of epitheliomas of the upper air passages, Laryngoscope **46:**407-414, 1936.

11 Dutta-Chaudhuri, R., Roy, H., and Sen Gupta, B. K.: Cancer of the larynx and hypopharynx; a clinicopathological study with special reference to aetiology, J. Indian Med. Ass. **32:**352-362, 1959.

12 Ennuyer, A., and Bataini, J. P.: Les tumeurs de l'amygdale et de la région vélopalatine; statistiques de la Fondation Curie; exploitation statistique: Dr. Fautrel, Paris, 1956, Masson et Cie.

13 Fletcher, G. H., and Jing, B.-B.: The head and neck (Hodes, P. J., editor-in-chief: Atlas of tumor radiology; sponsored by The American College of Radiology), Chicago, 1968, Year Book Medical Publishers, Inc.

14 France, C. J., and Lucas, R.: The management and prognosis of metastatic neoplasms of the neck with an unknown primary, Amer. J. Surg. **106:**835-839, 1963.

15 Friedman, M., and Daly, J. F.: The treatment of squamous cell carcinoma of the head and neck with methotrexate and irradiation, Amer. J. Roentgen. **99:**289-301, 1967.

16 Gárciga, C. E.: A new radiolaryngometric method, Radiology **57:**884-885, 1951.

17 Gary-Bobo, J., Pourquier, H., and Belotte, J.: La radiothérapie conventionnelle et la télécobalthérapie dans le traitement des cancers du sinus piriforme (comparaison de deux series

de 80 cas), J. Radiol. Electr. **44**:191-194, 1963.

18 Graham, J. M.: The surgery of the hypopharynx: post-cricoid carcinoma, Edinburgh Med. J. **49**:164-178, 1942.

19 Hollinger, P. H., and Rabbit, W. F.: Late development of laryngeal and pharyngeal carcinoma in previously irradiated areas, Laryngoscope **63**:105-112, 1953.

20 Hultberg, S.: Radiumhemmet method of treatment in hypopharyngeal cancer, Brit. J. Radiol. **26**:224-233, 1953.

21 Jacobsson, F.: Carcinoma of the hypopharynx; a clinical study of 322 cases, treated at Radiumhemmet, from 1939 to 1947, Acta Radiol. (Stockholm) **35**:1-21, 1951.

22 Jacobsson, F.: The Plummer-Vinson syndrome and post-cricoid carcinoma (unpublished data, 1962).

23 Jesse, R. H., and Fletcher, G. H.: Metastases in cervical lymph nodes from oropharyngeal carcinoma; treatment and results, Amer. J. Roentgen. **90**:990-996, 1963.

24 Jesse, R. H., and Neff, L. E.: Metastatic carcinoma in cervical nodes with an unknown primary lesion, Amer. J. Surg. **112**:547-553, 1966.

25 Jørgsholm, B.: Roentgen therapy in cancer of the extrathoracic portion of the oesophagus, Acta Radiol. (Stockholm) **38**:62-78, 1952.

26 Koop, C. E., Jordan, H. E., and Horn, R. C.: Neurilemmoma of the pharynx, Surg. Gynec. Obstet. **85**:641-645, 1947.

27 Lederman, M.: Epi-oesophageal cancer with special reference to tumours of the post cricoid region, Brit. J. Radiol. **28**:173-183, 1955.

28 Lederman, M.: Cancers of the hypo-pharynx; classification, results of radiotherapy, Ann. Otolaryng. (Paris) **72**:506-527, 1955.

29 Lederman, M.: The anatomy of cancer with special reference to tumours of the upper air and food passages, J. Laryng. **79**:181-208, 1964.

30 Lederman, M.: Role of irradiation in treatment of cancer of the hypopharynx, postcricoid, and cervical esophagus. In MacComb, W. S., and Fletcher, G. H.: Cancer of the head and neck, Baltimore, 1967, The Williams & Wilkins Co., pp. 347-365.

31 Leroux-Robert, J., and Ennuyer, A.: Cancer du sinus piriforme, Paris, 1952, Librairie Arnette.

32 Leroux-Robert, J., and Ennuyer, A.: Traitement des cancers de l'hypopharynx, Acta Un. Int. Cancr. **10**:296-324, 1954.

33 Letton, A. H., and Wilson, J. P.: Surgical management of carcinoma of the thyroid, (symposium on head and neck surgery), Southern Med. J. **56**:1388-1390, 1963.

34 MacComb, W. S., and Fletcher, G. H.: Cancer of the head and neck, Baltimore, 1967, The Williams & Wilkins Co.

35 McGavran, M. H., Bauer, W. C., Spjut, H. J., and Ogura, J. H.: Carcinoma of the pyriform sinus; the results of radical surgery, Arch. Otolaryng. (Chicago) **78**:826-830, 1963.

36 Martin, H. E.: Treatment of pharyngeal cancer, Arch. Otolaryng. (Chicago) **227**:661-691, 1938.

37 Ogura, J. H., Jurema, A. A., and Watson, R. K.: Partial laryngopharyngectomy and neck dissection for pyriform sinus cancer; conservation surgery with immediate reconstruction, Laryngoscope **70**:1399-1417, 1960.

38 Ogura, J. H., Watson, R. K., and Jurema, A. A.: Partial pharyngectomy and neck dissection for posterior hypopharyngeal cancer; immediate reconstruction with preservation of voice, Laryngoscope **70**:1523-1534, 1960.

39 Paymaster, J. C.: Some observations on oral and pharyngeal carcinomas in the State of Bombay, Cancer **15**:578-583, 1962.

40 Perez-Tamayo, R., and Soberon, M.: Methotrexate and radiotherapy in the treatment of advanced squamous cell carcinomas of the oral cavity and pharynx, Missouri Med. **65**:914-917, 1968.

41 Pietrantoni, L., Agazzi, C., and Fior, R.: Indications for surgical treatment of cervical lymph nodes in cancer of the larynx and hypopharynx, Laryngoscope **72**:1511-1527, 1962.

42 del Regato, J. A.: Roentgentherapy of carcinoma of the endolarynx, Laryngoscope **61**:511-516, 1951.

43 Rouvière, H.: Anatomie des lymphatiques de l'homme, Paris, 1933, Masson et Cie.

44 Scanlon, P. W.: The effect of mitotic suppression and recovery after irradiation on time-dose relationships and the application of this effect to clinical radiation therapy, Amer. J. Roentgen. **81**:433-455, 1959.

45 Slaughter, D. P., and dePeyster, F. A.: Pharyngeal neurilemmomas of cranial nerve origin, Arch. Surg. (Chicago) **59**:386-397, 1949.

46 Smith, R. R., Caulk, R., Russell, W., and Jackson, L. C.: End result of 600 laryngeal cancers using the American Joint Committee's method of classification and end-result reporting, Surg. Gynec. Obstet. **113**:435-444, 1961.

47 Strong, E. W., Henschke, U. K., Nickson, J. J., Frazell, E. L., Tollefsen, H. R., and Hilaris, B. S.: Preoperative x-ray therapy as an adjunct to radical neck dissection, Cancer **19**:1509-1516, 1966.

48 Sylvestre Begnis, C.: Los cánceres laringofaríngeos, Bol. Soc. Cir. Rosario **9**:649-658, 1942.

49 Turner, A. L.: Carcinoma of the post-cricoid region (pars laryngea pharyngis) and upper end of the oesophagus, Edinburgh Med. J. **25**:345-362, 1920.

50 Watts, M. McK.: The importance of the Plummer-Vinson syndrome in the aetiology of carcinoma of the upper gastro-intestinal tract, Postgrad. Med. J. **37**:523-533, 1961.

51 Willis, R. A.: The spread of tumors in the human body, London, 1934, J. & A. Churchill, Ltd.

52 Wookey, H.: The surgical treatment of carcinoma of the hypopharynx and the esophagus, Brit. J. Surg. **35**:249-266, 1948.

53 Wynder, E. L., Hultberg, S., Jacobsson, F., and Bross, I. J.: Environmental factors in cancer of the upper alimentary tract; a Swedish study with special reference to Plummer-Vinson (Paterson-Kelly) syndrome, Cancer **10**:470-487, 1957.

Endolarynx

There is unquestionable confusion in the medical literature as to the definition of a carcinoma of the larynx. Many carcinomas actually arising and developing inside the larynx are called extralaryngeal, and usually carcinomas that arise outside of the larynx itself are called laryngeal tumors.

Originally the terms *intrinsic* and *extrinsic* were meant to define tumors arising, respectively, inside or outside of the larynx but which in one way or another affected the laryngeal structures. Because the term *intrinsic* was made synonymous with operable carcinoma of the larynx, its significance varied with the concept of operability, and consequently it has not had the same meaning through time, nor does it mean the same thing to different authors. Most surgeons use the term *intrinsic* to define carcinomas of the glottis (i.e., actually of the vocal cord or the anterior commissure). It would be more logical to call those tumors carcinomas of the vocal cord than to give them the confusing term of intrinsic carcinomas.

It is reasonable to include in the same group all carcinomas of the endolarynx, whether operable or not, mainly because of the fact that, unlike laryngopharyngeal tumors, they rarely metastasize to the cervical nodes. Also, endolaryngeal carcinomas have a more favorable prognosis in general than tumors of the hypopharynx. The term carcinoma of the *endolarynx* includes all those tumors arising from the various laryngeal structures. The differentiation of the point of origin of these tumors is important in determining treatment and in establishing prognosis. In extensive cases it may be impossible to establish this point of departure, but the point of origin may make itself evident in the course of radiotherapy. These points of origin of carcinoma within the larynx present different clinical, pathologic, and diagnostic features that will be described separately. The following points of origin are recognized as separate clinical entities: the laryngeal wall of the epiglottis, the false cord, the laryngeal ventricle, the true cord, and the subglottis. Excluded from this group are tumors arising in the arytenoepiglottic fold

or free border of the epiglottis, which actually develop on both sides of the limiting lines of the endolarynx. These tumors have a different pathologic character and are considered separately in the discussions of laryngopharyngeal and oropharyngeal tumors.

Anatomy

The larynx is situated in front of, and just immediately below, the hypopharynx. The skeleton of the larynx is formed by three main cartilages: the epiglottis, the thyroid, and the cricoid, which are strongly interconnected by ligaments. In addition, just on the rim of the cricoid posteriorly and on both sides of the midline there are the arytenoid cartilages and the cartilages of Santorini, which are covered by numerous muscles and lined by a columnar ciliated epithelium. It is only on the free border of the true cord and on isolated areas of the false cords that the mucosa of the larynx is squamous in nature. The number of areas of squamous metaplasia increases with age.

The endolarynx is usually divided into three portions: the vestibule or supraglottic portion, the glottis, and the subglottic portion.

The *vestibule* is formed anteriorly by the laryngeal wall of the epiglottis. This is a triangular surface extending from the free border of the epiglottis to the anterior commissure of the vocal cords (Fig. 231). Laterally, the vestibule is formed by the false cords, which are made up of elastic tissue covered by mucous membrane and which extend from the laryngeal wall of the epiglottis to the arytenoids. Posterolaterally, the false cords are continuous with the arytenoepiglottic fold, which forms the posterolateral rim of the larynx. Just behind the false cords and on each side of the midline are the arytenoids two globular structures separated by a small space and composed of the arytenoid cartilages, ligaments, connective tissue, and the overlying mucous membrane (Fig. 232). Immediately below the false cords are the laryngeal ventricles or ventricles of Morgagni, the roof is formed by the false

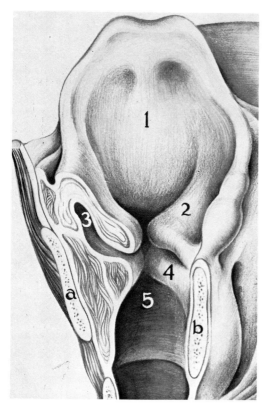 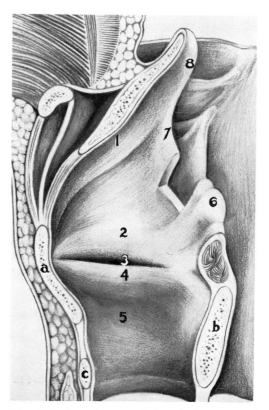

Fig. 231. Posterior view of larynx with frontal section through left half. 1, Laryngeal wall of epiglottis. 2, False cord. 3, Ventricle of Morgagni. 4, Buccal cord. 5, Subglottic area. a, Section of thyroid cartilage. b and c, Sections of cricoid cartilage at different levels.

Fig. 232. Lateral view of larynx. 1, Laryngeal wall of epiglottis and its close relationship with pre-epiglottic space. 2, False cord. 3, Opening of laryngeal ventricle. 4, True cord. 5, Subglottic area. 6, Arytenoid region. 7, Arytenoepiglottic fold with rectangular section to show its thickness and relationship to piriform sinus. 8, Free portion of epiglottis. a, Section at anterior midline of thyroid cartilage. b and c, Sections of cricoid cartilage.

cords and the floor by the upper surface of the true cords. Laterally, the ventricles lie very close to the wing of the thyroid cartilage. Posterolaterally, they are very near the anterior limits of the piriform sinus, separated only by a thin layer of muscle, connective tissue, and mucous membrane (Fig. 217).

The *glottis* is formed by the true vocal cords, which extend from the anterior angle of the thyroid cartilage to the arytenoids. Only their inner edge is visible on laryngeal examination. Laterally, they continue horizontally to form the floor of the ventricle. Below the glottis, the larynx has the shape of an inverted funnel.

The *subglottic* region is just immediately below the true cords. At this level, the lumen of the larynx is considerably smaller than in the supraglottic region, and it lacks the ability to expand because of the heavy cricoid cartilage that surrounds it.

Lymphatics. The lymphatics of the endolarynx are meager by contrast with those of the pharyngolarynx. The network of lymphatics is rather sparse, particularly at the level of the glottis. The lymphatics of the supraglottic region are richer, particularly on the superior surface of the false cords. Some of these lymphatics, after perforating the thyrohyoid membrane, end in the jugular nodes of the upper cervical region (Fig. 233). The few lymphatics of the subglottic region end in a pretracheal node in the lower anterior midline of the neck. Using radioactive gold in adult patients, Welsh[96] found cross-drainage to contralateral nodes to be "frequent."

Epidemiology

In the 1947 cancer survey in the United States, the age-adjusted incidence of cancer of the larynx was found to be 7.6 and 0.6, respectively, for male and female whites and 5.7 and 0.6, respectively, for male and female nonwhites per 100,000.

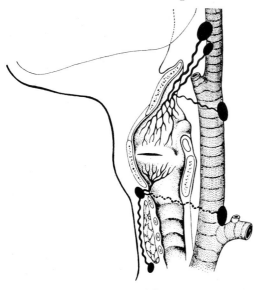

Fig. 233. Lymphatics of endolarynx. Note scarcity of lymphatics at level of glottis. Lymphatics of supraglottic area are richer, ending in nodes of anterior jugular chain. Lymphatics of subglottic area may end in pretracheal node of midline and rarely in lower cervical node.

For men 35 to 39 years of age, the incidence is only 0.7, but it rises rapidly thereafter to over 50.0 per 100,000 in those over 79 years of age. In recent years, there has been a reduction in the male-female ratio and a slight overall increase and a relative increase in the incidence rate among younger subjects (Bockmühl[17]; Jones and Gabriel[52]).

Epidemiologic studies have shown that the relative risk of having cancer of the larynx increases in proportion to the amount of tobacco smoked and, beyond that, by the amount of alcohol consumption by smokers (Wynder et al.[98]). Moore[69] studied 102 tobacco smokers who were cured of a carcinoma of the oral cavity, pharynx or larynx. Of sixty-five who continued to smoke, twenty-one developed a second carcinoma, whereas only two of the remaining thirty-seven developed a second lesion. Cahan and Montemayor[22] reported on sixty patients who had both carcinoma of the larynx and of the lung, in eighteen of whom the neoplastic manifestations were simultaneous.

Pathology
Gross pathology

Tumors of the endolarynx most frequently present a combination of ulceration and outgrowth. They infiltrate in dif-

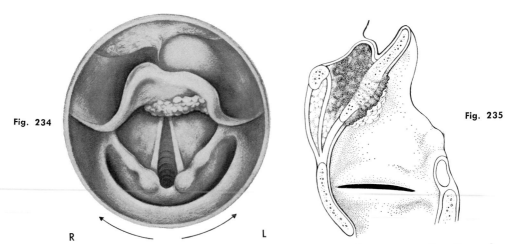

Fig. 234. Mirror view of tumor of laryngeal surface of epiglottis showing some distortion and tumefaction in left vallecula.

Fig. 235. Tumor of laryngeal wall of epiglottis with extension to pre-epiglottic area through epiglottic cartilage.

ferent directions and invade different structures, depending on their point of origin.

Carcinomas of the *laryngeal surface of the epiglottis* arise almost in direct contact with the epiglottic cartilage (Fig. 234). They easily invade and perforate this structure and extend without resistance into the pre-epiglottic space (Fig. 235).

Carcinomas of the *false cord* usually arise on the anterior half of its surface, close to the laryngeal wall of the epiglottis

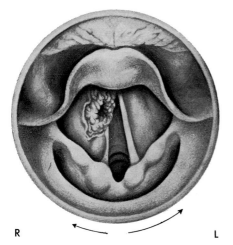

R ←——— **L**

Fig. 236. Mirror view of carcinoma of right false cord partially hiding true cord, with slight edema of arytenoid and diminution of mobility of right hemilarynx.

(Figs. 236 and 237). The base of the ulceration may be necrotic, and there will usually be some surrounding edema that may include the arytenoid. In their lateral extension, the tumors often reach the thyroid cartilage and may invade it (Fig. 238). They also may extend anteriorly toward the laryngeal wall of the epiglottis and to the false cord of the opposite side. In this process, the laryngeal ventricle becomes obliterated (Fig. 238), and the tumor may come in contact with the true cord, but actual invasion of the true cord occurs only in advanced disease.

Carcinomas of the *laryngeal ventricle* are probably more common than has been suspected. The ulceration is usually hidden within the ventricle (Fig. 239). The tumor extends toward the false cord, producing a bulky, nonulcerated tumefaction on the laryngeal vestibule (Fig. 240). Invasion of the thyroid cartilage occurs almost constantly and early in the development of these tumors (Fig. 241). The thin layer of muscles lying next to the lateral wing of the thyroid gland is also invaded and the skin ulcerated in late stages. Posterolateral extension of tumors of the laryngeal ventricle results in obliteration of the piriform sinus but seldom in ulceration of the mucous membrane in this area.

The *true cord* is the most common of all the single points of origin of carcinoma

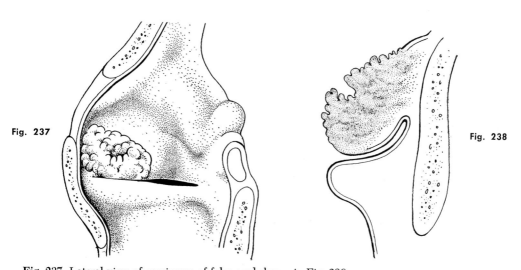

Fig. 237

Fig. 238

Fig. 237. Lateral view of carcinoma of false cord shown in Fig. 236.

Fig. 238. Frontal section of carcinoma of false cord illustrating obliteration of ventricle and infiltration close to thyroid cartilage.

within the larynx (Fig. 242). Early lesions appear as nonulcerated tumefactions of the anterior third of the cord or as papillary growths with a typical ragged appearance (Figs. 243 to 245). As the disease extends, there may be accompanying edema of the false cord. There is often extension to the opposite vocal cord through the anterior commissure. Infiltration of the subglottis

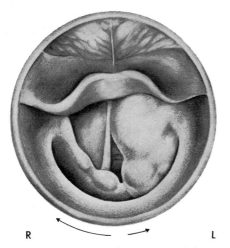

R → L

Fig. 239. Mirror view of carcinoma of laryngeal ventricle showing deformity of false cord, arytenoid, and arytenoepiglottic fold, with obliteration of piriform sinus and diminution of mobility of left hemilarynx. No ulceration is seen.

is not uncommon (Fig. 247). Carcinomas of the vocal cord may easily invade the thyroid cartilage at the lower half of its anterior midline. Fixation of the true cord is due to deep invasion of the intrinsic muscles by tumor rather than invasion of the arytenoid cartilage.

Carcinomas of the *subglottis* are usually submucous tumefactions adherent to the cricoid cartilage and with little superficial ulceration (Fig. 249). Deep infiltration of the cord is usually present but rarely results in an ulceration. Subglottic lesions usually develop on the anterior half of this narrow space. Infiltration of the wall may lead to eventual invasion of the thyroid gland or of the esophageal muscle. The arytenoid cartilage is practically never involved.

Microscopic pathology

Although the lining of the endolarynx is formed by columnar epithelium, the overwhelming majority of carcinomas arising in this area are epidermoid in nature, developing by metaplasia. The most highly differentiated of these carcinomas, however, are found to develop from the true cord, the free border of which is covered by a squamous epithelium. Most of the undifferentiated carcinomas of the larynx

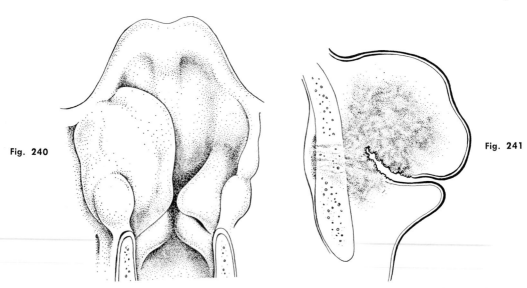

Fig. 240

Fig. 241

Fig. 240. Posterior view of carcinoma of laryngeal ventricle. Ulceration is hidden within ventricle, and nothing but considerable deformity can be observed.

Fig. 241. Frontal section of carcinoma of laryngeal ventricle showing marked deformity, infiltration of thyroid cartilage, and outside tumefaction.

arise in the supraglottic area. Intramucosal epithelioma (carcinoma in situ) can occur on the larynx. It may be present on the border of an invasive carcinoma or be present without invasion. It extends down the ducts of the mucous glands (Stout[90]).

Lane[56] reported polypoid, sarcoma-like masses (pseudosarcoma) in association with carcinoma of the larynx. Among non-squamous carcinomas arising in the larynx, the adenoid cystic carcinomas of salivary gland type predominate (Cady et al.[21]).

Metastatic spread

Carcinomas of the endolarynx produce a low proportion of metastatic lymph nodes as compared with hypopharyngeal carcinomas. The relative proportion of metastases from different laryngeal sites seems to follow the relative scarcity or

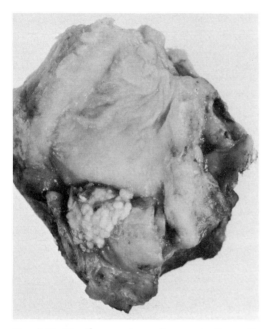

Fig. 242. Hemilaryngectomy for exophytic, well-differentiated squamous carcinoma of true vocal cord occurring in 74-year-old man. (WU neg. 67-10431.)

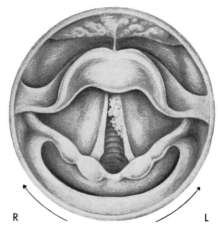

Fig. 243. Mirror view of early carcinoma of anterior half of true cord showing papillary outgrowth and perfect mobility of both sides of larynx.

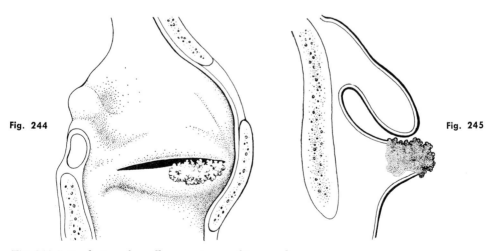

Fig. 244.

Fig. 245.

Fig. 244. Lateral view of papillary carcinoma of true cord.

Fig. 245. Frontal section of early carcinoma of vocal cord showing mostly papillary outgrowth and practically no infiltration.

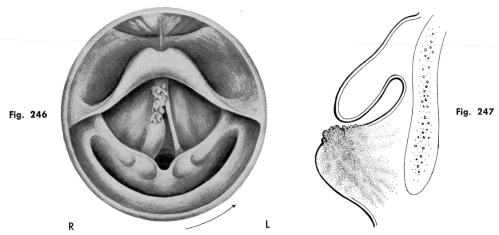

Fig. 246

Fig. 247

R   L

Fig. 246. Mirror view of carcinoma of true cord showing some papillary outgrowth on anterior half but also edema of posterior half with fixation of right hemilarynx. Presence of edema and fixation denotes infiltration beyond visible areas.

Fig. 247. Frontal section of infiltrating carcinoma of true cord showing some subglottic edema and diffuse infiltration of surrounding tissues.

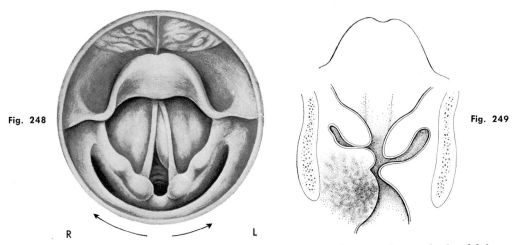

Fig. 248

Fig. 249

R   L

Fig. 248. Mirror view of carcinoma of subglottis showing no ulceration, having displaced left cord upward and diminished mobility of left hemilarynx. Such tumors usually cause marked dyspnea.

Fig. 249. Frontal section of carcinoma arising in subglottis. These are usually very infiltrating tumors showing submucosal extension and very little ulceration.

richness of lymphatics in the area. Mc-Gavran et al.,[67] in a report on ninety-six patients who had laryngectomies and neck dissections, noted that supraglottic carcinomas metastasized in one-third and subglottic carcinomas in one-fifth of the patients but that there were no instances of metastasis from glottic carcinomas. Contralateral metastases are observed in supra-glottic lesions. The variable tendency to produce metastases may also be related to the degree of undifferentiation of the carcinoma (Kuhn et al.[55]).

Clinical evolution

The most common presenting symptom in carcinoma of the endolarynx is *hoarseness*. The character of this hoarseness is an important factor in the clinical history. Patients with carcinomas of the vocal cord will usually have a progressively increasing hoarseness which may end in almost complete aphonia. Those with tumors of the supraglottic area will usually present an intermittent hoarseness with intervals of perfectly normal voice.

Dyspnea is often found in patients with carcinoma of the endolarynx. It is practically never present or important in those with supraglottic tumors. With tumors of the vocal cord, the intensity of the dyspnea will usually depend on the presence or absence of subglottic extension. With tumors of the subglottis, dyspnea is often a presenting symptom, and it rapidly becomes very marked.

Cough is not a common symptom. It may only occur after deglutition. Cough and associated expectoration may, however, be present in glottic and subglottic tumors. *Odynophagia* is more commonly associated with tumors of the laryngopharynx but may also be present with advanced endolaryngeal tumors. *Otalgia* occurs on the same side as the lesion when there is abundant secondary infection. *Local pain* is exceptionally present and is usually a sign of invasion of the cartilage. *Hemoptysis* is also uncommon but may be present in some vestibular tumors.

Left to themselves, carcinomas of the endolarynx will sooner or later occlude the air passage and necessitate a tracheotomy. Supraglottic tumors may extend to the free portion of the epiglottis and the arytenoepiglottic fold and, in their later stages, be unrecognizable from tumors that arise in these limiting areas. As has been stated, invasion of the skin in the anterior midline is not uncommon in advanced carcinomas of the ventricle. Death usually occurs because of pulmonary complications (Ackerman et al.[1]).

Diagnosis
Clinical examination

External inspection and palpation of the larynx is a very important factor that is usually disregarded. The larynx may be displaced and the symmetry of the thyroid cartilage disrupted when tumor, after invading the cartilage, has spread over its external surface. The tumefaction so pro-

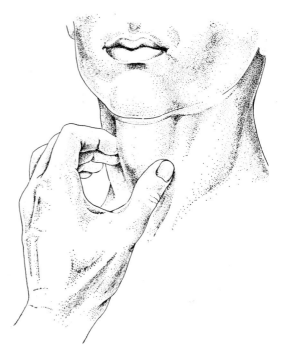

Fig. 250. Lateral mobilization of larynx produces crackle that is absent when tumor of larynx extends posteriorly.

duced by direct extension should not be confused with metastatic adenopathy.

The lateral mobilization of the larynx against the spine produces a noise, the *thyrovertebral crackle* (Fig. 250). This occurs on both sides of the midline by the contact of the posterior border of the thyroid cartilage and the cervical column. In carcinoma of the endolarynx, this crackle may not be present on the side of the lesion, which may be evidence that tumor has invaded posteriorly, interfering with the normal excursion of the thyroid cartilage. Neighboring edema may, in itself, suffice to give this impression, but the absence of the thyrovertebral crackle may be taken as a strong sign that tumor has extended beyond the limits for which a total laryngectomy would be successful.

Complete palpation of the neck will include the search for an adenopathy, a rare finding in carcinoma of the endolarynx. When a metastatic node is present, it will be found more commonly on the anterior jugular chain below the angle of the mandible. Less often, a node may be found on the anterior lower midline of the neck in front of the trachea.

Indirect laryngoscopy

When hoarseness is present, an indirect laryngoscopy should never be deferred. It is possible that the classic procedure for this examination, requiring a darkened room, a special floor lamp, and a head mirror, may account for the fact that few practitioners are ready to perform an indirect laryngoscopy. This examination requires no extraordinary skill, and in these times, when all senior medical students know how to use an ophthalmoscope, it is indeed paradoxical that an indirect laryngoscopy should be considered the gift of a specialist. Indirect laryngoscopic examination is greatly simplified by the use of a portable electric headlight.

For an indirect laryngoscopy the patient should be sitting in front of, and at a slightly lower level than, the examiner. In some instances, a better view may be obtained with the examiner standing and with the patient's head hyperextended. This permits a good view of the anterior commissure of the vocal cords. An anesthetic is not necessary as a general rule, and its use should be limited to those patients in whom complete relaxation is unobtainable.

In an indirect laryngoscopy the examiner should observe the symmetry of the laryngeal structures and also the movements of both sides of the larynx. This is achieved by requesting the patient alternately to breathe deeply and to produce the sounds *eh* and *ee*. Only after repeated alterations of breathing and phonation can the anterior commissure of the vocal cords be seen. When a tumor is discovered, the exact limits of its extension and its effect upon the mobility of the larynx should be noted, as well as the symmetry or asymmetry of the piriform sinuses. When there is respiratory difficulty, it is important to note whether the obstruction is glottic, supraglottic, or subglottic.

On indirect laryngoscopic examination it may sometimes be noted that the epiglottis is bent toward the posterior wall of the pharynx and that the cords are not entirely visible. This usually occurs in tumors of the laryngeal wall of the epiglottis and is a warning against examinations that are not thorough. In tumors of the supraglottic area, the mobility of the larynx is seldom impaired unless it be by the bulk of the tumor itself. In tumors of the glottis and subglottis, the mobility of the larynx may be considerably diminished or entirely abolished on one side. This usually occurs because of infiltration of muscles.

The direct laryngoscopy with its undeniable usefulness does not eliminate and, in fact, cannot substitute entirely for an indirect laryngoscopy. The indirect laryngoscopy permits a stereoscopic view of the larynx with greater sense of depth, and the movements of the larynx are better appreciated. The direct laryngoscopy gives a monocular view of the larynx. Because of the trauma of the instrument used and the corresponding reaction of the patient, the larynx becomes rigid and quickly edematous. A direct laryngoscopy, however, is sometimes necessary for proper visualization of certain tumors of the la-

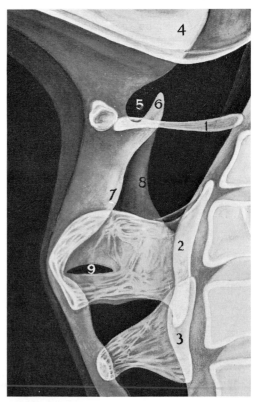

Fig. 251. Sketch of roentgenogram of normal adult male. 1, Hyoid bone. 2, Thyroid cartilage. 3, Cricoid cartilage. 4, Base of tongue. 5, Vallecula. 6, Free portion of epiglottis. 7, Laryngeal wall of epiglottis. 8, Arytenoepiglottic fold. 9, Laryngeal ventricle.

ryngeal wall of the epiglottis or anterior commissure and for obtaining certain biopsy specimens.

Roentgenologic examination

Coutard[28] introduced the radiographic examination of the larynx in 1922. This method of examination has become a valuable adjunct to the laryngoscopic examination in cancer of the endolarynx. A lateral roentgenogram of the soft tissues of the neck is taken, with the beam centered as accurately as possible at the level of the disease. This is a very important factor in the interpretation of the results, which requires a thorough knowledge of the radiographic appearance of a normal larynx as well as the chronology of calcification of laryngeal cartilages in the normal individual. The radiographic examination gives a better perception of the topography of the tumor than the simple laryngoscopic examination. Some apparently small carcinomas of the vocal cord may show extensive invasion of the subglottis (Fig. 252).

Some carcinomas of the laryngeal wall of the epiglottis may have invaded the pre-epiglottic space (Fig. 254). By direct invasion, destruction of the laryngeal cartilages may have taken place, but this is often difficult to interpret in view of the fact that the calcification of these cartilages is quite variable. However, definite decalcification at the midline of the thyroid cartilage is practically a sure sign of invasion by tumor. This may be observed in either advanced tumors of the vocal cord or in early carcinoma of the laryngeal ventricle (Fig. 255). Edema of the laryngeal structures may be difficult to interpret in the absence of a definite diagnosis of carcinoma. Postirradiation roentgenograms may be distorted by edema in the presence as well as in the absence of recurrence. Baclesse[6] made a very extensive and didactic presentation of this diagnostic procedure. A profile view of the soft tissue of the neck gives explicit information as to the spread of the tumor in the sagittal plane but is not of much value in describing the transverse spread.

Leborgne's exhaustive investigation[57] of the normal and pathologic larynx by means of tomography is a definite addition to our means of examining this region of the body (Flach[39]). The tomograms as a complement of the profile roentgenograms,

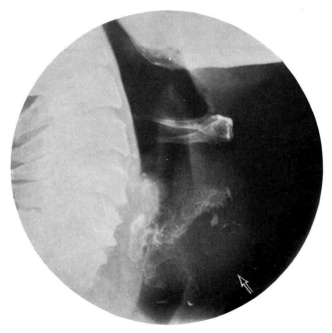

Fig. 252. Carcinoma of anterior commissure of vocal cords with invasion of thyroid cartilage and extension to anterior subglottic region. Note decalcification of thyroid cartilage anteriorly.

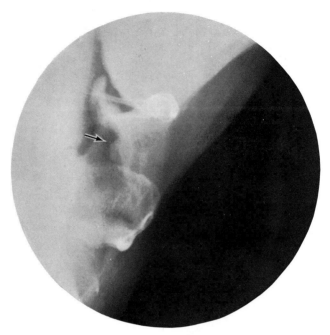

Fig. 253. Early carcinoma of laryngeal wall of epiglottis. (PCH 58-206.)

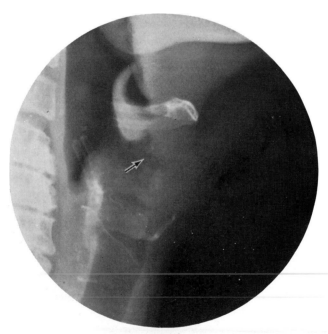

Fig. 254. Carcinoma of laryngeal wall of epiglottis. Note invasion of cartilage and extension in pre-epiglottic area as well as decalcification of thyroid cartilage anteriorly. (Courtesy Radium Institute, University of Paris, Paris, France.)

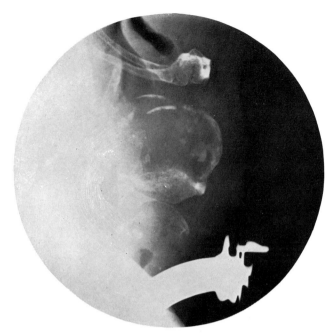

Fig. 255. Advanced carcinoma of laryngeal ventricle showing extensive destruction of thyroid cartilage and obstruction to air passages, necessitating tracheostomy. Note thickening of soft tissues around thyroid gland. Patient was living and well eight years after roentgentherapy.

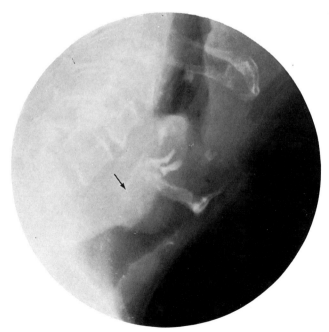

Fig. 256. Carcinoma of subglottis. Note almost complete obliteration of trachea and outstanding calcification of both arytenoid cartilages. (PCH 55-798.)

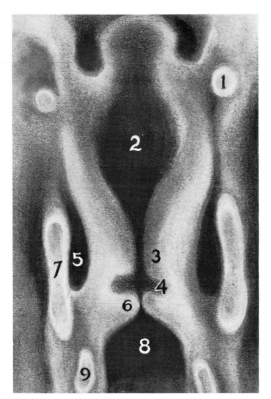

Fig. 257. Sketch of tomogram (laminagram) of normal adult male. 1, Cross section of hyoid bone. 2, Laryngeal vestibule. 3, False cords. 4, Laryngeal ventricle. 5, Piriform sinus. 6, True cord. 7, Cross section of thyroid cartilage. 8, Subglottis. 9, Cross section of cricoid cartilage.

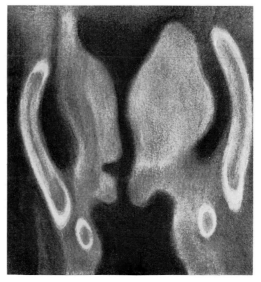

Fig. 258. Sketch of tomogram of larynx of patient with carcinoma of false cord. Note obliteration of laryngeal ventricle and bulging into piriform sinus.

permit evaluation of the spread of the tumor in all planes and are particularly useful in the tumors of the false cord and ventricle (Figs. 257 and 258).

The lateral roentgenogram and the simple tomogram of the larynx may be further enhanced by the use of a contrast medium in combination with either of these or a posteroanterior examination (Powers et al.[77, 78]; Lehman and Fletcher[60]; Fletcher and Jing[40]) (Fig. 259). The details obtained by contrast roentgenography have been utilized in staging (Howell et al.[49]). However, a contrast roentgenogram is not necessarily helpful nor is it a substitute for the basic radiographic examination of the soft tissues of the neck, anymore than tomograms or bronchography eliminate the basic roentgenogram of the chest. The interpretation of contrast roentgenograms lends itself to errors that

may be avoided (Holtz et al.[48]) by proper evaluation of all other diagnostic approaches.

Clinical classification

The International Union Against Cancer has proposed the use of the so-called TNM classification in these and various other tumors: T_1 to T_4 are variations of the primary tumor; N_0, N_1, and N_2 represent, respectively, absence of palpable or fixed adenopathy; M_0 and M_1 represent presence or absence of distant metastases. The use of these symbols does result in a convenient and rapid description permitting the grouping of like cases. The American Joint Committee on Cancer, representing various organizations, produced a set of definitions which have motivated various modified versions (MacComb[65]; Liegner and McCuaig[63]) or substitutions (Wang and Schulz[94]).

There are various points of contention: the relative importance of retained mobility and of fixation, whether or not fixation of one cord is graver than nonimmobilizing extension to both cords, whether or not extension beyond the endolarynx proper, regardless of structures involved, constitutes an extreme involvement. The obvious fact is that palpable adenopathy is not

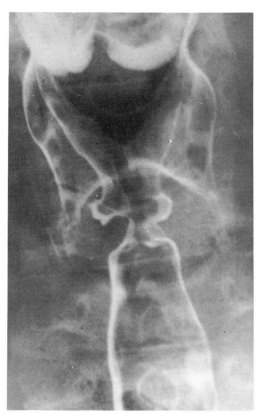

Fig. 259. Contrast posteroanterior roentgenogram of normal larynx showing contours of false cords, ventricles, true cords, and subglottis. (Courtesy Dr. G. H. Fletcher and Dr. B.-S. Jing, Houston, Texas; WU neg. 69-2412.)

always significant and that the actual development of an adenopathy is a significant transgression. The fact remains that, regardless of modifications, such classification may prove to be primarily an easy means of description and grouping of like cases. The prognostic value of the various classifications remains in doubt.

Biopsy

In most instances of carcinoma of the endolarynx, the diagnosis is clinically obvious. In every instance, nevertheless, microscopic proof is essential. Accordingly, a biopsy should be secured through indirect laryngoscopy. An effective local anesthesia is usually requisite. Biopsy of the larynx is often difficult, requiring special instruments and considerable experience. It should preferably be left to the specialist. At times, the obtention of a biopsy is impossible as,

for instance, in carcinomas of the laryngeal ventricle, where the ulceration is not visible, and consequently the biopsy on the smooth surface of the tumefaction will bring nothing but normal epithelium. Some advanced carcinomas of the vocal cord that infiltrate upward may be accompanied by so much edema of the false cord that the ulceration is not visible. In such cases, however, the biopsy is possible through direct laryngoscopy.

Differential diagnosis

Tuberculous lesions of the supraglottic area of the larynx may, at times, be confused with primary carcinomas. The tuberculous lesions are usually covered with abundant purulent material and mucus, are usually accompanied by abundant expectoration, and seldom interfere with the normal mobility of the larynx. They are secondary to pulmonary tuberculosis and are very rarely primary in the larynx. Radiographic examination of the lungs will consequently be of great value in establishing the differential diagnosis. At times, tumorlike tuberculous ulcerations may be observed in the space between the cords, posteriorly.

A *laryngocele* may be easily confused with a tumor of the laryngeal ventricle. Laryngoceles produce nonulcerated tumefactions of the false cord and usually have a long history with intermittent periods of remission. In some patients, percussion of the area of the larynx will result in a peculiar unilateral resonance. A lateral roentgenogram of the soft tissues of the neck may show an abnormal air bubble superimposed on the area of the false cord and the epiglottis (Fig. 260). In these cases, a tomogram of the larynx is very useful in revealing the existence of an air space lateral to the larynx. The laryngocele may be filled with mucus, in which case it will be more difficult to diagnose.

Keratosis (hyperkeratosis; leukoplakia; pachyderma laryngis) has long been considered a precancerous condition. It is not rare for laryngofissure, irradiation therapy, or laryngectomy to be suggested as therapy. We followed eighty-seven patients with this condition for a minimum of five and a maximum of fifteen years. In three, the cancer was missed at the first biopsy

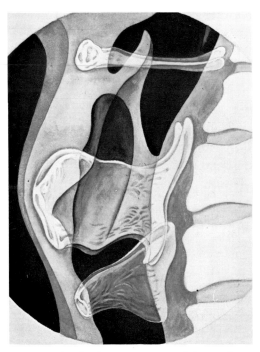

Fig. 260. Sketch of roentgenogram of larynx showing unusual, well-delimited, transparent air bubbles superimposed on areas of false cord and epiglottis. This should suggest laryngocele, which can be confirmed by tomogram of larynx.

and was found shortly thereafter. In the remaining eighty-four patients, three developed laryngeal cancer at intervals of nine months, six years, and eight years, respectively, after the diagnosis of keratosis. One of the patients died of laryngeal cancer, and the other two are living and well, one following surgery and the other following radiation therapy. Therefore, we believe that conservative therapeutic measures with careful follow-up and laryngeal examination and with biopsy as indicated are all that is necessary in this group of patients (McGavran et al.[66]). As far as we know, this is the only series of patients with keratosis that has been followed to determine the outcome. Consequently, we feel that the evidence that this is a precancerous lesion is not well established. Others agree with this concept (Lederman[59]; Derout et al.[34]).

Polyps of the vocal cords are a frequent cause of hoarseness. They appear as a glistening mass attached to the cord by a thin pedicle. In reality, these lesions are not tumors. They are formed by edema of the connective tissues, filled with varicosities (Cunning[31]). Laryngeal nodules, often called *singer's nodes,* are the result of a noninflammatory reaction to injury. They appear on the anterior third of the vocal cords, usually in persons who misuse their voices.

Papillomatosis usually presents as whitish grapelike growths, frequently pedunculated, extending to any surface within or outside the larynx: false cords, subglottis, artenoepiglottic folds, piriform sinus, epiglottis, tracheobronchial tree (Moore and Lattes[70]). Bronchioalveolar spread is rare and results in nodular densities in the roentgenogram (Rosenbaum et al.[83]). Björk and Weber[16] studied ninety-eight cases, almost half of which occurred in children under 5 years of age. Sex distribution was fairly equal in patients under the age of 40 years, but thereafter males predominated. Björk and Teir[15] did not confirm the frequent assertion that these lesions regress spontaneously after puberty. Transition of papillomas to carcinomas, if true, is a rare occurrence (Walsh and Beamer[93]). Practically all papillary carcinomas of the larynx are malignant from inception. Dmochowski et al.[35] found viral particles in the nuclei of cells of laryngeal papillomas. A viral origin has also been suggested by the transfer of papillomas from patients to laboratory animals.

A variety of treatments, including antibiotics and hormones, have been used with inconsistent results. Surgery is the treatment of choice, but radical treatment is justified only in the presence of anaplasia (Altmann et al.[3]). Rabbett[80] reported on eight children with laryngeal papillomas who received radiotherapy and developed carcinoma at a later date. Similar occurrences have both incriminated radiations for the "transformation" and developed the concept that radiotherapy is contraindicated in these lesions (Wlodyka[97]). In reality, papillomas recur after any form of treatment. It is difficult to ascertain whether or not these lesions "become" malignant or that their malignancy is recognized only after some time has elapsed and treatments have been unsuccessfully administered.

Oncocytic papillary cystadenomas of the

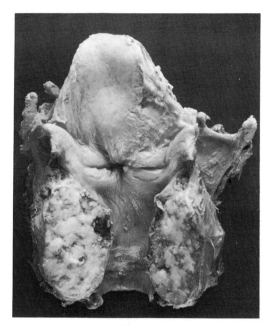

Fig. 261. Specimen of cartilaginous tumor arising from posterior one-half of cricoid cartilage. (From Goethals, P. L., et al.: Cartilaginous tumors of the larynx, Surg. Gynec. Obstet. **117**:77-82, 1963; by permission of Surgery, Gynecology & Obstetrics.)

larynx have been reported (Kroe et al.[54]). We have observed cases of *carcinoid, carcinosarcoma,* and *plasma cell myeloma.* About twenty-six cases of *granular cell myoblastoma* have been reported. *Pseudoepitheliomatous hyperplasia* is often mistaken for carcinoma (Ward and Oshiro[95]). *Neurofibromas* of the larynx may be observed as solitary lesions (Calvet and Claux[23]) or as part of a typical case of Recklinghausen's disease (Holinger and Cohen[46]).

Chondromas of the larynx usually arise from the inner aspect of the cricoid cartilage, infrequently from the thyroid cartilage, and rarely from the arytenoid. They cause dyspnea and appear as a submucous, smooth, nonulcerated lesion (Fig. 261). In 139 cartilaginous tumors studied by Van de Catsijne,[92] eighteen were *chondrosarcomas.* The treatment of choice is a surgical excision. In spite of the histologic appearance of chondrosarcoma, these tumors do not metastasize and are cured by local excision. Of eighteen cases of chondromatous tumors reported by Goethals et al.,[43] six recurred and necessitated further sur-

gery. Putney and Moran[79] reported two cases of chondrosarcoma of the larynx that recurred eight years after inadequate surgery.

Lymphosarcomas have rarely been seen in the larynx. Such cases are more likely to be manifestations of unsuspected chronic *lymphocytic leukemia.* A few cases of primary *malignant melanoma* of the larynx have been studied (Pantazopoulos[74]). Rare cases of *chemodectoma* have been recorded (Baxter[13]). Leroux-Robert[61] made a thorough clinical and surgical study of amyloid manifestations, or *"amyloid tumors"* of the larynx.

Treatment

The treatment of carcinomas of the endolarynx has always been the subject of circumstantial controversy, but vogues and unfounded partiality do not last. The favor once enjoyed by limited surgical procedures, such as laryngofissure (Jackson et al.[50]), has now waned. Although radiotherapy had previously shown good results in *early carcinomas of the vocal cord* (Regato[81]; Cantril[24]), it has now become evident that the results of cobalt[60] teletherapy and supervoltage roentgentherapy in these early lesions are rather consistently successful (Ennuyer and Bataini[37]; Buschke and Vaeth[20]; Hibbs and Hendrickson[45]; Chahbazian and Regato[27]). On the other hand, radiotherapy is no longer universally favored for the treatment of *early supraglottic carcinomas,* which may be controlled by partial laryngectomies. In general, in the treatment of *carcinomas of the subglottic region,* a total laryngectomy remains the treatment of choice (Fig. 262). Whether or not *advanced carcinomas* should be entrusted to radical surgery or radical radiotherapy remains a matter of the individual's convictions. Good results are not abundant in either case.

Radiotherapy

The treatment of carcinomas of the endolarynx by means of external irradiation is a delicate and fateful undertaking requiring careful planning and accurate performance. Lack of experience and skill usually spell failure. Cure lies between the narrow limits of enough to excessive irradiation, but the answer is not one of pre-

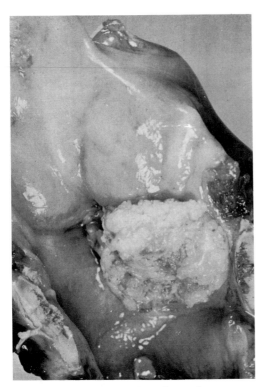

Fig. 262. Large verrucoid epidermoid carcinoma of subglottic area in 75-year-old man. Thirty-nine regional lymph nodes were negative. (WU neg. 57-5430.)

cise computing, for dosage is relative to the time in which it has been administered and to other circumstances of the treatment.

Conventional roentgentherapy required careful day-to-day observation of skin and mucous membrane reactions, of edema, etc., which permitted an appreciation of optimal daily dose and other details. The more precise field limits of supervoltage roentgentherapy and cobalt[60] teletherapy required better control, for it is relatively easy to fail to irradiate parts of an early lesion at the periphery of an inadequate field. With high-energy radiations, edema is seldom observed during the course of treatments and may only result subsequently when high daily doses and short courses of treatment are used.

Early carcinomas of the *vocal cord* are best suited for radiotherapy. Although they can be cured by conventional roentgentherapy, the high-energy radiations facilitate their adequate irradiation with greater impunity.

Moderately advanced lesions of the *glottic* region are also suitable for radiotherapy (Bryce et al.[18]). Fixation of the laryngeal musculature and subglottic infiltration are relatively unfavorable to radiotherapy. When radiotherapy fails in these lesions, a subsequent laryngectomy is not interfered with and often may be successful (Bryce et al.[18]), for irradiation may be limited to a small area within the larynx.

Carcinomas of the *supraglottic* region (or laryngeal vestibule) are curable by radiotherapy, but the conservative treatment is not so successful in these lesions except in early carcinomas of the laryngeal wall and false cords. Radiotherapy may be successful in carcinomas of the ventricle and in advanced carcinomas presenting destruction of the cartilages, but these results are not constant. The presence of a metastatic adenopathy does not, of necessity, eliminate the possibility of successful radiotherapy. Fletcher et al.[42] advocate laryngectomy and radical neck dissection for all large infiltrative carcinomas of the supraglottic region.

Carcinomas of the *subglottic* region may be controlled by radiotherapy but, in the past, the results have not warranted its practice as a treatment of choice. It is possible that dedicated efforts with cobalt[60] and supervoltage roentgentherapy may result in improvement of results in this area as well as in advanced carcinomas of any endolaryngeal origin.

Mucous membrane reactions and consequent dysphagia which resulted almost invariably from conventional roentgentherapy are seldom observed when high-energy radiations are utilized. The same is true of *skin reactions*, which are practically eliminated. *Edema* of the laryngeal structures depends primarily on the intensity of daily irradiation and on personal susceptibility. A preliminary *tracheostomy* is seldom necessary in supraglottic lesions, for the area allows for progressive adaptation. In the subglottic lesions, as well as in infiltrating lesions of the glottis, the opposite is true.

In the course of radiotherapy, the melting of the neoplasm may result in necrotic ulcerations that require careful attention. Early administration of antibiotics often minimizes the consequences. Chondronecrosis seldom occurs as a consequence of radiations alone except in cases of excessive irradiation or too short, intensive treatments. In advanced lesions with invasion of the cartilage, chondronecrosis is unavoidable but not necessarily serious or fatal, depending on location and management.

Surgery

The surgical removal of the larynx can be extended to include the upper part of the esophagus and to be carried out in continuity with neck dissection. A *total laryngectomy* is most successful in the treatment of early lesions of the vocal cords and supraglottic regions, which are also highly curable by radiotherapy. It has its best indication in the treatment of subglottic carcinomas that may invade the anterior wall of the esophagus and in the treatment of postirradiation recurrences (Arndt[4]; Baker[9]). A frequent cause of failure of total laryngectomies is the development of cervical lymph node metastases (Ogura et al.[73]; Carveth et al.[25]). For this reason, a prophylactic neck dissection in continuity is advisable. Stomal recurrences appear either in the soft tissues of the region of the stoma or in the submucosa of the trachea. The latter is due to subglottic extension and inadequate excision. Stomal recurrences often follow resection of advanced tumors, and very few can be recovered (Keim et al.[53]; Burnham and Hudson[19]). The price a patient must pay for a total laryngectomy is loss of voice, a permanent tracheostomy, and the necessity of learning to communicate by artificial means.

Following laryngectomy, an artificial voice may be acquired in various ways. The most satisfactory pseudovoice may be produced through coordination of respiration and aerophagia and the production of guttural, lingual, and labial sounds. This voice lacks variation in pitch and is usually monotonous. Acceptable speech is developed in 70% of the patients (Smith et al.[87]). Most patients adjust to important mutilations or dysfunctions necessitated by surgical treatment, but loss of speech requires emotional and intellectual adaptation which may not be possible in all patients (Bisi and Conley[14]; Barton[11]). The

extrovert, the enterprising optimist with a passion for salesmanship, seem to adapt best.

In an effort to avoid the complete loss of voice, *partial laryngectomies* of various kinds have been devised and used for carcinomas of the endolarynx in different locations. Once the most popular of these procedures, the laryngofissure, has fallen from favor mostly because of the success of radiotherapy in the early lesions of the cord, for which it was used. Ideally, the laryngofissure implies a block removal of the true cord with portions of the false cord, ventricle, and subglottis. A review by McGavran et al.[68] of seventy-nine specimens of laryngofissure for carcinoma of the true cord revealed that there was frequent extension of the tumor to the limits of excision. This procedure has narrow indications and limited success.

Sagittal hemilaryngectomies have never enjoyed great vogue. *Transverse hemilaryngectomies* have been advocated for the treatment of early supraglottic carcinomas that have not extended to the glottis, to the arytenoids, or to the pre-epiglottic space (Leroux-Robert and Ennuyer[62]; Alonso[2]; Ogura and Mallen[72]). The frequent association of the latter procedure with postoperative radiotherapy, although undeniably fruitful, makes it difficult to appreciate the true value of the surgical procedure itself.

In very selected patients with postirradiation recurrence of carcinoma of the vocal cord, the partial laryngectomy may prove fruitful (Ballantyne and Fletcher[10]). In recent years, there have been various reports of partial laryngectomy followed by radical radiotherapy with apparent good results. Ennuyer and Bataini[62] reported excellent five-year and ten-year survival rates yet did not advocate the routine use of the procedure.

Prognosis

In 1965, there were 2629 deaths from cancer of the larynx in the United States, a crude death rate of 1.4 per 100,000. Except for white females, a slight increase in death rates in the last three decades seems to have occurred.

The carcinoma of the larynx with the most favorable prognosis is that in the anterior two-thirds of the vocal cord. In a series of sixteen consecutive carcinomas of the vocal cord reported by Chahbazian and Regato,[27] five with some limitation of mobility and two with involvement of the anterior commissure and opposite cord, only one of the patients showed a recurrence after treatment with *cobalt*[60] *teletherapy*. In Buschke and Vaeth's series[20] of twenty-one patients with carcinomas of the vocal cord irradiated with one million volt roentgentherapy, there were six recurrences, all but one of which were controlled by subsequent laryngectomy. Perez et al.[75] reported a greater proportion of recurrences, following radiotherapy, in carcinomas with extension to the opposite cord. Of eighteen patients with recurrence, seven were salvaged by hemilaryngectomy and three had total laryngectomy. Wang and Schulz[94] had 140 five-year survivals (60%) in a series of 276 patients with carcinomas of the larynx in all stages treated by radiotherapy. Twelve of their failures were salvaged by laryngectomy. Ennuyer and Bataini[38] had eighteen survivals after cobalt[60] teletherapy in thirty-three patients with supraglottic carcinomas. Four out of eight with lymph node metastases were apparently controlled. Dahl et al.[33] obtained 123 survivals (64%) in a series of 790 patients irradiated for carcinomas in all stages.

Smith et al.[88] gathered and studied 600 cases of carcinoma of the larynx, in various stages, treated in seven institutions by surgery, radiotherapy, or both. In 135 tumors confined to the site of origin (T_1), the five-year survival rates were 92% and 87% for the glottic and the supraglottic lesions, respectively. In 283 carcinomas spreading beyond the site of origin, but still relatively confined (T_2), the five-year survival rate was 70%. In fifty-three more extensive lesions (T_3) and in ninety-eight tumors extending beyond the larynx (T_4), the five-year survival rates were 40% and 20%, respectively. Of 151 patients with a palpable adenopathy, only thirty-six (29%) survived five years. Shaw,[86] reporting on 306 patients with glottic carcinomas, noted that if the tumors were limited, the five-year survival rate following radiotherapy or surgery was 85%, whereas the crude five-year survival rate for all cases was 62%. Shaw[86]

advocates radiotherapy for the early lesions and surgery for the advanced ones or for those presenting a metastatic adenopathy.

Carveth et al.[25] reported on the results of radical surgery at the Mayo Clinic. Of 240 patients who had a *total laryngectomy* for endolaryngeal carcinoma, 147 (60%) survived five years. Of ninety patients who had a metastatic adenopathy and who were treated by laryngectomy and neck dissection, twenty-five (36%) survived. Barton[11] observed five cases of suicide in a series of fifty patients who had had a laryngectomy. The results of partial laryngectomies on selected patients are difficult to evaluate, partly because the limited operation is frequently associated with postoperative radiotherapy.

Leroux-Robert and Ennuyer[62] reported on a large series of carcinoma of the larynx treated by a combination of laryngectomy and postoperative radiotherapy at the Fondation Curie. Their results were impressive in view of the extensive material, the quality of both the surgery and the radiotherapy, and the excellent follow-up. In 159 patients so treated for supraglottic lesions, eighty-five (53%) were reported surviving five years. Ninety-six patients treated in this manner yielded a ten-year survival of 33% (Ennuyer and Bataini[36]).

REFERENCES

1 Ackerman, L. V., Wiley, H. M., and LeMone, D. V.: Necrotizing bronchopneumonia, Amer. J. Roentgen. 53:281-289, 1945.

2 Alonso, J. M.: Conservative surgery of cancer of the larynx, Trans. Amer. Acad. Ophthal. 51: 633-642, 1947.

3 Altmann, F., Basek, M., and Stout, A. P.: Papillomas of the larynx with intraepithelial anaplastic changes, Arch. Otolaryng. (Chicago) 62:478-485, 1955.

4 Arndt, J.: Zur Prognose und Therapie der inneren Larynxtumoren, Strahlentherapie 122: 27-36, 1963.

5 Baclesse, F.: Carcinomas of the larynx, Brit. J. Radiol. (suppl. 3), pp. 1-62, 1949.

6 Baclesse, F.: Tumeurs malignes du pharynx et du larynx; étude anatomo-topographique et radiographique, Paris, 1960, Masson et Cie.

7 Baclesse, F.: Comparative study of results obtained with conventional radiotherapy (200 KV) and cobalt therapy in the treatment of cancer of the larynx, Clin. Radiol. 18:292-300, 1967.

8 Baclesse, F., and Henry, R.: Les cancers glottiques anterieurs (considerations radiograph-

iques et radiothérapiques), J. Radiol. Electr. **31**:1-7, 1950.

9 Baker, H. W.: Surgical management of recurrent laryngeal cancer after irradiation, Cancer **16**:774-780, 1963.

10 Ballantyne, A. J., and Fletcher, G. H.: Preservation of the larynx in the surgical treatment of cancer, recurrent after radiation therapy, Amer. J. Roentgen. **99**:336-339, 1967.

11 Barton, R. T.: Life after laryngectomy, Laryngoscope **75**:1408-1415, 1965.

12 Bauer, W. C., Edwards, D. L., and McGavran, M. H.: A critical analysis of laryngectomy in the treatment of epidermoid carcinoma of the larynx, Cancer **15**:263-270, 1962.

13 Baxter, J. D.: Glomus tumor (chemodectoma) of the larynx, Ann. Otol. **74**:813-820, 1965.

14 Bisi, R. H., and Conley, J. J.: Psychologic factors influencing vocal rehabilitation of the postlaryngectomy patient, Ann. Otol. **74**:1073-1078, 1965.

15 Björk, H., and Teir, H.: Benign and malignant papilloma of the larynx in adults; a comparative clinical and histological study, Acta Otolaryng. (Stockholm) **47**:95-104, 1957.

16 Björk, H., and Weber, C.: Papilloma of the larynx, Acta Otolaryng. (Stockholm) **46**:499-516, 1956 (extensive bibliography).

17 Bockmühl, F.: Is the incidence of laryngeal cancer higher in women than in men at early ages? H.N.O. **14**:99-100, 1966.

18 Bryce, D. P., Ireland, P. E., and Rider, W. D.: Experience in the surgical and radiological treatment in 500 cases of carcinoma of the larynx, Ann. Otol. **72**:1-15, 1963.

19 Burnham, J. A., and Hudson, W. R.: Stomal recurrence of malignancy and evaluation and its significance in the post-laryngectomy patient, Southern Med. J. **60**:823-826, 1967.

20 Buschke, F., and Vaeth, J. M.: Radiation therapy of carcinoma of the vocal cord without mucosal reaction, Amer. J. Roentgen. **89**:29-34, 1963.

21 Cady, B., Rippey, J. H., and Frazell, E. L.: Non-epidermoid cancer of the larynx, Ann. Surg. **167**:116-120, 1968.

22 Cahan, W. G., and Montemayor, P. B.: Cancer of the larynx and lung in the same patients, a report of 60 cases, J. Thorac. Cardiovasc. Surg. **44**:309-320, 1962.

23 Calvet, J., and Claux, G.: Le neurinome du larynx, Rev. Laryng. (Bordeaux) **69**:47-60, 1948.

24 Cantril, S.: Radiation therapy in cancer of the larynx; a review, Amer. J. Roentgen. **81**:456-474, 1959.

25 Carveth, S. W., Devine, K. D., and ReMine, W. H.: Laryngectomy with radical neck dissection in extensive cancer of the larynx, Amer. J. Surg. **104**:705-707, 1962.

26 Caulk, R. M.: End results of radiotherapy in laryngeal cancer based upon clinical staging by the T.N.M. system, Amer. J. Roentgen. **96**:588-592, 1966.

27 Chahbazian, C. M., and del Regato, J. A.: Cobalt 60 teletherapy of early carcinoma of the vocal cords, Amer. J. Roentgen. **99**:333-335, 1967.

28 Coutard, Henri: Note preliminaire sur la radiographie du larynx normal et du larynx cancereux, J. Radiol. Electr., pp. 461-465, 1924.

29 Coutard, Henri, and Baclesse, F.: Roentgen diagnosis during the course of roentgen therapy of epitheliomas of the larynx and hypopharynx, Amer. J. Roentgen. **28**:293-312, 1932.

30 Cova, P. L.: Valutazione critica del metodo stratigrafico nel carcinoma laringeo, Radiol. Med. (Torino) **33**:505-533, 1947.

31 Cunning, D. S.: Diagnosis and treatment of laryngeal tumors, J.A.M.A. **142**:73-76, 1950.

32 Curtiss, C., and Kosinski, A. A.: Primary melanoma of the larynx, Cancer **8**:961-963, 1955.

33 Dahl, O., Jacobsson, F., and Walstam, R.: Telegamma therapy of laryngeal carcinoma, Acta Radiol. [Ther.] (Stockholm) **7**:81-87, 1968.

34 Derout, J., de Brux, J., and Leroux-Robert, J.: Étude histologique et statistique des dysplasies du larynx et leurs rapports avec les cancers, Ann. Otolaryng. (Paris) **81**:789-800, 1964.

35 Dmochowski, L., Grey, C. E., Sykes, J. A., Dreyer, D. A., Langford, P., Jesse, R. H. Jr., MacComb, W. S., and Ballantyne, J. A.: A study of submicroscopic structure and of virus particles in cells of human laryngeal papillomas, Texas Rep. Biol. Med. **22**:454-491, 1964.

36 Ennuyer, A., and Bataini, P.: Traitement du cancer du larynx; place actuelle de la radiothérapie, Gaz. Med. France **69**:3003-3013, 1962.

37 Ennuyer, A., and Bataini, P.: Télécobalthérapie des épithéliomas du vestibule laryngé, Ann. Otolaryng. (Paris) **81**:747-754, 1964.

38 Ennuyer, A., and Bataini, P.: Treatment of supra-glottic tumors by telecobalt therapy, Brit. J. Radiol. **38**:661-666, 1965.

39 Flach, M.: Zur Röntgenunlersuchung beim Kehlkapfkarzinom; Eine kritische Gegenüberstellung der Leistungsfähigkeit von Larynxtomographie und Laryngographie, Mschr. Ohrenheilk. **98**:397-412, 1964.

40 Fletcher, G. H., and Jing, B.-S.: The head and neck (Hodes, P. J., editor-in-chief: Atlas of tumor radiology; sponsored by The American College of Radiology), Chicago, 1968, Year Book Medical Publishers, Inc.

41 Fletcher, G. H., and Klein, R.: Dose-time-volume relationship in squamous-cell carcinoma of the larynx, Radiology **82**:1032-1042, 1964.

42 Fletcher, G. H., Jesse, R. H., Lindberg, R. D., and Koons, C. R.: The place of radiotherapy in the management of the squamous-cell carcinoma of the supraglottic larynx, Amer. J. Roentgen. **108**:19-26, 1970.

43 Goethals, P. L., Dahlin, D. C., and Devine, K. D.: Cartilaginous tumors of the larynx, Surg. Gynec. Obstet. **117**:77-82, 1963.

44 Harris, W., Kramer, R., and Silverstone, S. M.: Roentgen therapy for carcinoma of the larynx, Radiology **51**:708-716, 1948.

45 Hibbs, G. G., and Hendrickson, F. R.: Tele-

cobalt therapy of early malignant tumors of vocal cord, Radiology 86:447-449, 1966.

46 Holinger, P. H., and Cohen, L. L.: Neurofibromatosis (von Recklinghausen's disease) with involvement of the larynx; report of a case, Laryngoscope 60:193-196, 1950.

47 Holt, J. A. G.: Tumours of the larynx; the place of radiotherapy in the management of laryngeal cancer (the Nisbet symposium), J. Coll. Radiol. Aust. 9:199-203, 1965.

48 Holtz, S., Powers, W. E., McGavran, M. H., and Ogura, J.: Contrast examination of the larynx and pharynx; glottic, infraglottic and transglottic tumors, Amer. J. Roentgen. 89: 10-28, 1963.

49 Howell, T. J., Gildersleeve, G. A., and King, E. R.: The role of roentgenographic studies in the evaluation and staging of malignancies of the larynx and pharynx, Amer. J. Roentgen. 102:138-144, 1968.

50 Jackson, C. L., Blady, J. V., Norris, C. M., and Maloney, W. H.: Cancer of the larynx, J.A.M.A. 138:1080-1082, 1948.

51 Johnson, N. E., and Sisson, G. A.: Carcinoma of the larynx—review of 100 cases, Laryngoscope 74:710-722, 1964.

52 Jones, D. G., and Gabriel, C. E.: The incidence of carcinoma of the larynx in persons under twenty years of age, Laryngoscope 79: 251-255, 1969.

53 Keim, W. F., Shapiro, M. J., and Rosin, H. D.: Study of postlaryngectomy stomal recurrence, Arch. Otolaryng. (Chicago) 81:183-186, 1965.

54 Kroe, D. J., Pitcock, J. A., and Cocke, E. W.: Oncocytic papillary cystadenoma of the larynx; presentation of two cases, Arch. Path. (Chicago) 84:429-432, 1967.

55 Kuhn, A. J., Devine, K. D., and McDonald, J. R.: Cervical metastases from squamous cell carcinoma of the larynx, Laryngoscope 67: 169-190, 1957.

56 Lane, N.: Pseudosarcoma (polypoid sarcomalike masses) associated with squamous-cell carcinoma of the mouth, fauces, and larynx; report of ten cases, Cancer 10:19-41, 1957.

57 Leborgne, Felix: Tomographic study of cancer of the larynx, Amer. J. Roentgen. 43:493-499, 1940.

58 Lederman, M.: Cancer of the larynx. Classification: technique and results of teleradium treatment, Acta Un. Int. Cancr. 6:1249-1252, 1950.

59 Lederman, M.: Keratosis of the larynx, J. Laryng. 77:651-659, 1963.

60 Lehmann, Q. H., and Fletcher, G. H.: Contribution of the laryngogram to the management of malignant laryngeal tumors, Radiology 83:486-500, 1964.

61 Leroux-Robert, M. J.: "Tumeurs amyloides" du larynx, Ann. Otolaryng. (Paris) 79:249-270, 1962.

62 Leroux-Robert, J., and Ennuyer, A.: Resultats de l'association chirurgie-roentgenthérapie ou de la chirurgie seule dans les épithéliomas du larynx traités selon des indications thérapeutiques determinées (200 cas avec recul de plus de 5 Ans), Ann. Otolaryng. (Paris) 73: 521-545, 1956.

63 Liegner, L. M., and McCuaig, D.: Laryngeal cancer; primary treatment with cobalt 60 in a general hospital, Radiology 84:718-726, 1965.

64 Low-Beer, B. V. A.: Radiation therapy of cancer of the larynx, Laryngoscope 60:696-717, 1950.

65 MacComb, W. S.: Cancer of the larynx, Cancer 19:149-156, 1966.

66 McGavran, M. H., Bauer, W. C., and Ogura, J. H.: Isolated laryngeal keratosis; its relation to carcinoma of the larynx based on a clinicopathologic study of 87 consecutive cases with long-term follow-up, Laryngoscope 70:932-951, 1960.

67 McGavran, M. H., Bauer, W. C., and Ogura, J. H.: The incidence of cervical lymph node metastases from epidermoid carcinoma of the larynx and their relationship to certain characteristics of the primary tumor; a study based on the clinical and pathological findings in 96 patients treated by primary en bloc laryngectomy and radical neck dissection, Cancer 14: 55-66, 1961.

68 McGavran, M. H., Spjut, H. J., and Ogura, J.: Laryngofissure in the treatment of laryngeal carcinoma; a critical analysis of success and failure, Laryngoscope 69:44-53, 1959.

69 Moore, C.: Smoking and cancer of the mouth, pharynx, and larynx, J.A.M.A. 191:283-286, 1965.

70 Moore, R. L., and Lattes, R.: Papillomatosis of larynx and bronchi; case report with 34-year follow-up, Cancer 12:117-126, 1959.

71 Ogura, J. H.: Cancer of larynx, pharynx, and upper cervical esophagus, Arch. Otolaryng. (Chicago) 72:66-72, 1960.

72 Ogura, J. H., and Mallen, R. W.: Carcinoma of the larynx; diagnosis and treatment, Postgrad. Med. 34:493-498, 1963.

73 Ogura, J. H., Powers, W. E., Holtz, S., McGavran, M. H., Ellis, B., and Voorhees, R.: Laryngograms: their value in the diagnosis and treatment of laryngeal lesions, a study based on clinical, radiographic and pathologic findings on 99 patients with cancer of the larynx, Laryngoscope 70:780-809, 1960.

74 Pantazopoulos, P. E.: Primary malignant melanoma of the larynx, Laryngoscope 74:95-102, 1964.

75 Perez, C. A., Holtz, S., Ogura, J. H., Dedo, H. H., and Powers, W. E.: Radiation therapy of early carcinoma of the true vocal cords, Cancer 21:764-777, 1968.

76 Pietrantoni, L., Agazzi, C., and Fior, R.: Indications for surgical treatment of cervical lymphnodes in cancer of the larynx and hypopharynx, Laryngoscope 72:1511-1527, 1962.

77 Powers, W. E., Holtz, S., Ogura, J. H., Ellis, B. I., and McGavran, M. H.: Contrast examination of larynx and pharynx; accuracy and value in diagnosis, Amer. J. Roentgen. 86:651-660, 1961.

78 Powers, W. E., McGee, H. H., Jr., and Seaman, W. B.: Contrast examination of the larynx and pharynx, Radiology 68:169-178, 1957.

79 Putney, E. J., and Moran, J. J.: Cartilaginous tumors of the larynx, Ann. Otol. **73**:370-380, 1964.

80 Rabbett, W. F.: Juvenile laryngeal papillomatosis, Ann. Otol. **74**:1149-1164, 1965.

81 del Regato, J. A.: Symposium: carcinoma of the larynx; roentgen therapy of carcinoma of the endolarynx, Laryngoscope **61**:511-516, 1951.

82 Robbins, R.: Indications of radiation therapy in laryngeal cancer, Amer. J. Roentgen. **83**: 21-24, 1960.

83 Rosenbaum, H. D., Alavi, S. M., and Bryant, L. R.: Pulmonary parenchymal spread of juvenile laryngeal papillomatosis, Radiology **90**:654-660, 1968.

84 Rush, B. F., Jr., Reynolds, G., and Greenlaw, R.: Integrated irradiation and operation in treatment of cancer of the larynx and hypopharynx; a preliminary report, Amer. J. Roentgen. **102**:129-131, 1968.

85 Schall, L. A.: Cancer of the larynx; 5-year results, Laryngoscope **61**:517-522, 1951.

86 Shaw, H. J.: Glottic cancer of the larynx (1947-1956), J. Laryng. **79**:1-14, 1965.

87 Smith, J. K., Rise, E. N., and Gralnek, D. E.: Speech recovery in laryngectomized patients, Laryngoscope **76**:1540-1546, 1966.

88 Smith, R. R., Caulk, R., Jackson, L. C., and Russell, W.: End result of 600 laryngeal cancers using the American Joint Committee's method of classification and end-result reporting, Surg. Gynec. Obstet. **113**:435-444, 1961.

89 Som, M. L.: Surgical treatment of carcinoma of the epiglottis by lateral pharyngotomy, Trans. Amer. Acad. Ophthal. **63**:28-49, 1959.

90 Stout, A. P.: Intramucosal epithelioma of the larynx, Amer. J. Roentgen. **69**:1-13, 1953.

91 Taylor, H. M.: Ventricular laryngocele, Trans. Amer. Laryng. Ass. **66**:114-126, 1944.

92 Van de Catsijne, L.: Les tumeurs cartilagineuses du larynx, Acta Otorhinolaryng. Belg. **19**:875-912, 1965 (extensive bibliography).

93 Walsh, T. E., and Beamer, P. R.: Epidermoid carcinoma of the larynx occurring in two children with papilloma of the larynx, Laryngoscope **60**:1110-1124, 1950.

94 Wang, C. C., and Schulz, M. D.: Treatment of cancer of the larynx by irradiation, Ann. Otol. **72**:637-646, 1963.

95 Ward, P. H., and Oshiro, H.: Laryngeal granular-cell myoblastoma, Arch. Otolaryng. (Chicago) **76**:239-244, 1962.

96 Welsh, L. W.: The normal human laryngeal lymphatics, Ann. Otol. **73**:569-583, 1964.

97 Wlodyka, J.: The cancerogenic effect of x-ray on the larynx, Arch. Otolaryng. (Chicago) **76**: 372-388, 1962.

98 Wynder, E. L., Bross, I. J., and Day, E.: Epidemiological approach to the etiology of cancer of the larynx, J.A.M.A. **160**:1384-1391, 1956.

Lung

Anatomy

The lungs are half-cone-shaped organs appended to each of the two branches of bifurcation of the trachea, the main bronchi. They are separated in the midline by several organs which together are known as the mediastinum.

The lungs are divided externally into lobes by deep oblique fissures extending from above downward and from outside inward. The right lung has an additional transverse fissure and is thus divided into three lobes, the upper, the middle, and the lower, whereas the left lung has only two lobes. The external surface of the lung is covered by the pleura, a serous membrane that continues on to form the inner lining of the thoracic cage, thus forming a double envelope around the lungs on each side of the mediastinum.

Each lung contains the branches of successive subdivision of the bronchi until their termination in the pulmonary lobules. The bronchi are protected from collapse by incomplete rings of cartilage that become progressively spaced as the bronchi become smaller until they are merely wide plaques without annular shape. The bronchi are formed by three layers:

1 An inner layer of ciliated columnar epithelium with goblet cells resting on a lamina propria

2 The submucosa that contains numerous mucous glands and often lymphoid nodules

3 A muscular layer with an outer connective tissue lining that supports the bronchi

To designate the subdivisions of the bronchi we suggest the use of the international nomenclature accepted by the Thoracic Society (Table 20).

The lungs are supplied with blood by the bronchial arteries usually originating in the thoracic aorta and occupying a position posterior to the main bronchi. The branches of the bronchial artery within the lung accompany the divisions and subdivisions of the bronchi, extending to the pulmonary lobules without penetrating

Table 20. Designation of subdivisions of bronchi*

Lobe	Segments
Right lung	
Upper lobe	Apical bronchus
	Posterior bronchus
	Anterior bronchus
Middle lobe	Lateral bronchus
	Medial bronchus
Lower lobe	Apical bronchus
	Medial basal (cardiac) bronchus
	Anterior basal bronchus
	Lateral basal bronchus
	Posterior basal bronchus
Left lung	
Upper lobe	Apical bronchus
	Posterior bronchus
	Anterior bronchus
Lingula	Superior bronchus
	Inferior bronchus
Lower lobe	Apical bronchus
	Anterior basal bronchus
	Lateral basal bronchus
	Posterior basal bronchus

*Data from Thoracic Society: The nomenclature of broncho-pulmonary anatomy; an international nomenclature accepted by the Thoracic Society, Thorax 5:222-228, 1950.

them. The bronchial tree within the lobule and the lobule itself are irrigated by the branches of the pulmonary arteries. The oxygenated blood returning to the lungs travels through the pulmonary veins, which gather into two main trunks on each side, and finally travel to the base of the heart, where they open into the left auricle. In addition to the bronchi and the blood vessels, the lungs contain nerves, connective tissue, and lymphatics.

Lymphatics. The lymphatics of the lungs are a very rich intercommunicating network (Fig. 263). The superficial lymphatics of the visceral pleura and the deep lymphatics accompanying the bronchi and pulmonary veins are the most important. There are no lymphatics in the alveoli beyond the ductuli alveolaris. The rich plexus of lymphatics accompanying the pulmonary veins becomes more abundant as it flows toward the hilum. These lymphatics communicate with those of the bronchi and of the pleura. In each lung there are three areas of lymphatic drainage: the superior, the middle, and the inferior (Rouvière[236]).

In the *right lung*, the *superior area* is the anteromedial region of the superior lobe. Its lymphatics are drained by the right laterotracheal lymph nodes and particularly by the large node situated at the arch of the azygous vein. The *middle area* comprises the posterolateral region of the superior lobe, the middle lobe, and the superior region of the inferior lobe. It is drained by the right laterotracheal and intertracheobronchial lymph nodes. The *lower area* is drained by the lymph nodes of the bifurcation.

In the *left lung*, the *superior area* comprises the upper region of the superior lobe that is drained by the left laterotracheal nodes, the lymph node of the arterial canal, the anterior mediastinal chain of lymph nodes, and the subaortic lymph nodes. The *middle area* is formed by the lower region of the superior lobe and the superior and middle regions of the inferior lobe. It is drained by nodes in the anterior mediastinal and laterotracheal chains and also by the nodes at the bifurcation. The *inferior area* comprises the lower region of the inferior lobe and is drained by the lymph nodes at the bifurcation. Thus, the lymphatics of the left lower lobe may drain into the lymph nodes of the right upper mediastinum. The investigation of living patients using dyes has demonstrated that the lymphatic drainage of the left lower lobe is *predominantly* ipsilateral to the left prescalene lymph nodes (Baker et al.[13]).

The lymphatics of the *parietal pleura* can be divided into those of the diaphragm and those of the thoracic wall. The collecting trunks of the lymphatics of the diaphragm empty into the lateral precardiac and anterior mediastinal lymph nodes on the left and the posterior mediastinal lymph nodes on the right. The collecting trunks of the posterior region of the diaphragm communicate with the rich network of subperitoneal infradiaphragmatic lymphatics that terminate in intra-abdominal para-aortic nodes. They are also in communication with the lymphatics of the liver, the adipose capsule of the kidney, and the suprarenal gland. The lymphatics of the thoracic pleura are divided by Rouvière[236] into three regions:

1 Those of the first costal arch, first intercostal space, and entire pleural dome that are drained by the lymph nodes of the transverse cervical and

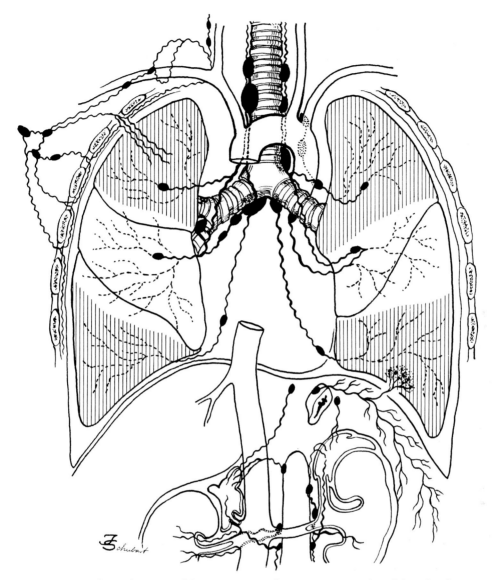

Fig. 263. Lymphatic drainage of lung. Drainage does not correspond to lobar distribution. Pleural symphysis leads to axillary and subdiaphragmatic metastases.

internal jugular chains; they may also drain into a subclavian or mediastinal trunk; at times, some of these collecting trunks may terminate in the upper axillary nodes.

2 Those located between the second and fourth ribs that are drained by the lymph nodes of the posterior intercostal and internal mammary chains, but some may occasionally end in axillary lymph nodes.

3 Those extending from the fourth to the sixth rib; the collecting trunks of

this region may also empty into axillary lymph nodes.

Rouvière[236] also pointed out that nodes of the tracheal bifurcation form a crossroad where lymphatic vessels that issue from the diaphragm, heart, cardia, esophagus, inferior part of the trachea, bronchi, and lungs meet directly or by means of lymphoid relays.

Epidemiology

Carcinoma of the bronchus has become the most frequent form of cancer in men

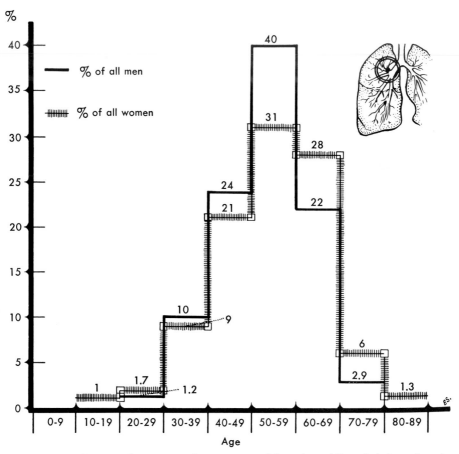

Fig. 264. Age of men and women with carcinoma of bronchus. (Compiled from data from Churchill et al.,[55] Ochsner et al.,[197] Overholt et al.,[204] and various other sources.)

in the United States and many other countries (Denoix and Gelle[75]). In 1912, Adler had difficulty in collecting 374 cases of cancer of the lung. In the 1947 cancer survey in the United States, the sex-age adjusted incidence of cancer of the lung was 29.2 for males and 6.43 for females per 100,000. There was a slightly greater incidence in whites than in nonwhites of both sexes. In the state of Connecticut, the incidence increased from 22.1 and 4.1 in 1945-1949 to 46.4 and 7.0 in 1960-1962 for males and females, respectively. A similar increase in incidence was observed in the state of New York. After 35 years of age, the incidence increases progressively so that it is over 200 per 100,000 in men of 60 to 64 years old.

In 1968, approximately 60,000 Americans developed cancer of the lung. The incidence in males doubled in Denmark from 1943-1947 to 1953-1957, whereas the incidence in females increased only two-thirds as much. Japan reported the next to the lowest rate in males in 1962-1963, yet this represented a fourfold increase since 1950-1951.

There is no doubt that this increase in cancer of the lung is real. The incidence rate for successively younger cohorts continues to increase. *Aging of the population* is not a prominent feature in the increase (Dunn[83]), for if crude mortality rates are corrected to relate them to a standard population of a fixed age distribution, the trend is not affected. Assuming some *faulty certification of deaths*, such errors could not possibly explain the magnitude of the increase (Gilliam[109]). It is not possible to assume that the increase is due to *better diagnosis* for, in view of the disproportionate increase in men, one would have to admit a difference in the diagnostic acumen according to sex (Shimkin[249]). Bonser and Thomas[35] made a study of the accuracy of the clinical diagnosis in the city of Leeds and found that false positive diagnoses were infrequent. There was no sex difference in the accuracy of certification.

This fantastic increase in cancer of the lung has resulted in the most extensive clinical, epidemiologic, and laboratory investigations ever attempted. Certain facts emerge from the welter of hundreds of articles written on this subject. There are many causes of cancer of the lung, although most of them share a minor part of the problem. All evidence suggests that these causes are environmental products of modern civilization. There are also variations in individual susceptibility. Carcinoma of the larynx may follow successful treatment of carcinoma of the bronchus (Lavelle[164a]).

The great influenza epidemic of 1918 with its metaplastic changes in the bronchi was thought to predispose to cancer of the lung (Winternitz et al.[297]). Proof of such relationship never developed. *Tuberculosis* may precede or coexist with bronchial carcinomas, but no relationship of cause to effect has been shown. Coincidence of pulmonary tuberculosis and carcinoma results from prolongation of life of patients with tuberculosis and increase in the incidence of pulmonary cancer. *Bronchiectasis* may be associated with squamous metaplasia of the bronchi, but this chronic lung disease does not appear to predispose to cancer. Previous pulmonary infection has nothing to do with lung cancer (McClung[173]). *Anthracosis* and *anthracosilicosis* are not related to carcinoma of the lung (Vorwald and Karr[285]). Ashley[10] found that individuals working in coal and textile industries had an excess of bronchitis and a deficit of lung cancer. He suggested that chronic lung disease associated with the inhalation of dust could confer protection on the lung against carcinogenic substances. There seems to be no doubt that cancer can develop within a preexisting *scar* within the lung. The number of such cases, however, is small (Raeburn and Spencer[216]; Yokoo and Suckow[204]). Primary adenocarcinoma may develop from bronchial atypia in a lung scar (Sasser et al.[240]). In congenital *cystic disease* of the lung, areas of atypical epithelium may be observed, either alone or associated with cancer, suggesting a possible causal relationship (Womack and Graham[298]).

There is adequate experimental and epidemiologic evidence to incriminate various organic and inorganic industry-related chemicals as causes of cancer of the lung (Hueper[139]), with definite risk to specific worker groups (Table 21). This is supported by experimental investigations in which cancer of the lung has been produced in animals exposed to radioactive metals, nickel, chromium, arsenic, etc. Occupational arsenic poisoning has been the cause of lung cancer in vine growers of Beaujolais. The use of arsenic on the vines was discontinued in 1944 (Galy et al.[105]). In the uranium miners on a Colorado plateau, there was an excess mortality from lung cancer—twenty-two observed as compared to 5.7 expected. Radiation, therefore, must have something to do with the production of lung cancer in this group of workers. Cancer of the lung has increased in uranium miners (Wagoner et al.[287]). Since these industries employ a small pro-

Table 21. Specific worker groups with specific respiratory cancer hazards*

Agent	Worker groups
Asbestos	Asbestos miners; textile workers
Arsenic	Manufacturers, handlers, and users of arsenical insecticides; arsenic smelter workers; taxidermists; sheep dip workers; copper smelter workers
Chromium	Chromate manufacturers, including plant maintenance workers; chrome pigment handlers
Nickel	Nickel-copper matte refinery workers
Iron	Iron ore (hematite) miners; iron foundry workers
Radioactive substances	Radioactive ore (pitchblende) miners; miners of nonradioactive ores working in radioactive mines
Isopropyl oil	Isopropyl alcohol manufacturers
Coal tar fumes	Coke oven operators; gas house retort workers
Petroleum oil mists	Paraffin pressers; mule spinners; metal lathe workers and drillers

*From Hueper, W. C.: Epidemiologic, experimental and histological studies on metal cancers of the lung, Acta Un. Int. Cancr. 15:424-436, 1959 (abst.).

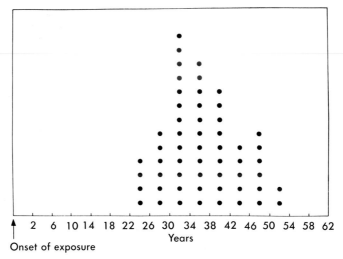

Fig. 265. Fifty-six cases of neoplasm of lung or pleura (each case represented by dot). Elapsed time from onset of exposure to death is shown on abscissa. (From Selikoff, I. J., et al.: Asbestosis and neoplasia [editorial], Amer. J. Med. **42**:487-496, 1967.)

portion of the population, the contribution to the occurrence of cancer of the lung would, therefore, be negligible.

It has become apparent that there is a risk of cancer of the lung, as well as of pleural and peritoneal mesotheliomas, in persons exposed to asbestos—not only workers in the asbestos industry, but also the population of the area in which the industry is located and relatives of workers who are exposed to the asbestos-loaded atmosphere, clothing, etc. There is an increase in the industrial production of asbestos. Russia, Canada, and Rhodesia produce about 90% of the world's supply. Selikoff et al.[245] have reported a study of asbestos workers who showed a risk of developing bronchial carcinoma seven or eight times greater than the expected rate (Fig. 265). They calculated that the risk for those workers who smoke is about ninety-two times that of those who neither worked with asbestos nor smoked. The clinical latency between exposure and the development of the neoplasm is about twenty years. Autopsy surveys in various locations, Pittsburgh (Cauna et al.[51]), Miami (Thomson et al.[272]), and Cape Town (Thomson et al.[272]) have shown that an increasing exposure results in a high proportion of carriers of asbestos bodies, which may be of the order of 34% to 47%. Accepting this as a greater risk

for cancer of the lung in the United States, we do not know how to evaluate its magnitude.

Clemmesen and Nielsen[57] demonstrated that the increase of cancer of the lung is particularly advanced in urban areas and in the poorer classes. In New Haven, Connecticut, Cohart[58] showed that the occurrence of cancer of the lung is 40% greater among the poor than among other economic classes. Stocks and Campbell[263] showed that there is a greater risk for men living in the cities than for those living in the country. *Industrial pollution* of the atmosphere, particularly of large cities, has been on the increase. Analysis of the air of industrial cities shows contamination by carcinogenic compounds such as benzpyrene (Kotin and Falk[158]; Stocks and Campbell[263]). Mills[184] showed twice the prevailing lung cancer incidence rates in urban residents driving over 12,000 miles per year in urban traffic.

Pathologic evidence that inhalation of carcinogenic agents might be a factor in the causation of cancer of the lung has been presented by Liebow.[169] In a study of 150 lungs resected for cancer, one-fifth presented honeycombing with atypical acinar proliferation confined to the upper portions of the pulmonary lobes. Emigrants from an industrial country seem to carry with them their greater risk. English immigrants in New Zealand have a higher incidence of cancer of the lung than native New Zealanders of the same stock. This is not true of other forms of cancer. Similarly, British immigrants in South Africa are more often subject to cancer of the lung than Caucasian South Africans. These facts are apparently unrelated to differences in smoking habits (Eastcott[84]; Dean[70]).

The evidence collected supports an important relationship between the *inhaling of tobacco smoke* and cancer of the bronchus (Oettlé[199]; Bocker[34a]). In the analysis of this relationship, it is important to recognize several factors. Evidence of the carcinogenic effect of tobacco (Roffo[234]) and tobacco smoke condensates (Wynder and Hoffmann[302]) on the skin of lower animals is clear. The complex chemical mixture in tobacco smoke has been found to contain known carcinogenic compounds (Van Duuren[280]). Production of bronchial carcinoma in lower animals fails in face of the impossibility to make such animals live for a long time in an atmosphere of tobacco smoke.

Uses of tobacco vary from one country to another, from urban to rural communities, from one age group to another, and from men to women. Cigar and pipe smokers infrequently inhale. Smokers of strong black cigarettes inhale much less than smokers of *blond* cigarettes. Outdoor workers smoke and inhale less than white collar workers. Most women smoke a lesser amount than men, and most women never learn to inhale (Doll and Hill[77]; Wynder et al.[301]; Stocks and Campbell[263]; Hammond and Garfinkel[128]). The present generation of young Americans of both sexes start smoking at a younger age, take to inhaling more frequently, and consume greater numbers of cigarettes than their parents. Between 1920 and 1955, cigarette consumption in the United States increased fourfold for all persons over 14 years of age. The use of other tobacco products decreased about two-thirds (Levin[168]). Dozens of retrospective studies have been made of the smoking habits of thousands of individuals and the occurrence of cancer of the lung and other diseases (Hammond and Horn[129]; Doll and Hill[77]; Dorn[82]; Levin[168]; Cornfield et al.[63]). Hammond[127] reported on a prospective study begun in 1959 and involving 36,975 matched pairs of smokers and nonsmokers with a total of 1,048,183 men and women. At the time of his report, 1385 smokers had died, 110 of lung cancer, whereas 662 nonsmokers had died, only twelve with cancer of the lung.

All of these studies have shown statistical correlation of cigarette smoking with the occurrence of squamous cell and undifferentiated carcinomas of the bronchus. These studies also show an increased risk with greater numbers of cigarettes smoked and with the length of the smoking habit. A man who smokes two packages of cigarettes daily has 1 chance in 10 of developing cancer of the lung. The rate of bronchial carcinoma in smokers of more than two packages of cigarettes daily was 217.3 per 100,000—*a rate sixty times greater than that for men who never smoked* (Shimkin[249]). In a comparison of 1040 men and 141 women with cancer of the lung and an equal number of nonsmokers, Lombard[170] found a thirtyfold increase of cancer in those having smoked over 18,000 packages of cigarettes. The occurrence seems to be twice as great in the smokers who cough as in those who do not (Boucot et al.[38]). In Israel, bronchial carcinomas are significantly fewer among smokers who utilize a water pipe than among cigarette smokers. The conclusion has been drawn that this has to do with differences in the temperature of the smoke (Rakower[217]), but it may have to do also with the washing of the smoke. In New York City, the occurrence of cancer of the lung in Jewish men is decidedly less than that among Catholics and Protestants. Also, the proportion of men who smoke cigarettes is lowest among Jewish men (Seidman[244]). The lower incidence of cancer in women may well be related to the lower proportion of smokers among women and the definite difference in the extent of inhaling among them in past generations.

Meticulous post-mortem studies of the bronchi have demonstrated that atypical changes and carcinoma in situ occurred much more frequently in smokers than in nonsmokers (Auerbach et al.[11]). Clemmesen and Nielsen[57] believe that there is a lapse of twenty years between exposure to a carcinogen and the development of cancer. He plotted the consumption of cigarettes per individual against mortality from cancer of the lung twenty years later and found close correlation. Cutler and Loveland[67] estimated that if 1000 men smoked more than a package of cigarettes a day, twenty-three would develop cancer by the age of 60 years, fifty-three by the age of 70 years, and eighty by the age of 80 years.

Kreyberg[161] divides cancer of the lung into three distinct etiologic groups: squamous cell, large cell, and small cell (oat cell) carcinomas, four out of five of which are related to smoking. At Barnes Hospital, practically all male patients with squamous or oat cell carcinoma smoked cigarettes. However, in a study of lung cancer in women with the same types of cancer, eleven of thirty-five did not smoke (Vincent et al.[284]). Adenocarcinomas, bronchiolar (alveolar cell) carcinomas, and various types of adenomas are not apparently related to smoking. Doll[76] confirmed this observation. In a group of nonsmokers with cancer of the lung, he found the occurrence to be the same in both sexes. He concluded also that 1 of every 5 deaths from cancer of the lung in patients 25 to 74 years of age (1950) could be attributed to causes other than smoking. Brisman et al.[41] reported cancer of the lung in four siblings. Familial aggregation of bronchial carcinomas is conspicuous in nonsmokers and probably is related to genetic factors (Burch[46]; Tokuhata and Lilienfeld[275]).

It is obvious that although there are numerous causes of cancer of the lung, the greatest risk appears to be related to tobacco inhaling and air pollution. Stocks[261] believes that the greater occurrence of lung cancer in urban communities must be attributed to air pollution. Buell et al.[45] reported a higher occurrence of pulmonary cancer in the Bay area of San Francisco, Los Angeles, and San Diego than in the remaining rural area. Bronchial carcinoma is rare in Ceylon, where cigarette consumption is low and there is no significant air pollution (Uragoda[279]). All individuals do not appear to be equally susceptible. Shimkin[249] estimated that of 29,000 individuals who died of cancer of the lung in 1956, 22,000 of the deaths were due to environmental factors, and 15,000 of these were due to smoking. The risk of smoking is great enough so that the English government has brought the facts to public attention, concluding that once the risks are known, responsible persons will act as it would seem best. The Departments of Health of Sweden and England have made public pronouncements of the relationship of smoking and cancer of the lung. In 1964, the Surgeon General of the United States Public Health Service made public a report[268] on smoking and cancer of the lung. Since then, millions of citizens, including 100,000 physicians, have given up smoking. In 1968, there were in the United States two million more individuals of smoking age, yet there were one million fewer smokers (15%) than in 1965. For the first time, in over thirty years, there was no appreciable increase in incidence of cancer of the lung. Prospective studies carried out in England (Doll and Hill[78]) and in the United States (Meighan and Weitman[181]) have shown a drastic reduction in death rates from cancer of the lung among those who have stopped smoking and that there is a definite relationship between the amount smoked and the incidence of cancer.

Bronchial carcinoid tumors occur in younger individuals of either sex. In a series of eighty-six patients with bronchial adenoma studied by Moersch and McDonald[186] (forty-five men and forty-one women), the ages ranged from 15 to 67 years. The average age of male patients was 42 years and that of female patients was 38 years (Fig. 266). The mean age in the series reported by Overholt et al.[203] was 40 years. A group of fifty-four patients with bronchial carcinoids studied at Barnes Hospital were 15 to 55 years of age, with the cases evenly distributed in the four decades. Carcinoid tumors, however, make up a relatively small percentage of all bronchial tumors. Of 175 patients with primary tumors of the bronchi seen at the Massachusetts General Hospital, 158 had carcinomas, and the remaining seventeen had adenomas (Adams[3]). A high percentage of tumors previously designated as bronchial adenomas are carcinoid tumors. The remaining neoplasms are adenoid cystic and mucoepidermoid tumors, adenomas of mucous glands, and mixed tumors.

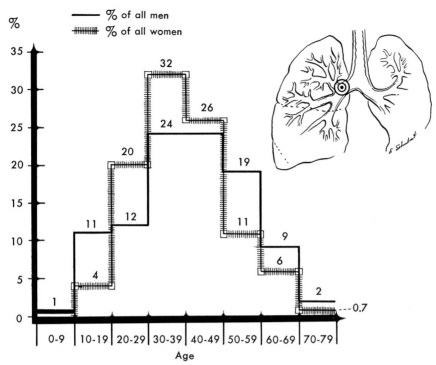

Fig. 266. Age of men and women with carcinoid tumors of bronchus. (Compiled from data from Graham and Womack,[114] Hazel et al.,[133a] Goldman,[110] Lampe,[163a] Meissner,[181a] and Som.[255a])

Pathology
Gross pathology

An overwhelming proportion of lung tumors arise within the bronchi (bronchogenic carcinoma, bronchial carcinoid), but a few malignant neoplasms arise from bronchiolar epithelium and pleural mesothelium.

Bronchogenic carcinoma is found more frequently in the right (60%) than in the left lung. It arises in the major bronchus in about 75% of the cases and in one of the peripheral bronchi in about 25%. The percentage arising from peripheral bronchi may be higher than 25%, but when the tumors reach a large size, it is hard to determine whether they arose peripherally or centrally. Rigler's retrospective radiologic study[224] demonstrated that many apparently central carcinomas arose years previously as small peripheral tumors. Tumors exhibiting definite squamous characteristics uniformly ulcerate the bronchi, whereas those arranged in the form of acini tend to invade and constrict the bronchi often without ulceration. The squamous carcinoma may remain fairly well localized, and foci of keratinization can be seen as small granular-like areas. Variable degrees of bronchial ulceration are seen. The more undifferentiated carcinomas are often large and can even replace an entire lobe of the lung. In these large tumors, areas of hemorrhage and necrosis are frequent. The adenocarcinomas can also be large and may, at times, show areas of mucoid degeneration.

Bronchogenic carcinomas tend to develop submucosal extension along the bronchi, but this extension often cannot be seen (Fig. 271). As the tumor grows within a major bronchus, it insinuates itself between and eventually destroys the bronchial cartilages (Fig. 267). With further extension, it may even reach the visceral pleura, grow through it, and become adherent to the thoracic wall or diaphragm. On the left, the tumor can spread to involve the pericardium and, in rare instances, the myocardium. Rarely, carcinomas of the lung may spread through the chest wall to form an ulcerating mass on the skin. In this

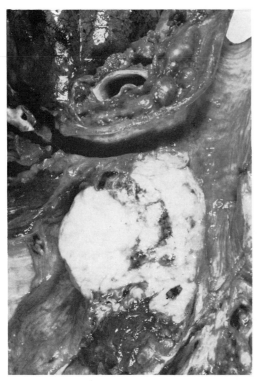

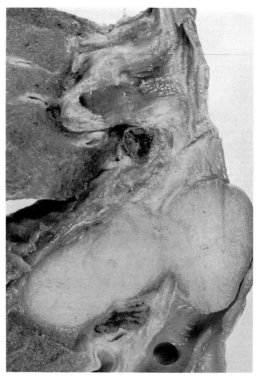

Fig. 267. Typical epidermoid carcinoma arising from main-stem bronchus with involvement of hilar lymph nodes and direct spread into adjoining lung.

Fig. 268. Dumbbell-shaped bronchial carcinoid occluding large bronchus, destroying bronchial cartilage, and pushing its way into lung parenchyma. This illustrates impossibility of bronchoscopic removal.

local spread, various nerves may be compressed or invaded (vagus, recurrent laryngeal, phrenic, sympathetic, and cervical ganglion nerves).

Other mediastinal structures such as pulmonary vessels can be surrounded, but usually the arteries are invaded only in their adventitial portion. Careful examination of 183 resected carcinomas revealed invasion of arteries and veins in over 40% of the cases, but this invasion was more common in peripheral tumors (Pryce and Walter[215]). Not too rarely, the tumor compresses the superior vena cava and partially or wholly obstructs it. True thrombosis is rare (Hussey et al.[141]). Occlusion of major bronchi, either partial or complete, often results in atelectasis and infection distal to the tumor. This infectious process may take the form of a diffuse necrotizing bronchopneumonia that may secondarily perforate the pleura to cause empyema. In other instances, the obstruc-

tion may initiate the formation of a lung abscess localized to a single lobe.

There is no doubt that *bronchial adenoma* is a misnomer, for these tumors do extend locally and can metastasize to regional lymph nodes and even, upon rare occasions, to distant organs such as the liver (Anderson[7]). However, they behave clinically in an entirely different fashion from bronchogenic carcinomas. They are very slow growing, and the best way to classify them is as *carcinoid tumors* in most instances. They certainly should be separated when groups of carcinomas treated surgically are reported.

Bronchial carcinoids arise predominantly in the main-stem bronchi, but sometimes they may develop in small bronchi not accessible to bronchoscopy (Maier and Fischer[177]). In a series of fifty-three patients, the tumors were found in the left lung in seventeen and in the right lung in thirty-six, with a preponderance (twen-

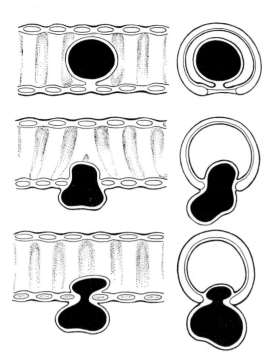

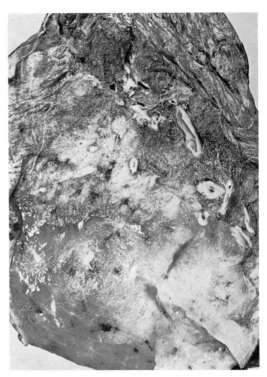

Fig. 269. Three morphologic types of bronchial adenoma (carcinoid): endobronchial, intramural, and extrabronchial.

Fig. 270. Cut section of bronchiolar tumor of lung. Note moist surface and resemblance to organizing pneumonia.

ty-four cases) for the right lower lobe. The tumors varied from 0.5 cm to 8 cm in diameter (Ackerman and Spjut[2]). Carcinoids are usually soft, well-vascularized tumors without areas of necrosis. They grow entirely within the bronchus (rare), assume a dumbbell shape (Fig. 268) with approximately equal growth inside and outside the lumen (fairly common), or present mainly extrabronchial growth (most common) (Fig. 269). On section, these tumors are well delineated, and often yellow in color. They may present superficial ulceration in the bronchial lumen and areas of hemorrhage. Local invasive qualities are the most prominent signs of their malignancy. They grow around the bronchial cartilages and may destroy them. They may directly invade the regional lymph nodes, although not rarely they grow around the nodes, leaving them free from tumor. These tumors can invade the submucosa for a short distance (Foster-Carter[94]) or even invade the heart (Black[30]). In their spread they may ramify within the bronchi and, if they grow into the lung parenchyma, they usually have a well-defined capsule.

The cylindromatous type of bronchial neoplasm is an adenoid cystic cancer arising from mucous glands. Moersch and McDonald[186] reported nine cases of this type among eighty-six adenomas. These cylindromatous tumors have a different prognosis. They seem to be identical with mucous and salivary gland tumors, presenting the same morphology. They arise in major bronchi beneath the intact epithelium but later may ulcerate through it and present an intraluminal polypoid mass. Bronchial tumors of the cylindromatous variety grow slowly, infiltrating contiguous structures. They frequently invade the trachea (McDonald et al.[176]) and eventually metastasize to regional lymph nodes. A true mucous gland adenoma of the bronchus was reported by Kroe and Pitcock.[162] Papillary neoplasms, which are rare, can involve the trachea and bronchial tree (Singer et al.[250]; Smith and Dexter[252]). Payne et al.[209] reported two tumors of the bronchus similar to mixed tumors of salivary gland origin.

We believe there are a few carcinomas of the lung that arise from *bronchiolar epithelium.* They present two gross patterns. In one, the lungs are studded with nodules up to 2 cm in diameter and the appearance is that of a metastatic tumor, whereas in the second type a lobe may be diffusely involved, simulating pneumonia (Fig. 270).

Microscopic pathology

Bronchogenic carcinoma is usually divided into three groups: squamous cell carcinoma, adenocarcinoma, and undifferentiated carcinoma. The undifferentiated carcinomas would include giant cell cancer, oat cell tumors, and those carcinomas that could not be classified as epidermoid carcinoma or adenocarcinoma (Fig. 271). Nash and Stout[193] reported fourteen cases of undifferentiated carcinoma that they designated as giant cell cancer. Individual tumor cells were extremely anaplastic and composed chiefly of pleomorphic giant cells. We are in agreement with Willis[295] that the degree of differentiation of a tumor may vary greatly in sections taken from different areas. Both adenocarcinoma and epidermoid carcinoma may be found in the same specimen, although such cases are few. The apparent evolution of a tumor from squamous metaplasia to carcinoma in situ and to infiltrating epidermoid carcinoma has been observed by us in a number of instances (Niskanen[196]; Black and Ackerman[31]).

The *bronchial carcinoid* has characteristic features and is often covered by an intact bronchial mucous membrane that may become stratified squamous in character. Beneath the epithelium, the extremely well-vascularized tumor has an appearance suggesting fetal lung. The epithelial cells of the tumor are uniformly regular, and mitotic figures are infrequent. The pattern of the tumor may or may not be uniform, and individual types are described as alveolar, medullary, or angiomatoid in character. Bone and cartilage (fragments of bronchial cartilage or bone due to metaplasia of the stroma) may be present. The carcinoid variant of bronchial

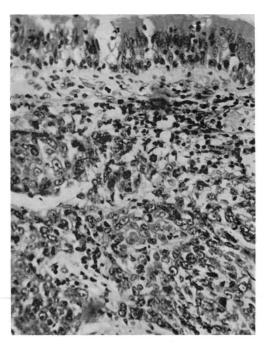

Fig. 271. Undifferentiated carcinoma growing beneath intact overlying columnar ciliated epithelium of bronchus. (Moderate enlargement.)

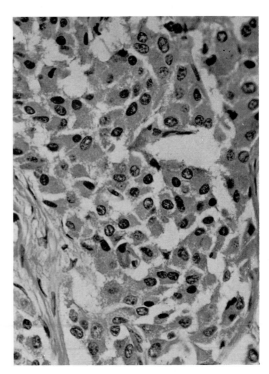

Fig. 272. Bronchial carcinoid tumor of oncocyte type. Note regularity of pattern, abscence of mitotic figures, and prominent vascularity. (High power.)

adenoma has been demonstrated to be similar in many respects to the carcinoid tumors of the gastrointestinal tract. They contain argentophilic material within their cells (Hamperl[130]; Feyrter[90]). Feyrter et al.[91] also isolated pharmacodynamically active substances, 5-hydroxytryptamine and epinephrine in relatively large amounts and norepinephrine and ascorbic acid in smaller amounts, in a bronchial carcinoid tumor. Hattori et al.[133] reported nine cases of oat cell carcinoma and one of bronchial carcinoid. They feel that oat cell carcinoma and bronchial carcinoids are specific tumors containing serotonin granules developing from argentaffin cells found in the bronchial mucous glands. The cylindromatous type of tumor is better designated as an adenocarcinoma originating from the mucous glands of the bronchus. The tumor cells may form glandular structures with a central lumen that often contains material staining as epithelial mucin. At times, the cells may form solid masses and grow in small nests that frequently invade nerve sheaths (Fig. 273). A rare benign mucoepidermoid tumor can arise from the surface epithelium of the bronchus (Sniffen et al.[255]).

The *alveolar cell tumor* probably has a bronchiolar origin (Herbut[134]). The tumor cells can be seen attached to the alveolar wall by very delicate connective tissue. The cells are cuboid or columnar, and papillary projections are common (Fig. 274). Cilia are only rarely present (Swan[270]; Vanek[282]). In the immediate vicinity of the tumor, fibrosis, chronic pneumonia, atelectasis, and emphysema are not infrequent. These changes may be related to the blockage of bronchi by tumor.

Metastatic spread

The profuse pulmonary network of lymphatics and the great vascularity and constant movements of the lung facilitate the spread of *bronchial carcinomas*. The regional lymphatic spread to mediastinal and

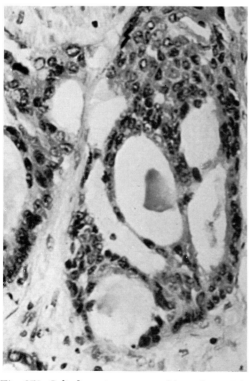

Fig. 273. Cylindromatous tumor of bronchus originating from bronchial mucous glands. This is slow-growing, metastasizing adenocarcinoma. (High power.)

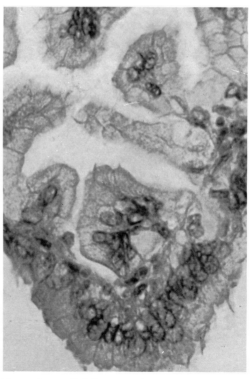

Fig. 274. Well-differentiated bronchiolar cell tumor with tall columnar cells.

peritracheal lymph nodes takes place in the majority of cases. In a series of 1176 autopsies on cases of bronchial carcinoma, 91% had regional lymph node metastases and 9% had none (Zschoch and Kober[305]). Well-differentiated carcinomas may remain localized or metastasize only to regional lymph nodes (Goldman[110]). The lymphatic spread becomes more extensive when pleural adhesions form and distant pathways of dissemination are facilitated. Through the diaphragm the tumor may involve the periesophageal, para-aortic, and pararenal nodes. Spread to the adrenal glands takes place through the lymphatics, remaining ipsilateral as long as the thoracic involvement is unilateral (Onuigbo[202]). Caranasos and Huebner[48] observed an increase in the thickness of the adrenal cortex in patients with bronchial carcinoma.

If the tumor erodes into the pulmonary veins, systemic dissemination becomes inevitable and brain, bone, and liver metastases do appear. The proportion of reported brain metastases at autopsy varies

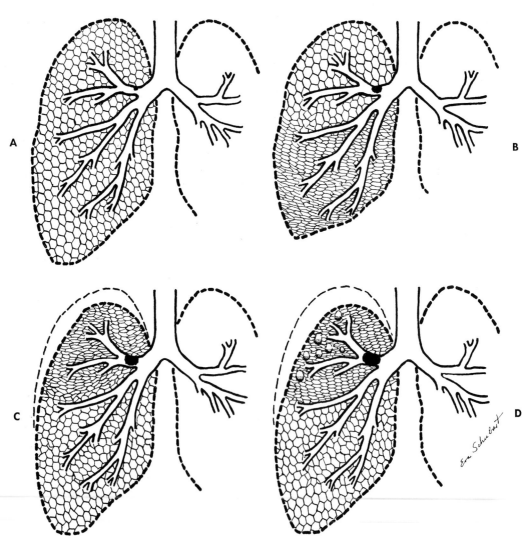

Fig. 275. Mechanism of bronchial obstruction by tumor developing in bronchial lumen. **A,** No obstruction with no change in peripheral lung. **B,** Ball-valve action with emphysema distal to partial obstruction. **C,** Almost complete obstruction with atelectasis. **D,** Complete obstructive atelectasis and abscess formation.

from 26% to 38% (Halpert et al.[126]). Metastases to the liver seldom coincide with brain metastases (Galluzzi and Payne[104]). The tumor may also spread through the vertebral vein plexus and reach the scalp.

The *bronchiolar carcinoma* (alveolar cell tumor) may not develop metastases or it may spread to the hilar lymph nodes. Distant metastases seldom occur. *Bronchial carcinoids* remain well localized and seldom metastasize. The cylindromatous type of so-called bronchial adenoma may involve the regional lymph nodes and may metastasize distantly (Belsey and Valentine[21]; McBurney et al.[172]).

Clinical evolution

Tumors of the lung are among the most insidious of all neoplasms. They may cause early or late symptoms in the course of their development, depending on their location, pathologic character, rate of growth, and other factors. In the majority of instances, the first symptoms are not alarming and, indeed, may be considered lightly even by the physicians consulted.

The earliest symptom is usually an irritative *cough*, sometimes nocturnal, accompanied by variable, increasing amounts of *mucoid expectoration*. Sometimes the sputum is tinged with blood, and *hemoptysis* may occur. *Paroxysmal hyperpnea* may rarely develop due to the presence of mucous plugs in secondary and tertiary bronchi (Rienhoff[220]). The patients sometimes notice the presence of a unilateral *wheeze,* which is due to partial obstruction of a bronchus (Fig. 275). Repeated attacks of *obstructive pneumonitis* (McDonald et al.[175]) with mild fever may develop over a period of weeks or months. *Pain,* often of a constrictive nature, usually results when the bronchus is entirely occluded and a sector of the lung becomes atelectatic. Marked symptoms of infection, suggesting pneumonia, may then occur. Pleural effusion and empyema may develop with consequent pain and *dyspnea. Loss of weight* is a rather constant symptom that may result simply from the presence of cough and accompanying *anorexia* but may be due also to the development of metastases (Table 22).

Tumors of the lung may produce symptoms apparently not due to a pulmonary lesion. Peripheral bronchogenic carcinomas, which make up about 25% of all bronchial carcinomas, are among these silently developing tumors (Thornton et al.[273]). Cases in which *dysphagia* is a predominant symptom have been described. *Dysphonia* due to compression of the recurrent laryngeal nerve often accompanies the dysphagic forms but also may be present without dysphagia. Tumors developing in the periphery of the upper lobes may produce an early Horner's syndrome (enophthalmia, myosis, and diminution of the palpebral fissure) due to compression of the cervical sympathetic plexus. They may also compress the brachial plexus and produce considerable pain in the region of the shoulder and arm.

Table 22. Initial and eventual symptoms of carcinoma of lung

	First symptom (%)		Eventual symptoms (%)	
*Symptoms**	*Björk[29a]* (342 patients)	*Ariel[9]* (1109 patients)	*Ochsner[197]* (129 patients)	*Rienhoff[220]* (327 patients)
Cough	58	21	92	71
Thoracic pain	11	36	67	50
Respiratory infection	10	7	60	18
Dyspnea	7	8	59	23
Hemoptysis	5	6	61	63
Loss of weight	—	1	79	39
Asthenia	3	7	7	—
Wheezing	—	1	17	—
Fever	2	—	—	13
Hoarseness	1	1	—	—
Dysphagia	—	1	—	—
Tightness of chest	1	1	—	3

*Only common symptoms connected with the primary lesion are listed.

Patients with bronchial carcinoma may present extrapulmonary manifestations not suggestive of the primary cause (Baker[14]). These may be metabolic, neuromuscular, vascular, hematologic, osseous, or connective tissue abnormalities (Knowles and Smith[155]). Patients with *osteoarthropathy* due to bronchial carcinoma may show a regression of these symptoms after removal of the tumor (Poletti and Riva[212]). Symptoms of *rheumatoid arthritis* may lead to an incorrect diagnosis and treatment by cortisone.

Hypercalcemia may be present and acquire striking proportions. It disappears with removal of the tumor (Myers[192]; Stone et al.[264]; Turkington et al.[277]). *Cushing's syndrome* may be associated with a rapid-growing carcinoma (Kovach and Kyle[159]; Friedman et al.[100]) or carcinoid tumor (Strott et al.[267]) (Fig. 276). *Idiopathic neuropathy* may accompany carcinoma of the lung (Ebaugh and Holt[86]). Morton et al.[189] reported twenty-three cases of bronchial carcinoma with ac-

companying myopathic myasthenic syndromes, polyneuropathies, sensory neuropathies, subacute cerebellar degeneration, and encephalomyelopathies which in fifteen instances preceded the diagnosis of carcinoma of the lung. There is a suggestive association of sensory neuropathies or encephalomyelitic forms of neuromyopathies and oat cell carcinoma (Dayan et al.[69]). Brain and Wilkinson[40] reported ten cases of subacute cerebellar degeneration associated with cancer of the lung.

The various tumors of the lung do not present distinctive signs and symptoms. However, the pattern of symptoms and signs may be distinctive of a particular neoplasm. *Bronchial carcinoid* develops slowly and becomes extremely vascularized. Thus, hemoptysis is often its first symptom and profuse hemorrhages and infectious complications may occur. When accompanied by metastases, it may give rise to a *carcinoid syndrome* (Williams and Azzopardi[294]; Schneckloth et al.[241]). Rare cases of oat cell carcinoma may cause the car-

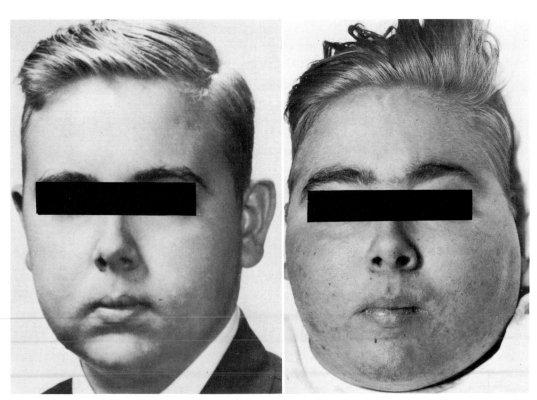

Fig. 276. Cushing's syndrome associated with ACTH-secreting bronchial carcinoid in 18-year-old youth. Note typical facies. (WU negs. 67-9059 and 68-8760.)

cinoid syndrome (Williams and Azzopardi[294]; Gowenlocken et al.[112]) or a hyponatremic syndrome (Ross[235]). Bensch et al.[26] presented objective information that both the bronchial carcinoid and the oat cell tumors are derived from Kulchitsky-type cells.

The clinical evolution of *alveolar carcinoma* is variable, with considerable cough, watery expectoration, dyspnea, and cyanosis (Delarue and Graham[72]).

At times, the first symptom of cancer of the lung may be related to its metastases and even dominate the clinical picture, relegating to second place the mild symptoms produced by the primary lesion. Not infrequently, a cerebral metastasis may strongly suggest a primary brain tumor. The pain caused by a bone metastasis may also call the attention to areas far removed from the primary source. Addison's disease may rarely occur as a consequence of extensive adrenal involvement. Metastatic brain abscesses also occur.

In the late stages of the disease there may be an aggregation of symptoms due to the extensive development of the tumor and its complications: excessive cough, abundant expectoration sometimes due to abscess formation, hemoptysis, dyspnea, pain due to pleural effusion, weight loss, anemia, and prominent cardiorespiratory symptoms. Death occurs frequently because of pulmonary insufficiency in alveolar carcinoma and pleural mesotheliomas. In bronchial carcinoma, death is frequently due to a combination of conditions, including widespread dissemination of the disease and cardiorespiratory failure.

Diagnosis

Routine roentgenographic chest surveys, adequate for the detection of pulmonary tuberculosis, have proved disappointing for the early discovery of cancer of the lung. Often these surveys contain a large proportion of women and of young individuals of both sexes who have little risk of having cancer of the lung (Guiss and Kuenstler[121]). This fact not only makes the surveys costly but also may contribute to carelessness in interpretation (Garland[106]; Guiss and Kuenstler[121]). Moreover, the lack of organization or the unwillingness of patients to follow up without delay the indications for further investigation or treatment usually annuls the gain of a few early discoveries.

Retrospective studies of the material of chest surveys usually lead to the conclusion that something would be gained if the films were read independently by two or more competent radiologists (Posner et al.[213]), that the surveys should be limited to men over 45 years of age, and that the procedure should be repeated at intervals of a few months (Guiss and Kuenstler[121]). The main difficulty, however, is the fact that peripheral tumors, which are likely to be asymptomatic for a longer time and can be more readily detected in the roentgenograms, are relatively infrequent. The cost of case finding by roentgenographic mass screening is prohibitive, but screening that is restricted to a high-risk group may prove more rewarding. Kubik et al.[163] recommend repeated radiographic screening in men 40 to 64 years of age in whom any two of the following circumstances coincide:

1 200,000 or more cigarettes consumed
2 Progressive cough
3 Repeated hemoptysis
4 Repeated pneumonic episodes

Overholt et al.[204] presented evidence that patients are cured in higher proportions when the diagnosis is made in the asymptomatic phase (Table 23). However, in a group of thirty-three patients with cancer of the lung discovered in a chest survey,

Table 23. Data in survey-detected and symptomatic cancer of lung*

Group	Cases	Explorations	Resections	Favorable cases†	3-yr survivals
Cancer detected by survey	30	26 (87%)	23 (77%)	13 (43%)	9 (30%)
Symptomatic cancer	263	168 (64%)	100 (38%)	40 (15%)	32 (12%)

*From Overholt, R. H., et al.: Surgical treatment of lung cancer found on x-ray survey, New Eng. J. Med. 252:429-432, 1955.
†No extension to lymph nodes and no metastases.

there was no significant improvement in the three-year survival (Greenberger[117]) despite the better apparent results at the end of one year. Posner et al.[214] compared a group of forty-eight cases of cancer of the lung discovered in mass survey with another of 190 cases discovered by general practitioners. Twenty-one (44%) of the first group were resected, whereas only fifty-seven (30%) of the second group were operated upon. However, at the end of two years, eight patients from the first group (16%) and twenty-five from the second group (13%) were apparently well, with no statistically significant advantage for the survey group.

Höst[137] also demonstrated that resection of lung cancer was performed about twice as frequently in cases detected by survey. However, the prognosis for this group of patients as compared with that of those not detected by survey was approximately the same. If surveys are done to detect lung cancer, they must be repeated at intervals of three to six months. Unfortunately, the fate of a patient with bronchial cancer probably depends more on the inherent malignancy of the tumor and its location than on the efficacy of diagnostic efforts. We may be able to improve the survival rate by earlier diagnosis and prompt surgical treatment in the biologically more favorable lesions (Höst[137]).

Boucot et al.[37] reported in some detail a survey of asymptomatic males in whom chest films were taken at six-month intervals. The results of treatment by surgery were depressing. They pointed out that the number of months gained by surgery in resectable cases must be balanced against immediate operative mortality in patients with operable lung cancer as well as shortened survival in patients shown to be inoperable at thoracotomy. It seems certain that present methods of screening have not significantly improved the results of treatment in lung cancer.

The development of successful surgical treatment of bronchial tumors has stimulated the efforts made toward the differentiation and the earlier diagnosis of these tumors. Unfortunately, they do not offer any characteristic physical findings. A mild persistent cough may appear. A label of "cigarette cough" should never be assigned

to this symptom merely because the patient is a smoker. The possibility of a tumor should be investigated in cases of hemoptysis, particularly in elderly patients. Early symptoms are, however, more often connected with various degrees of bronchial block. There may be unilateral wheezing, best heard at open mouth and near the end of forcible expiration. The air may become trapped, and zones of hyperresonance due to obstructive emphysema may be found distal to the point of obstruction. If the obstruction persists, atelectasis may develop later with resulting dullness to percussion. And persisting atelectasis results in retraction of the trachea or heart toward the involved side. There may also appear eventual cavitation of the lung, and after the tumor is no longer localized, the signs and symptoms may be due to infiltration. Spread to the pleura results in pleural effusion. A carcinoma involving the thoracic inlet may result in considerable pain and neurologic changes of the arm and in a Horner's syndrome (myosis, enophthalmos, narrowed palpebral fissure) on the side involved. Finally, cervical or axillary metastatic nodes or brain, liver, or bone metastases are not infrequently the source of initial or complicating symptoms of bronchial carcinomas.

It is important to know whether a bronchogenic tumor represents a bronchial carcinoid or a bronchogenic carcinoma. In most instances, a biopsy is the determining factor. Age of the patient, duration of the disease, and bronchoscopic observations are the most important differential points (Table 24). Whereas most carcinoid tumors arise in large bronchi, some may arise in regions not accessible to biopsy (Maier and Fischer[177]).

A bronchial tumor may suggest an unresolved pneumonia. The clinical picture may change due, for instance, to expectoration of a fragment of tumor and improved bronchial drainage, with consequent clearing of the radiographic appearance. *Any poorly explained pneumonic process with unusual clinical behavior and roentgenographic findings, particularly in an elderly patient, should be suspected of being due to a bronchial tumor.* A primary neoplastic obstruction of the main bronchus may also be diagnosed roentgenographically as a

Table 24. Differential characteristics of bronchial carcinomas and bronchial carcinoids

	Bronchial carcinoma	*Bronchial carcinoid*
Sex	90% male	50% female
Age	10% before 40 years	Average age, 40 years
Duration		
One year plus	2%	90%
Five years plus	0	80%
Metastases	Very frequent	Infrequent
Brain pathology	Metastases frequent	Abscess may occur
Hemoptysis	40%	80% (often repeated)
Pain	Often present	Frequently absent
Bronchoscopic observation	Often fixed; ulcerated; carina widened; mediastinum fixed	Usually nonulcerated; bleeds easily; mediastinum not fixed
Operability	Low	High

lung abscess. Such diagnosis should be taken with skepticism, especially in elderly men, if there is no other clear reason for the abscess.

Bronchial carcinomas rather frequently compress the superior vena cava. The symptoms of superior vena caval obstruction have been summarized by Ochsner and Dixon[198]:

1 Edema and cyanosis of the face, neck, and upper extremities (relieved when erect; aggravated when recumbent)
2 Venous hypertension in upper extremities
3 Normal venous pressure of lower extremities
4 Visible superficial collateral circulation on anterior chest wall
5 Development of deep collateral circulation

Bronchial carcinomas frequently metastasize to the brain and, in the absence of any symptoms from the primary lesion, may suggest a primary brain tumor. Most prominent neurosurgeons have at some time operated on the brain for a lesion thought to be primary but eventually found to be metastatic from an occult carcinoma of the lung. Therefore, a thorough roentgenologic examination of the lungs should be done routinely in every patient with suspected primary brain tumor (Parker[205]). Metastases to the suprarenal glands may rarely cause an addisonian syndrome.

Roentgenologic examination

The roentgenologic examination is the most important of all methods employed in the diagnosis of pulmonary tumors. Al-

though the information that it provides is not always decisive, the adequate utilization of the roentgenologic examination increases considerably the percentage of correct diagnoses (Robbins and Hale[230-232]). Adequate utilization implies not only roentgenograms in several projections (anteroposterior, posteroanterior, lordotic, lateral, oblique), roentgenograms in forced expiration, spot and overexposed roentgenograms, but also, advisedly, the use of air and opaque substances for contrast and of special roentgenography, such as stereography, planigraphy, and angiography. One must not overlook the fact that a great deal of the information offered by the roentgenologic examination is to be obtained by radioscopy, which sometimes yields the only positive findings.

The abnormalities observed in radioscopy and radiography may be due to the opaque mass of the tumor contrasting with the translucency of the lung. This type of otherwise asymptomatic lesion is often discovered in routine chest surveys. The evaluation of the "coin" lesion of the lung has been the subject of considerable discussion. The younger the patient, the less the chance that these well-delimited shadows may be malignant. Only 17% of lesions found in young men in military service proved to be cancer (Effler et al.[87]), whereas 58% of those found in a group of men over 50 years of age proved to be carcinoma (Wilkins[293]). The presence of calcification is an important finding supporting a diagnosis of benign lesion (Good and Wilson[111]). If the calcification is laminated, it is usually due to a granuloma (O'Keefe et al.[200]). The "popcorn" type of

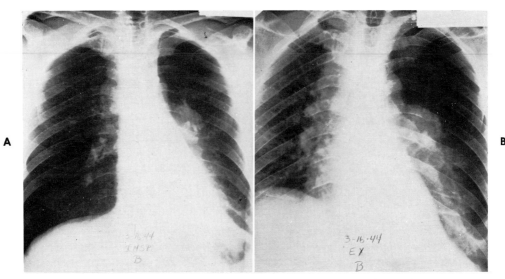

Fig. 277. **A,** Roentgenogram in inspiration showing no conspicuous abnormalities. **B,** Roentgenogram of same patient in expiration. Obstructive emphysema of left upper lobe now obvious due to early bronchial block. (Courtesy Dr. T. M. Berman, Miami Beach, Fla., and Dr. Leo G. Rigler, Los Angeles, Calif.)

calcification is usually associated with a hamartoma, but focal flecks of calcification within a nodule do not exclude carcinoma (Davis et al.[68]). O'Keefe et al.[200] demonstrated that 50% of the benign lesions and 14% of the malignant lesions showed calcification. It is also important to recognize that a calcified bronchial cartilage or a calcified Ghon complex may be included in the lesion. Focal necrosis with calcification may be present in a malignant tumor, but it is rare.

It may help to clarify issues to know that approximately 50% of bronchial tumors occur in the upper lobes, that they are rare in the middle areas of the lungs, and that only about 12% are observed in the left lower lobe. The roentgenographic appearance of a *bronchial carcinoma* may show bilateral well-defined nodules that are commonly interpreted as a metastatic carcinoma, whereas the localized form of this tumor suggests an inflammatory process. Often, however, *bronchial tumors,* by virtue of their location, produce cough or other symptoms before they are large enough to produce a shadow in the roentgenogram. When the obstruction of the bronchus is only partial, the roentgenogram taken on forced expiration may reveal an area of increased translucency, of obstructive emphysema, due to the trapping of air in the area of the lung corresponding to the obstructed bronchus. This phenomenon, first described by Westermark, is best observed in radioscopy (Rigler and Kelby[226]) (Fig. 277).

When complete obstruction of the bronchus occurs, the result is shrinkage of the corresponding part of the lung and atelectatic opacity with narrowing of intercostal spaces and deviation of the mediastinum toward the affected side (Fig. 278). The segmental collapse of the upper lobe is easily seen in routine roentgenograms, but lateral and oblique projections may be necessary to demonstrate the atelectasis elsewhere. Rigler et al.[227] feels that unilateral enlargement of the hilar shadow of the lung is the most commonly overlooked early sign of bronchogenic carcinoma. The obstruction may recede either spontaneously or under the influence of antibacterial medication, but in most instances it remains, and the atelectatic wedge becomes the site of inflammatory changes, showing in the roentgenogram variable degrees of opacity with eventual abscess formation (Fig. 279). Peripheral rapid-growing tumors with poor blood supply may show central necrosis and rarefaction (Thornton et al.[273]). Neoplastic abscesses may be

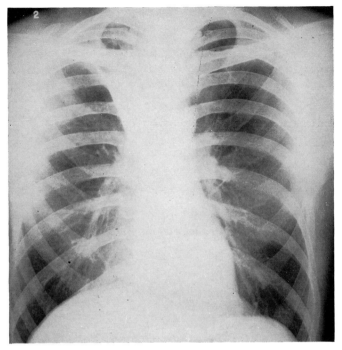

Fig. 278. Bronchogenic carcinoma with complete atelectasis of right upper lobe. Patient was found to be operable on exploratory thoracotomy. (Courtesy Dr. C. A. Brashear, Mount Vernon, Mo.)

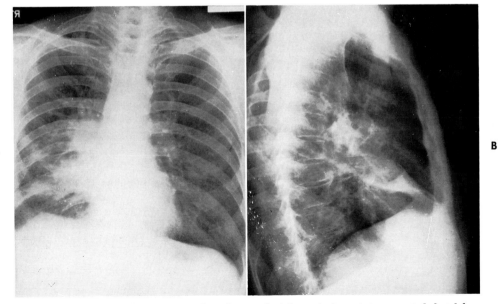

A

B

Fig. 279. A, Diffuse infiltration extending from right hilum. Atelectasis is suggested, but lobar distribution is not clear. B, Lateral roentgenogram clearly demonstrates complete atelectasis of right middle lobe due to carcinoma.

recognized by their ragged, inner contours and the irregularity in thickness of their walls (Isaac and Ottoman[144]). The radiologic diagnosis of enlarged mediastinal lymph nodes does not necessarily mean involvement by metastatic cancer. In a study made by Schröder and Eichorn,[242] only half the cases with enlarged mediastinal nodes showed metastases.

If the tumor is accompanied by pleural effusion or by any degree of thickening of the pleura, the resulting opacity may be rather ineloquent. Thoracentesis, followed by partial pneumothorax to replace the fluid, may reveal nodularities on the surface of the pleura.

Bronchography, or the visualization of all or part of the bronchial tree by means of the endotracheal injection of an opaque material, may help in localizing the point of bronchial obstruction, narrowing, or irregularity, the presence of bronchiectasis or abscess formation, or the independence of the bronchial tree from a tumor (di Rienzo[223]) (Fig. 280). The distinction between an inflammatory and a neoplastic narrowing of the bronchi may be difficult or impossible. But the introduction of iodized oil into the bronchial tree is objectionable, for it may cause a flare-up of a pneumonic process, may obscure subsequent examinations, and also may delay an operative procedure until it is eliminated, mostly through coughing.

Bronchography is being replaced by a wider use of *planigraphy* (tomography, laminagraphy, or body section roentgenography). Some have come to consider

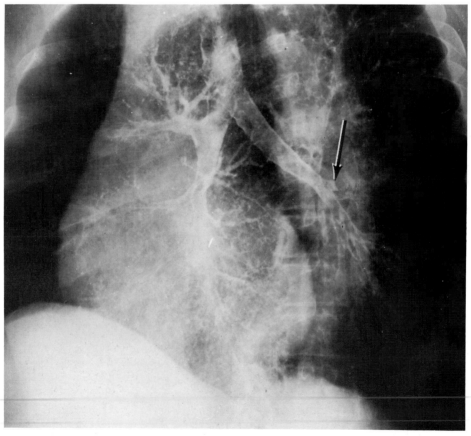

Fig. 280. Patient, 60-year-old man, had three positive cytologic examinations. Bronchoscopy and scalene node biopsy were negative. In this patient, posteroanterior film was not helpful but bronchogram showed block in superior segment of left lower lobe bronchus. At surgery, squamous carcinoma was found at this point. Regional lymph nodes were negative. (WU neg. 68-4202.)

planigraphy as a most important form of investigation in the diagnosis of tumors (Frimann-Dahl[101]; Rigler and Heitzman[225]). Eliminating superimposed shadows, it may reveal with great accuracy the site of a bronchial tumor and its extrabronchial extent. It is also very accurate in the important identification of calcification in a nodule. Rigler and Heitzman[225] believe that demonstration of cavitation or umbilication of a nodule constitutes strong evidence of cancer. In the past, planigraphy had the disadvantage of being a time-consuming procedure that could only be applied in special cases. The technique of planigraphy advocated by Frain and Gaucher[96] permits the routine performance of excellent tomograms following the plane of the bronchial tree (Figs. 281 and 282). In this technique, the beam of roentgen rays is horizontal and stationary. The patient and the film (in a parallel plane to the bronchial tree) turn synchronously on a vertical axis during the exposure. The resulting roentgenograms are of such value as to become indispensable in the investigation of pulmonary as well as mediastinal pathology.

Pulmonary arteriography has been capable of revealing diminished vascularity of the lung distal to the tumor. The procedure may be helpful in the diagnosis of cases of "unresolved pneumonia" (Keil et al.[152]).

Angiocardiographic studies may reveal involvement of the great vessels, precluding unnecessary operation (Steinberg and Finby[259]). The procedure also permits the precise evaluation of pulmonary circulation and the potential of the patient to stand

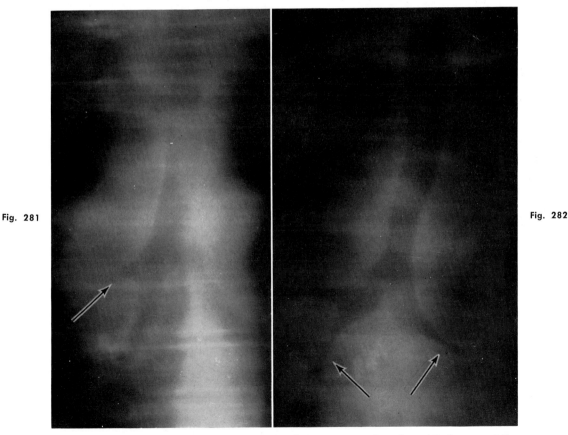

Fig. 281

Fig. 282

Fig. 281. Tomogram showing obstruction of right upper main bronchus. (Technique of Dr. C. Frain; courtesy Dr. P. Markovitz, Paris, France.)

Fig. 282. Tomogram showing narrowing of bronchi to right and to left by mediastinal growth. (Technique of Dr. C. Frain; courtesy Dr. P. Markovitz, Paris, France.)

impairment of his respiratory capacity. *Superior vena cavography* may give additional information in reference to the extent of the pulmonary carcinoma, and *azygography* has been found helpful in determining resectability.

As indicated before, the obstructive emphysema of some bronchial tumors may be best observed in radioscopy, which also facilitates the choice of those projections that are most advantageous for radiography. The radioscopic examination may reveal paradoxical movement of the diaphragm due to phrenic paralysis when that nerve is involved and may facilitate the taking of spot films. The routine radioscopic examination of the esophagus may also be helpful. Weiss et al.[292] indicated that six months after a chest film has been reported negative, the size of a carcinoma on the roentgenogram reflects the rate of its growth.

Pulmonary scintigram

The scanning of the lungs after injection of radioactive materials is a diagnostic procedure still under development. Ernst et al.[87a] tested the value of scintigrams, after injection of labeled macro-aggregated serum albumin, on 500 patients with various pulmonary diseases, including 138 with carcinomas. The method is primarily suited for the diagnosis of pulmonary embolism. In all patients with carcinomas located near the hilus ("central" tumors), the scan showed signs of abnormal pulmonary perfusion. Ernst et al.[87a] felt that the procedure showed greater diagnostic sensitivity than standard roentgenologic examination.

Bronchoscopy

Bronchoscopy is mandatory in every patient suspected of having a bronchial tumor. Since a great number of these tumors arise in the larger bronchi, the bronchoscopic examination will permit their visualization and biopsy, leading to the histopathologic verification of the diagnosis. The examination can be carried out with little discomfort by a skilled operator. But the examiner must possess knowledge of thoracic physiology and pathology as well as technical ability. A thorough bronchoscopic examination should provide information on the position of the tumor, but the bronchoscopist should also note the presence or absence of laryngeal paresis or paralysis and whether or not the carina is widened or fixed, which conditions are almost certain signs of mediastinal metastases. A detailed description of the gross appearance of the bronchial tumor should precede the taking of a biopsy. The presence of streaks of blood may be a lead toward the affected bronchus. Finally, whether growth is visualized or not, washings should be collected for cytologic examination.

Most bronchial carcinoids may be recognized at bronchoscopy. Biopsy may cause considerable bleeding because of the rich vascularity of these tumors, but they usually heal rapidly. A positive biopsy is obtainable preoperatively only in *about 30%* of cases of resectable bronchial carcinoma. In the more advanced lesions, the possibility of a positive biopsy increases progressively. A pulmonary tumor casting a well-circumscribed more or less circular shadow on the roentgenogram is invariably a peripheral lesion that cannot be visualized at bronchoscopy (Adams[3]).

Cytologic examination

The cytologic examination of sputum and of bronchial aspirations has proved to be a valuable adjunct in the diagnosis of bronchial carcinomas. This examination is an accurate and well-established laboratory procedure. It yields higher results than bronchial biopsy and scalene node biopsy combined. As a rule, sputum specimens are more adequate for diagnosis than bronchial washings. Sputum specimens taken immediately after bronchoscopy are least adequate, and those taken seventy-two hours after bronchoscopy proved best (Russell et al.[237]). Bean et al.[19] have utilized a bronchial brush to remove biopsy specimens. They reported thirty-nine cases of cancer identified by means of brush biopsy, thirty-two of which were negative by all other methods except by surgical biopsy. Peripheral pulmonary lesions often fail to yield a positive cytology. However, Frenzel and Papageorgiou,[98] using 10% saline aerosol to promote sputum and examining as many as ten specimens per patient, were able to diagnose fifteen out of thirty-eight coin lesions. Cytologic diagnosis may fail be-

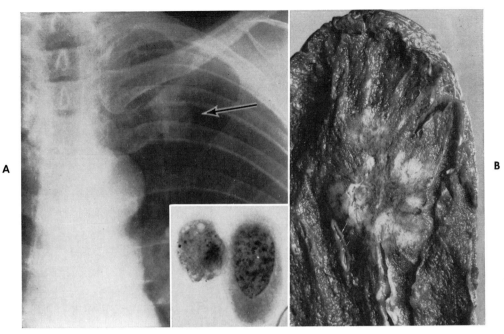

Fig. 283. **A,** Small, round shadow in left upper lung field, partially obscured by rib. Patient, 56-year-old man, had negative bronchoscopy, and tumor cells were found in sputum. **Inset,** Two cells found in sputum of patient. Large cell is cancer cell and other cell is macrophage. Nucleus of cancer cell shows pronounced aberrations from normal and emphasizes prominent nuclear-cytoplasmic relation. **B,** Gross specimen demonstrating small tumor found at radical left upper lobectomy. Regional lymph nodes were negative. Patient was alive and well three and one-half years after surgery. (**A,** WU neg. 58-373; **inset,** high power; WU neg. 58-386; **B,** WU neg. 58-81.)

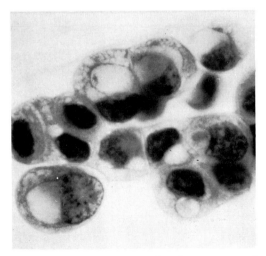

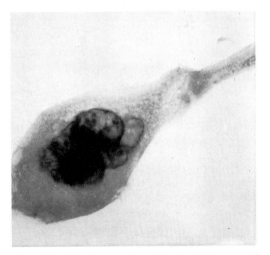

Fig. 284. Photomicrograph taken from imprint of bronchiolar cancer (alveolar cell tumor) demonstrating prominent vacuolation. (×1000; from Ackerman, L. V., and Spjut, H. J.: Exfoliative cytology and pulmonary cancer, Acta Un. Int. Cancr. **16:**371-376, 1960; WU neg. 57-2453.)

Fig. 285. Classic example of "tadpole" tumor cell seen in epidermoid cancer. Note prominent alterations of nucleus. (×1000; from Ackerman, L. V., and Spjut, H. J.: Exfoliative cytology and pulmonary cancer, Acta Un. Int. Cancr. **16:**371-376, 1960; WU neg. 57-2454.)

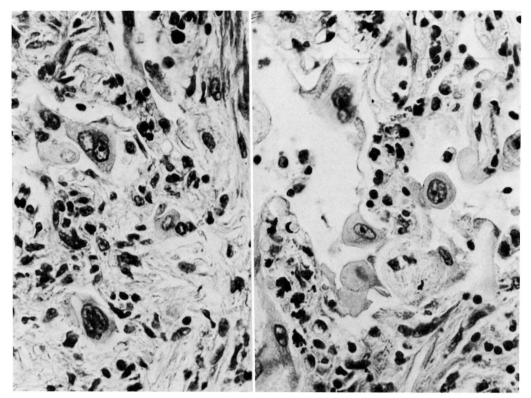

Fig. 286. Desquamated septal cells within alveoli mimic tumor cells. Such bizarre cells are rarely seen except following irradiation. (×440; from Bennett, D. E., et al.: Bilateral radiation pneumonitis, a complication of the radiotherapy of bronchogenic carcinoma, Cancer **23**:1001-1018, 1969; WU neg. 67-1398.)

cause of bronchial stenosis or because an insufficient number of specimens is examined, three specimens per patient being the optimum (Fig. 283). The exact diagnosis may be made in 80% of the cases (Figs. 284 and 285).

A positive cytologic diagnosis of cancer outweighs a negative bronchoscopic biopsy and authorizes a thoracotomy. In a series of forty-eight cases with positive cytologic diagnosis, a pulmonary resection was carried out in every patient without further confirmation of the diagnosis (Spjut et al.[257]). The cytologic examination is also of value in the follow-up of resected cases. It may reveal an early recurrence of the stump or evidence of a new carcinoma (Le Gal and Bauer[166]). Following irradiation of the lung, extremely atypical changes of the septate cells of the alveoli may be observed that may be impossible to differentiate from cancer (Bennett et al.[22]; Koss and Richardson[157]) (Fig. 286). A

false positive diagnosis may be rendered in patients with hypopharyngeal and esophageal tumors or with atypical pneumonia, pulmonary infarction, lipoid pneumonia, fungal diseases, or tuberculosis. A false positive diagnosis of adenocarcinoma is sometimes made, but a diagnosis of squamous cell carcinoma is quite reliable. In twelve patients who had negative chest roentgenograms, Melamed et al.[182] reported positive cytology—four had superficially invasive or in situ carcinoma and four had advanced carcinoma hidden in the mediastinal shadow. Pearson[210] reported forty-one patients with malignant cells in the sputum yet without visible tumor in the roentgenogram. At the time of reporting, carcinoma had been found in twenty-one patients, in two of them only at autopsy.

Biopsy

A bronchial biopsy asserts the diagnosis of bronchial neoplasm, but it does not

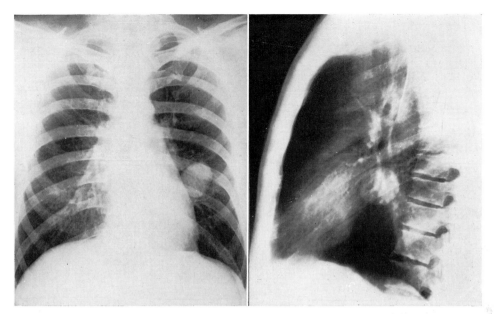

Fig. 287. Well-delineated peripheral lesion that proved to be bronchial carcinoid. (From Maier, H. C., and Fischer, W. W.: Adenomas arising from small bronchi not visible broncho-scopically, J. Thorac. Surg. **16:**392-398, 1947.)

permit an evaluation of the operability of the case. However, a positive biopsy from the carina usually indicates inoperability. Some surgeons conclude to inoperability if the biopsy shows a small cell carcinoma. The same may apply to demonstrable lymphatic permeation in the biopsy specimen. A positive biopsy from the supra-clavicular or scalene lymph nodes also indicates inoperability (Bansmer et al.[16]). A surgical exploration of the mediastinum for purposes of biopsy may also yield positive results and conclude to inoperability (Harken et al.[131]; Paulson[207]; Delarue and Starr[74]).

A *needle biopsy* is recommended only in advanced peripheral pulmonary tumors in order to obviate a thoracotomy or simply to establish a diagnosis before palliative procedures are instituted. Whenever curative procedures are contemplated, a thoracotomy and frozen section are preferable.

Pleural fluid sediment

A definite cytologic diagnosis of malignant pulmonary tumor may be obtained in cases with *pleural effusion* by centrifuging the fluid and sectioning the pellet obtained, but additional study of the smears

is fruitful. Such fluid is often bloody. Clear fluid seldom contains cancer cells.

Laboratory tests

Bioassay of oat cell carcinoma and of the pituitary gland in a case associated with Cushing's syndrome revealed significant corticotropic activity in the tumor but not in the pituitary gland (Marks et al.[179]). The adrenocortical function was studied in 100 patients with bronchial carcinoma, and 71% had elevated plasma corticoid levels. Anaplastic large cell carcinoma of the lung may produce gonadotropin (Fusco and Rosen[102]). Lebacq et al.[165] reported two patients with oat cell carcinoma with inappropriate ADH secretion. They had low plasma sodium and osmolarity and high urinary sodium and osmolarity. Unger et al.[278] identified insulin and glucagon in metastases from a bronchogenic carcinoma.

Differential diagnosis

Benign tumors of the bronchus are rarer than bronchial carcinoid or carcinoma. They grow slowly, they may or may not be accompanied by symptoms of bronchial block, and their nature may not be suspected unless a bronchoscopic biopsy is possible. Among the benign tumors are

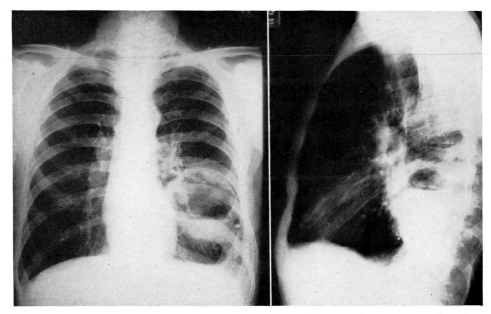

Fig. 288. Large unilateral abscess with fluid level in lower lobe secondary to primary broncho-genic carcinoma of main-stem bronchus. (Courtesy Dr. C. A. Brashear, Mount Vernon, Mo.)

fibromas, lipomas, hamartomas, neurofi-bromas, leiomyomas, and *xanthomas* (Scott et al.[243]).

Primary malignant tumors of the lung, other than carcinoma, are rare, and re-ported cases are often open to doubt. *Chondrosarcomas* arising from bronchial cartilage and capable of infiltrating along the branches of the pulmonary arteries have been reported (Lowell and Tuhy[171]). *Fibrosarcomas* occur in young individuals and have the same gravity as fibrosarcomas elsewhere (Carswell and Kraeft[50]; Black[30]). Rare cases of *carcinosarcoma* have been reported (Bergmann et al.[28]).

Granular cell myoblastoma can produce bronchial obstruction (Greenberg et al.[116]; Benson[27]). Primary *lymphosarcomas* of the lung do occur. Radiographically, they may appear to arise from the hilum without atelectases (Hutchinson et al.[142]), but they may present peripherally. They develop slowly and cause few symptoms (Van Hazel and Jensik[281]; Cooley et al.[62]; Hall and Blades[124]; Sternberg et al.[260]). Most lymphocytic tumors of the lung are prob-ably *pseudolymphomas* (Saltzstein[238]).

Primary *tumors of the trachea* are rare (Culp[64]). A good proportion of these are mucous and salivary gland type of tumors, often of the cylindromatous variety, which develop with preference in the upper half of the trachea. Epidermoid carcinomas are most commonly found in the proximity of the carina. Dyspnea and wheeze due to mechanical obstruction of the air passage are the prominent symptoms. Treatments usually meet with failure, for conservative attempts (Figi[92]) are often insufficient. The cylindromatous variety of tumor has been successfully treated by roentgen-therapy (Tinney et al.[274]). Clagett et al.[56] devised new techniques for the resection of tracheal tumors and in 1952 reported on four patients, three of whom were living.

Lung abscess has to be differentiated from both bronchial carcinoid and carci-noma, for the abscess may develop sec-ondarily to a bronchial block (Fig. 288). If the underlying cause of an abscess is not clear, the possibility of a bronchial tumor should be ruled out by bronchoscopy, if possible, particularly in elderly men.

Infrequently, *organizing pneumonia,* particularly in a man past 50 years of age, occurring in an upper lobe can exactly simulate bronchogenic carcinoma. The pa-tient may have weight loss and hemoptysis, and at operation the involved lobe will be firm. Frozen section is the only method of differentiating this lesion from cancer, al-though radiographic studies may be help-

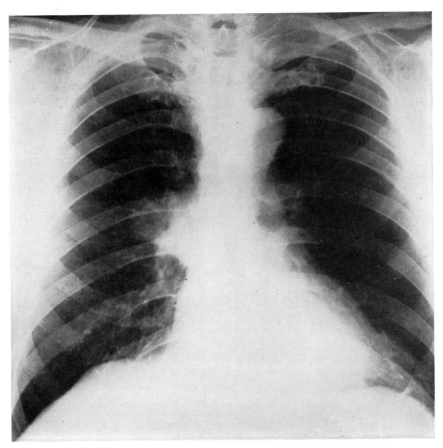

Fig. 289. Hilar mass of organizing pneumonia radiographically simulating bronchogenic carcinoma. (WU neg. 56-4249.)

ful at times. If a diagnosis of organizing pneumonia is made, the lobe is removed, and the bronchi are examined carefully in order to be certain that this organizing pneumonia is not secondary to carcinoma (Ackerman et al.[1]) (Fig. 289).

Tuberculosis of major bronchi usually presents no difficulty in diagnosis, for the sputum is invariably positive for acid-fast bacilli. The lesions are usually multiple, and there is no fixation of the mediastinum or widening of the carina. Of course, a sputum not showing bacilli does not eliminate the possibility of tuberculosis, and, on the other hand, cases of coexisting active tuberculosis and carcinoma may occur (Robbins and Silverman[229]). A *tuberculoma* casts a well-defined shadow on the roentgenogram that is usually impossible to differentiate from a primary peripheral tumor. Tuberculomas and other granulomas, particularly histoplasmosis, may

present concentric lines of calcification and are usually easily recognized at thoracotomy (Black and Ackerman[30a]) (Fig. 290). *Pulmonary infarction,* particularly when it involves the upper lobes, may be mistaken for carcinoma (Starzl et al.[258]).

An *aortic aneurysm* may be difficult to differentiate from carcinoma. The radioscopic examination may reveal an expansile pulsation that facilitates the diagnosis of aneurysm. However, a laminated clot may prevent the aneurysm from pulsating, and a diagnosis may not be reached until a thoracotomy is done.

The superior pulmonary sulcus syndrome of some bronchial carcinomas can be simulated by any other lesion located in the same area and involving the same structures, such as *bronchial cyst, carcinoma of the thyroid gland, Hodgkin's disease,* and *metastatic carcinoma* (Herbut[134]). The syndrome of obstruction of the superior

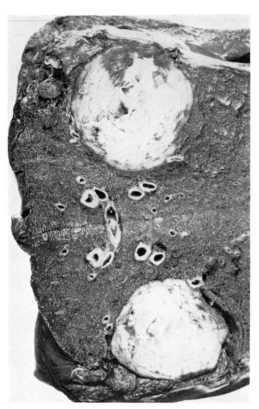

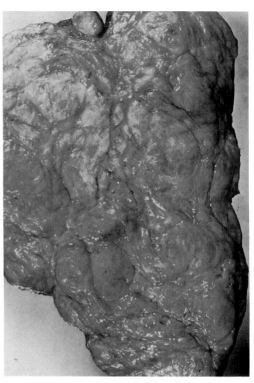

Fig. 291. Typical, extremely large, benign pleural mesothelioma. Note rather lobulated pattern of surface with no evidence of necrosis. Weight of tumor was 3500 gm, and it filled entire cavity. (From Foster-Carter, E. A., and Ackerman, L. V.: Localized mesotheliomas of the pleura; the pathologic evaluation of 18 cases, Amer. J. Clin. Path. 34:349-364, 1960; WU neg. 56-5725.)

Fig. 290. Large subpleural circumscribed granuloma. Presence of concentric rings of calcification was proof that it was benign.

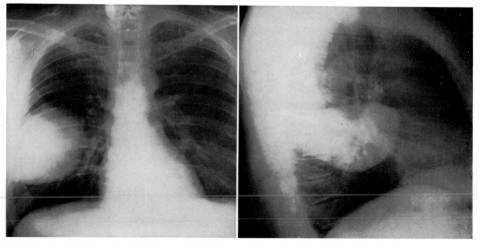

Fig. 292. Ovoid lesion in right lung field interpreted variously as interlobar effusion or peripheral pulmonary neoplasm. On exploratory thoracotomy, it was revealed to be benign solitary pleural mesothelioma. (From Benoit, H. W., Jr., and Ackerman, L. V.: Solitary pleural mesotheliomas, J. Thorac. Surg. 25:346-357, 1953; WU negs. 52-4478 and 52-4479.)

vena cava can also be due to *lymphosar-coma, Hodgkin's disease, metastatic carcinoma,* or *aortic aneurysm* (Hussey et al.[141]).

Hamartomas (chondromas) are tumor-like malformations (Albrecht[6]) arising in the pulmonary parenchyma, usually sub-pleurally, and are often asymptomatic but may impinge on the smaller bronchi and suggest the possibility of a peripheral bron-chial tumor (McDonald et al.[174]). Hamar-tomas vary in size from a few millimeters to 10 cm, are sharply delimited and fairly homogeneous, and may contain bone. Mi-croscopically, they are made up predomi-nantly of cartilage but invariably also con-tain fat, smooth muscle, and glandular, often ciliated, epithelium. They do not be-come malignant. Roentgenographically, a hamartoma appears as a dense, discrete, round or lobulated mass, sometimes con-taining scattered areas of calcification that facilitate the roentgenologic diagnosis. Large hamartomas not containing calcium may be confused with primary lung tumors (Hall[125]).

Metastatic carcinoma can rarely involve hilar lymph nodes and secondarily ulcerate through the bronchi to simulate a primary bronchogenic carcinoma. In our experi-ence, invasion of the bronchus by meta-static lesions has occurred mainly in cases of carcinoma of the breast, kidney, pan-creas, large bowel, or testis (Trinidad et al.[276]). King and Castleman[153] reported on twenty patients with metastatic carcinoma with involvement of the bronchus, four of whom presented blood-streaked expectora-tion. A single metastatic nodule within the lung is often impossible to differentiate from primary peripheral lung tumors. The diagnosis may be made easier by a thorough search for an occult primary lesion or by an inquiry into the past his-tory, which may reveal an almost forgot-ten, casually treated primary lesion.

Benign pleural mesotheliomas are usually asymptomatic. They have a variable microscopic pattern. Papillary areas or fibrous elements may predominate. Tissue cultures and electron microscopy have shown that even the fibrous type arises from mesothelium (Murray[191]; Luce and Spjut[171a]). Mesotheliomas may have a slow clinical onset with painless pleural effusion over a period of years but eventually

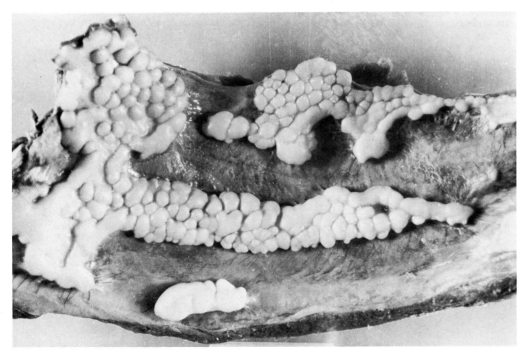

Fig. 293. Classic example of highly specific nodular pleural plaques in asbestosis. (Courtesy Dr. J. G. Thomson, Capetown, R.S.A.)

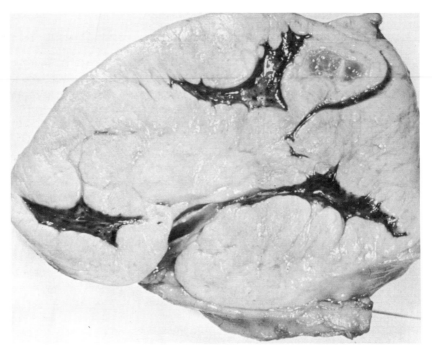

Fig. 294. Malignant pleural mesothelioma with extensive infiltration of lung parenchyma. Large bronchus totally surrounded by tumor is seen near one edge. (Courtesy Dr. I. Webster, Johannesburg, R.S.A.)

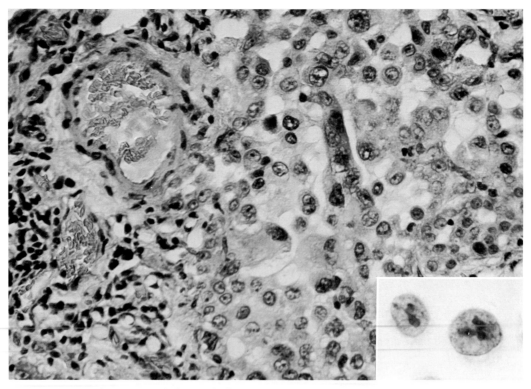

Fig. 295. Malignant mesothelioma of pleura. Note prominent nucleoli. **Inset,** Photomicrograph of cytology of malignant mesothelial cells. Note prominence of nucleoli. (×340; WU neg. 68-10950; **Inset,** ×1100; WU neg. 69-28.)

cause dyspnea. Others develop rapidly (Sano et al.[239]). Fibrous mesotheliomas may be accompanied by symptoms of hyperinsulinism that disappear after removal of the tumor. Pulmonary osteoarthropathy, equally reversible, has been observed also (Benoit and Ackerman[25]). It arises from the pleura, which becomes thickened and yellowish gray (Figs. 291 and 292). Pleural plaques may be present (Fig. 293). As the tumor becomes more diffuse, it may affect the entire pleura, invade between the fissures across the mediastinum, and involve the diaphragm, pericardium, thoracic wall, peritoneum, and even the opposite pleura (Foster-Carter and Ackerman[95]) (Fig. 294). These tumors may become very large and are usually confused with neurogenous tumors. At thoracotomy, the gross pattern and the frozen section are usually diagnostic.

The *malignant pleural mesothelioma* is associated with chest pain, dyspnea, and cough (Fig. 295). Malignant mesothelial cells are usually present and recognizable in the pleural fluid (Naylor[195]; Ratzer et al.[218]). Approximately one-fourth of the cases metastasize to hilar and bronchial lymph nodes and another one-fourth may metastasize to the liver. Schlienger et al.[240a] reported thirty-nine cases of malignant mesotheliomas, twenty-four of which metastasized. Wagner[286] diagnosed a total of eighty-seven pleural and peritoneal mesotheliomas. In only two of the patients it was not possible to establish a history of exposure to asbestos dust.

Treatment
Surgery

In 1933, Dr. Evarts A. Graham performed the first successful pneumonectomy for carcinoma of the lung (Fig. 296). His patient, a physician, lived twenty-nine years without evidence of cancer and outlived Dr. Graham, who succumbed to a carcinoma of the bronchus.

An *exploratory thoracotomy* is often necessary before deciding whether or not the patient is eligible for a resection. Obviously, a thoracotomy is not indicated in the presence of distant metastases. *Mediastinoscopy* has been practiced with increasing frequency (Paulson[207]). Whenever, by any of these means, mediastinal involvement is shown, the patient is inoperable. However, enlargement of nodes is no certainty of their involvement and biopsy should always be done. Delarue et al.[73] have also emphasized the great value of complementary pulmonary angiography and mediastinoscopy in assessing operability. In their hands, these procedures were done with no operative mortality and little morbidity. These procedures were important factors in selecting for surgery only those patients for whom cure was possible. A recurrent nerve paralysis also indicates inoperability, as does the presence of bloody pleural fluid containing tumor cells. Involvement of the pulmonary artery, vena cava, and azygos vein also indicates inoperability.

Only about one-third of patients with operable bronchial carcinoma may have a positive bronchoscopic biopsy, and an additional few may have a positive cytology. There remains an additional group of patients in whom the diagnosis has not been verified. In such patients, a frozen section is required at exploration. Small lesions should be excised rather than incised.

Pneumonectomies have been applied

Table 25. Operability and resectability of bronchial carcinomas at various institutions*

Source	*Tulane*	*Jefferson*	*Mayo*	*Overholt*	*Barnes*	*Total*
Period	1935-1953	1946-1953	1943-1949	1932-1951	1948-1955	
Cases	1170	532	767	733	1008	4210
Explored (%)	52	71	48	62	60	59
Resected (%)	33	39	24	37	35	34
Five-year survival:						
% all resections	14	22	—	21	21	19
% resected for cure	31	42	37	34	39	37
% total cases	8	9	8	8	9	8

*From Burford, T. H., and Ferguson, T. B.: Surgical treatment. In Fried, B. M.: Tumors of the lungs and mediastinum, Philadelphia, 1958, Lea & Febiger, pp. 266-283.

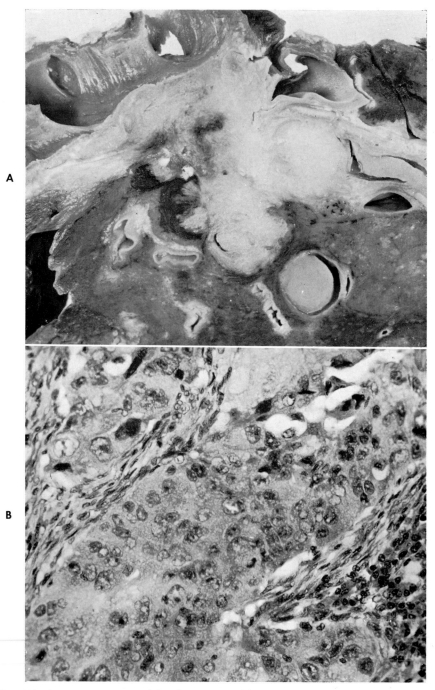

Fig. 296. **A,** Gross specimen of first lung successfully resected for carcinoma. Note extension to regional lymph nodes. This operation was done by Dr. Evarts A. Graham in 1933, and the patient died without evidence of cancer in 1962. **B,** Photomicrograph showing undifferentiated epidermoid carcinoma.

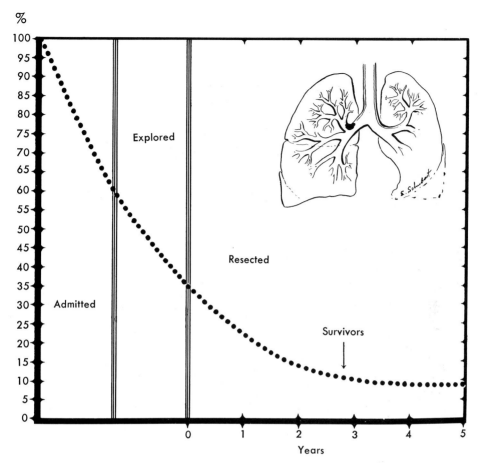

%

Fig. 297. Graphic illustration of survival of patients with carcinoma of bronchus. Patients who live two years following pneumonectomy and without evidence of recurrence usually remain well.

with improved skill to an increasing number of patients for thirty years. In the face of disappointing results, a still more radical approach has been advocated (Chamberlain et al.[52]), but not all thoracic surgeons have accepted the principles of *radical pneumonectomies* nor have raised their resectability rates. Increased resectability implies greater operative mortality without necessarily greater average survival (Johnson et al.[148]). The usually elderly patient who survives a pneumonectomy faces a diminishing pulmonary reserve (Adams et al.[4]). Extension of the operation to include involvement of contiguous organs, such as the pericardium, or massive lymph node metastases, in the hope of rescuing an occasional patient, has not proved to be worthwhile.

Lobectomies are well indicated in the treatment of peripheral carcinomas of the lung where they have proved to be successful (Churchill et al.[54]). Paulson et al.[208] also treat small hilar lesions by lobectomy combined at times with a bronchoplastic procedure to allow for wider excision of the major bronchi. Lobectomies are accompanied by lesser operative mortality. For these reasons there has been an increasing trend toward utilization of this procedure. The frequent occurrence of a second contralateral primary lesion and the feasibility of a second lobectomy become arguments in favor of lobectomy (Le Gal and Bauer[166]). Lobectomies are also used as compromise procedures in patients with low cardiac respiratory reserve or as a palliative procedure in patients with pulmonary suppuration or repeated hemoptysis (Robinson et al.[233]).

Pneumonectomy or lobectomy is the treatment of choice of rare primary tumors such as fibrosarcomas. Pleural mesotheliomas have been treated successfully by surgical resection (Stout and Himadi[265]; Stout and Murray[266]; Benoit and Ackerman[25]).

Metastatic lesions of the lung may be successfully resected particularly if they are single, if they result from primary lesions in the kidney, large bowel, or soft tissues, and if they are detected more than one year after control of the primary lesion. Of nineteen cases at risk, Johnson and Lindskog[149] reported nine patients surviving five years.

Endoscopic removal of bronchial tumors has been advocated. Mucoepidermoid tumors that appear as polypoid masses are not curable by this approach (Payne et al.[209]). Bronchial carcinoids cannot be treated by bronchoscopic removal, for the procedure leads to hemorrhage, bronchial stenosis, infection, and recurrence and, frequently, to death. Surgical resection is recommended (Carlens et al.[49]). In many cases, the location of the tumor and the secondary and inflammatory changes dictate the necessity for pneumonectomy. In the cylindromatous variety of these tumors, the possibility of lymph node involvement favors a pneumonectomy.

The operative mortality of pneumonectomies has steadily decreased. Operative deaths are mostly due to cardiovascular complications, pulmonary edema, hemorrhage, or pneumonia, to the development of pneumothorax, and, to a lesser extent, to the anesthesia. The most common complications of pneumonectomies are the bronchial fistulas, due to incomplete closure of the bronchial stump, and empyema.

Chemotherapy

Carcinoma of the lung has been the subject of numerous trials of chemotherapeutic agents as adjuvants to surgery (Curreri[65]; Curreri et al.[66]). *Nitrogen mustard,* a powerful alkylating agent, has been used extensively. This agent may temporarily relieve superior vena cava obstruction, particularly in the small cell type of lung cancer, but this is invariably only of short-term benefit. Neither has it proved advantageous to add a chemothera-

peutic agent at the end of an operative procedure (Slack[250a]). Chemotherapy has never been proved to prolong a life or cure a patient with lung cancer (Higgins and Wolf[135]). Chemotherapeutic agents are extremely helpful in malignant pleural effusions. Nitrogen mustard is much more simple to use than radioactive gold (Weisberger et al.[291]). Kinsey et al.[154] used mechlorethamine hydrochloride for malignant pleural effusion with excellent palliation. Unfortunately, when cancer cells appear in the pleural fluid in association with lung cancer, the duration of life is short.

Radiotherapy

Bronchial carcinomas are often rather radiosensitive. Their exposure to radiations frequently results in physical diminution, reestablishment of bronchial permeability and disappearance of atelectasis, consequent diminution of cough and pain, and improvement of the general condition. Irradiation by means of conventional roentgentherapy of 250 kv range has given worthwhile results and prolonged survival (Hughes et al.[140]) but, with rare exceptions (Euphrat[88]), this modality failed in its inability to deliver a homogeneously distributed and sufficiently high dose throughout the potential area of neoplastic involvement (Laval et al.[164]; Surmont et al.[269]). The advent of supervoltage roentgentherapy and cobalt[60] resulted in renewed interest in and unquestionably better results from radiotherapy of cancer of the lung. Haas et al.[123] pioneered in the use of betatron therapy. They reported improved results in apical tumors. Watson,[289] Wood,[299] and others reported on the initial advantages of supervoltage roentgentherapy. This highly penetrating modality not only eliminates concern of intense skin reactions, but also permits delivery of a large amount of radiations over a large volume of the lung and mediastinum, with greater field definition, with fewer systemic effects, and with greater possibilities of control of a reasonably limited tumor.

Adequate irradiation of a carcinoma of the bronchus and its potential metastatic manifestations in the mediastinum implies a rather heavy irradiation of a great part of the lung and probable untoward effects. Classically, the expected effect is pulmonary fibrosis, but irradiation actually results in an *acute pneumonitis* that, depending on complications, may result in greater or lesser fibrosis. If the radiation pneumonitis is anticipated during or shortly after the treatment, if the patient is hospitalized and subjected to medical management and early administration of antibiotics, the pneumonitis may be minimized with the resulting effect of only a progressive shrinkage of the lung and a minimum of fibrosis. There are considerable differences in the risks and in the patient's adaptation to a sudden fibrosis as compared to a progressive diminution of his respiratory capacity. At worst, the irradiation effects on the lung (Deeley[71]) should not discourage the radiotherapist from administering the necessary dose, for the patient would not be more of a respiratory cripple than if he had had a pneumonectomy.

Buschke[47] believes that patients with very undifferentiated carcinomas with marked hemorrhagic tendency or with prominent pulmonary involvement should be greatly benefited by radiotherapy. Superior vena caval obstruction, a syndrome more often connected with cancer of the lung than with any other condition, is often markedly affected by irradiation, lessening the distress of the patient's clinical course (Green and Spence[115]). Szur and Bromley[271] treated 107 patients with superior vena caval obstruction with improvement of the syndrome in thirty-seven. In patients with invasion of the ribs and compression of the brachial plexus, radiotherapy affords regression, recalcification, pain relief, and improvement of the general condition (Haas et al.[123]). Radiations are very effective in the palliation of pain caused by bone metastases. Attention has been called to the utilization of radiotherapy on limited postoperative recurrences of the bronchial stump (Pinsky and Emerson[211]). *Adenoid cystic carcinoma*, truly a malignant tumor, is highly radiosensitive (Vieta and Maier[283]). *Tracheobronchial papillomatosis* has also shown favorable response to radiatons (Blackman et al.[32]).

The poor results of pneumonectomy, the frequent marked clinical regressions, and a number of survivals following supervoltage or cobalt[60] therapy have brought about an enlargement of the attack of radio-

therapy on cancer of the lung. Smart and Hilton[251] indicated that in some instances radiotherapy was a reasonable alternative to surgery, in operable cases. The question arises of whether the extent of useful life afforded by radiotherapy alone equals, or betters, the results of surgery, considering also the relatively high operative mortality of pneumonectomies. Morrison et al.[189] detailed a clinical trial to compare the results of surgery and supervoltage roentgentherapy. All cases were diagnosed by biopsy, the patients were all under 70 years of age, in fairly good health, and with no evidence of mediastinal involvement or distant metastases, and random selection decided the modality of treatment. The immediate survival was better for patients undergoing radiotherapy, but the four-year survival was better for those undergoing surgery. Miller et al.[183] reported a five-year follow-up of a trial of surgery and radiotherapy for the primary treatment of small cell or oat cell carcinoma of the bronchus. The results were somewhat better with radical radiotherapy than with surgery. Radiation therapy has been combined with 5-fluorouracil and, compared with radiotherapy alone, with no apparent gain (Benninghoff and Alexander[24]).

A worthy approach appears to be that of administrating *preoperative* radiotherapy in operable patients in an effort to improve the survival; Manfredi et al.[178] reported that preoperative radiotherapy provides no advantage, but others have had a different experience (Bloedorn[33]). In order to resolve this dilemma, a group of clinical investigators conducted a randomized study in which no significant difference was found in the three-year survival of two groups of nearly 300 patients treated by either approach (Collaborative Study[59]). In this study, a group of inoperable patients was irradiated and later randomized to submit or not to surgery, with the result that there was no significant difference in the two subgroups. In a similar study, the same conclusions were reached (Medical Research Council[180]).

A randomized study of preoperative roentgentherapy was carried out in Veteran Administration Hospitals (Shields et al.[248]). The dosage administered, mostly with conventional voltage, varied considerably, and only about half of the patients irradiated subsequently underwent resection, ten to fifteen days after radiotherapy. In 27% (twenty-three) of those irradiated, no cancer was found at operation. Postoperative complications, however, were slightly greater in the irradiated group, but the operative mortality was the same as in the nonirradiated group. The three-year survival rate was better in the patients not receiving preoperative radiotherapy. Thus, the authors concluded that preoperative irradiation is contraindicated.

Prognosis

Between 1914 and 1950, the mortality rate of men with lung cancer increased twenty-five times (Dorn[81]) in the United States. In 1956 there were 29,000 deaths from cancer of the lung, and in 1965 there were 48,359 deaths, or a crude death rate of 24.9 per 100,000 population. The death rates were 44.2 and 7.9 for male and female whites and 33.0 and 5.7 for male and female nonwhites. The American Cancer Society[6a] estimates 68,000 deaths from cancer of the lung in the United States in 1970. The mortality from cancer of the lung among Mexican women in California is unusually high (Buechley et al.[43]). Contrarily, the death rate from cancer of the lung among Seventh-Day Adventists (a religious, essentially nonsmoking population) is very low. Scotland reported the highest death rates for both males and females in 1962-1963, twice that recorded in the United States. The lowest death rate is reported in Portugal.

Untreated cases of bronchial carcinoma develop rapidly toward death. Scarcely 1 out of 10 patients would be living at the end of three years, although some may live over five years (Buchberg et al.[42]).

Oat cell carcinomas have a consistently bad prognosis whether treated by surgery or radiotherapy. In a control study conducted by the National Research Council,[194] the results were poor following both methods of treatment. In a series of 120 patients with oat cell carcinoma reported by Hutzschenreuter and Schamaun,[143] the operability was 10% with an average survival of 1.8 months for inoperable patients and 1.6 months for those receiving pneumonectomy, and only 12% of those who received radiotherapy alone survived one year.

Eastridge et al.[85] reported 1284 cases of cancer of the lung, with surgical exploration in 34% and resection in 31% (lobectomy in 47% and pneumonectomy in 51%). The overall one-year survival was 23% and five-year survival was 3.5%. For the patients undergoing resection, the five-year survival for pneumonectomies was 24% and that for lobectomies 25%. The overall five-year survival rate for the United Kingdom has been estimated at 5% (Bignall et al.[29]). In a series of 6086 cases of bronchial carcinoma studied by Bignall et al.,[29] two-thirds of the patients died in the first year following admission. There were a few long-term survivors following radiotherapy, and between 20% and 35% of those who underwent resection survived five-years. In a series of 1613 cases reported by Bangma,[15] 828 patients were not subjected to resection, only eight of whom survived three years or more. *Radical* pneumonectomy does not seem to yield better results (Johnson et al.[148]). There is no apparent superiority of pneumonectomy over lobectomy (Belcher and Lond[20]).

The duration of symptoms is not related to prognosis. Patients with carcinoma of the left lung have been reported to have a better prognosis than those with carcinoma of the right lung because of a lesser proportion of metastases (Spjut et al.[257]), but the opposite has been reported by others (Gifford and Waddington[108]) for the same reasons. Evidence of vein invasion in the surgical specimen implies probability of distant metastases (Collier et al.[60]; Gagnon and Gelinas-Mackay[103]; Spjut et al.[257]) (Table 26). When a great proportion of nodes are found to be invaded or the tumor has been cut across, treatment will invariably fail (Gronqvist et al.[119]; Watkins and Gerard[288]). Epidermoid carcinomas have a relatively better prognosis (Gibbon et al.[107]). Primary adenocarcinoma of the lung is associated with a high rate of resection but a poor outlook for long-term survival (Sasser et al.[240]). Patients who survive resection may live in relative comfort and become reasonably active, but they all face a progressive degree of cardiopulmonary dis-

Table 26. Relationships of survival to presence or absence of lymph node metastases and blood vessel invasion*

Carcinoma in nodes	Carcinoma in blood vessels	Patients	Alive
Present	Present	94	10 (11%)
Present	Absent	45	11 (24%)
Absent	Present	50	12 (24%)
Absent	Absent	32	13 (41%)
Total		221†	46 (21%)

*From Spjut, H. J., et al.: Pulmonary cancer and its prognosis, Cancer 14:1251-1258, 1961.
†Five patients had no lymph nodes examined.

ability (Jones et al.[151]). Failure of treatment following lobectomy or pneumonectomy is unfortunately due to a high prevalence of local recurrence or persistent disease in the hemithorax from which the carcinoma was removed (Spjut and Mateo[256]).

In a series of 225 patients with inoperable bronchial carcinomas, 122 were given only supportive treatment and 103 were given roentgentherapy. All patients were dead in forty-two months, but the average survival was 1.9 months for the untreated and 5.2 months for the irradiated group (Barton et al.[17]). These figures do not reveal the great amount of worthwhile palliation that is obtained from radiotherapy. Cures are rarely obtained with the advanced cases that constitute the radiotherapist's material. Smithers[254] reported six of a series of 171 irradiated patients living over five years. Windeyer[296] reported four of a series of 200 patients living six years. A number of patients from various reported series appear to have lived over five years, particularly with the adequate use of supervoltage or cobalt[60] units (Morrison[188]). Smart and Hilton[251] submitted to radiotherapy thirty-three patients with apparently operable lesions. Of twelve followed for five years, four were living and well. As earlier cases are submitted to radiotherapy or to a combination of radiotherapy and surgery, the results may overshadow those of a purely surgical series.

Guttman[122] irradiated 103 patients after they were considered inoperable at thoracotomy. She used supervoltage roentgentherapy and large opposing fields and fractionated the total dose over five weeks. There was symptomatic relief in 75% of the patients; the survival was 57% at one year, 17% at three years, 11% at five years,

Table 27. Summary of follow-up of sixty patients with bronchial adenoma*†

Total dead		12
Dead of metastases	5	
Died postoperatively	3	
Died of intercurrent disease	4	
Total living (all apparently cured)		48
Living and well under five years	15	
Living and well five to ten years postoperatively	17	
Living and well eleven to twenty years postoperatively	13	
Living more than twenty years postoperatively	2	
		60

*From Overholt, R. H., et al.: Bronchial adenoma; a study of 60 patients with resections, Amer. Rev. Tuberc. 75:865-884, 1957.
†All surviving patients followed to January, 1956.

and 7% at ten years. Bignall et al.[29] reviewed a large group of patients with cancer of the lung who had been treated by radiotherapy over a period of twenty-five years, noting that the one-year survival was 17% in the years 1956-1961 and that it rose to 25% in 1962-1963, probably due to the use of supervoltage roentgentherapy. Not infrequently, however, even when the carcinoma of the lung is destroyed by radiotherapy, patients succumb to distant metastases. There is no convincing evidence that routine preoperative irradiation of operable lesions improves on the results of surgery alone (Collaborative Study[59]). In the series of seventeen patients reported by Baker et al.[12] in whom the resected specimen, following preoperative radiotherapy, showed no evidence of residual pulmonary tumor, only one was alive after 3.5 years.

Bronchial carcinoids have a good prognosis (Table 27). *Lymphosarcomas* have a much better prognosis than carcinomas.

REFERENCES

1 Ackerman, L. V., Elliott, G. V., and Alanis, M.: Localized organizing pneumonia: its resemblance to carcinoma; a review of its clinical, roentgenographic and pathologic features, Amer. J. Roentgen. **71**:988-996, 1954.

2 Ackerman, L. V., and Spjut, H. J.: Exfoliative cytology and pulmonary cancer, Acta Un. Int. Cancr. **16**:371-376, 1960.

3 Adams, R.: Primary lung tumors, J.A.M.A. **130**:547-553, 1946.

4 Adams, W. E., Perkins, J. F., Jr., Harrison, R. W., Buhler, W., and Long, E. T.: The significance of cardiopulmonary reserve in the late results of pneumonectomy for carcinoma of the lung, Dis. Chest **32**:380-388, 1957.

5 Adler, I.: Primary malignant growths of the lungs and bronchi, New York, 1912, Longmans, Green & Co., Inc.

6 Albrecht, E.: Ueber Hamartome, Verh. Deutsch. Ges. Path. **7**:153-157, 1904.

6a American Cancer Society: Cancer statistics, 1970, CA **20**:10-23, 1970.

7 Anderson, W. M.: Bronchial adenoma with metasis to the liver, J. Thorac. Surg. **12**:351-360, 1943.

8 Anlyan, A. K., Lovinggood, C. G., and Klassen, K. P.: Primary lymphosarcoma of the lung, Surgery **27**:559-563, 1950.

9 Ariel, I. M., Avery, E. E., Kanter, L., Head, J. R., and Langston, H. T.: Primary carcinoma of the lung, Cancer **3**:229-239, 1950.

10 Ashley, D. J. B.: The distribution of lung cancer and bronchitis in England and Wales, Brit. J. Cancer **21**:243-259, 1967.

11 Auerbach, O., Gere, J. B., Forman, J. B., Petrick, T. G., Smolin, H. J., Muesham, G. E., Kassourny, D. Y., and Stout, A. P.: Changes in the bronchial epithelium in relation to smoking and cancer of the lung; a report of progress, New Eng. J. Med. **256**:97-104, 1957.

12 Baker, N. H., Cowley, R. A., and Linberg, E.: A follow-up in patients with bronchogenic carcinoma "locally cured" by preoperative irradiation, J. Thorac. Cardiovasc. Surg. **40**:298-309, 1963.

13 Baker, N. H., Hill, L., Ewy, H. G., and Marable, S.: Pulmonary lymphatic drainage, J. Thorac. Cardiovasc. Surg. **54**:695-696, 1967.

14 Baker, R. R.: The clinical management of bronchogenic carcinoma, Johns Hopkins Med. J. **121**:401-411, 1967.

15 Bangma, P. J.: The results of the treatment of bronchogenic carcinoma; a study of 1,613 cases, Utrecht, 1963, Kemink & Zoon, N. V.

16 Bansmer, G., Lawrence, G. H., and Hill, L. D.: The scalene lymph node biopsy, J. Thorac. Cardiovasc. Surg. **37**:305-313, 1959.

17 Barton, H. L., McGranahan, G. M., Jr., and Jordan, G. L., Jr.: The evaluation of roentgen therapy in the management of non-sectable carcinoma of the lung, Dis. Chest **37**:170-175, 1960.

18 Batesman, E. M.: The solitary circumscribed bronchogenic carcinoma, Brit. J. Radiol. **37**:598-607, 1964.

19 Bean, W. J., Graham, W. L., Jordan, R. B., and Eavenson, L. W.: Diagnosis of lung cancer by the transbronchial brush biopsy technique, J.A.M.A. **206**:1070-1072, 1968.

20 Belcher, J. R., and Lond, M. S.: Lobectomy for bronchial carcinoma, Lancet **2**:639-642, 1959.

21 Belsey, H. R., and Valentine, J. C.: Cylindromatous mucous-gland tumors of the trachea and bronchi; a report of three cases, J. Path. Bact. **63**:377-387, 1951.

22 Bennett, D. E., Million, R. E., and Ackerman, L. V.: Bilateral radiation pneumonitis, a complication of the radiotherapy of bronchogenic carcinoma; report and analysis of 7 cases with autopsy, Cancer **23**:1001-1018, 1969.

23 Bennett, D. E., Sasser, W. F., and Ferguson, T. B.: Adenocarcinoma of the lung in men—a clinicopathologic study of 100 cases, Cancer **23**:431-439, 1969.

24 Benninghoff, D. L., and Alexander, L. L.: Treatment of lung carcinoma; radiation versus radiation combined with 5-fluorouracil, New York J. Med. **68**:532-534, 1968.

25 Benoit, H. W., Jr., and Ackerman, L. V.: Solitary pleural mesotheliomas, J. Thorac. Surg. **25**:346-357, 1953.

26 Bensch, K. G., Corrin, B., Pariente, R., and Spencer, H.: Oat cell carcinoma of the lung; its origin and relationship to bronchial carcinoid, Cancer **22**:1163-1172, 1968.

27 Benson, W. R.: Granular cell tumors (myoblastomas) of the tracheobronchial tree, J. Thorac. Cardiovasc. Surg. **52**:17-30, 1966.

28 Bergmann, M., Ackerman, L. V., and Kemler, R. L.: Carcinosarcoma of the lung; review of the literature and report of two cases treated by pneumonectomy, Cancer **4**:919-929, 1951.

29 Bignall, J. R., Martin, M., and Smithers, D. W.: Survival in 6,086 cases of bronchial carcinoma, Lancet **1**:1067-1070, 1967.

29a Bjork, V. O.: Bronchiogenic carcinoma, Acta Chir. Scand. **95**(suppl. 123):1-113, 1947.

30 Black, H.: Fibrosarcoma of the bronchus, J. Thorac. Surg. **19**:123-134, 1950.

30a Black, H., and Ackerman, L. V.: The clinical and pathologic aspects of tuberculoma of the lung; an analysis of 18 cases, Surg. Clin. N. Amer. **30**:1279-1297, 1950 (extensive bibliography).

31 Black, H., and Ackerman, L. V.: The importance of epidermoid carcinoma in situ in the histogenesis of carcinoma of the lung, Ann. Surg. **136**:44-54, 1952.

32 Blackman, J., Cantril, S. T., Lund, P. K., and Sparkman, D.: Tracheobronchial papillomatosis treated by roentgen irradiation, Radiology **73**:598-606, 1959.

33 Bloedorn, F. G., Cowley, A., Cuccia, C. A., and Mercado, R., Jr.: Combined therapy: irradiation and surgery in the treatment of bronchogenic carcinoma, Amer. J. Roentgen. **85**:875-885, 1962.

34 Blount, H. C., Jr.: Localized mesothelioma

of the pleura; a review with six new cases, Radiology **67**:822-833, 1956.

34a Bocker, D.: Smoking and health 1958-1963, National Library of Medicine, Oct., 1963 (extensive bibliography).

35 Bonser, G. M., and Thomas, G. M.: An investigation of the validity of death certification of cancer of the lung in Leeds, Brit. J. Cancer **13**:1-12, 1959.

36 Borow, M., Conston, A., Livornese, L. L., and Schalet, N.: Mesothelioma and its association with asbestosis, J.A.M.A. **201**:587-591, 1967.

37 Boucot, K. R., Cooper, D. A., and Weiss, W.: The role of surgery in the cure of lung cancer, Arch. Intern. Med. (Chicago) **120**:168-175, 1967.

38 Boucot, K. R., Cooper, D. A., Weiss, W., and Carnahan, W. J.: Cigarettes, cough and cancer of the lung, J.A.M.A. **198**:985-990, 1966.

39 Boucot, K. R., and Sokoloff, M. J.: Is survey cancer of the lung curable? Dis. Chest **27**:1-20, 1955.

40 Brain, L., and Wilkinson, M.: Subacute cerebellar degeneration associated with neoplasms, Brain **88**:465-478, 1965.

41 Brisman, R., Baker, R. R., Elkins, R., and Hartmann, W. H.: Carcinoma of the lung in four siblings, Cancer **20**:2048-2053, 1967.

42 Buchberg, A., Lubliner, R., and Rubin, E. H.: Carcinoma of the lung; duration of life of individuals not treated surgically, Dis. Chest **20**:257-276, 1951.

43 Buechley, R., Dunn, J. E., Jr., Linden, G., and Breslow, L.: Excess lung-cancer-mortality rates among Mexican women in California, Cancer **10**:63-66, 1957.

44 Buell, P., and Dunn, J. E.: Relative impact of smoking and air pollution on lung cancer, Arch. Environ. Health (Chicago) **15**:291-297, 1967.

45 Buell, P., Dunn, J. E., Jr., and Breslow, L.: Cancer of the lung and Los Angeles-type air pollution; prospective study, Cancer **20**:2139-2147, 1967.

46 Burch, P. R. J.: Genetic carrier frequency for lung cancer, Nature (London) **202**:711-712, 1964.

47 Buschke, F.: Roentgen therapy of carcinoma of the lung, Radiology **69**:489-493, 1957.

48 Caranasos, G., and Huebner, B. H.: Adrenal width and metastasis in bronchogenic carcinoma, Arch. Path. (Chicago) **76**:263-266, 1963.

49 Carlens, E., Wiklund, T., and Bergstrand, A.: Bronchial adenoma; a report of 70 cases and a critical analysis of the literature, Acta Chir. Scand. **185**(suppl.):1-55, 1954.

50 Carswell, J., Jr., and Kraeft, N. H.: Fibrosarcoma of the bronchus, J. Thorac. Surg. **19**:117-122, 1950.

51 Cauna, D., Totten, R. S., and Gross, P.: Asbestos bodies in human lungs at autopsy, J.A.M.A. **192**:371-373, 1965.

52 Chamberlain, J. M., McNeill, T. M., Parnassa, P., and Edsall, J. R.: Bronchogenic carcinoma; an aggressive surgical attitude, J. Thorac. Cardiovasc. Surg. **38**:727-745, 1959.

53 Churchill, E. D.: Report on medical progress; thoracic surgery, New Eng. J. Med. **223**:581-587, 1940.

54 Churchill, E. D., Sweet, R. H., Scannell, J. G., and Wilkins, E. W., Jr.: Further studies in the surgical management of carcinoma of the lung, J. Thorac. Surg. **36**:301-308, 1958.

55 Churchill, E. D., Sweet, R. H., Soutter, L., and Scannell, J. G.: The surgical management of carcinoma of the lung, J. Thorac. Surg. **20**:349-365, 1950.

56 Clagett, O. T., Moersch, H. J., and Grindlay, J. H.: Intrathoracic tracheal tumors, development of surgical technics for their removal, Ann. Surg. **136**:520-532, 1952.

57 Clemmesen, J., and Nielsen, A.: The geographical and racial distribution of cancer of the lung, Schweiz. Z. Allg. Path. **18**:803-819, 1955.

58 Cohart, E. M.: Socioeconomic distribution of cancer of the lung in New Haven, Cancer **8**:1126-1129, 1955.

59 Collaborative Study: Preoperative irradiation of cancer of the lung; preliminary report of a therapeutic trial, Cancer **23**:419-430, 1969.

60 Collier, F. C., Enterline, H. T., Kyle, R. H., Tristan, T. T., and Greenberg, R.: The prognostic implications of vascular invasion in primary carcinoma of the lung, Arch. Path. (Chicago) **66**:594-603, 1958.

61 Connelly, R. R., Cutler, S. J., and Baylis, P.: End results in cancer of the lung; comparison of male and female patients, J. Nat. Cancer Inst. **36**:277-287, 1966.

62 Cooley, J. C., McDonald, J. R., and Clagett, O. T.: Primary lymphoma of the lung, Ann. Surg. **143**:18-28, 1956.

63 Cornfield, J., Haensel, W., Hammond, E. C., Lilienfeld, A. M., Shimkin, M. B., and Wynder, E. L.: Smoking and lung cancer; recent evidence and a discussion of some questions, J. Nat. Cancer Inst. **22**:173-203, 1959.

64 Culp, O. S.: Primary carcinoma of the trachea, J. Thorac. Surg. **7**:471-487, 1938.

65 Curreri, A. R.: Nitrogen mustard as an adjunct to pulmonary resection in the treatment of carcinoma of the lung, Cancer Chemother. Rep. **16**:123-128, 1962.

66 Curreri, A. R., Ansfield, F. J., McIver, F. A., Waisman, H. A., and Heidelberger, C.: Clinical studies with 5-fluorouracil, Cancer Res. **18**:478-484, 1958.

67 Cutler, S. J., and Loveland, D. B.: The risk of developing lung cancer and its relationship to smoking, J. Nat. Cancer Inst. **15**:201-211, 1954.

68 Davis, E. W., Peabody, J. W., Jr., and Katz, S.: The solitary pulmonary nodule, J. Thorac. Surg. **32**:728-771, 1956 (extensive bibliography).

69 Dayan, A. D., Croft, P. B., and Wilkinson, M.: Association of carcinomatous neuromyopathy with different histological types of carcinoma of the lung, Brain **88**:435-449, 1965.

70 Dean, G.: Lung cancer among white South Africans, Brit. Med. J. 2:852-857, 1959.

71 Deeley, T. J.: The effects of radiation on the lungs in the treatment of carcinoma of the bronchus, Clin. Radiol. 11:33-39, 1960.

72 Delarue, N. C., and Graham, F. A.: Alveolar cell carcinoma of the lung, J. Thorac. Surg. 18:237-251, 1949.

73 Delarue, N. C., Sanders, D. E., and Silverberg, S. A.: The complimentary value of pulmonary angiography and mediastinoscopy in individualizing treatment for patients with lung cancer, Cancer 1970 (in press).

74 Delarue, N. C., and Starr, J.: A review of some important problems concerning lung cancer. Part II. The importance of complete preoperative assessment in bronchogenic carcinoma, Canad. Med. Ass. J. 96:8-20, 1967.

75 Denoix, P. F., and Gelle, X.: Estimation de l'importance comparée du cancer bronchopulmonaire en France et dans d'autres pays, Bull. Ass. Franc. Cancer 42:247-278, 1955.

76 Doll, R.: Mortality from lung cancer among non-smokers, Brit. J. Cancer 7:303-312, 1953.

77 Doll, R., and Hill, A. B.: Lung cancer and other causes of death in relation to smoking; a second report on the mortality of British doctors, Brit. Med. J. 2:1071-1081, 1956.

78 Doll, R., and Hill, A. B.: Mortality in relation to smoking; ten years' observations in British doctors, Brit. Med. J. 1:1399-1410, 1964.

79 Doll, R., Hill, A. B., Gray, P. G., and Parr, E. A.: Lung cancer mortality and the length of cigarette ends, Brit. Med. J. 1:322-325, 1959.

80 Doll, R., Hill, A. B., and Kreyberg, L.: The significance of cell type in relation to the aetiology of lung cancer, Brit. J. Cancer 11:43-48, 1957.

81 Dorn, H. F.: The increase in cancer of the lung, Indust. Med. 23:253-257, 1954.

82 Dorn, H. F.: Tobacco consumption and mortality from cancer and other diseases, Acta Un. Int. Cancr. 16:1653-1665, 1960.

83 Dunn, H. L.: Lung cancer in the twentieth century, J. Int. Coll. Surg. 23:326-342, 1955.

84 Eastcott, D. F.: The epidemiology of lung cancer in New Zealand, Lancet 1:37-39, 1956.

85 Eastridge, C. E., Hughes, E. A., Jr., and Greenberg, B. E.: Primary carcinoma of the lung; treatment of 1,284 cases, Amer. Surg. 33:700-705, 1967.

86 Ebaugh, F. G., and Holt, G. W.: Idiopathic neuropathy in cancer; a first sign in multiple system syndromes associated with malignancy, Amer. J. Med. Sci. 242:133-145, 1961.

87 Effler, D. B., Blades, B., and Markes, E.: Problem of solitary lung tumors, Surgery 24:917-928, 1948.

87a Ernst, H., Kruger, J., and Vessal, K.: Lung scanning as a screening method for cancer of the lung, Cancer 23:508-512, 1969.

88 Euphrat, E. J.: Long arrest of epidermoid carcinoma of the lung after irradiation, Cancer 9:453-458, 1956.

89 Ewing, James: Neoplastic diseases, Philadelphia, 1940, W. B. Saunders Co.

90 Feyrter, F.: Ueber das Bronchuscarcinoid, Virchow Arch. Path. Anat. 332:25-43, 1959.

91 Feyrter, F., Herttig, G., and Hornykiewicz, O.: Ueber die biologische Wirksamkeit von Extrakten aus Bronchuskarzinoiden, Wien. Klin. Wschr. 71:317-320, 1959.

92 Figi, F. A.: Primary carcinoma of the trachea, Arch. Otolaryng. (Chicago) 12:446-456, 1930.

93 Foot, N. C.: The identification of types of pulmonary cancer in cytologic smears, Amer. J. Path. 28:963-983, 1952.

94 Foster-Carter, A. F.: Bronchial adenoma, Quart. J. Med. 10:139-174, 1941.

95 Foster-Carter, E. A., and Ackerman, L. V.: Localized mesotheliomas of the pleura; the pathologic evaluation of 18 cases, Amer. J. Clin. Path. 34:349-364, 1960.

96 Frain, C., and Gaucher, M.: L'exploration tomographique en frontal oblique de l'arbre tracheobronchique, J. Radiol. Electr. 38:451-453, 1957.

97 Frantz, V. K.: Tumors of the pancreas. In Atlas of tumor pathology, Sect. VII, Fascs. 27 and 28, Washington, D. C., 1959, Armed Forces Institute of Pathology, pp. 142-149.

98 Frenzel, H., Papageorgiou, A.: Malignant cells in the sputum in coin lesions of the lung, German Med. Monthly 9:1-10, 1964.

99 Fried, B. M.: Bronchiogenic adenoma (benign tumor of the bronchus), Arch. Intern. Med. (Chicago) 79:291-306, 1947.

100 Friedman, M., Mikhail, J. R., and Bhoola, K. D.: Cushing's syndrome associated with carcinoma of the bronchus in a patient with normal plasma electrolytes, Brit. Med. J. 1:27-29, 1965.

101 Frimann-Dahl, J.: On the value of planigraphy in bronchial cancer, Acta Radiol. (Stockholm) 27:99-114, 1946.

102 Fusco, F. D., and Rosen, S. W.: Gonadotropin-producing anaplastic large-cell carcinomas of the lung, New Eng. J. Med. 275:507-515, 1966.

103 Gagnon, E. D., and Gelinas-Mackay, C.: Prognosis in lung cancer surgery based on blood vessel invasion, Canad. J. Surg. 2:156-160, 1959.

104 Galluzzi, S., and Payne, P. M.: Bronchial carcinoma; a statistical study of 741 necropsies with special reference to the distribution of blood-borne metastases, Brit. J. Cancer 9:511-529, 1959.

105 Galy, P., Touraine, R., Brune, J., Gallois, P., Boudier, R., Loire, R., Lhereux, P., and Wiesendanger, T.: Bronchopulmonary cancer secondary to chronic arsenic poisoning in vine-growers of Beaujolais, Lyon Med. 210:735-744, 1963.

106 Garland, L. H.: The detection of carcinoma of the lung by screening procedures, particularly photofluorography, Amer. J. Roentgen. 74:402-414, 1955.

107 Gibbon, J. H., Templeton, J. Y., and Nealon,

T. F., Jr.: Factors which influence the long term survival of patients with cancer of the lung, Ann. Surg. **145**:637-643, 1957.

108 Gifford, J. H., and Waddington, J. K. B.: Review of 464 cases of carcinoma of lung treated by resection, Brit. Med. J. **1**:723-730, 1957.

109 Gilliam, A. G.: Trends of mortality attributed to carcinoma of the lung; possible effects of faulty certification of deaths due to other respiratory diseases, Cancer **8**:1130-1136, 1955.

110 Goldman, A.: Carcinoma of the lung of long duration, J.A.M.A. **118**:359-364, 1942.

111 Good, C. A., and Wilson, T. W.: The solitary circumscribed pulmonary nodule, J.A.M.A. **166**:210-215, 1958.

112 Gowenlock, A. H., Platt, D. S., Campbell, A. C. P., and Wormsley, K. G.: Oat-cell carcinoma of the bronchus secreting 5-hydroxytryptophan, Lancet **1**:304-306, 1964.

113 Graham, E. A., and Singer, J. J.: Sucessful removal of entire lung for carcinoma of bronchus, J.A.M.A. **101**:1371-1374, 1933.

114 Graham, E. A., and Womack, N. A.: The problem of the so-called bronchial adenoma, J. Thorac. Surg. **14**:106-127, 1945.

115 Green, D., and Spence, W. F.: The role of radiotherapy in the palliation of advanced bronchogenic carcinoma, Dis. Chest **52**:57-61, 1967.

116 Greenberg, S. D., Beall, A. C., Jr., and Gonzales-Angulo, A.: Granular cell myoblastoma producing bronchial obstruction, Dis. Chest **44**:320-324, 1963.

117 Greenberger, R. A.: Mass survey detected lung cancer in Connecticut, Conn. Med. J. **20**:857-863, 1956.

118 Griswold, M. H.: Lung cancer in Connecticut on increase, Conn. Health Bull., vol. 69, 1955.

119 Gronqvist, Y. K. J., Clagett, O. T., and McDonald, J. R.: Involvement of the thoracic wall in bronchogenic carcinoma, J. Thorac. Surg. **33**:487-495, 1957.

120 Guiss, L. W.: A 5-year follow-up of roentgenographically detected lung cancer suspects, Cancer **13**:82-90, 1960.

121 Guiss, L. W., and Kuenstler, P.: A retrospective view of survey photofluorograms of persons with lung cancer, Cancer **13**:91-95, 1960.

122 Guttman, R. J.: Effectiveness of radiotherapy in explored inoperable carcinoma of the lung, Bull. N. Y. Acad. Med. **45**:657-664, 1969.

123 Haas, L. L., Harvery, R. A., and Melchor, C. F.: Radiation management of atypical lung tumors, J. Thorac. Surg. **33**:496-525, 1957.

124 Hall, E. R., Jr., and Blades, B.: Primary lymphosarcoma of the lung, Dis. Chest **36**:571-578, 1959.

125 Hall, W. C.: The roentgenologic significance of hamartoma of the lung, Amer. J. Roentgen. **60**:605-611, 1948.

126 Halpert, B., Erickson, E. E., and Fields, W. S.: Intracranial involvement from carcinoma of the lung, Arch. Path. (Chicago) **69**:93-103, 1960.

127 Hammond, E. C.: Smoking in relation to mortality and morbidity; findings in first thirty-four months of followup in a prospective study started in 1959, J. Nat. Cancer Inst. **32**:1161-1188, 1964.

128 Hammond, E. C., and Garfinkel, L.: Smoking habits of men and women, J. Nat. Cancer Inst. **27**:419-442, 1961.

129 Hammond, E. C., and Horn, D.: Smoking and death rates—report on forty-four months of followup of 187,783 men, J.A.M.A. **166**:1159-1172, 1294-1308, 1958.

130 Hamperl, H.: Ueber gutartige Bronchialtumoren (Cylindrome und Carcinoide), Virchow Arch. Path. Anat. **300**:46-88, 1937.

131 Harken, D. E., Black, H., Clauss, R., and Farrand, R. E.: A simple cervicomediastinal exploration for tissue diagnosis of intrathoracic disease, New Eng. J. Med. **251**:1041-1044, 1954.

132 Hattori, S., Matsuda, M., Sugiyama, T., Terazawa, T., and Wada, A.: Some limitations of cytologic diagnosis of small peripheral lung cancers, Acta Cytol. (Balt.) **9**:431-436, 1965.

133 Hattori, S., Matsuda, M., Tateishi, R., Tatsumi, N., and Terazawa, T.: Oat-cell carcinoma of the lung containing serotonin granules, Gann **59**:123-129, 1968.

133a Hazel, W. van, Holinger, P. H., and Jensik, R. J.: Adenoma and cylindroma of the bronchus, Dis. Chest **16**:146-166, 1949.

134 Herbut, P. A.: Bronchiolar origin of "alveolar cell tumor" of the lung, Amer. J. Path. **20**:911-929, 1944.

135 Higgins, G. A., Jr., and Wolf, J.: Chemotherapy and lung cancer—present status, J. Thorac. Cardiovasc. Surg. **51**:449-454, 1966.

136 Hood, R. H., Jr., Campbell, D. C., Jr., Dooley, B. N., and Dooling, J. A.: Bronchogenic carcinoma in young people, Dis. Chest **48**:469-470, 1965.

137 Höst, H.: The value of periodic mass chest roentgenographic surveys in the detection of primary bronchial carcinoma in Norway, Cancer **13**:1167-1184, 1960.

138 Hourihane, D. O., Lessof, L., and Richardson, P. C.: Hyaline and calcified pleural plaques as an index of exposure to asbestos—a study of radiological and pathological features of 100 cases with a consideration of epidemiology, Brit. Med. J. **1**:1069-1074, 1966.

139 Hueper, W. C.: Epidemiologic, experimental and histological studies on metal cancers of the lung, Acta Un. Int. Cancr. **15**:424-436, 1959 (abst.).

140 Hughes, F. A., Jr., Pate, J. W., and Campbell, R. E.: Bronchogenic carcinoma; comparison of natural course and treatment with resection, x-irradiation, and nitrogen mustard, J. Thorac. Cardiovasc. Surg. **39**:409-416, 1960.

141 Hussey, H. H., Katz, Sol, and Yater, W. M.: The superior vena caval syndrome; report of thirty-five cases, Amer. Heart J. **31**:1-26, 1946.

142 Hutchinson, W. B., Friedenberg, M. J., and Saltzstein, S.: Primary pulmonary pseudolymphoma, Radiology 82:48-56, 1963.

143 von Hutzschenreuter, P., and Schamaun, M.: Zur prognose des kleinzelligen Bronchuskarzinoms, Oncologia (Basel) 19:218-226, 1965.

144 Isaac, F., and Ottoman, R. E.: Cavitary form of pulmonary neoplasm, Radiology 52:662-668, 1949.

145 Janes, R. M.: Lipoid pneumonia simulating bronchiogenic carcinoma, J. Thorac. Surg. 16:451-457, 1948.

146 Jensen, H. E.: Exploratory thoracotomy; thoracotomy for pulmonary disease without preoperatively verified diagnosis, Thesis, Copenhagen, 1965.

147 Johnson, C. R., Clagett, O. T., and Good, C. A.: The importance of exploratory thoracotomy in the diagnosis of certain pulmonary lesions, Surgery 25:218-230, 1949.

148 Johnson, J., Kirby, C. K., and Blakemore, W. S.: Should we insist on "radical pneumonectomy" as a routine procedure in the treatment of carcinoma of the lung? J. Thorac. Surg. 36:309-315, 1958.

149 Johnson, R. M., and Lindskog, G. E.: 100 cases of tumor metastatic to lung and mediastinum; treatment and results, J.A.M.A. 202:94-98, 1967.

150 Jones, J. C.: Surgical aspects of bronchogenic carcinoma, J.A.M.A. 134:113-117, 1947.

151 Jones, J. C., Robinson, J. L., Meyer, B. W., and Motley, H. L.: Primary carcinoma of the lung, J. Thorac. Cardiovasc. Surg. 39:144-158, 1960.

152 Keil, P. G., Voelker, C. A., and Schissel, D. J.: Diagnostic value of pulmonary arteriography in bronchial carcinoma, Amer. J. Med. Sci. 219:301-306, 1950.

153 King, D. S., and Castleman, B.: Bronchial involvement in metastatic pulmonary malignancy, J. Thorac. Surg. 12:305-315, 1943.

154 Kinsey, D. L., Carter, D., and Klassen, K. P.: Simplified management of malignant pleural effusion, Arch. Surg. (Chicago) 89:389-392, 1964.

155 Knowles, J. H., and Smith, L. H., Jr.: Extrapulmonary manifestations of bronchogenic carcinoma, New Eng. J. Med. 262:505-510, 1960.

156 Konikov, N., Bleisch, V. R., and Piskie, V.: Prognostic significance of cytologic diagnoses of effusions, Acta Cytol. (Balt.) 10:335-339, 1966.

157 Koss, L. G., and Richardson, H. L.: Some pitfalls of cytological diagnosis of lung cancer, Cancer 8:937-947, 1955.

158 Kotin, P., and Falk, H. L.: The role and action of environmental agents in the pathogenesis of lung cancer. I. Air pollutants, Cancer 12:147-163, 1959.

159 Kovach, R. D., and Kyle, L. H.: Cushing's syndrome and bronchogenic carcinoma, Amer. J. Med. 24:981-988, 1958.

160 Kreyberg, L.: Occupational influences in a Norwegian material of 235 cases of primary epithelial lung tumours, Brit. J. Cancer 8:605-612, 1954.

161 Kreyberg, L.: Lung tumours: histology, aetiology and geographic pathology, Acta Un. Int. Cancr. 15:78-95, 1959 (abst.).

162 Kroe, D. J., and Pitcock, J. A.: Benign mucous gland adenoma of the bronchus, Arch. Path. (Chicago) 84:539-542, 1967.

163 Kubik, A., Gross, K., Helbich, P., Krivanek, J., Macik, G., Neumann, V., Ruzha, J., Stasek, V., Styblo, K., Svandova, E., and Tomanek, A.: An epidemiologic study of bronchial carcinoma in men of 40-64 years in the Kolin district, Rozhl. Tuberk. 27:75-83, 1967.

163a Lampe, I.: Personal communication, 1952.

164 Laval, P., Amalric, R., Clement, R., and Brunet, F.: Étude de la survie de 100 cancers pulmonaries inoperables traites par radiothérapie à 200 kv., J. Radiol. Electr. 40:301-307, 1959.

164a Lavelle, R. J.: Metachronous carcinoma of the larynx following successful treatment of carcinoma of the bronchus, Brit. J. Cancer 23:709-713, 1969.

165 Lebacq, E., Verberckmoes, R., and Maldague, P.: La secrétion inappropriée d'hormone antidiurétique dans le cas de tumeurs thoraciques anaplastiques de type oat-cell, Ann. Endocr. (Paris) 25:361-373, 1964.

166 Le Gal, Y., and Bauer, W. C.: Second primary bronchogenic carcinoma; a complication of successful lung cancer surgery, J. Thorac. Cardiovasc. Surg. 41:114-124, 1961.

167 Lemon, F. R., Walden, R. T., and Woods, R. W.: Cancer of the lung and mouth in Seventh-Day Adventists; preliminary report on a population study, Cancer 17:486-497, 1964.

168 Levin, M. L.: The cigarette smoker and lung cancer, CA 10:62-67, 1960.

169 Liebow, A.: Atypical proliferation in the lung in relation to neoplasia. In Proceedings of the Second Workshop Conference on Lung Cancer Research, Feb. 1959, American Cancer Society, Inc., Arden House, Harriman, N. Y., p. 18.

170 Lombard, H. L.: An epidemiological study in lung cancer, Cancer 18:1301-1309, 1965.

171 Lowell, L. M., and Tuhy, J. E.: Primary chondrosarcoma of the lung, J. Thorac. Surg. 18:476-483, 1949.

171a Luce, S. A., and Spjut, H. J.: An electron microscopic study of a solitary pleural mesothelioma, Cancer 17:1546-1554, 1964.

172 McBurney, R. P., Kirklin, J. W., and Woolner, L. B.: Metastasizing bronchial adenomas, Surg. Gynec. Obstet. 96:482-492, 1953.

173 McClung, J. P.: Previous pulmonary infection in lung cancer; a review, J. Chronic Dis. 20:65-78, 1967.

174 McDonald, J. R., Harrington, S. W., and Clagett, O. T.: Hamartoma (often called chondroma) of the lung, J. Thorac. Surg. 14:128-143, 1945.

175 McDonald, J. R., Harrington, S. W., and Clagett, O. T.: Obstructive pneumonitis of

neoplastic origin, J. Thorac. Surg. **18**:97-112, 1949.

176 McDonald, J. R., Moersch, H. J., and Tinney, W. S.: Cylindroma of the bronchus, J. Thorac. Surg. **14**:445-453, 1945.

177 Maier, H. C., and Fischer, W. W.: Adenomas arising from small bronchi not visible bronchoscopically, J. Thorac. Surg. **16**:392-398, 1947.

178 Manfredi, F., King, R., Behnke, R., and Heimburger, I.: Preoperative radiation in bronchogenic carcinoma, Amer. Rev. Resp. Dis. **94**:584-588, 1966.

179 Marks, L. J., Rosenbaum, D. L., and Russfield, A. B.: Cushing's syndrome on corticotropin-secreting carcinoma of the lung, Ann. Intern. Med. **58**:143-149, 1963.

180 Medical Research Council: Comparative trial of surgery and radiotherapy for the primary treatment of small-celled or oat-celled carcinoma of the bronchus. First report of the Medical Research Council by the Working-Party on the evaluation of different methods of therapy in carcinoma of the bronchus, Lancet **2**:979-986, 1966.

181 Meighan, S. S., and Weitman, M.: Smoking; habits and beliefs of Oregon physicians, J. Nat. Cancer Inst. **35**:893-898, 1965.

181a Meissner, W.: Personal communication, 1952.

182 Melamed, M. R., Koss, L. G., and Cliffton, E. E.: Roentgenologically occult lung cancer diagnosed by cytology; report of 12 cases, Cancer **16**:1537-1551, 1963.

183 Miller, A. B., Fox, Wallace, and Tall, R.: Five-year follow-up of the medical research council comparative trial of surgery and radiotherapy for the primary treatment of small-celled or oat-celled carcinoma of the bronchus, Lancet, **2**:501-505, 1969.

184 Mills, C. A.: Motor exhaust gases and lung cancer in Cincinnati, Amer. J. Med. Sci. **239**:316-319, 1960.

185 Mitchell, R. S., Vincent, T. N., and Filley, G. F.: Cigarette smoking, chronic bronchitis, and emphysema, J.A.M.A. **188**:12-15, 1964.

186 Moersch, H. J., and McDonald, J. R.: Bronchial adenoma, J.A.M.A. **142**:299-369, 1950.

187 Morandini, G. C., Gerna, G., Rossi, A., and Maestro, A.: Il trattamento del carcinoma del polmone con betatrone da 42 MeV. osservazioni preliminari su 56 casi, G. Ital. Mal. Torace **22**:391-404, 1968.

188 Morrison, R.: Inoperable cancer of the bronchus treated by megavoltage x-ray therapy, Lancet **2**:618-620, 1960.

189 Morrison, R., Deeley, T. J., and Cleland, W. P.: The treatment of carcinoma of the bronchus; a clinical trial to compare surgery and supervoltage therapy, Lancet **1**:683-684, 1963.

190 Morton, D. L., Itabashi, H. H., and Grimes, O. F.: Nonmetastatic neurological complications of bronchogenic carcinoma; the carcinomatous neuromyopathies, J. Thorac. Cardiovasc. Surg. **51**:14-19, 1966.

191 Murray, M. R.: See Stout and Murray.[266]

192 Myers, W. P.: Hypercalcemia in neoplastic disease, Arch. Surg. (Chicago) **80**:308-318, 1960.

193 Nash, A. D., and Stout, A. P.: Giant cell carcinoma of the lung, Cancer **11**:369-375, 1958.

194 National Research Council: London, England, 1966.

195 Naylor, B.: The exfoliative cytology of diffuse malignant mesothelioma, J. Path. Bact. **86**:293-298, 1963.

196 Niskanen, K. O.: Observations on metaplasia of the bronchial epithelium and its relation to carcinoma of the lung, Acta Path. Microbiol. Scand. (suppl. 80), pp. 1-80, 1949.

197 Ochsner, A., DeBakey, M., Dunlap, C. E., and Richman, I.: Primary pulmonary malignancy, J. Thorac. Surg. **17**:573-599, 1948.

198 Ochsner, A., and Dixon, J. L.: Superior vena caval thrombosis, J. Thorac. Surg. **5**:641-673, 1936.

199 Oettlé, A. G.: Cigarette smoking as the major cause of lung cancer, S. Afr. Med. J. **37**:957-963, 1963.

200 O'Keefe, M. E., Jr., Good, C. A., and McDonald, J. R.: Calcification in solitary nodules of the lung, Amer. J. Roentgen. **77**:1023-1033, 1957.

201 O'Neal, R. M., Lee, K. T., and Edwards, D. L.: Bronchogenic carcinoma; an evaluation from autopsy data, with special reference to incidence, sex ratio, histological type and accuracy of clinical diagnosis, Cancer **10**:1031-1036, 1957.

202 Onuigbo, W. I. B.: Some observations on the spread of lung cancer in the body, Brit. J. Cancer **11**:175-180, 1957.

203 Overholt, R. H., Bougas, J. A., and Morse, D. P.: Bronchial adenoma; a study of 60 patients with resections, Amer. Rev. Tuberc. **75**:865-884, 1957.

204 Overholt, R. H., Bougas, J. A., and Woods, F. M.: Surgical treatment of lung cancer found on x-ray survey, New Eng. J. Med. **252**:429-432, 1955.

205 Parker, H. L.: Involvement of central nervous system secondary to primary carcinoma of the lung, Arch. Neurol. Psychiat. **17**:198-213, 1927.

206 Paulson, D. L.: A philosophy of treatment for bronchogenic carcinoma, Trans. Southern Surg. Ass. **69**:73-80, 1958.

207 Paulson, D. L.: A philosophy of treatment of bronchogenic carcinoma, Ann. Thorac. Surg. **5**:289-299, 1968.

208 Paulson, D. L., Urshil, H. C., McNamara, J. J., and Shaw, R. B.: Bronchoplastic procedures for bronchogenic carcinoma, J. Thorac. Cardiovasc. Surg. **59**:38-48, 1970.

209 Payne, W. S., Ellis, F. H., Jr., Woolner, L. B., and Moersch, H. J.: The surgical treatment of cylindroma (adenoid cystic carcinoma) and muco-epidermoid tumors of the bronchus, J. Thorac. Cardiovasc. Surg. **38**:709-726, 1959.

210 Pearson, F. G.: Mediastinoscopy; a method of biopsy in the superior mediastinum, Canad. J. Surg. **6**:423-429, 1963.

211 Pinsky, H. J., and Emerson, G. L.: Radiation therapy for recurrent carcinoma of the bronchial stump, J. Thorac. Cardiovasc. Surg. **35:** 683-688, 1958.

212 Poletti, T., and Riva, G.: Le manifestazioni osteo-articolari precoci in corso di neoplasie polmonari, Minerva Med. **49:**750-758, 1958.

213 Posner, E., McDowell, L. A., and Cross, K. W.: Mass radiography and cancer of the lung, Brit. Med. J. **1:**1213-1218, 1959.

214 Posner, E., McDowell, L. A., and Cross, K. W.: Place of mass radiography in relation to lung cancer in men, Brit. Med. J. **5366:**1156-1160, 1963.

215 Pryce, D. M., and Walter, J. B.: The frequency of gross vascular invasion in lung cancer with special reference to arterial invasion, J. Path. Bact. **79:**141-146, 1960.

216 Raeburn, C., and Spencer, H.: Lung scar cancers, Brit. J. Tuberc. **51:**237-245, 1957.

217 Rakower, J.: Smoking habits and lung cancer in Israel, Harefuah **68:**115-119, 1965.

218 Ratzer, E. R., Pool, J. L., and Melamed, M. R.: Pleural mesotheliomas; clinical experiences with 37 patients, Amer. J. Roentgen. **99:**863-880, 1967.

219 Rienhoff, W. F., Jr.: The present status of the surgical treatment of carcinoma of the lung, Ann. Surg. **125:**541-565, 1947.

220 Rienhoff, W. F., Jr.: A clinical analysis and follow-up study of five hundred and two cases of carcinoma of the lung, Dis. Chest **17:**33-53, 1950.

221 Rienhoff, W. F., Jr.: Pneumonectomy; a preliminary report of the operative technique in two successful cases, Bull. Hopkins Hosp. **53:**390-393, 1933.

222 Rienhoff, W. F., Jr.: Discussion of paper by Jones, J. C.: Surgical aspects of bronchogenic carcinoma, J.A.M.A. **134:**113-117, 1947.

223 di Rienzo, S.: Radiologic exploration of the bronchus (translation by Tomas A. Hughes), Springfield, Ill., 1949, Charles C Thomas, Publisher.

224 Rigler, L. G.: A roentgen study of the evolution of carcinoma of the lung, J. Thorac. Surg. **34:**283-297, 1957.

225 Rigler, L. G., and Heitzman, E. R.: Planigraphy in the differential diagnosis of the pulmonary nodule, Radiology **65:**692-702, 1955.

226 Rigler, L. G., and Kelby, G. M.: Emphysema; early roentgen sign of bronchogenic carcinoma, Radiology **49:**578-585, 1947.

227 Rigler, L. G., O'Laughlin, B. J., and Tucker, R. C.: Significance of unilateral enlargement of the hilus shadow in the early diagnosis of carcinoma of the lung, Radiology **59:**683-692, 1952.

228 Rinker, C. T., Templeton, A. W., MacKenzie, J., Ridings, G. R., Almond, C. H. and Kiphart, R.: Combined superior vena cavography and azygography in patients with suspected lung carcinoma, Radiology **88:**441-465, 1967.

229 Robbins, E., and Silverman, G.: Coexistent bronchogenic carcinoma and active pulmonary tuberculosis, Cancer **2:**65-97, 1949.

230 Robbins, L. L., and Hale, C. H.: Roentgen appearance of lobar and segmental collapse of the lung; collapse of entire lung or major part thereof, Radiology **45:**23-26, 1945.

231 Robbins, L. L., and Hale, C. H.: Roentgen appearance of lobar and segmental collapse of lung; collapse of right middle lobe, Radiology **45:**260-266, 1945.

232 Robbins, L. L., and Hale, C. H.: Roentgen appearance of lobar and segmental collapse of the lung; collapse of upper lobes, Radiology **45:**347-355, 1945.

233 Robinson, J. L., Jones, J. C., and Meyer, B. W.: Indications for lobectomy in the treatment of carcinoma of the lung, J. Thorac. Surg. **32:**500-507, 1956.

234 Roffo, A. H.: Developments of carcinoma in rabbits from effects of tobacco, Bol. Inst. Med. Exper. **7:**501-538, 1930.

235 Ross, E. J.: Hyponatraemic syndrome associated with carcinoma of the bronchus, Quart. J. Med. **32:**297-320, 1963.

236 Rouvière, H.: Anatomie des lymphatiques de l'homme, Paris, 1932, Masson et Cie.

237 Russell, W. O., Neidhardt, H. W., Mountain, C. F., Griffith, K. M., and Chang, J. P.: Cytodiagnosis of lung cancer, Acta Cytol. (Balt.) **7:**1-44, 1963 (extensive bibliography).

238 Saltzstein, S. L.: Pulmonary malignant lymphomas and pseudolymphomas; classification, therapy and prognosis, Cancer **16:**928-955, 1963.

239 Sano, M. E., Weiss, E., and Gault, E. S.: Pleural mesothelioma, J. Thorac. Surg. **19:** 783-788, 1950.

240 Sasser, W. F., Bennett, D. E., Ferguson, T. B., and Burford, T. H.: Primary adenocarcinoma of the lung in men, Ann. Thorac. Surg. **5:**508-516, 1968.

240a Schlienger, M., Eschwege, F., Blanche, R., and Depièrre, R.: Mesothéliomes pleuraux malins; étude de 39 cas dont 25 autopsies, Bull. Cancer (Paris) **56:**265-308, 1969.

241 Schneckloth, R. E., McIsaac, W. M., and Page, I. H.: Serotonin metabolism in carcinoid syndrome with metastatic bronchial adenoma, J.A.M.A. **170:**1143-1147, 1959.

242 Schröder, H. G., and Eichorn, H. -J.: Chest radiography including tomography for the visualization of intrathoracic lymph node metastasis, Radiol. Diagn. (Berlin) **7:**355-360, 1966.

243 Scott, H. W., Marrow, A. G., and Payne, T. P. B.: Solitary xanthoma of the lung, J. Thorac. Surg. **17:**821-825, 1948.

244 Seidman, H.: Lung cancer among Jewish, Catholic, and Protestant males in New York City, Cancer **19:**185-190, 1966.

245 Selikoff, I. J., Bader, R. A., Bader, M. E., Churg, J., and Hammond, E. C.: Asbestosis and neoplasia (editorial), Amer. J. Med. **42:** 487-496, 1967.

246 Selikoff, I. J., Churg, J., and Hammond, E. C.: Asbestos exposure and neoplasia, J.A.M.A. **188:**142-146, 1964.

247 Selikoff, I. J., Hammond, E. C., and Churg,

J.: Asbestos exposure, smoking and neoplasia, J.A.M.A. **204**:106-112, 1968.

248 Shields, T. W., Higgins, G. A., Lawton, R., Heilbrunn, A., and Keehn, R.: Preoperative x-ray therapy as an adjuvant in the treatment of bronchogenic carcinoma, J. Thorac. Cardiovasc. Surg. **59**:49-61, 1970.

248a Shields, T. W., and Shocket, E.: Preoperative evaluation of patients with clinically resectable bronchogenic carcinoma, Arch. Surg. (Chicago) **76**:707-712, 1958.

249 Shimkin, M. B.: On the etiology of bronchogenic carcinoma (extensive bibliography). In Spain, D. M., editor: The diagnosis and treatment of tumors of the chest, New York, 1960, Grune & Stratton, Inc.

250 Singer, D. B., Greenberg, S. D., and Harrison, G. M.: Papillomatosis of the lung, Amer. Rev. Resp. Dis. **94**:777-783, 1966.

250a Slack, N. H.: Bronchogenic carcinoma: nitrogen mustard as a surgical adjuvant and factors influencing survival; University Surgical Adjuvant Lung Project, Cancer **25**:987-1002, 1970.

251 Smart, J., and Hilton, G.: Radiotherapy of cancer of the lung, Lancet **6**:880-881, 1956.

252 Smith, J. F., and Dexter, D.: Papillary neoplasms of the bronchus of low-grade malignancy, Thorax **18**:340-349, 1963.

253 Smither, W. J.: Asbestos, asbestosis and mesothelioma of the pleura, Proc. Roy. Soc. Med. **59**:57-61, 1966.

254 Smithers, D. W.: Facts and fancies about cancer of the lung, Brit. Med. J. **1**:1235-1239, 1953.

255 Sniffen, R. C., Soutter, L., and Robbins, L. L.: Muco-epidermoid tumors of the bronchus arising from surface epithelium, Amer. J. Path. **34**:671-683, 1958.

255a Som, M. L.: Personal communication, 1951.

256 Spjut, H. J., and Mateo, L. E.: Recurrent and metastatic carcinoma in surgically treated carcinoma of lung, Cancer **18**:1462-1466, 1965.

257 Spjut, H. J., Roper, C. L., and Butcher, H. R., Jr.: Pulmonary cancer and its prognosis, Cancer **14**:1251-1258, 1961.

258 Starzl, T. E., Brittain, R. S., Herrman, G., Marchioro, T. L., and Waddell, W. R.: Pseudotumors due to pulmonary infarction, Amer. J. Surg. **106**:619-627, 1963.

259 Steinberg, I., and Finby, N.: Great vessel involvement in lung cancer; angiographic report on 250 consecutive proved cases, Amer. J. Roentgen. **81**:807-818, 1959.

260 Sternberg, W. J., Sidransky, H., and Ochsner, S.: Primary malignant lymphomas of the lung, Cancer **12**:806-819, 1959.

261 Stocks, P.: Recent epidemiological studies of lung cancer mortality, cigarette smoking and air pollution, with discussion on a new hypothesis of causation, Brit. J. Cancer **20**:595-623, 1966.

262 Stocks, P.: Lung cancer and bronchitis in relation to cigarette smoking and fuel consumption in twenty countries, Brit. J. Prev. Soc. Med. **21**:181-185, 1967.

263 Stocks, P., and Campbell, J. M.: Lung cancer death rates among non-smokers and pipe and cigarette smokers; an evaluation in relation to air pollution by benzpyrene and other substances, Brit. Med. J. **2**:923-929, 1955.

264 Stone, G. E., Waterhouse, C., and Terry, R.: Hypercalcemia of malignant disease; case report and a proposed mechanism of etiology, Ann. Intern. Med. **54**:977-985, 1961.

265 Stout, A. P., and Himadi, G. H.: Solitary (localized) mesothelioma of the pleura, Ann. Surg. **133**:50-64, 1951.

266 Stout, A. P., and Murray, M. R.: Localized pleural mesothelioma, Arch. Path. (Chicago) **34**:951-964, 1942.

267 Strott, C. A., Nugent, C. A., and Tyler, F. H.: Cushing's syndrome caused by bronchial adenomas, Amer. J. Med. **44**:97-104, 1968.

268 Surgeon General's Report: Health consequences of smoking, Washington, D. C., 1964, United States Department of Health, Education and Welfare.

269 Surmont, J., Pierquin, B., Lemoine, J. M., and Fauvet, J.: Irradiation en haute-energie (betatron 22 mev.) dan le traitment des cancers bronchiques, Bronches **9**:388-401, 1959.

270 Swan, L. L.: Pulmonary adenomatosis of man, Arch. Path. (Chicago) **47**:517-544, 1949.

271 Szur, L., and Bromley, L. L.: Obstruction of the superior vena cava in carcinoma of bronchus, Brit. Med. J. **2**:1273-1281, 1956.

272 Thomson, J. G., Path, F. C., and Graves, W. M., Jr.: Asbestos as an urban air contaminant, Arch. Path. (Chicago) **81**:458-464, 1966.

273 Thornton, T. F., Adams, W. E., and Bloch, R. G.: Solitary circumscribed tumors of the lung, Surg. Gynec. Obstet. **78**:364-370, 1944.

274 Tinney, W. S., Moersch, H. J., and McDonald, J. R.: Tumors of trachea, Arch. Otolaryng. (Chicago) **41**:284-290, 1945.

275 Tokuhata, G. K., and Lilienfeld, A. M.: Familial aggregation of lung cancer in humans, J. Nat. Cancer Inst. **30**:289-312, 1963.

276 Trinidad, S., Lisa, J. R., and Rosenblatt, M. B.: Bronchogenic carcinoma simulated by metastatic tumors, Cancer **16**:1521-1529, 1963.

277 Turkington, R. W., Goldman, J. K., Ruffner, B. W., and Dobson, J. L.: Bronchogenic carcinoma simulating hyperparathyroidism, Cancer **19**:406-414, 1966.

278 Unger, R. H., Lochner, J. deV., and Eisentraut, A. M.: Identification of insulin and glucagon in a bronchogenic carcinoma, J. Clin. Endocr. **24**:823-831, 1964.

279 Uragoda, C. G.: Incidence of bronchial carcinoma in a Ceylon chest clinic, Brit. J. Dis. Chest **61**:154-158, 1967.

280 Van Duuren, B. L.: Identification of some polynuclear aromatic hydrocarbons in cigarette-smoke condensate, J. Nat. Cancer Inst. **21**:1-16, 1958.

281 Van Hazel, W., and Jensik, R. J.: Lymphoma of the lung and pleura, J. Thorac. Surg. **31**:19-44, 1956.

282 Vanek, J.: Multinodular carcinoma of the lung, Acta Radiol. Cancer. Bohemoslov. **4:** 97-119, 1949.

283 Vieta, J. O., and Maier, H. C.: The treatment of adenoid cystic carcinoma (cylindroma) of the respiratory tract by surgery and radiation therapy, Dis. Chest **31:**1-19, 1957.

284 Vincent, T. N., Satterfield, J. V., and Ackerman, L. V.: Carcinoma of the lung in women, Cancer **18:**559-570, 1965.

285 Vorwald, A. J., and Karr, J. W.: Pneumoconiosis and pulmonary carcinoma, Amer. J. Path. **14:**49-58, 1938.

286 Wagner, J. C.: Epidemiology of diffuse mesothelial tumors; evidence of an association from studies in South Africa and United Kingdom, Ann. N. Y. Acad. Sci. **132:**575-578, 1965.

287 Wagoner, J. K., Archer, V. E., Carroll, B. E., Holaday, D. A., and Lawrence, P. A.: Cancer mortality patterns among U. S. uranium miners and millers, 1950 through 1962, J. Nat. Cancer Inst. **32:**787-801, 1964.

288 Watkins, E., Jr., and Gerard, F. P.: Malignant tumors involving the chest wall, J. Thorac. Cardiovasc. Surg. **39:**117-129, 1960.

289 Watson, T. A.: Supervoltage roentgen therapy in cancer of the lung, Amer. J. Roentgen. **75:**525-539, 1954.

290 Watson, W. L., and Farpour, A.: Terminal bronchiolar or "alveolar cell" cancer of the lung, Cancer **19:**776-780, 1966.

291 Weisberger, A. S., Levine, B., and Storaasli, J. P.: Use of nitrogen mustard in treatment of serous effusions of neoplastic origin, J.A.M.A. **159:**1704-1707, 1955.

292 Weiss, W., Boucot, K. R., and Cooper, D. A.: The survival of men with measurable proved lung cancer in relation to growth rate, Amer. J. Roentgen. **98:**404-414, 1966.

293 Wilkins, E. W., Jr.: The asymptomatic isolated pulmonary nodule, New Eng. J. Med. **252:**515-520, 1955.

294 Williams, E. D., and Azzopardi, J. G.: Tumors of the lung and the carcinoid syndrome, Thorax **15:**30-36, 1960.

295 Willis, R. A.: Pathology of tumours, St. Louis, 1948, The C. V. Mosby Co.

296 Windeyer, B.: Personal communication to Buschke, F.: Roentgen therapy of carcinoma of the lung, Radiology **69:**489-493, 1957.

297 Winternitz, M. C., Wason, I. M., and McNamara, F. P.: The pathology of influenza, New Haven, Conn., 1920, Yale University Press.

298 Womack, N. A., and Graham, E. A.: Epithelial metaplasia in congenital cystic disease of the lung, Amer. J. Path. **17:**645-654, 1941.

299 Wood, C. A. P.: The treatment of carcinoma bronchus by supervoltage therapy, Acta Un. Int. Cancr. **15:**514-519, 1959.

300 Woolner, L. B., Anderson, H. A., and Bernatz, P. E.: "Occult" carcinoma of the bronchus; a study of 15 cases of in situ or early invasive bronchogenic carcinoma, Dis. Chest **37:**278-288, 1960.

301 Wynder, E. L., Bross, I. J., Cornfield, J., and O'Donnell, W. E.: Lung cancer in women, New Eng. J. Med. **255:**1111-1121, 1956.

302 Wynder, E. L., and Hoffmann, D.: A study of tobacco carcinogenesis. VII. The role of higher polycyclic hydrocarbons, Cancer **12:** 1079-1086, 1959.

303 Wynder, E. L., Lemon, F. R., and Bross, I. J.: Cancer and coronary artery disease among Seventh-Day Adventists, Cancer **12:** 1016-1028, 1959.

304 Yokoo, H., and Suckow, E. E.: Peripheral lung cancers arising in scars, Cancer **14:** 1205-1215, 1961.

305 Zschoch, H., and Kober, B.: Autopsy statistics on the metastases of lung carcinoma, Arch. Geschwulstforsch. **30:**126-134, 1967.

Chapter 8

Tumors of the thyroid gland

Anatomy

The thyroid gland lies in front of the trachea at the lower anterior midline of the neck. It consists of two rounded pyramidal lobes extending from the thyroid cartilage to the sixth tracheal ring and of a connecting median isthmus near the lower pole of the lobes that covers the second, third, and fourth tracheal rings. Each lateral lobe is related posteriorly to the carotid sheath and the esophagus and medially to the tracheal wall and recurrent laryngeal nerve (Fig. 298). The gland is enveloped in a connective tissue capsule, and the pretracheal fascia firmly fixes it to the cricoid and thyroid cartilages.

An arterial anastomosis between the capsule and the fascial sheath is supplied to each lobe by the superior thyroid branch of the external carotid artery, an inferior thyroid branch of the thyrocervical trunk, and, rarely, a single small branch from the innominate artery at the midline. Three sets of venous channels are present: the superior and the middle thyroid veins draining into the internal jugular veins and the inferior thyroid veins draining into the respective innominate veins.

Lymphatics. The lymphatics of the thyroid gland originate around the thyroid follicles and form a delicate but rich network that extends into the gland (Fig. 299). The collecting trunks gather into six main groups (Rouvière[89]):

1 The *median superior trunks* arise in the superior portion of the isthmus and adjacent areas of the lateral lobe. They travel upward in front of the larynx and then laterally to end in the subdigastric group of nodes of the internal jugular chain. In about half of the cases, some of these trunks are interrupted by an intercricothyroid lymph node.

2 The *median inferior trunks* descend along the inferior thyroid vein and usually drain into the lymph nodes of the transverse pretracheal chain. Some of these lymphatics may fail to make this first stop and continue onward to drain directly into a large lymph node at the junction of the brachiocephalic trunks. A group of lymphatics arising from the posterior surface of the lower pole of the lateral lobes, the *posteroinferior collecting trunks*, drain into the recurrent chain of lymph nodes of the same side and thus constitute a lateral continuation of the inferior median collecting trunks.

3 and 4 The *right* and *left lateral trunks* arise from the lateral lobes. Some of them follow an upward direction to drain into the anterosuperior nodes of the internal jugular chain, and others follow a transverse direction to end either in the inferior and external nodes of the internal jugular chain or in the central nodes of this same chain.

5 and 6 The *posterosuperior trunks* are present in only about one-fifth of the cases. They arise from the posterosuperior region of the lateral lobes, ascend past the lateral border of the pharynx, and terminate in the lateral retropharyngeal node.

In summary, the lymphatics of the thyroid gland are drained by the lymph nodes of the internal jugular chain and recurrent chain and by the pretracheal and retropharyngeal lymph nodes.

Epidemiology

The sex-age-adjusted incidence rates for malignant tumors of the thyroid gland in the 1947 United States survey were 1.0 and 3.4 per 100,000 for males and females, respectively. The age-adjusted rates for

377

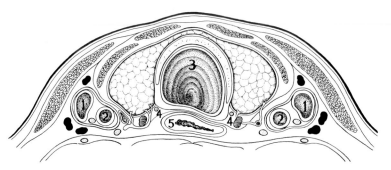

Fig. 298. Transverse section of neck at level of third tracheal ring. Note intimate relationship of thyroid gland to jugular vein, **1**; carotid artery, **2**; trachea, **3**; recurrent laryngeal nerve, **4**; esophagus, **5**.

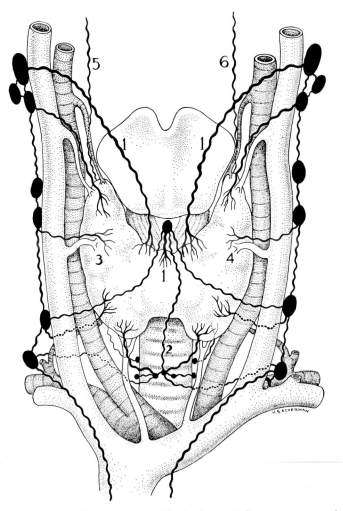

Fig. 299. Lymphatic trunks that drain thyroid gland. **1**, Median superior trunk. **2**, Median inferior trunk. **3** and **4**, right and left lateral trunks. **5** and **6**, Posterosuperior trunks. All of these are drained by lymph nodes of internal jugular chain and recurrent chain and by pretracheal and retropharyngeal lymph nodes.

white males and females were 1.2 and 3.4, whereas for nonwhites they were 0.2 and 3.3, respectively. In the state of New York there was an increase in incidence from 0.8 and 1.9 for males and females in 1949-1951 to 1.0 and 2.9 in 1958-1960. The increase affected individuals under 55 years of age almost exclusively (Carroll et al.[10]). There was a similar increase in the state of Connecticut from a rate of 0.6 and 1.5 per 100,000 for males and females in 1945-1949 to 1.2 and 3.4 in 1960-1962. The incidence rates increase with age. In males past 55 years of age and in females past the age of 65 years, the rates are more than double the average rate and gradually increase, from three to five times the average rates, in patients past 80 years of age. Geographic areas of endemic goiter, where carcinoma of the thyroid gland has been more frequent, are disappearing through the general use of iodized salt; this has happened in Switzerland. In Hawaii, carcinoma of the thyroid gland shows one of the highest frequencies (Haber and Lipkovic[41a]). In Cali, Colombia, there is a statistically significant excess of follicular carcinoma (Cuello et al.[22a]).

Although carcinoma of the thyroid gland predominates in elderly patients, it may be found also in children, particularly in females. Of fifty-nine children with thyroid gland cancer seen by Hayles et al.,[46] forty were girls.

The proportion of carcinoma of the thyroid gland found in patients with toxic diffuse goiter, toxic nodular goiter, nontoxic nodular goiter, and nontoxic single thyroid nodules progressively increases in the order listed, although carcinoma very rarely arises in toxic diffuse goiter and rarely in toxic nodular goiter. The proportion of carcinoma found in nontoxic nodular goiter and in single thyroid nodules varies considerably with the selection of groups. In a series of 218 patients with nontoxic nodular goiter followed for ten years, there was no case of cancer (Vander et al.[116]). In another series of 241 patients operated upon for nodular goiter, only 1.7% had carcinoma (Watt and Foushee[123]) Cole et al.[16] found a high proportion of carcinomas—17% in nontoxic nodular goiter and 25% in single nontoxic nodules. Any suspicion as to the

accuracy of the diagnosis of carcinoma was dispelled by the eventual fatal outcome of thirteen of the sixteen patients in whom carcinoma was discovered.

There is evidence to suggest that even mild irradiation of the thyroid gland in early life results in changes that may lead, directly or indirectly, to the development of cancer of the gland (Clark[14]; Wilson et al.[126]). In a series of 1502 children who had been irradiated shortly after birth (for supposed enlargement of the thymus) and who were followed for the next twenty years, eighteen cases of malignant tumors, mostly of the thyroid gland, were found (Simpson et al.[105]). Hempelmann[50] has pointed out that nodularities in the previously irradiated thyroid gland of young adults probably represent radiation-induced thyroid changes that may later develop into carcinoma. The mean interval between the irradiation and the diagnosis of cancer in a series of 528 such patients was 10.9 years (Raventos and Winship[84]). Carcinoma of the thyroid gland does not develop in adults who have received therapeutic irradiation for cancer of the larynx or for other reasons (DeLawter and Winship[24]), yet it is said to be prevalent in individuals exposed to atomic bomb irradiation (Socolow et al.[109]) as compared with nonexposed ones. At autopsy, carcinoma of the thyroid gland in the Japanese was higher in women and in those who had been exposed to 50 rads or more of direct atomic radiation (Sampson et al.[91]).

Pathology
Gross and microscopic pathology

A histologic classification of tumors of the thyroid gland has proved practical, for it clarifies treatment and prognosis. The following histologic classification is used as a basis for discussion.

Adenoma
  Simple
  Hürthle cell
  Atypical
Adenocarcinoma
  Papillary
  Follicular (alveolar)
Carcinoma
  Small cell
  Giant cell
  Hürthle cell

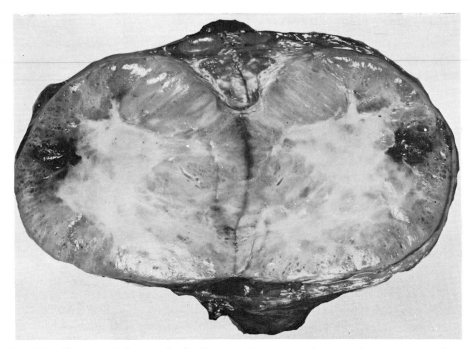

Fig. 300. Adenoma of thyroid gland. Note complete encapsulation with compression of contiguous thyroid gland and typical central fibrosis and hemorrhage.

Carcinoma—cont'd
  Medullary
  Epidermoid
Plasmacytoma
Lymphosarcoma
Fibrosarcoma
Teratoma

The adenoma is the most common of the thyroid tumors, presenting a discrete, well-encapsulated nodule weighing from 25 gm to 200 gm. It arises from the epithelium of preexisting follicles rather than from rests of embryonal epithelium. It has a definite complete connective tissue capsule that becomes more fibrotic as the lesion grows and that shells out easily. It compresses the adjacent thyroid tissue (Fig. 300). The benign adenoma should be differentiated from the nodules so frequently found in the adenomatous goiter which do not have a complete connective tissue capsule. Grossly, evidence of blood vessel invasion should be searched for, but we have seen this only a few times. The cellular neoplastic adenomas probably do not function (Dobyns and Lennon[27]).

Microscopically, adenomas show variable patterns, but division in several small

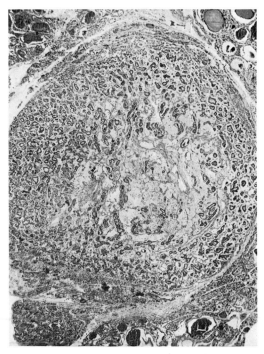

Fig. 301. Adenoma of thyroid gland. Note complete encapsulation, central degeneration, and striking difference between histology of adenoma and contiguous, compressed thyroid gland. (Low power.)

Table 28. Relative incidence of 500 benign tumors of thyroid gland*

Type	No.	% of total	Average age	Females (%)
Follicular	433	86.6	43	83
Embryonal	65	13.0	43	89
Fetal	262	52.3	45	79
Simple	61	12.2	39	90
Colloid	19	3.8	41	84
Hürthle	26	5.2	44	92
Papillary	24	4.8	46	83
Unclassified	43	8.6	43	81

*From Meissner, W. A., and McManus, R. G.: A comparison of the histologic pattern of benign and maligant thyroid tumors, J. Clin. Endocr. 12:1474-1479, 1952.

Table 29. Age and sex distribution in 198 carcinomas of thyroid gland*

Type	Females	Males	Total	Average age	Age range
Differentiated carcinoma					
Follicular adenocarcinoma	62	11	73	44.5	9-72
Papillary adenocarcinoma	74	12	86	45.5	9-80
Undifferentiated carcinoma					
Small cell carcinoma	26	4	30	46.5	9-72
Giant cell carcinoma	8	1	9	59.4	36-70

*Modified from Warren, S., and Meissner, W. A.: Tumors of the thyroid gland. In Atlas of tumor pathology, Sect. IV, Fasc. 14, Washington, D. C., 1953, Armed Forces Institute of Pathology.

groups is not warranted, for these variants often blend with each other. The use of the terms embryonal or fetal to designate adenomas is particularly unfortunate. The *colloid adenoma* is a rare but definite entity in our opinion. The microscopic appearance of an adenoma may suggest a malignant character, but if encapsulation is present and there is no evidence of blood vessel invasion, the tumor must be classified as benign. By contrast, a regular microscopic pattern may suggest a benign character, but if blood vessel invasion is present or if there is diffuse invasion of the capsule, the tumor must be classified as malignant.

We do not believe that *papillary cyst-adenoma* exists, for all of these tumors, in our opinion, are malignant. It is true that their evolution often is long and may even be measured in decades. We have now seen several instances of the most innocuous-appearing papillary tumors that have finally metastasized and demonstrated their malignant character.

Hürthle cell adenoma is a rare form of adenoma made up of large cells with acidophilic granular cytoplasm. Some adenomas may be extremely atypical microscopically, with highly cellular zones, and may even be considered to be cancer. However, a follow-up of thirty-one *atypical*

cellular adenomas over more than a five-year period showed no evidence of recurrence or distant metastasis (Hazard and Kenyon[49]).

Meissner and McManus[67] and Warren and Meissner[122] have tabulated their experience with large series of adenomas and carcinomas (Tables 28 and 29).

Grossly, a *papillary adenocarcinoma* may be so small that only a small gray nodule is seen (Fig. 302). Our smallest tumor measured 4 mm. The larger tumors have papillary processes that can be identified by the use of a hand lens. Microscopically, the papillary adenocarcinomas have well-defined papillary fronds, and there may or may not be layering of the cells. Frequently, they are extremely well differentiated, with the formation of psammoma bodies (small calcific spherules).

The psammoma body is extremely important in the diagnosis of papillary adenocarcinoma of the thyroid gland. The presence of such bodies is almost diagnostic of papillary adenocarcinoma. These bodies apparently arise at the site of degenerating or dead epithelium (Klinck and Winship[62]). Psammoma bodies do not occur in chronic thyroiditis or in metastatic cancer to the thyroid gland. Psammoma bodies were found only once in a nontoxic nodular

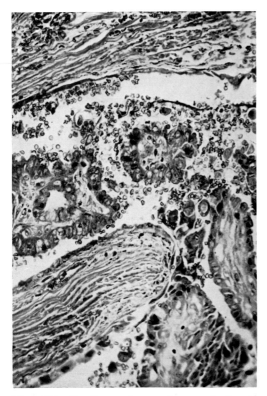

Fig. 302. Papillary adenocarcinoma of thyroid gland showing blood vessel invasion. (Low power.)

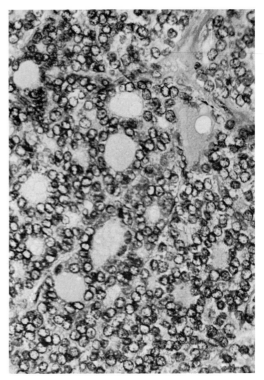

Fig. 303. Follicular adenocarcinoma of thyroid gland. Note well-defined follicles. This section is taken from metastatic focus in humerus. (High power.)

goiter out of 2153 noncancerous thyroid glands. Furthermore, these psammoma bodies are often present in normal thyroid tissue adjacent to the carcinoma. It is common to have some portion of a papillary cystadenocarcinoma show a follicular pattern. Spindle and giant cell metaplasia can be associated with papillary cancer of the thyroid gland (Hutter et al.[53]).

Primary *aberrant thyroid tumors* do not exist. If aberrant thyroid tumors arose from the lateral anlage of the thyroid gland, they would lie between the carotid sheath and the thyroid lobe laterally and the esophagus and the trachea medially (Weller[124]). Almost all so-called lateral aberrant thyroid tumors, however, lie superficial or external to the carotid sheath. In fifty-one supposedly lateral aberrant thyroid tumors in which the thyroid gland itself was examined, the primary source was found in the gland in thirty-one cases (King and Pemberton[60]). Crile et al.[22] reported six-

teen consecutive patients with lateral cervical metastases in whom exploration revealed the primary tumor to be in the thyroid gland. Histopathologic study further substantiated the evidence that the thyroid tumor was primary and that the neck nodules were lymph node metastases. Although in most instances a node is completely replaced by cancer, partial replacement of a node or evidence of tumor in peripheral sinuses can be demonstrated by cutting numerous sections. In 55% of the supposedly aberrant thyroid tumors reported by King and Pemberton,[60] lymphoid tissue was present. This evidence substantiates the concept that *so-called aberrant thyroid tumors are metastatic implants rather than primary tumors.* This view is now generally accepted (Black[8]; Crile et al.[22]; Warren and Feldman[121]). Gerard-Marchant[37] and Roth[87] have shown that inclusions of normal thyroid follicles may be found in cervical lymph nodes. No more than a dozen such cases have been seen. This finding does not represent metastatic carcinoma of the thyroid gland.

Rarely carcinoma can arise from a lingual thyroid (Ashhurst and White[1]), or from within the thyroglossal duct (Fish and Moore[30]).

In the *follicular adenocarcinoma,* the better differentiated the tumor, the more closely it resembles normal thyroid. We have seen metastases in bone, liver, and kidney in which the tumor looked exactly like normal thyroid tissue (Fig. 303). Microscopically, these tumors form well-differentiated follicles which, in some instances, may resemble normal thyroid tissue. The recognition of this tumor in the thyroid gland as a carcinoma depends on evidence of infiltration of remaining gland, capsule, and/or adjoining soft tissue.

The *small cell carcinoma* and the *giant cell carcinoma* are highly malignant but fortunately infrequent carcinomas of the thyroid gland. These tumors do not arise from preexisting adenomas. The small cell carcinomas have more variation in size and shape than malignant lymphoma (Walt et al.[119]). The giant cell carcinoma is extremely pleomorphic with pseudo-fibrosarcomatous areas and takes its name from the tumor giant cells that are present. This tumor progresses rapidly to replace the gland.

Tumors of a high degree of malignancy show a greater and more rapid local invasion. The local spread of a carcinoma of the thyroid gland may involve the recurrent laryngeal and vagus nerves, subcutaneous tissues, and muscle. The only muscle in the thyroid area that escapes complete destruction is the sternocleidomastoid. Tumor may surround or invade the trachea down to the submucosa, causing edema and sometimes ulceration, but its cartilaginous rings and fibrous sheaths make the trachea somewhat resistant to involvement. It may also invade and even ulcerate the esophagus. Spread to neighboring bones, particularly the clavicle and the sternum, is not unusual.

Hürthle cell carcinomas make up 5% to 10% of all malignant tumors of the thyroid gland (Frazell and Duffy[33]) and appear predominantly in women (Gardner[36]). They are encapsulated tumors simulating adenomas, but diffuse infiltration of surrounding structures may be present. Microscopically, the cells are large, opaque, and acidophilic (Fig. 304).

Medullary carcinoma is an unusual form of neoplasm. Hazard et al.[47] reported twenty-one out of 600 carcinomas of the thyroid gland. Fourteen occurred in women and seven in men. Lymph node metastases are relatively common. The microscopic pattern shows undifferentiated neoplasm with masses of amyloid (Fig. 305). This amyloid is present both in the primary tumor and in the metastases. It probably arises from parafollicular cells, may be familial, and is associated, at times, with pheochromocytomas and parathyroid adenomas (Sarosi and Doe[92]; Davis[23]). Meyer and Abdel-Bari[68] demonstrated by bioassay that this tumor secretes thyrocalcitonin.

Epidermoid carcinomas are rare tumors that probably arise from metaplasia of normal thyroid epithelium (Jaffé[54]).

Extramedullary *plasmacytomas* have been reported by Shaw and Smith[98] and Barton and Farmer.[5] We believe that most of these are not true neoplasms but rather extensive replacement of the thyroid gland by plasma cells.

Lymphosarcomas of the thyroid gland have been infrequently reported (Kellett and Sutherland[58]; Dinsmore et al.[25]). They must be differentiated from small cell carcinomas. Lymphosarcoma infrequently arises from or is associated with Hashimoto's disease (Kenyon and Ackerman[59]; Ranstrom[83]). The response to irradiation may be a helpful differentiating point.

Fibrosarcomas may arise from the stroma, but few authentic cases have been reported (Zeckwer[133]). The demonstration of fibroglia fibrils is strong confirmatory evidence.

Teratomas are few even among the exceptional cases of teratomas of the neck (Potter[80]; Bale[3]).

The microscopic diagnosis of carcinoma of the thyroid gland is usually not difficult. The extreme hyperplasia of the gland in Graves' disease may infiltrate surrounding muscle, but invariably the patient has profound clinical signs and symptoms to correlate with this hyperplasia. Adenomas can be recognized as malignant only when

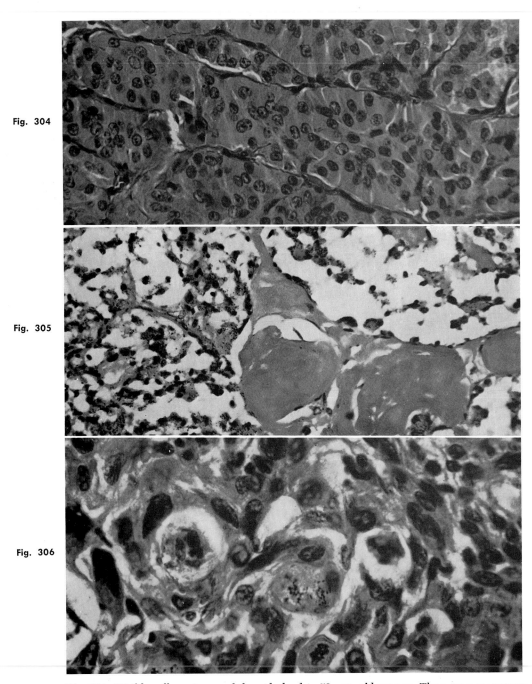

Fig. 304

Fig. 305

Fig. 306

Fig. 304. Hürthle cell carcinoma of thyroid gland in 59-year-old woman. There were metastases to regional lymph nodes. Individual cells are large with uniform nuclei. It would be difficult on microscopic pattern alone to call this cancer. (×70; WU neg. 60-789.)

Fig. 305. Undifferentiated medullary carcinoma with amyloid. (×300; WU neg. 59-4732.)

Fig. 306. Highly undifferentiated carcinoma of thyroid gland with numerous bizarre mitotic figures and giant cells. This type of tumor would often be designated as giant cell carcinoma. This slide comes from metastasis in lung. (×600; WU neg. 60-7823.)

they locally infiltrate surrounding thyroid tissue or show evidence of true tumor venous thrombi. The papillary cystadeno-carcinoma with psammoma bodies is always a malignant tumor no matter how benign its pattern. The greatest difficulty is in the recognition of extremely well-differentiated follicular carcinoma. This can be recognized with certainty only when it infiltrates the tissues outside the thyroid gland or grows within veins. This neoplasm is rarely pure in its morphologic expression. More often it is mingled with an obvious papillary adenocarcinoma.

Metastatic spread

The regional metastases of the well-differentiated tumor of the thyroid gland may be slow to appear. It is not unusual for metastases to remain in the cervical and mediastinal nodes or the lungs for five years or more. Regional lymph node metastases are commonly present particularly in the papillary adenocarcinomas. The nodes along the larynx, trachea, and external jugular vein are commonly invaded, and later the submaxillary, retropharyngeal, supraclavicular, mediastinal, and retrosternal nodes may become involved. Posteromediastinal lymph node involvement is rare.

The organs most frequently affected by metastatic disease are lymph nodes, lungs, bone, liver, kidneys, and brain. Pulmonary metastases are usually multiple and often subpleural. There is a striking tendency for thyroid tumors to metastasize to bone. In 110 cases collected by Bérard and Dunet,[6] the bones of the skull were involved in 25.6%, the vertebral column in 21%, the humerus, femur, sternum, ribs, and pelvic bones in from 7% to 10% each, and the clavicle in 4%. These metastases usually appear in the spongy portion of the bone, are richly vascularized, and may pulsate. Tumor appears between the compact tissue of the flat bones of the skull, in the body of the vertebrae, in the manubrium, in the epiphysis, or in the medullary cavity of the long bones. Spontaneous fractures can occur.

Clinical evolution

Most tumors of the thyroid gland develop slowly over a period that sometimes has extended to twenty-five years. This slow development is not indicative of benignity of the process, for it is present in definitely metastasizing tumors. The first sign is usually a *nodule* or *goiter* noticed by the patient or found on physical examination. As the tumor expands, pressure symptoms may develop. *Hoarseness* may be due to displacement of the larynx by any tumor but also results from *recurrent laryngeal paralysis* in malignant tumors. *Dysphagia* is observed due to malignant infiltration of the esophagus. Invasion of the trachea may result in *hemoptysis*, which has been the first symptom of alarm in patients with long-standing goiter (Grimes and Bell[40]). *Choking attacks* or a sensation of fullness in the neck may result from obstruction of the superior vena cava due to direct invasion of cervical veins. *Loss of weight* seldom occurs early in the course of the disease unless it is due to dysphagia.

The appearance of a cervical adenopathy is often the first sign of a nonpalpable papillary cystadenocarcinoma of the thyroid gland. This fact originally led to the concept of *lateral aberrant thyroid tumors*, a misconception due to the fact that patients appeared cured for years following extirpation of what were actually metastases. It is now generally accepted that tumors believed to have developed from aberrant thyroid tissue are actually metastatic lesions even though at times they present a benign morphologic pattern. Metastatic neck nodes in the jugular, transverse supraclavicular, and spinal chains may appear in the course of development of an otherwise symptomless goiter or after fixation or other symptoms of extracapsular infiltration have taken place. Axillary and mediastinal lymph node metastases may also occur.

Adenomas present as single nodules. Well-delimited carcinomas also present as single nodules. *Papillary adenocarcinomas* have the most benign clinical course and are also the most frequent malignant form among young patients (Frazell and Foote[34]). Frequently, a lymph node metastasis is the initial sign, and patients often live for years with obvious evidence of disease even after lung metastases have occurred. *Follicular adenocarcinomas* (alveolar) are usually large when first seen and may present bone metastases. The first symptom may be bone pain or fracture. Regional lymph node involvement is infrequent. Long survivals have been observed. In general, however, length of life is not so long as in patients with papillary lesions. *Small cell carcinomas* are highly malignant, usually arise from a nonadenomatous gland, and rapidly infiltrate and metastasize. Life expectancy is short as a rule. *Giant cell carcinomas* occur most frequently in elderly patients. They develop rapidly and often compress the esophagus and the trachea. Distant metastases are infrequent, probably because the rapid local development of the primary lesion almost invariably leads to a rapid death (Frazell and Foote[34]). *Hürthle cell carcinomas* are frequently small when first seen and are more common in women than in men. They have a tendency to remain localized to the neck. Life expectancy is long even in the presence of lung and bone metastases. *Epidermoid carcinomas*, fortunately rare, are highly malignant. *Fibrosarcomas* also develop rapidly and are usually fatal. *Lymphosarcomas* are said to originate in the thyroid gland. About 175 such cases have been reported (Mikal[71]). Most of the patients are elderly women with a large "goiter" of recent development (Dinsmore et al.[25]).

Metastases from thyroid tumors show a predilection for bones. A bone metastasis may be the first clinical manifestation of cancer of the thyroid gland. These metastases often cause fractures of the humerus, femur, or ribs. When the bone metastases are superficial and large, they may pulsate. Lung metastases are second in frequency but may not appear until late in the development of the disease. Metastases to brain and other organs have been observed but are not the rule. Long periods of survival are common in patients with well-differentiated tumors even in the presence of bone and lung metastases.

Diagnosis

Thyroid tumors predominate in women. They occur in young individuals. Actually, in patients under the age of 20 years a single nontoxic thyroid nodule has a greater chance of being malignant than of being benign. The growth is easily palpable or

even visible. In the presence of metastatic cervical lymph nodes from an unknown primary tumor, a search for the primary lesion implies careful investigation of the thyroid gland. Skillful palpation is necessary if small thyroid nodules are to be detected. About one-half of all thyroid tumors escape the most careful clinical search and may be found only on microscopic examination of the gland.

Palpation of the region of the thyroid gland may fail to detect a small tumor situated behind the lower borders of the sternocleidomastoid muscles. To bring out the thyroid lobe on each side and to be able to palpate it between the fingers of one hand, the patient should be seated in front of the examiner with the chin slightly rotated toward the side to be palpated (Fig. 307). With the thumb of one hand, the examiner displaces the larynx laterally toward the side to be examined, permitting palpation of one lobe of the thyroid between the index finger and thumb of the opposite hand. This procedure may then be complemented by

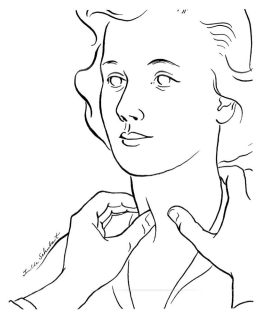

Fig. 307. Palpation of thyroid gland, with patient's chin slightly to side to be palpated and neck muscles relaxed. Examiner pushes larynx and thyroid gland with thumb of one hand while he feels thyroid lobe between thumb and index finger of opposite hand.

palpation of the gland while the patient swallows. Palpation of the thyroid gland may also be done with the physician standing behind the seated patient with head in hyperextension.

Adenomas are usually felt as discrete, oval-shaped nodules not adherent to skin and slipping easily from under the palpating fingers. If a mass is cancer and not an adenoma, it presents less well-defined limits and a certain degree of fixation and greater induration. A tendency to fixation may be found, however, in benign adenomas that have been subject to hemorrhage. Sudden tenderness and enlargement often mark the development of hemorrhage and distention of the capsule. This is often followed by surrounding reaction and a tendency to fixation. In highly malignant tumors, usually more bulky, the tumefaction is diffuse, and the induration may extend beyond the anatomic limits of the gland. Palpation of the neck should include search for possible metastatic lymph nodes in the jugular and spinal, as well as in the transverse (supraclavicular), chain of nodes. The transformation of an adenoma into carcinoma is a rare event and a difficult one to prove. Careful histologic examination should demonstrate benign areas with gradual transition to carcinoma (Silverberg and Vidone[104]).

Roentgenologic examination

Every patient suspected of having a thyroid tumor must have a lateral roentgenogram of the soft tissues of the neck. This examination may prove of value in demonstrating calcification within the tumor or compression of the trachea. Barium as a contrast material will help the study of the adjacent esophagus. Soft tissue roentgenography may identify characteristic calcifications in or around the thyroid gland. These calcifications are undoubtedly due to psammoma bodies in papillary carcinoma (Segal et al.[94]). The routine examination of the chest may reveal the presence of unsuspected upper mediastinal and pulmonary metastases. Pulmonary metastases are most often diffuse and nodular. Osseous metastases are most often observed in the bones of the spine, pelvis, ribs, and skull. They occur less often in the humerus and the femur. Bone lesions are osteolytic,

resulting in considerable destruction and eventual fractures of long bones. There is usually no periosteal reaction. A few cases show new bone formation, but there is often extension of the tumor to the surrounding soft tissues and even extension through a joint to the adjacent bone (Sherman and Ivker[100]).

Radioactive scanning

The normal thyroid gland has great avidity for iodine[131]. Tumors of the thyroid gland take up iodine less well and may not take it up at all. Under these circumstances, careful scanning for radioactivity will reveal negative uptake by a thyroid nodule, indicating its probable malignant nature. In general, the better differentiated the tumor, the more orderly the follicles, and the more abundant the colloid, the greater the relative uptake of radioactive iodine (Fitzgerald et al.[31]). The poorly differentiated neoplasms, the papillary tumors, and the Hürthle cell carcinoma, with few exceptions, show little or no uptake of the radioactive material. The same finding

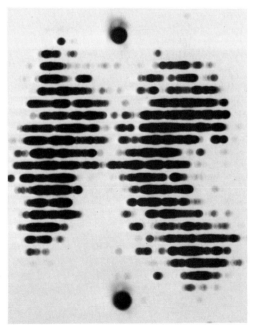

Fig. 308. Scintigram of thyroid gland demonstrating "cold" nodule in 41-year-old euthyroid patient. Pathologic examination of this nodule showed focal area of cystic degeneration in nodular goiter. (Courtesy Dr. Paul W. Palmer, Colorado Springs, Colo.; WU neg. 68-7633.)

may be due, however, to a colloid cyst or a nonfunctioning adenoma (Dobyns and Lennon[27]) (Fig. 308). So-called "hot" nodules are most often found to be benign (Attie[2]; Greene[39]; Perlmutter and Slater[77]), whereas a good proportion of "cold" nodules prove to be carcinoma (Shimaoka and Sokal[101]). The chances of a single "cold" nodule being cancer rise if the rest of the thyroid gland is entirely normal.

In preparing for scintiscanning, it is important to eliminate any thyroid medication that may block the uptake of radioiodine. The administration of thyroid-stimulating hormone may, on the contrary, increase the uptake. If radioiodine is detected in the neck, outside the thyroid gland, this may be taken for evidence of lymph node metastases. However, thyroid gland anomalies and lingual thyroid tissue may also be responsible. Distant metastases in lung, liver, or bone may also be detected, but in the myxedematous patients there may be debatable findings due to failure of the radioactive iodine to enter the organic iodine pool (Saenger et al.[90]).

Differential diagnosis

Thyroid tumors have to be differentiated from three types of thyroiditis: subacute thyroiditis, invasive thyroiditis, and Hashimoto's disease.

In *subacute thyroiditis* (struma fibrosa), the gland is usually symmetrically enlarged and tender following a respiratory infection. Fixation to the trachea is minimal. Subacute thyroiditis runs a variable course of weeks or months without significant interference with the function of the thyroid gland, although the basal metabolic rate may be slightly elevated (Schilling[93]). Odynophagia and otalgia are rather characteristic symptoms but, in addition, there may be nervousness, asthenia, and loss of weight. Subacute thyroiditis is identical with pseudotuberculosis or giant cell thyroiditis (Crile[18]). It does not respond to roentgentherapy but does respond to steroids.

Invasive thyroiditis is a rare lesion that usually involves a single lobe of the thyroid gland and invades surrounding muscle (Woolner et al.[130]). It is a rare, painful, slowly developing, unilateral process appearing predominantly in women over 20 years of age. It has a tendency to prominent fixation with pressure symptoms such as laryngeal paralysis and dysphagia. At operation, the fibrous tissue extends to involve the surrounding muscles. Surgical treatment is preferable. Crile and Fisher[21] reported on the rare association of thyroiditis and papillary carcinoma.

Hashimoto's disease (struma lymphomatosa) is most often observed in elderly women and rarely in men. It has been reported in children (Lasser and Grayzel[63]). In Marshall and Meissner's series[65] of 114 patients, all but two were women. The entire gland may become indurated and enlarged, but it usually retains its normal configuration. There is seldom any pain or tenderness to palpation, and fixation is minimal (Joll[55]). The disease is not frequently diagnosed before surgery is done. Grossly, the thyroid gland is enlarged, the capsule is thin and nonadherent, and the cut surface is lobular, reddish yellow, and without evidence of fibrosis. Microscopically, the follicles are small, lined by eosinophilic epithelium, and colloid is scanty. ACTH and cortisone are apparently of value in the treatment of Hashimoto's disease. Carcinoma of the thyroid gland associated with Hashimoto's disease has been observed (Shands[97]).

Parathyroid adenomas may be associated with bone lesions and a variety of clinical conditions including duodenal ulcers, pancreatitis, and a syndrome of multiple adenomas arising in various endocrine organs. Parathyroid carcinoma is usually functioning, and about fifty cases have been reported. Clinically, the presence of palpable cervical lymph nodes in a patient with hypercalcemia suggests the presence of a parathyroid carcinoma (Holmes et al.[52]). *Pseudohyperparathyroidism* can occur in a number of malignant tumors in the absence of any changes in the bone—carcinoma of the kidney, small cell carcinomas of the lung, breast, cervix, and prostate, and malignant lymphomas. The explanation for this is still not available (Snedecor and Baker[108]).

Functioning *carcinomas of the parathyroid gland* are extremely rare. They are often associated with nephrolithiasis and fibrocystic disease of the bone. Tange[112] collected and studied two dozen such cases. Tumors of the parathyroid gland may be considered malignant if there is invasion of surrounding tissues and/or involvement of regional lymph nodes. The microscopic patterns of tumors of the parathyroid gland are difficult to interpret, for benign adenomas may show great variation in size and shape of cells with many bizarre nuclei without mitotic activity (Black and Ackerman[7]). Carcinoma of the parathyroid gland has a trabecular pattern, and mitotic figures are present (Castleman[11]). In one of our cases, true tumor thrombi and nerve sheath invasion were present. Removal of these tumors may result in regression of symptoms of hyperparathyroidism and of bone lesions. Recurrence of the tumor results in recurrence of signs and symptoms of hyperparathyroidism (Meyer and Ragins[69]).

Metastatic lesions in the thyroid glands from primary tumors elsewhere are unusual but may occur from carcinomas of the breast, lung, bladder, or prostate or from melanocarcinomas (Mortensen et al.[73]). If a metastasis is present in the thyroid gland, it is usually only part of a generalized process (Silverberg and Vidone[104]). Hodgkin's disease may rarely involve the thyroid gland.

Treatment
Surgery

The early manifestations of various malignant tumors of the thyroid gland are clinically indistinguishable from the more frequent benign manifestations of nontoxic nodular goiter. The gravity of the actual circumstances may not be known before operation. The eventual success of the treatment of the malignant neoplasms depends not only on the technical ability of the surgeon, but more on his understanding of the process and the natural history of these tumors.

In the presence of a *single nodule*, simple "enucleation" is dangerous, for if the nodule proves to be malignant, the danger of tumor implantation is present and the procedure may actually preclude subsequent adequate surgery. If there is no gross evidence of infiltration or lymph node enlargement, the nodule should be excised with a good margin of normal thyroid tissue for *frozen section*. In most instances, the compliance with these prerequisites means the performance of a lobectomy. Usually, the microscopic examination reveals an adenomatous thyroid, an adenoma, or a malignant tumor. Difficulties in the microscopic diagnosis of carcinoma arise only if there is no infiltration outside the nodule. If the nodule represents a carcinoma or a Hürthle cell tumor, most surgeons would do or recommend no more. If the nodule is found to contain a papillary carcinoma, the evidence is that, in a large proportion of cases, other foci will be found in the thyroid gland (Clark et al.[15]), yet local recurrence seldom occurs after adequate lobectomy. This fact leads some surgeons to perform a total thyroidectomy in such cases. In patients reoperated upon because of local recurrence, Rose et al.[88] demonstrated contralateral metastases in 24.4%. Other surgeons would recommend an ipsilateral *prophylactic neck dissection* (Frazell and Foote[34]) as a complement to the lobectomy or thyroidectomy. In a variable proportion of one-third to one-half of these cases, microscopic involvement of the jugular nodes may be found. In young women and children, the chain of jugular nodes may be removed without resection of the sternocleidomastoid muscle, for it is seldom involved (Pollock and Juler[79]). Further study by Hutter et al.[52a] indicated that there is no risk in abstention—that a therapeutic neck dissection may be done successfully when the metastases develop clinically.

In the presence of *gross infiltration* of the surrounding tissues or of *lymph node involvement*, a frozen section will simply confirm the suspicion of malignant tumor. Under these circumstances, at least a total thyroidectomy and neck dissection would be required. It must be pointed out that a classical neck dissection fails to remove retrothyroid and pretracheal lymph nodes which are often involved. Removal of upper mediastinal nodes would require sternostomy (Welti[125]). Often such surgical attempts are futile, and a number of experienced surgeons prefer to admit their impotence under such circumstances. Moreover, the radical removal of the entire thyroid gland in such cases often implies development of occult, or overt, hypoparathyroidism (Michie et al.[70]). This important dysfunction develops not necessarily because of removal of the parathyroid glands but because of trauma or injury to their blood supply and perhaps hormonal causes. Hypoparathyroidism is subject to prolonged and costly medical management.

The finding of accessory thyroid nodules in the region of the gland, and not connected with it, is not rare. Such detached nodules are not necessarily evidence of metastatic carcinoma (Hathaway[44]). Hemorrhage is the most common complication of surgery of the thyroid gland. Paralysis of the laryngeal nerves is a definite risk.

Radiotherapy

Malignant tumors of the thyroid gland may exhibit remarkable radiosensitivity which may lead, under given circumstances of the case, to radiocurability.

Irradiation by means of *radioactive iodine* may be very useful in some instances. However, the avidity of thyroid tumors for iodine[131] is unpredictable. This uptake may be increased by thyroidectomy or the administration of thyrotropic hormones or of an obliterating dose of radioactive iodine. If the uptake of iodine[131] is good, the irradiation of the tumor is considerable but not necessarily uniform. The administration of large amounts of radioactive iodine may result in untoward irradiation of male and female gonads with an obvious hazard to young patients (Kammer and Goodman[57]; Trunnell et al.[115]). The results are rather unpredictable. Relatively, the best results are obtained in the highly differentiated metastatic carcinomas. In the undifferentiated tumors, for lack of uptake, the results are consistently bad (Smithers et al.[107]).

External irradiation is definitely a more adequate means of irradiating tumors of the thyroid gland, their cervical and mediastinal lymph node metastases, and the distant implants of the tumor. Irradiation of inoperable or residual carcinomas of the thyroid gland, and of the adjacent frequently involved lymph nodes can be accomplished with success. Irradiation of the entire potential area of regional involvement in the neck and mediastinum offers a delicate problem of radiotherapeutic planning and dosimetry, but it can be achieved successfully, particularly with cobalt[60] or supervoltage roentgentherapy (Halnan[42]). We have cases of long-standing control of undifferentiated inoperable or recurrent tumors. Others have reported similar experiences in papillary and differentiated tumors (Smedal et al.[106]). It is in the undifferentiated tumors, usually abandoned by the surgeon (Burn and Taylor[9]) and not showing great avidity for iodine[131] (Pochin[78]), that the radiotherapist has a frequent opportunity to put in practice the advantages of external irradiation (Mabille[64]). The palliative effects in metastatic lesions of the lung, bone, and other organs are often long lasting (Trevor and Pack[114]). In the management of lymphosarcomas, external irradiation is the treatment of choice (Sheline et al.[99]).

Hormonotherapy

It is now definitely established that many tumors of the thyroid gland, particularly the well-differentiated ones, are thyrotropin dependent. Thus, the administration of thyroid hormone has resulted in regression of tumors (Root[86]). Appreciable palliation may sometimes be obtained by the administration of thyroid extract in papillary and follicular carcinomas (Crile[20]).

Prognosis

It is frequently pointed out that institutions that report a relatively large number of cases of carcinoma of the thyroid gland also report a relatively small proportion of deaths and few autopsies of patients dying from its consequences. The answer is, of course, in the natural history of the disease, which frequently results in patients dying with, but not necessarily of, cancer of the thyroid gland. Cancer of the thyroid gland discovered at autopsy is a rare occurrence (Silverberg and Vidone[104]). In 1965, there were in the United States 1052 deaths reportedly due to cancer of the thyroid gland, or a crude rate of 0.5 per 100,000 population. Only sixteen of these deaths occurred in patients under 35 years of age. The rates for white females and nonwhite males were 0.7 and 0.2, respectively. There is no clear evidence of regional differences in mortality from carcinoma of the thyroid gland in the United

States. Austria reports the highest age-adjusted death rates, over three times greater than the United States rates. In Cali, Colombia, there is an apparent greater death rate from carcinoma of the thyroid gland in the goiter areas as compared with nongoiter areas (Wahner et al.[117]).

The most important single factor in the prognosis of thyroid tumors is the patient's age. Nearly all patients under 20 years of age are likely to show a ten-year survival. The proportion of patients surviving a decade diminishes considerably in the successive decades of life (Halnan[42]). Winship and Rosvoll[128] collected 526 cases of carcinoma of the thyroid gland in children, 18% of whom eventually died of cancer. The extent of the disease when first seen was the most important factor in relation to survival.

The prognosis of *adenomas* of the thyroid gland is excellent except when microscopic examination reveals invasion of blood vessels (Hazard and Kenyon[48]). Patients with *papillary carcinoma* also have an excellent prognosis. Woolner et al.[129] reported on a series of 140 patients with *occult* papillary carcinomas, fifty-eight of whom presented lymph node metastases and none of whom had died of cancer. Often, on the basis of limited experience, the feeling is expressed that patients with papillary carcinoma do not die of their disease. Tollefsen et al.[113] reported seventy deaths in a series of 700 patients seen at the Memorial Hospital in New York. The most common cause of death was recurrent carcinoma in the neck. Patients with *follicular carcinoma* have almost as good a prognosis as those with papillary carcinoma. These two histologic characters are often mixed and some consider the preponderance of papillary character as particularly favorable.

Hürthle cell carcinomas are considered as differentiated tumors and also offer a favorable outlook, varying only in reference to their extent when treated (Chesky et al.[13]; Gardner[36]). The evidence as to the role of coexisting thyroiditis is divided (Hirabayashi and Lindsay[51]; Prior and Fairchild[81]). The occult *sclerosing carcinoma* has been shown to possess the ability to metastasize (Klinck and Win-

Table 30. Survival of patients with carcinoma of thyroid gland

Type of tumor	Cumulative survivial to		
	5 yr (%)	10 yr (%)	20 yr (%)
Papillary	73	60	45
Follicular	71	48	24
Undifferentiated	17	17	17

ship[61]), but it still has a good outlook. Patients with *medullary carcinoma* have a moderately favorable prognosis. Freeman and Lindsay[35] reported on thirty-three patients, of whom eighteen were living for a mean 8.7 years. *Giant cell carcinomas* of the thyroid gland are seldom cured.

Although age and the inherent character of the tumor seem to be the stronger factors in predicting the survival of patients with tumors of the thyroid gland, the treatment applied also influences the length of survival and, in a few, cure. *Surgery* is the treatment of choice of the majority of these tumors, but it is futile in the undifferentiated or advanced tumors. *Radioiodine therapy* is also futile in undifferentiated tumors but may be of lasting palliative value in differentiated residual or metastatic carcinomas. *External irradiation* has gained an increasingly large place in the treatment of these tumors. Results obtained by radiotherapy in advanced cases, either beyond surgery or those recurring after surgery, have encouraged its use as a systematic routine complement of moderate surgery (Mabille[64]; Smedal et al.[106]) or as the only treatment of undifferentiated and advanced tumors. Definitely external irradiation is the treatment of choice of *lymphosarcomas* (Sheline et al.[99]). Good results have also been obtained with irradiation of anaplastic carcinomas (Rafla[81a]). The prognosis is particularly favorable when the tumor has not extended outside the gland (Woolner et al.[131]).

REFERENCES

1 Ashhurst, A. P. C., and White, C. Y.: Carcinoma in an aberrant thyroid at the base of the tongue, J.A.M.A. **85**:1210-1220, 1925.
2 Attie, J. N.: The use of radioactive iodine in the evaluation of thyroid nodules, Surgery **47**:611-614, 1960.

3 Bale, G. F.: Teratoma of the neck in the region of the thyroid gland; a review of the literature and report of four cases, Amer. J. Path. 26:565-579, 1950.

4 Barrie, H. J.: Interstitial emphysema and pneumothorax after operations on the neck, Lancet 1:996-998, 1940.

5 Barton, F. E., and Farmer, D. A.: Plasmacytoma of the thyroid gland, Ann. Surg. 132: 304-309, 1950.

6 Bérard, L., and Dunet, C.: Le cancer thyroidien, Paris, 1924, Gaston Doin.

7 Black, B. K., and Ackerman, L. V.: Tumors of the parathyroid, Cancer 3:415-444, 1950.

8 Black, B. M.: Papillary adenocarcinoma of the thyroid gland, so-called lateral aberrant thyroid tumors, Trans. Amer. Ass. Study Goiter, pp. 34-50; Western J. Surg. 56:134-144, 1948.

9 Burn, J. I., and Taylor, S. F.: Natural history of thyroid carcinoma; a study of 152 treated patients, Brit. Med. J. 2:1218-1223, 1962.

10 Carroll, R. E., Haddon, W., Jr., Handy, V. H., and Wieben, E. E., Sr.: Thyroid cancer: cohort analysis of increasing incidence in New York State, 1941-1962, J. Nat. Cancer Inst. 33:277-283, 1964.

11 Castleman, B.: Tumors of the parathyroid glands. In Atlas of tumor pathology, Sect. IV, Fasc. 15, Washington, D. C., 1952, Armed Forces Institute of Pathology.

12 Catz, B., Petit, D. W., Schwartz, H., Davis, F., McCammon, C., and Starr, P.: Treatment of cancer of the thyroid postoperatively with suppressive thyroid medication, radioactive iodine and thyroid-stimulating hormone, Cancer 12:371-383, 1959

13 Chesky, V. E., Dresse, W. C., and Hellwig, C. A.: Hurthle cell tumors of the thyroid gland; a report of 25 cases, J. Clin. Endocr. 11:1535-1548, 1951.

14 Clark, D. E.: Association of irradiation with cancer of the thyroid in children and adolescents, J.A.M.A. 159:1007-1009, 1955.

15 Clark, R. L., Jr., White, E. C., and Russell, W. O.: Total thyroidectomy for cancer of the thyroid; significance of intraglandular dissemination, Ann. Surg. 149:858-866, 1959.

16 Cole, W. H., Majarkis, J. D., and Slaughter, D. P.: Incidence of carcinoma of the thyroid in nodular goiter, J. Clin. Endocr. 9:1007-1011, 1949.

17 Cole, W. H., Slaughter, D. P., and Majarkis, J. D.: Carcinoma of the thyroid gland, Surg. Gynec. Obstet. 89:349-356, 1949.

18 Crile, G., Jr.: Thyroiditis, Ann. Surg. 127: 640-654, 1948.

19 Crile, G., Jr.: The endocrine dependency of certain thyroid cancers and the danger that hypothyroidism may stimulate their growth, Cancer 10:1119-1137, 1957.

20 Crile, G., Jr.: Endocrine dependency of papillary carcinomas of the thyroid, J.A.M.A. 195:101-104, 1966.

21 Crile, G., Jr., and Fisher, E. R.: Simultaneous occurrence of thyroiditis and papillary carcinoma; report of two cases, Cancer 6:57-62, 1953.

22 Crile, G., Jr., McNamara, J. M., and Hazard, J. B.: Results of treatment of papillary carcinoma of the thyroid, Surg. Gynec. Obstet. 109:315-320, 1959.

22a Cuello, C., Correa, P., and Eisenberg, H.: Geographic pathology of thyroid carcinoma, Cancer 23:230-239, 1969.

23 Davis, P. W.: A review of 17 cases of medullary carcinoma of the thyroid gland, Proc. Roy. Soc. Med. 60:743-744, 1967.

24 DeLawter, D. S., and Winship, T.: Follow-up study of adults treated with roentgen rays for thyroid disease, Cancer 16:1028-1031, 1963.

25 Dinsmore, R. S., Dempsey, W. S., and Hazard, J. B.: Lymphosarcoma of the thyroid, J. Clin. Endocr. 9:1043-1047, 1949.

26 Dische, S.: The radioisotope scan applied to the detection of carcinoma in thyroid swellings, Cancer 17:473-479, 1964.

27 Dobyns, B. M., and Lennon, B.: A study of the histopathology and physiologic function of thyroid tumors, using radioactive iodine and radioautography, J. Clin. Endocr. 8:732-748, 1948.

28 Dobyns, B. M., Skanse, B., and Maloof, F.: A method for the preoperative estimation of function in thyroid tumors; its significance in diagnosis and treatment, J. Clin. Endocr. 9: 1171-1184, 1949.

29 Dobyns, B. M., Vickery, A. L., Maloff, F., and Chapman, E. M.: Functional and histologic effects of therapeutic doses of radioactive iodine on the thyroid of man, J. Clin. Endocr. 13:548-567, 1953.

30 Fish, J., and Moore, R. N.: Ectopic thyroid tissue and ectopic thyroid carcinoma; a review of the literature and report of a case, Ann. Surg. 157:212-222, 1963.

31 Fitzgerald, P. J., Foote, F. W., Jr., and Hill, R. F.: Concentration of I^{131} in thyroid cancer, shown by radioautography, Cancer 3: 86-105, 1950.

32 Frantz, V. K., Quimby, E. H., and Evans, T. C.: Radioactive iodine studies of functional thyroid carcinoma, Radiology 51:532-552, 1948.

33 Frazell, E. L., and Duffy, B. J.: Hurthle-cell cancer of the thyroid: a review of forty cases, Cancer 4:952-956, 1951.

34 Frazell, E. L., and Foote, F. W., Jr.: Papillary cancer of the thyroid, Cancer 11:895-922, 1958.

35 Freeman, D., and Lindsay, S.: Medullary carcinoma of the thyroid gland, Arch. Path. (Chicago) 80:575-582, 1965.

36 Gardner, L. W.: Hürthle-cell tumors of the thyroid, Arch. Path. (Chicago) 59:372-381, 1955.

37 Gerard-Marchant, R.: Inclusions thyroidiennes dans les ganglions lymphatiques du cou, Bull. Cancer (Paris) 49:190-195, 1962.

38 Graham, A.: Malignant epithelial tumors of the thyroid, Surg. Gynec. Obstet. 39:781-790, 1924.

39 Greene, R.: Discrete nodules of the thyroid gland, with special reference to carcinoma, Ann. Roy. Coll. Surg. Eng. 21:73-89, 1957.

40 Grimes, O. F., and Bell, H. G.: The significance of hemoptysis in carcinoma of the thyroid gland, Surgery 24:401-408, 1948.

41 Grisham, J. W.: Personal communication, 1961.

41a Haber, M. H., and Lipkovic, P.: Thyroid cancer in Hawaii, Cancer 25:1224-1227, 1970.

42 Halnan, K. E.: The place of non-surgical methods in diagnosis and management, and the long-term value of treatment of thyroid cancer, Brit. J. Surg. 52:736-739, 1965.

43 Hashimoto, H.: Zur Kenntnis der lymphomatosen Veranderung der Schliddruse (Struma lymphomatosa), Arch. Klin. Chir. 97:219-248, 1912.

44 Hathaway, B. M.: Innocuous accessory thyroid nodules, Arch. Surg. (Chicago) 90:222-227, 1965.

45 Hawk, W. A., and Hazard, J. B.: Needle biopsy of the thyroid gland, Surg. Gynec. Obstet. 122:1053-1065, 1966.

46 Hayles, A. B., Kennedy, R. L. J., Beahrs, O. H., and Woolner, L. B.: Management of the child with thyroidal carcinoma, J.A.M.A. 173:21-28, 1960.

47 Hazard, J. B., Hawk, W. A., and Crile, G., Jr.: Medullary (solid) carcinoma of the thyroid—a clinicopathologic entity, J. Clin. Endocr. 19:152-161, 1959.

48 Hazard, J. B., and Kenyon, R.: Encapsulated angioinvasive carcinoma (angioinvasive adenoma) of the thyroid gland, Amer. J. Clin. Path. 24:755-756, 1954.

49 Hazard, J. B., and Kenyon, R.: Atypical adenoma of the thyroid, Arch. Path. (Chicago) 58:554-563, 1954.

50 Hempelmann, L. H.: Risk of thyroid neoplasms after irradiation in childhood, Science 160:159-163, 1968.

51 Hirabayashi, R. N., and Lindsay, S.: The relation of thyroid carcinoma and chronic thyroiditis, Surg. Gynec. Obstet. 121:243-252, 1965.

52 Holmes, E. C., Morton, D. L., and Ketcham, A. S.: Parathyroid carcinoma; a collective review, Ann. Surg. 169:631-640, 1969.

52a Hutter, R. V. P., Frazell, L., and Foote, F. W., Jr.: Elective radical neck dissection: an assessment of its use in the management of papillary thyroid cancer, CA 20:87-93, 1970.

53 Hutter, R. V. P., Tollefsen, H. R., DeCosse, J. J., Foote, F. W., Jr., and Frazell, E. L.: Spindle and giant cell metaplasia in papillary carcinoma of the thyroid, Amer. J. Surg. 110:660-668, 1965.

54 Jaffé, R. H.: Epithelial metaplasia of the thyroid gland, Arch. Path. (Chicago) 23:821-830, 1937.

55 Joll, C. A.: The pathology, diagnosis and treatment of Hashimoto's disease (struma lymphomatosa), Brit. J. Surg. 27:351-389, 1939 (classic article).

56 Kalderon, A. D., and Cohn, J. D.: Papillary adenocarcinoma in a thyroglossal duct, Cancer 19:839-843, 1966.

57 Kammer, H., and Goodman, M. J.: Sterility after radioiodine therapy for metastatic thyroid carcinoma, J.A.M.A. 171:1963-1965, 1959.

58 Kellett, H. S., and Sutherland, T. W.: Reticulosarcoma of the thyroid gland, J. Path. Bact. 61:233-244, 1949.

59 Kenyon, R. and Ackerman, L. V.: Malignant lymphoma of the thyroid, Cancer 8:964-969, 1955.

60 King, W. L. M., and Pemberton, J. deJ.: So-called lateral aberrant thyroid tumors, Surg. Gynec. Obstet. 74:991-1001, 1942.

61 Klinck, G. H., and Winship, T.: Occult sclerosing carcinoma of the thyroid, Cancer 8:701-706, 1955.

62 Klinck, G. H., and Winship, T.: Psammoma bodies and thyroid cancer, Cancer 12:656-662, 1959.

63 Lasser, R. P., and Grayzel, D. M.: Subacute thyroiditis, struma fibrosa, struma lymphomatosa; a clinical-pathological study, Amer. J. Med. Sci. 217:518-529, 1949.

64 Mabille, J. P.: Resultats therapeutiques des cancers thyroïdiens; statistique de la Fondation Curie, Ann. Radiol. (Paris) 4:477-491, 1961.

65 Marshal, S. F., and Meissner, W. A.: Struma lymphomatosa (Hashimoto's disease), Ann. Surg. 141:737-746, 1955.

66 Meissner, W. A., and Legg, M. A.: Persistent thyroid carcinoma, J. Clin. Endocr. 18:91-98, 1958.

67 Meissner, W. A., and McManus, R. G.: A comparison of the histologic pattern of benign and malignant thyroid tumors, J. Clin. Endocr. 12:1474-1479, 1952.

68 Meyer, J. S., and Abdel-Bari, W.: Granules and thyrocalcitonin-like activity in medullary carcinoma of the thyroid gland, New Eng. J. Med. 278:523-529, 1968.

69 Meyer, K. A., and Ragins, A. B.: Carcinoma of the parathyroid gland, Surgery 14:282-295, 1943.

70 Michie, W., Stowers, J. M., Frazer, S. C., and Gunn, A.: Thyroidectomy and the parathyroids, Brit. J. Surg. 52:503-514, 1965.

71 Mikal, S.: Primary lymphoma of the thyroid gland, Surgery 55:233-239, 1964.

72 Mortensen, J. D., Woolner, L. B., and Bennett, W. A.: Gross and microscopic findings in clinically normal thyroid glands, J. Clin. Endocr. 15:1270-1280, 1955.

73 Mortenson, J. D., Woolner, L. B., and Bennett, W. A.: Secondary malignant tumors of the thyroid gland, Cancer 9:306-309, 1956.

74 Morton, J. J.: Interinnomino-abdominal (hindquarter) amputation, Ann. Surg. 115:628-646, 1942.

75 Mustacchi, P., and Cutler, S. J.: Survival of patients with cancer of the thyroid gland, J.A.M.A. 173:1795-1798, 1960.

76 Newton, T. H., and Eisenberg, E.: Angiography of parathyroid adenomas, Radiology 86:843-850, 1966.

77 Perlmutter, M., and Slater, S. L.: Which nodular goiters should be removed? A physiologic plan for the diagnosis and treatment of nodular goiter, New Eng. J. Med. **255**:65-71, 1956.

78 Pochin, E. E.: Prospects from the treatment of thyroid carcinoma with radioiodine, Clin. Radiol. **28**:113-125, 1967.

79 Pollock, W. F., and Juler, G.: Thyroid carcinoma in children; a plea for conservation of functions, Amer. J. Dis. Child. **105**:243-248, 1963.

80 Potter, E. L.: Teratoma of the thyroid gland, Arch. Path. (Chicago) **25**:689-693, 1938.

81 Prior, J. T., and Fairchild, R. D.: Thyroid neoplasms and coexistent thyroiditis; observations on fifteen cases, Amer. J. Surg. **106**:57-63, 1963.

81a Rafla, S.: Anaplastic tumors of the thyroid, Cancer **23**:668-677, 1969.

82 Rall, J. E., Alpers, J. B., Lewallen, C. G., Sonenberg, M., Berman, M., and Rawson, R. W.: Radiation pneumonitis and fibrosis; a complication of radioiodine treatment of pulmonary metastases from cancer of the thyroid, J. Clin. Endocr. **17**:1263-1276, 1967.

83 Ranström, S.: Malignant lymphoma of the thyroid and its relation to Hashimoto's and Brill-Symmers' disease, Acta Chir. Scand. **113**:185-193, 1957.

84 Raventos, A., and Winship, T.: The latent interval for thyroid cancer following irradiation, Radiology **83**:501-508, 1964.

85 Rawson, R. W., Marinelli, L. D., Skanse, B. N., Trunnell, J., and Fluharty, R. C.: The effect of total thyroidectomy on the function of metastatic thyroid cancer, J. Clin. Endocr. **8**:826-841, 1948.

86 Root, A. W.: Cancer of the thyroid in childhood and adolescence, Amer. J. Med. Sci. **246**:734-749, 1963.

87 Roth, L. M.: Inclusions of nonneoplastic thyroid tissue within cervical lymph nodes, Cancer **18**:105-111, 1965.

88 Rose, R. G., Kelsey, M. P., Russell, W. O., Ibanez, M. L., White, E. C., and Clark, R. L.: Follow-up study of thyroid cancer treated by unilateral lobectomy, Amer. J. Surg. **106**:494-500, 1963.

89 Rouvière, H.: Anatomie des lymphatiques de l'homme, Paris, 1933, Masson et Cie.

90 Saenger, E. L., Barrett, C. M., Passino, J. W., Seltzer, R. A., and Dooley, W. D.: Experiences with I¹³¹ in the management of carcinoma of the thyroid, Radiology **83**:892-901, 1964.

91 Sampson, R. J., Key, C. R., Buncher, C. R., and Iijima, S.: Thyroid carcinoma in Hiroshima and Nagasaki. I. Prevalence of thyroid carcinoma at autopsy, J.A.M.A. **209**:65-70, 1969.

92 Sarosi, G., and Doe, R. P.: Familial occurrence of parathyroid adenomas, pheochromocytoma, and medullary carcinoma of the thyroid with amyloid stroma (Sipple's syndrome), Ann. Intern. Med. **68**:1305-1309, 1968.

93 Schilling, J. A.: Struma lymphomatosa, struma fibrosa and thyroiditis, Surg. Gynec. Obstet. **81**:533-550, 1945.

94 Segal, R. L., Zuckerman, H., and Friedman, E. W.: Soft tissue roentgenography, J.A.M.A. **173**:1890-1894, 1960.

95 Seidlin, S. M., Rossman, I., Oshry, E., and Siegel, E.: Radioiodine therapy of metastases from carcinoma of the thyroid; a six-year progress report, J. Clin. Endocr. **9**:1122-1137, 1949.

96 Selzman, H. M., and Fechner, R. E.: Oxyphil adenoma and primary hyperparathyroidism; clinical and ultrastructural observations; J.A.M.A. **199**:109-111, 1967.

97 Shands, W. C.: Carcinoma of the thyroid in association with struma lymphomatosa (Hashimoto's disease), Ann. Surg. **151**:675-682, 1960.

98 Shaw, R. C., and Smith, F. B.: Plasmocytoma of the thyroid gland, Arch. Surg. (Chicago) **40**:646-657, 1940.

99 Sheline, G. E., Galante, M., and Lindsay, S.: Radiation therapy in the control of persistent thyroid cancer, Amer. J. Roentgen. **97**:923-930, 1966.

100 Sherman, R. S., and Ivker, M.: The roentgen appearance of thyroid metastases in bone, Amer. J. Roentgen. **63**:196-203, 1950.

101 Shimaoka, G., and Sokal, J. E.: Differentiation of benign and malignant thyroid nodules by scintiscan, Arch. Intern. Med. (Chicago) **114**:36-39, 1964.

102 Silliphant, W. M., Klinck, G. H., and Levitin, M. S.: Thyroid carcinoma and death; a clinicopathological study of 193 autopsies, Cancer **17**:513-525, 1964.

103 Silverberg, S. G., and Vidone, R. A.: Adenoma and carcinoma of the thyroid, Cancer **19**:1053-1062, 1966.

104 Silverberg, S. G., and Vidone, R. A.: Carcinoma of the thyroid in surgical and postmortem material; analysis of 300 cases at autopsy and literature review, Ann. Surg. **164**:291-299, 1964.

105 Simpson, C. L., Hempelmann, L. H., and Fuller, L. M.: Neoplasia in children treated with x-rays in infancy for thymic enlargement, Radiology **64**:840-845, 1955.

106 Smedal, M. I., Salzman, F. A., and Meissner, W. A.: The value of 2 Mv. roentgenray therapy in differentiated thyroid carcinoma, Amer. J. Roentgen. **99**:352-364, 1967.

107 Smithers, D. W., Howard, N., and Trott, N. G.: Treatment of carcinoma of the thyroid with radioiodine, Brit. Med. J. **2**:969-974, 1965.

108 Snedecor, P. A., and Baker, H. W.: Pseudohyperparathyroidism due to malignant tumors, Cancer **17**:1492-1496, 1964.

109 Socolow, E. L., Hashizume, A., Neriishi, S., and Niitani, R.: Thyroid carcinoma in man after exposure to ionizing radiation; a summary of the findings in Hiroshima and Nagasaki, New Eng. J. Med. **268**:406-410, 1963.

110 Sokal, J. E.: The problem of malignancy in

nodular goiter—recapitulation and a challenge, J.A.M.A. **170**:405-412, 1959.

111 Soley, M. H., Lindsay, S., and Dailey, M. E.: The clinical significance of a solitary nodule in the thyroid gland, Western J. Surg. **56**: 96-104, 1948.

112 Tange, J. D.: Carcinoma of the parathyroid, Brit. J. Surg. **66**:254-259, 1958.

113 Tollefsen, H. R., DeCosse, J. J., and Hutter, R. V. P.: Papillary carcinoma of the thyroid; a clinical and pathological study of 70 fatal cases, Cancer **17**:1035-1044, 1964.

114 Trevor, W., and Pack, G. T.: The treatment of metastatic cancer of the thyroid; a report of unusual cases, Southern Surg. **15**:9-17, 1949.

115 Trunnell, J. B., Marinelli, L. D., Duffy, B. J., Hill, R., Peacock, W., and Rawson, R. W.: The treatment of metastatic thyroid cancer with radioactive iodine; credits and debits, J. Clin. Endocr. **9**:1138-1152, 1949.

116 Vander, J. B., Gaston, E. A., and Dawber, T. R.: Significance of solitary nontoxic thyroid nodules; preliminary report, New Eng. J. Med. **251**:970-973, 1954.

117 Wahner, H. W., Cuello, C., Correa, P., Uribe, L. F., and Gaitan, E.: Thyroid carcinoma in an endemic goiter area, Cali, Columbia, Amer. J. Med. **40**:58-66, 1966.

118 Walt, A. J., Woolner, L. B., and Black, B. M.: Primary malignant lymphoma of the thyroid, Cancer **10**:663-677, 1957.

119 Walt, A. J., Woolner, L. B., and Black, B. M.: Small-cell malignant lesions of the thyroid gland, J. Clin. Endocr. **17**:45-60, 1957.

120 Warren, S.: The significance of invasion of blood vessels in adenomas of the thyroid gland, Arch. Path. (Chicago) **11**:255-257, 1931.

121 Warren, S., and Feldman, J. D.: The nature of lateral "aberrant" thyroid tumors, Surg. Gynec. Obstet. **88**:31-44, 1949.

122 Warren, S., and Meissner, W. A.: Tumors of the thyroid gland. In Atlas of tumor pathology, Sect. IV, Fasc. 14, Washington, D. C., 1953, Armed Forces Institute of Pathology, p. 93.

123 Watt, C. H., and Foushee, J. C.: The incidence of carcinoma in nodular thyroids in southwest Georgia, J. Med. Ass. Georgia **40**: 414-417, 1951.

124 Weller, G. L.: Development of the thyroid, parathyroid and thymus glands in man, Contr. Embryol. **24**:95-139, 1933, Carnegie Institute of Washington.

125 Welti, H.: Malignant tumors of the thyroid; a study of 233 cases, Trans. Amer. Goiter Ass., pp. 313-322, May, 1953.

126 Wilson, G. M., Kilpatrick, R., Eckert, H., Curran, R. C., Jepson, R. P., and Blomfield, G. W.: Thyroid neoplasms following irradiation, Brit. Med. J. **2**:929-934, 1958.

127 Winship, T., and Greene, R.: Reticulum cell sarcoma of the thyroid gland, Brit. J. Cancer **9**:401-408, 1955.

128 Winship, T., and Rosvoll, R. V.: Childhood thyroid carcinoma, Cancer **14**:734-743, 1961 (extensive bibliography).

129 Woolner, L. B., Lemmon, M. L., Beahrs, O. H., Black, B. M., and Keating, F. R., Jr.: Occult papillary carcinoma of the thyroid gland; a study of 100 cases observed in a 30 year period, J. Clin. Endocr. **20**:89-105, 1960.

130 Woolner, L. B., McConahey, W. M., and Beahrs, O. H.: Invasive fibrous thyroiditis, J. Clin. Endocr. **17**:201-220, 1957.

131 Woolner, L. B., McConahey, W. M., Beahrs, O. H., and Black, B. M.: Primary malignant lymphoma of the thyroid; review of forty-six cases, Amer. J. Surg. **111**:502-523, 1966.

132 Wozencraft, P., Foote, F. W., Jr., and Frazell, E. L.: Occult carcinomas of the thyroid; their bearing on the concept of lateral aberrant thyroid carcinoma, Cancer **1**:574-583, 1948.

133 Zeckwer, I. T.: Fibrosarcoma of the thyroid, Arch. Surg. (Chicago) **12**:561-570, 1926.

Chapter 9

Tumors of the mediastinum

Anatomy

The mediastinum forms a septum between the pleural cavities. Its walls are formed laterally by the parietal pleura, anteriorly by the sternum with attached muscles, and posteriorly by thoracic vertebral bodies. Its lower limit is the diaphragm, and the upper limit is the first thoracic vertebra and the manubrium. The heart, the pericardium, and great vessels divide the mediastinum into an anterior and a posterior portion. The anterior portion contains the thymus, branches of the internal mammary arteries, lymph nodes, and fibro-areolar tissue. The posterior portion contains the bifurcation of the trachea with the esophagus and then the descending portion of the aorta behind and to the left of it. The vagus nerves run laterally. The thoracic duct is found between the azygos vein and the aorta in the lower portion of the mediastinum. Above the fifth thoracic vertebra, the duct crosses to the left and ascends to the cervical region.

Epidemiology

Primary tumors of the mediastinum are rare. The majority of these, about 75%, are benign. *Teratomas* are seldom manifested in patients under 30 years of age. *Neurogenous tumors* occur at any age and are equally divided between sexes (Ackerman and Taylor[4]). *Thymomas,* in general, occur in the young or old of both sexes. But whereas thymic carcinomas predominate in elderly individuals, thymic lymphosarcomas are found most often in young patients. A variety of other mediastinal tumors, including tumors of the heart, make up a very small proportion of the total.

Pathology

Gross and microscopic pathology

The most common tumor of the *anterior* portion of the mediastinum is the teratoma, often designated as a dermoid cyst. Teratoma, however, is the more accurate name, for multiple sections usually show the presence of tissues arising from all three layers. These tumors vary in size and are well-delineated structures. On section, they are cystic and may contain cloudy fluid and grumous material similar to that seen in teratomas of the ovary. Calcification of the wall may be present. In a review of 233 cases of teratoid tumors, all but three were found in the anterior part of the mediastinum (Blades[8]). They are usually located in front of the pericardium and great vessels. Teratomas have a well-defined wall that may be lined by squamous or columnar epithelium. They contain hair, sebaceous material, and, frequently, bone, cartilage, and teeth. Numerous other tissues, such as muscle, lipoid, nerve, pancreatic, intestinal, salivary gland, sweat gland, and mucous gland, may be present.

Most of these tumors are benign, but a few are malignant. Laipply[37] found that of 245 reported teratoid tumors, twenty-eight (11%) were malignant. These are usually epidermoid carcinomas, but malignant tumors can arise from any of the structures found within a teratoma. By pressure teratomas can erode through the pleura or into the bronchi. At times, because of communication with bronchi, infection results. The epidermoid carcinomas metastasize to regional lymph nodes, lungs, and other distant organs.

Neurogenous tumors are the neoplasms most frequently found in the *posterior* portion of the mediastinum, but they may rarely be found anteriorly situated. They vary considerably in size and may weigh as much as 1000 gm. They are usually firm and grayish white, presenting cystic areas and a tendency to encapsulation. Fatty degeneration within them is common. If they arise from nerve elements near the intervertebral foramina, they may assume a dumbbell shape. If they arise from an intercostal nerve, erosion of the inferior margin of the rib can occur. Neurogenous tumors of the mediastinum can be divided into two main groups: those arising from the nerve cells of the sympathetic system and those arising from nerve sheaths. Among thirty-six tumors of the sympathetic nervous system studied at Barnes Hospital, seventeen were neuroblastomas, sixteen were ganglioneuroblastomas, and three were ganglioneuromas (Perez et al.[59]).

Thymic tumors are the most common neoplasms found in the upper part of the anterior mediastinum. In patients with a thymic lesion, hyperplasia of the thymus or a tumor may be present. The borderline between a hyperplasia and a benign adenoma may be difficult to define. In clinical myasthenia gravis, Kreel et al.[35] found that if a thymic tumor was present it was malignant in three out of four instances. Thymic tumors are often large, encapsulated, without evidence of necrosis, and with separation by fibrous trabeculae. In the large tumors (Fig. 314), the dominant cell type is often spindle in appearance, intermingled with a variable degree of lymphoid tissue supported by connective stroma, but the dominant cell also may be lymphoid, lymphoepithelial, or vesicular in type. Locally invasive thymomas may extend through the chest wall and diaphragm (Katz[32]). Malignant thymomas may infiltrate neighboring tissues and implant on pleural surfaces, but distant metastases are practically unknown.

Other primary tumors of the mediastinum, rarely observed, include *lipomas*, which may become very large and may have an extrathoracic extension. A large benign tumor made up mainly of fat but also containing thymus can occur. *Liposarcomas* have also been reported (Cicciarelli et al.[15]). *Nonchromaffin paragangliomas* occur in the mediastinum (Pachter[54]; Mendelow and Slobodkin[49]). *Pheochromocytomas* may arise in the posterior portion of the mediastinum. Over twenty cases of *hemangiomas* have been reported (Ellis et al.[17]). They may be part of a teratoma (Schlumberger[66]). *Choriocarcinomas* apparently arising in the mediastinum have been reported (Magovern and Blades[42]). More often, they are a metastasis from an occult testicular lesion (Laipply[36]) that may be represented only by a scar on the testis. Mediastinal seminomas have

been reported (Oberman and Libcke[52]). Mediastinal carcinoids without connection to the bronchial tree can occur and behave like those arising within the lung (Rosai and Higa[64]). An account of other rare tumors of the mediastinum may be found in the works of Schlumberger[66] and Pachter and Lattes.[55, 56]

Primary tumors of the heart are rare but may be subdivided in various categories as follows (Manion*):

1 Tumors arising from or as result of faulty embryologic development
  A Teratomas and dermoid cysts
    (1) Benign
    (2) Malignant
  B Sequestrated lung (accessory lung) and bronchogenic cysts
  C Thyroid rest tumors
  D Thymic rest tumors
  E Adenomatoid tumors
  F Inclusion cysts
2 Benign pericardial and cardiac tumors
  A Pericardiac cysts and diverticuli
  B Mesotheliomas
  C Angiomas and lymphangiomas
  D Fibromas
  E Lipomas
  F Leiomyomas
  G Neuromas, neurofibromas, and ganglioneuromas
  H Granular cell myoblastomas
3 Benign heart tumors
  A Rhabdomyomas
  B Lymphangioendotheliomas
  C Myxomas
  D Valve tumors
    (1) Fibromas
    (2) Myxomas
4 Malignant tumors of the heart
  A Mesotheliomas
  B Sarcomas
    (1) Angiosarcoma
    (2) Fibrosarcoma
    (3) Rhabdomyosarcoma
    (4) Leiomyosarcoma
    (5) Liposarcoma
    (6) Neurosarcoma
    (7) Lymphosarcoma
    (8) Malignant mesenchymoma
    (9) Osteoclastoma
5 Tumors arising from major vessels
  A Benign
    (1) Fibroma
    (2) Angioma
    (3) Hemangiopericytoma
  B Malignant
    (1) Fibrosarcoma
    (2) Myxosarcoma
    (3) Chondrosarcoma
    (4) Osteogenic sarcoma

*From Manion, W. C.: Personal communication, 1969.

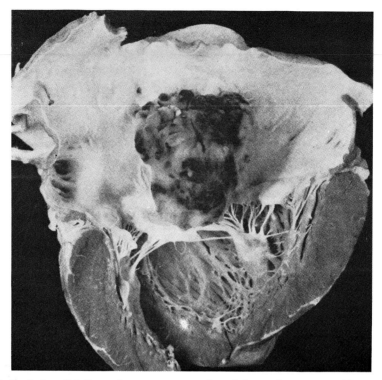

Fig. 309. Typical well-delineated myxoma arising from left auricle. Because of location, it was erroneously thought that patient had rheumatic heart disease. (From Dexter, R., and Work, J. L.: Myoxma of the heart, Arch. Path. [Chicago] 32:995-999, 1941.)

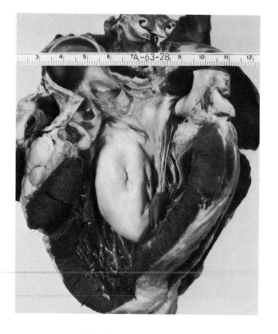

Fig. 310. Large delimited lipoma of heart that apparently arose in tricuspid valve and infiltrated papillary muscles and myocardium of septum. (From Estevez, J. M., et al.: Lipoma of the heart; review of the literature and report of two autopsied cases, Arch. Path. [Chicago] 77:638-642, 1964.)

The majority of these are benign, and the most common is the *myxoma*, which arises frequently as a polypoid mass from the left atrium (Fig. 309). *Fibrous hamartomas* may involve the atria, the ventricle, or the interventricular septum. They are often large and poorly demarcated. *Rhabdomyomas*, solitary or multiple, are congenital and are frequently associated with tuberous sclerosis of the brain (Prichard[60]; Farber[20]). A similar association has been reported in a few cases of *lipoma* (Fig. 310). *Malignant cardiac tumors* are in the minority but may be of practically every type of sarcoma (Whorton[79]). *Metastatic tumors* of the heart are about thirty times as common as primary neoplasms (Sterns et al.[73]). *Mesotheliomas of the pericardium* are usually malignant (Thomas and Phython[76]), but benign proliferation of the mesothelium may be mistaken for a true neoplasm. Tumors may also arise from any of the major vessels (Manion[46]; Ali and Lee[5]).

Metastatic spread

Malignant teratomas metastasize to mediastinal lymph nodes and to the lungs. Distant metastases are sometimes observed. Malignant neurogenous tumors may metastasize to the lungs, liver, and other organs after they infiltrate directly neighboring organs. Distant metastases from malignant thymomas are practically never observed. Pleural surface nodules are actual implants from contiguous development of the tumor (Rachmaninoff and Fentress[61]).

Clinical evolution

In their development, mediastinal tumors produce symptoms that are due to pressure and that depend on their location. In the anterior portion of the mediastinum, the most common symptoms produced are retrosternal pain, dyspnea, and respiratory complications. In the posterior portion, the symptoms vary greatly, depending on the level at which pressure develops. There may be compression of the trachea or bronchi with resulting cough and dyspnea, compression of the brachial plexus or intercostal nerves with resulting pain, or compression of the phrenic or recurrent nerves with consequent paralysis of the diaphragm or of the larynx. Compression of the esophagus results in dysphagia, compression of the sympathetic nerve produces a Horner's syndrome, and compression of the superior vena cava produces the typical clinical syndrome of superior vena caval obstruction. Compression of the azygos vein or the inferior vena cava may result in hydrothorax or ascites, respectively.

Teratomatous tumors may rupture into the pleura, lung, or bronchus, and secondary infection and fever follow. Expectoration of blood, grumous material, or hair may be observed in these cases. Pain is often a prominent sign. Weight loss may occur in terminal stages.

Neurogenous tumors may develop without symptoms or may be accompanied by pain along nerve roots or intercostal nerves. Occasionally, there is bone pain in a rib or vertebra. In the malignant forms, pain is particularly severe. Symptoms of posterior mediastinal compression develop as the tumor becomes sufficiently large. Horner's syndrome or paralysis of the diaphragm is not necessarily a sign of malignant transformation in neurogenous tumors. Malignant schwannomas may be associated with clinical manifestations of Recklinghausen's disease.

Thymic tumors show variable rate of growth and produce symptoms of anterior mediastinal compression. If the dominant cell type is lymphoid, the patients may present myasthenia gravis (Lattes[38]). Myasthenia gravis also may develop before or even after removal of a vesicular type of thymoma (Castleman[13]). Suppression of erythrogenesis with occasional agammaglobulinemia and splenomegaly has been observed (Bayrd and Bernatz[7]). Thymic lymphosarcomas occur usually in children, develop rapidly, and produce respiratory embarrassment and superior vena cava obstruction.

Choriocarcinomas may manifest themselves by gynecomastia and overpigmentation of the nipples. *Chemodectomas* are slow and indolent in behavior (Mendelow and Slobodkin[49]). *Pheochromocytomas* may be associated with intermittent, or sustained, hypertension (Pampari and Lacrenza[57]). Most other rare tumors of the mediastinum, benign or malignant, produce only symptoms of compression or are discovered in routine roentgenograms.

Benign tumors of the heart may develop without production of clinical symptoms (Estevez et al.[18]). Atrial myxomas may cause pulmonary hypertension and low cardiac output (Goodwin et al.[26]). Sudden death may occur as a result of occlusion of cardiac orifices by a pedunculated tumor (Yater[81]). *Malignant tumors of the heart* can also cause congestive heart failure. Symptoms of angina pectoris may result from invasion of the coronary arteries, abnormalities of rhythm from involvement of the conduction system (Fishberg[22]), and pericardial effusion from extension to the pericardium (Whorton[79]).

Diagnosis

Frequently, the diagnosis of a mediastinal tumor is made by routine roentgenographic examination before the development of symptoms. But, whether in the presence or absence of symptoms, and except for the probability suggested by location, rate of growth, etc., the exact diagnosis must await biopsy. Benign tumors of the mediastinum occur about four times as frequently as malignant tumors. When the symptoms of a mediastinal tumor have been present for more than one year, the likelihood is that the tumor is benign. Fever, pain, and superior vena caval obstruction are more often observed in patients with malignant tumor.

Teratomatous tumors may cause cough and expectoration of sebaceous oily material or hair. Cholesterol crystals found in the pleural fluid should arouse suspicion of a ruptured teratomatous cyst.

Neurogenous tumors seldom produce characteristic signs except for their location in the posterior portion of the mediastinum and nerve compression. Association with Recklinghausen's disease may be an eloquent sign. A bloody pleural effusion is not necessarily an indication of malignancy in a neurogenous tumor (Parish[58]).

Thymic tumors may be accompanied by myasthenia gravis, particularly when the tumor is encapsulated. However, cases have been reported of apparent benign thymoma with infiltration of adjacent structures that were accompanied by myasthenia gravis (Katz[32]). Nonencapsulated thymic tumors seem to follow a more malignant course (O'Gara et al.[53]). The overall occurrence of the association with myasthenia gravis is of the order of 25% (Legg and Brady[39]). Anemia is present in a good number of patients with thymic tumors, and in some it may be accompanied by leukopenia and thrombocytopenia and agammaglobulinemia (Hirst et al.[30]). An associated immunopathy, with depressed synthesis of gamma globulins, may be rarely observed (Korn et al.[33]). Thymoma may be associated with lupus erythematosus (Singh[70]).

Choriocarcinomas, besides gynecomastia and pigmentation of nipples, may cause a positive Friedman's test and evidence of increased gonadotropin production. Pheochromocytomas may be associated with paroxysmal or sustained hypertension. Signs of tricuspid valvular lesion with right auricular enlargement or pulmonary stenosis should suggest a tumor of the heart because tricuspid stenosis is rare and pulmonary stenosis usually congenital (Yater[81]). Relentless cardiac failure in young patients, in the absence of the usual etiologic factors, should raise the suspicion that the symptoms are due to a myxoma of the heart. Atrial myxomas often occur in females and may be thought to be rheumatic heart disease. Sudden attacks of extreme dyspnea and cyanosis may occur because of changes in position. Myxomas may produce multiple emboli. Histopathologic examination of these may lead to the diagnosis (Newman et al.[51]).

Roentgenologic examination

Roentgenologic examination of the chest, which often is responsible for the discovery of these tumors, is the most important investigative procedure toward the establishment of a presumptive diagnosis. Of 155 mediastinal tumors and cysts reported by Ringertz and Lidholm,[62] ninety-five (61%) were found by routine mass radiography studies. Adequate utilization of this means of exploration implies radioscopic examination which permits observation of mobility of the tumor during respiration and transmission of cardiovascular pulsations. Paralysis of the diaphragm could pass unnoticed on a roentgenogram, but it is easily noticed in radioscopy. Observation of the passage of barium through the esophagus yields useful information as to its infiltration or change of position due to tumor expansion. Lateral, oblique, and special roentgenographic views may be necessary in addition to conventional ones. Kymography may be helpful in revealing the inherent or transmitted character of pulsations. Planigraphy (tomography) may help establish the relationship of the tumor to adjacent organs (Markovits and Desprez-Curley[47]). Angiocardiography may also be used to advantage in the differential diagnosis.

Teratomas are invariably located in the anterior portion of the mediastinum and are clearly delineated on lateral films (Fig.

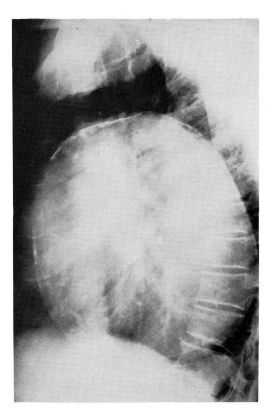

Fig. 311. Huge mediastinal teratoma that had been present for many years in 60-year-old man. Tumor was well delineated with partially calcified wall.

311). They may contain teeth or irregular calcifications. Neurogenous tumors may project their shadow at the costovertebral angle or may produce an enlargement of the intercostal space when they arise from intercostal nerves. Ragged destruction of a rib and lobulation or irregularity of outline (Gregg[28]) usually indicate a malignant neurogenous tumor. They generally occur in the posterior mediastinum (Fig. 312).

Thymic tumors are usually situated in the upper part of the mediastinum but can be seen in a lower situation (Figs. 313 and 314). They rarely present peripheral calcification. They are best seen in a frontal projection and are difficult to discern in lateral views. Lymphosarcomas form voluminous polylobated masses in the superior and anterior mediastinum and may be accompanied by retrosternal infiltration (Fleischner et al.[23]). Lipomas are peculiarly more translucent than other tumors of the mediastinum. Rare malignant tumors of the mediastinum may betray their nature by signs of direct extension, ragged bone destruction, or metastases to the lungs. In benign tumors of the heart, the left auricle may appear enlarged, whereas in the malignant ones the right auricle is usually enlarged, and there may be pericardial effu-

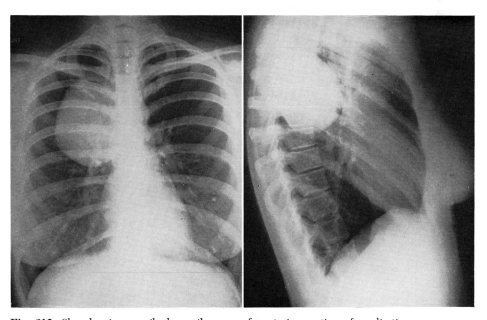

Fig. 312. Sharply circumscribed neurilemoma of posterior portion of mediastinum.

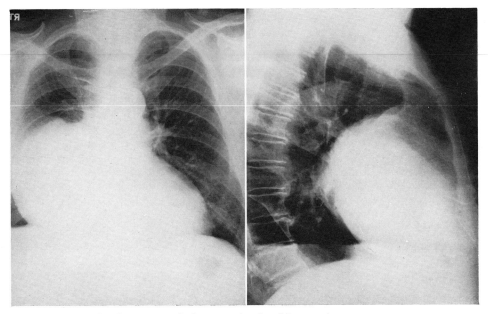

Fig. 313. Large, sharply circumscribed, anteriorly placed benign thymoma.

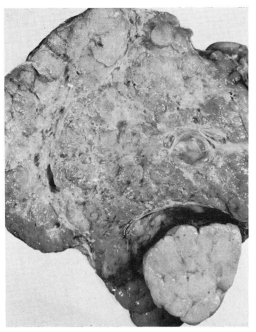

Fig. 314. Cross section of firm, yellowish white, encapsulated thymoma shown in Fig. 313.

sion. In the diagnosis of tumors of the heart, angiocardiography has become a powerful tool (Goodwin et al.[26]; Schlienger et al.[65a]). In many instances, a lobulated filling defect lying against the wall of the atrium has been observed. Steinberg et al.[72] reported three such cases showing an attachment to the interatrial wall.

Endoscopy

Bronchoscopy may be indicated as an additional investigative procedure. It may exclude the possibility of a bronchial tumor and, in addition, may contribute valuable information concerning the mobility or compression of the trachea and bronchi, signs of inflammation, etc. Bronchoscopy is not helpful in posteriorly situated tumors, but esophagoscopy is indicated. An esophagoscopy may eliminate the possibility of a hidden primary lesion or may contribute information as to the displacement or secondary infiltration of the esophagus.

Biopsy

In most cases of mediastinal tumor, a thoracotomy becomes necessary for the establishment of a histopathologic diagnosis. When a surgical extirpation is not indicated, or possible, biopsy should be done. A needle biopsy is seldom advisable except after surgical exposure.

Differential diagnosis

Mediastinal tumors must be differentiated from a variety of other conditions. *Plunging goiters* are often toxic and adenomatous, may occupy the upper portion of the anterior mediastinum, and are accompanied by dyspnea, cough, and dysphagia. The thyroid mass is usually felt above the sternal notch, and it can be seen in radioscopy moving with the trachea on deglutition. Mediastinal goiters may be found in the posterior portion of the mediastinum, where they may be confused with neurogenous tumors (Sweet[74]). Six of Lindskog and Kausel's cases[40] were retrotracheal or retroesophageal. Calcifications observed radiographically are nonspecific. They may occur in substernal thyroid tissue but also in bronchogenic cysts, neurofibromas, etc. (Arbuckle[6]). In these cases, scanning with the help of radioactive iodine is of considerable help in the differential diagnosis.

Mediastinal *parathyroid adenomas* may occur in the anterior or posterior portion of the mediastinum. As many as 18% of all such tumors are found there but are rarely large enough to be seen roentgenographically. An unexplained high serum calcium level and low serum phosphorus level may accompany such a tumor.

Aortic aneurysms may be difficult to differentiate. Detailed history, blood serology, careful radioscopic observation, kymography (Scott and Moore[68]; Fabricius[19]), and lateral and oblique roentgenographic studies will all contribute to the diagnosis of aneurysms. In a few instances, however, the diagnosis is difficult due to a laminated clot within the aneurysm that prevents pulsation. Dissecting aneurysms may cause progressively intense pain that suggests the presence of a malignant tumor because of the absence of cardiac signs. Kinking of the aortic arch is a rare condition that may simulate a mediastinal tumor.

Mediastinal granulomas are usually due to replacement of a lymph node by a granulomatous process. The identification of a specific cause may be impossible (Kunkel et al.[36]). In some areas, a common cause may be histoplasmosis (Ferguson and Burford[21]). A *mediastinal abscess* is rare and usually accompanied by a history of trauma or signs of acute infection. A radiographic fluid level in the mediastinum is usually diagnostic (Brewer and Dolley[10]). *Hydatid cysts,* of frequent occurrence in South America, may present the appearance of a mediastinal tumor. The precipi-

tin and skin tests are a great help in the differential diagnosis. *Spinal tuberculosis* with formation of abscess may give the impression of a tumor on routine roentgenograms, but lateral views will show the characteristic changes in the vertebrae.

Large *hyperplastic lymph nodes* found in the mediastinum (Castleman[13]; Veneziale et al.[78]), sometimes designated as *lymphoid hamartomas* (Abell[2]), may be erroneously diagnosed as thymomas. They are usually found in the paratracheal region, and their rupture may cause abscesses, fistulas, and mediastinal fibrosis. Practically all *highly undifferentiated tumors* of the mediastinum are *not* thymic tumors. They may represent mediastinal involvement by carcinoma of the bronchus or of the esophagus (Heuer and Andrus[29]). *Metastatic tumors* of the mediastinum occur more frequently than primary tumors. The granulomatous type of thymoma described by Lowenhaupt and Brown[41] is, in reality, not a thymoma but *Hodgkin's disease* of the nodular sclerosing type (Burke et al.[11]).

Bronchial cysts arise in children or young adults as a result of a developmental aberration of the primitive foregut. The term bronchial (or bronchogenic) is applied to cysts arising from the respiratory system most commonly located in the anterior portion of the mediastinum near the tracheal bifurcation, but these cysts are analogous to those arising in the lower mediastinum usually designated as gastroenterogenous. Although a majority of these cysts are found accidentally, they may grow to promote cough, dyspnea, wheezing, and pain. Maier[44] divides them into paratracheal, carinal, hilar, paraesophageal, and miscellaneous groups. The roentgenograms may not show some of these cysts, but in other instances they may suggest the diagnosis. In radioscopy, the lesions can be seen moving with the trachea upon deglutition. In the lateral roentgenogram, their situation in front of the spine distinguishes them from the more posteriorly situated neuromas and, unlike teratomas, they do not present a very definite outline.

Gastroenterogenous cysts (esophageal, gastric) are more often found in the posterior mediastinum of children, usually to the right of the midline. *Pericardial cysts* (celomic, mesothelial) develop in the cardiophrenic angle adjacent to the pericardium, and they are filled with clear fluid (spring water cysts). They are usually asymptomatic and may be confused with teratomas, angiomas, and lipomas developing in the same region. They have been found predominantly in middle-aged patients. Pericardial cysts are seldom diagnosed roentgenologically. They appear as well-circumscribed, homogeneous, not very dense shadows. In nineteen of our cases, only five were radiographically diagnosed before intervention. At operation, they are found to be unrelated to the pericardium (Drash and Hyer[16]).

Abell[1] described thirty-six developmental cysts of the mediastinum. Tracheobronchial cysts were the most common (seventeen cases), and pericardial cysts were second in frequency (eight cases). *Lymphangiomas* (cystic hygromas) are most often found in young children and are usually cervicomediastinal, but they can be entirely in the mediastinum (Skinner and Hobbs[71]). *Intrathoracic meningoceles* are rare and are usually associated with congenital anomalies. They present as uniformly radiopaque well-defined masses in the posterior portion of the mediastinum that can be taken for neurogenous tumors. Intraspinal injection of an opaque medium may help to establish the differential diagnosis (Byron et al.[12]).

Because of the rarity of primary tumors of the heart, either benign or malignant, other more common conditions such as *heart failure* and mediastinal tumor are thought responsible for their symptoms. A diagnosis of a *valvular lesion* may be made because of the murmurs present (mitral stenosis, tricuspid stenosis, aortic insufficiency). If auricular fibrillation or flutter or heart block is present, it is often thought to be due to the common types of heart disease. In some instances, angina pectoris may be present. *Metastases to the heart* are by far more common than primary tumors of this organ, but metastatic lesions are seldom diagnosed during life. Metastatic lesions occur most frequently in the region of the right auricle. Malignant melanomas are among the most frequent offenders (Moragues[50]).

The tumors that arise from the chest wall, such as *chondromas* and *chondrosarcomas* (costal cartilage origin), may project into the anterior or posterior portion of the mediastinum. *Large solitary mesotheliomas of the pleura* may be confused with a neurogenous tumor. Even tumors of the spinal cord may extend into the mediastinum.

Treatment

It is often impossible to establish the benign or malignant nature of a mediastinal lesion without resort to a thoracotomy. When all investigative procedures have been exhausted, an intervention should be decided upon. Except in a few instances of secondary infection, heart disease, etc., this course is justified, for procrastination increases the risk of complications while reducing the chance of cure. The operative risk is outweighed by that of postponement. A so-called radiotherapeutic trial, for the purposes of testing the radiosensitivity of the tumor before ascertaining its nature, is not justifiable. For even when radiotherapy would be the treatment of choice, adequate irradiation requires advance knowledge of the histopathologic nature of the tumor.

Surgery

In the majority of instances of mediastinal tumors, surgery is the treatment of choice, and the exploratory thoracotomy is extended to surgical extirpation. The usual surgical approach of these tumors is posterolateral. In the hands of competent surgeons, the operative risk is minimal. Blades reported on 109 mediastinal tumors (ninety-four benign and fifteen malignant) removed by various surgeons without a single death. A series of twenty-two consecutive interventions for neurogenous tumors resulted in no operative mortality (Godwin et al.[24]). Thanks to the advances of vascular surgery, it is possible to remove benign tumors of the heart successfully (Robertson[63]). Unfortunately, few cases are diagnosed in time for a successful intervention. Extracorporeal circulation has been utilized for the removal of intrapericardial teratomas. This has been done successfully in a large number of cases (Manion[46]), even when removal of a segment of the involved heart muscle is necessary.

Radiotherapy

In various tumors of the mediastinum the patient may best be treated by irradiation either for palliation or cure. In such instances, there is no advantage in the surgical effort to remove "most" of the tumor. The surgical intervention should be confined to the removal of a specimen for biopsy and to ascertain, when possible, the extent of the tumor. In addition, radiotherapy may be well indicated in the treatment of extensive tumors for which the surgical attempt has proved fruitless. This may be the case of *thymic tumors* and *malignant teratomas*. Benign *neurogenous tumors* are seldom responsive to irradiation. Radiosensitivity and radiocurability, however, are not always predictable. Mediastinal *neuroblastomas* and *ganglioneuroblastomas* may be cured by radiotherapy (Perez et al.[59]). Bagshaw et al.[6a] reported three patients surviving six to seven years in a series of six cases of mediastinal seminoma treated by radiotherapy.

Prognosis

Patients with *benign teratomas* have an excellent prognosis when surgically treated. Even without treatment, patients may live for years without discomfort. The outlook of patients with neurogenous tumors that are surgically removed is, in general, good. Neuroblastomas are known to mature into a ganglioneuroma. Both tumors have been cured by radiotherapy alone (Perez et al.[59]) or in combination with surgery (Pachter and Lattes[56]).

Thymic tumors are curable by surgical excision (Sellors et al.[69]). Legg and Brady[39] reported a 61% five-year survival in a series of fifty-one patients with thymic tumors. The ten-year survival rate for patients with thymic tumors without myasthenia gravis was 67%, whereas that for patients with myasthenia gravis was only 32% (Wilkins et al.[80]).

In the presence of erythroblastopenic anemia, surgical removal often fails (Hirst and Robertson[30]). *Seminoma-like tumors* have an excellent prognosis. Kountz et al.[34] collected nine cases in which the patients received radiotherapy, with eight survivals. *Benign tumors of the heart* may be successfully resected (Maurer[48]; Goodwin et al.[26]).

REFERENCES

1 Abell, M. R.: Mediastinal cysts, Arch. Path. (Chicago) **61**:360-379, 1956.

2 Abell, M. R.: Lymphoid hamartoma, Radiol. Clin. N. Amer. **6**:15-24, 1968.

3 Abbott, O. A., Warshawski, F. E., and Cobbs, B. W., Jr.: Primary tumors and pseudotumors of the heart, Ann. Surg. **155**:855-872, 1962.

4 Ackerman, L. V., and Taylor, F. H.: Neurogenous tumors within the thorax; a clinicopathological evaluation of forty-eight cases, Cancer **4**:669-691, 1951 (extensive bibliography).

5 Ali, M. Y., and Lee, G. S.: Sarcoma of the pulmonary artery, Cancer **17**:1220-1224, 1964.

6 Arbuckle, R. K.: Solitary tumors of the chest; the differential diagnosis in fifty proved cases, Amer. J. Roentgen. **62**:52-64, 1949.

6a Bagshaw, M. A., McLaughlin, W. T., and Earle, J. D.: Definitive radiotherapy of primary mediastinal seminoma, Amer. J. Roentgen. **105**:86-94, 1969.

7 Bayrd, E. D., and Bernatz, P. E.: Benign thymoma and agenesis of erythrocytes, J.A.M.A. **163**:723-727, 1957.

8 Blades, B.: Relative frequency and site of predilection of intrathoracic tumors, Amer. J. Surg. **54**:139-148, 1941.

9 Blades, B.: Mediastinal tumors, Ann. Surg. **123**:749-765, 1946.

10 Brewer, L. A., III, and Dolley, F. S.: Tumors of the mediastinum; a discussion of diagnostic procedure and surgical treatment based on experience with forty-four operated cases, Amer. Rev. Tuberc. **60**:419-438, 1949.

11 Burke, W. A., Burford, T. H., and Dorfman, R. F.: Hodgkin's disease of the mediastinum, Ann. Thorac. Surg. **3**:287-296, 1967.

12 Byron, F. X., Alling, E. E. and Samson, P. C.: Intrathoracic meningocele, J. Thorac. Surg. **18**:294-303, 1949.

13 Castleman, B.: Tumors of the thymus gland. In Atlas of tumor pathology, Sect. V, Fasc. 19, Washington, D. C., 1953, Armed Forces Institute of Pathology.

14 Castleman, B., and Norris, E. H.: The pathology of the thymus in myasthenia gravis, Medicine (Balt.) **28**:27-58, 1949.

15 Cicciarelli, F. E., Soule, E. H., and McGoon, D. C.: Lipoma and liposarcoma of the mediastinum; a report of 14 tumors including one lipoma of the thymus, J. Thorac. Cardiovasc. Surg. **47**:411-429, 1964.

16 Drash, E. C., and Hyer, H. J.: Mesothelial mediastinal cysts, J. Thorac. Surg. **19**:755-768, 1950.

17 Ellis, F. H., Jr., Kirklin, J. W., and Woolner, L. B.: Hemangioma of the mediastinum; review of the literature and report of case, J. Thorac. Surg. **30**:181-186, 1955.

18 Estevez, J. M., Thompson, D. S., and Levinson, J. P.: Lipoma of the heart; review of the literature and report of two autopsied cases, Arch. Path. (Chicago) **77**:638-642, 1964.

19 Fabricius, B.: The value of kymography for the differential diagnosis between aneurysm of

the aorta and mediastinal tumor, Acta Radiol. (Stockholm) **26**:89-98, 1945.

20 Farber, Sidney: Congenital rhabdomyoma of the heart, Amer. J. Path. **7**:105-130, 1931.

21 Ferguson, T. B., and Burford, T. H.: Mediastinal granuloma; a 15-year experience, Ann. Thorac. Surg. **1**:125-141, 1965.

22 Fishberg, A. M.: Auricular fibrillation and flutter in metastatic growths of the right auricle, Amer. J. Med. Sci. **180**:629-634, 1930.

23 Fleischner, F. G., Bernstein, C., and Levine, B. E.: Retrosternal infiltration in malignant lymphoma, Radiology **51**:350-358, 1930.

24 Godwin, J. T., Watson, W. L., Pool, J. L., Cahan, W. G., and Nardiello, V. A., Jr.: Primary intrathoracic neurogenic tumors, J. Thorac. Surg. **20**:169-194, 1950.

25 Goodwin, J. F.: Diagnosis of left atrial myxoma, Lancet **7279**:464-467, 1963.

26 Goodwin, J. F., Stanfield, C. A., Steiner, R. E., Bentall, H. H., Sayed, H. M., Bloom, V. R., and Bishop, M. B.: Clinical features of left atrial myxoma, Thorax **17**:91-110, 1962.

27 Greenberg, M., and Angrist, A.: Primary vascular tumors of the pericardium, Amer. Heart J. **35**:623-634, 1948.

28 Gregg, D. McC.: Some radiological aspects of primary intrathoracic neurogenic tumors; based on a review of 19 cases, J. Fac. Radiol. **8**:385-393, 1957.

29 Heuer, George J., and Andrus, William DeWitt: The surgery of mediastinal tumors, Amer. J. Surg. **50**:146-224, 1940.

30 Hirst, E., and Robertson, T. I.: The syndrome of thymoma and erythroblastopenic anemia; a review of 56 cases including 3 case reports, Medicine (Balt.) **46**:225-264, 1967.

31 Iverson, L.: Thymoma; a review and reclassification, Amer. J. Path. **32**:695-719, 1956.

32 Katz, J. H.: Malignant thymoma in myasthenia gravis, New Eng. J. Med. **248**:1059-1064, 1953.

33 Korn, D., Gelderman, A., Cage, G., Nathanson, D., and Strauss, A. J. L.: Immune deficiencies, aplastic anemia and abnormalities of lymphoid tissue in thymoma, New Eng. J. Med. **276**:1333-1339, 1967.

34 Kountz, S. L., Connolly, J. E., and Cohn, R.: Seminoma-like (or seminomatous) tumors of the anterior mediastinum, J. Thorac. Cardiovasc. Surg. **45**:289-301, 1963.

35 Kreel, I., Osserman, K. E., Genkins, G., and Kark, A. E.: Role of thymectomy in the management of myasthenia gravis, Ann. Surg. **165**:111-117, 1967.

36 Kunkel, W. M., Clagett, O. T., and McDonald, J. R.: Mediastinal granulomas, J. Thorac. Surg. **27**:565-574, 1954.

37 Laipply, T. C.: Cysts and cystic tumors of the mediastinum, Arch. Path. (Chicago) **39**:153-161, 1945.

38 Lattes, R.: Thymoma and other tumors of the thymus; an analysis of 107 cases, Cancer **15**:1224-1260, 1962.

39 Legg, M. A., and Brady, W. J.: Pathology and clinical behavior of thymomas; a survey of 51 cases, Cancer **18**:1131-1144, 1965.

40 Lindskog, G. E., and Kausel, H. W.: Diagnostic and therapeutic problems in benign mediastinal tumors, New Eng. J. Med. **244**:250-252, 1961.

41 Lowenhaupt, E., and Brown, R.: Carcinoma of the thymus of granulomatous type, a clinical and pathological study, Cancer **4**:1193-1209, 1951.

42 Magovern, G. J., and Blades, B.: Primary extragenital chorioepithelioma in the male mediastinum, J. Thorac. Surg. **35**:378-383, 1958.

43 Mahaim, I.: Les tumours et les polypes du coeur, étude anatomoclinique, Paris, 1945, Masson et Cie (extensive bibliography).

44 Maier, H. C.: Bronchogenic cysts of the mediastinum, Ann. Surg. **127**:476-502, 1948.

45 Maier, H. C.: Intrathoracic pheochromocytoma with hypertension, Ann. Surg. **130**:1059-1065, 1949.

46 Manion, W. C.: Personal communication, 1969.

47 Markovits, P., and Desprez-Curley, J. P.: Inclined frontal tomography in the examination of the mediastinum, Radiology **78**:371-380, 1962.

48 Maurer, E. R.: Successful removal of tumor of the heart, J. Thorac. Surg. **23**:479-485, 1952.

49 Mendelow, H., and Slobodkin, M.: Aortic-body tumor (chemodectoma) of the mediastinum, Cancer **10**:1008-1014, 1957.

50 Moragues, V.: Cardiac metastases from malignant melanoma, Amer. Heart J. **18**:579-588, 1939.

51 Newman, H. A., Cordell, A. R., and Prichard, R. W.: Intracardiac myxomas; literature review and report of six cases, one successfully treated, Amer. Surg. **32**:219-230, 1966.

52 Oberman, H. A., and Libcke, J. H.: Malignant germinal neoplasms of the mediastinum, Cancer **17**:498-507, 1964.

53 O'Gara, R. W., Horn, R. C., and Enterline, H. T.: Tumors of the anterior mediastinum, Cancer **11**:562-590, 1958.

54 Pachter, M. R.: Mediastinal non-chromaffin paraganglioma; a clinicopathologic study based on eight cases, J. Thorac. Cardiovasc. Surg. **45**:152-160, 1963.

55 Pachter, M. R., and Lattes, R.: Uncommon mediastinal tumors; report of two parathyroid adenomas, one nonfunctional parathyroid carcinoma and one "bronchial-type-adenoma," Dis. Chest **43**:519-529, 1963.

56 Pachter, M. R., and Lattes, R.: Neurogenous tumors of the mediastinum; a clinicopathologic study based on 50 cases, Dis. Chest **44**:79-87, 1963.

57 Pampari, D., and Lacrenza, C.: Intrathoracic pheochromocytoma, J. Thorac. Surg. **36**:174-181, 1958.

58 Parish, C.: The clinical features of intrathoracic neurogenic tumor, J. Fac. Radiol. **8**:381-384, 1957.

59 Perez, C. A., Vietti, T., Ackerman, L. V., Eagleton, M. D., and Powers, W. E.: Tumors of the sympathetic nervous system in children, Radiology **88**:750-760, 1967.

60 Prichard, R. W.: Tumors of the heart; review of the subject and report of one hundred and fifty cases, Arch. Path. (Chicago) **51**:98-128, 1951.

61 Rachmaninoff, N., and Fentress, V.: Thymoma with metastasis to the brain, Amer. J. Clin. Path. **41**:618-625, 1964.

62 Ringertz, N., and Lidholm, S. O.: Mediastinal tumors and cysts, J. Thorac. Surg. **31**:458-487, 1956.

63 Robertson, R.: Primary cardiac tumors—surgical treatment, Amer. J. Surg. **94**:183-193, 1957.

64 Rosai, J., and Higa, E.: Primary mediastinal carcinoid tumor; clinicopathologic study of seven cases, Lab. Invest. **22**:507, 1970.

65 Santy, P., Berard, M., Galy, P., and Minette, A.: Les tumeurs nerveuses du mediastin; reflexions sur une statique de 48 observations, Acta Chir. Belg. **46**(suppls. 1-3):674-715, 1954.

65a Schlienger, R., Gravier, J., and Dolloz, C.: Angiocardiographie des myxomes intracardiaques, J. Radiol. Electr. **50**:663-668, 1969.

66 Schlumberger, H. E.: Tumors of the mediastinum. In Atlas of tumor pathology, Sect. V, Fasc. 18, Washington, D. C., 1951, Armed Forces Institute of Pathology.

67 Schweisguth, O., Renault, M. P., and Binet, J. P.: Intrathoracic neurogenic tumors in infants and children, Ann. Surg. **150**:29-41, 1959.

68 Scott, W. G., and Moore, S.: Roentgen kymographic studies of aneurysms and mediastinal tumors, Amer. J. Roentgen. **40**:165-172, 1938.

69 Sellors, T. H., Thackray, A. C., and Thomson, A. D.: Tumours of the thymus; a review of 88 operation cases, Thorax **22**:193-220, 1967.

70 Singh, B. N.: Thymoma presenting with polyserositis and the lupus erythematosus syndrome; case report, Aust. Ann. Med. **18**:55-58, 1969.

71 Skinner, G. F., and Hobbs, M. E.: Intrathoracic cystic lymphangioma, J. Thorac. Surg. **6**:98-107, 1936.

72 Steinberg, I., Dotter, C. T., and Glenn, G.: Myxoma of the heart; roentgen diagnosis during life in three cases, Dis. Chest **24**:509-520, 1953.

73 Sterns, L. P., Eliot, R. S., Varco, R. L., and Edwards, J. E.: Intracavitary cardiac neoplasms; a review of fifteen cases, Brit. Heart J. **28**:75-83, 1966.

74 Sweet, R. H.: Intrathoracic goiter located in the posterior mediastinum, Surg. Gynec. Obstet. **89**:57-66, 1949.

75 Thomas, G. I., Edmark, K. W., Jones, T. W., and Eyer, K. M.: Myxoma of the left ventricle, J. Thorac. Cardiovasc. Surg. **46**:220-226, 1963.

76 Thomas, J., and Phythyon, J. M.: Primary mesothelioma of the pericardium, Circulation **15**:385-390, 1957.

77 Toch, H., Hagstrom, J. W. C., and Steinberg, I.: Hemangioma of the mediastinum; report of a case with compression of the spinal cord, Amer. J. Roentgen. **94**:580-583, 1965.

78 Veneziale, C. M., Sheridan, L. A., Payne, W. S., and Harrison, E. G., Jr.: Angiofollicular lymph-node hyperplasia of the mediastinum, J. Thorac. Cardiovasc. Surg. **47**:111-121, 1964.

79 Whorton, C. M.: Primary malignant tumors of the heart, Cancer **2**:245-260, 1949.

80 Wilkins, E. W., Jr., Edmunds, L. H., and Castleman, B.: Cases of thymoma at the Massachusetts General Hospital, J. Thorac. Cardiovasc. Surg. **52**:322-330, 1966.

81 Yater, W. M.: Tumors of the heart and pericardium, Arch. Intern. Med. (Chicago) **48**:627-666, 1931.

Chapter 10

Cancer of the digestive tract

Esophagus

Stomach

Small bowel

Appendix

Large bowel

Anus

Accessory

organs

Esophagus

Anatomy

The esophagus is a muscular tube, 25 cm in length, extending from the lower border of the cricoid cartilage to the stomach. The upper limit corresponds to the level of the sixth cervical vertebra, and the lower limit is at the level of the tenth or eleventh thoracic vertebra posteriorly or the junction of the seventh rib cartilage with the sternum anteriorly. The esophagus has three normal constrictions: the narrowest and most rigid, about 1.5 cm, at the level of the cricoid; the longest, 4 to 6 cm, at the level of the crossing of the aorta and of the left main stem bronchus; the diaphragmatic constriction, about 1 to 2 cm in height.

The anterior surface of the cervical esophagus is in contact with the trachea. In the thorax, it is placed deep in the posterior portion of the mediastinum, separated from the spine by the muscles. Laterally, it is in relation on the right side with the azygos vein and the pleura and on the left side with the recurrent nerve, the common carotid artery, the subclavian artery, the thoracic duct, and the aortic arch. After the crossing of the bronchus at the level of the fourth or fifth dorsal vertebra, the esophagus progressively becomes separated from the spine by the descending aorta and also by the thoracic duct and the azygos vein. The vagus nerves take a lateral position to the esophagus. Anteriorly, this lower thoracic portion of the esophagus is in relation with the pleura and the left lung (Fig. 315).

Lymphatics. The two main lymphatic networks of the mucosa and submucosa and of the muscular layers of the esophagus gather on the external surface in three groups of lymphatic trunks:

1 The *upper trunks*, which end in the cervical lymph nodes along the internal jugular vein and in the supraclavicular lymph nodes

2 The *middle trunks*, which end in the posteromediastinal lymph nodes and in the retrotracheal lymph nodes

3 The *lower trunks*, which go to the lymph nodes of the cardia and to those of the lesser curvature of the stomach (Fig. 316)

There is a rich intercommunication between the mucosal, submucosal, and muscular lymphatic networks. These networks may extend directly from the mucosa or the submucosa or from the muscularis to the closest node, or the collecting vessels in the submucosa may ascend or descend in the muscularis and then traverse it to empty into nodes. The collecting vessels in the muscularis parallel this. In other words, the lymphatic vessels from any one segment of the esophagus may drain directly into the closest node or empty into nodes at considerable distance either above or below the lesion.

Epidemiology

The incidence of carcinoma of the esophagus exhibits wide variations from one country to another. The 1947 survey in the United States revealed an age-adjusted rate of 8.3 and 1.9 per 100,000 population for male and female whites and

9.7 and 2.2 for male and female nonwhites. A slight decrease seems to have taken place in later years as evidenced by the comparison of age-adjusted rates in Connecticut state surveys of 1945-1949 and 1960-1962 (7.6 and 6.7 for males) and the New York state surveys of 1949-1951 and 1958-1960 (5.05 and 4.66 for males). In contrast, Marcial et al.[42] have reported a remarkably high crude incidence of car-

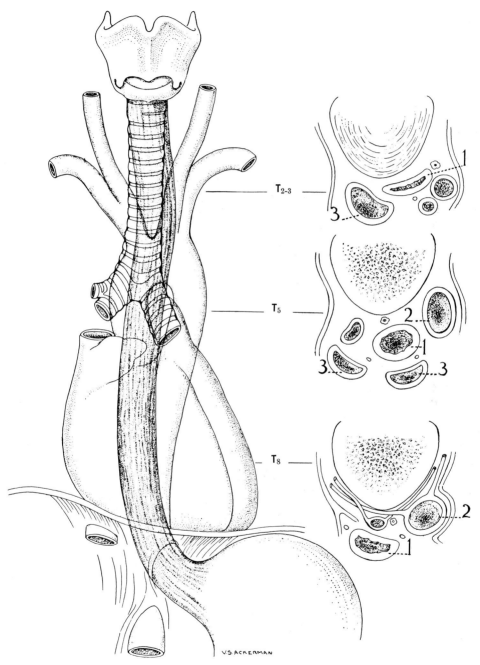

Fig. 315. Relationship of esophagus, **1,** to aorta, **2,** and to tracheobronchial tree, **3.** Three cross sections give levels of spine, demonstrating intimate relationship of esophagus to other structures. (After Testut, L.: Traité d'anatomie humaine, ed. 8, vol. 4, Paris, 1931, Gaston Doin.)

cinoma of the esophagus in Puerto Rico (13.7 for males and 5.6 for females per 100,000). When corrected for age differences in the populations, this is an incidence rate three to four times as high as that in Continental United States. Over 90% of all cases are found among patients over 50 years of age, with a peak incidence between 60 and 69 years of age. The male/female ratio for the United States

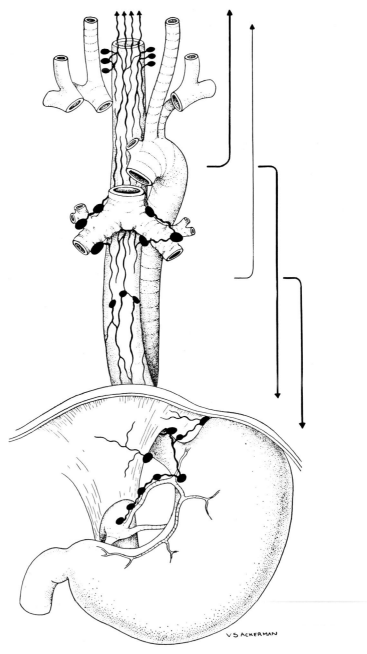

Fig. 316. Lymphatics of esophagus demonstrating drainage to cervical, mediastinal, and subdiaphragmatic lymph nodes. Curved arrows indicate possible areas of drainage toward cervical or subdiaphragmatic regions. Chances of subdiaphragmatic spread increase from upper third downward.

has remained practically unchanged at about 4.4 for whites and nonwhites.

The prevalence of carcinoma of the esophagus among Chinese has been long accepted. This seems to be true for Chinese residents of Java (Kouwenaar[34]). An unexplained increase of carcinoma of the esophagus among the Bantu of the Transkei region of South Africa has been observed in recent years (Burrell[12]; Burrell et al.[13]; Higginson and Oettlé[28]). Hartz[26] reported an unusually high incidence among Negroes of Curaçao. In Scandinavia, the proportion of women among patients with carcinoma of the esophagus has repeatedly been found to be rather high (Ahlbom[2]; Kiviranta[32]; Voutilainen and Koulumies[85]), whereas in the Chinese the proportion of men is higher than in other races (Lang[36]).

The cause or causes of cancer of the esophagus are not known. Heavy consumption of strong alcoholic beverages (China, Russia, and Japan) has been thought to play a role in the etiology of this form of cancer. In the Transkei region of South Africa, an illegal beverage is brewed with unknown ingredients, often in asphalt barrels. It is possible that this beverage could have some relation to the high incidence of cancer of the esophagus in that region. A history of heavy alcohol consumption, of cirrhosis of the liver, and of heavy use of tobacco is often encountered in patients with esophageal carcinoma (Steiner[73]; Wynder and Bross[93]). In England, Scotland, and Scandinavia, the occurrence of this form of cancer among underprivileged women has long been connected with the occurrence of the Plummer-Vinson syndrome (Ahlbom[2]), a nutritional deficiency now being corrected by the addition of iron and vitamins to the baking flour. Burrell et al.[13] have attempted to explain the recently increased incidence among the Bantus by the presence of a carcinogenic substance in their food. Wright and Richardson[91] reported four cases of carcinoma of the thoracic esophagus in patients with a malabsorption syndrome. Mason et al.[44] found higher incidence rates in communities with high population density in the state of Connecticut and suggested that investigation of etiologic factors should be sought among cases found in an industrial environment. It seems likely that differences in sex ratios and racial incidences may be explained by nutritional variations as influenced by other factors such as alcoholism.

Pathology
Gross pathology

Ochsner and DeBakey[52] collected 8572 cases of esophageal cancer from the medical literature and found that 20% developed in the upper third, 37% in the middle third, and 43% in the lower third of the esophagus.

Some carcinomas of the esophagus develop in the form of a bulky, fungating growth that rapidly closes the lumen (Fig. 317). Others are superficially ulcerated

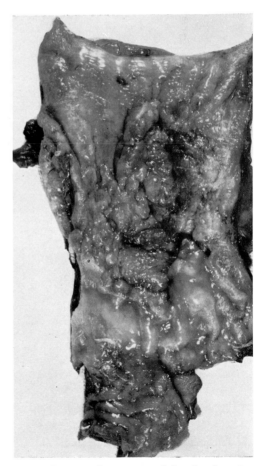

Fig. 317. Surgical specimen of deeply ulcerating, constricting, undifferentiated carcinoma of esophagus. Pathologic examination revealed metastases to many regional lymph nodes, and death from distant metastases followed within year.

and spread in surface without much obstruction. Not infrequently, they extend over a wide area (10 cm or more). Submucosal infiltration may sometimes be the cause of pallor of the mucous membrane and a verrucous appearance. The tumor may be associated with considerable formation of connective tissue, and for that reason it is designated as scirrhous. Mathews and Schnabel,[45] in a review of 237 autopsies on patients with cancer of the esophagus, found twenty-two with no obstruction (Fig. 318). These lesions usually show deep ulceration with even dilatation of the lumen. More often, however, as the obstruction of the esophagus progresses, a compensating dilatation that may reach tremendous proportions occurs on the segment of normal esophagus proximal to the tumor. Because of the lack of serosal covering of this organ, the ability of tumors to spread outside of it is enhanced, and because of the intimate association of the esophagus with important structures within the thorax, various organs may be directly invaded even at an early stage of the disease (Table 31). Tumors of the upper third of the esophagus may involve the carotid arteries, pleura, recurrent laryngeal nerves, and trachea.

Tumors of the middle third may invade the left main-stem bronchus, thoracic duct, aortic arch, subclavian artery, intercostal arteries, azygos vein, and right pleura. Tumors of the lower third may invade the pericardium, left auricle, left pleura, and descending aorta. In addition, the tumor may simply spread into the mediastinum, producing a mediastinitis, or extend to the pleura and lung and be the cause of empyema. Invasion of a large artery may occur. Veins are less frequently perforated than arteries and are more usually effaced by compression (Bérard and Sargnon[9]).

Necrotizing bronchopneumonia and gangrene are very commonly found because of the frequent invasion of the trachea, left main bronchus, and the lung itself.

Microscopic pathology

The overwhelming majority of carcinomas of the esophagus are epidermoid, usually rather undifferentiated. Submucous infiltration, not noticeable grossly, may be found 4 cm to 7 cm beyond the apparent borders of the lesion. Epidermoid carcinomas of the esophagus are, as a rule, much less differentiated than carcinomas of the oral cavity, and they metastasize

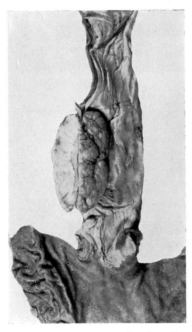

Fig. 318. Autopsy specimen of polypoid, nonobstructing, undifferentiated carcinoma of esophagus in patient operated on for metastatic brain lesion thought to be primary brain tumor. Primary lesion was not clinically suspected.

Table 31. Organs invaded by carcinoma of esophagus at different levels*

Level	Cases	Thyroid gland	Aorta and great arteries	Trachea and bronchi	Pleural cavity	Great veins	Lung and lung hilus	Peri-cardium	Liver
Upper third	122	15	4	90	5	3	0	0	0
Middle third	358	0	25	216	15	7	65	13	0
Lower third	154	0	10	35	24	1	38	16	5
Total	634	15	39	341	44	11	103	29	5

*From Dormanns, E.: Das Oesophaguscarcinom; Ergebnisse der unter Mitarbeit von 39 pathologischen Instituten Deutschlands durchgeführten Erhebung über das Oesophaguscarcinom (1925-1933), Z. Krebsforsch. 49:86-108, 1939.

earlier. Their submucosal spread may be recognized only microscopically.

Many adenocarcinomas of the terminal third of the esophagus represent secondary involvement from a primary gastric tumor. It is less common for epidermoid carcinoma of the esophagus to invade the stomach (Garlock[21]). Rarely, true adenocarcinomas are observed in the middle third of the esophagus with squamous epithelium proximal and distal to the lesion. The association of adenocarcinomas of the esophagus with hiatal hernia requires a reappraisal of the concept of hiatal hernia itself (Gould and Barnhard[23]).

Carcinomas showing both squamous and glandular elements may occur at the junction of the esophagus and the stomach. Polypoid tumors of the esophagus, previously designated as *carcinosarcomas*, may, in reality, be carcinomas in a spindle-like stroma (Scarpa[64]). Frequently, they are unaccompanied by metastases and are susceptible to surgical cure (Stener et al.[74]).

Metastatic spread

In the upper third of the esophagus, dissemination through the lymphatics may lead to lymph nodes of the anterior jugular chain or of the supraclavicular region. Tumors of the middle third may metastasize to the mediastinum and also to the subdiaphragmatic lymph nodes. Tumors of the lower third metastasize predominantly to abdominal lymph nodes. In a study of seventy-two cases of carcinoma of the

esophagus Churchill and Sweet[15] found only one of twenty-four carcinomas of the upper third that metastasized to the subdiaphragmatic lymph nodes, whereas eleven of thirty-two of the middle third presented abdominal metastases, and eight of sixteen carcinomas of the lower third were found to metastasize to the subdiaphragmatic lymph nodes. Metastases through the blood vessels may occur. Tumor emboli enter the caval system and are the cause of direct pulmonary metastases. Mediastinal lymph nodes may secondarily invade any of the surrounding structures. Distant metastases to liver, bones, and kidneys are not infrequent. The distribution of lymph nodes and distant metastases in relation to the level of origin of the carcinomatous lesion is shown in Table 32.

Clinical evolution

The early symptoms of carcinoma of the esophagus may cause no alarm. There may be a sensation of fullness or of substernal pressure or distress. *Dysphagia* is the most frequent symptom and may be progressive or may appear suddenly or spasmodically. As the dysphagia progresses, the patient unconsciously masticates more thoroughly or gradually changes to soft and liquid foods. With marked dysphagia, there may be regurgitation of saliva and mucus that accumulate in the dilated portion of the esophagus above the tumor. A rapid *weight loss* inevitably follows dysphagia due to dehydration and

Table 32. Distribution of metastases according to level of origin of carcinoma of esophagus*

Organ	Upper third (121)	Middle third (418)	Lower third (285)	All (824)
Lymph nodes				
Supraclavicular	6	20	12	38
Infraclavicular	1	5	1	7
Peritracheal and periesophageal	84	99	37	220
Mediastinal	28	231	147	406
Abdominal	11	104	121	236
Liver	20 (16%)	122 (29%)	122 (43%)	264 (32%)
Lungs and pleura	38 (31%)	82 (20%)	56 (20%)	176 (21%)
Bone	11 (9%)	31 (7%)	26 (9%)	68 (8%)
Kidneys	5	30	24	59
Omentum and peritoneum	2	15	27	44
Suprarenal glands	4	10	21	35

*From Dormanns, E.: Das Oesophaguscarcinom; Ergebnisse der unter Mitarbeit von 39 pathologischen Instituten Deutschlands durchgeführten Erhebung über das Oesophaguscarcinom (1925-1933), Z. Krebsforsch. 49:86-108, 1939.

undernourishment. *Pain* may be present, but it is not a constant symptom. It may be felt diffusely below the sternum and spread toward the neck. *Cough* may appear because of regurgitation of food or because of a bronchoesophageal fistula. Because of the fistula, *fever* may also appear. *Sialorrhea* may occur and is attributed to a reflex resulting from the esophageal obstruction. *Laryngeal paralysis* may result from involvement or compression of a recurrent nerve. *Anemia* is not uncommon. The rapid loss of weight leads to *asthenia* and cachexia, and *fetid odor* may emanate from fermentations in the dilated esophagus. Patients may die of starvation or of necrotizing bronchopneumonia, empyema, mediastinitis, or hemorrhage from a large thoracic vessel.

Diagnosis

The early symptoms of carcinoma of the esophagus may be so trivial as to be disregarded even by the physician. Very frequently, the early sensation of substernal distress or pressure is dismissed as a neurotic disorder or globus hystericus. Spasmodic dysphagia may be attributed to a swallowed object. In a review of over 3000 cases of carcinoma of the esophagus, there was an average delay of 4.3 months between the onset of the first symptom and the establishment of the diagnosis. This average delay had not changed in a period of thirteen years (Kiviranta[32]). Merendino and Mark[46] found that there was an average delay of 108 days before therapy was instituted after the patient had consulted a physician.

There are a few instances in which the clinical onset of carcinoma of the esophagus is disguised by the appearance first of a metastatic lesion, usually in the supraclavicular region or on the skin. The verification of metastatic squamous cell carcinoma of the supraclavicular region should always indicate the need for investigation of the esophagus.

A relatively early diagnosis of cancer of the esophagus implies investigation of minor symptoms that are not usually clinically impressive: dull retrosternal pressure, burning or pain, mild dysphagia, or spasmodic dysphagia. A diagnosis is only obtained usually by the performance of special procedures, of which esophagoscopy and roentgenologic examinations are the most important. In advanced cases, the presence of other symptoms and of supraclavicular or other metastases makes the diagnosis of the primary site simply of secondary interest.

Roentgenologic examination

A radioscopic examination should always precede the taking of roentgenograms and is, at times, considerably more eloquent. When the patient swallows a small amount of thick barium meal, the barium is delayed shortly at the level of the cricopharyngeus and then falls in the form of a continuous stream and passes rapidly into the stomach. In the presence of an obstruction the barium falls sluggishly and stops at the level of the constriction. In carcinoma of the esophagus, as Souttar so succinctly stated, "There may be a very moderate degree of dilatation above, giving a solid shadow which terminates in a cone pointing downwards, and from the apex of this cone a fine twisted stream of barium can be seen threading the tortuous channel of the growth"* (Fig. 319). If there is a stenotic obstruction, the barium may stop at this point altogether and pass no further. The examination may have to be repeated after the administration of antispasmodics. If there is a bronchoesophageal fistula, the barium usually passes into the bronchial tree. The barium may conceal the lower limits of the tumor. In the diagnosis of esophagogastric lesions, the gastric air bubble should be observed before introducing any opaque material. Tumors in this area may be seen protruding in the air bubble and contrasting with it (Sherman[68]).

A permanent record of the roentgenologic findings is, of course, always desirable. It might be easier in the differential diagnosis to study certain irregularities on the film and to compare them with previous studies. Moreover, the roentgenograms help in establishing evidence of a tumor shadow around the obstruction and in marking the limits of the lesion when

---

*From Souttar, H. S.: Treatment of carcinoma of the oesophagus; based on 100 personal cases and 18 post-mortem reports, Brit. J. Surg. **15:**76-94, 1927.

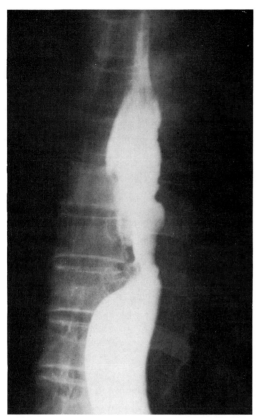

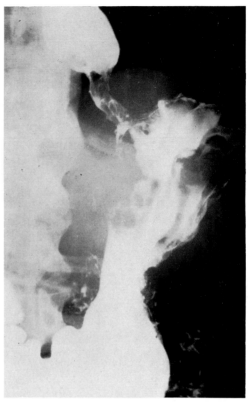

Fig. 319. Irregular filling defect of middle third of esophagus in 73-year-old man who complained of substernal heartburn. This proved to be squamous cell carcinoma of esophagus. (WU neg. 60-3331.)

Fig. 320. Adenocarcinoma of terminal portion of esophagus and cardia showing typical filling defect and dilatation of esophagus above lesion.

treatment is contemplated. The radiographic examination is also of value in establishing evidence of mediastinal and pulmonary metastases.

Esophagoscopy

A laryngoscopic examination should always be carried out before esophagoscopy. It may reveal a hemiparalysis of the larynx or, rarely, a bilateral paralysis. The esophagoscopy should carry little danger in experienced hands, but perforation is always possible in the presence of cancer. The tumor may be seen as an ulcer, as a polypoid, exophytic lesion, or as submucous nodules. An early carcinoma may be masked behind a benign-appearing "leukoplakia." The tumor may not be seen at all due to a constriction above the ulceration. The apparent gross limits of a carcinoma of the esophagus may be quite misleading.

Microscopic examination may reveal tumor several centimeters away from the apparent borders of the lesion. A bronchoscopic examination is a necessary complement, particularly in such patients in whom surgical intervention is contemplated.

Biopsy and exfoliative cytology

At the time of esophagoscopy, a biopsy is frequently, but not always possible. When not possible, a cytologic examination of aspirated fluid may be successful in establishing the diagnosis (Klayman[33]). In the presence of severe esophagitis, there is the possibility of error in the cytologic interpretation (Johnson et al.[29]). A liver scan and needle biopsy are well indicated when liver metastases are suspected (Marcial et al.[42]).

Differential diagnosis

In establishing a differential diagnosis of carcinoma of the esophagus with other forms of tumor, it should be remembered that a *postcricoid carcinoma* (more frequent in women) may invade the upper fourth of the esophagus and be considered as a lesion of this organ. Also, very frequently *adenocarcinomas of the stomach* invade the lower third of the esophagus. The differences are only of importance for purposes of classification. *Metastatic lesions* secondarily involving the esophagus are rather infrequently observed. Toreson[81] reported twenty-six such instances from primary lesions in the bronchus, stomach, larynx, breast, etc.

Achalasia, a functional abnormality, offers the greatest difficulty in differential diagnosis because of obstruction and dilatation of the esophagus which seem identical with those of carcinoma. Achalasia, however, occurs in younger individuals and is often associated with hypertrophic gastritis. The history of dysphagia may be considerably longer, and, because of retention of food and chronic irritation, there may be marked chronic esophagitis. Very rarely, a carcinoma of the esophagus may develop in a patient with achalasia. In patients with proved achalasia, a carcinoma should be suspected if there is recurrence of dysphagia with retrosternal pain and marked loss of weight (Baer and Sicher[6]).

Esophageal varices are often accompanied by hematemesis (Higgins[27]) and rarely may simulate carcinoma (Lawson et al.[37]). Typical irregularities of the lower third of the esophagus are evidenced in radiographic examination, particularly if the patient is examined in a horizontal position. Esophageal varices are often associated with portal hypertension. *Peptic ulcers* of the terminal portion of the esophagus may be the cause of stenosis. They are frequently associated with hiatal hernia of the stomach. On esophagoscopic examination, the esophageal ulcer is characteristically flat without accompanying constriction of the lumen and is easily diagnosed (Allison[3]) (Fig. 321). Infrequently, the presence of *heterotopic gastric mucosa* in the esophagus may cause ulceration and may be confused with carcinoma (Bosher and Taylor[11]).

A *hypopharyngeal diverticulum* may cause dysphagia and regurgitation as well as cough during sleep, all of which may

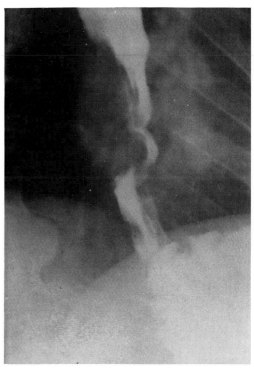

Fig. 321. Area of tortuous defect of lower end of esophagus in 66-year-old man who complained of painless dysphagia. Abnormality was due to extensive area of benign ulceration and scarring. (WU neg. 60-3751.)

suggest a carcinoma of the esophagus, particularly in an elderly man. The diagnosis is easily established in radiographic and esophagoscopic examinations. A single case of epidermoid carcinoma was observed by Riberi et al.[61] in such a diverticulum.

Benign tumors of the esophagus are rare and are encountered most often in elderly men (Totten et al.[82]). They are usually symptomless but may cause dysphagia. In a few instances, there may be ulceration into the lumen of the esophagus, bleeding, and secondary infection. The most common benign tumors are the leiomyomas (Storey and Adams[75]; Glanville[22]), but neurofibromas and paragangliomas (Taylor[79]) have been seen simulating a malignant tumor. Pedunculated polyps, fibromas, and hemangiomas may appear in the mouth during vomiting, to disappear again (Adams[1]), but the majority of these tumors are intramural (Myers and Bradshaw[47]). Fibrous polyps and polypoid fibromas can occur in an intraluminal posi-

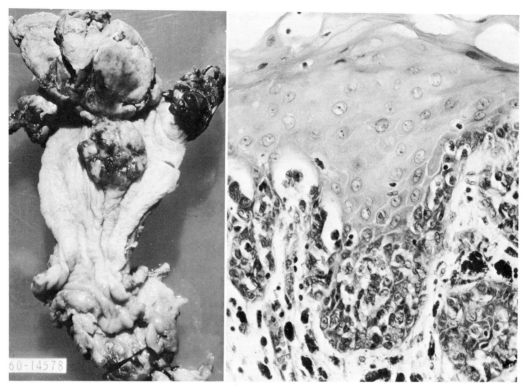

Fig. 322   **Fig. 323**

Fig. 322. Large polypoid malignant melanoma of esophagus. (Courtesy California Tumor Tissue Registry, Los Angeles County–University of Southern California Medical Center, Los Angeles, Calif.; from Waken, J. K., and Bullock, W. K.: Primary melanocarcinoma of the esophagus, Amer. J. Clin. Path. 38:415-421, 1962; © 1962, The Williams & Wilkins Co., Baltimore, Md., U.S.A.)

Fig. 323. Malignant melanoma of esophagus with junctional change. (High power; courtesy California Tumor Tissue Registry, Los Angeles County–University of Southern California Medical Center, Los Angeles, Calif.; from Waken, J. K., and Bullock, W. K.: Primary melanocarcinoma of the esophagus, Amer. J. Clin. Path. 38:415-421, 1962; © 1962, The Williams & Wilkins Co., Baltimore, Md., U.S.A.)

tion (Totten et al.[82]). When the benign tumors are large enough to present within the lumen, they have rather characteristic roentgenologic features: abrupt angle at edge of tumor, sharply outlined lobulated surface, spherical or ovoid shape, motion with esophagus during swallowing, and obliterated mucosal pattern due to stretching (Schatzki and Hawes[65]). *Leiomyosarcomas* present a fairly typical radiographic appearance (Palazzo and Schulz[53]). They are rare and may be curable by surgical resection (Rainer and Brus[60]). *Malignant melanomas* of the esophagus have also been encountered (Garfinkle and Cahan[20]) and may have a polypoid appearance (Figs. 322 and 323). *Aortic aneurysms* may compress the esophagus. Evidence of this compression will be clear on roentgenologic examination because of the site and shape of the compression and the displacement of the esophagus. *Mediastinal cysts* and *metastatic nodes* from carcinomatous lesions elsewhere may also give an extrinsic deformity of the esophagus, but here, as in the preceding example, the mucosal pattern will not be modified, and there will be no evidence of irregularities. *Diverticula* may also result in dysphagia, but the differential diagnosis will be easily solved on roentgenologic examination. *Foreign bodies* are easily seen because of their density or because they become coated with barium.

Treatment

Despite discouraging risks and results, there have been continued diligent efforts, surgical as well as radiotherapeutic, to minimize or solve the problems presented by carcinoma of the esophagus.

Surgery

Beyond pioneer surgical efforts, there has been, in the past three decades, increased interest in the surgical approach to this form of cancer. Progress has been primarily due to better anesthesia, better understanding of esophageal anastomosis, antibiotics, fortified liquid diet, etc. In spite of this progress, however, operative mortality remains high. Franklin et al.[19] performed fifty-eight resections, with twenty-two of the patients (38%) dying within the first month. The mortality is greater for resections of the upper third of the esophagus. Sturdy[76] reported on seventy-one resections with 23 patients dying within one month, with an operative mortality of 32%. The mortality for resection of the lower third of the esophagus only is variously reported to be around 10% (Sweet[78]).

In order to achieve a complete removal of a carcinoma of the *cervical esophagus,* a laryngoesophagectomy plus neck dissection are usually required (Turner[83]; Wookey[90]). Pharyngeal reconstructions are plagued by postoperative strictures and salivary fistulae as well as by failures due to local recurrences and metastases. Gastric and colonic transplants have been routed through retrosternal or subcutaneous tunnels, but these formidable procedures increase, prohibitively, the operative mortality.

Surgical removal of carcinomas of the *thoracic esophagus* (middle two-thirds) may be done through various abdominothoracic approaches, with resection and gastric or colonic interposition done as a one-stage procedure (Sturdy[76]; Belsey[8]). For these procedures, the esophagus is mobilized and transected 5 cm or more from the apparent limits of the tumor. A frozen section may be utilized to assure the adequacy of the margin (Sturdy[76]; Ushigome et al.[84]). Sun and Wu[77] demonstrated atypical epithelial proliferation and carcinoma in situ in the periphery of twenty-two of 100 sur-

gical specimens. Sturdy[76] reported an operative mortality of 32% for these procedures.

First to receive the attention of surgeons, the *esophagogastric* carcinomas, or those arising in the terminal third of the esophagus, have been widely accepted as a surgical problem. Surgical treatment of these lesions usually implies adequate resection of adjacent metastatic lymph nodes. The operative mortality is acceptable in view of the relatively better results.

Palliative procedures

A bypass *esophagogastrostomy* or *esophagojejunostomy* above an unresectable tumor is considered worthy by some surgeons. The value of palliative *gastrostomy* or *jejunostomy* is rather controversial. These procedures do not relieve the distress occasioned by the inability to swallow saliva, and there is no evidence that they prolong life. *Intubation* by means of a Souttar or plastic tube creates a passage for liquids and soft foods as well as for saliva. These prostheses may be placed through the esophagoscope sometimes combined with a gastrostomy. *Bouginage* may be dangerous and is rarely employed.

The main complications of surgery are massive hemorrhage, leakage of anastomosis, pulmonary collapse, and embolism.

Radiotherapy

Squamous cell carcinomas of the esophagus are radiosensitive and potentially radiocurable (Figs. 324 and 325). Early attempts to irradiate carcinomas of the esophagus by means of a *radium bougie,* placed in the esophageal lumen, were only rarely reported successful. Such an approach, as well as the *interstitial implantation* of radioactive sources through the esophagoscope, would not permit a homogeneous irradiation of the primary lesion and of its metastatic lymph nodes with a satisfactorily high daily dose to assure successful radiotherapy. Except for expeditious palliation of patients with carcinomas of the cervical esophagus (Lederman[39]), intracavitary irradiation has lost its indications.

The *external irradiation* of carcinoma of the esophagus and its potential lymph node metastases presents a number of difficulties: the tumor is deeply situated,

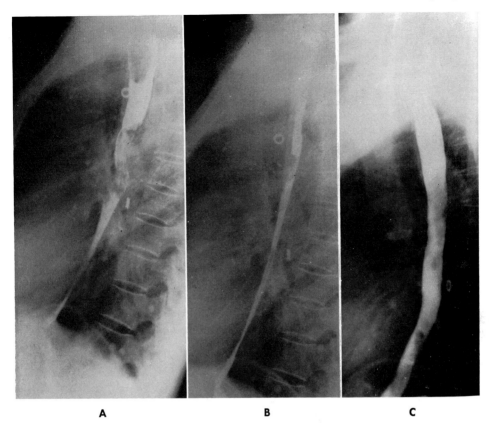

A　　　　　　**B**　　　　　　**C**

Fig. 324. Patient, 65-year-old man, had dysphagia. **A,** First film showed filling defect 3 cm in length in middle third of esophagus. In August, 1957, patient was explored. Squamous carcinoma of esophagus was fixed to posterior wall of mediastinum, aortic arch, and left main-stem bronchus. Metal markers were placed to localize neoplasm. On Aug. 28, 1957, cobalt[60] teletherapy was started, with tumor receiving dose of 6500 R in seven weeks. **B,** Second film taken little over month after completion of therapy. **C,** Third film taken Dec. 29, 1960. Patient died in March, 1963. (Courtesy Dr. Victor Marcial, San Juan, P. R.)

often involving vital structures, and a thorough irradiation of the potential areas of tumor involvement implies large fields and the irradiation of normal radiosensitive structures, with consequent complications and hazards.

The physical challenge of bringing to the depth of the tumor as high a dose as possible with *conventional roentgentherapy* stimulated the use of a clever artifice well justified under the circumstances: *rotational roentgentherapy* (Nielsen[51]; Krebs et al.[35]). This technologic approach increased the ratio of depth-to-surface dosage and encouraged a more adequate irradiation of the primary lesion. Although the method fired the imagination of physicists and clinicians, and influenced the manufacture of modern radiotherapeutic equipment, it has its limitations and disadvantages. It

may be possible, under exceptional circumstances of size and position, to rotate a source of radiations around the primary esophageal tumor but not, at the same time, around its metastases. Even in moderately sized tumors, the amount of lung surface to be irradiated becomes prohibitive (Borgstrom and Gynning[10]). Moreover, with *cobalt[60] teletherapy* and *supervoltage roentgentherapy* it is perfectly possible, and more accurate, to irradiate the potential area of involvement through two or more fields, leaving most of the lung areas outside of the fields of irradiation (Watson[88, 89]; Pearson[56, 57]; Marcial et al.[42]). Some radiotherapists still prefer rotational techniques with cobalt[60] or supervoltage roentgentherapy, but few would use them in the treatment of carcinomas of the cervical esophagus.

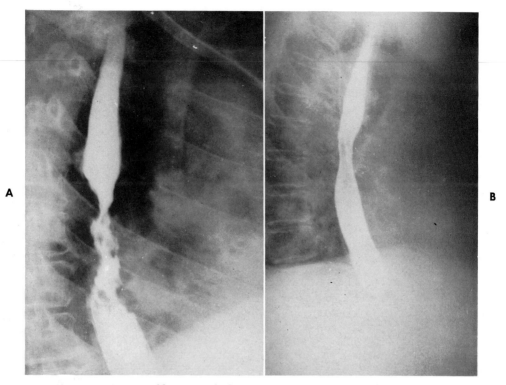

Fig. 325. Patient, 63-year-old woman, had history of dysphagia of several months' duration. **A,** Film taken April 20, 1960, showed lesion 12 cm in length. Patient received dose of 6500 R in forty-seven days. **B,** Second film shows regression of neoplasm. Patient died in March, 1967. (Courtesy Dr. Victor Marcial, San Juan, P. R.)

Details of dosimetry are beyond the scope of this book. It is enough to point out that the administration of the necessary high and homogeneous irradiation over a wide area is further complicated by the considerably different absorption of radiation through bone, muscle, and lungs. Calculations on the basis of conventional depth-dose charts may result in gross errors. In this, as in other such problems of clinical radiotherapy, the only safeguard is the planning for a long fractionation of treatments that results in a lesser daily dose and a greater degree of impunity.

An improvement of the dysphagia takes place in the majority of patients, with consequent improvement of nutrition and gain in weight. Most of the experienced radiotherapists in this field prefer not to do a preliminary gastrostomy when radiotherapy is contemplated. Some favor the introduction of a Souttar tube to facilitate and accelerate improvement of nutrition. Radiation pneumonitis, medically manageable, may occur during the latter course of the treatments or after their completion. Mediastinitis, hemorrhage, etc., which occur in untreated patients, may also take place, though rarely, in the course of radiotherapy.

Palliative radiotherapy usually implies as much planning, skill, and dedication as the curative efforts (Pearson[56, 57]). The best palliation is obtained in patients who, though candidates for cure, fail to be permanently benefitted. Patients with verified sterilization of the primary lesion frequently succumb to the development of metastases (Watson[88, 89]). Dysphagia is eliminated in many patients who will subsequently die of their disease. Elimination of dysphagia and of bleeding reestablishes nutrition and temporary well-being (Walker[86]).

Preoperative radiotherapy plus surgery

In view of the persistently poor results of surgery, there has been, in recent years, an increasing interest in the utilization of

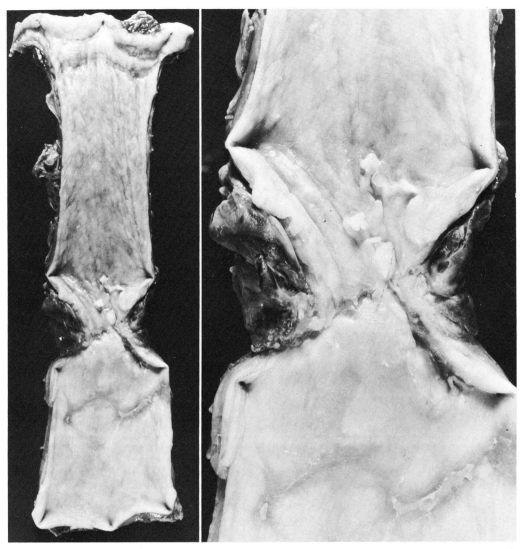

Fig. 326. Patient, a Bantu, had extensive circumferential carcinoma of esophagus that was treated by preoperative irradiation. Although there is no obvious residual tumor, thorough sectioning did show profound irradiation effect and persistent tumor. (Courtesy South African Institute for Medical Research, Johannesburg, R.S.A.; SA negs. 4889-38 and 4889-41A.)

radiations as a surgical adjuvant (Cliffton et al.[17]) (Fig. 326). Nakayama et al.[49] have proposed a method that presents several original departures from conventional procedures, and it is carried out in various steps:

1 A celiotomy with removal of celiac nodes and gastrostomy
2 Preoperative irradiation through fields intended to cover only the primary lesion, with a dose of 2000 to 3000 rads in four to five days
3 Total thoracic esophagectomy within four or five days of completion of irradiation, bringing out of the neck the remaining cervical esophagus
4 Connection of cervical esophagus and gastrostomy through a rubber tube
5 Antethoracic esophagogastrostomy, six months later, to replace the rubber tubing

By proceeding in several stages rather than in one, Nakayama et al.[49] claim to have reduced the operative mortality from 9.7% to 2.5%. They justify the short administration of a relatively small total dose of radiations on the basis of clinical studies and animal experiments which are unconvincing, not to say irrelevant. The entire method is advocated on the basis of a "difference" in five-year survivors of three out of eight irradiated patients compared with four out of twenty-one patients undergoing surgery without preoperative irradiation.

Preoperative radiotherapy should ideally aim at the irradiation of the entire potential area of involvement, including adjacent lymph node metastases. Whereas any amount of radiations is capable of destroying portions of a tumor and preoperative irradiation does not aim at complete destruction, the devitalization of neoplastic tissues which is sought is best accomplished when all of the tumor is irradiated rather than the primary lesion only and when the dose administered is as large as possible and administered over a moderately long time. Doses two or three times larger than those administered by Nakayama et al.,[49] delivered over volumes two or three times greater, in periods of several weeks, contribute a greater benefit and are perfectly compatible with subsequent surgery (Anabtawi et al.[4]; Parker and Gregorie[55]; Seymour and Pettit[67]; Watson[89]).

Prognosis

The average life expectancy of patients with carcinoma of the esophagus is only a few months (Shimkin[69]) (Fig. 327), with about 25% dying within six months and 75% within one year (Greenwood[24]). In 1965, there were 5542 deaths from cancer of the esophagus in the United States, or a crude mortality rate of 2.9 per 100,000. Whereas the mortality rates for whites remained the same, that of nonwhites increased considerably from 1930 to 1960. Cancer of the esophagus accounted for 11% of all deaths from cancer in Puerto Rico from 1950 to 1961, with the age-adjusted mortality of men for 1956-1959 ranking above France, Switzerland, Finland, Japan, and twenty other countries (Martínez[43]).

Statistics of limited scope have shown that a greater proportion of patients have received treatment in recent years than previously. But although not all patients

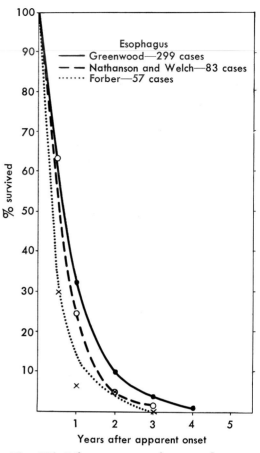

Fig. 327. Life expectancy of untreated patients with carcinoma of esophagus. (From Shimkin, M. B.: Duration of life in untreated cancer, Cancer **4**:1-8, 1951.)

die with metastases, their theoretical curability contrasts with the meager results obtained (Merendino and Mark[46]). Despite the relative results of any advocated modality of treatment, the overall survival of these patients remains dismally low—only 1.4% of Nakayama's 2382 patients[48] survived five years and only 1.7% of 1109 patients registered from 1950 to 1958 at the Puerto Rico Cancer Registry survived five years.

From 1951 to 1960, Franklin et al.[19] studied 129 patients with carcinoma of the esophagus at the Hammersmith Hospital in London. Ninety-one of these patients were explored, but only fifty-eight had a resection, with thirty-six of them dying within one month and the remaining twenty-two living over one year. At the time of their report (1964), only one patient, a woman, had lived five years after operation and had, in fact, lived ten years. In another series of 208 patients seen by Sturdy[76] at the Royal Gwent Hospital in Newport, England, seventy-one were submitted to radical surgery, with nine surviving two years and six surviving five years. Sturdy[76] pointed out that the average survival of the unsuccessfully resected patients was fourteen months, that patients with palliative surgical bypass survived an average of ten months, that patients who were only explored survived one and one-half months, that those who underwent a jejunostomy lived one month as an average, and that those who had only intubation or bouginage lived three months. In a small group of nine patients with negative nodes and adequate resection reported by Robertson et al.,[62] seven patients had long survivals.

Of 541 patients seen at the Pereira-Rossell Hospital in Montevideo between 1950 and 1959, Leborgne et al.[38] irradiated 431 (80%). Although 79% of those treated showed clinical improvement, only 9.2% survived two years and 3.1% survived five years. None of the survivors in this series had lesions in the upper two-thirds of the esophagus, and six of the seven survivors were women. In another series of 413 patients seen at the Gonzalez-Martinez Hospital in San Juan between 1956 and 1964, Marcial et al.[42] reported 100 (24%) surviving one year. In 173 patients eligible for five-year analysis, the total five-year survival was 8.7%; in ninety-two of these patients who received complete surgical or radiologic treatment, the five-year survival was 16%. Six of eighteen patients who had resections only survived. Nine of seventy-four patients who received radiotherapy survived five years; two of these had been surgically explored but did not have resections. There were, among the five-year survivors, two patients with carcinoma of the upper third of the esophagus (out of fourteen treated), six with lesions of the middle third (out of eighty-two), and seven with carcinomas of the lower third (out of thirty-five treated).

Pearson[57] reported on 429 patients seen at the Royal Infirmary of Edinburgh between 1956 and 1962: 174 were resected with a five-year survival (actuarial method) of 9%. Ninety-nine patients received radical megavoltage radiotherapy, with twenty surviving five years, without the handicaps of radical surgery. The overall five-year survival in the entire series of patients was two and one-half times better for women than for men.

Palliative surgery is obviously beneficial but only to a small group of patients. To accept a prohibitive surgical mortality to end in only an occasional patient being cured (Franklin et al.[19]) is to deny a great proportion of all patients a reasonable chance of palliation by radiotherapy. Radiotherapy which is applied for curative purposes affords considerable palliation to a large proportion of patients in the form of temporary or permanent relief of dysphagia and pain (Watson[89]). In a few patients, radiotherapy may shorten the duration of life by precipitating hemorrhage or perforation (Papillon and Goyon[54]). It has been shown that such procedures as jejunostomy and gastrostomy result in very little palliation and practically no extention of survival.

It is difficult to reach very definite conclusions at the present time. We would be inclined to favor surgery alone for lesions of the lower third of the esophagus, radiotherapy alone for lesions of the cervical esophagus and thoracic inlet, and preoperative radiotherapy combined with surgery for lesions of the middle half of the esophagus.

REFERENCES

1 Adams, R.: Fibroma of the esophagus, Lahey Clin. Bull. 3:72-81, 1943.
2 Ahlbom, H. E.: Simple achlorhydric anaemia, Plummer-Vinson syndrome, and carcinoma of the mouth, pharynx, and oesophagus in women; observations at Radiumhemmet, Stockholm, Brit. Med. J. 2:331-333, 1936.
3 Allison, P. R.: Peptic ulcer of the esophagus, Thorax 3:20-42, 1948.
4 Anabtawi, I. N., Brackney, E. L., and Ellison, R. G.: Carcinoma of the esophagus treated by combined radiation and surgery, J. Thorac. Cardiovasc. Surg. 48:205-210, 1964.
5 Armstrong, R. A., Blalock, J. B., and Carrerra, G. M.: Adenocarcinoma of the middle third of the esophagus arising from ectopic gastric mucosa, J. Thorac. Surg. 37:398-403, 1959.
6 Baer, P., and Sicher, K.: The association of achalasia of the cardia with oesophageal carcinoma, Brit. J. Radiol. 20:528-532, 1947.
7 Baker, R. R., and Lott, S.: Carcinoma of the thoracic esophagus, Johns Hopkins Med. J. 121:153-161, 1967.

8 Belsey, R.: Reconstruction of the esophagus with cleft colon, J. Thorac. Cardiovasc. Surg. 49:33-55, 1965.

9 Bérard, L., and Sargnon, A.: Cancer de l'oesophage, Paris, 1927, Gaston Doin.

10 Borgstrom, K. -E., and Gynning, I.: Roentgenographic changes in the lungs and vertebrae following intense rotation roentgen therapy of esophageal cancer, Acta Radiol. (Stockholm) 47:281-288, 1957.

11 Bosher, L. H., Jr., and Taylor, F. H.: Heterotopic gastric mucosa in the esophagus with ulceration and stricture formation, J. Thorac. Surg. 21:306-312, 1951.

12 Burrell, R. J. W.: Esophageal cancer among Bantu in the Transkei, J. Nat. Cancer Inst. 28:495-514, 1962.

13 Burrell, R. J. W., Roach, W. A., and Shadwell, A.: Esophageal cancer in the Bantu of the Transkei associated with mineral deficiency in garden plants, J. Nat. Cancer Inst. 36:201-209, 1966.

14 Buschke, F.: Surgical and radiological results in the treatment of esophageal carcinoma, Amer. J. Roentgen. 71:9-24, 1954.

15 Churchill, E. D., and Sweet, R. H.: Transthoracic resection of tumors of the stomach and esophagus, Ann. Surg. 115:897-920, 1942.

16 Clarke, C. A., and McConnell, R. B.: Six cases of carcinoma of the oesophagus occurring in one family, Brit. Med. J. 2:1137, 1955.

17 Cliffton, E. E., Goodner, J. T., and Bronstein, E.: Preoperative irradiation for cancer of the esophagus, Cancer 13:37-45, 1960.

18 Dormanns, E.: Das Oesophaguscarcinom; Ergebnisse der unter Mitarbeit von 39 pathologischen Instituten Deutschlands durchgeführten Erhebung über das Oesophaguscarcinom (1925-1933), Z. Krebsforsch. 49:86-108, 1939.

19 Franklin, R. H., Burn, J. I., and Lynch, G.: Carcinoma of the oesophagus; a review of 129 treated patients, Brit. J. Surg. 51:178-183, 1964.

20 Garfinkle, J. M., and Cahan, W. G.: Primary melanocarcinoma of the esophagus; first histologically proved case, Cancer 5:921-926, 1952.

21 Garlock, J. H.: Treatment of carcinoma of the esophagus (editorial), Gastroenterology 29:684-686, 1955.

22 Glanville, J. N.: Leiomyomata of the esophagus, Clin. Radiol. 16:187-190, 1965.

23 Gould, D. M., and Barnhard, H. J.: Changing concepts in the structure, function and disease of the lower esophagus, Amer. J. Med. Sci. 233:581-595, 1957.

24 Greenwood, Major: Natural duration of cancer, British Ministry of Health Reports on Public Health and Medical Subjects, no. 33, London, 1926, His Majesty's Stationery Office.

25 Gynning, I.: Roentgen rotation therapy in cancer of the esophagus, Acta. Radiol. (Stockholm) 35:428-442, 1951.

26 Hartz, P. H.: The incidence of malignant tumors in unselected autopsy material at Curaçao, Netherlands, West Indies, Amer. J. Cancer 40:355-358, 1940.

27 Higgins, W. H., Jr.: The esophageal varix;

a report of one hundred and fifteen cases, Amer. J. Med. Sci. 214:436-441, 1947.

28 Higginson, J., and Oettlé, A. G.: Cancer incidence in the Bantu and "Cape colored" races of South Africa; report of a cancer survey in the Transvaal (1953-55), J. Nat. Cancer Inst. 24:589-671, 1960.

29 Johnson, W. D., Koss, L. G., Papanicolaou, G. N., and Seybold, J. F.: Cytology of esophageal washings; evaluation of 364 cases, Cancer 8:951-957, 1955.

30 Jørgsholm, B.: Roentgentherapy in cancer of the extrathoracic portion of the esophagus, Acta Radiol. (Stockholm) 38:61-78, 1952.

31 Joske, R. A., and Benedict, E. B.: The role of benign esophageal obstruction in the development of carcinoma of the esophagus, Gastroenterology 36:749-755, 1959.

32 Kiviranta, U. K.: Carcinoma of the esophagus; its incidence, age and sex distribution and prognosis in Finland, Acta Otolaryng. (Stockholm) 42:73-88, 1952.

33 Klayman, M. I.: The diagnosis of esophageal carcinoma by exfoliative cytology, including two cases of cardiospasm associated with carcinoma of the esophagus, Ann. Intern. Med. 43:33-44, 1955.

34 Kouwenaar, W.: On cancer incidence in Indonesia; symposium on geographical pathology and demography of cancer; sponsored by the World Health Organization, 1950.

35 Krebs, C., Nielsen, H., and Andersen, P. E.: Rotation treatment of cancer of the esophagus; a clinical material, Acta Radiol. (Stockholm) 32:304-316, 1949.

36 Lang, K. C.: Report of 59 cases of esophageal carcinoma, Chin. Med. J. (Peking) 53:57-63, 1938.

37 Lawson, T. L., Dodds, W. J., and Sheft, D. J.: Carcinoma of the esophagus simulating varices, Amer. J. Roentgen. 107:83-85, 1969.

38 Leborgne, R., Leborgne, F., and Barlocci, L.: Cancer of the oesophagus; results of radiotherapy, Brit. J. Radiol. 36:806-811, 1963.

39 Lederman, M.: Carcinoma of the oesophagus, with special reference to the upper third, Brit. J. Radiol. 39:193-204, 1966.

40 Lott, J. S., and Smith, I. H.: Cobalt-60 beam therapy in carcinoma of the esophagus, Radiology 71:321-326, 1958.

41 Maleki, A., Hashemian, H., and Afchari, R.: Cancer of the esophagus in Iran, J. Radiol. Electr. 46:135-141, 1965.

42 Marcial, V. A., Tomé, J. M., Ubiñas, J., Bosch, A., and Correa, J. N.: The role of radiation therapy in esophageal cancer, Radiology 87:231-239, 1966.

43 Martínez, I.: Cancer of esophagus in Puerto Rico; mortality and incidence analysis, 1950-1961, Cancer 17:1278-1288, 1964.

44 Mason, M. J., Bailar, J. C., III, and Eisenberg, H.: Geographic variation in the incidence of esophageal cancer, J. Chronic Dis. 17:667-676, 1964.

45 Mathews, R. W., and Schnabel, T. G.: Primary esophageal carcinoma, with especial reference

to nonstenosing variety, J.A.M.A. **105**:1591-1595, 1935.

46 Merendino, K. A., and Mark, V. H.: An analysis of 100 cases of squamous-cell carcinoma of the esophagus. I. With special reference to the delay periods and delay factors in diagnosis and therapy, contrasting state and city and county institutions, Cancer **5**:52-61, 1952.

47 Myers, R. T., and Bradshaw, H. H.: Benign intramural tumors and cysts of the esophagus, J. Thorac. Surg. **21**:470-482, 1951.

48 Nakayama, K.: Pre-operative irradiation in the treatment of patients with carcinoma of the oesophagus and some other sites, Clin. Radiol. **15**:232-241, 1964.

49 Nakayama, K., Orihata, H., and Yamaguchi, K.: Surgical treatment combined with pre-operative concentrated irradiation for esophageal cancer, Cancer **20**:778-788, 1967.

50 Nakayama, K., Yanagisawa, F., Nabeya, K., Tamiya, T., Kobayashi, S., and Makino, K.: Concentrated preoperative irradiation therapy, Arch. Surg. (Chicago) **87**:1003-1018, 1963.

51 Nielsen, J.: Clinical results with rotation therapy in cancer of the esophagus, Acta Radiol. (Stockholm) **26**:361-391, 1945.

52 Ochsner, A., and DeBakey, M.: Surgical aspects of carcinoma of the esophagus, J. Thorac. Surg. **10**:401-445, 1941 (extensive bibliography).

53 Palazzo, W. L., and Schulz, M. D.: Spindle-cell tumors of the gastro-intestinal tract, Radiology **51**:779-789, 1948.

54 Papillon, J., and Goyon, M.: Le traitement radiothérapique du cancer de l'oesophage d'après 225 observations, Bull. Ass. Franc. Cancer **43**:331-340, 1956.

55 Parker, E. F., and Gregorie, H. B., Jr.: Combined radiation and surgical treatment of carcinoma of the esophagus, Ann. Surg. **161**:710-722, 1965.

56 Pearson, J. G.: The radiotherapy of carcinoma of the oesophagus and post cricoid region in south east Scotland, Clin. Radiol. **17**:242-257, 1966.

57 Pearson, J. G.: The value of radiotherapy in the management of esophageal cancer, Amer. J. Roentgen. **105**:500-513, 1969.

58 Pierquin, B., Wambersie, A., and Tubiana, M.: Cancer of the thoracic oesophagus; two series of patients treated by 22 MeV betatron, Brit. J. Radiol. **39**:189-192, 1966.

59 Plachta, A.: Benign tumors of the esophagus; review of the literature and report of 90 cases, Amer. J. Gastroent. **38**:639-652, 1962.

60 Rainer, W. G., and Brus, R.: Leiomyosarcoma of the esophagus; review of the literature and report of 3 cases, Surgery **58**:343-350, 1965.

61 Riberi, A., Battersby, J. S., and Vellios, F.: Epidermoid carcinoma occurring in a pharyngo-esophageal diverticulum, Cancer **8**:727-730, 1955.

62 Robertson, R., Coy, P., and Mokkhavesa, S.: The results of radical surgery compared with radical radiotherapy in the treatment of squamous carcinoma of the thoracic esophagus;

the case for preoperative radiotherapy, J. Thorac. Cardiovasc. Surg. **53**:430-440, 1967.

63 Rouvière, H.: Anatomie des lymphatiques de l'homme, Paris, 1933, Masson et Cie.

64 Scarpa, F. J.: Polypoid squamous carcinoma of the esophagus; report of a case and its implications for the histogenesis of "carcinosarcoma" of the esophagus, Cancer **19**:861-866, 1966.

65 Schatzki, R., and Hawes, L. E.: Tumors of the esophagus below the mucosa and their roentgenological differential diagnosis, Rev. Gastroent. **17**:991-1014, 1950.

66 Seaman, W. B., and Ackerman, L. V.: The effect of radiation on the esophagus; a clinical and histological study of the effects produced by the betatron, Radiology **68**:534-541, 1957.

67 Seymour, E. Q., and Pettit, H. S.: Preoperative x-ray therapy in cancer of the esophagus, Radiology **85**:952-955, 1965.

68 Sherman, R. S.: The roentgen diagnosis of cancer of the cardiac region of the stomach, Surgery **23**:874-883, 1948.

69 Shimkin, M. B.: Duration of life in untreated cancer, Cancer **4**:1-8, 1951.

70 Smithers, D. W.: Adenocarcinoma of the esophagus, Thorax **11**:257-267, 1956.

71 Smithers, D. W.: The treatment of carcinoma of the oesophagus, Ann. Roy. Coll. Surg. Eng. **20**:36-49, 1957.

72 Souttar, H. S.: Treatment of carcinoma of the oesophagus; based on 100 personal cases and 18 post-mortem reports, Brit. J. Surg. **15**:76-94, 1927.

73 Steiner, P. E.: The etiology and histogenesis of carcinoma of the esophagus, Cancer **9**:436-452, 1956.

74 Stener, R., Kock, N. G., Pettersson, S., and Zetterlund, B.: Carcinosarcoma of the esophagus, J. Thorac. Cardiovasc. Surg. **54**:746-750, 1967.

75 Storey, C. F., and Adams, W. C., Jr.: Leiomyoma of the esophagus; a report of four cases and review of the surgical literature, Amer. J. Surg. **91**:3-23, 1956 (extensive review of literature).

76 Sturdy, D. E.: Surgical management of carcinoma of the oesophagus, Brit. J. Surg. **52**:245-251, 1965.

77 Sun, S.-C., and Wu, H.: Squamous cell carcinoma of the esophagus; early carcinomatous changes of the epithelium adjacent to the principal lesion, Chin. Med. J. (Peking) **81**:558-567, 1962.

78 Sweet, R. H.: The results of radical surgical extirpation in the treatment of carcinoma of the esophagus and cardia with five year survival statistics, Surg. Gynec. Obstet. **94**:46-52, 1962.

79 Taylor, F. H.: Paraganglioma simulating carcinoma of the esophagus, J. Thorac. Surg. **21**:189-193, 1951.

80 Testut, L.: Traité d'anatomie humaine, ed. 8, vol. 4, Paris, 1931, Gaston Doin.

81 Toreson, W. E.: Secondary carcinoma of the esophagus as a cause of dysphagia, Arch. Path. (Chicago) **38**:82-84, 1944.

82 Totten, R. S., Stout, A. P., Humphreys, G. H., II, and Moore, R. L.: Benign tumors and cysts of the esophagus, J. Thorac. Surg. **25**:606-622, 1953 (extensive bibliography).

83 Turner, G. G.: Henry Jacob Bigelow Lecture: Some experiences in the surgery of the oesophagus, New Eng. J. Med. **205**:657-674, 1931.

84 Ushigome, S., Spjut, H. J., and Noon, G. P.: Extensive dysplasia and carcinoma in situ of esophageal epithelium, Cancer **20**:1023-1029, 1967.

85 Voutilainen, A., and Koulumies, M.: Results of radiation therapy of cancer of the oesophagus, Ann. Chir. Gynaec. Fenn. **54**:40-51, 1965.

86 Walker, J. H.: Carcinoma of the esophagus-cobalt 60 teletherapy; experience and comparison with surgical results, Amer. J. Roentgen. **92**:67-76, 1964.

87 Waken, J. K., and Bullock, W. K.: Primary melanocarcinoma of the esophagus, Amer. J. Clin. Path. **38**:415-421, 1962.

88 Watson, T. A.: Radiation treatment of cancer of the esophagus, Surg. Gynec. Obstet. **117**:346-354, 1963.

89 Watson, T. A.: Radiotherapy in the treatment of cancer of the oesophagus, Radiol. Clin. (Basel) **36**:1-14, 1967.

90 Wookey, H.: Surgical treatment of carcinoma of the hypopharynx and esophagus, Brit. J. Surg. **35**:249-266, 1948.

91 Wright, J. T., and Richardson, P. C.: Squamous carcinoma of the thoracic oesophagus in malabsorption syndrome, Brit. Med. J. **4**:540-542, 1967.

92 Wu, Y. K., and Loucks, H. H.: Carcinoma of the esophagus or cardia of the stomach, Ann. Surg. **134**:946-956, 1951.

93 Wynder, E. L., and Bross, I. J.: A study of etiological factors in cancer of the esophagus, Cancer **14**:389-413, 1961.

94 Wynder, E. L., Hultberg, S., Jacobsson, F., and Bross, I. J.: Environmental factors in cancer of the upper alimentary tract; a Swedish study with special reference to Plummer-Vinson (Paterson-Kelly) syndrome, Cancer **10**:470-487, 1957.

95 Zuppinger, A.: Die Behandlung der Oesophaguskarzinome; Zucher Erfahrungen, Ergebn. Med. Strahlenforsch. **7**:389-456, 1936.

Stomach

Anatomy

The stomach is a peritoneal organ situated in the left hypochondrial region and epigastrium. It is slightly flattened anteroposteriorly and thus has a posterior and an anterior wall, a right lateral border (the lesser curvature), and a left lateral border (the greater curvature). From the esophageal opening called the cardia to the duodenal opening called the pylorus, the stomach is arbitrarily divided into the fundus, corpus, pyloric antrum, and pyloric canal. It is attached, or rather suspended, by several peritoneal folds: the gastrohepatic ligament arising from the lesser curvature and the gastrocolic, gastrolineal, and gastrophrenic ligaments arising from the greater curvature.

The anterior relationships of the stomach vary with the distention of the organ. They include the left lobe of the liver, the diaphragm, and the anterior abdominal wall. Posteriorly, the stomach is in relation with the diaphragm, spleen, left suprarenal gland and kidney, pancreas, fourth portion of the duodenum, mesocolon, and, with distention, the transverse colon.

The arterial supply of the stomach is derived from the celiac axis. The lesser curvature derives its blood supply from the left gastric artery and the right gastric branch of the hepatic artery. The greater curvature is primarily supplied by both the right and the left gastroepiploic branches of the gastroduodenal artery and by the gastric branches of the splenic artery. The venous drainage of the stomach goes into the portal system directly or via the superior mesenteric and splenic veins.

The stomach is a muscular organ made up of an inner circular and an outer longitudinal layer. It is covered on its surface by serosa and is lined by velvety mucosa thrown up into rugal folds. The gastric glands are densely arranged, penetrate the whole thickness of the mucosa, and contain four types of cells: chief, parietal, mucous, and argentaffin. The distribution of these cells varies in different portions of the stomach. Beneath the mucosa, the submucosa contains abundant blood vessels, lymphatics, and loose connective tissue.

Lymphatics. The stomach has several networks of lymphatics: mucosal, submucosal, intermuscular, and subserosal. These networks freely intercommunicate with each other and, to a lesser extent, with those of the esophagus and the duo-

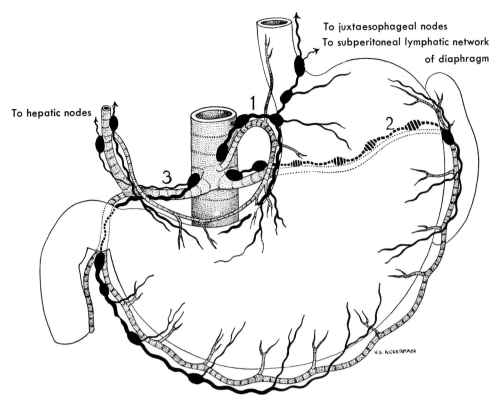

To juxtaesophageal nodes
To subperitoneal lymphatic network
of diaphragm

To hepatic nodes

V.5. ACKERMAN

Fig. 328. Lymphatic drainage of stomach showing collecting trunks of left gastric artery, **1**; splenic artery, **2**; hepatic artery, **3**.

denum. The subserosal lymphatics, which collect the lymph from all the other networks, are themselves drained by several lymphatic trunks (Fig. 328) that more or less follow the trajectory of the blood vessels:

1 The *left gastric artery collecting trunks* drain an extensive area comprising the medial two-thirds of the vertical portion of the stomach and drain into the lymph nodes that are generally grouped at the upper extremity of the lesser curvature. Some of the lymphatics of the anterior wall and those of the fundus may be interrupted by juxtacardiac lymph nodes, which are not always present.

2 The *splenic artery collecting trunks* drain all the remaining area outside of the left gastric artery chain, from the fundus to the middle portion of the greater curvature. They converge toward the lower pole of the spleen and end in the lymph nodes of the splenic artery chain which are found along the course of the gastroepiploic vessels and upper border of the spleen.

3 The *hepatic artery collecting trunks* drain the remaining area—i.e., the lower half of the greater curvature, the pyloric and the gastroepiploic areas. These end in the gastroepiploic lymph nodes, the infrapyloric lymph nodes, the retropancreaticoduodenal lymph nodes, and sometimes the superior mesenteric nodes (Rouvière[172]).

Epidemiology

In the 1947 cancer survey in the United States, the sex-age-adjusted incidence rates for cancer of the stomach were 34.8 and 18.8 for males and females, respectively, per 100,000 population. These rates have gradually declined in subsequent surveys. In 1962, the sex-age-adjusted rates in the state of Connecticut were 15.8 and 7.8 for males and females per 100,000. There is no reasonable explanation for this remarkable decrease in incidence, which has now become one of the lowest reported from any

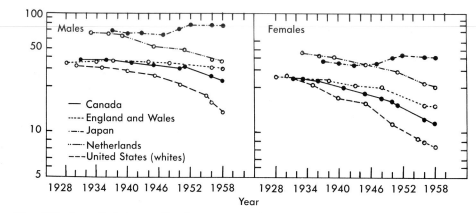

Fig. 329. Age-adjusted mortality from cancer of stomach.[78] (From Wynder, E. L., et al.: An epidemiological investigation of gastric cancer, Cancer **16**:1461-1496, 1963; WU neg. 69-2888.)

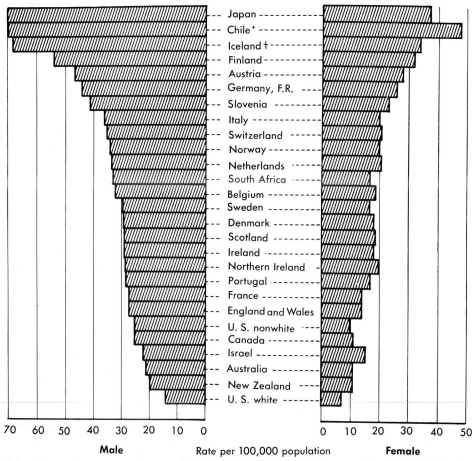

Fig. 330. Mortality from cancer of stomach, 1956-1957 (*1954-1955; †crude rate).[169a] (From Wynder, E. L., et al.: An epidemiological investigation of gastric cancer, Cancer **16**:1461-1496, 1963; WU neg. 69-187.)

country (Fig. 329). A low incidence also prevails in Canada, as well as in Africa and Southeast Asia. The highest incidence is reported in Japan, Iceland, Finland, the Soviet Union, Central Europe, and Chile (Fig. 330). In the United States, the incidence rates are relatively higher for both male and female nonwhites. Seldom observed in the United States in individuals under 35 years of age, the rates in 1960-1962 were 9.4 and 8.5 per 100,000 for males and females 40 to 44 years of age and 282 and 157 for those over 85 years of age.

The incidence of carcinoma of the stomach among Japanese living in the American West and Hawaii (Quisenberry[160]) is strikingly higher than that observed in other racial groups of the same community (Steiner[197]) and similar to the equally high incidence reported in Japan. There is also an excess of gastric cancer in foreign-born Americans from high-risk European countries. The tumor is relatively frequent among Chinese living in Java, whereas it is infrequent among native Indonesians (Kouwenaar[107]). The incidence seems also to be higher in European than in Asian immigrants in Israel (Tulchinsky and Modan[220]).

Sarcomas of the stomach make up 1% to 5% of all gastric neoplasms, and about 60% are lymphosarcomas. Taylor[217] found that the average age of patients with sarcomas of the stomach was about a decade less than that of patients with carcinomas.

Since cancer of the stomach has been observed among members of low socioeconomic groups (Terris and Hall[218]), it has been thought that it may be related to "inadequate" *diet* (Cramer[41]), yet it occurs infrequently among the indigenous people of Java (Sutomo[212]) and of North Africa in spite of subnormal diets. The incidence of gastric cancer has been related to diets low in fresh vegetables, fruits, and vitamins (Wynder et al.[232]). Stocks and Davies[202] have drawn apparent relationships between the zinc-copper ratio of garden soils and the householder's death from cancer of the stomach. Dungal and Sigurjonsson[48] found the amount of 3,4-benzopyrene obtainable from smoked and singed food to be greater in a northern district of Iceland where the relative occurrence of cancer of the stomach is higher.

In a study of genetic factors, Woolf[230] found that blood relatives of patients with cancer of the stomach exhibited a significantly greater frequency of gastric cancer than expected for the general population (Macklin[125]). Blood type A seems to be associated with a high risk (Berndt and Pietschker[17]; Hogg and Pack[90]).

Pernicious anemia is associated with a high occurrence of gastric cancer (Rubin[173]; Blackburn[21]), as are *achlorhydria* and *hypochlorhydria*. Shearman et al.[183] showed that the latter conditions and a low serum–vitamin B_{12} are observed before pernicious anemia develops and are often associated with cancer of the stomach. In a nine-year follow-up of 1747 patients with hypochlorhydria, achlorhydria, or pernicious anemia, Hitchcock et al.[88] observed carcinoma in nineteen and *gastric polyps* in forty-five. It is not possible to determine whether or not carcinomas arise from gastric polyps (Monaco et al.[136]). Cancer seems to be associated more often with multiple polyps (Pearl and Brunn[156]) than with single polyps (Stewart[199]). The relationship to *chronic gastritis* is controversial (Konjetzny[106]; Hurst[94]).

The remarkable decrease in the incidence of cancer of the stomach in the United States in the past thirty years is the best proof that its main causes are environmental, but the true cause or causes remain to be identified.

The relationship of *chronic gastric ulcer* to carcinoma of the stomach is also debated, but the majority of writers believe that benign chronic gastric ulcers show definite malignant transformation in a small number of patients. Mallory[126] presented the strongest dissenting opinion mainly on histologic grounds. At autopsy, the advanced stage of the tumor in most instances precludes study and obscures evidence of its development from an ulcer. But when gastrectomies are done for chronic gastric ulcers, a number of carcinomas, apparently arising from benign ulcers, are found. In a series of 362 resected carcinomas reported by Stout,[207] twenty-six (7%) had apparently developed in the margin of a preexisting chronic ulcer. Jordan[96] reported recurrence of ulcerlike lesions eight, fourteen, and twenty-three years after the original ulcer had apparently been healed, and a study of these recurrent ulcers showed that they had apparently become malignant.

Pathology
Gross and microscopic pathology

In practically all instances, carcinoma of the stomach arises from mucus-secreting cells. This adenocarcinoma has different patterns. Most clinicians, surgeons, and pathologists use a morphologic classification, for this bears some relation to prognosis. The following modified classification of carcinoma of the stomach is adapted from Borrmann[25]:

Superficial spreading carcinoma (carcinoma in situ, muco érosif à marche lente)

Gastric carcinoma apparently arising from previous chronic ulceration

Ulcerating carcinoma

Polypoid carcinoma

Linitis plastica

Advanced carcinomas (no specific type)

The number of cases found in each category will, to a large extent, depend on the source of the material. If postmortem material is studied, a high percentage of cases will be of no specific type. If the surgical material is from a hospital in which the clinical staff is cancer conscious, the roentgenologist is expert, and the surgical staff technically skilled and disposed to resect chronic gastric ulcers, this naturally will be reflected by an increased proportion of carcinomas apparently arising on the basis of preexisting ulcer and an increased number of small ulcerated or superficial carcinomas.

Carcinomas of the stomach usually arise in the pyloric region, pars media, or cardiac area. In 837 cases summarized by Oppolzer,[144] there were 456 in the pyloric region, 244 in the pars media, sixty-one in the cardiac area, fourteen in the region of the greater curvature, and in sixty-two instances the involvement was total. We have not seen carcinomas arising from parietal or chief cells. Squamous cell carcinoma of the stomach usually appears in the pyloric area. There have been only about twenty-five cases reported (Dreyer and Louw[45]). Squamous metaplasia can occur in the gastric mucosa. We have seen only one instance in the pyloric area. Morson[139] be-

lieves that about one-third of all carcinomas of the stomach arise from areas of metaplasia. Correa et al.[40a] believe the risk of gastric cancer is directly related to the prevalence of intestinal metaplasia. Squamous metaplasia can occur in gastric cancer. McPeak and Warren[124] presented evidence that more well-differentiated glandular tumors occur in the cardioesophageal junction than in other parts of the stomach. Squamous carcinoma arising in the esophagus can invade the stomach (Altschuler and Shaka[5]).

Superficially spreading carcinoma. The superficially spreading type of carcinoma, or, as Gutmann et al.[79] designate it, the *muco érosif à marche lente*, is usually limited to the mucosa but can involve the submucosa. This lesion often originates near the pylorus and frequently is associated with irregular, superficial, serpiginous ulcerations that have been known to reach 5 cm or 6 cm in diameter. The base of the ulcer has a diffuse reddish tint, and the mucosa frequently presents a slight nodulation. The pyloric ring muscles frequently show hypertrophy (Fig. 331). The muscularis is not involved (Gutmann et al.[79]). It shows multiple microscopic areas of change in the overlying epithelium with disturbances of architecture and replacement by the glandular type of carcinoma. At times, there is normal epithelium between the areas of disease that, as Mallory[126] indicated, may have multiple foci of origin. The two most common gross characteristics of the disease are its wide extension and its superficiality (Stout[206]). Externally, the stomach appears normal, and even when it is open, there may be doubt as to the presence of tumor, especially if there is no obvious ulceration. It is not known just how often carcinoma begins in this fashion, but superficially spreading carcinomas are seen with increasing frequency in clinics where patients are referred for early gastrointestinal study and where surgical resection is frequently done. Golden and Stout[73] were able to collect thirty-one cases of this type of gastric tumor between 1937 and 1947 at the Presbyterian Hospital in New York City.

Gastric carcinoma arising on basis of previous chronic ulceration. We believe

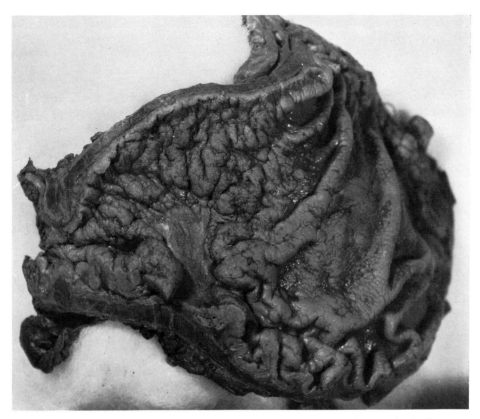

Fig. 331. Superficially spreading type of carcinoma of stomach with superficial ulceration, wide submucosal extension, and hypertrophy of muscles of pylorus. (Courtesy Dr. A. P. Stout, New York, N. Y.)

that an extremely small number of gastric ulcers can undergo carcinomatous changes and that the validity of such an assumption depends primarily upon the pathologic study. Benign chronic gastric ulcers occur on the lesser curvature and at the pylorus, whereas carcinoma is most frequently found in the prepyloric and cardiac areas. The typical chronic ulcer has punched-out, well-defined margins with overhanging edges. Small benign chronic ulcers are circular, but large ones are oval and are parallel to the long axis of the stomach. On section, the ulcer shows diffuse fibrosis of its wall with replacement of the muscularis and fibrosis and thickening of the serosal surface. Partially obliterated blood vessels may be seen. An ulcer of this variety that has recently become carcinomatous seldom shows enough macroscopic changes to justify a definite diagnosis of cancer. At times, near the margins of the ulcer there is, poorly defined, slightly elevated submucosal thickening. As the carcinoma grows, it tends to obliterate the old ulcer, but replacement of the base of the ulcer is delayed until last. Stoerk[203] believes that radiating gastric folds extending around a carcinoma are evidence of a preexisting benign ulcer.

The histologic criteria for making a diagnosis of carcinoma arising on the basis of a preexisting chronic ulceration are as follows: The base of the ulcer is devoid of carcinoma, and there is invariably destruction of the muscularis with replacement by dense fibrous tissue. The ulcer floor is made up of scar and granulation tissue. The free ends of the muscle are bent upward into the ulcer margin and are sharply demarcated against the connective tissue of the base (Klein[105]). Often there is fibrous thickening on the serosal surface that is continuous with the base of the ulcer. Small arterioles are often obliterated. These signs indicate a process of long duration. Carcinoma usually occurs in the margins of the ulcer in single or multiple zones and presents a disorderly glandular pattern. As the disease spreads, it extends out to the serosal surface, and only in an advanced stage is the base of the ulcer invaded. Fusion of the muscularis mucosae and the muscularis propria is said by Newcomb[141] to occur in 100% of the patients with chronic peptic ulceration. Gomori[75] felt that the presence of this sign depends predominantly upon the stage of the ulceration and found actual fusion in only thirty-four of sixty-four cases. Carcinoma only rarely occurs on the basis of a healed scar due to preexisting ulcer. A primary carcinoma may ulcerate, but the loss of substance rarely transgresses the true muscular coat except in superficial spreading carcinoma. In this type, peptic ulceration with destruction of the entire wall of the stomach is not unusual (Bralow and Collins[27]).

Ulcerating carcinoma. The primary ulcerating carcinoma has shallow rather than overhanging edges, with fairly extensive and sometimes nodular submucosal infiltration around the borders of the ulcer (Fig. 332, *A*). Sections of the ulcer show partial or complete replacement of the muscularis by tumor, but there is no fibrosis. As this tumor becomes larger, the ulceration becomes deeper and the submucosal extent becomes greater (Fig. 332, *B*). Vascular changes are not present. Ulcerating carcinoma shows no microscopic evidence of

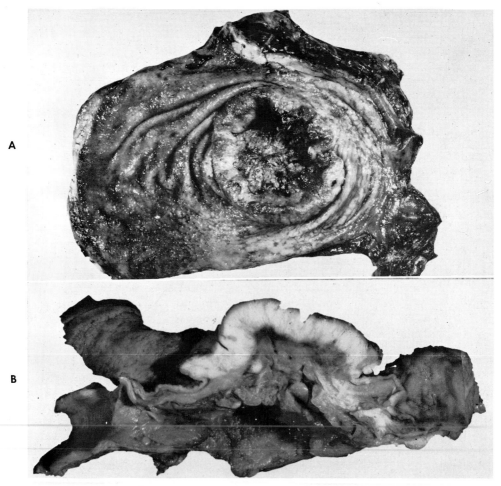

Fig. 332. A, Primary ulcerating carcinoma, fairly well delineated, with nodular infiltration around periphery. **B,** Cross section showing invasion of entire wall of stomach by grayish white tumor.

a previously existing chronic process. The tumor infiltrates all layers of the stomach, tends to spread submucosally, and is present throughout the entire ulcer bed.

Polypoid carcinoma. Pearl and Brunn[156] divided polyps into two varieties:

1 The neoplastic variety with a definite stalk freely movable on the submucosa, with the muscularis mucosa within this stalk and normal mucous membrane between the polyps

2 The inflammatory hyperplasias or pseudopolyps, which are flatter, do not present a definite stalk, are immovable on the submucosa, and have no invagination of the muscularis mucosae

Polypoid carcinomas are well delineated, grow mainly within the lumen of the stomach, and may become very large, particularly if they are in areas such as the cardia, where obstruction can only occur late.

Linitis plastica. Linitis plastica is a rare variant of carcinoma which, because of its rarity and its somewhat bizarre nature, has

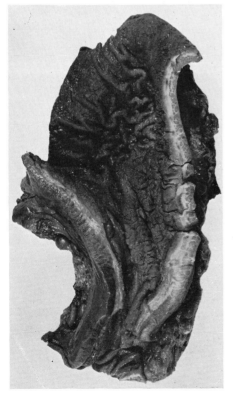

Fig. 333. Carcinoma of stomach, linitis plastica type. Note small size of stomach and hypertrophy of muscularis.

been the subject of profuse writings and frequent illustrations far beyond its merit. Stomachs affected by these tumors are often referred to as the leather-bottle type because of shrinkage of the organ. In an advanced stage, the wall of the stomach is markedly thickened, and fibrous nodules may be seen on its serosal surface. A cross section of the stomach reveals considerable hypertrophy of the muscularis, which is particularly prominent in the pyloric area (Fig. 333). Bands of fibrous tissue can be seen coursing through the wall of the stomach, which is rigid with a cartilaginous consistency, and the submucosa is thickened. Fairly frequently, there is an associated ulcer in the pyloric region. The mucosa is invariably firmly fixed to the submucosa and later, in the more advanced stages, to the muscularis (Saphir and Parker[175]).

Microscopically, there may be a great deal of difficulty in diagnosing linitis plastica because of the overproduction of connective tissue. A mucin stain may be helpful. This fibrosis is hyaline in some areas and is accompanied by large numbers of inflammatory cells, particularly plasma and mononuclear cells. The fibrosis extends not only to the submucosa but replaces areas of muscularis and is also present on the serosal surface. There is hypertrophy of the muscularis, and areas of superficial ulceration may be present. Because of the inflammation and fibrosis and the small number of tumor cells present, this lesion was thought for many years to be only inflammatory (Saphir and Parker[175]).

Advanced carcinoma. Advanced carcinoma unfortunately makes up the greatest proportion of tumors of the stomach. Its frequency is naturally extremely high in postmortem studies. The tumor is usually very large, replacing wide areas in the stomach, and is often a combination of the fungating and the invasive types. Its appearance depends on its mucin production, cellularity, and the connective tissue content.

• • •

All carcinomas of the stomach are adenocarcinomas, varying only in degree of differentiation from very well-differentiated (Fig. 334) to disorderly, bizarre patterns. If multiple sections are taken, the pattern

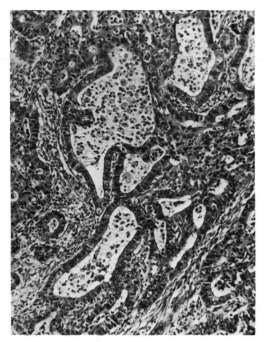

Fig. 334. Typical fairly well-differentiated adenocarcinoma of stomach. (Moderate enlargement.)

often varies from section to section. The amount of connective tissue in the tumor will also vary from minimal to extreme desmoplasia. The same may be said of mucin production, which is variable. With mucin stains, however, practically every case will reveal small amounts of mucin in a few cells, or perhaps the entire lesion will contain an overwhelming amount of mucus with only a few carcinoma cells floating within it. At times, blood vessel invasion may be seen.

A study of the local spread of carcinoma of the stomach is important, particularly from the standpoint of treatment and prognosis. The superficially spreading variety may involve as much as 50 sq cm of the mucosa and submucosa. The linitis plastica also may involve large areas by direct extension. Grossly, this extension is manifested by nodular thickening and fixation of the mucosa. It was once thought that the spread of carcinoma of the stomach stopped at the pylorus, but study of resected specimens (Castleman[34]) and of autopsy material in carcinomas originating close to the pylorus has demonstrated invasion (in 25% to 30% of the cases) of as much as 6 cm (Zinninger and Collins[235])

of the duodenum. Extension takes place mostly through lymphatics, and tumor can involve any layer of the duodenum (Paramananandhan[153]). A rare instance of extensive spread to the entire length of the small and large bowels has been reported (Lumb[116]). In advanced carcinoma, tumor nodules are often seen on the serosal surface of the stomach, and not infrequently there is direct extension to the liver, diaphragm, transverse colon, pancreas, and hilus of the spleen.

Gastritis probably should not be divided into hypertrophic or atrophic varieties but should simply be called *chronic gastritis*. When associated with advanced carcinoma, gastritis is usually found either surrounding the tumor or as a pangastritis. It has an inflammatory and an epithelial component. The inflammatory element is made up of an increased number of plasma cells and lymphocytes, with focal accumulations of lymphocytes that at times form germinal follicles. Along with these changes there is interglandular fibrosis. The epithelial changes (most important) are related to dedifferentiation of the specific cells to nonspecific mucous glands and the formation of epithelium resembling that in the large bowel. Large cystic glands are often present. However, the association of achlorhydria, hypochlorhydria, pernicious anemia, and gastric atrophy is well established. Frequently, gastric atrophy is accompanied by polyps and/or cancer. At times, the carcinomas may show multiple foci of origin. The relationship between atrophy and cancer appears well established.

Lymphosarcoma of the stomach has several gross variants—it may form a large, lobulated, soft tumor mass growing within the lumen of the stomach (Fig. 335), it may form disclike areas, or, rarely, it may have diffuse involvement with giant rugae resembling cerebral convolutions. It commonly shows ulceration, which is the reason it is mistaken grossly and roentgenographically for carcinoma (Thorbjarnarson et al.[219]). These tumors gradually increase in size, invade the muscularis, form a subserosal tumor, infrequently obstruct the lumen with polypoid masses, and occasionally form diffuse thickenings of the stomach wall. They most often involve the cur-

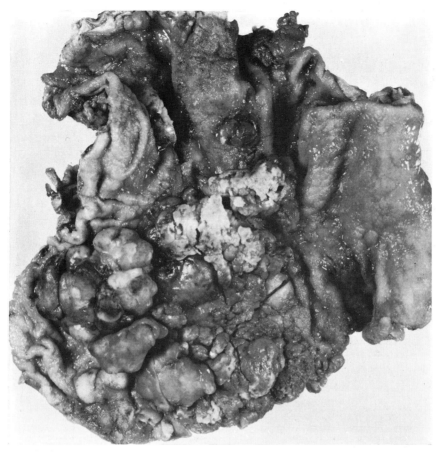

Fig. 335. Huge polypoid lymphosarcoma of stomach in 62-year-old woman. There were two involved lymph nodes. (WU neg. 50-496.)

vatures of the stomach. Of seventy-four cases in which there were available data (Taylor[217]), there was involvement of one or both curvatures in fifty-five, diffuse involvement in ten, and pyloric stenosis in only six.

The same microscopic types of lymphosarcoma occur in the stomach as are found elsewhere. There is no difficulty in establishing the diagnosis when tumor is present in the stomach (Figs. 336 and 337) and also in the regional lymph nodes. It has been shown that ulcerated and polypoid lesions of the stomach involving all layers, but without involvement of lymph nodes, may represent *pseudolymphosarcoma* of the stomach. These lesions can be recognized microscopically by the intermingling of plasma cells, the formation of germinal centers, and, most important, the *absence of lymph node involvement* (Faris and Saltzstein[60]). Obviously, lymphosarcoma of the stomach may exist in the absence of lymph node involvement, but the pathologist must be wary of the diagnosis of lymphosarcoma under such circumstances.

The second most common form of malignant mesenchymal tumors of the stomach is the *leiomyosarcoma*. These tumors arise from the gastric muscularis and present the same gross characteristics as the leiomyomas except that they may be softer and more cellular. The microscopic evidence of malignancy in a leiomyoma is the presence of numerous mitotic figures, necrosis, and a bizarre cellular pattern. Highly undifferentiated leiomyosarcomas are rare (Marshall[130]). Conversely, on rare occasion, a smooth muscle tumor appearing perfectly benign microscopically may metastasize. Other types of sarcomas are rare.

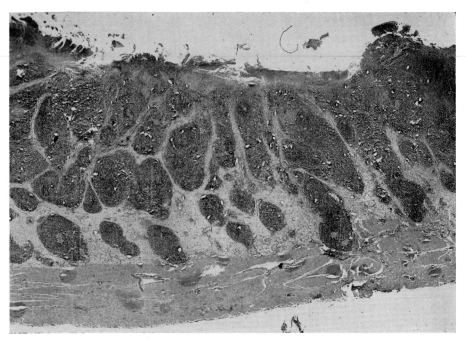

Fig. 336. Diffuse infiltration of stomach wall. (Low power; from Snoddy, W. T.: Primary lymphosarcoma of the stomach, Gastroenterology **20:**537-553, 1952.)

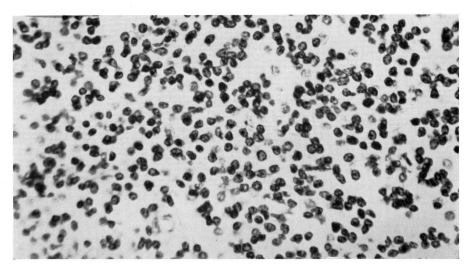

Fig. 337. Characteristic lymphosarcoma of lymphatic type of stomach. (High-power enlargement.)

Metastatic spread

Depending greatly upon the care with which surgical specimens are examined, the largest proportion of operable carcinomas of the stomach show evidence of lymph node metastases. Coller et al.[39] demonstrated metastases in 75% of their patients. Eker[53] found a greater proportion of metastases accompanying the total than the partial gastric resections. About 25% of all surgical specimens (Meissner[134]) and 10% of all cases observed at autopsy (Stout[204]) do not present lymph node metastases. Most metastases are found in the inferior gastric, subpyloric, and celiac axis nodes whenever the carcinoma arises in the distal portion (Berry and Rott-schafer[19]), whereas the pancreaticolineal, pericardial, and superior gastric nodes are most often invaded when the primary lesion arises in the proximal portion of the stomach (Sunderland et al.[210]). In advanced stages, the para-aortic and supra-diaphragmatic nodes become implicated; peritoneal implants appear and gravitation of neoplastic cells may create a rectal shelf. Liver metastases are frequent. Lymphangitic metastases of the lung are not infrequently observed, and the proportion of bone and ovarian metastases found is relatively small.

Of thirty-one cases of *superficially spreading* carcinoma studied by Golden and Stout,[73] only fifteen showed lymph node metastases. *Polypoid carcinomas* metastasize less frequently than *sessile carcinomas.* Carcinomas of the *linitis plastica* type may spread through submucosal, intramuscular, and subserosal tissue spaces and lymphatic channels. They are accompanied by fibrosis and give rise to an extensive thickening of the esophagus, small intestine, and colon (Fernet et al.[62]).

Lymphosarcoma commonly involves the perigastric and adjacent retroperitoneal lymph nodes, and metastases to spleen, pancreas, and liver are common. Generalized spread occurs late in the disease. *Leiomyosarcomas* metastasize only rarely to regional lymph nodes but metastasize frequently to lungs, liver, and other distant organs.

Clinical evolution
Nonpainful gastrointestinal symptoms

In the majority of instances, the patient with carcinoma of the stomach notices a vague epigastric uneasiness after meals with moderate distention and a sense of heaviness in the epigastrium. Most patients give no history of previous gastrointestinal disturbances. The indefinite symptoms may be accompanied by relatively easy physical and mental fatigue and an inexplicable distaste for food, particularly meat. With the continuation of the symptoms, a slow but progressive weight loss may ensue, accompanied by a minimal degree of secondary anemia. Unfortunately, during this period the diagnosis of cancer of the stomach is seldom considered. The patient is classed as neurotic, given symptomatic medication for the anorexia, and treated for the anemia without resort to diagnostic roentgenology. As the disease progresses, the diagnosis is clarified by symptoms due to pyloric obstruction, extreme weight loss, or some other easily recognizable clinical finding.

Ulcer variety (painful)

The ulcer type of symptoms occurs much less frequently. Sometimes gastrointestinal symptoms are present for a number of years. These occur periodically and are relieved by alkaline powders, food, or other symptomatic remedies. Pain occurs shortly after eating and may be relatively severe, but the character of this pain may change to become more persistent and oppressive and be associated with weight loss. In 6.4% of 1000 cases of proved carcinoma reported by LaDue et al.,[109] an ulcer syndrome appeared. The administration of an ulcer regimen may engender considerable clinical improvement, but if the symptoms are caused by carcinoma, they eventually recur. In 25% of a series of 274 patients with carcinomas, Eker and Efskind[54] found a long history of gastric distress. In 15% there was great probability of a previous ulcer, and in 8% there was unquestionable histopathologic evidence of previous ulcer. Pain and dysphagia are often the first symptoms of carcinomas of the proximal third of the stomach (Eisenbud and Finby[51]).

Ihre et al.[95] operated on 593 patients with gastric ulcers that had been diagnosed as benign and found 6.2% to be malignant. They also treated medically 473 patients with gastric ulcers and, after a follow-up of from ten to twenty-five years, found that 1.9% developed carcinoma. Of 278 patients treated for gastric ulcer and followed for five to twelve years, Rønnov-Jessen et al.[171] reported that one case of lymphosarcoma and ten of carcinoma developed and estimated that nine of these were present from the beginning.

A follow-up study of 222 patients who had had a partial gastrectomy for gastric or duodenal ulcer revealed eleven cases of cancer in the gastric stump occurring, on an average, twenty years after the operation (Helsingen and Hillestad[85]). In the gastric ulcer group, the subsequently observed occurrence of gastric cancer was three times higher than expected. Gray and Lofgren[77] reported on fifty-two patients who developed gastric ulcers after gastroenterostomy, with eleven of forty-one operated upon for duodenal ulcer developing cancer and six of eleven operated upon for gastric ulcer developing carcinoma. In Liavaag's series,[115] the occurrence of subsequent carcinoma was the same as expected for the general population.

Occult carcinoma

Unfortunately, in a number of instances carcinoma of the stomach may cause no complaints that could lead to an early diagnosis. The patient may not present weight loss or pain, and the first symptoms are due to metastatic disease. This may be manifested by an enlargement of the abdomen due to a nodular liver or the presence of fluid. Rarely, dyspnea will ensue due to lymphangitic lung metastases. In other instances, jaundice or anemia or a supraclavicular metastasis develops.

• • •

Whatever their clinical type of onset, carcinomas of the stomach resemble each other in their terminal stages. The patients lose a great deal of weight and may develop considerable pain, and symptoms and signs of obstruction may occur due to the tumor occluding the esophagus or pylorus which, in itself, may cause death. Without obstruction, bleeding from a large ulcerating lesion occurs, and obstinate, progressive, severe anemia with palpitation and weakness is apparent. Ascites may occur, and in a few instances the tumor may metastasize to lymph nodes around the bile ducts and cause a terminal jaundice. In relatively rare instances, the tumor may perforate, and a terminal peritonitis follows. Often bronchopneumonia is the immediate cause of death.

Lymphosarcoma of the stomach may be very slow or rapid in evolution. The patients very frequently have pain of the ulcer type (Joseph and Lattes[97]). Dyspepsia, anorexia, and weight loss are common. It is interesting that *obstructive phenomena in lymphosarcoma of the stomach are infrequent.* As the disease progresses, sec- ondary clinical signs such as weakness and profound weight loss appear. Hematemesis may be the first symptom of a lymphosarcoma (Stout[207]). Bleeding into the gastrointestinal tract, persistent diarrhea, and melena are common. Lymphosarcoma may perforate, causing an acute abdominal syndrome that suggests a benign condition. *Leiomyosarcoma* may also cause hematemesis and bleeding into the intestinal tract with consequent anemia.

Diagnosis
Early diagnosis

The appalling extent of carcinomas found after a short clinical history, the high proportion of cases that have metastasized at the time of operation, and the rather poor results obtained by radical treatment naturally demand that efforts be made to diagnose cancer of the stomach before its presence has made itself obvious. The systematic radioscopic examination of asymptomatic individuals, promising in theory, has met with discouraging practical difficulties. The periodic radioscopic examination of symptomless individuals past 40 years of age is a painstaking, prohibitively costly task even in a limited group (Kirklin and Hodgson[102]). St. John et al.[174] reported on a series of 2432 individuals over the age of 50 years with no digestive symptoms in whom two carcinomas and one lymphosarcoma of the stomach were discovered in routine radioscopic examination. But the radioscopic examination of such a large number of individuals to find a few tumors makes this method of attack unrealistic. The theoretical yield of an examination of 1000 men 65 years of age or older is only one case of cancer of the stomach (Levin[114]). As a protective measure, the procedure would have to be repeated periodically.

A simplification of the roentgenologic examination in order to make it more applicable to mass surveys cannot be done without sacrificing a great part of its merits. To limit the examination to radioscopy alone is not a simplification or saving, for this would take more of the roentgenologist's time, which is the major expense involved (Rigler[167]). Roentgenographic examination alone would be simpler, but the results would lack precision. *Photofluorog-*

raphy has the advantages of saving the roentgenologist's time and of being relatively inexpensive. Roach reported on a total of 10,000 photofluorographic gastrointestinal examinations and asserted the usefulness of the method but questioned its practical value in increasing the curability of carcinoma of the stomach.

A number of carcinomas of the stomach are found in the periodic roentgenologic examination of patients presenting mild symptoms, patients with atrophic gastritis, pernicious anemia, achlorhydria, hypochlorhydria (less than 20% free acid), unexplained anemia (less than 11 gm % of hemoglobin), and repeated occult blood in feces, and patients with known gastric polyps. Such patients should have periodic examinations by competent roentgenologists (Rigler[167]), and when possible gastroscopy and exfoliative cytology should be done. State et al.[194] reported on a series of 1540 patients who were found to be achlorhydric or hypochlorhydric: 1832 roentgenologic examinations were made, yielding seven carcinomas and thirty-two gastric polyps, and three other carcinomas were missed through error.

It is of paramount importance that the clinician direct his efforts to diagnose carcinoma of the stomach when the symptomatology is still uncertain and the diagnosis difficult. Early symptoms, when present, are often mild and frequently attributed to less serious causes. The delay that takes place between the onset of symptoms and proper diagnosis is, in part, due to self ministrations of remedies possibly encouraged by advertisements of "relief for acid indigestion" (Welch[227]; Welch and Allen[228]), with the result that many carcinomas of the stomach are "buried under mounds of powder" (Finch[64]). The wishful-thinking attitude of the patient is sometimes matched only by that of his physician, who may try to eliminate all other possible explanations for the common symptoms before arriving at the diagnosis of cancer. The problem of cancer of the stomach will not show any favorable change unless the physician confronted with anorexia, dyspepsia, slow digestion, or asthenia in a patient over 40 years of age *thinks of cancer first* and appropriately eliminates that possibility before embarking on medical management. One important type of case is the patient with an apparently typical history of gastric ulcer. If the patient has no previous history of ulcers, the physician should be particularly careful in establishing a roentgenologic diagnosis. But even when there has been previous successful medical management of a gastric ulcer and when the ulcer is found in the lesser curvature, the possibility of carcinoma is not entirely eliminated, and close observation of the patient, repeated roentgenologic study, exploration, and surgical treatment should be decided upon without delay. The fact that patients may not return until symptoms have persisted for too long is a reflection on the physician, for the patient should be properly warned from the beginning of the various possibilities and of the necessity for a close follow-up.

Clinical examination

Some carcinomas of the stomach may be diagnosed at a fairly early stage because of symptoms of esophageal or pyloric obstruction. The diagnosis of advanced carcinoma of the stomach can be made at a glance. The emaciated elderly patient, usually a man with marked loss of weight, with a large palpable mass, and with ascites, is familiar. In a few instances, the clinical signs and symptoms of metastases will be noticed first.

On inspection of a patient with early carcinoma of the stomach, usually nothing is observed. However, if obstruction exists, there may be evidence of weight loss, and in certain instances the mucous membranes may appear pale due to anemia. The patient should be scrutinized carefully for the presence of mild jaundice. If this is present, it very frequently means obstruction of the biliary tree due to metastatic lymph nodes. At times, the falciform ligament is involved by tumor that spreads down to implicate the umbilicus. Peristaltic waves going from left to right may be seen in early obstruction. If the lesion is in the region of the pylorus and the patient has lost any considerable amount of weight, a large dilated stomach can be visualized easily. The supraclavicular and axillary regions should be palpated in search of enlarged lymph nodes. At times, a firm, painless mass may be felt within the abdomen.

It is not rare to find a large nodular liver also. A rectal palpation is imperative, for the presence of a rectal shelf means advanced disease. A rectal shelf is due to peritoneal metastases in the cul-de-sac. These metastases produce some connective tissue and form a mass. This is felt on rectal examination as a poorly defined, extramucosal, constricting nodular mass. It is usually associated with ascites.

Patients with *lymphosarcoma* of the stomach are generally young, although not infrequently aged (McNeer and Berg[120]), and may present a good general condition. Epigastric tenderness or rigidity may be the only physical finding (Redd[163]), but a palpable mass is felt in a number of other patients. In those with advanced disease there may be striking weight loss, melena, and generalized adenopathy. Nonlymphomatous sarcomas of the gastric wall are seldom palpable, and they may be entirely silent. They may be accompanied by symptoms of obstruction, melena, and pain.

Roentgenologic examination

The roentgenologic examination is the most important step toward the diagnosis of cancer of the stomach (Fig. 338). However, the procedure does not yield its full usefulness unless the technique is adequate and thorough *and unless it is carried out by a competent roentgenologist.* Faulty technique, inadequate use of radioscopy, or the entrusting of the examination to inexperienced or unsupervised personnel is dangerous. In the roentgenologic exploration of the stomach, radioscopy is a much more important procedure than radiography. Radioscopic study of mucosal patterns, of the mobility and distensibility of the entire stomach, of the flexibility and pliability of its walls, and of the progress of peristaltic waves is of paramount importance. In addition, radioscopy offers the opportunity of observation from different angles and of observing the changes imposed on the apparent abnormality by pressure from outside. Spot films are chosen during the course of radioscopy for careful study, for purposes of comparison or reproduction, and for permanent records.

The early roentgenologic signs caused by carcinoma of the stomach may be limited to changes in the mucosal pattern, or the lesion may be exophytic and produce a filling defect (Fig. 339). Rarely, infiltrating lesions produce only rigidity of

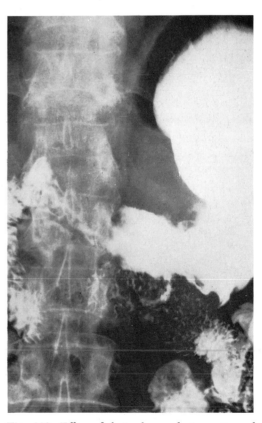

Fig. 339. Filling defect of prepyloric portion of stomach produced by carcinoma.

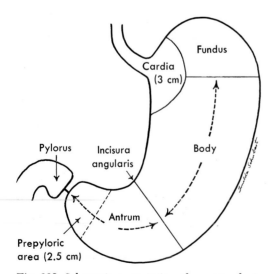

Fig. 338. Schematic presentation of roentgenologic appearance of stomach with arbitrary subdivisions.

the stomach wall and, more rarely, they are ulcerated and show a defect. Superficially spreading carcinomas usually obliterate the mucosal folds of the pyloric region, smoothing the surface and changing the wave form, and there may be spasm in the immediate neighborhood of the lesion (Gutmann et al.[79]; Golden and Stout[73]; Sherman and Wilner[185]). The discovery of this early lesion is definitely the exclusive domain of roentgenology and depends on wise utilization of radioscopy. Carcinomas of the cardiac region of the stomach may sometimes be seen to fungate into the air bubble (Fig. 341). Examination of this area is handicapped by its inaccessibility to palpation and pressure, but difficulties encountered elsewhere, such as peristalsis, tone changes, etc., do not interfere with the examination in this area (Sherman[184]). A review of 269 cases of carcinoma of the proximal third of the stomach showed that only 72% had been

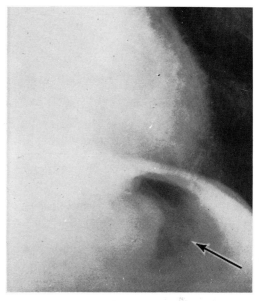

Fig. 341. Routine chest film of male adult. Air in fundus of stomach demonstrated shadow of unsuspected carcinoma. (WU neg. 56-538.)

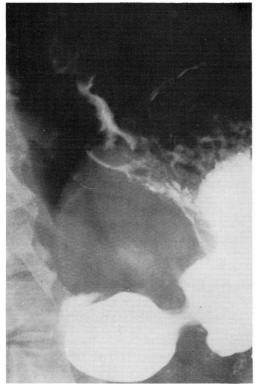

Fig. 340. Carcinoma of esophagogastric junction with only three weeks' history proved to have extensive lymph node and pulmonary metastases. (Courtesy Dr. R. R. Anderson, Colorado Springs, Colo.)

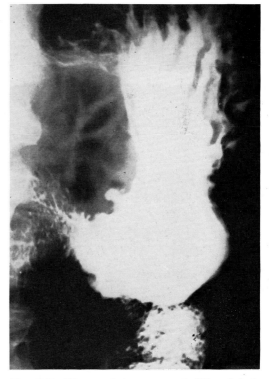

Fig. 342. Characteristic extramural filling defect of lesser curvature due to benign chronic ulcer.

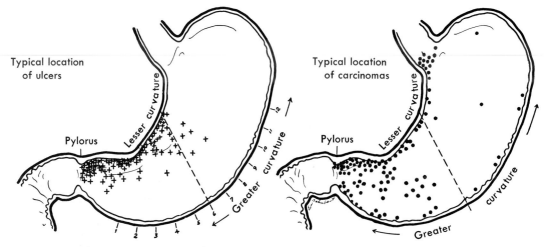

Fig. 343. Note concentration of benign lesions on lesser curvature. Malignant ulcers are common in prepyloric area and occur high on lesser curvature and almost exclusively on greater curvature. (Adapted from Stout, A. P.: Tumors of stomach, Bull. N. Y. Acad. Med. **23:** 101-108, 1947.)

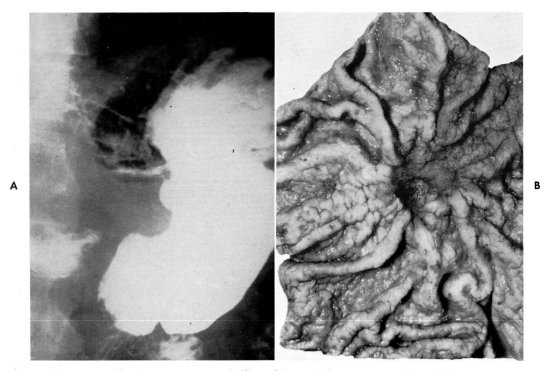

Fig. 344. A, Characteristic extramural filling defect of chronic gastric ulcer of lesser curvature. **B,** Convergence of folds into bed of ulcer shown in **A.**

correctly diagnosed (Finby and Eisenbud[63]). A division or splashing of the stream of barium in its passage from the esophagus to the stomach may indicate the presence of a tumor in this zone.

The changes are often present both in the esophagus and in the stomach.

If too much barium is used or if the examination is not methodical and careful, a lesion in the cardia may pass unsuspected.

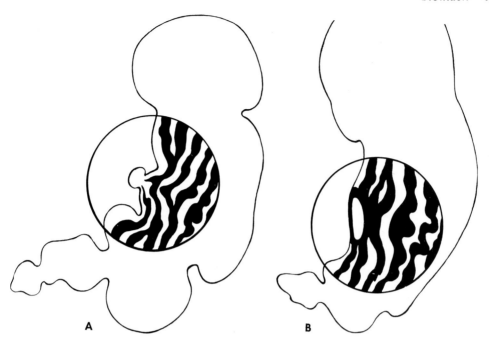

Fig. 345. A, Chronic gastric ulcer, extramural in character, with rugae extending into ulcer. **B,** Intramural malignant ulcer with effacement of rugae and meniscus sign.

Carcinoma of the stomach may present in the form of an ulcer. The prepyloric area is an extremely common site of cancer, so that ulcers in that area should be considered with extreme suspicion (Fig. 339). The majority of ulcers in the lesser curvature are benign (Figs. 342 to 344). Halolike margins surrounding an ulcer signify carcinoma almost without exception (Carman[33]). A markedly irregular or ragged crater invariably denotes cancer (Palmer[151]). Rugal patterns are often effaced around malignant ulcers (Fig. 345).

The roentgenologic diagnosis of advanced carcinoma is relatively easy, for often a palpable mass is felt, and fluoroscopy shows an extensive filling defect with ragged outline and perhaps an extragastric mass with delay in the passage of barium through the pyloric area. The leather-bottle shape of the stomach in linitis plastica is typical (Fig. 346). The accuracy of the roentgen diagnosis of carcinoma of the stomach varies, of course, according to institutions. In a review of 861 cases, Amberg[6] found 7.8% false positive diagnoses and 8.4% false negative diagnoses.

The filling defect caused by *lymphosarcomas* of the stomach may present smooth

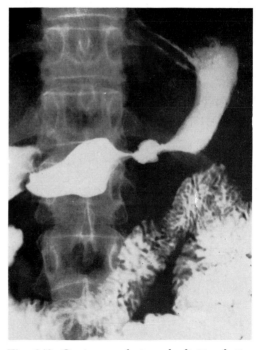

Fig. 346. Carcinoma of stomach, linitis plastica type, with leather-bottle-shape deformity and prepyloric ulceration.

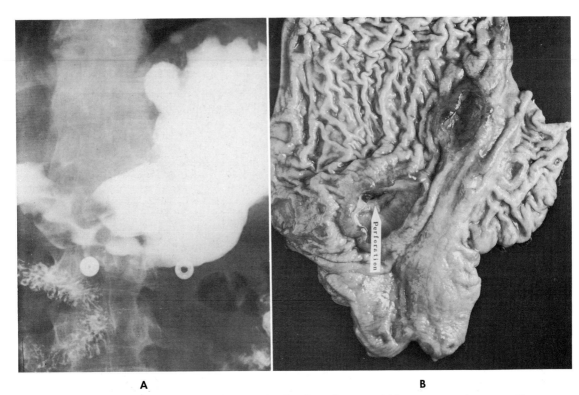

A　　　　　　　　　　　　　　　　　　　　**B**

Fig. 347. **A,** Multiple gastric ulcerations and enlarged gastric folds in region of antrum. **B,** Surgical specimen of lesion shown in **A** illustrating gross appearance of lymphosarcoma of stomach with perforation of gastric wall. (From Sherrick, D. W., et al.: The roentgenologic diagnosis of primary gastric lymphoma, Radiology **84:**925-932, 1965.)

margins (Förssman[67]). A roentgenologic diagnosis of lymphosarcoma is usually associated with the presence of giant rugae with pliable walls (Horst and Lessman[93]), but this tumor can also produce a large superficial ulcer on the posterior wall or lesser curvature, a large tumor with dilatation rather than obstruction of the pyloric area, and separate polypoid lesions in combination with giant rugae (Sherrick et al.[186]) (Fig. 347).

The problems of roentgenologic diagnosis of cancer of the stomach are various (Shanks[182]). A *small lesion* may be missed because of excess barium or insufficient study of mucosal patterns. An *unusual* carcinoma may appear as a local rigidity of the wall, simulating a healed ulcer. A lesion arising in *inaccessible sites,* such as the cardia, may be missed because of difficulty in palpation. *Previous deformity* of the stomach due to surgical interventions or concomitant pathology may be the cause of confusion. Ulcerlike lesions and those

situated in the pyloric area may be most difficult to interpret. But by far the greatest problems are the expense of the procedure plus the necessity for unusual skill. Consequently roentgenographic examination is not utilized often or early enough. Selective celiac trunk arteriography has been used in stomach lesions. It does not have too much practical value, but in malignant tumors it can define the shape and extent of the neoplasm.

Often lung metastases from carcinoma of the stomach are of the lymphangitic variety which may be so uniform as to be misinterpreted as pulmonary fibrosis. The roentgenologic appearance of these metastases is that of a stringlike design radiating from the hilus toward the periphery and branching to become a fine webbing of delicate striations punctuated by denser miliary nodules. The pattern is more marked in the middle and lower lobes (Wu[231]; Schattenberg and Ryan[178]) (Fig. 348).

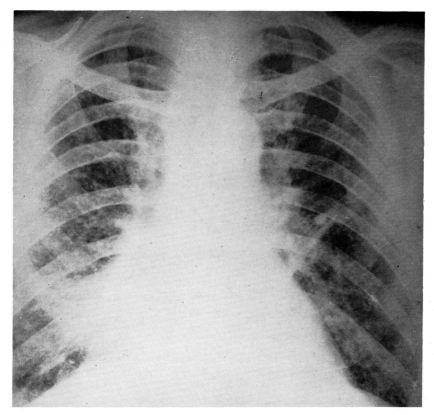

Fig. 348. Lymphangitic metastases from carcinoma of stomach. Note radiating bands extending from hilum to periphery and prominent mediastinal shadows due to implicated lymph nodes.

Gastroscopic examination

With the advent of the flexible gastroscope, gastroscopic examination of the stomach has become widely used (Morrissey et al.[138]). Furthermore, the fiberscope permits taking biopsy and cytologic specimens under direct vision with increased accuracy (Gear et al.[72]). It should be emphasized that while this examination is technically simple and usually without danger in skillful hands, there are contraindications to the procedure, such as esophageal varices, esophageal obstruction, and aortic aneurysm. While the technical ability to perform this examination is important, it is not nearly so important as the ability to recognize and interpret the various lesions seen.

Comparisons are often made between gastroscopic and roentgenologic examination. Such comparisons are not helpful, for gastroscopy is another examination that supplements roentgenologic study but does not compete with it. It should be emphasized that in considering one or the other of these procedures the quality of results obtained depends greatly on the caliber of the men who do the work. Certain areas of the stomach cannot be visualized through the gastroscope: the upper part of the greater curvature, the portion of the fundus that infringes on the diaphragm, and the part of the posterior wall on which the gastroscope rests. The prepyloric area can be visualized only if there is favorable peristalsis, but a good part of the lesser and greater curvatures may be satisfactorily studied in most cases.

The gastroscopic examination may be of value in the differentiation of chronic gastritis from neoplasms. Also, in a few instances, it may discover tumors that were not seen roentgenologically. In the presence of obvious carcinoma, the gastroscopist is not capable of determining the extent of the involvement nor can he evaluate operability. The gastroscopic examination in *lymphosarcoma* may reveal hypertrophy of rugal folds with intact, though somewhat stiffened, mucous membrane (Rafsky et al.[161]), but when ulceration occurs, the appearance is indistinguishable from that of carcinoma (Renshaw and Spencer[164]).

Biopsy through an operating gastroscope is possible. Benedict[12, 13] reported on sixty-three gastroscopic biopsies without complications, but the specimens obtained may be inadequate for histologic diagnosis. Gastroscopic examination should be reserved for difficult diagnostic problems. Gastroscopic biopsy is most helpful in the differential diagnosis of gastritis, lymphoma, and diffuse carcinoma (Benedict[14]). Positive microscopic diagnoses of malignant tumors are conclusive (Shallenberger et al.[181]). Debray et al.[43] reported on gastric biopsy by means of a suction apparatus. There were no complications but a high proportion of false negative results.

Gastric photography

The diagnosis of gastric lesions is definitely aided by the skillful use of intragastric photography with a specially designed camera (Hoon[91]) and the flexible fiberscope (Hara et al.[81]). With the available equipment, twenty to thirty photographs of excellent quality may be obtained. The procedure is particularly fruitful in visualizing the area and lesions of the fundus (Milton and Lynch[135]). Often, a correct differentiation might be made between a benign and a malignant ulcer (Carandang et al.[32]). Blendis et al.[22] believe that the combination of roentgenology, cytology, and gastric photography permits earlier diagnosis.

Exfoliative cytology

Exfoliative cytology has reached a high level of accuracy in diagnosing carcinomas of the stomach (Raskin et al.[162]; Cantrell[31]). The cytologic diagnosis may, in some instances, be more accurate than the roentgenologic examination in determining whether or not a given lesion is benign or malignant. In a few patients in whom the radiologic findings were apparently negative in the face of gastric symptoms, cytology showed malignant cells (Schade[177]).

MacDonald et al.[119] identified malignant cells in the gastric contents of eighty-three of eighty-nine patients with gastric cancer. Gastric cytology was utilized in 301 patients by Bach-Nielsen,[9] who found suspected or definite tumor cells in 84% of the patients with malignant gastric tumors. In another series of fifty-eight malignant and eighty-one benign lesions, the correct diagnosis was made radiologically in ninety-one patients (70%), on cytologic findings in 117 (85%), and by a combination in 94% or 130 patients (Dor[44]). Taebel et al.[215] reported positive cytology in 81% of 282 patients with proved malignant gastric lesions and negative cytology in 99% of 1584 patients with benign lesions or normal stomachs. Reported false negative results range from 2% to 20% (Table 33), usually in heavily infected ulcerated lesions, and false positive results range from 1% to 5% (Kernen and

Table 33. Review of literature relative to accuracy of exfoliative gastric cytology in diagnosis of cancer*

Date	Reported by	Total cases	*False negatives (proved gastric cancer)*			*False positives (proved or apparently benign)*		
			Cases	False	% False	Cases	False	% False
1960	Schade	558	282	6	2	276	13	5.0
1962	Van Haam	1050	50	7	14	1000	14	1.4
1963	MacDonald	380	89	6	7	291	1	0.3
1964	Yamada	337	181	34	19	156	5	3.0
1964	Henning	380	227	39	17	153	6	4.0
1965	Taebal	1866	282	53	19	1584	4	0.25
1967	Present report	184	29	5	17	155	1	0.6

*From Kernen, J. A., and Bales, C.: Cytologic diagnosis of gastric cancer, Calif. Med. 108:104-108, 1968.

Bales[100]). Exfoliative cytology, however, is too time consuming to be of value as a screening procedure.

Gastric analysis

Gastric analysis should be done routinely in patients suspected of having cancer of the stomach. Achlorhydria and marked hypochlorhydria are found in about 70% of patients with carcinoma of the stomach (Hurst[94]). Vanzant et al.[222] showed that the proportion of cases of achlorhydria among normal individuals increases with age and that about 26% of persons examined at the age of 70 years have achlorhydria. The mean free acidity of men also decreases with age but remains constant in women. Comfort et al.[40] reviewed 277 cases in which there had been gastric analysis at least two years before the diagnosis of cancer of the stomach and noted that the secretory activity was below normal regardless of the age of the patient when the test was done. In this group there were 127 cases (46%) with anacidity; the number had increased to 191 (69%) when the diagnosis of cancer was made. Comfort et al.[40] assumed that it is the atrophy of the gastric mucosa that is responsible for this depression of secretory activity. In cases of cancer developing on an ulcer, Stewart[200] found a certain degree of gastric acidity in most patients.

Free hydrochloric acid is absent in about 70% of the patients with advanced carcinoma of the stomach. However, in early carcinoma of the stomach, where a diagnostic test is of utmost importance, the gastric analysis is often of no value. This is particularly true when cancer is engrafted upon a previously existing ulcer, for there may be a normal or even elevated amount of hydrochloric acid. Taylor studied thirty-three patients with *lymphosarcoma,* 17 of whom showed normal or elevated free hydrochloric acid. This is probably explained by the fact that these tumors arise in the submucosa, and the function of the mucosa continues for an appreciable time before there is diminution or cessation in the output of hydrochloric acid.

Other laboratory procedures

Patients with, or suspected of having, a gastric lesion should have multiple stool examinations for *occult blood.* Frequently, a strongly positive reaction is found in patients with carcinomas as well as in those with lymphosarcomas, but negative reactions may be obtained which, of course, are of no diagnostic value. In many instances, there is normochromic anemia, and the differential cell count may show an elevation rather than a depression of white cells and no lymphocytosis. Studies of the bone marrow in patients with cancer of the stomach may show a tendency toward erythropoietic hyperplasia (Cheney[35]), and infrequently a leukemoid reaction may be present (Kugelmeier[108]).

Differential diagnosis

Benign tumors of the stomach are often silent and are found in variable proportions at autopsy, depending on the thoroughness of the search (Rieniets[166]). The proportion found in surgical specimens is always smaller (Dudley et al.[46]), and they are seldom present as a problem of clinical diagnosis. Benign gastric tumors may be epithelial or mesenchymal.

Polyps are the most common benign epithelial growths encountered in the stomach. They are adenomatous, pedunculated, and sometimes multiple (Stewart[199]) (Figs. 349 and 350). Gastric polyps occur predominantly in men past 50 years of age but are also found in women and in young individuals (Hardt et al.[82]). Three-fourths of them are found in the pyloric area and may prolapse into the duodenum, giving obstructive symptoms, and symptoms of gastritis may also be present. Polyps less than 2 cm in diameter are invariably benign. Larger lesions should be excised for, although they may be benign, they may also be carcinomatous. Irregular contour of a polyp should be considered as a suspicious sign of carcinoma (Marshak and Feldman[129]). Ulceration is not necessarily a sign of malignancy (Yarnis et al.[233]). Monaco et al.[136] studied 153 patients with adenomatous polyps of the stomach. A few of the polyps showed changes of carcinoma in situ but none of these metastasized. Achlorhydria is frequently found in these patients, particularly in those with multiple polyposis (Pearl and Brunn[156]). The so-called inflammatory fibroid polyp (Helwig and Ranier[86]) is not a true neo-

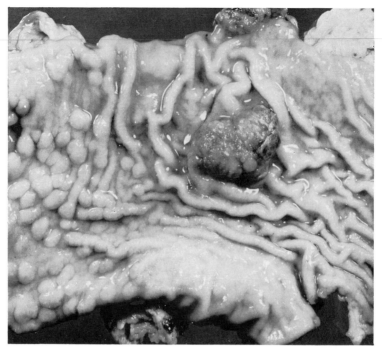

Fig. 349. Two pedunculated adenomatous polyps may be seen. Focal carcinoma was present in both. Regional nodes were negative.

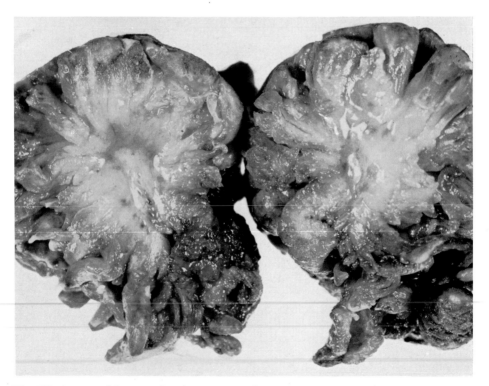

Fig. 350. Section of large single adenomatous polyp.

plasm. It may be associated with anemias.

The most common among the benign mesenchymal tumors are the *leiomyomas,* which are often found near the cardioesophageal junction, on the posterior wall of the corpus in close proximity to the lesser curvature, but rarely near the pyloric area. Leiomyomas arise from the internal and external musculature of the stomach and may consequently present as submucous, intramural, or subserous masses. They are seldom pedunculated. Most leiomyomas are symptomless and are discovered only at autopsy. However, the submucous variety may become ulcerated and infected, causing anorexia and epigastric discomfort. They may bleed severely, causing hematemesis, tarry stools, anemia, and weight loss. Pedunculated leiomyomas may cause signs of pyloric obstruction with epigastric pain and vomiting. The roentgenologic picture is rather characteristic with a well-circumscribed defect, a normal mucosa adjacent to the lesion, possible mucosal ulceration over the tumor, and normal peristalsis and pliability of the wall without signs of spasm (Baker and Good[11]). The leiomyosarcomas can enlarge and excavate and be diagnosed radiographically as carcinoma (Figs. 351 and 352). Ochsner and Janetos[142] reported eighty benign gastric tumors, thirty-eight adenomas, and twenty-six leiomyomas; indigestion, abdominal pain, and bleeding were common symptoms. A special type of benign smooth muscle tumor characterized as leiomyoblastoma may be mistaken microscopically for a malignant lesion, but these tumors behave almost without exception as benign tumors (Tallqvist et al.[216]).

Neurogenous tumors are often described within the stomach (Manrique and Halliburton[127]), but most of these neoplasms are in reality of smooth muscle origin. We have yet to see a neurogenous tumor of the stomach except once in association with extensive Recklinghausen's disease. Most articles dealing with neurogenous tumors present gross and microscopic illustrations more compatible with smooth muscle than neurogenous origin (West and Knox[229]). *Lipomas* are rare, are usually submucosal, and occur predominantly in the pyloric area, giving obstructive symptoms that may be thought to be due to carcinoma (Paaby[145]). They may be multiple and hemorrhagic (Fawcett et al.[61]). *Glomus tumors* (Kay et al.[98]), *carcinoids* (Black and Haffner[20]), and *plasma cell tumors* (Ende et al.[57]) have also been found in the stomach and confused with cancer. *Eosinophilic gastroduodenitis* may produce pyloric obstruction and be mistaken for carcinoma (McCune et al.[117]). *Benign lymphoid hyperplasia* may give rise to a large mass with ulceration or with enlarged gastric rugae and may be confused with carcinoma (Perez and Dorfman[157]). *Hypertrophic pyloric stenosis* may occur in the adult and may be secondary to other gastric lesions or may be primary. In the latter case, there is a deficiency of the longitudinal muscles along the pyloric canal (DuPlessis[49]).

The most common problem of differential diagnosis is *gastric ulcer.* In the first place, a typical history of gastric ulcer may be due to the presence of carcinoma of the stomach. It is true that most ulcers in the lesser curvature are benign, but some malignant ulcerations may be found there (Fig. 343). Ulcers situated below the incisura angularis, in the horizontal portion, should be regarded with greater suspicion (Sussman and Lipsay[211]; Marshall[130]). On the other hand, ulcers in the greater curvature (Matthews[132]) and the prepyloric area (Hampton[80]) have a greater chance of being malignant. However, in a series of forty-four ulcers of the greater curvature reported by Findley,[65] only five proved to be malignant. Benign and malignant ulcers alike may present no irregularities in their outline, but benign ulcers are extramural in contrast with the intramural situation of malignant ulcers. In benign ulcers there is tenderness to palpation and no accompanying palpable mass. Tone and peristalsis are usually increased. The rugal patterns often converge into the ulcer crater, whereas they are usually effaced in cases of cancer. In some benign ulcers there may be widespread rigidity surrounding the ulcer because of fibrosis. Under these circumstances, a benign ulcer is called malignant (Harper and Gree[83]). Under medical treatment, the acute and subacute benign ulcers usually disappear. Chronic ulcers may not heal because of fibrosis. In

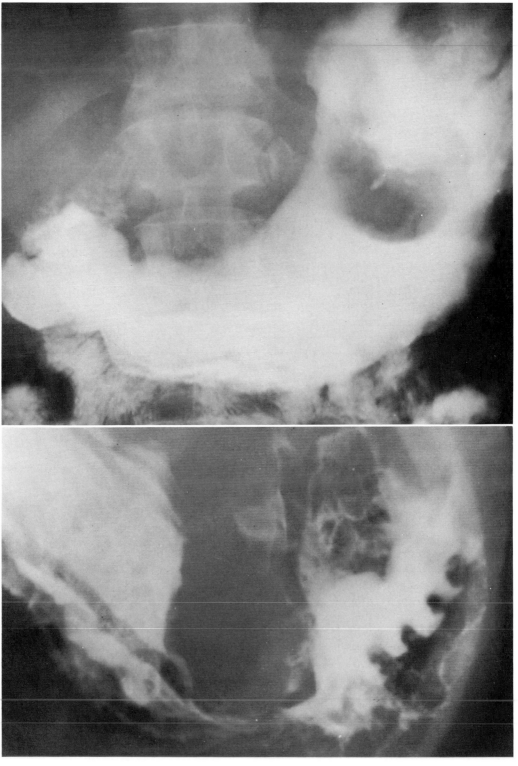

Fig. 351. Huge ulcerating and cavitating leiomyosarcoma of stomach. (WU negs. 68-7811 and 68-7810.)

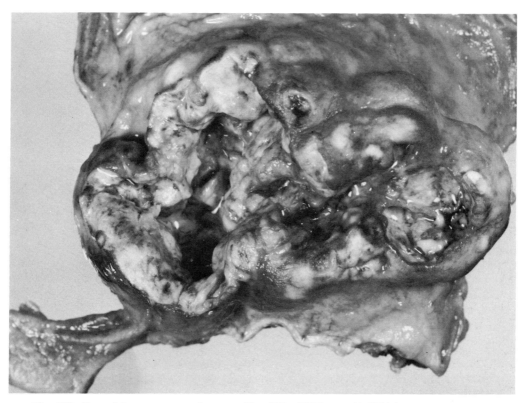

Fig. 352. Same leiomyosarcoma shown in Fig. 351. (WU neg. 68-7870.)

a series of 145 cases of benign gastric ulcer that were frequently re-examined roentgenologically, only nine were not completely healed with eight weeks of medical treatment (Smith and Jordan[190]). Patients with malignant ulcers may undergo symptomatic improvement under medical treatment. The ulceration may be filled in by continued growth, or the defect may appear larger in spite of apparent clinical improvement. If the roentgenologic study reveals the presence of a concomitant active *duodenal ulcer,* the chances are overwhelming that both ulcerations are benign (Fischer et al.[66]). Among 45,000 cases of duodenal ulcer and 13,000 cases of carcinoma of the stomach observed at the Mayo Clinic between 1911 and 1945, there were only forty-eight instances of coexistence of both.

In *chronic gastritis* there may be intermittent spasms that produce filling defects on the roentgenogram. These lesions may be easily mistaken for carcinoma unless frequent examinations are made after ad-

ministration of antispasmodics until peristaltic waves may be seen radioscopically to pass through the area of apparent rigidity. Gastroscopic examination may help in the diagnosis. Acidity rises as the gastritis undergoes improvement under symptomatic treatment. The presence of a *hiatal hernia* does not eliminate the possibility of an associated carcinoma of the stomach (Smithers[191]).

Metastases to the stomach from malignant tumors developing elsewhere are extremely rare. It is not infrequent, however, for the stomach to be invaded by carcinoma arising in the pancreas, gallbladder, large bowel, etc. In generalized lymphosarcoma, involvement of the stomach is not rare. Metastasis from an unsuspected *melanoma* elsewhere may have its manifestation in the stomach and produce a rather characteristic radiographic appearance, the so-called bull's-eye sign (Potchen et al.[158]). *Hodgkin's disease,* thought to be primary in the stomach, is rarely encountered (Bloch[23]).

Treatment
Surgery

The only chance for complete cure of carcinoma of the stomach is surgical resection of the lesion and its regional metastatic implants. The accomplishment of this aim requires institution of surgical treatment to early lesions and radicality of the performance without compromising the principles of cancer surgery. Horn[92] studied seventy-four cases of gastric carcinoma at autopsy and found that 17.6% of the tumors for which gastric resection was not done were theoretically curable.

A great deal of the effectiveness of the surgical treatment depends on its application to early lesions. This implies judgment of the nature of ulcers on the basis of their radioscopic and radiographic appearance, size, location (Kirsh[104]), chronicity, etc. At the Massachusetts General Hospital a diagnosis of benign ulcer was made in 221 patients; cancer was found in sixteen of them. It used to be considered that all ulcers more than 2.5 cm in *size* were malignant. In a review by Cohn et al.[38] of 533 patients with ulcers larger than 2.5 cm, 72% proved to be benign and only 37% of 136 ulcers larger than 4 cm proved to be malignant. *Chronicity* of gastric ulcers points to a greater chance of malignancy. Strode[208] found this to be particularly true in the Japanese. *Obstruction* in the presence of an ulcer is more often due to cancer than to a benign ulcer. Hemorrhage and perforation are more often associated with benign ulcers. Other relative findings favoring a diagnosis of cancer are *achlorhydria* and positive *cytologic examination*.

The decision to submit an assumed benign ulcer to a medical regimen implies a small chance that the lesion may be malignant, and thus its proper treatment may be delayed (Table 34). We feel that this chance is minimized and its consequences greatly reduced if the patient is made aware from the start of this possibility and of the necessity for his submitting to close follow-up and repeated radiologic examinations. Failure to respond to a controlled *short* medical treatment constitutes one of the indications for surgical treatment.

Any patient suspected of having cancer of the stomach should be subjected to surgical exploration except for reasons of noncorrectable poor general condition or definite direct or indirect evidence of metastases (rectal shelf, jaundice, ascites, skin nodules, etc.). An effort should always be made to establish a histopathologic diagnosis. The presence of an epigastric palpable mass does not containindicate operation. A palpable mass was present in 28% of the operable group reported by Lahey et al.[111] The roentgenologist cannot determine with exactitude whether or not any given lesion is inoperable.

The preoperative preparation of patients with cancer of the stomach should attempt to reestablish, as much as possible, a good general physical condition. At exploration, it may be found that resection is inadvisable because of peritoneal implants, liver metastases, or wide direct extension to nonresectable structures. However, the most common cause for inability to resect is metastases to nodes along the celiac axis. Biopsy should always be done to establish a definite diagnosis for the record.

Subtotal gastrectomy. Most types of subtotal gastric resections are modifications of the original Billroth II operation, varying in respect to site and fashion of the anastomosis. McNeer et al.[123] collected ninety-two cases of subtotal gastrectomy with autopsy studies and reported fourteen deaths from distant metastases without regional recurrence and four deaths due to unrelated causes and forty-six gastric recurrences, nine duodenal recurrences, and nineteen perigastric node metastases. Admittedly, these were subtotal gastrec-

Table 34. Results of medical treatment of gastric ulcer*

Type of result	Cases	%
Cure	68	46.0
Symptoms disappeared under medical regimen	23	16.0
Gastric ulcer persisted roentgenologically	7	5.0
Surgical treatment	16	11.0
Definite evidence of carcinoma developed	14	10.0
Death from hemorrhage	1	0.7
Deaths from unrelated causes	17	12.0
Total	146	

*After Judd, E. S., and Priestley, J. T.: Treatment of gastric ulcer, Surg. Gynec. Obstet. 77:21-25, 1943.

tomies of varied quality and extent. The subtotal gastrectomy of today is a much more radical procedure. The results of subtotal gastrectomy are improved when the operation includes extensive resection of the lesser curvature and of a good margin of the duodenum, excision of the greater omentum and the gastrohepatic omentum (State et al.[195]), and a radical removal of regional lymph nodes (Walters et al.[224]). Such a radical subtotal procedure diminishes the incidence of local recurrences.

In the treatment of carcinomas of the cardiac end of the stomach, a proximal subtotal gastrectomy and esophagectomy may be done by the abdominal approach. The transthoracic esophagogastrectomy, followed by an intrathoracic esophagogastric anastomosis, has gained considerable favor (Payne and Clagett[155]). An almost complete excision of the lesser curvature and its adjacent nodes may be carried out, leaving a tubelike distal stomach that facilitates anastomosis (Kirklin and Clagett[103]).

Total gastrectomy. A radical removal of the entire stomach and adjacent structures is recommended by some in an effort to reduce local recurrences. The operation implies removal of the duodenum to the lowest possible level, removal of all of the gastrohepatic omentum, careful separation of the great omentum from its point of origin in the hepatic flexure to well past the splenic flexure, removal of the spleen with the nodes in the splenic hilum, and mobilization of the esophagus and removal of an esophageal cuff with the paracardial nodes (Lahey and Marshall[110]). The operation may be extended to include portions of the pancreas, liver, transverse colon, and esophagus (McNeer and James[121]). In the treatment of carcinomas of the cardiac end of the stomach, the transthoracic esophagogastrectomy may be extended to include a complete gastrectomy and to be completed by an esophagojejunostomy (Reynolds and Young[168]).

A subtotal gastrectomy is adequate for carcinomas of the gastric antrum (Mayo et al.[133]). A total gastrectomy should be reserved for lesions of the upper portions of the stomach or for those involving the entire stomach (Herter and Auchincloss[87]).

There is no doubt that total gastrectomy is followed by profound physiologic changes. There is decreased capacity for ingesting food, which makes frequent small feedings necessary. There are profound nutritional and metabolic changes, resulting steatorrhea, inability to digest complex carbohydrates, attacks of postprandial hypoglycemia and hypokalemia (dumping syndrome), and failure to gain weight. The cured patients develop macrocytic anemia and have to be treated with parenteral vitamin B_{12} (Allison[4]). There are chronic inflammatory changes of the lower esophagus and jejunum about the anastomotic site. A characteristic radiographic appearance shows a dilatation of the esophagus and the contiguous duodenum or jejunum with changes in the intestinal pattern. All of these changes are sufficiently characteristic to be called a *total gastrectomy syndrome* (Paulson and Harvey[154]).

Goligher and Riley[74] studied 224 patients after various forms of partial and total gastrectomy. Six months after operation, 168 patients (75%) had dumping that in twenty-eight (12%) was severe. One year later, sixty-seven patients (47%) still had dumping, but it was severe only in ten (7%). In total gastrectomies, the syndrome appeared more frequently and severe. Objections to total gastrectomy are often based on the fairly high proportion of patients who fail to adapt to the new circumstances (Stammers[193]).

Operative mortality. As the operability and resectability of carcinoma of the stomach have increased, the operative mortality has steadily decreased (State et al.[195]). The operative mortality of subtotal resections has decreased from 33% in 1933 to 10% in 1946 (Pack[147]). The operative mortality of total gastrectomies was about 37% in 1933 (Pack[147]), but in recent years it has diminished to less than 10% (Lahey and Marshall[110]; Scott and Longmire[179]). However, it must be recognized that such a low operative mortality is achieved only by highly experienced surgeons. Sweet[213] reported 147 cases of esophagogastrectomy with seventeen resulting operative deaths, or 11.5%. The operative mortality for the United States for subtotal gastrectomy done by a competent surgeon is 7% (Watman[226]).

Palliative interventions. Gastrostomies and jejunostomies for obstructive inoperable carcinoma of the stomach are attended by a relatively high mortality, very little, if any, prolongation of life (Pack and McNeer[148]), and no relief of symptoms. The same is true of gastroenterostomies except that the operative mortality is still higher. A palliative subtotal gastric resection is preferable when possible. It alleviates obstructive symptoms and gives freedom from distress, a sense of well-being, and, often, an ability to return to fairly active life. Total gastrectomy should not be done as a palliative procedure because of the excessive operative mortality and morbidity (Fretheim[70]).

Recurrences that take place after a short interval are usually the result of persistent tumor. If the interval is long, a new carcinoma may have developed (Bernhard et al.[18]; Fortner and Booher[68]). Recurrences following gastrectomy can rarely be controlled by further surgery.

Radiotherapy

Considering the small proportion of patients who eventually benefit by the surgical treatment of cancer of the stomach, the contributions, however small, of any other form of treatment would be welcome. Sauerbrey and Reinhold[176] demonstrated that radiation therapy can give good palliation to patients with inoperable carcinoma of the stomach. The best results occur in those in whom the general condition is good, the disease is well localized, and there is no clinical evidence of remote metastases. But radiotherapy usually fails because of the biologic character of adenocarcinomas of the stomach, their mode of extension, and widespread metastases. The reasons for the failure are qualitative, not quantitative.

Radiotherapy has found widespread usefulness in the treatment of *lymphosarcomas*. Whereas there may be doubts as to the claims of control, either by surgery or by radiotherapy, of lymphosarcomas that appear limited to the stomach, there is ample evidence of the value of radiotherapy as a single procedure, or as a postoperative measure, in the control of lymphosarcomas with proved metastases (Redd[163]; Burnett and Herbert[29]). If a diagnosis of lymphosarcoma is suspected before resection, it is preferable to biopsy both the lesion and the nodes rather than to subject the patient to unnecessary surgery. Radiotherapy must be extensive and thorough, though not necessarily intensive. Supervoltage roentgentherapy and cobalt[60] teletherapy permit this to be done with a greater degree of impunity. Of course, whenever a diagnosis of lymphosarcoma is made after resection, if the tumor is incompletely excised or if lymph nodes are involved, radiotherapy is indicated.

Chemotherapy

The application of various antineoplastic drugs to the treatment of cancer of the stomach has met with systematic failure. A cooperative study of thio-tepa as a surgical adjuvant revealed an increase in the operative mortality of patients who had a gastrectomy plus splenectomy (Veterans Administration Surgical Adjuvant Cancer Chemotherapy Study Group[223]). A combination of 5-fluorouracil and radiotherapy in the treatment of unresectable carcinomas of the stomach has been found encouraging (Childs et al.[36]).

Medical treatment

Palliative medical measures should be instituted for advanced carcinoma of the stomach. Gastric lavage, together with a high-protein, high-vitamin diet, may be helpful, and sometimes small, frequent feedings will be of value. The anemia that may accompany even small carcinomas of the stomach may be profound but can profitably be treated with iron (Cheney[35]). Medication to relieve pain should be given as indicated.

Prognosis

In 1965, there were 18,027 deaths in the United States from cancer of the stomach, a crude mortality rate of 9.3 per 100,000 population. The relative mortality rate of nonwhite males was 15.0, whereas that of whites was only 11.2. White and nonwhite females showed a mortality of 7.4 and 7.0, respectively. These death rates have been diminishing in the United States in the past few years, and a similar decrease has been reported in Canada, England, and other countries (Sigurjonsson[188];

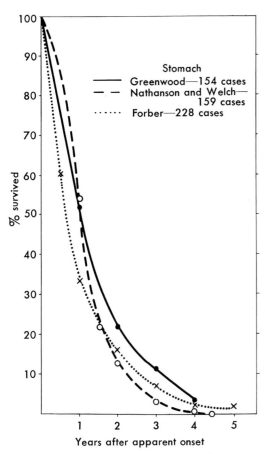

Fig. 353. Life expectancy of untreated patients with carcinoma of stomach. (From Shimkin, M. B.: Duration of life in untreated cancer, Cancer 4:1-8, 1951.)

Wynder et al.[232]). The American Cancer Society estimates at 17,000 the total number of deaths from cancer of the stomach to occur during 1970 in the United States.[7a] There seems to be no difference in prognosis according to race (Strudwick et al.[209]). A rather large proportion of cases is found in stages not justifying any attempt to curative treatment (45%), and the five-year survivals have remained at a low level (Cutler[42]).

In spite of greater operability and resectability, the overall prognosis for carcinoma of the stomach is shockingly poor (Fig. 353). Diagnosis is made in a great proportion of patients only where there is no hope for cure. An additional number of patients are explored but the lesions are not resected, and a large proportion of those resected recur. A review of 1983 cases of cancer of the stomach seen at the University of Minnesota from 1936 to 1963 revealed a decrease in the overall five-year survival from 12% in 1950-1958 to 8.8% in 1958-1963 (Gilbertsen[72a]).

There is no doubt but that where cancer education is widespread, where the medical profession is alert, and where diagnostic roentgenology is available, a greater number of cases are diagnosed in the operable stage. A statistical study of patients seen at the Mayo Clinic from 1940 to 1949 revealed that for every 100 patients examined, there were eighty laparotomies and forty-four resections, with fourteen five-year survivals (Berkson et al.[116]). For every 100 patients with carcinoma of the stomach seen at Hines Veterans Hospital from 1931 to 1947, there were sixty-three explorations and thirty-two resections, with four five-year survivals (Lawton et al.[113]). Mayo et al.[133] reported their five-year survival rates in a group of 129 patients with gastric carcinoma. The percentage of survivals ranges from 7.7 to 66.7 according to how it is calculated. The discouraging fact remains that no matter how figured, there were only ten survivors in the entire group (Fig. 355). This group of patients is not, of course, representative of the whole population, where the estimated results are even lower. Slungaard and Weber-Laumann[189] studied all the cases of carcinoma of the stomach that occurred in a single county in Norway over a period of five years. Of the 372 patients, 141 were explored, and 111 carcinomas were resected. Of the latter group, twenty-five patients, ten of whom had presented lymph node involvement, were alive at the end of five years.

Paradoxically, patients with a short *clinical history* present a greater proportion of inoperable lesions than those with a long history. Edwards[50] reported thirty-one patients with a history not exceeding three months, of whom only eight had operable lesions, whereas in another group of thirty-one patients with histories of from three to ten years, ten had resectable lesions. The survival rate of patients operated on has also been found to be greater for the group with longer histories (Swynnerton and Truelove[214]; Brookes et al.[28]). There is apparently definite correlation between the

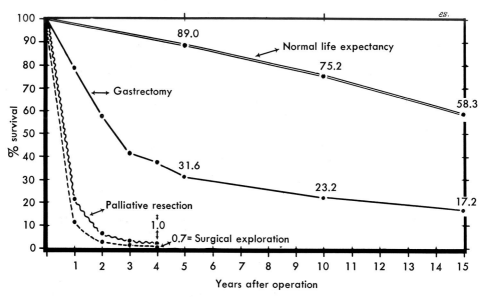

Fig. 354. Carcinoma of stomach. Survival rates in successive years after operation. These figures had changed little in 1961. (Modified from Berkson, J., et al.: Mortality and survival in cancer of the stomach; a statistical summary of the experience of the Mayo Clinic, Proc. Staff Meet. Mayo Clin. **27**:137-151, 1952.)

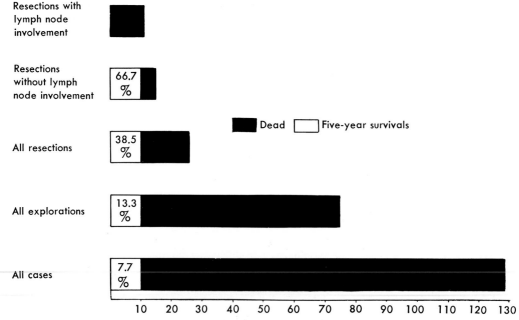

Fig. 355. One hundred twenty-nine cases of gastric carcinoma (1940-1949). Note that percentage of survivals varies from 7.7 to 66.7, depending on how calculations are made. (From Mayo, H. W., Jr., et al.: A critical evaluation of radical subtotal gastric resection as a definite procedure for antral gastric carcinoma, Trans. Southern Surg. Ass. **66**:289-298, 1955.)

degree of *gastric acidity* and the prognosis—the lower the acidity, the worse the prognosis. The *age* of the patient does not seem of prognostic importance (Guiss[78a]). Women are slightly less curable than men (Berkson et al.[16]).

The *degree of differentiation* of the carcinoma has a definite bearing on the prognosis, the survival rate being more than double for patients with the most differentiated tumors than for those with the undifferentiated tumors. There appears to be correlation in the prognosis of the different *gross varieties* of tumor, for the superficially spreading type is highly curable (Bragg et al.[26]), and the linitis plastica type has a very unfavorable outlook. The polypoid tumors have a smaller percentage of metastases than the invasive type. Steiner et al.[108] reviewed thirty cases with survival of over five years. They found that the tumors often presented well-circumscribed margins and a certain microscopic appearance (the blue cell type), and some showed degenerative changes. In a series reported by Urban and McNeer,[221] the five-year survivors had small superficial tumors with circumscribed borders. We had 180 patients treated by gastric resection who were followed more than five years. Twenty-three (13%) survived

five or more years. The most favorable group was associated with tumors possessing a pushing growth pattern, often with degeneration of neoplastic cells at the advancing margin of the tumor. Only a small percentage of the patients had such changes, but a surprising proportion of this small percentage survived (Monafo et al.[137]). It is probable that these changes determine, to a great extent, the prognosis in a given patient. In Japan, the end results of treatment of gastric cancer have improved mainly because of the increased finding of cancers still limited to mucosa and submucosa (Muto et al.[140]).

The presence or absence of *metastases,* which is related to some of the gross and microscopic variations, is the most decisive factor in the prognosis (Harvey et al.[84]). Approximately one-half of patients without metastases survive five years after adequate resection. *Extension* of the tumor outside the stomach carries the same connotation as does the presence of metastases. Following extensive gastric resection with splenectomy, Šerý and Dvoracek[180] found that when the nodes in the lineal area were involved no patients were saved. Of ten patients with these nodes involved, only two lived three years, and none survived five years. If metastatic tumor in the lymph

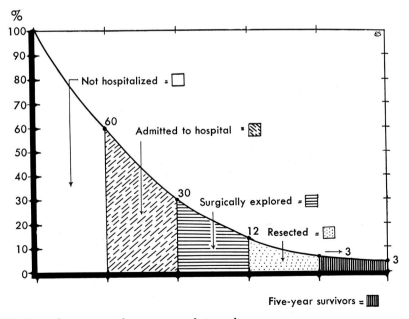

Fig. 356. Fate of patients with carcinoma of stomach.

node extends beyond the capsule of that node, the prognosis is much worse (Zacho et al.[234]).

Marshall[130] reviewed 1078 cases of carcinoma of the stomach seen at the Lahey Clinic between 1932 and 1954. The percentage of curative resections remained between thirty-eight and forty-one each year. In spite of the importance given to early diagnosis, the five-year survival rate did not prove this point, for it remained the same whether the patients had symptoms for three months, six months, or even longer. Of 856 of these patients who had a resection, 529 (61.8%) presented lymph node involvement and, of these, only 7.2% survived five to ten years, whereas the five-year to ten-year survival rate was 34.8% for those who had no lymph node involvement. In a selected group of thirty-nine patients whose cases were diagnosed under favorable circumstances, Amberg and Rigler[7] found that thirty-five of the lesions were operable and twenty-eight were resectable, but eighteen (64%) already presented lymph node metastases—yet, unquestionably, the presence or the absence of lymph node involvement is the factor of greatest significance in the prognosis.

Eker and Efskind[54] studied exhaustively 1314 patients who had a resection for carcinoma of the stomach. They found excellent correlation of the degree of differentiation of the carcinoma and the rate of survival, but unfortunately three-fourths of the gastric carcinomas were in a highly undifferentiated category. Patients with Grade III or Grade IV carcinomas and without demonstrable metastases had a worse prognosis than patients with well-differentiated carcinomas with metastases. Small tumors are more readily curable, and diffuse infiltrative tumors have a very bad outlook. Eker and Efskind[54] also demonstrated that lesions less than 1 cm distant from the pyloric sphincter have a poorer prognosis than those at a greater distance.

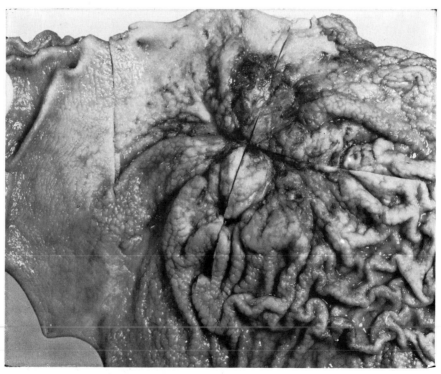

Fig. 357. Pseudolymphosarcoma of stomach. Note areas of ulceration with prominent rugal folds. (From Ackerman, L. V.: Is it cancer? Will it become cancer? Proceedings of Fourth National Cancer Conference, Philadelphia, 1960, J. B. Lippincott Co., pp. 97-112; WU neg. 55-4180.)

The prognosis of *sarcomas* of the stomach is surprisingly good. Of forty-one patients with sarcoma of the stomach treated by surgery at the Lahey Clinic, eighteen (44%) survived five years or longer (Marshall and Meissner[131]). Joseph and Lattes[97] reported forty-six patients with primary lymphosarcomas of the stomach with cure in twenty-seven. In 145 patients with lymphosarcoma treated by radiation therapy, Ennuyer and Bataini[59] reported fifty-seven (39%) well five or more years. It appears evident that a proportion of reported lymphosarcomas of the stomach without lymph node involvement are, in reality pseudolymphomatous formations, but verified cases of lymphosarcoma with metastases have been cured by radiotherapy (Redd[163]; Burnett and Herbert[29]) (Fig. 357).

REFERENCES

1 Albot, G., Hernandez, C., Boisson, J., Veyne, S., Chaput, J.-C., and Farias, L.: Apport diagnostique de l'artériographie sélective du tronc coeliaque dans quelques cas d'épaississement bénin ou malin de la muqueuse gastrique, Sem. Hop. Paris **43**:1192-1206, 1967.

2 Allen, A. W.: Gastric ulcer and cancer, Surgery **17**:750-754, 1945.

3 Allen, A. W., and Welch, C. E.: Gastric ulcer, Ann. Surg. **114**:498-509, 1941.

4 Allison, P. R.: Radical total gastrectomy for carcinoma of the stomach, Lancet **1**:1014-1016, 1963.

5 Altshuler, J. H., and Shaka, J. A.: Squamous cell carcinoma of the stomach; review of the literature and report of a case, Cancer **19**:831-838, 1966.

6 Amberg, J. R.: Accuracy of roentgen diagnosis in carcinoma of the stomach, Amer. J. Dig. Dis. **5**:259-263, 1960.

7 Amberg, J. R., and Rigler, L. G.: Results of surgery in carcinoma of the stomach discovered by periodic roentgen examination, Surgery **39**:760-775, 1956.

7a American Cancer Society: Cancer statistics, 1970, CA **20**:10-23, 1970.

7b Appelman, H. D., and Helwig, E. B.: Glomus tumors of the stomach, Cancer **23**:203-213, 1969.

8 Bachman, A. L., and Parmer, E. A.: Radiographic diagnosis of recurrence following resection for gastric cancer, Radiology **84**:913-924, 1965.

9 Bach-Nielsen, P.: Gastric cytology, with special reference to the diagnosis of malignant disease, Danish Med. Bull. **13**:88-91, 1966.

10 Bachrach, W. H.: Observations upon the complete roentgenographic healing of neoplastic ulcerations of the stomach, Surg. Gynec. Obstet. **114**:69-82, 1962.

11 Baker, H. L., Jr., and Good, C. A.: Smooth-

muscle tumors of the alimentary tract; their roentgen manifestations, Amer. J. Roentgen. **74**:246-254, 1955.

12 Benedict, E. B.: Value of gastric biopsy specimens obtained through the flexible operating gastroscope, Arch. Path. (Chicago) **49**:538-542, 1950.

13 Benedict, E. B.: The differential diagnosis of benign and malignant lesions of the stomach by means of the flexible operating gastroscope, Gastroenterology **14**:275-279, 1950.

14 Benedict, E. B.: Positive stomach diagnosis by gastroscopic biopsy, Surg. Clin. N. Amer. **37**:1239-1247, 1957.

15 Benedict, E. B., and Allen, A. W.: Adenomatous polypi of the stomach, with special reference to malignant degeneration, Surg. Gynec. Obstet. **58**:79-84, 1934.

16 Berkson, J., Walters, W., Gray, H. K., and Priestley, J. T.: Mortality and survival in cancer of the stomach; a statistical summary of the experience of the Mayo Clinic, Proc. Staff Meet. Mayo Clin. **27**:137-151, 1952.

17 Berndt, H., and Pietschker, H.: Magenkrebs und Blutgruppe, Deutsch. Gesundh. **21**:1864-1869, 1966.

18 Bernhard, A., Kuss, B., and Bartsch, W. M.: Das Karzinom im Restmagen, Med. Klin. **59**:1413-1417, 1964.

19 Berry, R. E. L., and Rottschafer, W.: The lymphatic spread of cancer of the stomach observed in operataive specimens removed by radical surgery including total pancreatectomy, Surg. Gynec. Obstet. **104**:269-279, 1957.

20 Black, W. C., and Haffner, H. E.: Diffuse hyperplasia of gastric argyrophil cells and multiple carcinoid tumors, Cancer **21**:1080-1099, 1968.

21 Blackburn, E. K.: Possible association between pernicious anaemia and leukaemia; a prospective study of 1,625 patients with a note on the very high incidence of stomach cancer, Int. J. Cancer **3**:163-170, 1968.

22 Blendis, M., Beilby, J. O. W., Wilson, J. P., Cole, M. J., and Hadley, G. D.: Carcinoma of the stomach; evaluation of individual and combined diagnostic accuracy of radiology, cytology and gastrophotography, Brit. Med. J. **1**:656-659, 1967.

23 Bloch, C.: Roentgen features of Hodgkin's disease of the stomach, Amer. J. Roentgen. **99**:175-181, 1967.

24 Block, M., Griep, A. H., and Pollard, H. M.: The occurrence of gastric neoplasms in youth, Amer. J. Med. Sci. **215**:398-404, 1948.

25 Borrmann, R.: Geschwulste des Magens. In Henke, F., and Lubarsch, O., editors: Handbuch der speziellen pathologischen Anatomie und Histologie, vol. 4, Berlin, 1926, Julius Springer, pp. 812-1000.

26 Bragg, D. G., Seaman, W. B., and Lattes, R.: Roentgenologic and pathologic aspects of superficial spreading carcinoma of the stomach, Amer. J. Roentgen. **101**:437-446, 1967.

27 Bralow, S. P., and Collins, M.: Relationship of peptic ulceration to superficial spreading

carcinoma of the stomach, Gastroenterology **32**:1152-1161, 1957.

28 Brookes, V. S., Waterhouse, J. A. H., and Powell, D. J.: Carcinoma of the stomach; a 10-year survey of results and of factors affecting prognosis, Brit. Med. J. **1**:1577-1583, 1965.

29 Burnett, H. W., and Herbert, E. A.: The role of irradiation in the treatment of primary malignant lymphoma of the stomach, Radiology **67**:723-728, 1956.

30 Buschke, Franz, and Cantril, S. T.: Secondary lymphosarcoma of the stomach, Amer. J. Roentgen. **49**:450-454, 1943.

31 Cantrell, E. G.: Why use gastric cytology? Gut **10**:763-766, 1969.

32 Carandang, N., Schuman, B. M., and Priest, R. J.: The gastrocamera in the diagnosis of stomach disease J.A.M.A. **204**:717-722, 1968.

33 Carman, R. D.: New roentgen-ray sign of ulcerating gastric cancer, J.A.M.A. **77**:990, 1921.

34 Castleman, B.: Extension of gastric carcinoma into the duodenum, Ann. Surg. **103**:348-352, 1936.

35 Cheney, Garnett: The anemia of gastric cancer—its response to therapy, Folia Haemat. **52**:51-63, 1934.

36 Childs, D. S., Jr., Moertel, C. G., Holbrook, M. A., Reitemeier, R. J., and Colby, M., Jr.: Treatment of unresectable adenocarcinomas of the stomach with a combination of 5-Flurorouracil and radiation, Amer. J. Roentgen. **102**:541-544, 1968.

37 Chusid, E. L., Hirsch, R. L., and Colcher, H.: Spectrum of hypertrophic gastropathy, giant rugal folds, polyposis, and carcinoma of the stomach, Arch. Intern. Med. (Chicago) **114**:621-628, 1964.

38 Cohn, I., Jr., Sartin, J., and Sudduth, P.: Giant ulcers of the stomach, Amer. J. Gastroent. **32**:121-135, 1959.

39 Coller, F. A., Kay, E. B., and MacIntyre, R. S.: Regional lymphatic metastases of carcinoma of the stomach, Arch. Surg. (Chicago) **43**:748-761, 1941.

40 Comfort, M. W., Kelsey, M. P., and Berkson, J.: Gastric acidity before and after the development of carcinoma of the stomach, J. Nat. Cancer Inst. **7**:367-374, 1947.

40a Correa, P., Cuello, C., and Duque, E.: Carcinoma and intestinal metaplasia of the stomach in Colombian migrants, J. Nat. Cancer Inst. **44**:297-306, 1970.

41 Cramer, W.: On aetiology of cancer of mamma in mouse and in man, Amer. J. Cancer **30**:318-331, 1937.

42 Cutler, S. J.: Cancer illness among residents of Atlanta, Georgia, Cancer morbidity, series 1, P.H.S. pub. 13, Washington, D. C., 1950, United States Federal Security Agency, National Institutes of Health, National Cancer Institute.

43 Debray, C., Housset, P., and Nicolaidis, C. L.: La gastro-biopsie dirigée. Nouvel appareillage à aspiration-section. Appareillage; technique; résultats globaux (A propos de 112 cas), Sem. Hop. Paris **40**:133-153, 1964.

44 Dor, P.: Le diagnostic cytologique du cancer gastrique, Bull. Ass. Franc. Cancer **50**:243-249, 1963.

45 Dreyer, B., and Louw, J. H.: Squamous-cell carcinoma of the stomach, Brit. J. Surg. **44**:425-426, 1956.

46 Dudley, G. S., Miscall, Laurence, and Morse, S. F.: Benign tumors of the stomach, Arch. Surg. (Chicago) **45**:702-726, 1942.

47 Dungal, N.: The special problem of stomach cancer in Ireland, J.A.M.A. **178**:789-198, 1961.

48 Dungal, N., and Sigurjonsson, J.: Gastric cancer and diet; a pilot study on dietary habits in two districts differing markedly in respect of mortality from gastric cancer, Brit. J. Cancer **21**:270-276, 1967.

49 DuPlessis, D. J.: Primary hypertrophic pyloric stenosis in the adult, Brit. J. Surg. **53**:485-492, 1966.

50 Edwards, H. C.: Carcinoma of the stomach, Brit. Med. J. **1**:973-978, 1950.

51 Eisenbud, M., and Finby, N.: Carcinoma of the proximal third of the stomach; a critical study of clinical observations in 74 cases, Ann. Intern. Med. **46**:43-52, 1957.

52 Eker, R.: Carcinoma ventriculi; a pathological examination of 225 operated carcinomata ventriculi, Acta Chir. Scand. **88**:556-572, 1943.

53 Eker, R.: Carcinomas of the stomach; Investigation of the lymphatic spread from gastric carcinomas after total and partial gastrectomy, Acta Chir. Scand. **101**:112-126, 1951.

54 Eker, R., and Efskind, J.: The pathology and prognosis of gastric carcinoma, Acta Chir. Scand. (suppl. 264), pp. 1-182, 1960 (exhaustive study, excellent bibliography).

55 Ekström, T.: On the development of cancer in gastric ulcer and ulcer symptoms in gastric cancer, Acta Chir. Scand. **102**:387-401, 1952.

56 Elliott, G. V., Wald, S. M., and Benz, R. I.: A roentgenologic study of ulcerating lesions of the stomach, Amer. J. Roentgen. **77**:612-622, 1957.

57 Ende, N., Daron, P. B., Richardson, L. K., Raider, L., and Ziskind, J.: Plasma-cell tumor of the stomach, Radiology **55**:207-213, 1950.

58 Engel, G. C.: Reducing mortality in gastric carcinoma, J.A.M.A. **135**:687-690, 1947.

59 Ennuyer, A., and Bataini, P.: Lympho-réticulo-sarcomes de l'estomac et de l'intestin, Bull. Ass. Franc. Cancer **52**:215-240, 1965.

60 Faris, T. D., and Saltzstein, S. L.: Gastric lymphoid hyperplasia; a lesion confused with lymphosarcoma, Cancer **17**:207-212, 1964.

61 Fawcett, N. W., Bolton, V. L., and Geever, E. F.: Multiple lipomas of the stomach and duodenum, Ann. Surg. **129**:524-527, 1949.

62 Fernet, P., Azar, H. A., and Stout, A. P.: Intramural (tubal) spread of linitis plastica along the alimentary tract, Gastroenterology **48**:419-424, 1965.

63 Finby, N., and Eisenbud, M.: Carcinoma of the proximal third of the stomach; a critical study of roengenographic observations in

sixty-two cases, J.A.M.A. **154**:1155-1160, 1954.

64 Finch, E.: Treatment of cancer; the problem of organization, Lancet **1**:803-806, 1948.

65 Findley, J. W., Jr.: Ulcers of the gastric curvature of the stomach, Gastroenterology **40**:183-187, 1961.

66 Fischer, A., Clagett, F., and McDonald, J. R.: Coexistent duodenal ulcer and gastric malignancy, Surgery **21**:175-183, 1947.

67 Förssman, Gosta: Ueber die Röntgendiagnostik und Strahlenbehandlung von Magensarkomen insbesondere Lymphosarkomen und Retikulumzellensarkomen, Acta Radiol. (Stockholm) **24**:343-373, 1943.

68 Fortner, J. G., and Booher, R. J.: The problem of clinically recurrent gastric cancer, New York J. Med. **64**:1971-1974, 1964.

69 France, C. J., and Brines, O. A.: Mesenchymal tumors of the stomach, Arch. Surg. (Stockholm) **61**:1019-1035, 1950.

70 Fretheim, B.: Gastric carcinoma treated with abdominothoracic total gastrectomy, Arch. Surg. (Chicago) **71**:24-32, 1955.

71 Garlock, J. H.: Radical surgical treatment for carcinoma of the cardiac end of the stomach, Surg. Gynec. Obstet. **74**:555-560, 1942.

72 Gear, M. W. L., Truelove, S. C., Williams, D. G., Massarella, G. R., and Boddington, M. M.: Gastric cancer simulating benign gastric ulcer, Brit. J. Surg. **56**:739-742, 1969.

72a Gilbertsen, V. A.: Results of treatment of stomach cancer; an appraisal of efforts for more extensive surgery and a report of 1,983 cases, Cancer **23**:1305-1308, 1969.

73 Golden, R., and Stout, A. P.: Superficial spreading carcinoma of the stomach, Amer. J. Roentgen. **59**:157-167, 1948.

74 Goligher, J. C., and Riley, T. R.: Incidence and mechanism of the early dumping syndrome after gastrectomy, Lancet **1**:630-636, 1952.

75 Gomori, G.: Carcinoma arising from chronic gastric ulcer, Surg. Gynec. Obstet. **57**:439-450, 1933.

76 Graham, R. M., Ulfelder, H., and Green, T. H.: The cytologic method as an aid in the diagnosis of gastric carcinoma, Surg. Gynec. Obstet. **86**:257-259, 1948.

77 Gray, H. K., and Lofgren, K. A.: The significance of an ulcerating lesion in the stomach after gastro-enterostomy, Proc. Staff Meet. Mayo Clin. **23**:454-460, 1948.

78 Guiss, L. W., and Stewart, F. W.: Chronic atrophic gastritis and cancer of the stomach, Arch. Surg. (Chicago) **46**:823-843, 1943.

78a Guiss, L. W.: End results for gastric cancer; 2,891 cases, Surg. Gynec. Obstet. **93**:313-331, 1951.

79 Gutmann, R. A., Bertrand, I., and Peristiany, T. J.: Le cancer de l'estomac au debut, Paris, 1939, Gaston Doin.

80 Hampton, A. O.: The incidence of malignancy in chronic prepyloric gastric ulceration, Amer. J. Roentgen. **30**:473-479, 1933.

81 Hara, Y., Tobita, Y., Tsunoda, H., Sugiyama, K., Arakawa, M., Ansfield, F. J., and Hoon, J. R.: Intragastric photography; gastrocamera

with fiberscope, Arch. Surg. (Chicago) **94**:337-343, 1967.

82 Hardt, L. L., Steigmann, F., and Milles, C.: Gastric polyps, Gastroenterology **11**:629-639, 1948.

83 Harper, R. A. K., and Gree, B.: Malignant gastric ulcer, Clin. Radiol. **12**:95-108, 1961.

84 Harvey, H. D., Titherington, J. B., Stout, A. P., and St. John, F. B.: Gastric carcinoma, Cancer **4**:717-725, 1951.

85 Helsingen, N., and Hillestad, L.: Cancer development in the gastric stump after partial gastrectomy for ulcer, Ann. Surg. **143**:173-179, 1956.

86 Helwig, E. B., and Ranier, A.: Inflammatory fibroid polyps of the stomach, Surg. Gynec. Obstet. **96**:355-367, 1953.

87 Herter, F. P., and Auchincloss, H., Jr.: Total gastrectomy, Cancer **10**:320-331, 1957.

88 Hitchcock, C. R., MacLean, L. D., and Sullivan, W. A.: The secretory and clinical aspects of achlorhydria and gastric atrophy as precursors of gastric cancer, J. Nat. Cancer Inst. **18**:795-811, 1957.

89 Hitchcock, C. R., Sullivan, W. A., and Wangensteen, O. H.: The value of achlorhydria as a screening test for gastric cancer, Gastroenterology **29**:621-632, 1955.

90 Hogg, L., Jr., and Pack, G. T.: The controversial relationship between blood group A and gastric cancer, Gastroenterology **32**:797-806, 1957.

91 Hoon, J. R.: Operation of the gastrocamera in intragastric photography, Int. Surg. **46**:118-124, 1966.

92 Horn, R. C., Jr.: Carcinoma of the stomach; autopsy findings in untreated cases, Gastroenterology **29**:515-525, 1955.

93 Horst, H., and Lessman, F. P.: Objawy radiologiczne mięsaków limfatycznych zoladka, Pol. Przegl. Radiol. **29**:161-168, 1965.

94 Hurst, A. F.: Gastritis, Clin. J. **66**:89-100, 1937.

95 Ihre, B. J. E., Barr, H., and Havermark, G.: Ulcer-cancer of the stomach, Gastroenterologia (Basel) **102**:78-91, 1964.

96 Jordan, S. M.: Gastric ulcer and cancer, Gastroenterology **34**:254-268, 1958.

97 Joseph, J. I., and Lattes, R.: Gastrolymphosarcoma; clinicopathologic analysis of 71 cases and its relation to disseminated lymphosarcoma, Amer. J. Clin. Path. **45**:653-669, 1966.

98 Kay, S., Callahan, W. P., Jr., Murray, M. R., Randall, H. T., and Stout, A. P.: Glomus tumors of the stomach, Cancer **4**:726-736, 1951.

99 Keefer, C. S., and Bloomfield, A. L.: The significance of gastric anacidity, Bull. Johns Hopkins Hosp. **39**:304-329, 1926.

100 Kernen, J. A., and Bales, C.: Cytologic diagnosis of gastric cancer, Calif. Med. **108**:104-108, 1968.

101 Kirklin, B. R., and Harris, M. T.: Hypertrophy of the pyloric muscle of adults; a distinctive roentgenologic sign, Amer. J. Roentgen. **29**:437-442, 1933.

102 Kirklin, B. R., and Hodgson, J. R.: Carci-

noma of the stomach; its incidence and detection, Amer. J. Roentgen. **60**:600-602, 1948.

103 Kirklin, J. W., and Clagett, O. T.: Some technical aspects of esophagogastrectomy for carcinoma of lower part of esophagus and cardiac end of stomach, Surg. Clin. N. Amer. **31**:959-964, 1951.

104 Kirsh, I. E.: Benign and malignant ulcers of the greater curvature of the stomach; a study of 8 cases, 6 proved benign, Amer. J. Roentgen. **75**:318-332, 1956.

105 Klein, S. H.: Origin of carcinoma in chronic gastric ulcer, Arch. Surg. (Chicago) **37**:155-174, 1938.

106 Konjetzny, Georg E.: Der Magenkrebs, Stuttgart, 1938, Ferdinand Enke.

107 Kouwenaar, W.: On cancer incidence in Indonesia; symposium on geographical pathology and demography of cancer; sponsored by the World Health Organization, 1950.

108 Kugelmeier, L. M.: Leukämoide Reaktionen bei Carcinom, Folia Haemat. **53**:370-381, 1935.

109 LaDue, J. S., Murison, P. J., McNeer, G., and Pack, G. T.: Symptomology and diagnosis of gastric cancer, Arch. Surg. (Chicago) **60**:305-335, 1950.

110 Lahey, F. H., and Marshall, S. F.: Should total gastrectomy be employed in early carcinoma of the stomach? Experience with 139 total gastrectomies, Ann. Surg. **132**:540-565, 1950.

111 Lahey, F. H., Swinton, N. W., and Peelen, Matthew: Cancer of the stomach, New Eng. J. Med. **212**:863-868, 1935.

112 Laurén, P.: The two histological main types of gastric carcinoma: diffuse and so-called intestinal-type carcinoma; an attempt at a histo-clinical classification, Acta Path. Microbiol. Scand. **64**:31-49, 1965.

113 Lawton, S. E., Fildes, C. E., and Seidman, L.: Cancer of the stomach, Amer. J. Surg. **81**:221-226, 1951.

114 Levin, M. L.: Personal communication.

115 Liavaag, K.: Cancer development in gastric stump after partial gastrectomy for gastric ulcer, Ann. Surg. **155**:103-106, 1962.

116 Lumb, G.: A case of gastric carcinoma with spread exclusively to the remainder of the bowel and perianal skin, Brit. J. Surg. **37**:41-45, 1949.

117 McCune, W. S., Gusack, M., and Newman, W.: Eosinophilic gastroduodenitis with pyloric obstruction, Ann. Surg. **142**:510-518, 1955.

118 MacDonald, I., and Kotin, P.: Biologic predeterminism in gastric carcinoma as the limiting factor of curability, Surg. Gynec. Obstet. **98**:148-152, 1954.

119 MacDonald, W. C., Brandborg, L. L., Taniguchi, L., and Rubin, C. E.: Gastric exfoliative cytology, Lancet **2**:83-86, 1963.

120 McNeer, G., and Berg, J. W.: The clinical behavior and management of primary malignant lymphoma of the stomach, Surgery **46**:829-840, 1959.

121 McNeer, G., and James, A.: Resection of stomach and adjacent organs in continuity for advanced cancer, Cancer **1**:449-454, 1948.

122 McNeer, G., Sunderland, D. A., McInnes, G., Vanderberg, H. J., Jr., and Lawrence, W., Jr.: A more thorough operation for gastric cancer, anatomical basis and description of technique, Cancer **4**:957-967, 1951.

123 McNeer, G., Vandenberg, H., Jr., Donn, F. Y., and Bowden, L.: A critical evaluation of subtotal gastrectomy for the cure of cancer of the stomach, Ann. Surg. **134**:2-7, 1951.

124 McPeak, E., and Warren, S.: Histologic features of carcinoma of the cardio-esophageal junction and cardia, Amer. J. Path. **24**:971-1001, 1948.

125 Macklin, M. T.: The role of heredity in gastric and intestinal cancer, Gastroenterology **29**:507-511, 1955.

126 Mallory, T. B.: Carcinoma in situ of the stomach and its bearing on the histogenesis of malignant ulcers, Arch. Path. (Chicago) **30**:348-362, 1940.

127 Manrique, J., and Halliburton, J. C.: Recopilación y estudio de la casuística nacional sobre tumores benignos del estómago, Bol. Inst. Clin. Quir. **25**:131-144, 1949.

128 Marks, J. H.: Leiomyosarcoma of the stomach with excavation of the center of the tumor, Amer. J. Roentgen. **67**:76-79, 1952.

129 Marshak, R. H., and Feldman, F.: Gastric polyps, Amer. J. Dig. Dis. **10**:909-935, 1965.

130 Marshall, S. F.: Treatment of cancer of the stomach; end result, Gastroenterology **34**:34-46, 1958.

131 Marshall, S. F., and Meissner, W. A.: Sarcoma of the stomach, Ann. Surg. **131**:824-837, 1950.

132 Matthews, W. B.: Peptic ulcers involving the greater curvature of the stomach, Ann. Surg. **101**:844-855, 1935.

133 Mayo, H. W., Jr., Owens, J. K., and Weinberg, M.: A critical evaluation of radical subtotal gastric resection as a definite procedure for antral gastric carcinoma, Trans. Southern Surg. Ass. **66**:289-298, 1955.

134 Meissner, W. A.: Malignancy of gastric cancer, J. Nat. Cancer Inst. **10**:533-543, 1949.

135 Milton, G. W., and Lynch, A.: The diagnosis of gastric lesions; an assessment of the role of the gastro-camera, Brit. J. Surg. **52**:607-612, 1965.

136 Monaco, A. P., Roth, S. I., Castleman, B., and Welch, C. E.: Adenomatous polyps of the stomach; a clinical and pathological study of one hundred and fifty-three cases, Cancer **15**:456-467, 1962.

137 Monafo, W. W., Jr., Krause, G. L., Jr., and Guerra Medina, J.: Carcinoma of the stomach; morphological characteristics affecting survival, Arch. Surg. (Chicago) **85**:754-762, 1962.

138 Morrissey, J. F., Tanaka, Y., and Thorsen, W. B.: Gastroscopy; a review of the English and Japanese literature, Gastroenterology **53**:456-476, 1967.

139 Morson, B. C.: Carcinoma arising from areas of intestinal metaplasia in the gastric mucosa, Brit. J. Cancer **9**:377-385, 1955.

140 Muto, M., Maki, T., Majima, S., and Yamaguchi, I.: Improvement in the end-results of

surgical treatment of gastric cancer, Surgery 63:229-235, 1968.

141 Newcomb, W. D.: The relationship between peptic ulceration and gastric carcinoma, Brit. J. Surg. 20:279-308, 1932.

142 Ochsner, S. F., and Janetos, G. P.: Benign tumors of the stomach, J.A.M.A. 191:881-887, 1965.

143 Olsson, O., Westerborn, A., and Endresen, R.: Results of treatment of gastric cancer; 15 years' experience with 201 resections, Acta Chir. Scand. 111:1-15, 1956.

144 von Oppolzer, R.: Ueber das Magencarcinom. Lebensdauer und Schicksal von 859 Fallen der Jahre 1926-1935 der Klinik v. Eiselsberg Ranzi, Arch. Klin. Chir. 192:55-93, 1938.

145 Paaby, H.: Benign tumors of the stomach; a case of lipoma submucosa ventriculi simulating cancer of the stomach, Acta Chir. Scand. 97:381-388, 1948.

146 Pack, G. T., and McNeer, G.: Total gastrectomy for cancer, Int. Abst. Surg. 77:265-299, 1943; in Surg. Gynec. Obstet. Oct., 1943.

147 Pack, G. T., and McNeer, G.: End results in the treatment of cancer of the stomach, Surgery 24:769-778, 1948.

148 Pack, G. T., and McNeer, G.: Palliative operation for gastric cancer, Rev. Gastroent. 16:291-321, 1949.

149 Palmer, E. D.: Syphilis of the stomach and the stomach in syphilis; a review of the literature with particular reference to gross pathology and gastroscopic diagnosis, Amer. J. Syph. Gonor. Ven. Dis. 33:481-496, 1949.

150 Palmer, E. D.: Benign intramural tumors of the stomach; a review with special reference to gross pathology, Medicine (Balt.) 30:81-181, 1951.

151 Palmer, W. L.: Benign and malignant gastric ulcers; their relation and clinical differentiation, Ann. Intern. Med. 13:317-338, 1939.

152 Palumbo, L. T.: Esophagoduodenal anastomosis in selected cases of total gastrectomy, J. Int. Coll. Surg. 14:267-279, 1950.

153 Paramanandhan, T. L.: The duodenal spread of gastric carcinoma, Brit. J. Surg. 54:169-174, 1967.

154 Paulson, M., and Harvey, J. C.: Hematological alterations after total gastrectomy; evolutionary sequences over a decade, J.A.M.A. 156:1556-1560, 1954.

155 Payne, J. H., and Clagett, O. T.: Transthoracic gastric resection for lesions of cardia of stomach and lower part of esophagus, Surgery 23:912-920, 1948.

156 Pearl, F. L., and Brunn, H.: Multiple gastric polyposis, Surg. Gynec. Obstet. 76:257-281, 1943.

157 Perez, C. A., and Dorfman, R. F.: Benign lymphoid hyperplasia of the stomach and duodenum, Radiology 87:505-510, 1966.

158 Potchen, E. J., Khung, C. L., and Yatsuhashi, M.: X-ray diagnosis of gastric melanoma, New Eng. J. Med. 271:133-136, 1964.

159 Pygott, F.: Long survival after carcinoma of the stomach, Gut 3:118-125, 1964.

160 Quisenberry, W. B.: The epidemiologic approach to the problem of gastric cancer, Proceedings of the Third National Cancer Conference, Philadelphia, 1957, J. B. Lippincott Co., pp. 721-729.

161 Rafsky, H. A., Katz, H., and Krieger, C. I.: Varied clinical manifestations of lymphosarcoma of the stomach, Gastroenterology 3:297-305, 1944.

162 Raskin, H. F., Kirsner, J. B., Palmer, W. L., Pleticka, S. and Yarema, W. A.: Gastrointestinal cancer; definitive diagnosis by exfoliative cytology, Arch. Surg. (Chicago) 76:507-516, 1958.

163 Redd, B. L.: Lymphosarcoma of the stomach; review and case reports, Amer. J. Roentgen. 82:634-650, 1959.

164 Renshaw, J. F., and Spencer, F. M.: Gastroscopy and lymphoma of the stomach, Gastroenterology 9:1-5, 1947.

165 Reynolds, J. T., and Young, J. P., Jr.: The use of the Roux Y in extending the operability of carcinoma of the stomach of the lower end of the esophagus, Surgery 24:246-263, 1948.

166 Rieniets, J. H.: The frequency and pathologic aspects of gastric leiomyoma, Proc. Staff Meet. Mayo Clin. 5:364-366, 1930.

167 Rigler, L. G.: Roentgen examination of stomach in symptomless persons, J.A.M.A. 137:1501-1507, 1948.

168 Rigler, L. G., Blank, L., and Hebbel, R.: Granuloma with eosinophils; benign inflammatory fibroid polyps of the stomach, Radiology 66:169-176, 1956.

169 Roach, J. F., Sloan, R. D., and Morgan, R. H.: The detection of gastric carcinoma by photofluorographic methods. Part III. Findings, Amer. J. Roentgen. 67:68-75, 1952.

169a Roberts, J. A. F.: Some associations between blood groups and disease, Brit. Med. Bull. 15:129-133, 1959.

170 Rojel, K.: On linitis plastica and on sclerosing carcinoma of the stomach (carcinoma disseminatum Krompecher; carcinoma fibrosum Konjetzny), Acta Chir. Scand. 97:451-469, 1948.

171 Rønnov-Jessen, V., Ahlgren, P., and Qvist, C. F.: Incidence of gastric cancer in medically treated patients with gastric ulcer, Acta Med. Scand. 178:141-153, 1965.

172 Rouvière, H.: Anatomie des lymphatiques de l'homme, Paris, 1932, Masson et Cie.

173 Rubin, C. E.: The diagnosis of gastric malignancy in pernicious anemia, Gastroenterology 29:563-584, 1955.

174 St. John, F. B., Swenson, P. C., and Harvey, H. D.: An experiment in the early diagnosis of gastric carcinoma, Ann. Surg. 119:225-231, 1944.

175 Saphir, Otto, and Parker, M. L.: Linitis plastica type of carcinoma, Surg. Gynec. Obstet. 76:206-213, 1943.

176 Sauerbrey, R., and Reinhold, H.: Über den Wert der Röntgentiefentherapie beim inoperablen Magenkarzinom, Deutsch. Gesundh. 18:1527-1530, 1963.

177 Schade, R. O. K.: The cytological diagnosis of gastric carcinoma, Gastroenterologia (Basel) 85:190-194, 1956.

178 Schattenberg, H. J., and Ryan, J. F.:

Lymphangitic carcinomatosis of the lung, case report with autopsy findings, Ann. Intern. Med. **14**:1710-1721, 1941.

179 Scott, H. W., and Longmire, W. P., Jr.: Total gastrectomy, Surgery **26**:488-498, 1949.

180 Šerý, Z., and Dvoracek, C.: Evaluation of splenectomy as an aid in improving the radicality and results of abdominothoracic operations for cancers of the stomach and gastric cardia, Ann. Surg. **151**:29-36, 1960.

181 Shallenberger, P. L., DeWan, C. H., Weed, C. B., and Reganis, J. C.: Biopsy through the flexible operating gastroscope, Gastroenterology **16**:327-340, 1950.

182 Shanks, S. C.: Problems in the x-ray diagnosis of cancer of the stomach, Proc. Roy. Soc. Med. **43**:117-128, 1950.

183 Shearman, D. J. C., Finlayson, N. D. C., Wilson, R., and Samson, R. R.: Carcinoma of the stomach and early pernicious anaemia, Lancet **2**:403-405, 1966.

184 Sherman, R. S.: The roentgen diagnosis of cancer of the cardiac region of the stomach, Surgery **23**:874-883, 1948.

185 Sherman, R. S., and Wilner, D.: Superficial spreading gastric carcinoma; is it detectable roentgenologically? Amer. J. Roentgen. **79**:781-785, 1958.

186 Sherrick, D. W., Hodgson, J. R., and Dockerty, M. B.: The roentgenologic diagnosis of primary gastric lymphoma, Radiology **84**:925-932, 1965.

187 Shimkin, M. B.: Duration of life in untreated cancer, Cancer **4**:1-8, 1951.

188 Sigurjonsson, J.: Trends in mortality from cancer, with special reference to gastric cancer in Iceland, J. Nat. Cancer Inst. **36**:899-907, 1966.

189 Slungaard, U., and Weber-Laumann, A.: Prognosis of gastric carcinoma; analyzed in a Norwegian county, Acta Chir. Scand. **129**:425-433, 1965.

190 Smith, F. H., and Jordan, S. M.: Gastric ulcer; a study of 600 cases, Gastroenterology **11**:575-597, 1948.

191 Smithers, D. W.: The association of cancer of the gastric cardia with partial thoracic stomach, short oesophagus and peptic ulceration, Brit. J. Radiol. **23**:261-269, 1950.

192 Snoddy, W. T.: Primary lymphosarcoma of the stomach, Gastroenterology **20**:537-553, 1952.

193 Stammers, F. A. R.: Discussion on resectable carcinoma of the stomach, Proc. Roy. Soc. Med. **42**:667-671, 1949.

194 State, D., Gaviser, D., Hubbard, T. B., and Wangensteen, O. H.: Early diagnosis of gastric cancer, J.A.M.A. **142**:1128-1132, 1950.

195 State, D., Moore, G., and Wagensteen, O. H.: Carcinoma of the stomach; a ten-year survey (1936 to 1945, inclusive) of early and late results of surgical treatment at the University of Minnesota Hospitals, J.A.M.A. **135**:262-267, 1947.

196 Steiner, C. A., and Palmer, L. H.: Polyposis of the stomach treated by total gastrectomy, Amer. J. Surg. **76**:211-214, 1948.

197 Steiner, P. E.: Etiologic implications of the racial incidences of gastric cancer, J. Nat. Cancer Inst. **10**:429-437, 1949.

198 Steiner, P. E., Maimon, S. N., Palmer, W. L., and Kirsner, J. B.: Gastric cancer; morphologic factors in five-year survival after gastrectomy, Amer. J. Path. **24**:947-969, 1948.

199 Stewart, M. J.: Observations of the relation of malignant disease to benign tumors of the intestinal tract, Brit. Med. J. **2**:567-569, 1929.

200 Stewart, M. J.: Cancer of the stomach; some pathological considerations, Brit. J. Radiol. **20**:505-507, 1947.

201 Stewart, M. J., and Taylor, A. L.: Adenomyoma of the stomach, J. Path. Bact. **28**:195-202, 1925.

202 Stocks, P., and Davies, R. I.: Zinc and copper content of soils associated with the incidence of cancer of the stomach and other organs, Brit. J. Cancer **18**:14-24, 1964.

203 Stoerk, O.: Ulcer-cancer of the stomach, Wien. Klin. Wschr. **38**:347-352, 1925.

204 Stout, A. P.: Pathology of carcinoma of the stomach, Arch. Surg. (Chicago) **46**:807-822, 1943.

205 Stout, A. P.: Gastric mucosal atrophy and carcinoma of the stomach, New York J. Med. **45**:973-977, 1945.

206 Stout, A. P.: Superficial spreading type of carcinoma of the stomach, J. Nat. Cancer Inst. **5**:363, 1945.

207 Stout, A. P.: The relationship of gastric ulcer to gastric cancer: panel discussion, Cancer **3**:515-552, 1950.

208 Strode, J. E.: In support of surgical removal of small ulcerating lesions of the stomach without benefit of medical treatment, Surg. Gynec. Obstet. **98**:607-618, 1954.

209 Strudwick, W. J., Ewing, J. B., and White, J. E.: Carcinoma of the stomach in American Negroes, Surg. Gynec. Obstet. **119**:580-582, 1964.

210 Sunderland, D. A., McNeer, G., Ortega, L. A., and Pearce, L. S.: The lymphatic spread of gastric cancer, Cancer **6**:987-996, 1953.

211 Sussman, M. L., and Lipsay, J. J.: The roentgen differentiation of benign and malignant ulcers, Surg. Clin. N. Amer. **27**:273-287, 1947.

212 Sutomo, T.: Additional data on cancer incidence in Indonesia; symposium of geographical pathology and demography of cancer; sponsored by the World Health Organization, 1950.

213 Sweet, R. H.: The treatment of carcinoma of the esophagus and cardiac end of the stomach by surgical extirpation; two hundred three cases of resection, Surgery **23**:952-975, 1948.

214 Swynnerton, B. F., and Truelove, S. C.: Carcinoma of the stomach, Brit. Med. J. **1**:287-292, 1952.

215 Taebel, D. W., Prolla, J. C., and Kirsner, J. B.: Exfoliative cytology in the diagnosis of stomach cancer, Ann. Intern. Med. **63**:1018-1026, 1965.

216 Tallqvist, G., Salmela, H., and Lindstrom, B. L.: Leiomyoblastoma of the stomach; a

clinicopathological study of 10 cases, Acta Path. Microbiol. Scand. **71**:194-202, 1967.

217 Taylor, E. S.: Primary lymphosarcoma of the stomach, Ann. Surg. **110**:200-221, 1939.

218 Terris, M., and Hall, C. E.: Decline in mortality from gastric cancer in native-born and foreign-born residents of New York City, J. Nat. Cancer Inst. **31**:155-162, 1963.

219 Thorbjarnarson, B., Beal, J. M., and Pearce, J. M.: Primary malignant lymphoid tumor of the stomach, Cancer **9**:712-717, 1956.

220 Tulchinsky, D., and Modan, B.: Epidemiological aspects of cancer of the stomach in Israel, Cancer **20**:1311-1317, 1967.

221 Urban, C. H., and McNeer, G.: The relation of the morphology of gastric carcinoma to long and short term survival, Cancer **12**:1158-1162, 1959.

222 Vanzant, F. R., Alvarez, W. C., Eustermann, G. B., Dunn, H. L., and Berkson, J.: The normal range of gastric acidity from youth to old age; an analysis of 3,746 records, Arch. Intern. Med. (Chicago) **49**:345-359, 1932.

223 Veterans Administration Surgical Adjuvant Cancer Chemotherapy Study Group (O. Serlin, chairman): Use of thio-TEPA as an adjuvant to the surgical management of carcinoma of the stomach, Cancer **18**:291-297, 1965.

224 Walters, W., Gray, H. K., Priestley, J. T., and Waugh, J. M.: Report on surgery of stomach and duodenum for 1947, Proc. Staff Meet. Mayo Clin. **23**:554-562, 1948.

225 Wang, C. C., and Petersen, J. A.: Malignant lymphoma of the gastrointestinal tract; roentgenographic considerations, Acta Radiol. (Stockholm) **46**:523-532, 1956.

226 Watman, R.; quoted by Welch, C. E., and Burke, J. F.: An appraisal of the treatment of gastric ulcer, Surgery **44**:943-958, 1958.

227 Welch, C. E.: Carcinoma of the stomach, Surg. Clin. N. Amer. **27**:1100-1105, 1947.

228 Welch, C. E., and Allen, A. W.: Carcinoma of the stomach, New Eng. J. Med. **238**:583-589, 1948.

229 West, J. P., and Knox, G.: Neurogenic tumors of the stomach, Surgery **23**:450-466, 1948.

230 Woolf, C. M.: Investigations on genetic aspects of carcinoma of the stomach and breast, Univ. Calif. Pub. Public Health **2**:265-349, 1955.

231 Wu, T. T.: Generalized lymphatic carcinosis ("lymphangitic carcinomatosa") of lungs, J. Path. Bact. **43**:61-76, 1936.

232 Wynder, E. L., Kmet, J., Dungal, N., and Segi, M.: An epidemiological investigation of gastric cancer, Cancer **16**:1461-1496, 1963.

233 Yarnis, H., Marshak, R. H., and Friedman, A. I.: Gastric polyps, J.A.M.A. **148**:1088-1094, 1952.

234 Zacho, A., Fischermann, K., and Sørensen, B. L.: Prognostic role of breach of lymph node capsule in nodal metastases from gastric carcinoma, Acta Chir. Scand. **125**:365-369, 1963.

235 Zinninger, M. M., and Collins, W. T.: Extension of carcinoma of the stomach into the duodenum and esophagus, Ann. Surg. **130**:557-566, 1949.

Small bowel

Anatomy

The small intestine extends from the pyloric ring of the stomach to the ileocecal valve and consists of a small-caliber musculomembranous tube divided into three portions: the duodenum, the jejunum, and the ileum. The limits between the last two portions are arbitrary.

The duodenum starts at the pyloric ring of the stomach and follows an upward direction toward the neck of the gallbladder to form its first portion, the duodenal bulb. Then it descends as a retroperitoneal structure between the head of the pancreas and the hilus of the right kidney. This second descending portion is intimately associated with the head of the pancreas, and into it open the pancreatic and the common biliary ducts. At the level of the third lumbar vertebra, the duodenum bends to form the third horizontal portion which extends to the mesenteric vessels, and the fourth portion extends from these vessels to the duodenojejunal angle. This sharp bend in the small intestine is situated on the left side of the second lumbar vertebra. From there on, the small intestine has a variable length and is divided into loops that occupy mostly the left side of the abdomen and finally open into the large bowel at the level of the ileocecal valve. The jejunoileum is attached to the posterior abdominal wall by the mesentery. The mesentery inserts in an oblique line measuring about 12 cm in length and extends from the duodenojejunal angle on the left side of the second lumbar vertebra, crosses the midline in a downward direction, and ends to the right of the sacrolumbar disk. The free border of the mesentery spreads like a fan and measures about twenty feet in length. The blood supply of the small intestine comes from the superior mesenteric artery.

The mucosal surface of the small intestine is increased by circular folds (valves of Kerckring) and the villi. These folds are of maximum development in the distal half of the duodenum and the proximal half of the jejunum. They gradually become less prominent in the ileum and disappear at about its midportion. The folds are made up of all layers of the mucosa, including muscularis mucosae. The villi are formed by mucous membrane, and their openings are designated as the crypts of Lieberkühn. The lining epithelium is made up of columnar cells, goblet cells, and argentaffin cells.

Lymphatic tissue is present throughout the small intestine, but it becomes most prominent in the ileum, where aggregations of follicles are designated as Peyer's patches (thirty to forty in number). The submucosa contains the muscularis mucosae and numerous blood vessels. The external and internal layers of the muscular wall are well developed. The outer surface is covered by serosa.

Lymphatics. The lymphatics of the *duodenum* converge behind the head of the pancreas to end in the posterior pancreaticoduodenal lymph nodes. The lymphatics of the *jejunum* and the *ileum* run through the mesentery in greater number than the blood vessels and are drained by the mesenteric lymph nodes. Those arising from the terminal segment of the ileum drain into the lymph nodes of the ileocolic chain and, at times, into a posterior cecal lymph node.

Epidemiology

Tumors of the small bowel are astonishingly infrequent considering the area of vulnerability. The 1947 United States survey revealed an age-adjusted incidence of 1.0 and 0.6 per 100,000 population for white males and females and of 0.7 and 0.2 for nonwhite males and females. The largest proportion of tumors of the small intestine encountered at surgery are malignant (Darling and Welch[14]), but autopsy series show that benign tumors occur more frequently.

In a study of 1399 benign tumors of the small intestine, River et al.[47] found that

adenomas, lipomas, and leiomyomas are the most frequent. Polyposis involving the small intestine and, at times, the stomach may be associated with the presence of melanin spots of the oral mucosa, lips, and digits. This latter condition is inherited as a simple mendelian dominant trait (Jeghers et al.[34]). Burdick et al.[11] recorded a family group of ten patients with the Peutz-Jeghers syndrome. About 40% of patients with this syndrome have relatives with both pigment changes and polyps and another 15% have pigment without polyps. Carcinoid tumors seem to occur in patients of all ages, but those arising in the small intestine occur in patients considerably older, as an average, than do those arising in the appendix (Barclay and Robb[2a]). Instances of more than one case of carcinoma of the small intestine in members of the same family have been reported (Pridgen et al.[45]). Lymphosarcoma of the small bowel may be associated with the malabsorption syndrome (Williams et al.[62]; Spence and Ritchie[54a]).

Pathology
Gross and microscopic pathology

Tumors can arise from any of the tissues normally present within the small bowel but very rarely originate in aberrant pancreatic tissue or within a Meckel's diverticulum (Albright and Sprague[1]). The classification shown in Table 35 has proved useful. In a series of 199 tumors studied by Ostermiller et al.,[40] 122 were malignant and seventy-seven were benign. Pagtalunan et al.[41] reported 327 malignant tumors —18% in the duodenum, 36% in the jejunum, and 41% in the ileum. There were 129 adenocarcinomas, one-third in the duodenum and one-half in the jejunum. Of the sixty-eight carcinoids, 85% were found in the ileum, and of the sixty-one lymphosarcomas, 31% were in the jejunum and 52% in the ileum. The distribution of benign and malignant tumors found in surgical specimens at Barnes Hospital in St. Louis is shown in Table 36. Barnett[3] reviewed benign duodenal tumors and found seventy-eight adenomas, twenty-eight leiomyomas, seventeen lipomas, and eight hemangiomas, all of which were more often found in the first half of the duodenum.

Table 35. Classification of tumors of small bowel according to tissue of origin

Tissue of origin	Benign	Malignant
Smooth muscle	Leiomyoma	Leiomyosarcoma
Glandular epithelium	Adenoma	Adenocarcinoma
Chromaffin cells of crypts of Lieberkühn		Carcinoid
Lymphoid tissue	Pseudolymphoma	Lymphosarcoma
Fat	Lipoma	Not reported
Connective tissue	Fibroma	Fibrosarcoma
Nerve sheath	Neurofibroma (also neurilemoma)	Malignant schwannoma
Blood vessels	Hemangioma	Angiosarcoma
Lymph vessels	Lymphangioma	Not reported

Table 36. Benign and malignant small bowel tumors, 1952-1968 (Barnes Hospital, St. Louis, Mo.)

	Duodenum	Jejunum	Ileum	Total
Adenomatous polyp	8	2	0	10
Villous adenoma	2	1	0	3
Lipoma	3	3	3	9
Liposarcoma	0	1	0	1
Leiomyoma	5	10	7	22
Leiomyosarcoma	2	3	6	11
Carcinoid	0	0	14	14
Islet cell tumor or carcinoid tumor	12	0	0	12
Carcinoma	4	5	3	12
Lymphoma	2	13	25	40
Miscellaneous	4	1	0	5
Total	42	39	58	139

The smooth muscle tumor, the *leiomyoma*, is a common benign tumor of the small intestine. About 80% occur with equal frequency in the jejunum and ileum and the remaining 20% in the duodenum. Rarely, the appendix and Meckel's diverticulum may be a primary site (Golden and Stout[23]). A small percentage of these tumors arise from the muscularis mucosae but more frequently from the subserosa or from the muscular wall. Those that arise from the muscularis mucosae grow toward the lumen, those from the subserosa grow away from the lumen, and those from the muscular wall can grow in either direction. These tumors are of variable size. Those discovered at autopsy as incidental findings are usually very small, whereas those that produce clinical signs and symptoms are much larger, weighing as much as 1000 gm. They are rather firm, and if they grow toward the lumen or invaginate from the subserosal area, they may finally centrally ulcerate. Grossly, it may be impossible to tell whether the lesion is a leiomyoma or a *leiomyosarcoma*. The malignant smooth muscle tumors may have cellular areas with zones of necrosis, and excavation of the central portion of the tumor with fistula formation can occur (Weinstein and Roberts[60]). A fairly low proportion of all the cases are malignant. The various gross patterns are well illustrated by Wald[59] (Figs. 358 and 359).

Microscopically, the leiomyoma is fairly cellular, often with areas of hyaline change, and if the tumor has ulcerated, there is considerable inflammation. Myofibrils may be difficult to identify. At times, because of the bizarre appearance of the cells and the innumerable mitotic figures, a diagnosis of leiomyosarcoma may be made. Unfortunately, some of the tumors that appear benign microscopically rarely metastasize, whereas those that appear malignant may remain localized. The leiomyoma, in contrast to the tumors of neural origin, is nonencapsulated (Stout[55]).

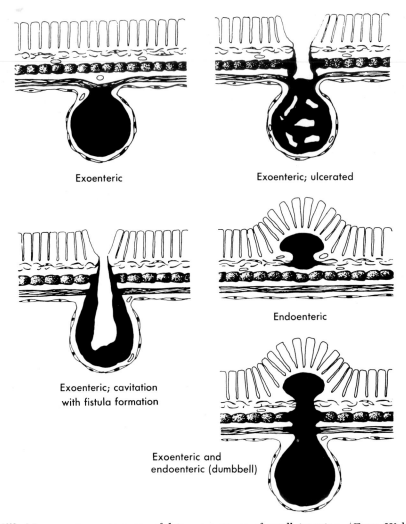

Exoenteric

Exoenteric; ulcerated

Exoenteric; cavitation
with fistula formation

Endoenteric

Exoenteric and
endoenteric (dumbbell)

Fig. 358. Macroscopic appearances of leiomyosarcomas of small intestine. (From Wald, M.: Leiomyosarcoma of the jejunum, Aust. New Zeal. J. Surg. **33**:147-154, 1963; WU neg. 68-7990.)

Polyps or *adenomas* arising from glandular epithelium may occur anywhere in the small bowel and, at times, may be multiple. Microscopically, the benign polyps are similar to polyps found elsewhere. Bartholomew et al.[4] reported that polyps in the Peutz-Jeghers syndrome are unusual in that they contain columnar cells, goblet cells, and Paneth cells. They lack a well-defined stalk and present bands of smooth muscle throughout, suggesting that they are hamartomas. Malignant changes have been reported in these polyps. Erroneous interpretation is possible due to the intermingling of smooth muscle and glands.

Rarely, such polyps are malignant and can metastasize and cause death (Horn et al.[33]; Williams and Knudsen[61]).

Carcinomas of the first and third portions of the duodenum are uncommon, but they arise in the periampullary area. Pridgen et al.[45] reported forty-four carcinomas of the jejunum and nineteen of the ileum. The most common locations were the upper third of the jejunum and the lower third of the ileum. These carcinomas are often constricting, form an annular ring with involvement of the entire lumen of the bowel, and completely obstruct the bowel proximal to the lesion. At times, the

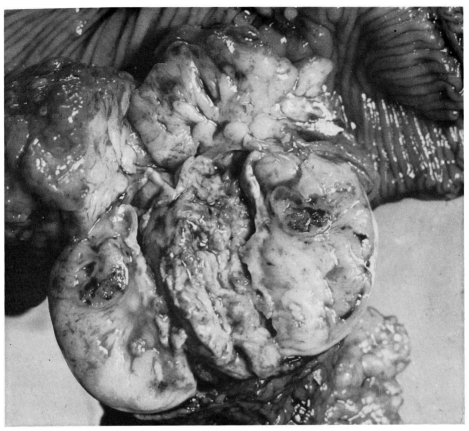

Fig. 359. Large, soft, ulcerating leiomyosarcoma of small intestine. Patient living and well six years after operation. (WU neg. 54-1566.)

tumor is fungating and nonobstructing and shows hypertrophy of its muscularis with considerable dilatation.

Carcinoid tumors can arise in any part of the small bowel but in most instances appear in the terminal ileum or the appendix. They can even occur in a Meckel's diverticulum (Herena and Schraft[28]). These tumors are frequently multiple, often appear to be submucosal, and usually present only very small areas of superficial ulceration. On section, they are orange-yellow in color due to the large amount of cholesterol present. This color is present not only in the primary tumor but also in the metastases. A carcinoid tumor may have multiple foci of origin, frequently causes partial obstruction of the bowel, and often invades the entire width of the bowel wall to implicate the serosal surface. With this involvement, a buckling of the bowel may result. Along with these changes, there is

frequently hypertrophy of the muscularis (Fig. 360). Microscopically, carcinoid tumors arise from the enterochromaffin system. This system includes a number of cell types distributed throughout the intestinal tract. Carcinoid tumors tend to correspond cytologically to the type of enterochromaffin cell that is dominant in a given region (Black[6]); they form well-ordered acini with practically no mitotic figures. All the cells appear similar—they are rather small with fine nucleoli. Tumor cells are frequently present within lymphatics. All of these tumors are of low-grade malignancy. In a case reported by Campbell et al.,[13] in which there were associated peptic ulcers, the cells were argyrophil but not argentaffin. The tumor was found to contain notable quantities of histamine and 5-hydroxytryptophan but not 5-hydroxytryptamine.

The *lymphosarcoma* of the small bowel

is almost as common as the adenocarcinoma. It occurs particularly in the ileum and often in young male adults. In a series of 109 lymphosarcomas of the intestine collected by Ullman and Abehouse,[58] seventy-seven occurred in the small bowel, thirty-six of these in the ileum. In seventy-nine resected isolated malignant lymphomas of the gastrointestinal tract, forty-four involved the stomach, twenty-five the small

bowel, nine the large bowel, and one the esophagus. The tumor may diffusely infiltrate the ileum over a fairly long distance (15 cm to 20 cm) and replace the wall with lymphoid masses. This lymphosarcoma of the small bowel may present disklike areas of involvement, diffuse involvement of the submucosa, or giant rugae (Fig. 361). In the terminal ileum, it may rarely intussuscept.

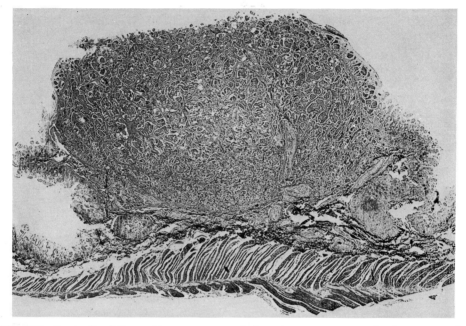

Fig. 360. Carcinoid of ileum. Note restriction of the tumor to mucosa and submucosa with hypertrophy of muscularis. (Very low-power enlargement.)

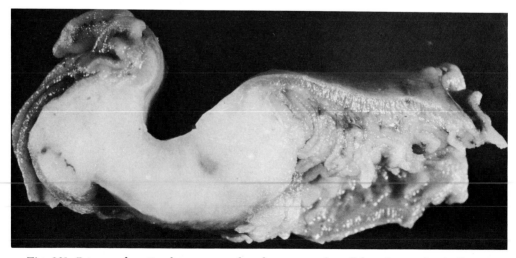

Fig. 361. Primary ulcerating homogeneous lymphosarcoma of small bowel occurring in Bantu. (Courtesy South African Institute for Medical Research, Johannesburg, R.S.A.; SA neg. 4893.)

The *lipoma* is another common benign tumor of the small bowel, and it most frequently (approximately one-third) appears in the ileum (Schottenfeld[50]). Lipomas are often submucosal (about 90%) and form a fairly well-defined tumor mass usually with an intact overlying mucosa. They are occasionally found in the subserosa and may be multiple. They are of variable size and may be pedunculated. On section, lipomas are soft, light yellow in color, and homogeneous. Due to impaired blood supply, necrosis or hemorrhage may occur within them. Microscopically, they are composed of normal fat with a variable amount of connective tissue stroma. *Liposarcomas* of the small intestine have not been reported.

The *fibromas, neurofibromas,* and *neurilemomas* of the small bowel are relatively few in number as compared with leiomyomas but present very similar gross characteristics. Microscopically, the neural tumors are encapsulated (the leiomyomas are nonencapsulated). Fibromas are rare and are made up purely of connective tissue cells. At times, *fibrosarcomas* and *malignant schwannomas* occur. *Hemangiomas* are extremely rare and usually single but can be multiple (Hansen[26]). They are often submucosal in nature. Microscopically, they can be capillary or cavernous. They can invade the muscularis and even perforate retroperitoneally. The malignant variant is extremely rare. *Lymphangiomas* are equally rare, polypoid, soft, and velvety and are made up of small nodules. There may be yellowish zones in the folds of the mucous membrane (Puppel and Morris[46]). Taylor and Helwig[56] have reported nine tumors arising in the second portion of the duodenum that they identify as benign *nonchromaffin paragangliomas.* These lesions are usually pedunculated and may have symptoms suggesting peptic ulcer.

Metastatic spread

Leiomyomas, fibrosarcomas, and *malignant schwannomas* metastasize to the liver and lungs but infrequently to lymph nodes. Adenocarcinomas, on the contrary, first metastasize to the regional lymph nodes and sometimes to the liver, lungs, and bone. *Carcinoid* tumors vary in their ability to metastasize—those arising in the ileum do so more frequently than those from the appendix. *Lymphosarcomas* frequently extend to the regional lymph nodes and later to distant ones.

Clinical evolution

Many of the tumors of the small bowel reported in the medical literature were found at autopsy and were, for the most part, symptomless. Darling and Welch[14] reported on 132 patients, nineteen of whom had symptomless tumors, all but one of which were benign. Of the 113 patients who presented symptoms, eighty-five (75%) had malignant tumors with the following major patterns: obstruction (67%), bleeding (53%), palpable mass (31%), and perforation (11%).

Bleeding into the intestinal tract is present in a rather large proportion of patients. The amount of bleeding varies with the cases. Leiomyomas often are accompanied by bleeding which, at times, is profuse and alarming. Carcinoid tumors, by contrast, rarely bleed. The subserosal tumors tend to grow to large dimensions. Liquefaction necrosis may result, followed by hemorrhage. Hemorrhage also occurs in patients with cavernous hemangioma, adenocarcinoma, and lymphosarcoma. Free perforation into the peritoneal cavity occurs in about 10% of patients with leiomyosarcomas, 3% with malignant lymphomas, and 1% with carcinomas. Carcinoid tumors do not usually perforate (Higgins et al.[30]).

Symptoms of small bowel obstruction are intermittent pain, nausea, occasional vomiting, peristaltic rushes, and borborygmi. As the obstruction becomes complete, the distention becomes marked, and vomiting, at times fecal, becomes persistent. Obstruction was present in twenty-seven of thirty-nine patients with submucosal myomas reported by Smith.[54] *Intussusception* is a fairly frequent complication of small bowel tumors and is much more common with benign than with malignant tumors. The development of intussusception depends on the location of the tumor and on whether or not it is polypoid or pedunculated in character. Patients with submucous lipomas, pedunculated leiomyomas, and polyps are most prone to intussusception. In most instances, intussusception is sudden and painful, but in some patients only mild recurrent symptoms may be present.

Milder symptoms of intestinal irritation may be present and suggest peptic ulcer, indigestion, or constipation. Such vague symptomatology may often be found in those with adenomatous tumors. Intermittent episodes of small bowel obstruction, associated with pain, diarrhea, and weight loss, are frequently observed in patients with carcinoid tumors. Carcinoids that have already produced metastases often cause symptoms (Pearson and Fitzgerald[42]).

A case of unusual cyanosis in a patient with pulmonary stenosis was published by Biörck et al.[5] in 1952. In 1954 Thorson et al.[57] described a clinical *syndrome of carcinoid* of the small intestine with metastases to the liver, characterized by cutaneous flushes and cyanosis, chronic diarrhea and peristaltic rushes, respiratory distress, and valvular disease of the right heart. They suggested that the syndrome was due to the production and release of serotonin (5-hydroxytryptamine) by the tumor. Lembeck[35] analyzed a carcinoid tumor and found it rich in serotonin. Erspamer[19] believes that serotonin is produced by the chromaffin cells of the intestinal tract from which carcinoids arise. It is interesting that blood histamine is also increased, either directly or as a secondary release by 5-hydroxytryptamine, a serotonin precursor. Increases in the urinary excretion of 5-hydroxyindolacetic acid during severe flushing episodes suggest that they are due to increased serotonin release (Sjoerdsma et al.[52]). But patients with metastatic carcinoids do not necessarily present this syndrome, not all patients with the carcinoid syndrome exhibit all of the typical features, and questions have been raised as to the specificity of gross lesions of the left heart. Some cases of carcinoid have been reported that were accompanied by pruritus or associated with multiple peptic ulcers (Campbell et al.[13]). The variability of the clinical pattern may be due to the elaboration of different biologically active substances (Gardner et al.[22]).

Bleeding results in secondary anemia. Benign tumors are seldom the cause of death unless intestinal obstruction or intussusception develops with secondary peritonitis. A few of the patients, particularly those with leiomyomas, may die of hemorrhage. The spread of adenocarcinomas and other malignant tumors causes weight loss and other signs of deterioration of the general condition.

Diagnosis
Clinical examination

Examination of a patient with a tumor of the small bowel usually reveals little of significance. Benign small bowel tumors are usually freely movable, and only the very large ones can be palpated. Cameron,[12] in reviewing 200 malignant tumors of the small bowel, found that 65% of the sarcomas and 29% of the carcinomas were palpable. A small bowel obstruction may cause distention and visible peristaltic waves. Intussusception may cause the formation of a firm, tender mass. Intussusception in the adult frequently indicates a small bowel tumor (Lowman and Mendelsohn[36]). Repeated intestinal hemorrhages, not otherwise explained, may be a sign of tumor of the small intestine.

Lymphosarcoma is difficult to diagnose. This tumor often causes considerable dilatation of the affected bowel, and it is very common to find regional lymph node involvement. If the tumor begins in the region of the ileum, inguinal lymph node metastases may mark the clinical onset, and later there will be generalization of the process. The symptomatology may be either very slow or very rapid in its evolution. Signs of intestinal obstruction, weakness, weight loss, and anorexia may appear. Bleeding into the gastrointestinal tract often results in a rather profound secondary anemia. Diarrhea, which does not respond to medication, is fairly common. Nodular lymphoid hyperplasia of the small intestine may be associated with hypogammaglobulinemia (Hermans[29]). The malabsorption syndrome may be associated with or followed by lymphosarcoma.

Roentgenologic examination

The radiologic investigation of the small bowel is usually done after other segments of the gastrointestinal tract have been eliminated as possible sites of origin of the symptoms. Occasionally, a thorough exam-

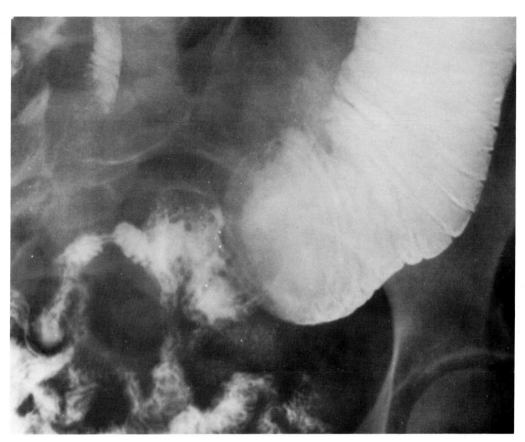

Fig. 362. Classic roentgenogram of typical circumferential adenocarcinoma of jejunum. Regional lymph nodes were negative. (WU neg. 68-8031.)

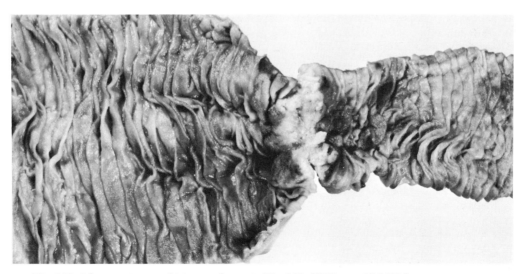

Fig. 363. Adenocarcinoma of jejunum shown in Fig. 362. (WU neg. 68-3431.)

ination is suggested by the incidental find-ing of air or fluid levels in roentgenograms taken for other purposes. The efficiency of the roentgenologic diagnosis decreases from the duodenum to the jejunum and ileum. The length and pliability of the small intestine and the unavoidable over-lap of its different portions are the natural causes. But much is also due to the fact that the technique of examination is sel-dom mastered due to infrequent utilization. Numerous techniques have been advocated for the examination of the small intestine. In the *intestinal series* utilized with minor variations in different institutions, the pa-tient is given a certain amount of barium, and roentgenograms are taken at estab-lished intervals to observe the progress of the barium toward the colon. Fluoroscopic observation is essential in many cases (Good[24]). The complete examination re-quires repeated periods of study at inter-vals of thirty to forty-five minutes. There is usually need for careful manipulation during fluoroscopy. But, whereas dedica-tion and skill may make the difference, the radiologic exploration of the small intestine is not so fruitful as that of other regions of the gastrointestinal tract.

The roentgenologic diagnosis of small bowel tumors is made on the basis of alter-ations in the mucosal patterns and the presence of obstruction, intussusception, or extraluminal defects. Carcinomas may pro-duce a typical napkin-ring constriction with proximal dilatation (Figs. 362 and 363). The involved area is usually short, and the mucosal pattern through it is destroyed. Polypoid carcinomas are rare. A similar constriction may be found in carcinoids. A number of tumors of the small bowel are extraluminal and nonob-structing. The roentgenologic examination may reveal only irregularity of outline with obliteration of the mucosa and dilatation of the lumen. Ulcerated lesions may make themselves visible by retaining a small amount of barium. In the diagnosis of car-cinomas of the duodenum, the radiologic examination, carried out thoroughly and expertly, offers the most important oppor-tunity for service to the patient (Freed-man et al.[21]; Brenner and Brown[9]).

In lymphosarcomas, the roentgenograph-ic findings are extremely variable and none

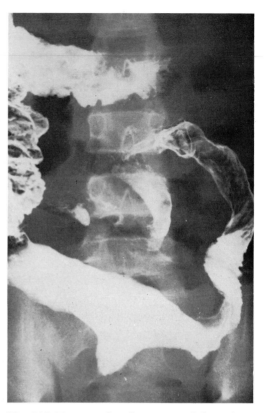

Fig. 364. Extensive lymphosarcoma of ileum (gar-den hose effect.)

are diagnostic (Fig. 364). Diffuse lympho-sarcoma can mimic the sprue pattern or it can be polypoid with intussusception or be associated with ulceration and perforation (Marshak et al.[38]). Furthermore, dysgam-maglobulinemia may occur with nodular lymphoid hyperplasia of the small intestine (Grise[25]).

Intramural smooth muscle tumors may not alter the normal roentgenologic ap-pearance of the gut. Submucosal tumors may present a well-circumscribed defect, adjacent normal mucosal pattern, and pos-sible nichelike ulceration in the center of the tumor. Fluoroscopically, the stream of the opaque material may be split and normal peristalsis may be observed (Baker and Good[2]). Adenomatous polyps of the duodenum have been reported and, at times, are large (Fig. 365) (Deutschber-ger et al.[16]).

If there are multiple tumors with mini-mal ulceration and buckling in the region of the terminal ileum, then a diagnosis of multiple carcinoid should be considered

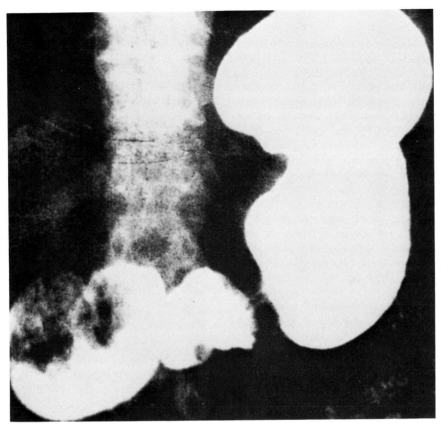

Fig. 365. Roentgenogram of stomach and duodenum with patient in prone position showing lobulation of defect within tremendously enlarged duodenal bulb due to large adenomatous polyp. (From Deutschberger, O., et al.: Benign duodenal polyp; review of literature and report of a giant adenomatous polyp of the duodenal bulb, Amer. J. Gastroent. **38**:75-84, 1962.)

(Miller and Herrmann[39]). It is not infrequent for intussusception to take place between the ileum and the cecum. A case reported by Botsford and Seibel[8] showed valvulae conniventes of the small bowel inside the large bowel after evacuation. Nonmalignant lesions tend to extend over longer segments of the bowel and demarcation between the involved and the uninvolved areas is gradual rather than abrupt, but it is impossible, in many instances, to determine roentgenologically whether a given lesion of the small bowel is benign or malignant. Some lesions are well circumscribed and regular in contour but, on microscopic examination, may show evidence of malignancy. Debray et al.[15] utilized selective arteriography of the upper mesenteric vessels to diagnose a leiomyoma and a malignant schwannoma of the small intestine.

Laboratory examination

Patients suspected of having tumors of the small bowel should have examinations of the stools for the presence of occult blood. *Serotonin* may be chemically demonstrated in the surgical specimens of some malignant carcinoids, particularly of small intestine origin, but it may be absent in others. There are difficulties in determining plasma serotonin. Sjoerdsma et al.[53] developed a simplified test that is dependent upon a high titer of serotonin in the urine. This test is positive only in cases with metastases to the liver. Serotonin is absent in the cerebrospinal fluid.

Differential diagnosis

Any lesion of the small bowel that gives signs suggesting small bowel obstruction may exactly simulate a tumor. A *duodenal ulcer* is the most common such lesion. The diverticula, a *Meckel's diverticulum, complications from an appendicitis*, and *regional ileitis* may all simulate small bowel tumor. However, Hofbert et al.[32] reported an adenocarcinoma of the terminal ileum in a patient with coexisting active regional ileitis. Other lesions in close proximity to the duodenum may cause defects in the bowel wall, and thus an erroneous diagnosis of primary duodenal neoplasm may be made. These lesions include *cysts* and *tumors of the pancreas, carcinoma of the hepatic flexure*, and *metastatic lesions of the retroperitoneal lymph nodes*. Specific infections such as *tuberculosis* should be ruled out. Tuberculosis, however, is most prominent in the region of the ileum, and invariably there is roentgenologic evidence of pulmonary disease. Enteric-coated potassium chloride may cause segmental ulcerative lesions of the small intestine due to venous infarction (Boley et al.[7]). *Cicatrizing enteritis* occurs in young men and often shows multiple lesions and typical roentgenologic signs (Figs. 366 and 367). Various intestinal anomalies and infections may be the cause of bleeding (Hodes and Edeiken[31]). Eosinophilic granuloma may rarely develop in the small intestine (Polayes and Kreiger[44]). Coincident occurrence of large bowel carcinoma with carcinoids of the small intestine has been reported.

Pernow and Waldenström[43] reported a patient who presented clinical symptoms of a *carcinoid syndrome* and high values of 5-hydroxyindolacetic acid (5-HIAA) in the urine. Surgical exploration revealed a benign ovarian teratoma with large numbers of argentaffin cells. Removal of the tumor brought the urine 5-HIAA to normal, and all symptoms except those of cardiac origin disappeared.

Secondary invasion of the small bowel by carcinomas arising in other organs is particularly frequent. Carcinoma of the stomach can transgress the pylorus and involve the first portion of the duodenum. Carcinoma of the gallbladder, transverse colon, pancreas, and common bile ducts can also invade the duodenum to ulcerate its surface and at times completely occlude it. Carcinoma of the large bowel may

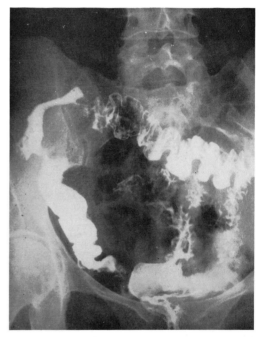

Fig. 366. Cicatrizing enteritis involving terminal ileum and ascending colon.

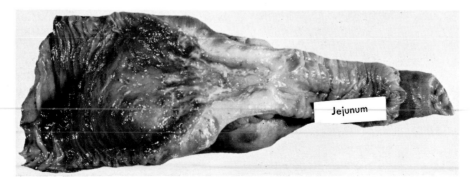

Fig. 367. Cicatrizing enteritis involving jejunum showing narrowing of lumen, hypertrophy of muscularis, and dilatation of proximal segment.

secondarily involve the small bowel. *Implantation on the surface of the small bowel* from primary lesions of the stomach, pancreas, and gallbladder and peritoneal implants, even from breast and bronchus, can buckle the serosal surface, invade the wall, and ulcerate the mucosa. True metastases to the small bowel, particularly in the submucosa, are rare. The most frequent metastatic carcinomas are from squamous cell carcinomas of the cervix, adenocarcinomas of the kidney, and malignant melanomas of the skin. The commonest sites of metastases are the jejunum and ileum, and the symptoms may suggest a primary tumor of the small bowel (Farmer and Hawk[20]). Melanomas of the small intestine are invariably metastatic (Herbut and Manges[27]) from unsuspected primary lesions.

Treatment

If a small bowel tumor is diagnosed from the clinical history, physical findings, and roentgenologic examination, an exploratory laparotomy should be done. Before exploration, however, if there has been any degree of obstruction, the electrolyte balance should be restored by appropriate measures, and if there has been any degree of bleeding, transfusions should be given. At times, frozen section can determine whether the tumor is benign or malignant. If the lesion is located in the terminal ileum and there are large, yellow metastases in the liver, frozen section usually shows the lesion to be a carcinoid tumor. Even in the presence of liver metastases, extensive surgical procedures are justified. If the tumor is malignant or there is any question of neoplastic change, then a radical rather than a conservative operation should be done with removal of the accompanying mesentery and draining lymph node areas (Shorb and McCune[51]).

The long natural history of carcinoids and the debilitating effects of serotonin demand some approach to palliative management. Radiotherapy has shown definite palliative effects on metastatic carcinoid. Numerous serotonin antagonists have been used clinically. In general, as soon as these drugs are discontinued, the carcinoid syndrome recurs. In addition, many of these drugs introduce difficulties of their own.

Nevertheless, the use of drugs has contributed to relief in many of these patients.

Prognosis

In 1965, there were 745 deaths from cancer of the small bowel in the United States, or a crude rate of 0.4 per 100,000 population.

If a *benign tumor* of the small bowel is completely resected, the prognosis is excellent. *Leiomyomas* may appear benign histologically, but metastases can occur. Therefore, a guarded prognosis should be given because clinically silent metastases may exist.

Adenocarcinomas of the small bowel give a poor prognosis because, in practically every instance, by the time the tumor is discovered, metastases to regional nodes and distant areas already exist. Of forty-nine patients with adenocarcinoma of the small bowel reported by Pridgen et al.,[45] eleven lived five or more years after surgical treatment. Those tumors arising in the jejunum and ileum seem to have a relatively better prognosis than those of the duodenum (Brookes et al.[9a]). If a *lymphosarcoma* is well localized to one segment of the bowel and to a few regional nodes, cure is possible. Marcuse and Stout[37] reported on a series of thirteen patients with lymphosarcoma, of whom three were living and well from six to fourteen years after treatment. Three others were well from twenty months to four years. In adenocarcinoma and lymphosarcoma with regional lymph node involvement, the prognosis is extremely poor. In a series reported by Dorman et al.,[18] no patient with carcinoma or sarcoma with regional lymph node metastases survived five years.

Carcinoids of the small bowel have an excellent prognosis even if regional metastases are already present at the time of treatment. Brookes et al.[9a] reported a series of thirty-one patients with carcinoid of the small intestine who were treated surgically, with thirteen (42%) surviving five years. With resection of the primary lesion, these patients may live ten or more years.

REFERENCES

1 Albright, H. L., and Sprague, J. S.: Primary adenocarcinoma Meckel's diverticulum, New Eng. J. Med. **226**:142-146, 1942.
2 Baker, H. L., and Good, C. A.: Smooth-muscle

tumors of the alimentary tract; their roentgen manifestations, Amer. J. Roentgen. 74:246-254, 1955.

2a Barclay, F. T., and Robb, W. A. T.: A clinicopathologic study of carcinoid tumors, Surg. Gynec. Obstet. 126:483-496, 1968.

3 Barnett, W. O.: Benign tumors of the duodenum, Amer. Pract. 13:625-632, 1962.

4 Bartholomew, L. G., Dahlin, D. C., and Waugh, J. M.: Intestinal polyposis associated with mucocutaneous melanin pigmentation (Peutz-Jeghers syndrome), Proc. Staff Meet. Mayo Clin. 32:675, 1957.

5 Biörck, G., Axen, O., and Thorson, A.: Unusual cyanosis in a boy with congenital pulmonary stenosis and tricuspid insufficiency; fatal outcome after angiocardiography, Amer. Heart J. 44:143-148, 1952.

6 Black, W. C., III: Enterochromaffin cell types and corresponding carcinoid tumors, Lab. Invest. 19:473-486, 1968.

7 Boley, S. J., Allen, A. C., Schultz, L., and Schwartz, S.: Potassium-induced lesions of the small bowel. I. Clinical aspects, J.A.M.A. 193:81-84, 1965.

8 Botsford, T. W., and Seibel, R. E.: Benign and malignant tumors of the small intestine, New Eng. J. Med. 236:683-694, 1947.

9 Brenner, R. L., and Brown, C. H.: Primary carcinoma of the duodenum, Gastroenterology 29:189-198, 1955.

9a Brookes, V. S., Waterhouse, J. A., and Powell, D. J.: Malignant lesions of the small intestine, Brit. J. Surg. 55:405-410, 1968.

10 Brunt, P. W., Sircus, W., and Maclean, N.: Neoplasm and the celiac syndrome in adults, Lancet 1:180-184, 1969.

11 Burdick, D., Prior, J. T., and Scanlon, G. T.: Peutz-Jeghers syndrome; a clinical-pathological study of a large family with a 10-year follow-up, Cancer 16:854-867, 1963.

12 Cameron, A. L.: Primary malignancy of the jejunum and ileum, Ann. Surg. 108:203-220, 1938.

13 Campbell, A. C. P., Gowenlock, A. H., Platt, D. S., and Snow, P. J. D.: A 5-hydroxytryptophan-secreting carcinoid tumour, Gut 4:61-67, 1963.

14 Darling, R. C., and Welch, C. E.: Tumors of the small intestine, New Eng. J. Med. 260:397-408, 1959.

15 Debray, C., Morin, G., Leymarios, J., Hernandez, C., Pironneau, A., Validire, J., Marche, C., and Haas, R.: Tumeurs de l'intestin grêle diagnostiquées exclusivement par l'arteriographie sélective de la mésentérique supérieure. A propos de 2 cas, Arch. Mal. Appar. Dig. 54:593-602, 1965.

16 Deutschberger, O., Tchertkoff, V., Daino, J., and Vieira, E. F.: Benign duodenal polyp; review of the literature and report of a giant adenomatous polyp of the duodenal bulb, Amer. J. Gastroent. 38:75-84, 1962.

17 Dockerty, M. B., and Ashburn, F. E.: Carcinoid tumors (so-called) of the ileum, Arch. Surg. (Chicago) 47:221-246, 1943.

18 Dorman, J. E., Floyd, C. E., and Cohn, I., Jr.: Malignant neoplasms of the small bowel, Amer. J. Surg. 113:131-136, 1967.

19 Erspamer, V.: Pharmacology of indolealkylamines, Pharmacol. Rev. 6:426-487, 1954.

20 Farmer, R. G., and Hawk, W. A.: Metastatic tumors of the small bowel, Gastroenterology 47:496-504, 1964.

21 Freedman, E., Rabwin, M. H., and Sava, M.: Benign and malignant tumors of the duodenum, Radiology 65:557-568, 1955.

22 Gardner, B., Dollinger, M., Silen, W., Back, N., and O'Reilly, S.: Studies of carcinoid syndrome; its relationship to serotonin, bradykinin and histamine, Surgery 61:846-852, 1967.

23 Golden, R., and Stout, A. P.: Smooth muscle tumors of the gastrointestinal tract and retroperitoneal tissues, Surg. Gynec. Obstet. 73:784-810, 1941.

24 Good, C. A.: Tumors of the small intestine, Amer. J. Roentgen. 89:685-705, 1963.

25 Grise, J. W.: Dysgammaglobulinemia with nodular lymphoid hyperplasia of the small intestine, Radiology 90:579-580, 1968.

26 Hansen, P. S.: Hemangioma of the small intestine, Amer. J. Clin. Path. 18:14-42, 1948.

27 Herbut, P. A., and Manges, W. E.: Melanoma of the small intestine, Arch. Path. (Chicago) 39:22-27, 1945.

28 Herena, R., and Schraft, W. C., Jr.: Carcinoid tumor of Meckel's diverticulum, New York J. Med. 64:1208-1210, 1964.

29 Hermans, P. E.: Nodular lymphoid hyperplasia of the small intestine and hypogammaglobulinemia; theoretical and practical considerations, Fed. Proc. 26:1606-1611, 1967.

30 Higgins, P. M., Lehman, G., and Morton, H. S.: Perforation of jejunal and ileal neoplasm, a survey of the literature and case reports, Canad. J. Surg. 6:338-347, 1963.

31 Hodes, P. J., and Edeiken, J.: Roentgen manifestations of small intestinal bleeding, J.A.M.A. 141:1284-1290, 1949.

32 Hofbert, P. W., Weingarten, B., Friedman, L. D., and Morecki, R.: Adenocarcinoma of the terminal ileum in a segment of bowel with coexisting active ileitis, New York J. Med. 63:1567-1571, 1963.

33 Horn, R. C., Jr., Payne, W. A., and Fine, G.: The Peutz-Jeghers syndrome, Arch. Path. (Chicago) 76:29-37, 1963.

34 Jeghers, H., McKusick, V. A., and Katz, K. H.: Generalized intestinal polyposis and melanin spots of the oral mucosa, lips, and digits; a syndrome of diagnostic significance, New Eng. J. Med. 241:993-1005; 1031-1036, 1949.

35 Lembeck, F.: 5-hydroxytryptamine in a carcinoid tumor, Nature (London) 172:910, 1953.

36 Lowman, R. M., and Mendelsohn, W.: Intussusception in adults with small bowel tumors, Gastroenterology 12:290-301, 1949.

37 Marcuse, P. M., and Stout, A. P.: Primary lymphosarcoma of the small intestine; analysis of thirteen cases and review of the literature, Cancer 3:459-474, 1950.

38 Marshak, R. H., Wolf, B. S., and Eliasoph, J.: The roentgen findings in lymphosarcoma

of the small intestine, Amer. J. Roentgen. **86:** 682-692, 1961.

39 Miller, E. R., and Herrmann, W. W.: Argentaffin tumors of the small bowel; roentgen sign of malignant change, Radiology **39:**214-220, 1942.

40 Ostermiller, W., Joergenson, E. J., and Weibel, L.: A clinical review of tumors of the small bowel, Amer. J. Surg. **111:**403-410, 1966.

41 Pagtalunan, R. J. G., Mayo, C. W., and Dockerty, M. G.: Primary malignant tumors of the small intestine, Amer. J. Surg. **108:**13-18, 1964.

42 Pearson, C. M., and Fitzgerald, P. J.: Carcinoid tumors—a re-emphasis of their malignant nature; review of 140 cases, Cancer **2:** 1005-1026, 1949.

43 Pernow, B., and Waldenström, J.: Determination of 5-hydroxytryptamine, 5-hydroxyindole acetic acid and histamine in thirty-three cases of carcinoid tumor (argentaffinoma), Amer. J. Med. **23:**16-25, 1957.

44 Polayes, S. H., and Krieger, J. L.: Eosinophilic granuloma of the jejunum, a hitherto undescribed lesion of the intestines, J.A.M.A. **143:** 549-551, 1950.

45 Pridgen, J. E., Mayo, C. W., and Dockerty, M. B.: Carcinoma of the jejunum and ileum exclusive of carcinoid tumors, Surg. Gynec. Obstet. **90:**513-524, 1950.

46 Puppel, I. E., and Morris, L. E., Jr.: Lymphangioma of the jejunum, Arch. Path. (Chicago) **38:**410-412, 1944.

47 River, L., Silverstein, J., and Tope, J. W.: Collective review; benign neoplasms of the small intestine, Int. Abstr. Surg. **102:**1-38, 1956; in Surg. Gynec. Obstet., Jan., 1956 (extensive bibliography).

48 Rouvière, H.: Anatomie des lymphatiques de l'homme, Paris, 1932, Masson et Cie.

49 Sanders, R. J., and Axtell, H. K.: Carcinoid of the gastrointestinal tract, Surg. Gynec. Obstet. **119:**369-380, 1964 (extensive bibliography).

50 Schottenfeld, L. E.: Lipomas of the gastrointestinal tract, Surgery **14:**47-72, 1943.

51 Shorb, P. E., and McCune, W. S.: Carcinoid tumors of the gastrointestinal tract, Amer. J. Surg. **107:**329-336, 1964.

52 Sjoerdsma, A., Weissbach, H., and Udenfriend, A.: A clinical physiologic and biochemical study of patients with malignant carcinoid (argentaffinoma), Amer. J. Med. **20:**520-532, 1956.

53 Sjoerdsma, A., Weissbach, H., Terry, L. L., and Udenfriend, S.: Further observations on patients with malignant carcinoid, Amer. J. Med. **34:**5-15, 1957.

54 Smith, O. N.: Leiomyoma of the small intestine, Amer. J. Med. Sci. **194:**700-707, 1937.

54a Spence, W. J. E., and Ritchie, S.: Lymphomas of small bowel and their relationship to idiopathic steatorrhea, Canad. J. Surg. **12:**207-209, 1969.

55 Stout, A. P.: The peripheral manifestations of specific nerve sheath tumor (neurilemoma), Amer. J. Cancer **24:**751-796, 1935.

56 Taylor, H. B., and Helwig, E. B.: Benign nonchromaffin paragangliomas of the duodenum, Virchow Arch. Path. Anat. **335:**356-366, 1962.

57 Thorson, A., Biörck, G., Bjorkman, G., and Waldenstrom, J.: Malignant carcinoid of the small intestine with metastases to the liver, valvular disease of the right side of the heart (pulmonary stenosis and tricuspid regurgitation without septal defects), peripheral vasomotor symptoms, bronchoconstriction, and an unusual type of cyanosis, Amer. Heart J. **47:** 795-817, 1954.

58 Ullman, A., and Abeshouse, B. S.: Lymphosarcoma of the small and large intestines, Ann. Surg. **95:**878-915, 1932.

59 Wald, M.: Leiomyosarcoma of the jejunum, Aust. New Zeal. J. Surg. **33:**147-154, 1963.

60 Weinstein, M., and Roberts, M.: Leiomyosarcoma of the duodenum, Arch. Surg. (Chicago) **66:**318-328, 1953.

61 Williams, J. P., and Knudsen, A.: Peutz-Jeghers syndrome with metastasizing duodenal carcinoma, Gut **6:**179-184, 1965.

62 Williams, M. J., Sutherland, D. H., and Clark, C. G.: Lymphosarcoma of the small intestine with a malabsorption syndrome and pneumatosis intestinalis; report of a case with peroral jejunal biopsy, Gastroenterology **45:**550-557, 1963.

Appendix

Anatomy

The appendix is a flexuous cylindrical structure 8 cm to 10 cm in length that is implanted on and communicates with the cecum. It has a mesenteric attachment, the mesoappendix, which carries in its free border the appendiceal artery, a terminal branch of the superior mesenteric artery. Because of the considerable variation in the development of the cecal area, the normal position of the appendix is variable.

The appendix is formed from the outside by a serous layer, muscular layer, submucosa, and mucosa. It has several points where the longitudinal and the circular muscle fibers are deficient so that the submucosa and the serosa may be continuous. The mucous membrane is composed of columnar epithelium with numerous large and small lymphatic nodules. Argentaffin cells are regularly present in the base of the glands.

Lymphatics. The lymphatics of the appendix gather into several collecting trunks that may terminate in the inferior nodes of the ileocolic chain or the posterior cecal nodes, or even in lymph nodes situated on the anterior surface of the third portion of the duodenum.

Epidemiology

Tumors of the appendix are rare. The *carcinoids* make up approximately 90% of the entire group. Four out of five appendiceal tumors are found in women, and the greater number occur in the third decade of life. Most carcinoids of the gastrointestinal tract originate in the appendix (MacDonald[12]). *Mucoceles* make up about 7% to 8% of tumors of the appendix. They are more common in men than in women. Adenocarcinomas are rare and lymphosarcomas rarer still (Knox[10]).

Pathology
Gross and microscopic pathology

The *carcinoid* usually occurs in the distal end of the appendix, forms a submucosal mass, and quickly obliterates the lumen. This tumor tends to remain localized, but it can metastasize. The *adenocarcinoma* occurs more frequently at the base of the appendix and forms polypoid masses usually growing within the lumen. Preinvasive adenocarcinoma of the appendix has been reported (McCollum and Pund[11]). We have observed villous tumors of the appendix, both primary lesions and secondary involvement from the cecum, and one associated with an adenocarcinoma (Fig. 368) (Goldfarb and Kempson[6]).

The *mucocele* occurs primarily in the appendix and, when localized there, should be considered a benign lesion. If the appendix ruptures and tumor escapes into the peritoneal cavity, this tumor can grow and produce mucin and, because of secondary changes produced, can cause death. In this sense, a mucocele might be con-

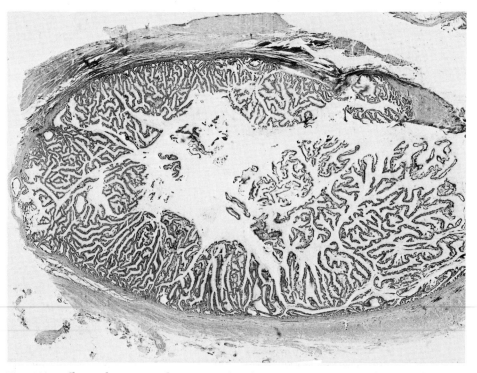

Fig. 368. Villous adenoma involving appendix showing characteristic villous fronds almost filling lumen of appendix. (WU neg. 63-4147; from Goldfarb, W. G., and Kampson, R.: Villous adenomas of the appendix, Surgery **55:**769-772, 1964.)

sidered malignant. Woodruff and McDonald[23] believe that the pseudomyxoma peritonei of appendiceal origin derives from a slowly growing cystadenocarcinoma of the appendix and that it cannot result from a benign mucocele. Others, however, do not agree with this concept. In 43,000 appendectomies performed at the Mayo Clinic, 146 mucoceles were found (Woodruff and McDonald[23]). The mucocele results from obliteration of the distal portion of the appendiceal lumen, probably by an inflammatory process. In eighty-one patients with mucocele of the appendix reported by Hughes,[8] nine had a walled-off cyst adjacent to the cecum, eleven had a carcinoma of the cecum, and two had carcinoids of the appendix. Mucoceles may be associated with carcinoma in situ (Hellsten[7]). Even after obstruction, the lining epithelium continues to secrete mucus which gradually increases the size of the appendix and results in atrophy of the lining epithelium and thinning of the wall (Fig. 369). The average size of a mucocele when first discovered is about 5 cm, but it may attain a huge size. Perforation may occur, and the mucoid material may escape into the retroperitoneal area and form cysts or into the peritoneal cavity with formation of

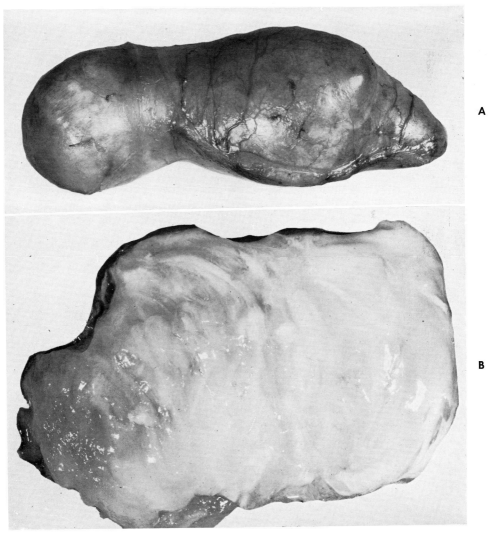

A

B

Fig. 369. **A,** Large unruptured mucocele of appendix with uniform enlargement. **B,** Same specimen on cut section showing mucoid surface and obliteration of normal mucosal markings.

gelatinous implants. Following perforation, the appendix may collapse, the perforated area may heal, and a reaccumulation of mucus may form, followed by a second perforation. Other complications such as gangrene or periappendiceal abscesses result. With growth of the peritoneal implants, intestinal obstruction may occur. Local invasion of other tissues, such as bladder and bowel, is not infrequent, but metastases to the regional lymph nodes do not occur. Acute peritonitis very frequently develops when pseudomyxoma peritonei is present. A comparison of the three main types of appendiceal lesions is given in Table 37.

Lymphosarcomas arise from the appendix. Their histopathologic appearance is no different from that of lymphosarcomas in other locations (Knox[10]). We have seen a pseudolymphoma of the appendix in a patient with epilepsy who was receiving mephenytoin (Mesantoin).

Metastatic spread

Few cases of carcinoid actually metastasize. When they do, they infrequently involve the regional lymph nodes (Knowles et al.[9]). Mucoceles of the appendix may give rise to peritoneal pseudomyxoma. Adenocarcinomas spread in the same fashion as other carcinomas of the gastrointestinal tract. Lymphosarcomas may show widespread extension.

Clinical evolution

The evolution of most tumors of the appendix is frequently silent. A good proportion of carcinoids is discovered during abdominal operations, but others produce pain that suggests a diagnosis of appendicitis. *Carcinoids* located in the tip of the appendix may not cause any symptoms, but those located at the base may cause an obstructive appendicitis (Miller and Kerr[15]). Carcinoids, particularly those with metastases to the liver, may give rise to a *carcinoid syndrome* characterized by cutaneous flushes, cyanosis, chronic diarrhea, peristaltic rushes, respiratory distress, and valvular disease of the right side of the heart (Thorson et al.[21]; Branwood and Bain[2]; Markgraf and Dunn[14]).

Mucoceles of the appendix are frequently symptomless, and very few are suspected preoperatively. Some may cause pain in the right lower quadrant and epigastrium. If the mucocele ruptures in the peritoneal cavity, the resulting process may cause intestinal obstruction. Symptoms of appendicitis often accompany cancer of the cecum. Ruderman and Strawbridge[17] found seventy-one such cases in the literature. *Adenocarcinomas* and *lymphosarcomas* may also cause pain. All of these tumors may rarely become palpable.

Diagnosis

Clinical examination

Clinical examination usually reveals signs suggesting acute or subacute appendicitis. The mucocele presents a palpable mass, and if pseudomyxoma peritonei is present, nodular abdominal masses may be evident. The diagnosis of any neoplasm of the appendix is rarely made before exploratory laparotomy.

Even at exploration, carcinoid tumors and adenocarcinomas are very seldom even considered unless obvious tumor metastases have appeared. A metastatic carcinoid in a regional lymph node may be yellow on section. The mucocele can be diagnosed on its very characteristic appearance. It is uniformly swollen, and the wall is thinned out. A lymphosarcoma is practically never recognized at exploration.

Roentgenologic examination

A radiographic diagnosis of mucocele is suggested by a well-circumscribed shadow and the displacement of the cecum. Calcium deposits may also be observed within the tumor or on its wall (Euphrat[5]; Bonann and Davis[1]).

Laboratory examination

There are difficulties in the demonstration of serum serotonin in carcinoids. However, a simplified urine test is available (Sjoerdsma et al.[20]) that is positive in the presence of hepatic metastases.

Differential diagnosis

The most important differential diagnosis is *appendicitis*. The only differentiating feature is that the mucocele may form a mass, which, however, may be confused with a periappendiceal abscess. At times, roentgenologic examination reveals calci-

Table 37. Differential character of three types of carcinoma of appendix*

	Carcinoid type	*Cystic type*	*Colonic type*
Location	Usually tip	Tip or base	Tip or base, more frequently base
Incidence	89%	8%	3%
Gross character	Yellowish solid	Cystic, frequently on basis of mucocele	Grayish, polypoid, or ulcerating
Microscopic structure	Poorly formed acini, mucosa intact over tumor; reduction of silver salts; affinity for chrome salts	Papillary projections originating in cyst; comparable to cystadenocarcinoma of ovary; epithelial cells few because of destruction by mucus	Frequently well-formed acini; mucous membrane ulcerated; comparable to carcinoma of colon
Mitoses	Few	Few	Variable
Mucus	None	Secretes large quantities	Secretes variable quantities
Metastasis	To regional nodes in less than 1%	So-called pseudomyxoma peritonei	To lymph nodes and liver

*From Uihlein, A., and McDonald, J. R.: Primary carcinoma of the appendix resembling carcinoma of the colon, Surg. Gynec. Obstet. **76**:711-714, 1943; by permission of Surgery, Gynecology & Obstetrics.

fication within a mucocele. A pseudomucinous tumor of the ovary may be associated with a mucocele.

Treatment

A simple appendectomy may be sufficient treatment for a *carcinoid* of the appendix without evidence of metastases (Moertel et al.[16]). But when examination reveals that the tumor has extended through the wall to the appendiceal fat, the question is often raised as to whether or not an ileocolectomy is indicated. Symptoms of carcinoid syndrome may be alleviated by serotonin antagonists (Dubach and Gsell[3]).

With *adenocarcinomas* of the appendix, it is necessary to do an ileocolectomy in order to remove all potential regional lymph node metastases (Sieracki and Tesluk[19]). Of forty-three patients with adenocarcinoma of the appendix treated by appendectomy, twenty died with metastases, whereas only eight of forty-five treated by colectomy and appendectomy died with metastases (Edmondson and Hobbs[4]).

Mucoceles should be carefully resected. When pseudomyxoma peritonei is present, as much as possible of the gelatinous tumor should be removed. Saegesser[18] uses surgery and proteolytic enzymes for this purpose. Long et al.[10a] found alkylating agents useful in association with repeated surgical interventions.

Prognosis

The prognosis of the well-localized carcinoid and the unperforated mucocele is excellent. An adenocarcinoma of the appendix with no regional metastases also has a good prognosis. If pseudomyxoma peritonei is present, the prognosis is poor, although the duration of life may be long. Lymphosarcomas of the appendix also have a relatively poor prognosis except for the polypoid group, which are often relatively benign.

REFERENCES

1 Bonann, L. J., and Davis, J. G.: Retroperitoneal mucocele of the appendix; a case report with characteristic roentgen features, Radiology **51**:375-382, 1948.
2 Branwood, A. W., and Bain, A. D.: Carcinoid tumour of the small intestine with hepatic metastases, pulmonic stenosis, and atypical cyanosis, Lancet **2**:1259-1261, 1954.
3 Dubach, U. C., and Gsell, O. R.: Carcinoid syndrome: alleviation of diarrhoea and flushing with "Deseril" and Ro 5-1025, Brit. Med. J. **1**:1390-1391, 1962.
4 Edmondson, H. T., Jr., and Hobbs, M. L.: Primary adenocarcinoma of the appendix, Amer. Surg. **33**:717-732, 1967.
5 Euphrat, E. J.: Roentgen features of mucocele of the appendix, Radiology **48**:113-117, 1947.
6 Goldfarb, W. G., and Kempson, R.: Villous adenomas of the appendix, Surgery **55**:769-772, 1964.
7 Hellsten, S.: Mucocele and carcinoma of the appendix, Acta Path. Microbiol. Scand. **60**:473-482, 1964.
8 Hughes, J.: Mucocele of the appendix with pseudomyxoma peritonei; a benign or malignant disease? Ann. Surg. **165**:73-76, 1967.

9 Knowles, C. H. R., McCrea, A. N., and Davis, A.: Metastasis from argentaffinoma of the appendix, J. Path. Bact. **72**:326-329, 1956.

10 Knox, G.: Lymphosarcoma primary in the appendix, Arch. Surg. (Chicago) **50**:288-292, 1945.

10a Long, R. T. L., Spratt, J. S., Jr., and Dowling, E.: Pseudomyxoma peritonei; new concepts in management with a report of seventeen patients, Amer. J. Surg. **117**:162-169, 1969.

11 McCollum, W., and Pund, E. R.: Preinvasive adenocarcinoma of the appendix; report of sixteen cases, Cancer **4**:261-264, 1951.

12 MacDonald, R. A.: A study of 356 carcinoids of the gastrointestinal tract; report of four new cases of the carcinoid syndrome, Amer. J. Med. **21**:867-878, 1956.

13 McVay, J. R.: The appendix in relation to neoplastic disease, Cancer **17**:929-937, 1964.

14 Markgraf, W. H., and Dunn, T. M.: Appendiceal carcinoid with carcinoid syndrome, Amer. J. Surg. **107**:730-732, 1964.

15 Miller, S. E. P., and Kerr, I. F.: Argentaffin tumours of the appendix, Brit. J. Surg. **54**:781-783, 1967.

16 Moertel, C. G., Dockerty, M. B., and Judd, E. S.: Carcinoid tumors of the vermiform appendix, Cancer **21**:270-278, 1968.

17 Ruderman, R. L., and Strawbridge, H. T. G.: Carcinoma of the cecum; presenting as acute appendicitis; case report and review of the literature, Canad. Med. Ass. J. **96**:1327-1329, 1967.

18 Saegesser, F.: Mucocèle appendiculaire et pseudomyxome péritonéal, Lyon Chir. **61**:641-660, 1965.

19 Sieracki, J. C., and Tesluk, H.: Primary adenocarcinoma of the vermiform appendix, Cancer **9**:997-1011, 1956.

20 Sjoerdsma, A., Weissbach, H., Terry, L. L., and Udenfriend, S.: Further observations on patients with malignant carcinoid, Amer. J. Med. **34**:5-15, 1957.

21 Thorson, A., Biörck, G., Bjorkman, G., and Waldenstrom, J.: Malignant carcinoid of the small intestine with metastases to the liver, valvular disease of the right side of the heart (pulmonary stenosis and tricuspid regurgitation without septal defects), peripheral vasomotor symptoms, bronchoconstriction, and an unusual type of cyanosis, Amer. Heart J. **47**:795-817, 1954.

22 Uihlein, A., and McDonald, J. R.: Primary carcinoma of the appendix resembling carcinoma of the colon, Surg. Gynec. Obstet. **76**:711-714, 1943.

23 Woodruff, R., and McDonald, J. R.: Benign and malignant cystic tumors of the appendix, Surg. Gynec. Obstet. **71**:750-755, 1940.

Large bowel

Anatomy

The terminal portion of the gastrointestinal tract, the *large bowel,* extends from the ileocecal valve to the anus. It originates in the right iliac fossa as a peritoneal portion, the *cecum,* which extends from the appendix to the level of the iliac crest and continues vertically, and retroperitoneally, as the *ascending colon,* toward the lower surface of the liver, to which it is attached. At this point, the bowel changes direction, at the *hepatic flexure,* to become the *transverse colon,* a peritoneal portion, attached posteriorly at about the level of the second lumbar vertebra. At the level of the spleen, the bowel makes a right angle turn, at the *splenic flexure,* to become again retroperitoneal as the *descending colon.* At the point where the attachment of the mesosigmoid begins, in the left iliac fossa, the bowel curves upon itself to form the *sigmoid colon.* The *rectum* begins at the termination of the mesosigmoid on the anterior aspect of the sacrum and occupies the sacrococcygeal curvature; the peritoneum covers only the anterior surface of its upper portion.

The blood supply of the large bowel comes from three major sources: (1) the superior mesenteric artery, (2) the inferior mesenteric artery, and (3) the branches of the internal iliac artery (middle hemorrhoidal, inferior hemorrhoidal, and pudic arteries).

The ascending colon, the hepatic flexure, and most of the transverse colon are supplied by the superior mesenteric artery through its right colic and middle colic branches. The splenic flexure, the descending colon, the sigmoid, and the upper half of the rectum are supplied by the left colic and sigmoid branches of the inferior mesenteric artery. The superior hemorrhoidal artery is a terminal branch of the inferior mesenteric artery. The lower half of the rectum and the anus are supplied by the middle hemorrhoidal artery (from the internal iliac) and the inferior hemorrhoidal artery (from the internal pudic branch of the internal iliac).

Branches of the mesenteric arteries form a continuous vessel within the circle of the colon, forming a marginal arch at a fairly constant distance from the mesenteric border. From this arch, the vasa rectae originate to pursue a straight course, entering the mesenteric border of the bowel without anastomosing with one another. The anastomosis of blood vessels within the bowel wall is not very frequent, and consequently the part of the colon located between the taenia is very poorly supplied but does receive some blood from the terminal vessels on either side.

Lymphatics. The lymphatics of the *cecum* are divided into anterior and posterior groups which empty into the nodes of the ileocolic chain.

The abundant subserous network of lymphatics of the *colon* is drained, for the most part, by the paracolic lymph nodes, but some do not stop at this first relay and continue to the intermediate group of lymph nodes or even directly to the mesenteric or lateroaortic nodes. The segment of the colon that is supplied by the superior mesenteric artery drains its lymph into the satellite lymph nodes of the right colic artery or into the central superior mesenteric group of lymph nodes. The part of the colon that is supplied by the inferior mesenteric artery has two different lymphatic connections: (1) a superior segment drained by the central superior mesenteric group of lymph nodes and (2) an inferior segment drained by the lateroaortic nodes.

The lymphatics of the *ascending colon* empty into the paracolic lymph nodes, but a few may communicate with the perirenal lymphatic pathways. The lymphatics of the right side of the *transverse colon* (the right two-thirds or three-fourths) terminate in the paracolic lymph nodes. Some empty into the nodes accompanying the middle colic artery and thence into the central group of the superior mesenteric chain. The lymphatics of the remaining one-third or one-fourth of the transverse colon drain into the paracolic chain and finally into the central nodes of the superior mesenteric artery. The lymphatics of the *descending colon* are drained by the lymph nodes

along the left colic artery and then by the nodes of the inferior mesenteric chain. The collecting trunks of the *sigmoid colon* empty into the lymph nodes accompanying it and the inferior mesenteric artery to terminate in the para-aortic lymph nodes.

The lymphatics of the *rectum* have numerous anastomoses with those of the prostate, seminal vesicles, vagina, bladder, and levator ani muscles. They are divided into inferior, middle, and superior trunks. The *inferior collecting trunks* originate in the cutaneous part of the anus and drain into the superficial inguinal lymph nodes. The *middle collecting trunks* usually follow the middle hemorrhoidal vessels and terminate in the hypogastric lymph nodes. They may also accompany the lateral and medial sacral arteries and drain into the nodes of the promontory and sacrum (Fig. 370). The *superior collecting trunks* extend through the *entire length* of the rectum and empty into the anorectal lymph nodes that are found along the course of the superior hemorrhoidal blood vessels. They finally terminate in the nodes found at the level of the bifurcation of the inferior mesenteric artery. These are by far the most important lymph nodes draining the rectum. Some of these trunks may end in a node in the region of the inferior mesenteric artery, near the point of origin of its lower sigmoid branch, without stopping at the nodes of the bifurcation. These are also long collecting trunks that arise from the lower portion of the rectum and terminate without interruption in lymph nodes at the summit of the pelvic mesocolon or preaortic and lateroaortic lymph nodes (Rouvière[140]).

Epidemiology

In the United States, the large bowel is the most frequent site of carcinoma in the gastrointestinal tract, cancer of the stomach having decreased in recent years. In the survey of 1947, the sex-age adjusted incidence of cancer of the *colon* was 25.1 for males and 26.8 for females per 100,000 population. In the state of Connecticut, the incidence in males rose 18% from 1945-1949 to 1960-1962. An increase of 15% incidence in males was also observed in the state of New York from 1949-1951 to 1958-1960. The incidence in females re-

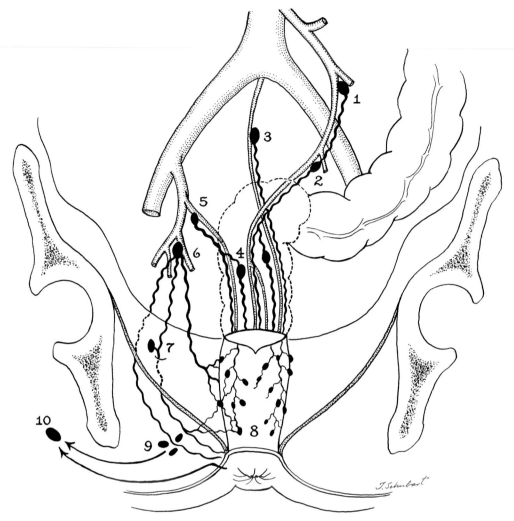

Fig. 370. Lymphatics of rectum. Superior collecting trunks may lead to nodes at point of origin of inferior mesenteric artery or at point of origin of sigmoid vessels, **1** and **2**. Middle collecting trunks follow medial sacral arteries and lead to nodes of promontory, **3**, but may also follow middle hemorrhoidal vessels and go to sacral nodes, **4**, or empty into a hypogastric node, **5**. Inferior trunks may lead to hypogastric group of nodes, **6**, or, after passing through ischiorectal nodes, **9**, to inguinal nodes, **10**. Lymphatics of lower part of rectum may also empty into external iliac nodes, **7**, and nodes at wall of rectum, **8**.

mained unchanged in both instances. The sex-age adjusted incidence rates per 100,000 for cancer of the *rectum* were 21.2 for males and 15.0 for females in the 1947 survey. There was a considerable difference between the incidence in nonwhite (12.7) and in white (22.1) males, whereas the incidence in females was much closer— 13.6 for nonwhite and 15.2 for white females. There has been no important variation in the incidence of cancer of the rectum, and consequently the ratio of can-

cer of the colon to cancer of the rectum has increased from 1942 to 1962 (Axtell and Chiazze[3]). Cancer of the colon or rectum is rare in young individuals (Sessions et al.[144]; Miller and Liechty[119]). It has rarely been reported in children (Williams[181]; Kern and White[105]; Middlekamp and Haffner[117]). Of 7837 patients with carcinoma of the large bowel reported by Ederer et al.,[50] only thirty-one were under 45 years of age, whereas the actual incidence for individuals under 40 years of age

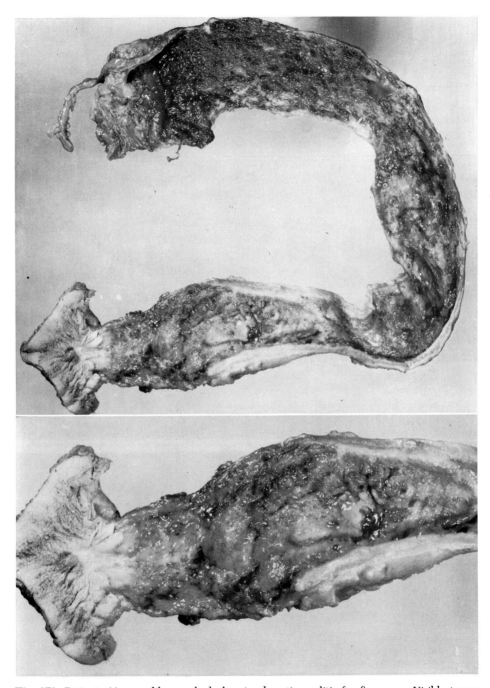

Fig. 371. Patient, 44-year-old man, had chronic ulcerative colitis for five years. Visible tumor replaced all layers of bowel and involved twenty-two of forty-seven lymph nodes. Gross pattern of neoplasm is atypical. (WU negs. 60-2966 and 60-2967.)

is of the order of 5 per 100,000. The incidence of cancer of the colon gradually rises to over 300 per 100,000 for both males and females and that of cancer of the rectum to 180 for males and 100 for females in the age group 80 to 84 years. Berg et al.[10a] found a prevalence of 2% undiagnosed carcinomas of the colon and rectum in autopsies of individuals over 70 years of age.

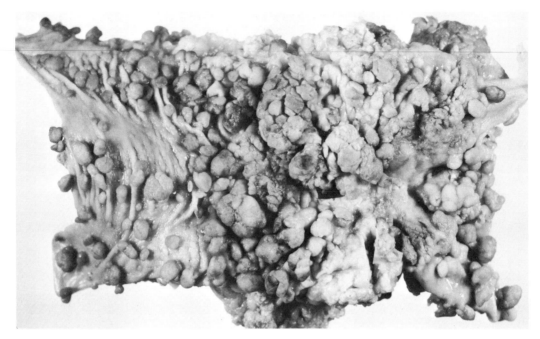

Fig. 372. Extensive polyposis of colon at hepatic flexure with flat ulcerating carcinoma in lower right-hand corner. Twenty-six lymph nodes submitted with specimen were involved by tumor. (WU neg. 68-1574.)

The incidence of cancer of the colon and rectum is lower in most countries of the world than in the United States. It is very low in Finland and relatively uncommon in Puerto Rico. In Japan, the incidence of cancer of the colon is much lower, but that of cancer of the rectum is about the same as in the United States; the rare cases of cancer of the colon occur in patients with a significantly higher economic status than those with cancer of the rectum (Wynder et al.[188]). In countries of Africa, most of the relatively few cases observed occur in the rectum or rectosigmoid (Davies[35]). It is of interest that immigrants in the United States tend to acquire the overall incidence of the country rather than that of their country of origin (Haenszel[87]; Staszewski[160]; Stemmermann[162]). This, of course, suggests an exogenous cause. In the South African Bantu, the occurrence of cancer of the large bowel is very low, and it is not associated with polyps. It has been suggested that this low occurrence may be due to diet, to rapid transit through the bowel, and to the bacterial flora (Bremner and Ackerman[15]).

In patients with *chronic ulcerative colitis,*

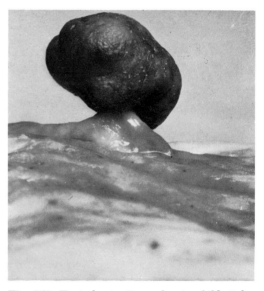

Fig. 373. Typical retention polyp in child. Polyp was dark red in color, with ulcerated surface and short pedicle. (WU neg. 59-4574.)

there is a definite increased risk of carcinoma of the colon, more so than of the rectum (Goldgrabber et al.[74]), and the carcinoma is often multicentric (Fig. 371).

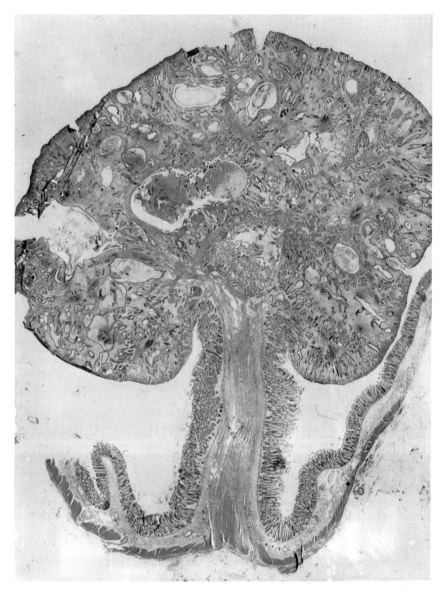

Fig. 374. Polyp shown in Fig. 373 demonstrating ulcerated surface and lakes of mucin in cystic spaces. (WU neg. 59-5594.)

The highest risk of cancer is in those patients with a chronic, continuous form of the disease and in those in whom the ulcerative colitis begins at an early age (Holowach and Thurston[98]). The longer a patient has ulcerative colitis, the greater the risk of developing cancer—twenty times greater in those patients with a twenty-year history than for those with a five-year history (Edwards and Truelove[52, 53]). Histologically, characteristic precancerous changes were recognized by rectal biopsy in nine patients with chronic ulcerative colitis. One or more foci of invasive carcinoma together with widespread precancerous changes were found in the colon or rectum of five of these patients (Morson and Pang[124]).

Familial polyposis of the colon, a widespread adenomatous proliferation leading to the formation of multiple adenomas, is a hereditary disease transmitted in accordance with mendelian laws (Dukes[45]) that is associated with a very high occurrence

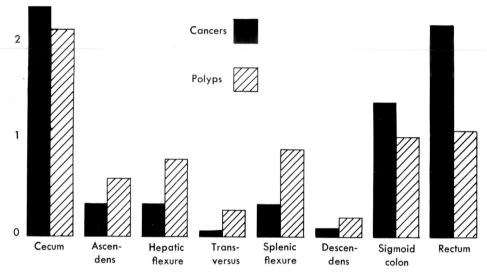

Fig. 375. Percentile distributions of 100 carcinomas and polyps of colon per centimeter length of segment of fixed colon. Note that cancer is concentrated in rectosigmoid and cecal areas and polyps are distributed more uniformly throughout bowel. (From Spratt, J. S., Jr., et al.: Relationships of polyps of the colon to colonic cancer, Ann. Surg. **148:**682-698, 1958; WU neg. 58-2476.)

of carcinoma at a relatively early age (Fig. 372). Polyposis can also be associated with exostoses, osteomas, sebaceous cysts, and desmoid tumors (Gardner's syndrome) (Belleau and Braasch[9]). The Peutz-Jeghers syndrome is a rare hereditary condition consisting of gastrointestinal polyposis and melanin pigmentation of the skin and the oral mucosa (Rintala and Nylund[138]). Hull-siek[100] collected 128 cases of polyposis of the colon and noted that carcinoma developed in forty-six. *Retention* polyps occurring in children often under 6 years of age, and infrequently in adults, are probably not true neoplasms (Figs. 373 and 374) and do not become malignant (Horrilleno et al.[99]; Roth and Helwig[139]). There are also families in which cancer of the large bowel develops frequently in the absence of polyps (Lynch and Krush[112]).

It has been thought for a long time that *adenomatous polyps* of the large bowel become malignant and thus their removal would reduce the incidence of cancer. This point of view has prevailed because adenomatous polyps are often found together with carcinoma and also because microscopic focal areas of apparent carcinoma have been seen within polyps. Hult-born[101] pointed out that the apparent rela-tionship in the distribution of polyps and carcinomas of the large bowel was based on clinical material, whereas in autopsy material the distribution of polyps throughout the colon is unlike that of carcinoma, with 50% of carcinomas but only 20% of polyps occurring in the rectosigmoid area (Fig. 375). Moreover, there is no difference in the age at which the two lesions occur. If the number of polyps and the number of carcinomas for each decade are estimated, there results a very large number of polyps for each carcinoma. It is, therefore, rather exaggerated to assume that every polyp is destined to become cancer. A subserial section study of twenty small carcinomas (2 cm or less) showed no evidence of pre-existing adenomatous polyp (Spratt and Ackerman[158]). A large proportion of carcinomas of the large bowel, about 88%, occur in an otherwise apparently normal bowel without polyps, and 12% are associated with adenomatous polyps, but 12% is also the occurrence rate of adenomatous polyps in persons without cancer. Regression of polyps and carcinoma has been reported in a few cases of diversion colostomy (Dunphy et al.[48]).

The case of *villous adenomas* is completely different from that of adenomatous

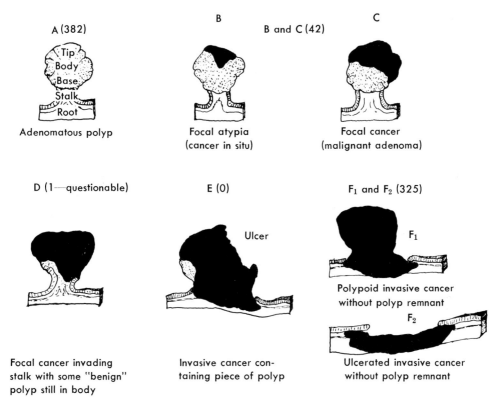

A (382)

Tip
Body
Base
Stalk
Root

Adenomatous polyps

B   B and C (42)   C

Focal atypia
(cancer in situ)

Focal cancer
(malignant adenoma)

D (1—questionable)   E (0) F_1 and F_2 (325)

F_1

Polypoid invasive cancer
without polyp remnant

F_2

Ulcer

Focal cancer invading
stalk with some "benign"
polyp still in body

Invasive cancer con-
taining piece of polyp

Ulcerated invasive cancer
without polyp remnant

Fig. 376. Sequential types of lesions theoretically depicting development of cancer of colon from adenomatous polyps. (WU neg. 58-2767.)

polyps. They present or develop zones of invasive carcinoma that are often observed when first encountered and are found in equal proportions in men and women and found primarily in the rectosigmoid area (Ewing[54]; Wheat and Ackerman[179]).

Pathology
Gross pathology

Carcinoma of the large bowel has a fairly characteristic distribution. It is mostly concentrated in the rectosigmoid and cecal areas, whereas polyps of the large bowel are more evenly distributed (Fig. 375).

Adenomas of the large bowel, usually called polyps, have many gross and microscopic variants. Polyps found in children are usually single, from 1 cm to 4 cm in diameter, and have a well-defined pedicle. On section, they present cystic areas of retained mucus and, microscopically, the glands show no epithelial alteration. They do not become malignant. Two other types of polyps are known as adenomatous polyps

and villous adenomas. They are described in the following paragraphs.

Adenomatous polyps are usually small (less than 1 cm) and show no evidence of carcinomatous changes. A few show focal epithelial alterations from normal, and still a smaller number show microscopic changes that may be considered as focal carcinoma (Fig. 376). But when such changes are confined to the adenomatous polyp, without invasion of the stalk, they usually have no clinical significance. If there is a polyp with focal microscopic cancer or if there is a polypoid cancer above the level of the muscularis mucosae, metastasis to regional lymph nodes is an extreme rarity (Kraus[106]; Lane and Kaye[108]).

Villous adenomas are frequently large tumors arising in the rectosigmoid area in elderly individuals. They are usually single and form a soft papillary mass. Microscopically, delicate, fingerlike processes spring directly from the mucosa, forming a distinctive pattern (Figs. 377 and 378). A high percentage of these lesions are asso-

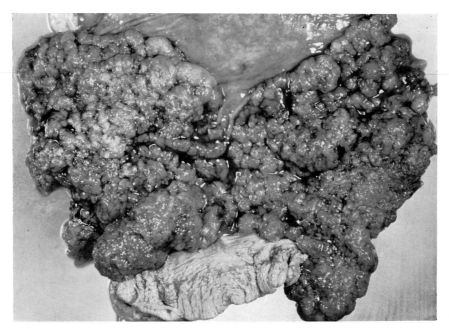

Fig. 377. Extensive villous adenoma of rectum necessitating radical surgical removal because of its large size. It showed no deep invasion or lymph node metastases. (Courtesy Dr. F. Leidler, Houston, Texas.)

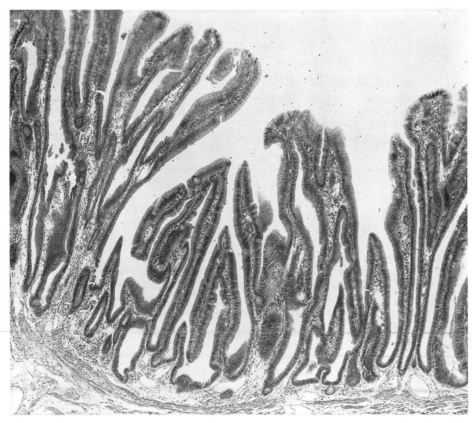

Fig. 378. Villous adenoma. Note pattern with villi springing directly from mucosal surface. (WU neg. 54-2858A.)

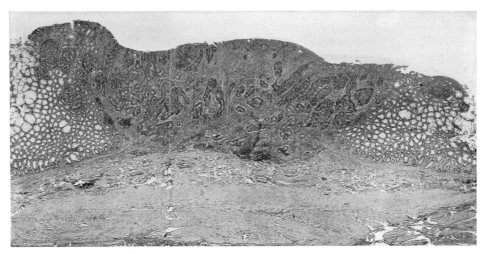

Fig. 379. Flat, ulcerating, small (less than 1.5 cm) cancer of colon springing directly from mucosal surface. (Low power; WU neg. 60-792.)

ciated with infiltrating carcinoma (Wheat and Ackerman[179]; Ewing[54]; Bensaude[10]).

Carcinoma can spring directly from the mucosal surface, as Helwig[90] demonstrated (Fig. 379). The typical carcinoma of the large bowel is a well-delimited lesion more frequently fungating than deeply ulcerating. It shows a sharp delimitation between the normal mucosa and the carcinoma.

These carcinomas have a classic gross pattern. They tend to grow the largest in areas in which there is the greatest space for their development, such as in the cecum. Their surface is usually ulcerated, and as they enlarge in size they tend to show a deep central ulceration with overhanging margins. They may become completely circumferential and produce partial or complete obstruction of the bowel. With obstruction, the proximal large bowel may dilate, and the muscularis becomes hypertrophied. On section, grayish yellow tumor can often be seen replacing the muscular layers of the bowel. These carcinomas can also be flat and deeply ulcerating. The mucinous type of carcinoma of the bowel may show a rather pebbly overlying mucosa with some degree of submucosal extension (Fig. 384). On section, mucoidlike material often can be observed. Rarely, a gross variant of carcinoma of the large bowel exactly resembling the linitis plastica of the stomach may occur (Sizer et al.[150]).

Multiple carcinomas of the large bowel are not too uncommon. Berson and Ber-

ger[11] found seventy-nine patients with two carcinomas and nine with three. The frequency of multiple carcinomas in this group was 4.6%. This new carcinoma may be successfully treated in spite of the fact that the symptoms caused by the second primary lesion may suggest an inoperable recurrence (Ginzburg et al.[68]).

Carcinomas of the large bowel tend to spread locally and to reach the serosal surface of the bowel where infection plus tumor causes adherence to neighboring organs. Fixation often means tumor extension. Rarely, submucosal intramural spread can take place. In 103 specimens studied by Black and Waugh,[13] the greatest extension of any tumor beyond its apparent gross limits was only 12 mm. There were only four in which the spread was more than 5 mm. These figures are rather conservative. Dunphy[47] emphasized that shrinkage occurs in fixed specimens and alters the measurement. We have seen intramural spread over 7 cm in length. Carcinoma of the cecum may directly invade the lateral abdominal gutter and, at times, the anterior abdominal wall. Involvement of the pancreas, gallbladder, liver, spleen, and wall of the stomach may also occur. Fixation, however, is most common in the region of the rectum and the sigmoid. In men, bladder invasion is common, but only rarely does true invasion of the prostate occur. Denonvilliers' fascia usually provides a protective check to intraprostatic invasion. In both sexes, local extension usually first develops anteriorly. Posterior extension to the sacrum invariably means advanced disease. In women, tumor rather frequently invades the vagina, where it may present as an ulcerating mass. Bladder invasion in women is relatively infrequent, for the pelvic organs form an effective but vulnerable barrier.

Microscopic pathology

The microscopic appearance of carcinoma of the large bowel is that of a usually fairly well-differentiated adenocarcinoma that shows variable degrees of mucoid degeneration (Fig. 385). The few very undifferentiated adenocarcinomas of the colon may be hard to recognize. In rare cases, the tumor may show mucin production within its cells (signet ring type), and in these instances the tumor tends to extend submucosally, grows quickly through the wall, often obstructs, and develops early metastases. Squamous cell carcinoma of the colon has been reported by Hicks and Cowling.[95] Perineural space invasion is seen as small nests of tumor cells lying within the distended sheath of nerves. Blood vessel invasion should also be searched for, particularly in submucosal and serosal areas. The more undifferentiated the tumor, the higher the proportion of blood vessel invasion.

Vein invasion is invariably demonstrated microscopically when there is metastatic carcinoma within the liver. Grinnell[81] reported that vessel invasion before complete penetration of the muscular wall of the large bowel is rare. Such invasion was present in a little over one-fourth of the cases examined by Sunderland[164] and was present most frequently in the lowest 1 cm of the rectum, probably because the submucosa of this area is richly endowed with veins of the hemorrhoidal plexus. This invasion should be substantiated by special stains to prove that tumor is within a vessel.

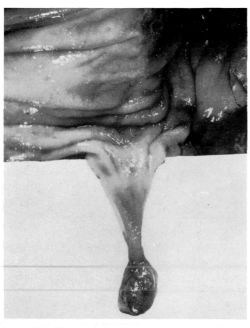

Fig. 380. Benign adenomatous polyp (pedunculated type) found in surgical specimen from abdominoperineal resection for carcinoma of rectum.

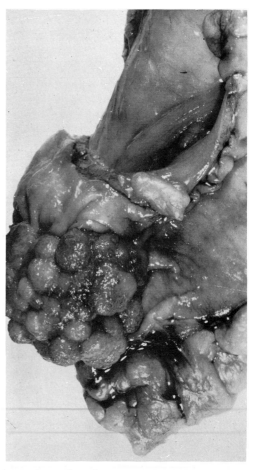

Fig. 381. Polypoid carcinoma in same specimen shown in Fig. 380.

Metastatic spread

The *lymphatic* spread of carcinomas of the large bowel proceeds in a rather orderly fashion from lymph node to lymph node, progressing along the aorta as far as the mesenteric and pancreatic lymph node areas (Coller and MacIntyre[26]). Rarely does a tumor bypass a lymph node group. Retrograde lymph node involvement only takes place if the ascending node areas are completely filled (Gilchrist and David[66]). Once the thoracic duct has been reached by the tumor, metastases may present themselves in the supraclavicular lymph nodes.

Carcinomas of the large bowel can be divided into two distinct clinical types: those with metastases and those without metastases. This distinction can usually be made by paying attention to the advancing margin of the tumor. Tumors seldom metastasize if the advancing margin has a pushing border with inflammatory infiltrate, made up of plasma cells and lymphocytes, at the interface between the tumor and the surrounding tissue. This is the type of tumor that may push its way into other organs but, no matter how large it becomes, there will be no metastases, and cure can still be effected if adequate excision is possible. By contrast, infiltrating tumors without such infiltrate metastasize in a high percentage of instances no matter what their size. This pushing border with inflammatory infiltrate is an expression of immune host response (Ackerman[1]).

Venous spread of carcinomas of the large bowel is rather frequent, with consequent metastases to the liver in most cases but also to the lungs, kidneys, adrenal glands, and brain. Bone metastases are observed rarely. Grossly visible vein invasion is observed most frequently in cases of undifferentiated carcinomas with extensive local spread and lymph node involvement (Carroll[20]).

There seems to be no relationship between the size of a primary tumor and the presence or absence of metastases, but infiltrating and highly undifferentiated tumors do metastasize more frequently (Fig. 386). The occurrence of visceral metastases is related to the extent of the local spread and to the site of the primary le-

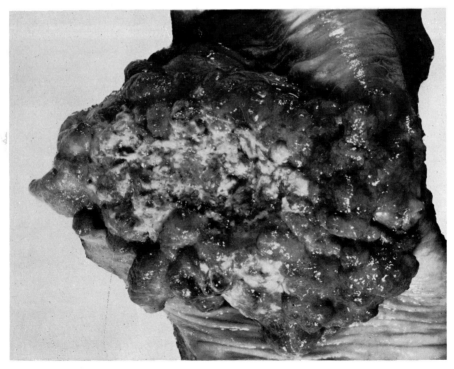

Fig. 382. Advanced fungating carcinoma of rectum. Same surgical specimen shown in Figs. 380 and 381. Patient living over eight years after operation.

sion (Dionne[37]). The deeper the infiltration of the wall and the higher the situation of the lesion in the large bowel, the greater the relative chance of visceral metastases. Microscopic evidence of vein and of perineural space invasion imply probability of visceral metastases (Seefeld and Bargen[143]).

Clinical evolution

The symptoms produced by large bowel polyps are rectal bleeding, diarrhea, and rectal discharge of mucus. When the tumor develops in the rectal ampulla near the anus, there may be tenesmus, sensation of foreign body, or even self-palpated evidence of growth. Symptoms may be present for as long as several years before a diagnosis is made. Large pedunculated polyps may protrude or cause obstruction and pain. They may become ulcerated and secondarily infected, with consequent pain and discharge. Rarely, large villous adeno-

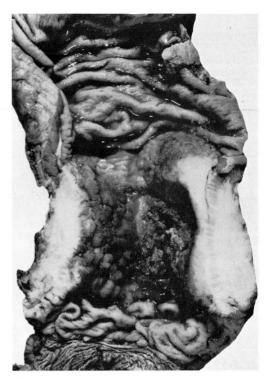

Fig. 384. Signet-ring carcinoma of bowel with hypertrophy of muscularis and pebbly overgrowth of involved mucosa. Patients with this type of cancer are hopeless.

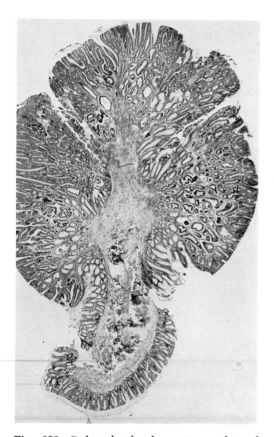

Fig. 383. Pedunculated adenomatous polyp of large bowel. (Low-power enlargement.)

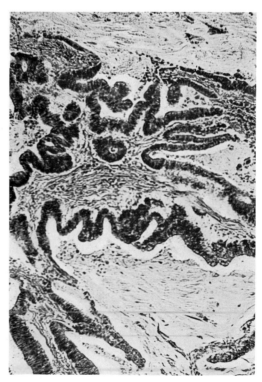

Fig. 385. Adenocarcinoma of rectum with prominent mucin production. (Moderate enlargement.)

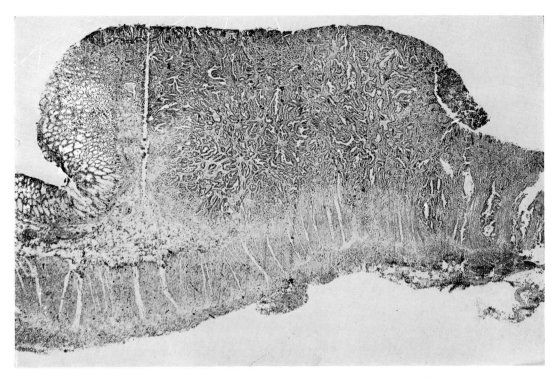

Fig. 386. Flat, small carcinoma of large bowel that has already invaded all layers of bowel and metastasized to regional lymph nodes. (Low-power enlargement.)

mas cause a syndrome of circulatory collapse due to excessive loss of potassium from the surface of the tumor (Findlay and O'Connor[59]).

The clinical development of carcinoma in the different sections of the colon and rectum offers nuances within the syndrome common to all carcinomas of the large bowel. In almost every instance, it produces an insidious alteration in bowel habits (constipation or diarrhea), pain and nausea from obstruction, or blood in the stool. Rectal tenesmus may coexist with the constipation. A minimal obstruction may cause some distention, but as the obstruction progresses, peristaltic waves attempt to pass fecal material through the opening, causing spasmodic attacks of pain, "gas pain," and constipation and alternate attacks of mucinous diarrhea. At times, there may be a complete block with distention and fecal vomiting. The obstruction is usually progressive, but it may occur suddenly as a consequence of intussusception or ingestion of barium. The growth rate of colonic carcinomas is variable. By measuring the size on sequential roentgenographic films, it can be observed that each carcinoma reveals its own growth rate, and this growth rate does not change with time. In one instance in a poor-risk patient, we were able to take measurements over a period of seven and one-half years and found that the growth rate did not change (Spratt and Ackerman[157]) (Fig. 387). Welin et al.[178] studied the rate and patterns of growth of 375 tumors of the large intestine and rectum as seen by repeated films using the double contrast enema method. This study demonstrated some overlap between growth rates of carcinomas and benign tumors. However, many benign lesions showed no growth or even regression. Villous tumors often grew at the same rate as carcinomas. The knowledge of the doubling time of the tumor of the large bowel may contribute to determining the treatment.

Gius[69] emphasized that in the development of obstruction of the large bowel, compensatory hypertrophy of the muscle coat may delay the onset of significant symptoms. Without obstruction, the patient looks and feels well. Rectal bleeding

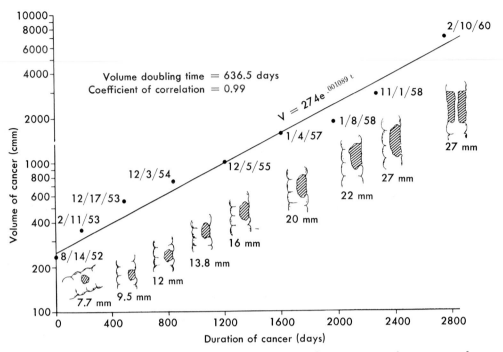

Fig. 387. Observed growth in primary well-differentiated adenocarcinoma of transverse colon. Note constancy of growth rate of this cancer over period of observation (seven and one-half years). (From Spratt, J. S., Jr., and Ackerman, L. V.: The growth of a colonic adenocarcinoma, Amer. Surg. **27**:23-28, 1961; WU neg. 60-2191.)

Table 38. Symptoms of carcinoma of colon and rectum (300 cases)*

| | Location of carcinoma (% of patients) | | | |
Symptom	Rectum	Left colon	Right colon	Total %
Blood in stool	86	46	9	46
Altered bowel function	79	82	81	80
Abdominal cramps or pain	7	77	87	57
None	2	2	3	2

*From Swinton, N. W., et al.: Diagnosis of cancer of the large bowel, J.A.M.A. **140**:463-469, 1949.

may be observed early, usually following defecation but sometimes in the intervals between stools. Then again the blood may pass unnoticed, mixed with fecal material. Bleeding may be marked with cecal lesions. Anemia and asthenia may result from prolonged bleeding. Persistent pain, not related to obstruction, may develop as a cause of direct extension of the tumor within the pelvis or because of metastases. Marked weight loss usually results from visceral metastases. Bleeding is the most frequent initial symptom of rectal lesions, obstruction in carcinomas of the splenic flexures, and pain in tumors arising in the

transverse colon. In the cecal area, a palpable mass is the most common finding. Swinton et al.[166] reported a study on symptoms of carcinoma of the colon and rectum (Table 38).

The lesions in the various parts of the large bowel do show some differences. The tumors in the descending colon, particularly the sigmoid and the rectum, frequently give symptoms of obstruction. Obstruction of the left colon is about eight times more frequent than that of the right colon. The carcinomas of the right colon obstruct only when they become large, and this obstruction most frequently causes abdominal pain. The pain is usually intermittent, tends to become more constant, and is typically not severe. Weakness is often also associated with carcinoma of the right colon. Changes in bowel habits are present in about two-thirds of the patients. Carcinomas arising in the cecum tend to grow very large and often produce no symptoms of obstruction but may present an obscure profound anemia, related perhaps to the large bleeding surface of a fungating tumor.

The spread of carcinomas of the large bowel may result in spread of pain to the perineum and down the thigh. Obstruction of the ureters may occur, with death due to uremia. In other instances, complete bowel obstruction may appear, and death may follow because of perforation and terminal peritonitis. The formation of fistulas with growth of the carcinoma into the bladder, peritoneal cavity, or abdominal wall occurs very rarely. In a few patients in whom extensive local and distant spread of the disease has developed, death may supervene from a combination of factors. Hypoproteinemia, anemia, hemorrhage, and bronchopneumonia often contribute to the terminal picture. Long survivals in spite of liver metastases have been reported (Solomon and Kreps[154]).

Diagnosis
Symptomatology

The patient with a benign or a malignant tumor of the large bowel often disregards the early symptoms or ascribes them to a benign cause. To be sure, rectal bleeding may be due to a variety of benign causes, but its cause should always be investigated and removed (Swinton and Pyrtek[167]). Bleeding may be noticed only during constipation and may disappear with the use of laxatives or lubricants, so that the patient is naturally inclined to consider constipation as the primary cause of the bleeding. Diarrhea is often attributed to "indigestion." On the other hand, it is not infrequent to find rather advanced lesions, nearing obstruction, producing few, if any symptoms. Anemia and weight loss in aged persons should evoke suspicion of an intestinal tumor. Symptoms of large bowel polyps and carcinoma may not differ greatly.

Clinical examination

The inspection and external palpation of a large bowel tumor may reveal few positive findings. In eighty-one of 102 patients with carcinoma of the cecum reported by Vynalek et al.,[172] a palpable mass was felt. A mass could also be palpated in twenty of twenty-seven patients with carcinoma of the hepatic flexure and in twenty-six of fifty-five patients with carcinomas of the transverse colon. In cases of obstruction, a palpable mass may be due only to retention of feces. Meteorism usually centers well above the lesion, not infrequently in the cecal region. Hemorrhoids often coexist (Carstam[21]) or develop because of cancer of the rectum, so that although they offer an easy explanation of rectal bleeding, they should not deter the examiner from making a complete investigation.

Rectal palpation is a valuable and easy means that should be resorted to in all instances. Shedden[147] feels that the examining finger can reach higher if the patient is in the lateral decubitus position rather than in the knee-chest or dorsal decubitus position. A squatting position may, at times, bring down a prolapsing lesion. Vaginorectal palpation may give additional information in women with tumors on the anterior wall of the rectum. In a group of 817 cases of carcinoma of the large bowel reported by Jackman[102] from the Mayo Clinic, 444 could be felt by the examining finger, and an additional 132 were visible by sigmoidoscopy. Often, however, rectal palpation is not done in the presence of symptoms, with consequent delay in diagnosis and adequate treatment (Fig. 388).

In the presence of carcinoma, a thorough palpation should attempt to determine whether or not there is fixation and the relative position of the lesion in respect to the cervix or the prostate. The ulcerative or polypoid character of the lesion should be recorded.

Proctosigmoidoscopy. An adequate preparation of the patient is required for proctosigmoidoscopy. The presence of feces or mucus may mask a small lesion or hinder thorough investigation. Whether the lateral decubitus, the lithotomy, or the knee-chest position is chosen for the examination depends on the patient and the lesion. Lesions situated low on the posterior wall of

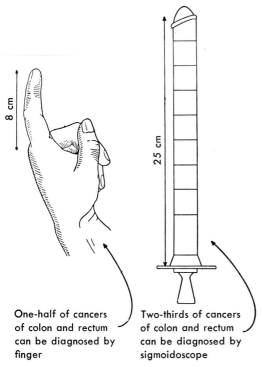

8 cm

25 cm

One-half of cancers
of colon and rectum
can be diagnosed by
finger

Two-thirds of cancers
of colon and rectum
can be diagnosed by
sigmoidoscope

Fig. 388. Length and diagnostic possibilities of index finger and proctoscope in cancer of rectum. (From Welch, C. E., and Giddings, W. P.: Carcinoma of colon and rectum, New Eng. J. Med. **244:**859-867, 1951.)

the rectum may be easier to palpate than to see, and higher lesions may escape detection unless the examiner is aware that on a routine examination all of the rectal wall should be visualized. Although it is not always possible to introduce the proctoscope into the sigmoid, it usually can be done without difficulty. Proctosigmoidoscopy may be carried to all of the large bowel within 25 cm to 30 cm from the anus, increasing considerably the chances of discovering additional lesions. One-half of the carcinomas of the colon and rectum can be diagnosed by the finger, and two-thirds of the carcinomas of the colon and rectum can be diagnosed by the sigmoidoscope (Fig. 388).

Biopsy

In frank carcinomas of the rectum and rectosigmoid, removal of specimens for histopathologic confirmation of the diagnosis is an easy procedure. In large ulcerated carcinomas, it is possible to remove a specimen from the border of the lesion showing only hyperplastic epithelium. In polypoid lesions, whenever possible, it is preferable to remove the entire tumor to permit careful orientation and sectioning (Turell and Haller[168]). With large papillary tumors, the surgeon must look for zones of ulceration and fixation, for it is extremely easy to miss an infiltrating carcinoma concealed within the papillary fronds. The size of the tumor, as well as the condition of the stalk, must be recorded. In polyps that have been biopsied previously and not entirely removed, fixation may result from secondary infection and inflammation. It is important that the surgeon and the pathologist discuss these and all details before a definite diagnosis is made and a course of action taken.

Cytologic examination is of little practical value in the diagnosis of cancer of the large bowel. In a few instances of lesions not radiographically demonstrable, of association with diverticulitis, etc., the procedure may prove of some help. Cytology, however, may be helpful in association with a silicone-foam enema (Cook and Margulis[27]).

Roentgenologic examination

For lesions beyond reach of the examining finger or the proctoscope, roentgenologic examination is the most significant diagnostic procedure. This examination may also contribute additional information even when the lesions are accessible or are discovered by other methods. It is important to recognize that a great deal of useful information may be obtained by the expert observation and control of the progress of the barium enema in *radioscopy*. Roentgenograms taken without benefit of radioscopy imply insufficient skill or lack of proper understanding of their different diagnostic value. Unless the patient is mobilized during radioscopy, some rectosigmoid lesions, such as those of a particular segment of the bowel in lateral and oblique projections, may be missed. Spot roentgenograms can be wisely chosen only when the examiner studies the course of the barium column to a point of obstruction or filling defect. Some rectosigmoid lesions cannot be visualized in a regular anteroposterior view. A posteroanterior view,

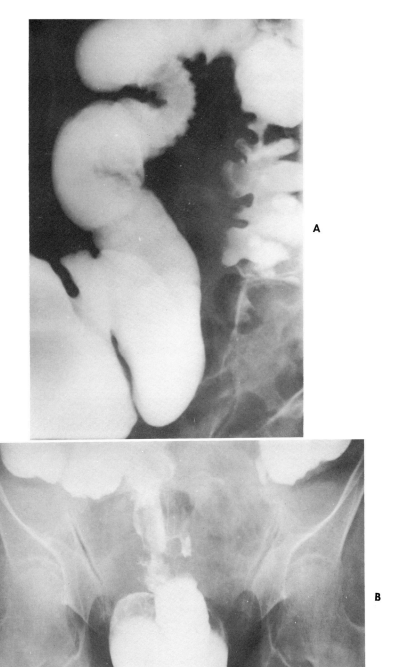

Fig. 389. A, Roentgenogram of patient with carcinoma of rectosigmoid in anteroposterior projection. **B,** Roentgenogram of same patient in Chassard-Lapine position. (**A,** PCH 61-2346; **B,** PCH 61-2346.)

taken with the patient sitting on the film and bending forward (Chassard and Lapine[23]) may offer a good projection of the area (Fig. 389).

Lack of proper preparation may cause errors in the interpretation of a barium enema. Fecal material, air, or oil in the bowel may simulate the rounded images of apparent polyps. A repetition of the procedure is preferable to a hasty decision. Many roentgenologists put great emphasis on the postevacuation roentgenogram which is done routinely. Figiel et al.[57] recommend compression and high-kilovoltage techniques in order to identify accurately small polypoid lesions. Cook and Margulis[27] have devised a silicone-foam diagnostic enema that results in actual casts of the bowel through polymerization. These molds are easily passed and may provide an accurate diagnosis of carcinomas, polyps, diverticulosis, ulcerative colitis, etc.

The usual barium enema, even in expert hands, does not permit detection of all small or large lesions of the colon. The air contrast method used routinely by Welin[177] is extremely accurate in demonstrating small tumors, whether they be polyps or cancer (Fig. 390). This method is also

used as a routine procedure at St. Marks Hospital in London. If a patient has symptoms suggesting a lesion of the large bowel, we believe that an air contrast enema must be used, although it may be time consuming. It is accurate and also reassuring if the results are reported to be within normal limits. With a negative air contrast enema, a repetition of the examination would not be necessary for at least three years, and perhaps longer, in view of the slow doubling time of the cancer of the large bowel (400 to 600 days). If a conventional barium enema is used, a negative finding has only limited value. If small carcinomas are to be identified, then *air contrast enemas must be routine.*

The roentgenologic demonstration of polypoid lesions may require additional qualifications: a polypoid tumor more than 1 cm in diameter has a 1 in 3 chance of being malignant. Sessile polyps showing a dimpling or indentation of the colonic wall often prove to be malignant (Fig. 392). Also, if the breadth of the polyp is greater

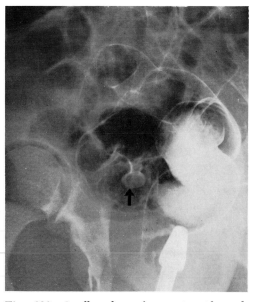

Fig. 390. Small polyp of rectosigmoid made visible by double contrast and rotation during examination. (Courtesy Dr. C. W. Yates and Dr. L. Crowell, Houston, Texas.)

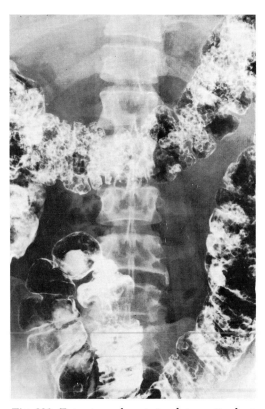

Fig. 391. Extensive polyposis involving entire large bowel which was treated by total colectomy.

than its height, the lesion is likely to be malignant. According to Wolf,[185] villous tumors can be recognized radiographically by their surface pattern or their changes in shape.

Carcinomas of the large bowel are usually visualized as an intraluminal filling defect breaking the smooth continuity of the bowel wall (Figs. 393 and 394). There is a variable degree of obstruction to the barium enema but, even when it appears complete, the bowel is still permeable to feces traveling in the opposite direction (Fig. 395). Spasms and proximal hypermotility may be associated with carcinomas, particularly when they are still small. Intussusception may be associated with small lesions of the cecum near the ileocecal valve. Beyond identifying the location and extent of the tumor and revealing other associated lesions, the roentgenologic examination may contribute additional infor-

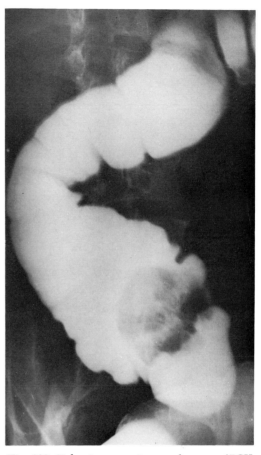

Fig. 393. Voluminous carcinoma of cecum. (PCH 68-088.)

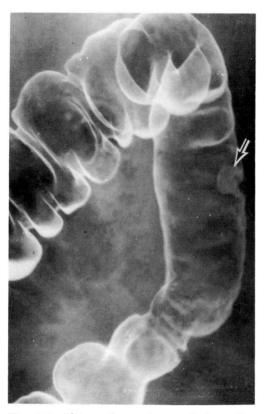

Fig. 392. Flat sessile carcinoma of descending colon with indentation of serosa. This film illustrates value of air contrast in detecting small carcinomas. (WU neg. 60-1110.)

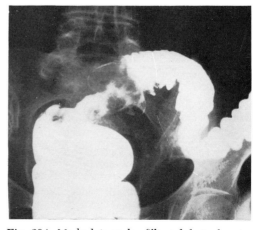

Fig. 394. Marked irregular filling defect of rectosigmoid due to carcinoma.

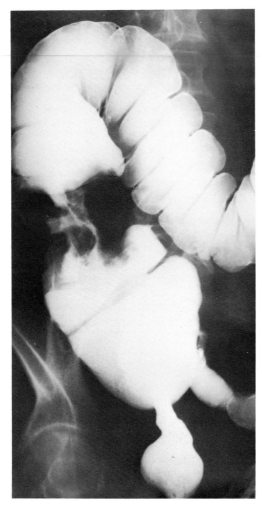

Fig. 395. Carcinoma of ascending colon. (PCH 50-251.)

mation concerning the fixation or mobility of the lesion (Levene and Bragg[110]).

Follow-up reexaminations may reveal postoperative recurrences at the site of anastomosis or adjacent areas. These recrudescences may have to be differentiated from suture granulomas, spasms, or edema of the bowel wall (Fleischner and Berenberg[60]).

Laboratory examination

An investigation of occult blood can easily be done in every patient suspected of harboring an intestinal tumor. The small amount of feces adhering to the examiner's glove is usually sufficient for this test. A blood count and hemoglobin determination may reveal secondary anemia. Villous tumors may cause considerable loss of fluid and potassium, placing the patient in electrolyte imbalance. Further laboratory tests may be necessary to evaluate surgical risk.

Differential diagnosis

Carcinoma of the large bowel may not be suspected if there are no specific symptoms pointing to it, but when suggestive evidence of its presence is encountered, there are various specific lesions of the large bowel with which it must be differentiated. The clinical points of differentiation are often vague, and the roentgenologic examination is by far the best method of distinguishing the various lesions.

If a carcinoma arises in the cecum, the symptoms suggest *appendicitis* with right lower quadrant pain and perhaps tenderness. About 25% of the patients with cecal carcinoma are operated upon with this preoperative interpretation. *A man over 50 years of age with symptoms suggesting appendicitis should be examined carefully.* If a mass is present and there is evidence of anemia, weight loss, and occult blood in the stool, carcinoma rather than appendicitis should be considered, and a barium enema should be given (Burt[17]).

Carcinoma of the cecum may also suggest *peptic ulcer, gallbladder disease, or kidney tumor.* A peptic ulcer and gallbladder disease may be ruled out by roentgenologic study and the history. A kidney tumor extends toward the retroperitoneal region and usually cannot be moved laterally. A carcinoma of the cecum can be palpated to the side and is felt in a lower region than the kidney tumor. The retrograde pyelograms may show displacement of the ureter by a cecal mass, but the kidney itself and its pelvis are normal.

The usual *tuberculosis* of the large bowel does not mimic carcinoma inasmuch as it involves both the ileum and the cecum, with multiple areas of ulceration and considerable spasm. Tuberculosis in the ileocecal region can cause obstructive symptoms in rare instances when the tuberculosis is hyperplastic. The roentgenologic examination may also demonstrate involvement of the ileum, and this indirect sign is often helpful in the differential diagnosis. Active tuberculosis of the lungs may or may not be shown on roentgenologic ex-

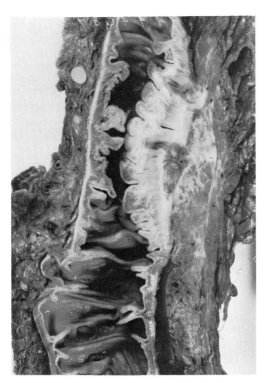

Fig. 396. Multiple diverticula of sigmoid colon with adjacent diverticulitis producing tumorlike swelling of bowel wall and pericolic abscess. (From Golden, R.: Diverticulosis, diverticulitis and carcinoma of the colon; a roentgenological discussion, New Eng. J. Med. **211**:614-623, 1934.)

amination, but when it is not present, the diagnosis becomes more difficult.

If a *foreign body*, particularly in the region of the cecum, ulcerates and obstructs the bowel, it may form a mass that is difficult to differentiate from carcinoma. A prominent, edematous ileocecal valve may partially intussuscept into the cecum and be diagnosed radiographically as a cancer of the cecum.

Diverticulitis and *diverticulosis* occur particularly in the region of the sigmoid and may give symptoms and signs suggesting large bowel carcinoma. Diverticulitis may also occur in the cecal region, suggesting carcinoma of the cecum (Anderson[1a]; Henry[93]). Bleeding sometimes occurs, and the diverticula may become infected. With infection, a pericolic abscess may form to cause the development of inflammatory masses that may be thought to be malignant (Svane[165]). Diverticulitis may give symptoms in either side of the abdo-

men, and in a few instances it is extremely difficult to differentiate from carcinoma roentgenologically (Schatzki[142]). The roentgenologic demonstration of diverticula does not rule out carcinoma. When there is constriction of the lumen due to secondary infection and inflammation (Fig. 396), the constriction varies from moment to moment, unlike that of a malignant lesion; in addition, the mucosal contours persist or are exaggerated, producing a very irregular, jagged, sawtooth margin (Golden[73]).

The acute variety of ulcerative colitis is not hard to diagnose. Chronic localized areas of *ulcerative colitis* and pericolic inflammatory masses may present filling defects and inflammatory masses resembling carcinoma. The carcinomatous changes in long-standing cases of ulcerative colitis may occur at any point of the colon and not necessarily in the rectosigmoid (Edling et al.[51]). They occur at an earlier age than the usual carcinoma of the colon (Goldgraber et al.[74]). Conversely, there may be in obstructing carcinomas a proximal ulceration grossly simulating ulcerative colitis. It is important to recognize the difference (Glotzer et al.[72]). *Colitis cystica profunda* can be confused radiographically and grossly with a polyp (Fig. 397). It can occur in association with ulcerative colitis or effects of irradiation. Microscopically, this lesion invariably presents a defect of the mucosa (Wayte and Helwig[175]) with submucosal lakes of mucin indirectly associated with glands. This pattern may lead to an incorrect diagnosis of mucinous carcinoma. *Oleogranulomas* of the rectal wall may result from the injection of sclerosing solutions for the treatment of internal hemorrhoids and also from the injection of foreign lipids in oily anesthetics. Hernandez et al.[94] reported a case in which there was an annular constricting lesion of the rectum simulating carcinoma (Fig. 398).

Endometriosis may manifest itself as a constricting lesion of the rectosigmoid that could be mistaken for a carcinoma. The endometrioma may appear polypoid on radiologic examination, but there is usually an abrupt change from the normal to the abnormal segment of bowel (Fig. 399). The serosal and deep structures of the bowel wall are usually affected (Boles and Hodes[14]), whereas the mucosa is intact.

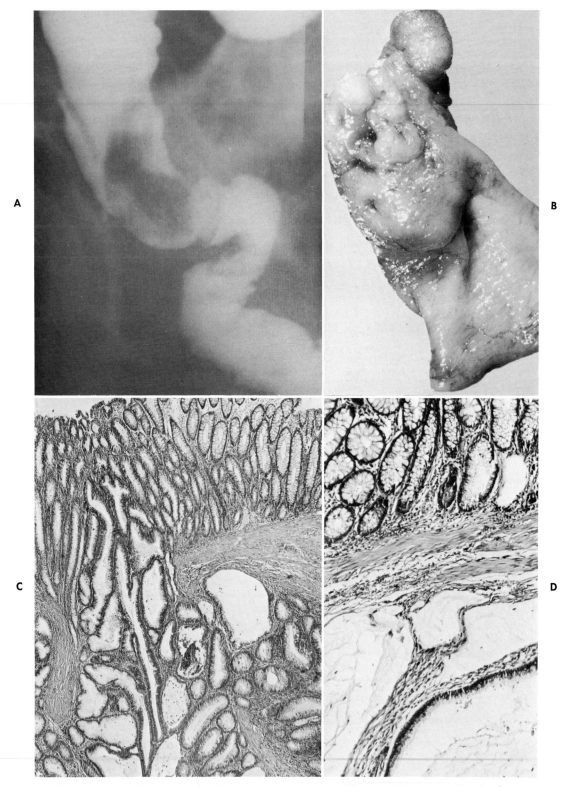

Fig. 397. A and **B,** Polypoid lesion in region of sigmoid flexure. This is example of colitis cystica profunda with polypoid shape. **C** and **D,** Displacement of mucous glands into submucosa with formation of lakes of mucin. (**A** and **B,** From Fechner, R. E.: Polyps of the colon possessing features of colitis cystica profunda, Dis. Colon Rectum **10:**359-364, 1967; **C** and **D,** slide contributed by Dr. R. E. Fechner, Houston, Texas; low power; WU negs. 68-7299 and 68-7300.)

Endometriosis should be suspected in women of childbearing age in whom the clinical manifestation of pain or tenderness is periodically related to menses. At exploration, a frozen section may solve the problem of differential diagnosis (Spjut and Perkins[155]). The rare condition known as *pneumatosis cystoides intestinalis* may be mistaken radiologically for carcinoma of the large bowel (Ramos and Powers[137]; Smith and Welter[153]).

Metastatic carcinomas in the large bowel from primary lesions elsewhere may also

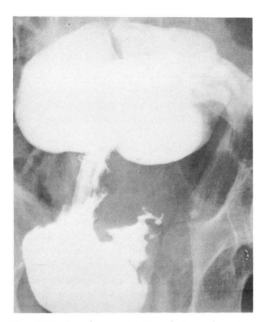

Fig. 398. Annular contricting lesion of rectum which strongly suggests carcinoma but proved to be oleogranuloma. (From Hernandez, V., et al.: Oleogranuloma simulating carcinoma of the rectum, Dis. Colon Rectum 10:205-209, 1967.)

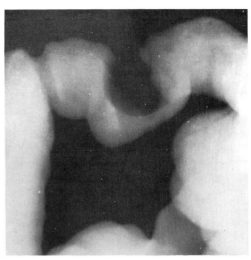

Fig. 399. Polypoid filling defect demonstrated in proximal sigmoid colon illustrating intact mucosa and submucosal appearance of endometriosis. (From Spjut, H. J., and Perkins, D. E.: Endometriosis of the sigmoid colon and rectum, Amer. J. Roentgen. 82:1070-1075, 1959.)

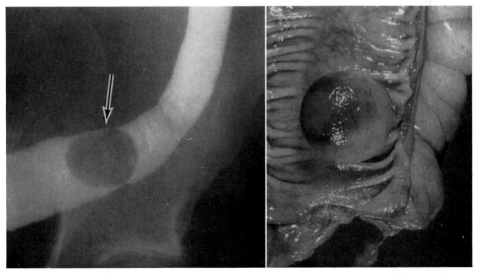

Fig. 400. Sharply circumscribed lipoma of large bowel. These lesions are radiolucent. (From Ochsner, S. F., and Ray, J. E.: Submucosal lipomas of the colon, Dis. Colon Rectum 3:1-8, 1960.)

be confused with primary carcinomas. The metastatic lesions are usually multiple and extrinsic and present other characteristics that may permit their radiologic diagnosis (Wigh and Tapley[180]).

Benign tumors of the large bowel, other than adenomas, develop relatively infrequently. *Lipomas* are usually located in the submucosa of the cecum and ascending colon (Helwig and Hansen[91]) but are also found in the left colon (Mayo and Griess[115]). Pain is a frequent symptom, possibly due to intussusception when the tumor is located in the mobile portions of the colon. Constipation, diarrhea, and bleeding may occur. Roentgenologic recognition is relatively easy because of the characteristic radiolucent, sharply defined defect (Ochsner and Ray[128]) (Fig. 400).

Carcinoids of the large bowel may be found most frequently in the cecum and rectum, for the most part in elderly individuals of both sexes (Peskin and Orloff[134]). They are frequently symptomless and are not accompanied by the carcinoid syndrome. Microscopically, they do not show reduction of silver salts. The smaller of these lesions seldom are found to have metastasized, but those more than 2 cm in diameter show a high proportion of metastases (Freund[62]; Bates[7]). As a consequence, although a wide local excision may be sufficient for the former lesions, an abdominoperineal resection may be required for the latter. *Leiomyosarcomas* of the colon (Meszaros[116]) and rectum (Quan and Berg[136]) are rare. They may present large palpable masses and ulcerations and are surgically curable.

Benign lymphomas are often polypoid and resemble the adenomatous polyps (Li[111]; Cornes et al.[28]). Usually such polyps are found near the anus, have a broad base, show a lobular pattern with follicle formation and reaction centers, and may be as large as 5 cm in diameter (Helwig and Hansen[91]). Benign lymphomas remain confined to the mucosa and the submucosa. Local excision is often successful. Hemangiomas of the colon are rare (Babcock and Jones[4]), and so are the leiomyomas (Stout[163]). Dermoid cysts, neurofibromas, teratomas, chordomas, etc. may develop in the presacral space and displace the rectum forward (McCarty[113]; Oppenheim and O'Brien[129]).

Lymphosarcomas, primary in the large bowel, are relatively infrequent (Ullman and Abeshouse[171]). They are usually reported in very young patients or in the elderly of both sexes. The most common location of reported lesions in the large bowel is the cecum, with the rectum, sigmoid, and transverse colon being less frequent sites (Delahaye et al.[36]; Glick and Soule[71]). The patients are usually in good general condition and symptomless. The tumors may be polypoid or form large palpable masses. The radiographic appearance may suggest their nature to an experienced observer (Winkelstein and Levy[184]). Microscopically, the appearance of lymphosarcoma in the large bowel is the same as elsewhere and, of course, does not permit the assertion that it is primary there. Frequently, in spite of their bulk, there may not be any associated lymph node metastases. A diagnosis of lymphosarcoma in the large bowel requires thorough investigation for a primary lesion elsewhere. A bone marrow biopsy is *de rigueur*. The prognosis of these lesion is rather poor (Culp and Hill[30]).

Melanomas of the anorectal mucocutaneous junction tend to involve the submucosa of the rectum and present as polypoid or sessile tumors of the ampulla, covered by normal mucosa or superficially ulcerated. The tumor may not be darkly pigmented, and frequently it presents satellite nodules. Melanomas may be limited to the area of the sphincter or rectal ampulla or metastasize to the inguinal nodes. Blood-borne metastases to the liver and lungs are frequent.

The *sacrococcygeal chordoma* is a relatively rare tumor that occurs most frequently in men between the ages of 45 and 50 years. At times, it may be confused with carcinoma of the rectum or the rectosigmoid area. It begins in the sacrococcygeal area and may slowly surround and obstruct the large bowel. However, it practically never ulcerates the lumen. Roentgenographic examination invariably shows destruction of the sacrum. A biopsy will reveal the typical microscopic picture (Mabrey[114]) (Fig. 401). A chordoma of this region can, at times, be successfully re-

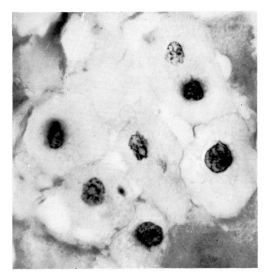

Fig. 401. Typical physaliferous (*physallis,* bubble) cells of sacrococcygeal chordoma. Patient was referred with diagnosis of carcinoma of rectum. Note cytoplasmic vacuolation due to glycogen.

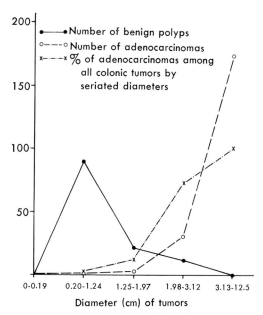

Fig. 402. Distribution of 228 adenocarcinomas and 124 benign polyps of colon and rectum according to seriated diameters of tumors. Note that after size has reached 3 cm, practically all polypoid lesions are cancer. (WU neg. 59-4938.)

sected (Dahlin and MacCarty[33]). Often, however, because of extensive invasion of the sacrum and the surrounding soft tissue, that is impossible. Under such circumstances, well-planned radiotherapy may occasionally give palliation (Wood and Himadi[186]). Patients with sacrococcygeal chordomas usually die from local invasion rather than from distant metastases.

Superficially ulcerated *hidradenomas* close to the anal orifice may cause confusion in diagnosis. It is not too unusual for other inflammatory lesions such as lymphogranuloma venereum or amebic granuloma to simulate carcinoma. An infectious granuloma that destroys the mucosa cannot be differentiated roentgenologically from carcinoma (Gunn and Howard[86]).

Hemorrhoids are often unfortunately considered the sole cause of rectal bleeding. They may have preceded the carcinoma and may have been aggravated by the development of tumor, or they may appear as a consequence of regional interference with the return circulation. The most frequent cause of delay in diagnosis is the assumption by patients or by physicians that rectal bleeding is due to hemorrhoids (Shallow et al.[145]). *A diagnosis of hemorrhoids alone should not be made in an aged patient without a thorough rectal palpation and proctoscopic examination.*

Treatment
Prevention and detection

The rising incidence of cancer of the large bowel in the United States imposes considerations of earlier detection and treatment. Under diagnosis we have discussed the adequate procedures of examination of symptomatic patients. Proctosigmoidoscopy and barium enemas are not easy to establish as screening procedures for asymptomatic individuals. Moreover, for the detection of early lesions, these procedures would require a greater sophistication than in the usual symptomatic patient and should be repeated at reasonable intervals. These efforts have proved to be impractical.

On the assumption that carcinomas arise from preexisting adenomatous polyps, the removal of all polyps has been advocated. However, the number of persons with large bowel polyps is in wide disproportion to the occurrence of cancer in these areas (Table 39). Assuming that carcinomas do arise from adenomas, Arminski and McLean[2] estimated that it would require eradication of all polyps in 500 individuals to prevent the occurrence of one carci-

Table 39. Age-adjusted incidences of carcinomas and polyps of colon and rectum in standard population of 1 million

Age groups (yr)	Frequency distribution		Ratio of carcinomas to polyps
	Carcinomas of colon	*Polyps of colon*	
20-39	21	11,300	1:538
40-59	148	24,000	1:162
60-79	244	23,500	1:96
80+	40	1,500	1:40
Total	453	60,300	1:133

noma. Removal of *villous* growths is always justified on the basis of the fact that their benign or malignant nature is not predictable. Thus any villous growth accessible through proctosigmoidoscopy should be resected. Radiographic demonstration of polyps in the colon presents a difficult problem. In a series of over 1000 tumors less than 1.5 cm in diameter, only thirteen were malignant (Grinnell[84]), whereas in another series all lesions more than 3 cm in diameter proved malignant (Spratt and Ackerman[156]). In view of the fact that there is always a chance of cancer in the smallest lesions, the remaining question is whether or not the individual case deserves close observation for growth or can run the risk of surgical intervention.

The exciting work of Gold and Freedman,[72a] Krupey et al.,[106a] and Thompson et al.[167a] has demonstrated specific antigens of the human digestive system which they can identify through radioimmunoassay. In the presence of a carcinoma of the large bowel, such antigens will be present in the serum and may remain positive after surgery because of the presence of persistent tumor. Such evidence of persistence has directed surgeons to reexplore the patients in some instances and tumor has been found. In a series of eighteen patients without clinical manifestations in whom the radioimmunoassay was positive, cancer of the large bowel was eventually found in sixteen. The carcinoembryonic antigen (CEA), so named because similar constituents are found in the embryonic gut, offers a means of detection of cancer of the large bowel early in its development and a basis for screening the susceptible population. The procedure is being thoroughly tested to facilitate its utilization. It is hoped that histopathologic evidence of host immunity may be correlated with sophisticated immunologic techniques.

Surgery

The treatment of carcinoma of the large bowel is radical surgical excision. No other treatment is so successful. The operability of these tumors has increased in recent years, whereas the operative risk has decreased. In a series of 1000 cases reported by Ginzburg et al.,[68] the resectability rate was 91% and the operative mortality 4.2%. The improved five-year survival is related to reduced operative mortality, expanded operability, and increased resectability. The reduction in operative mortality followed the use of multiple blood transfusions and a reduction in the frequency of anastomotic dehiscence. The use of antibacterial drugs appeared to exert no effect upon operative mortality and the incidence of postoperative sepsis, as shown in the study made by Polk et al.[135]

Operability. Few cases with carcinoma of the large bowel should be considered inoperable. Even in the presence of inoperable metastases, palliative resections are warranted (Bacon and Martin[6]). However, surgical intervention may be contraindicated in the presence of a terminal state of the patient, cardiac failure not correctable by preoperative therapy, a recent myocardial infarction, etc. Fixation of the tumor does not preclude operation, for it may be due to the accompanying inflammation rather than to the tumor. The possibility of peritoneal spread, as indicated by a doughy consistency of the abdomen, ascites, enlarged liver, or the presence of bone metastases does not necessarily contraindicate an exploration of the abdomen because resection of the tumor still may be beneficial. The presence of distant intra-abdominal metastases should always be confirmed by frozen section. Miller et al.[120] emphasize the necessity of resections in all patients with perforation of the colon due to cancer. They reported forty-three patients with localized perforation and abscess formation, thirty-eight of whom were operated with an operative mortality of 9.3%.

The one-stage *abdominoperineal resection* of Miles[118] is the procedure of choice for carcinoma of the rectum, rectosigmoid, and low sigmoid colon. This operation is applicable to over 90% of the resectable cases and can be done with a low operative mortality. Preliminary transverse colostomy is indicated in the presence of colonic obstruction or a perforation with extracolic abscess.

Sphincter-saving operations appeal to the patient, but they should not be done at great risk of local recurrence. The incidence of local recurrence is very high when less radical operations are done for lesions located at the peritoneal reflection or below. In all such cases an abdominoperineal resection should be done. *Anterior resections* are followed by excellent functional results (Goligher[76]), but they should not replace abdominoperineal resections in any patient under circumstances that would decrease the chances of cure. The recent trend has been toward a greater proportion of anterior resections. They should not be done on lesions that can be palpated through the anus.

Another conservative approach, the so-called *"pull-through"* operation, has been popularized by Bacon,[5] Waugh and Turner,[174] and Black and Botham.[12] This procedure is advocated for lesions of the midrectum, at least 5 cm above the anal margin. In this procedure, part or all of the rectum, the rectosigmoid, and part of the sigmoid may be removed. The distal end of the sigmoid is brought down, through the sphincteric apparatus, to present in the perineum, where it is allowed to heal in place without anastomosis by suture. This operation does imply a greater risk of local recurrence and less adequate excision of potentially metastatic nodes.

Local recurrences. Recurrences of carcinoma of the colon in the area of previous end-to-end anastomosis have been reported increasingly (Goligher et al.[77]). Speck et al.[154a] reported 13% recurrences at the suture line in patients operated upon. The recurrence rate seems to be greater in the left portion of the colon than in the right (Beal and Cornell[8]). There seems to be no relation between the amount of bowel removed below and above the tumor and the rate of recurrence if there is a margin of at least 6 cm on both sides. Local recurrences possibly are due to free cancer cells within the lumen of the bowel that may implant at the point of transection or of surgical trauma (clamps). The frequency of recurrence at the suture line has also been interpreted as a lymphatic return of cancer cells to the barrier area (Gricouroff[79]). This may be reduced by ligating the bowel some distance proximal and distal to the neoplasm before transection, as little handling of the tumor as possible, and ligation of the vascular trunks leading to the segment to be removed. Wright et al.[187] studied seventy-one instances of recurrences at the suture line. They pointed out that such occurrences were common in colocolic but rare in ileocolic anastomosis. Pelvic recurrences following abdominoperineal resections are most frequently found in the posterior vaginal wall and lateral ligaments in women and in the prostate, bladder, and presacral region in men (Gilbertsen[64]; Morson et al.[125]). Recurrences may also appear in the abdominal scar (Tyndal et al.[170]).

The frequent adherence of carcinoma of the large bowel to adjacent structures (bladder, vagina, uterus, small bowel) has determined the necessity for *enlarged resections*. It is not possible to determine at operation whether adherence is inflammatory or neoplastic. Rather than risk cutting through tumor, resection of the involved structure is indicated. Pelvic exenteration is well indicated for locally advanced carcinoma of the rectum or the sigmoid. Naturally this operation is contraindicated if there is objective evidence of disease outside the pelvis. This would include frozen section proof of cancer within para-aortic lymph nodes, liver, or peritoneal implants (Butcher and Spjut[19]). Extension of the operation can also be done when the tumor becomes fixed to the liver, gallbladder, stomach, or anterior abdominal wall. Such direct extension is not always accompanied by distant metastases. The removal of adjacent organs naturally increases the operative mortality, but the risk is well justified by the final results. In the mucoid carcinomas arising within longstanding fistula in ano, there is often local invasion of the buttocks. Because of this local spread, often without lymph node involvement, radical local removal of the tumor must be done (Rundle and Hales[141]).

Palliative resections are well indicated in patients in fairly good condition. These resections alleviate the distress of an ulcerating mass, relieve disturbing bowel symptoms, and diminish toxicity. The relief of bowel symptoms alone makes the operation worthwhile. Modlin and Walker[121] showed that although patients live much more comfortably, life as a whole is not prolonged. Rarely with lung or liver metastases patients may survive several years. Recurrent carcinomas of the colon

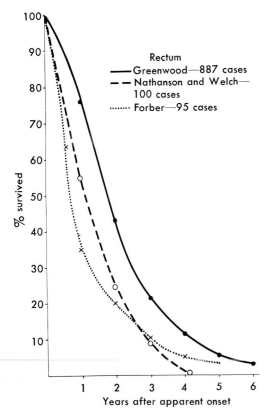

Fig. 403. Life expectancy of untreated patients with cancer of rectum. (From Shimkin, M. B.: Duration of life in untreated cancer, Cancer 4:1-8, 1951.)

and rectum have been resected and occasionally long periods of freedom from recurrence may follow (Dunphy[47]).

Palliative colostomy is an unsatisfactory procedure, for while it relieves impending obstruction, the patient continues to have distressing symptoms (passage of blood, secondary infection, and pain).

Complications of abdominoperineal resection have been reduced. Coronary thrombosis, pulmonary embolus, and thrombophlebitis occur in a variable number of patients. Urinary infection accounts for most of the morbidity, and renal failure accounts for the highest mortality (Shallow et al.[145]). Paralytic ileus develops in almost 10% of the patients (Jones et al.[103]). There are also occasional postoperative hemorrhages, peritonitis, and frequent infection of the perineal wound. Peritonitis may occur because of continuous leakage following resection and anastomosis. In spite of these complications, the operative mortality attending the abdominoperineal resection is almost negligible. The Miles resection[118] carries the disadvantage, when applied to men, that it usually results in impotence.

Radiotherapy

Adenocarcinomas of the colon and rectum, together with other adenocarcinomas, were long considered to be "radioresistant." Few pursued the possibilities of radiotherapy in this field except with an aim of *palliation* in the hopeless patients with postoperative recurrences or metastases. In the treatment of *perineal recurrences* following abdominoperineal resections, radiotherapy has been fruitfully utilized for pain relief (Murdock and Kramer[126]).

With the use of cobalt[60] and supervoltage roentgentherapy, attempts have been made to irradiate, thoroughly and judiciously, the *inoperable* carcinomas of the sigmoid and rectum and the *pelvic recurrences*. Williams and Horwitz[182] demonstrated the usefulness, as well as the complications of, radiotherapy in these patients. Smedal et al.,[152] Murphy and Castro,[127] Gremmel and Schulte-Brinkmann,[78] and Fajbisowicz et al.,[55] also have reported on the palliative results of their efforts. Wang and Schulz[173] irradiated a series of 111 inoperable or recurrent cases. A great

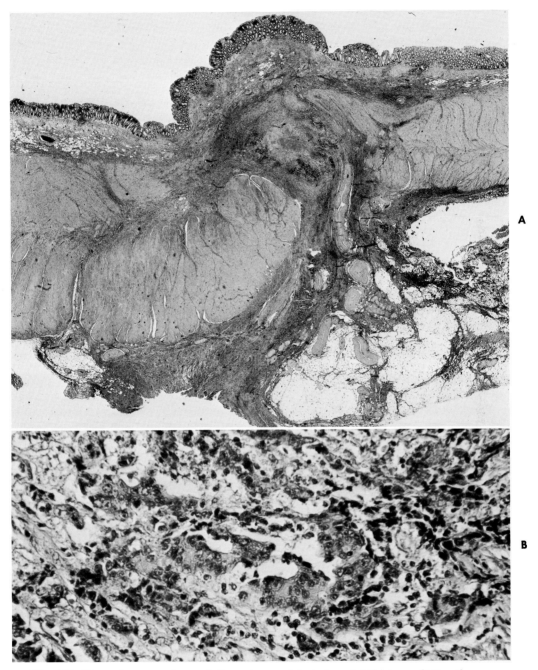

Fig. 404. Biopsy demonstrating typical carcinoma of large bowel following radiation therapy with cobalt[60] from May to June, 1967. Patient had abdominoperineal resection in August, 1967. Regional lymph nodes were negative, and there were profound radiation changes present. A small focus of residual carcinoma was seen. (**A,** ×300; WU neg. 68-10444; **B,** ×5; WU neg. 68-10445.)

proportion of the patients received good palliation. In eighty-four cases of postoperative recurrence which were irradiated, there were four patients surviving from six to nine years without evidence of cancer; of twenty-seven inoperable patients who were irradiated, two survived eight years without evidence of cancer. These results imply considerable dedication and skill; all patients have to be given the same time and effort in order that a few may benefit. Whiteley et al.[179a] found that 80% of patients benefited, particularly when the disease was localized to the pelvis.

Leaming et al.[109] reported on a series of 1786 patients with carcinoma of the rectum who had received *preoperative* irradiation by means of conventional roentgentherapy. There was a significant improvement in the results obtained, compared with the nonirradiated, particularly in those with Dukes' Type C lesions. This early report re-awoke the interest in radiotherapy as a surgical adjuvant. Obviously, what may be expected from preoperative radiotherapy is perhaps a slight increase in the operability and a reduction of the proportion of local and regional recurrences, but preoperative radiotherapy cannot interfere with failures due to metastases that may be present at the time of operation. It remains to be shown whether or not adequate irradiation does result in any complications or increased operative mortality for the frankly operable cases (Fig. 404).

Trials of this approach have been varied. A preliminary report on a randomized study in Veterans Administration Hospitals by Higgins et al.[96] has shown no apparent improvement of results in the irradiated group. A low-dosage regimen through large fields was chosen by the surgeons in the study, with immediate intervention.

Fletcher et al.[61] reported their experience with preoperative irradiation to a higher total dose. Not only was the irradiation well tolerated, but the operation was carried out without complications or operative mortality in twenty-seven patients. Two of the irradiated cases were converted from inoperable to operable, and a 10 cm tumor completely disappeared.

Stearns et al.[161] have made a report of a recent randomized study (1957-1962) and its comparison with the retrospective study of 1939-1951. The early results indicate an overall improvement of the irradiated as well as the nonirradiated groups which they attribute to better surgical techniques.

Preoperative irradiation consumes skill and talent as well as time. The operation must be postponed for weeks for the treatments to be administered and a proper lapse before operation. Unless serious efforts are made in treatment planning, patients and surgeons are not likely to think of this approach except when surgery alone is likely to be ineffective. Optimum results cannot be expected under these circumstances.

Postoperative irradiation is sought whenever the surgeon is conscious of having left tumor behind or whenever the histopathologic examination of the specimen suggests it. This is usually the case after operation of locally extensive tumors in spite of surgical precautions. Few have embarked on a study of this approach (Morson and Bussey[123]).

Chemotherapy

The administration of alkylating agents and antimetabolites has not proved encouraging in the treatment of patients with recurrent or inoperable tumors of the colon and rectum except for occasional ephemeral palliation. *Perfusion* of drugs after isolation of pelvic circulation has shown some response but has not become very popular (Pace and Knoernschild[133]). Use of the drugs as a *surgical adjuvant* has received greater attention (Curreri and Mackman[31]). A report of the Veterans Administration Adjuvant Study Group revealed that a randomized trial of TSPA as a surgical adjuvant, as well as a palliative procedure, showed no significant results (Dwight[49]). In another cooperative study in university hospitals, no difference in survival was observed with the use of Thio-TEPA (Holden et al.[97]). Combinations of chemotherapy and irradiation also have been probed for possibilities of useful sensitization but mostly for additive effects (Childs et al.[24]; Henderson et al.[92]).

Prognosis

In 1965, there were 32,000 deaths from cancer of the colon and 10,533 from cancer

Table 40. Variability of five-year survival rates on basis of selection of material*

Basis of calculation	Total cases	5-yr survivals		5-yr survivals without disease	
		Cases	%	Cases	%
All cases	735	94	13	58	8
All proved cases	515	85	16	58	11
All proved determinate cases	503	85	17	58	11
All cases of resection	237	60	25	37	16
All cases of resection except those with remote metastases	214	57	27	37	17
All cases of resection surviving operation	178	57	32	37	21
All cases of resection surviving operation except those with remote metastases	161	57	35	37	23

*Slightly modified from Ottenheimer, E. J.: Cancer of the rectum, New Eng. J. Med. 237:1-7, 1947.

of the rectum in the United States, comprising 10.8% and 3.5%, respectively, of all deaths from cancer and a crude mortality rate of 16.5 and 5.4 per 100,000 population. The mortality rates are higher for male and female whites (16.5 and 18.3) than for nonwhites (9.3 and 10.5) with cancer of the colon, whereas they are much closer for cancer of the rectum (6.6 and 4.9 for whites as compared with 4.0 and 3.0 for nonwhites). The highest mortality rate for cancer of the colon is found in Scotland, where it is 1.3 times the United States rate for whites, and the lowest rate is reported from Japan and Chile. The highest mortality rate for cancer of the rectum is reported from Denmark, where it is 2.1 times the United States rate for whites, and the lowest rate is reported from Chile. There seems to be an unquestionably greater mortality rate from cancer of the colon and rectum among city dwellers in the United States (Haenszel and Dawson[88]) as well as in some other countries.

In a series of 100 patients with untreated carcinoma of the rectum studied by Daland et al.,[34] the mean duration of life after diagnosis was fourteen months, with 45% living less than one year and 90% living fewer than three years. Five-year survival rates of treated patients vary greatly, depending on the factors included in the calculations. Using all cases of cancer of the rectum reported in Connecticut from 1935 to 1945, Ottenheimer[131] figured that a five-year survival rate of from 8% to 35% could be shown, depending on the basis of the computation (Table 40).

There is some indication that the results

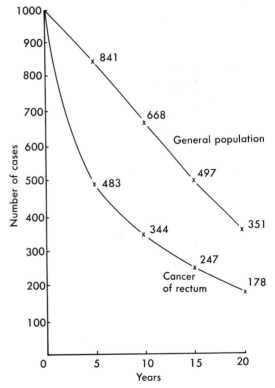

Fig. 405. From comparison of survival rate of patients treated surgically for cancer of rectum at St. Mark's Hospital with that of group of general population of similar age and sex distribution. (From Bussey, H. J. R.: The long-term results of surgical treatment of cancer of the rectum, Proc. Roy. Soc. Med. 56:494-496, 1963.)

of the surgical treatment of carcinoma of the large bowel have improved in recent years. The five-year survival rates have increased for patients with localized carcinoma of the colon for the three periods of 1940-1949, 1950-1954, and 1955-1959.

The same is not true, however, for carcinoma of the rectum (Cutler et al.[32]). Glenn and McSherry[70] reviewed the results of the treatment of 1026 patients with carcinoma of the large bowel from 1932 to 1959. Over 90% of the patients were considered operable, and in 65% a curative operation was attempted. The operative mortality declined over the years to 2.4%, and the five-year survival rate was 40%. Bussey[18] reported on the results of the surgical treatment of cancer of the rectum during a twenty-five-year period (1928-1952) at St. Mark's Hospital in London: 2083 patients survived the operation with about half of all patients cured. Local recurrences took place mostly during the first five years and were negligible after ten years (Figs. 405 to 407).

Turnbull et al.[169] have objective information that strongly suggests that operative manipulation of a cancer-bearing segment of the colon will increase the incidence of fatal metastases. They reported on a series of cases in which the lymphovascular pedicles were divided before manipulating and resecting the cancer. In their patients with Stage C lesions, the five-year survival rate was greatly improved when compared with a group of patients in whom a conventional technique was used (Fig. 408).

Various factors may have a bearing on the prognosis of carcinomas of the large bowel. *Location* of the lesion is of some relative importance. Carcinomas of the right colon have a better prognosis than those of the left colon, and those of the proximal rectum fare better than the distal ones (Osnes[130]). The *size* of the primary lesion seems to bear no relationship to the presence or absence of metastases (Butcher and Spjut[19]) or to the results. A clinical impression of *fixation* of the

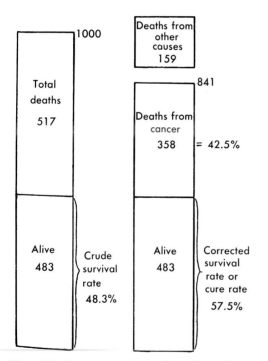

Fig. 406. From comparison of crude and corrected five-year survival rates of patients treated surgically for cancer of rectum. (From Bussey, H. J. R.: The long-term results of surgical treatment of cancer of the rectum, Proc. Roy. Soc. Med. **56**: 494-496, 1963.)

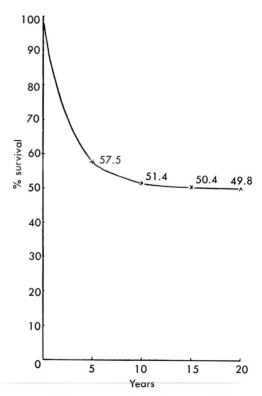

Fig. 407. From corrected survival rate of "cure" rate of patients treated surgically for cancer of rectum—St. Mark's Hospital series 1928-1952 (2083 operation survivors). (From Bussey, H. J. R.: The long-term results of surgical treatment of cancer of the rectum, Proc. Roy. Soc. Med. **56**:494-496, 1963.)

tumor carries a more serious implication in the male than in the female. There are indications of a *sex* difference in results, favorable to women (Cutler et al.[32]). Carcinoma of the colon in *children* has a very bad prognosis. The lesions are recognized late and are often undifferentiated and of the signet-ring type (Middlekamp and Haffner[117]).

The degree of *differentiation* of the tumor is of definite prognostic value. The degree of invasion and the proportion of metastases definitely increase with the degree of undifferentiation of the tumor. Signet-ring carcinomas are considered as highly undifferentiated in contrast to colloid carcinomas. The character of the *advancing edges* of the tumor, as observed microscopically, is important. The chances of lymph node involvement and visceral metastases are greater for the tumors with "infiltrating" rather than "pushing" edges (Fig. 409). *Retrograde* intramural spread confers a very poor prognosis (Grinnell[83]). *Vein invasion* by the tumor may imply serious consequences because of the increased chance of metastases to the liver, the lungs, etc. (Brown and Warren[16]). Sunderland[164] found that the five-year survival of patients with lymph node metastases but without vein invasion was three times higher (58%) than when vein invasion was demonstrated. Lahey[107] found that the best prognosis was that of carcinomas without vein invasion and without lymph node metastases—90% five-year survivals. *Nerve sheath space invasion* usually means a large proportion of metastases and of local recurrences (Seefeld and Bargen[143]).

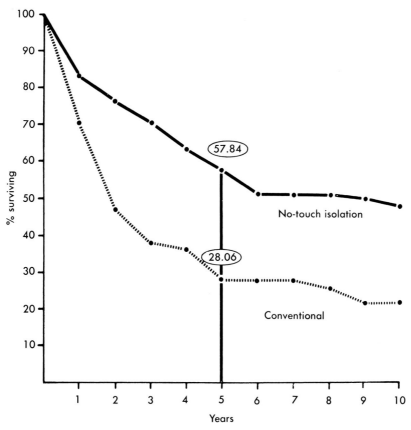

Fig. 408. Life table (not corrected for age) for Stage C cancers, 1950-1964. Note almost 30% variation in five-year survival of patients with Stage C cancers when no-touch isolation technique is compared to conventional technique. (From Turnbull, R. B., Jr., et al.: Cancer of the colon: the influence of the no-touch isolation technic on survival rates, Ann. Surg. **166:**420-427, 1967.)

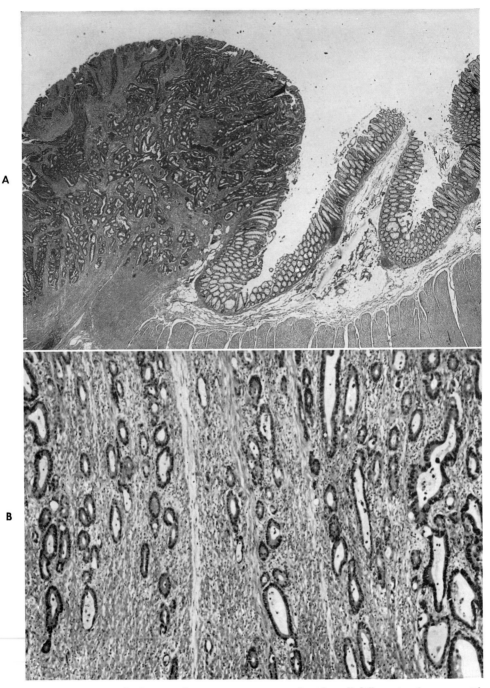

Fig. 409. Cancer with sharp pushing margins contrasted with well-differentiated cancer with infiltrating margins. There is a much higher incidence of metastases in carcinomas with infiltrating margins than in those with pushing margins. (**A**, ×12; WU neg. 60-2530; **B**, ×85; WU neg. 60-2316.)

The presence or absence of *lymph node metastases* (Dukes and Bussey[46]) is the most important single factor in the prognosis of patients with carcinoma of the large bowel (Table 41). The relative *number* and *position* of the lymph node metastases may also influence the prognosis. Spratt and Spjut[159] showed that when more than sixteen mesenteric nodes appeared to be involved, all patients died within five years and that when more than six lymph nodes were involved, the five-year survival was under 10%. Node involvement *adjacent* to the primary lesion is not so serious as involvement at the point of ligature of the vessels. *Retrograde* lymph node involvement has serious connotations.

The combined study of the local extension and of the metastatic involvement may yield the best information toward the prognosis. Dukes[38] divided his cases into three groups: Type A presented wall involvement but no spread beyond the serosa (Fig. 410). Type B had involvement of the wall and spread beyond the serosa but no regional lymph node involvement. Type C revealed spread through the wall, involvement of the serosa, and metastases to the regional lymph nodes. Gabriel[63] found that of his patients in Type A, 90% survived over five years; of those in Type B, 65% lived for five years; of those in Type C, only 20% survived five years. In Grinnell's series,[80] also using Dukes' classification, the patients in Types A, B, and C had 100%, 43%, and 23% five-year survivals, respectively.

The *type of operation* performed may have a bearing on the prognosis. Judd and Bellegie[104] studied the results of 282 an-

Table 41. Prognosis of carcinoma of large bowel on basis of clinical and pathologic factors

Outlook	Clinical findings		Pathology	
			Gross	*Microscopic*
Excellent	No symptoms	Tumor movable and small	Polypoid; limited to bowel wall; not circumferential	Type A (Dukes); no metastases; no vein invasion; no perineural sheath invasion; low-grade tumors
Fair to good	No symptoms except local; weight loss less than 25 pounds; no perineal pain	Tumor fixed or not	Partial circumferential lesion; polypoid	No perineural sheath invasion; no vessel invasion; type A, B, or C (Dukes); no node involvement or only node involvement in immediate vicinity of tumor
Poor	Weight loss greater than 25 pounds; pain in perineal region and thighs	Tumor fixed	Circumferential lesion—deeply excavating; submucosal extension; vessel invasion; lymph node metastases	Perineural sheath invasion; vessel invasion; lymph node metastases; signet-ring type; type B and C (Dukes); high percentage high-grade tumors
Hopeless	Distant metastases	Lungs Bone Liver Peritoneal implants Para-aortic lymph nodes Pancreatic Inguinal		

Secondary involvement of contiguous organs does not necessarily give a bad prognosis but does increase operative mortality. The organ involved and the degree of invasion are important. Compromise surgical procedures influence long-time results. The type of preoperative and postoperative care, the presence or absence of obstruction, and the ability of the surgeon influence immediate operative mortality.

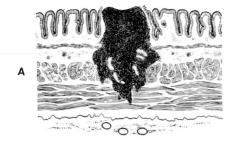

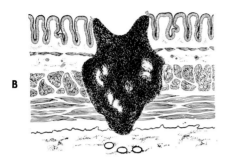

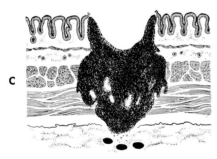

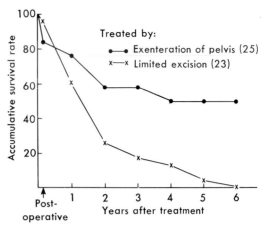

Fig. 411. Chart dramatically demonstrating value of pelvic exenteration in patients with locally advanced carcinoma of large bowel. (From Butcher, H. R., Jr., and Spjut, H. J.: An evaluation of pelvic exenteration for advanced carcinoma of the lower colon, Cancer **12**:681-687, 1959; (WU neg. 58-4990.)

Fig. 410. Schematic representation of Dukes' classification of carcinoma of large bowel. **A** represents invasion of muscle only, **B** represents invasion to serosa, and **C** represents invasion through serosa and involvement of regional lymph nodes.

terior resections: for lesions 16 cm to 20 cm above the dentate line, the recurrence rate was only 16%; for those 11 cm to 15 cm from the dentate line, the recurrences rose to 30%; for those within 10 cm of the dentate line, the rate of recurrence was 42%. Butcher and Spjut[19] compared the results of pelvic exenteration with those of more limited resections in cases of advanced tumors, showing favorable results for the more radical operation (Fig. 411). Palliative colostomies are attended by a high operative mortality and do not prolong life.

REFERENCES

1 Ackerman, L. V.: Pathologic evidence of host immunity in cancer: lymphocyte plasma cell infiltrate in malignant neoplasms (presented at the Tenth International Cancer Congress, Houston, Texas, May, 1970), Int. J. Cancer (in press).

1a Anderson, L.: Acute diverticulitis of the cecum, Surgery **22**:479-488, 1947.

2 Arminski, T. C., and McLean, D. W.: Incidence and distribution of adenomatous polyps of the colon and rectum based on 1,000 autopsy examinations, Dis. Colon Rectum **7**:249-261, 1964.

3 Axtell, L. M., and Chiazze, L., Jr.: Changing relative frequency of cancer of the colon and rectum in the United States, Cancer **19**: 750-754, 1966.

4 Babcock, W. W., and Jones, K. C.: Hemangioma of the colon, Amer. J. Surg. **80**:854-859, 1950.

5 Bacon, H. E.: Abdominoperineal proctosigmoidectomy with sphincter preservation; five-year and ten-year survival after "pull-through" operation for cancer of rectum, J.A.M.A. **160**: 628-634, 1956.

6 Bacon, H. E., and Martin, P. V.: The rationale of palliative resection for primary cancer of the colon and rectum complicated by liver and lung metastasis, Dis. Colon Rectum **7**: 211-217, 1964.

7 Bates, H. R., Jr.: Carcinoid tumors of the rectum, Dis. Colon Rectum **5**:270-280, 1962.

8 Beal, J. M., and Cornell, G. N.: A study of the problem of recurrence of carcinoma at the anastomotic site following resection of the colon for carcinoma, Ann. Surg. **143**:1-7, 1956.

9 Belleau, R., and Braasch, J. W.: Genetics and polyposis, Med. Clin. N. Amer. 50:379-392, 1966.

10 Bensaude, A.: L'évolution cancéreuse des tumeurs bénignes du rectum, Paris, 1937, Masson et Cie.

10a Berg, J. W., Downing, A., and Lukes, R. J.: Prevalence of undiagnosed cancer of the large bowel found at autopsy in different races, Cancer 25:1076-1080, 1970.

11 Berson, E. J., and Berger, L.: Multiple carcinomas of the large intestine, Surg. Gynec. Obstet. 80:75-84, 1945.

12 Black, B. M., and Botham, R. J.: Combined abdominoendorectal resection for lesions of the mid and upper parts of the rectum, Arch. Surg. (Chicago) 76:688-696, 1958.

13 Black, W. A., and Waugh, J. M.: The intramural extension of carcinoma of the descending colon, sigmoid, and recto-sigmoid, Surg. Gynec. Obstet. 87:457-469, 1948.

14 Boles, R. S., and Hodes, P. J.: Endometriosis of the small and large intestine, Gastroenterology 34:367-380, 1958.

15 Bremner, C. G., and Ackerman, L. V.: Polyps and cancer of the large bowel in the South African Bantu, Cancer 1970 (in press).

16 Brown, C. E., and Warren, Shields: Visceral metastasis from rectal carcinoma, Surg. Gynec. Obstet. 66:611-621, 1938.

17 Burt, C. A. V.: Carcinoma of the cecum complicated by appendicitis or para-cecal abscess, Surg. Gynec. Obstet. 88:501-508, 1949.

18 Bussey, H. J. R.: The long-term results of surgical treatment of cancer of the rectum, Proc. Roy. Soc. Med. 56:494-496, 1963.

19 Butcher, H. R., Jr., and Spjut, H. J.: An evaluation of pelvic exenteration for advanced carcinoma of the lower colon, Cancer 12:681-687, 1959.

20 Carroll, S. E.: The prognostic significance of gross venous invasion in carcinoma of the rectum, Canad. J. Surg. 6:281-288, 1963.

21 Carstam, N.: Hemorrhoids and cancer, Acta Chir. Scand. 97:71-82, 1948.

22 Chalier, A., and Perrin, E.: De la resection, transvaginale du rectum cancereux, Rev. Gynec. Chir. Abd. (Paris) 19:101-146, 1912.

23 Chassard and Lapine: Étude radiographique de l'arcade pubienne chez la femme enceinte; une nouvelle méthode d'appréciation du diamètre bi-ischiatique, J. Radiol. Electr. 7:113-124, 1923.

24 Childs, D. S., Jr., Moertel, C. G., Holbrook, M. A., Reitemeier, R. J., and Colby, M. Y., Jr.: Treatment of malignant neoplasms of the gastrointestinal tract with a combination of 5-fluorouracil and radiation; a randomized double-blind study, Radiology 84:843-848, 1965.

25 Colcock, B. P.: Prognosis in carcinoma of the colon and rectum, Surg. Gynec. Obstet. 85:8-13, 1947.

26 Coller, F. A., and MacIntyre, R. S.: Regional lymphatic metastases of carcinoma of the colon, Ann. Surg. 114:56-67, 1941.

27 Cook, G. B., and Margulis, A. R.: The use of silicone foam for examining the human sigmoid colon, Amer. J. Roentgen. 87:633-643, 1962.

28 Cornes, J. S., Wallace, M. H., and Morson, B. C.: Benign lymphomas of the rectum and anal canal; a study of 100 cases, J. Path. Bact. 82:371-382, 1961.

29 Crowder, V. H., and Cohn, I.: Perforation in cancer of the colon and rectum, Dis. Colon Rectum 10:415-420, 1967.

30 Culp, C. E., and Hill, J. R.: Malignant lymphoma involving the rectum, Dis. Colon Rectum 5:426-436, 1962.

31 Curreri, A. R., and Mackman, S.: Reoperation in carcinoma of the colon following resection and adjuvant chemotherapy, Surg. Gynec. Obstet. 123:274-276, 1966.

32 Cutler, S. J., et al.: End results in cancer, Report no. 3, National Cancer Institute, End Results Section of Biometry Branch, Washington, D. C., 1968, U. S. Government Printing Office.

33 Dahlin, D. C., and MacCarty, C. S.: Chordoma, Cancer 5:1170-1178, 1952.

34 Daland, E. M., Welch, C. E., and Nathanson, I.: One hundred untreated cancers of the rectum, New Eng. J. Med. 214:451-458, 1936.

35 Davies, J. N. P.: Cancer in Africa. In Collins, D. H.: Modern trends in pathology, New York, 1959, Hoeber Medical Division, Harper & Row, Publishers, pp. 132-160.

36 Delahaye, R. P., Isnard, J., and Pyard, M.: Les lymphosarcomes du caecum, J. Radiol. Electr. 44:625-634, 1963.

37 Dionne, L.: The pattern of blood-borne metastasis from carcinoma of rectum, Cancer 18:775-781, 1965.

38 Dukes, C. E.: The classification of cancer of the rectum, J. Path. Bact. 35:323-332, 1932.

39 Dukes, C. E.: Histological grading of rectal cancer, Proc. Roy. Soc. Med. 30:371-376, 1937.

40 Dukes, C. E.: Cancer of the rectum; an analysis of 1,000 cases, J. Path. Bact. 50:527-539, 1940.

41 Dukes, C. E.: Discussion on the pathology and treatment of carcinoma of the colon, Proc. Roy. Soc. Med. 38:381-384, 1945.

42 Dukes, C. E.: Familial intestinal polyposis, J. Clin. Path. 1:34-38, 1947.

43 Dukes, C. E.: The significance of the unusual in the pathology of intestinal tumours, Ann. Roy. Coll. Surg. Eng. 4:90-103, 1949.

44 Dukes, C. E.: The etiology of cancer of the colon and rectum, Dis. Colon Rectum 2:27-32, 1959.

45 Dukes, C. E.: The control of precancerous conditions of the colon and rectum, Canad. Med. Ass. J. 90:630-635, 1964.

46 Dukes, C. E., and Bussey, H. J. R.: The spread of rectal cancer and its effect on prognosis, Brit. J. Cancer 12:309-320, 1958.

47 Dunphy, J. E.: Recurrent cancer of the colon and rectum, New Eng. J. Med. 237:111-113, 1947.

48 Dunphy, J. E., Patterson, W. B., and Legg,

M. A.: Etiologic factors in polyposis and carcinoma of tne colon, Ann. Surg. **150**:488-498, 1959.

49 Dwight, R. W.: Adjuvant chemotherapy in cancer of the large bowel, Amer. J. Surg. **107**:609-613, 1964.

50 Ederer, F., Cutler, S. J., Eisenberg, H., and Keogh, J. R.: Survival of patients with cancer of the large intestine and rectum, J. Nat. Cancer Inst. **26**:489-510, 1961.

51 Edling, N. P. G., Lagercrantz, R., and Rosenqvist, H.: Roentgenologic findings in ulcerative colitis with malignant degeneration, Acta Radiol. (Stockholm) **52**:124-128, 1959.

52 Edwards, F. C., and Truelove, S. C.: The course and prognosis of ulcerative colitis, Gut **4**:299-315, 1963.

53 Edwards, F. C., and Truelove, S. C.: The course and prognosis of ulcerative colitis. III. Complications, Gut **5**:1-22, 1964.

54 Ewing, M. R.: Villous tumours of the rectum, Ann. Roy. Coll. Surg. Eng. **6**:413-441, 1950.

55 Fajbisowicz, S., Lalanne, C. M., Sarrazin, D., and Juillard, G.: La télécobalthérapie du cancer du rectum à l'Institut Gustav-Roussy, Ann. Radiol. (Paris) **9**:833-836, 1966.

56 Fechner, R. E.: Polyp of the colon possessing features of colitis cystica profunda, Dis. Colon Rectum **10**:359-364, 1967.

57 Figiel, L. S., Figiel, S. J., and Hennessey, A.: Carcinoma of the colon; incidence of error in the roentgen diagnosis, Amer. J. Gastroent. **40**:487-503, 1963.

58 Figiel, L. S., Figiel, S. J., and Wietersen, F. K.: Roentgenologic observations of growth rates of colonic polyps and carcinoma, Acta Radiol. (Stockholm) **3**:417-429, 1965.

59 Findlay, C. W., Jr., and O'Connor, T. F.: Villous adenomas of the large intestine with fluid and electrolyte depletion, J.A.M.A. **176**:404-408, 1961.

60 Fleischner, F. G., and Berenberg, A. L.: Recurrent carcinoma of the colon at the site of the anastomosis; roentgen observations, Radiology **66**:540-547, 1956.

61 Fletcher, W. S., Allen, C. V., and Dunphy, J. E.: Preoperative irradiation for carcinoma of the colon and rectum; a preliminary report, Amer. J. Surg. **109**:76-83, 1964.

62 Freund, S. J.: Carcinoid tumor of the rectum, Amer. J. Surg. **93**:67-73, 1957.

63 Gabriel, W. B.: Prognosis in cancer of the rectum, Lancet **2**:1055-1057, 1111-1112, 1936.

64 Gilbertsen, V. A.: Adenocarcinoma of the rectum; incidence and locations of recurrent tumor following present-day operations performed for cure, Ann. Surg. **151**:340-348, 1960.

65 Gilbertsen, V. A.: Improving the prognosis for patients with intestinal cancer, Surg. Gynec. Obstet. **124**:1253-1259, 1967.

66 Gilchrist, R. K., and David, V. C.: Lymphatic spread of carcinoma of the rectum, Ann. Surg. **108**:621-642, 1938.

67 Ginsburg, L., and Dreiling, D. A.: Successive independent (metachronous) carcinomas of the colon, Ann. Surg. **143**:117-120, 1956.

68 Ginsburg, L., Freund, S., and Dreiling, D. A.: Mortality and major complications following resection for carcinoma of the large bowel, Ann. Surg. **150**:913-927, 1959.

69 Gius, J. A.: The role of hypertrophy of the muscularis in the delayed onset of symptoms in cancer of the colon, Surgery **24**:221-230, 1948.

70 Glenn, F., and McSherry, C. K.: Carcinoma of the distal large bowel; 32-year review of 1,026 cases, Ann. Surg. **163**:838-849, 1966.

71 Glick, D. D., and Soule, E. H.: Primary malignant lymphoma of colon or appendix; report of 27 cases, Arch. Surg. (Chicago) **92**:144-151, 1966.

72 Glotzer, D. J., Roth, S. I., and Welch, C. E.: Colonic ulceration proximal to obstructing carcinoma, Surgery **56**:950-956, 1964.

72a Gold, P., and Freedman, S. O.: Specific carcinoembryonic antigens of the human digestive system, J. Exp. Med. **122**:467-481, 1965.

73 Golden, R.: Diverticulosis, diverticulitis and carcinoma of the colon; a roentgenological discussion, New Eng. J. Med. **211**:614-623, 1934.

74 Goldgraber, M. B., Humphreys, E. M., Kirsner, J. B., and Palmer, W. L.: Carcinoma and ulcerative colitis, Gastroenterology **34**:809-839, 1958.

75 Goldgraber, M. B., and Kirsner, J. B.: Carcinoma of the colon in ulcerative colitis, Cancer **17**:657-666, 1964.

76 Goligher, J. C.: Preservation of the anal sphincters in the radical treatment of rectal cancer, Ann. Roy. Coll. Surg. Eng. **22**:311-329, 1958.

77 Goligher, J. C., Dukes, C. E., and Bussey, H. J. R.: Local recurrences after sphincter-saving excisions for carcinoma of the rectum and recto-sigmoid, Brit. J. Surg. **39**:199-211, 1951.

78 Gremmel, H., and Schulte-Brinkmann, W.: Ergebnisse bei Bestrahlung des Rektumkarzinoms 1952 bis 1963, Strahlentherapie **133**:321-330, 1967.

79 Gricouroff, G.: La récidive sur l'anastomose après exérèse des cancers coliques, Bull. Cancer (Paris) **53**:409-414, 1966.

80 Grinnell, R. S.: The grading and prognosis of carcinoma of the colon and rectum, Ann. Surg. **109**:500-533, 1939.

81 Grinnell, R. S.: The lymphatic and venous spread of carcinoma of the rectum, Ann. Surg. **116**:200-216, 1942.

82 Grinnell, R. S.: Results in the treatment of carcinoma of the colon and rectum; an analysis of 2,341 cases over a 35-year period with 5-year survival results in 1,667 patients, Surg. Gynec. Obstet. **96**:31-43, 1953.

83 Grinnell, R. S.: Distal intramural spread of carcinoma of the rectum and rectosigmoid, Surg. Gynec. Obstet. **99**:421-430, 1954.

84 Grinnell, R. S.: The rationale of subtotal and total colectomy in the treatment of cancer

and multiple polyps of the colon, Surg. Gynec. Obstet. **106**:288-292, 1958.

85 Grinnell, R. S.: Lymphatic block with atypical and retrograde lymphatic metastasis and spread in carcinoma of the colon and rectum, Ann. Surg. **163**:272-280, 1966.

86 Gunn, H., and Howard, N. J.: Amebic granulomas of the large bowel, J.A.M.A. **97**:166-170, 1931.

87 Haenszel, W.: Cancer mortality among the foreign-born in the United States, J. Nat. Cancer Inst. **26**:37-132, 1961.

88 Haenszel, W., and Dawson, E. A.: A note on mortality from cancer of the colon and rectum in the United States, Cancer **18**:265-272, 1965.

89 Helwig, E. B.: Benign tumors of the large intestine, Surg. Gynec. Obstet. **76**:419-426, 1943.

90 Helwig, E. B.: The evolution of adenomas of the large intestine and their relation to carcinoma, Surg. Gynec. Obstet. **84**:36-49, 1947.

91 Helwig, E. B., and Hansen, J.: Lymphoid polyps (benign lymphoma) and malignant lymphoma of the rectum and anus, Surg. Gynec. Obstet. **92**:233-243, 1951.

92 Henderson, I. W. D., Lipowska, B., and Lougheed, M. N.: Clinical evaluation of combined radiation and chemotherapy in gastrointestinal malignancies, Amer. J. Roentgen. **102**:545-551, 1968.

93 Henry, F. C.: Acute diverticulitis of the cecum, Ann. Surg. **129**:109-118, 1949.

94 Hernandez, V., Hernandez, I. A., and Berthrong, M.: Oleogranuloma simulating carcinoma of the rectum, Dis. Colon Rectum **10**:205-209, 1967.

95 Hicks, J. D., and Cowling, D. C.: Squamous-cell carcinoma of the ascending colon, J. Path. Bact. **70**:205-212, 1955.

96 Higgins, G. A., Jr., Dwight, R., Walsh, W. S., and Humphrey, E. W.: Preoperative radiation therapy as an adjuvant to surgery for carcinoma of the colon and rectum, Amer. J. Surg. **115**:241-246, 1968.

97 Holden, W. D., Dixon, W. J., and Kuzma, J. W.: The use of triethylenethiophosphoramide as an adjuvant to the surgical treatment of colorectal carcinoma, Ann. Surg. **165**:481-503, 1967.

98 Holowach, J., and Thurston, D. L.: Chronic ulcerative colitis in childhood, J. Pediat. **48**:279-291, 1956.

99 Horrilleno, E. G., Eckert, G., and Ackerman, L. V.: Polyps of the rectum and colon in children, Cancer **10**:1210-1220, 1957.

100 Hullsiek, H. E.: Multiple polyposis of the colon, Surg. Gynec. Obstet. **47**:346-356, 1928.

101 Hultborn, K. A.: The casual relationship between benign epithelial tumors and adenocarcinoma of the colon and rectum, Acta Radiol. (Stockholm) **113**(suppl.):5-17, 1954.

102 Jackman, R. J.: Diagnostic errors in carcinoma of the large intestine, Proc. Staff Meet. Mayo Clin. **22**:447-450, 1947.

103 Jones, T. E., Robinson, J. R., and Meads, G.

B.: One hundred and thirty-seven consecutive combined abdominoperineal resections without mortality, Arch. Surg. (Chicago) **56**:109-116, 1948.

104 Judd, E. S., Jr., and Bellegie, N. J.: Carcinoma of rectosigmoid and upper part of rectum; recurrence following low anterior resection, Arch. Surg. (Chicago) **64**:697-706, 1952.

105 Kern, W. H., and White, W. C.: Adenocarcinoma of the colon in a 9-month-old infant, Cancer **11**:855-857, 1958.

106 Kraus, F. T.: Pedunculated adenomatous polyp with carcinoma in the tip and metastasis to lymph nodes, Dis. Colon Rectum **8**:283-286, 1965.

106a Krupey, J., Gold, P., and Freedman, S. O.: Physicochemical studies of the carcinoembryonic antigens of the human digestive system, J. Exp. Med. **128**:387-398, 1968.

107 Lahey, Frank H.: In discussion of Hayden, E. P.: The surgical treatment of carcinoma of the rectum, New Eng. J. Med. **233**:83-84, 1945.

108 Lane, N., and Kaye, G. I.: Pedunculated adenomatous polyp of the colon with carcinoma, lymph node metastasis, and suture-line recurrence, Amer. J. Clin. Path. **48**:170-182, 1967.

109 Leaming, R. H., Stearns, M. W., Jr., and Deddish, M. R.: Pre-operative irradiation in rectal carcinoma, Radiology **77**:257-263, 1961.

110 Levene, G., and Bragg, E. A.: Mobility of the rectosigmoid, Radiology **54**:717-725, 1950.

111 Li, I. Y.: Benign lymphoma of the rectum, Surgery **23**:814-820, 1948.

112 Lynch, H. T., and Krush, A. J.: Heredity and adenocarcinoma of the colon, Gastroenterology **53**:517-527, 1967.

113 McCarty, R. B.: Presacral tumors, Ann. Surg. **131**:424-432, 1950.

114 Mabrey, R. E.: Chordoma; a study of 150 cases, Amer. J. Cancer **25**:501-517, 1935.

115 Mayo, C. W., and Griess, D. F.: Submucous lipoma of the colon, Surg. Gynec. Obstet. **88**:309-316, 1949.

116 Meszaros, W. T.: Leiomyosarcoma of the colon, Amer. J. Roentgen. **89**:766-770, 1963.

117 Middlekamp, J. N., and Haffner, H.: Carcinoma of the colon in children, Pediatrics **32**:558-571, 1963.

118 Miles, W. E.: Cancer of the rectum, London, 1926, Harrison & Sons.

119 Miller, F. E., and Liechty, R. D.: Adenocarcinoma of the colon and rectum in persons under thirty years of age, Amer. J. Surg. **113**:507-510, 1967.

120 Miller, L. D., Boruchow, I. B., and Fitts, W. T.: An analysis of 284 patients with perforative carcinoma of the colon, Surg. Gynec. Obstet. **123**:1212-1218, 1966.

121 Modlin, J., and Walker, H. S. K.: Palliative resections in cancer of the colon and rectum, Cancer **2**:767-776, 1949.

122 Moore, G. E., and Sako, K.: The spread of carcinoma of the colon and rectum; a study

of invasion of blood vessels, lymph nodes and the peritoneum by tumor cells, Dis. Colon Rectum 2:92-97, 1959.

123 Morson, B. C., and Bussey, H. J. R.: Surgical pathology of rectal cancer in relation to adjuvant radiotherapy, Brit. J. Radiol. **40:** 161-165, 1967.

124 Morson, B. C., and Pang, L. S. C.: Rectal biopsy as an aid to cancer control in ulcerative colitis, Gut 8:423-431, 1967.

125 Morson, B. C., Vaughan, E. G., and Bussey, H. J. R.: Pelvic recurrence after excision of rectum for carcinoma, Brit. Med. J. **2:**13-18, 1963.

126 Murdock, M. G., and Kramer, S.: Cobalt 60 therapy in the management of perineal recurrence from carcinoma of rectum and colon, Amer. J. Roentgen. **91:**149-154, 1964.

127 Murphy, W. T., and Castro, L.: Irradiation of cancer of the rectum and rectosigmoid, Dis. Colon Rectum 7:102-105, 1964.

128 Ochsner, S. F., and Ray, J. E.: Submucosal lipomas of the colon, Dis. Colon Rectum 3: 1-8, 1960.

129 Oppenheim, A., and O'Brien, J. P.: Unusual anal, rectal and perirectal tumors palpable by rectal examination, Amer. J. Surg. **79:**302-311, 1950.

130 Osnes, S.: Carcinoma of the colon and rectum; a study of 353 cases with special reference to prognosis, Acta Chir. Scand. **110:**378-388, 1955.

131 Ottenheimer, E. J.: Cancer of the rectum, New Eng. J. Med. **237:**1-7, 1947.

132 Ottenheimer, E. J., and Oughterson, A. W.: Observations on cancer of the colon and rectum in Connecticut; an analysis based on 5572 proved cases, New Eng. J. Med. **252:**561-567, 1955.

133 Pace, W. G., and Knoernschild, H.: Pelvic perfusion and carcinoma of the rectum, Amer. J. Surg. **109:**52-56, 1964.

134 Peskin, G. W., and Orloff, M.: A clinical study of 25 patients with carcinoid tumors of the rectum, Surg. Gynec. Obstet. **109:**673-682, 1959.

135 Polk, H. C., Jr., Spratt, J. S., Jr., and Butcher, H. R., Jr.: Frequency of multiple primary malignant neoplasms associated with colorectal carcinoma, Amer. J. Surg. **109:**71-75, 1965.

136 Quan, S. H. Q., and Berg, J. W.: Leiomyoma and leiomyosarcoma of the rectum, Dis. Colon Rectum 5:415-425, 1962.

137 Ramos, A. J., and Powers, W. E.: Pneumatosis cystoides intestinalis; report of a case, Amer. J. Roentgen. **77:**678-683, 1957.

138 Rintala, A., and Nylund, C. E.: Familial polyposis of the intestine and pigmentation, Acta Chir. Scand. **114:**110-123, 1957.

139 Roth, S. I., and Helwig, E. B.: Juvenile polyps of the colon and rectum, Cancer **16:** 468-479, 1963.

140 Rouvière, H.: Anatomie des lymphatiques de l'homme, Paris, 1932, Masson et Cie.

141 Rundle, F. F., and Hales, K. B.: Mucoid carcinoma supervening on fistula-in-ano, its sur-

gical pathology and treatment, Ann. Surg. **137:**215-219, 1953.

142 Schatzki, R.: The roentgenologic differential diagnosis between cancer and diverticulitis of the colon, Radiology 34:651-662, 1940.

143 Seefeld, P. H., and Bargen, J. A.: The spread of carcinoma of the rectum; invasion of lymphatics, veins and nerves, Ann. Surg. **118:** 76-90, 1943.

144 Sessions, R. T., Riddell, D. H., Kaplan, H. J., and Foster, J. H.: Carcinoma of the colon in the first two decades of life, Ann. Surg. **162:**279-284, 1965.

145 Shallow, T. A., Wagner, F. B., and Colcher, R. E.: Clinical evaluation of 750 patients with colon cancer diagnostic survey and follow-up convering a fifteen-year period, Ann. Surg. **142:**164-175, 1955.

146 Shedden, W. M.: Carcinoma of the rectum and sigmoid with particular reference to the disease as seen in youth, New Eng. J. Med. **209:**528-539, 1933.

147 Shedden, W. M.: Cancer of the rectum and sigmoid, New Eng. J. Med. **223:**801-808, 1940.

148 Shimkin, M. B.: Duration of life in untreated cancer, Cancer 4:1-8, 1951.

149 Singleton, A. O.: The blood supply of the large bowel with reference to resection (symposium on surgical management of malignancy of colon), Surgery 14:328-341, 1943.

150 Sizer, J. S., Frederick, P. L., and Osborne, M. P.: Primary linitis plastica of the colon; report of a case and review of the literature, Dis. Colon Rectum 10:339-343, 1967.

151 Slaughter, D. P.: Symposium on abdominal surgery; polyposis of the colon, Surg. Clin. N. Amer. 24:161-174, 1944.

152 Smedal, M. I., Wright, K. A., and Siber, F. J.: The palliative treatment of recurrent carcinoma of rectum and rectosigmoid with 2 mv. radiation, Amer. J. Roentgen. **100:**904-908, 1967.

153 Smith, B. G., and Welter, L. H.: Pneumatosis intestinalis, Amer. J. Clin. Path. **48:** 455-465, 1967.

154 Solomon, H. A., and Kreps, S. I.: Twenty-six years of survival following carcinoma of sigmoid with prolonged liver metastasis, J.A.M.A. **144:**221-224, 1950.

154a Speck, R. L., Thomas, W. H., Larson, R. A., Wright, H. K., and Cleveland, J. C.: Analysis of 860 patients with carcinoma of the transverse and descending colon, Surg. Gynec. Obstet. **130:**259-262, 1970.

155 Spjut, H. J., and Perkins, D. E.: Endometriosis of the sigmoid colon and rectum, Amer. J. Roentgen. **82:**1070-1075, 1959.

156 Spratt, J. S., Jr., and Ackerman, L. V.: The relationship of the size of colonic and rectal tumors to their biological characteristics, Surg. Forum 10:56-61, 1960.

157 Spratt, J. S., Jr., and Ackerman, L. V.: The growth of a colonic adenocarcinoma, Amer. Surg. 27:23-28, 1961.

158 Spratt, J. S., Jr., and Ackerman, L. V.: Small

primary adenocarcinomas of the colon and rectum, J.A.M.A. **179**:337-346, 1962.

159 Spratt, J. S., and Spjut, H. J.: Prevalence and prognosis of individual clinical and pathologic variables associated with colorectal carcinoma, Cancer **20**:1976-1985, 1967.

160 Staszewski, J.: Cancer in Poland in 1959, Brit. J. Cancer **18**:1-13, 1964.

161 Stearns, M. W., Jr., Deddish, M. R., and Quan, S. H. Q.: Preoperative irradiation for cancer of the rectum and rectosigmoid; preliminary review of recent experience (1957-1962), Dis. Colon Rectum **11**:281-284, 1968.

162 Stemmermann, G. N.: Cancer of the colon and rectum discovered at autopsy in Hawaiian Japanese, Cancer **19**:1567-1572, 1966.

163 Stout, A. P.: Carcinoid tumors of the rectum derived from Erspamer's pre-enterochrome cells, Amer. J. Path. **18**:993-1009, 1942.

164 Sunderland, D. A.: The significance of vein invasion by cancer of the rectum and sigmoid, Cancer **2**:429-437, 1949.

165 Svane, S.: Non-specific inflammatory tumors of the colon simulating neoplasms; a report on 12 cases, Acta Chir. Scand. **129**:537-546, 1965.

166 Swinton, N. W., Hare, H. F., and Meissner, W. A.: Diagnosis of cancer of the large bowel, J.A.M.A. **140**:463-469, 1949.

167 Swinton, N. W., and Pyrtek, L. J.: Rectal bleeding, Surg. Clin. N. Amer. **28**:793-799, 1948.

167a Thompson, D. M. P., Krupey, J., Freedman, S. O., and Gold, P.: The radioimmunoassay of circulating carcinoembryonic antigen of the human digestive system, Proc. Nat. Acad. Sci. U.S.A. **64**:161-167, 1969.

168 Turell, R., and Haller, J. C.: A re-evaluation of the malignant potential of colorectal adenomas, Surg. Gynec. Obstet. **119**:867-887, 1964.

169 Turnbull, R. B., Jr., Kyle, K., Watson, F. R., and Spratt, J.: Cancer of the colon: the influence of the no-touch isolation technic on survival rates, Ann. Surg. **166**:420-427, 1967.

170 Tyndal, E. C., Dockerty, M. B., and Waugh, J. M.: Pelvic recurrence of carcinoma of the rectum, Surg. Gynec. Obstet. **118**:47-51, 1964.

171 Ullman, A., and Abeshouse, B. S.: Lymphosarcoma of the small and large intestines, Ann. Surg. **95**:878-915, 1932.

172 Vynalek, W. J., Saylor, L. L., and Schrek, R.: Carcinoma of the colon, Surg. Gynec. Obstet. **84**:669-677, 1947.

173 Wang, C. C., and Schulz, M. D.: The role of radiation therapy in the management of carcinoma of the sigmoid rectosigmoid, and rectum, Radiology **79**:1-5, 1962.

174 Waugh, J. M., and Turner, J. C., Jr.: A study of 268 patients with carcinoma of the mid-rectum treated by abdominoperineal re-section with sphincter preservation, Surg. Gynec. Obstet. **107**:777-783, 1958.

175 Wayte, D. M., and Helwig, E. B.: Colitis cystica profunda, Amer. J. Clin. Path. **48**:159-169, 1967.

176 Welch, C. E., and Giddings, W. P.: Carcinoma of colon and rectum, New Eng. J. Med. **244**:859-867, 1951.

177 Welin, S.: Results of the Malmö technique of colon examination, J.A.M.A. **199**:369-371, 1967.

178 Welin, S., Youker, J., and Spratt, J. S., Jr.: The rate and patterns of growth of 375 tumors of the large intestine and rectum observed serially by double contrast enema study (Malmö technique), Amer. J. Roentgen. **90**:673-687, 1963.

179 Wheat, M. W., Jr., and Ackerman, L. V.: Villous adenomas of the large intestine (clinico-pathologic evaluation of 50 cases of villous adenomas with emphasis on treatment), Ann. Surg. **147**:476-487, 1958.

179a Whiteley, H. W., Jr., Stearns, M. W., Jr., Leaming, R. H., and Deddish, M. R.: Palliative radiation therapy in patients with cancer of the colon and rectum, Cancer **25**:343-346, 1970.

180 Wigh, R., and Tapley, N. DuV.: Metastatic lesions to the large intestine, Radiology **70**:222-229, 1958.

181 Williams, C., Jr.: Carcinoma of the colon in childhood, Ann. Surg. **139**:816-825, 1954.

182 Williams, I. G., and Horwitz, H.: The primary treatment of adenocarcinoma of the rectum by high voltage roentgen rays (1,000 kv.), Amer. J. Roentgen. **76**:919-928, 1956.

183 Williams, I. G., Shulman, I. M., and Todd, I. P.: The treatment of recurrent carcinoma of the rectum by supervoltage x-ray therapy, Brit. J. Surg. **44**:506-508, 1957.

184 Winkelstein, A., and Levy, M. H.: Lymphosarcoma of the intestines, Gastroenterology **1**:1093-1099, 1943.

185 Wolf, B. S.: Roentgen diagnosis of villous tumors of the colon, Amer. J. Roentgen. **84**:1093-1104, 1960.

186 Wood, E. H., and Himadi, G. M.: Chordomas; a roentgenological study of sixteen cases previously unreported, Radiology **54**:706-716, 1950.

187 Wright, H. K., Thomas, W. H., and Cleveland, J. C.: The low recurrence rate of colonic carcinoma in ileocolic anastomoses, Surg. Gynec. Obstet. **129**:960-962, 1969.

188 Wynder, E. L., Kajitani, T., Ishikawa, S., Dodo, H., and Takano, A.: Environmental factors of cancer of the colon and rectum, Cancer **23**:1210-1220, 1969.

189 Zinninger, M. M., and Hoxworth, P. I.: Cancer of the colon, Surgery **14**:366-377, 1943.

Anus

Anatomy

The anus is a short canal 15 mm to 20 mm in length that extends from the semilunar valves to the outer surface of the posterior perineum, ending the digestive tract.

Most important among the constituents of the anus are its muscular fibers which form the internal and external anal sphincters. Between these sphincters there are ductlike structures that sometimes empty into the fibers of the internal sphincter or into the crypts of Morgagni and that are lined, for the most part, by columnar epithelium which, in the presence of infection, can undergo metaplasia to squamous epithelium. The anus is covered by a stratified squamous epithelium that extends up to the mucocutaneous junction, where abrupt transition to columnar epithelium takes place. Externally, the skin of the anus is continuous with the skin of the posterior perineum. The outer anatomic limits of the anus are formed by a circle 6 cm in diameter, centering in the orifice. The skin of the margin of the anus is slightly more pigmented than the surrounding skin and has numerous folds. The venous return of the anal region ends in the caval circulation, through the inferior hemorrhoidal plexus which originates as a group of small venules surrounding the anal canal, and in the portal circulation, through anastomosis with the superior hemorrhoidal plexus which is situated in the submucosa above the anorectal line.

Lymphatics. The lymphatics of the anus communicate above with those of the rectal ampulla and below with the lymphatics of the perineum (pp. 485 and 486). Some of the upper lymphatics of the anus communicate above with those of the rectal ampulla leading into the sacral, the upper mesocolic, and the paraortic nodes (Fig. 412). The inferior portion of the anus has a large subdermic network of lymphatics which sweep upward along the inner aspect of the thigh to end in the superficial inguinal lymph nodes (Fig. 413).

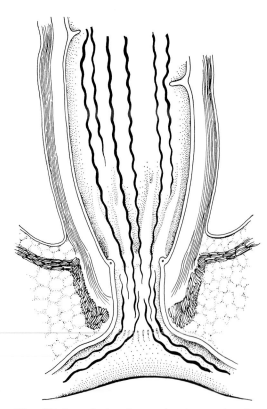

Fig. 412. Lymphatics of anus showing overlapping of perineal and rectal lymphatics.

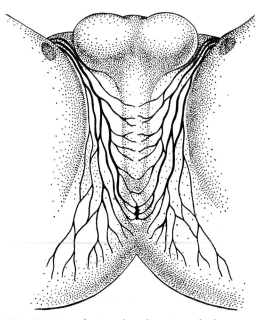

Fig. 413. Lymphatics of anal region, which sweep upward to end in inguinal lymph nodes.

Epidemiology

Carcinomas of the anus are relatively uncommon. When they are included in the same group with carcinomas of the rectum, they make up only about 5% of the entire group. The occurrence of carcinoma of the anus is highest in women (about 65%), whereas carcinoma of the rectum is most frequent in men (60% to 70%). There seems to be some difference in the sex distribution, depending on whether the tumor arises in the perineal or the rectal aspect of the anus.

Wolfe and Bussey[25] found thirty-six men among fifty patients with carcinoma of the anal margin, whereas the proportion of men and women was about the same in 102 patients with carcinoma of the anal canal. Gabriel[7] had previously reported a preponderance of women with carcinoma of the anal canal. The largest numbers of patients are found to be in the fifth and sixth decades of life, but there seems to be no difference in the age occurrence between the two sites nor with the occurrence of adenocarcinoma of the rectum.

Preexisting lesions of the anus have been reported in a great number of patients. These preexisting lesions include anal fistulas (Winkelman et al.[23]; Bretlau[1]), condylomas, and hemorrhoids, but although they might contribute to the development

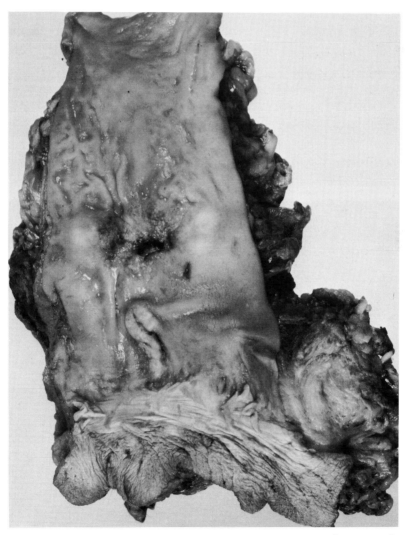

Fig. 414. Squamous carcinoma arising at mucocutaneous junction extending upward to form ulcer in rectum. (WU neg. 68-9208.)

of carcinoma, they cannot always be called precancerous lesions. In a series of sixty-four anal carcinomas in the female, eleven patients had multiple primary lesions in the anal region and genital tract, five of whom had had previous radiotherapy to the area (Cabrera et al.[2]).

Pathology

Gross pathology

Early carcinoma of the anus is often represented by a small nodule, superficially ulcerated, accompanied by evident secondary infection found within the anal margin. Carcinomas arising within the canal are often submucous and nonulcerated (Zimberg and Kay[26]), whereas those arising from the perianal skin are exophytic and spread considerably more in surface than do those on the anal margin. Internally, the tumor may extend beneath the intact rectal mucosa and become ulcerated farther above in the form of an apparently separate rectal tumor (Fig. 414). It is perhaps interesting to note that carcinomas of the rectum seldom show retrograde submucosal extension to the anus. When carcinoma of the rectum arises near the mucocutaneous junction, it not infrequently fungates and ulcerates at the anus (Fig. 415). Most carcinomas of the anus arise on the anterior or posterior anal quadrants. Very few are seen in the lateral quadrants. They invade the perianal skin, muscles of the sphincter, and ischiorectal fat rather frequently. Further extension may result in invasion of the levator ani, prostate, pelvic peritoneum, bladder, cervix, and broad ligaments.

Microscopic pathology

Most tumors of the anus are epidermoid carcinomas and, as a rule, are poorly differentiated. Some have the appearance of basosquamous carcinoma. Most undifferentiated anal tumors seem to arise high in the anal canal. Basal cell carcinomas arising from the anal skin have been reported (Lott and Alexander[12]). They appear predominantly in men (Wittoesch et al.[24]). Basaloid tumors characteristically arise in the upper anal canal (Pang and Morson[18]).

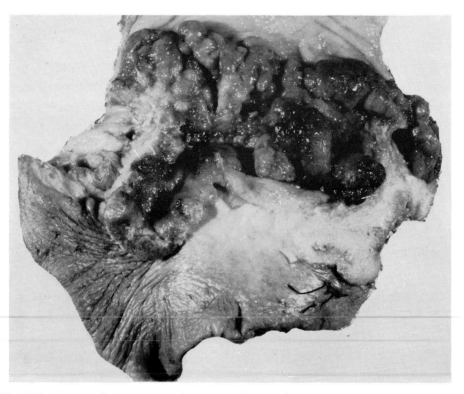

Fig. 415. Primary adenocarcinoma of rectum with typical burgeoning growth, retrograde invasion, and ulceration of anus.

It appears certain that some carcinomas presenting within the anus arise from the anal ducts. Epidermoid carcinomas involving the rectum independent of the anorectal junction may be explained by the cephalad course that anal ducts take beneath the rectal mucosa with origin from the transitional epithelium lining these ducts (Grinvalsky and Helwig[8]). Klotz et al.[10] collected 373 carcinomas of the anal canal which they designated as transitional cloacogenic carcinomas. Many of these had the same gross appearance as large bowel carcinoma, but a smaller group presented no intraluminal lesion.

Metastatic spread

Tumors that develop within the anal canal metastasize via the lymphatics of the rectum to the perirectal and also to the inguinal nodes, whereas carcinomas of the perineal aspect of the anus metastasize more frequently to the inguinal regions. Stearns[22] studied seventy-four cases of epidermoid carcinoma of the anal region and found the proportion of lymph node involvement to be 47% in the pelvic lymph nodes, 47% in the inguinal nodes, and 23% in the mesenteric nodes. Blood-borne

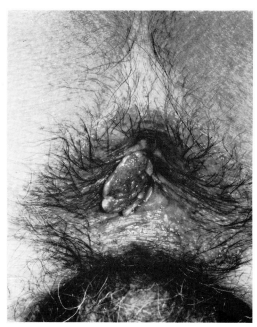

Fig. 416. Early carcinoma of anus. (Courtesy Dr. M. Greenberg, Milwaukee, Wis.)

metastases do occur in the liver and lungs (Kuehn et al.[11]).

Clinical evolution

Carcinoma of the anus develops unobtrusively and is usually not discovered until a year or eighteen months after onset. One of the first symptoms observed is *pruritus*, which may be associated with most of the benign conditions of the anus (condyloma, fissures, leukoplakia). As the tumor grows in size, *tenesmus*, not relieved by evacuation, may appear. *Pain* and a heavy sensation in the lower rectum, not relieved by defecation, may become increasingly noticeable, and there may be small repeated rectal hemorrhages (Sawyers et al.[21]). Incontinence is frequently observed.

Common constitutional symptoms such as fever, weight loss, anemia, and asthenia are usually absent unless the lesion is far advanced and is associated with considerable infection or distant metastases. The tumor will present itself in the form of an ulcerating lesion with raised, greatly indurated edges (Fig. 416) or, on the contrary, in the form of an exophytic, rather soft, papillary growth extending both on the perineal and rectal aspects of the anus and obstructing the lumen. Often, inguinal lymph nodes will be enlarged only because of secondary infection, but their metastatic involvement is not infrequent.

Diagnosis
Clinical examination

In most cases of carcinoma of the anus, the clinical findings are such that the diagnosis may be made on clinical inspection. However, biopsy will be necessary to differentiate an epidermoid carcinoma of the anus from an adenocarcinoma of the rectum that has invaded the anus. An early submucous lesion may be detected only by palpation. Moreover, examination should include exploration of the rectal ampulla by endoscopy whenever possible in order to establish the upper limits of the tumor. There is, of course, no possibility of detecting internal metastases. Thorough inguinal palpation should always be done, however, for involvement in that region may be discovered. Aspiration biopsy of the inguinal lymph nodes may be useful in resolving uncertainties in diagnosis.

Gabriel[7] divided carcinomas of the anus into two groups: carcinomas of the *anal margin* and carcinomas of the *anal canal*. Morson[15] further defined as anal canal tumors all those lying entirely above, mainly above, or astride the line of the anal canal valves, whereas those lying mainly below or entirely below that line were regarded as marginal tumors.

On occasion, biopsy of the anal region may reveal changes in the epithelium that can be interpreted as *carcinoma in situ*. At times, such changes are an incidental finding in hemorrhoidectomy specimens. We have seen three such cases, and in all three, invasive carcinoma developed within a period of four years, necessitating abdominoperineal resection.

Differential diagnosis

Melanocarcinomas arising in the region of the anus are rare. About 190 cases have been reported (Mason and Helwig[13]). They arise from the anorectal junction and are often polypoid in character (Chalier and Bonnet[3]). Junctional change may be present at the anal-squamous mucosa. These tumors can masquerade as thrombosed hemorrhoids. No matter how radical the treatment, practically no patient is cured (Quan et al.[17]; Morson and Volkstadt[16]).

Hemorrhoids that have become thrombosed and indurated may offer difficulty in differential diagnosis, but they are rarely ulcerated. *Tuberculous ulcers* are shallow, present soft borders, and may be associated with fistulas. They occur most often in young patients who have evidence of tuberculosis elsewhere. *Condyloma acuminatum*, which is probably of viral origin, may grow very large about the anus, is rather soft, and microscopically shows localized papillary overgrowth but without invasion of underlying tissue.

The *lymphogranuloma venereum* may also offer some difficulty in differentiation clinically, but this most often occurs in young blacks in the United States who present a positive Frei test. In every case, a biopsy should be done in order to eliminate the possibility that an early carcinoma of the anus does exist, though masked by a preexisting chronic inflammatory lesion.

Treatment

Evaluation of therapy is difficult, for usually the number of cases reported is small, the treatment variable, and the follow-up short.

Surgery

The surgical treatment of carcinoma of the anus ranges from a simple conservative excision to an abdominoperineal resection sometimes associated with an inguinal dissection. From the standpoint of surgery, the relative position of the tumor in respect to the dentate line is a useful reference. *Marginal anal tumors* arising below the canal are often well delimited and differentiated and can be treated by local excision (Hohm and Jackman[9]). In contrast, carcinomas of the *anal canal* proper may invade the sphincter muscles and regional lymph nodes and may have to

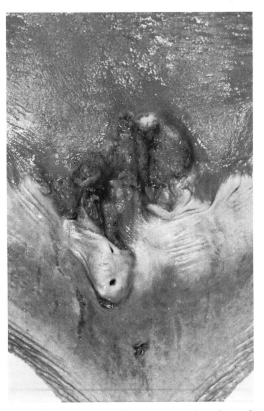

Fig. 417. Squamous cell carcinoma of anal canal. Tumor is arising from epithelium entirely above level of anal valves. (From Morson, B. C.: The pathology and results of treatment of squamous cell carcinoma of the anus and anal canal, Proc. Roy. Soc. Med. **53:**416-420, 1960.)

be treated by an abdominoperineal resection (Fig. 417). Because of their lateral invasive spread, *transitional cloacogenic carcinomas* must be treated by an abdominoperineal resection with particular attention to be paid to the adequate excision of the primary tumor (Klotz et al.[10]). However, an abdominoperineal resection does not resect the hemorrhoidal, obturator, iliac, or inguinal lymph nodes that may often be involved. A complete extirpation of these nodes requires an additional abdominal lymphadenectomy that has not been found justified (Wolfe and Bussey[25]). Whereas an inguinal dissection is indicated in all suspected cases of inguinal metastases, we do not feel that there is justification for a *prophylactic* inguinal dissection in any case. Similarly, confirmation of metastases in one groin does not justify a bilateral inguinal dissection. In a series of forty-one patients treated by abdominoperineal resection, only three, among those whose primary lesion was controlled, subsequently developed inguinal metastases. These three patients had a therapeutic inguinal dissection and were all controlled. In another nine patients in whom a prophylactic inguinal dissection was done, no metastases were found (Dillard et al.[4]).

Radiotherapy

Early attempts to treat anal carcinomas by radiotherapy were mostly in the form of interstitial curietherapy or surface applications of radium with the help of specially made molds (Meland[14]). Curietherapy offers the advantage of possible control without permanent colostomy. Significantly, however, in a series of eighteen patients who were cured of carcinoma of the anal canal by means of curietherapy, seven subsequently needed a colostomy (Roux-Berger and Ennuyer[20]). Since lymphatic spread toward the pelvis and the abdomen is uncommon and prognosis depends greatly on the surgical control of inguinal metastases, a conservative approach is justifiable for the treatment of the primary lesion. The trend has been away from radiumtherapy and very low voltage contact roentgentherapy toward well-filtered, higher voltage, fractionated roentgentherapy. Radiotherapy does not seem

to have many partisans mainly because of its duration and epidermal reactions. These are, as a general rule, rather radiosensitive epidermoid carcinomas that, like other such tumors, should benefit by radiotherapy, but the great radiosensitivity of the moist skin of the area requires protraction of the treatment to avoid untoward effects.

Supervoltage or cobalt[60] irradiation does permit a more homogeneous distribution of radiations throughout the anal and ischiorectal regions and diminishes the superficial reactions. Conservative treatment of the primary lesion does not preclude a prophylactic or a therapeutic inguinal dissection, but it does eliminate the possibility of early radical excision of mesenteric nodes. Thus, radiotherapy in any form should be limited to early differentiated, not too extensive, or deep lesions.

Indications

Following is a summary of indications for either surgery or roentgentherapy.

Group I—tumors restricted to anal margin. These tumors are usually well differentiated and the chances of their having lymph node metastases are remote. Adequate local excision is the indicated treatment. These lesions also respond well to irradiation. If such a lesion is poorly differentiated, then abdominoperineal resection must be done because of the considerable risk of mesenteric lymph node metastases.

Group II—tumors of anal canal. In these tumors, an abdominoperineal resection gives the patient the best chance of cure. If the inguinal lymph nodes are not palpable, we do not believe that there is good evidence to do a prophylactic dissection. If, on follow-up, nodes on one side become enlarged, a unilateral therapeutic dissection should be done.

Group III—extensive, inoperable tumors. These lesions, because of obstruction, may require colostomy and relief of symptoms by means of roentgentherapy.

Prognosis

The prognosis of epidermoid carcinoma of the anus depends upon the location of the tumor and its microscopic differentiation. Well-differentiated tumors of the anal margin do well. If the tumor of the anal margin is poorly differentiated or if the tumor is arising from the anal canal, a fair percentage of the patients will be salvaged by abdominoperineal resection even if the mesenteric lymph nodes are involved.

Wolfe and Bussey[25] reported on forty-nine patients with inguinal metastases in whom twenty-eight inguinal dissections were done: seven of eighteen patients with carcinomas of the anal canal and two of nine patients with carcinomas of the anal margin were living and well after five years. In seventy-nine cases of epidermoid carcinoma of the anus treated at Barnes Hospital in St. Louis and Ellis Fischel State Cancer Hospital in Columbia, Mo., during the years 1940 to 1957, there was an overall survival of 39%. Gabriel[7] reported eighty-seven cases of carcinoma of the anal canal. In the period 1941 to 1954, the five-year survival for fifty-six patients was 51%. In the same time period, there were twenty-eight patients with carcinoma of the anus with seventeen five-year survivals.

Roux-Berger and Ennuyer[20] reported the results of radiotherapy at the Radium Institute of the University of Paris (1921 to 1940). Of fifty-one patients treated for carcinoma of the anal canal, eighteen (34%) lived five years or more without recurrence or metastases. The results were in definite relationship to the extent of the lesion. Six additional patients with carcinoma of the anal margin yielded three five-year survivals. Fajbisowicz et al.[5] reported on fifty-five patients with carcinoma of the anal canal, without previous treatment, irradiated with cobalt[60] at the Institut Gustave-Roussy of France, with nineteen (35%) living and well after a minimum of three years.

REFERENCES

1 Bretlau, P.: Carcinoma arising in anal fistula, Acta Chir. Scand. **133**:496-500, 1967.

2 Cabrera, A., Tsukada, Y., Pickren, J. W., Moore, R., and Bross, I. D. J.: Development of lower genital carcinomas in patients with anal carcinoma; a more than casual relationship, Cancer **19**:470-480, 1966.

3 Chalier, A., and Bonnet, P.: Les tumeurs mélaniques primitives du rectum, Rev. Chir. Paris **46**:914-957, 1912; **47**:64-103, 235-255, 372-391, 563-588, 1913.

4 Dillard, B. M., Spratt, J. S., Jr., Butcher, H.

R., Jr., and Ackerman, L. V.: Epidermoid cancer of anal margin and canal; review of 79 cases, Arch. Surg. (Chicago) **86**:727-777, 1963.

5 Fajbisowicz, S., Lalanne, C. M., Sarrazin, D., and Juillard, G.: La télécobalthérapie du cancer du canal anal à l'Institut Gustave-Roussy, Ann. Radiol. (Paris) **9**:825-832, 1966.

6 Gabriel, W. B.: Squamous-cell carcinoma of the anus and anal canal, Proc. Roy. Soc. Med. **34**:139-157, 1941.

7 Gabriel, W. B.: Discussion on squamous cell carcinoma of the anus and anal canal, Proc. Roy. Soc. Med. **53**:403-409, 1960.

8 Grinvalsky, H. T., and Helwig, E. B.: Carcinoma of the anorectal junction, Cancer **9**:480-488, 1956.

9 Hohm, W. H., and Jackman, R. J.: Anorectal squamous-cell carcinoma; conservative or radical treatment? J.A.M.A. **188**:241-244, 1964.

10 Klotz, R. G., Pamukcoglu, T., and Souilliard, D. H.: Transitional cloacogenic carcinoma of the anal canal; a clinicopathologic study of 373 cases, Cancer **20**:1727-1745, 1967 (extensive bibliography).

11 Kuehn, P. G., Beckett, R., Eisenberg, H., and Reed, J. F.: Hematogenous metastases from epidermoid carcinoma of the anal canal, Amer. J. Surg. **109**:445-449, 1965.

12 Lott, B. D., and Alexander, C. M.: Basal cell carcinoma of the anus, Ann. Surg. **130**:1101-1103, 1949.

13 Mason, J. K., and Helwig, E. B.: Ano-rectal melanoma, Cancer **19**:39-50, 1966 (extensive bibliography).

14 Meland, O. N.: Carcinoma of the anus, Amer. J. Roentgen. **57**:199-204, 1947.

15 Morson, B. C.: The pathology and results of treatment of squamous cell carcinoma of the anus and anal canal, Proc. Roy. Soc. Med. **53**:416-420, 1960.

16 Morson, B. C., and Volkstadt, H.: Malignant melanoma of the anal canal, J. Clin. Path. **16**:126-132, 1967.

17 Quan, S. H. Q., White, J. E., and Deddish, M. R.: Malignant melanoma of the anorectum, Dis. Colon Rectum **2**:275-283, 1959.

18 Pang, L. S., and Morson, B. C.: Basaloid carcinoma of the anal canal, J. Clin. Path. **20**:128-135, 1967.

19 Richards, J. C., Beahrs, O. H., and Woolner, L. B.: Squamous cell carcinoma of the anus, anal canal, and rectum in 109 patients, Surg. Gynec. Obstet. **114**:474-482, 1962.

20 Roux-Berger, J. L., and Ennuyer, A.: Carcinoma of the anal canal; statistics of the Foundation Curie, Paris, Amer. J. Roentgen. **60**:807-815, 1948.

21 Sawyers, J. L., Herrington, J. L., Jr., and Main, F. B.: Surgical considerations in the treatment of epidermoid carcinoma of the anus, Ann. Surg. **157**:817-824, 1963.

22 Stearns, M. W., Jr.: Epidermoid carcinoma of the anal region; inguinal metastases, Amer. J. Surg. **90**:727-733, 1955.

23 Winkelman, J., Grosfeld, J., and Bigelow, B.: Colloid carcinoma of anal-gland origin; report

of a case and review of the literature, Amer. J. Clin. Path. **42:**395-401, 1964.
24 Wittoesch, J. H., Woolner, L. B., and Jackman, R. J.: Basal cell epithelioma and basaloid lesions of the anus, Surg. Gynec. Obstet. **104:** 75-80, 1957.

25 Wolfe, H. R. I., and Bussey, H. J. R.: Squamous-cell carcinoma of the anus, Brit. J. Surg. **55:**295-301, 1968.
26 Zimberg, Y. H., and Kay, S.: Anorectal carcinomas of extramucosal origin, Ann. Surg. **145:**344-354, 1957.

Accessory organs

Salivary glands
Pancreas
Liver

Gallbladder
Extrahepatic ducts and
   periampullary region

Salivary glands

Anatomy

The *parotid gland,* so designated because of its relationship with the external auditory canal, is the largest of the major salivary glands. It has an irregular form and is found molded around the vertical branch of the mandible. Its borders are in relation to the external acoustic meatus, the sternocleidomastoid muscle, and the mandible. The deep portion of the gland occupies the retromandibular fossa. Its posterior surface is in relation to the sternocleidomastoid muscle, the mastoid process, the posterior belly of the digastric muscle, and the styloid process and muscles. The anterior surface is in relation to the masseter muscle, the mandibular ramus, and the internal pterygoid muscle. Frequently, the medial extremity of the gland extends beyond the styloid process and comes in relationship with the carotid sheath and the lateral pharyngeal recess. The entire gland is enclosed in an enveloping sheath of superficial cervical fascia which is attached to the external acoustic meatus, zygomatic process, and glenoid fossa. Anteriorly, this space is closed by the fused layers of fascia that cover the masseter muscle and join the buccopharyngeal fascia.

The secretion of the parotid gland is gathered through an abundant network of channels emptying into the canal of Stensen, which carries the saliva to the oral cavity. This canal originates in the substance of the gland, follows an upward direction to about 1.5 cm to 2 cm from the zygomatic arch, then turns forward and travels horizontally over the external surface of the masseter muscle, perforates it, and opens into the buccal mucosa.

The parotid gland contains in its substance the external carotid artery with its terminal branches, the posterior facial vein, and, lateral to these, the facial nerve and its pes anserinus (Fig. 418). The facial nerve emerges from the skull through the stylomastoid foramen and immediately enters the substance of the parotid gland. Within the gland the main trunk breaks into two divisions: temporocervical and the cervicofacial. The point of bifurcation of the facial nerve lies posteriorly and slightly medial to the ascending ramus of the mandible, two-thirds of the distance between the angle of the mandible and the condyloid process. Variations of facial nerve branching and anastomosis are common.

The *submaxillary gland* is about one-fourth the size of the parotid gland. It extends from the lower border of the mandible to the hyoid bone. It is also in relation to the posterior belly of the digastric, stylohyoid, and mylohyoid muscles. The secretion of the submaxillary gland is canalized by the canal of Wharton which, after traveling for 4 cm to 5 cm, opens on the anterior midline of the floor of the mouth.

The *sublingual gland,* which is 2 cm thick and 2 cm to 3 cm in length, is less than one-tenth the size of the parotid

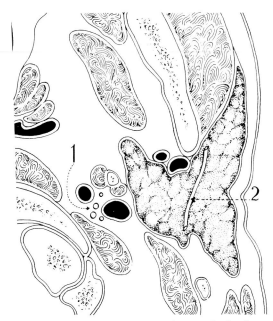

Fig. 418. Transverse section of parotid gland to illustrate its pharyngeal prolongation and close relationship to last four cranial nerves, **1**, and approximate level at which parotid gland is crossed by facial nerve, **2**.

gland. It is enclosed in a fascial covering and lies in the floor of the mouth immediately beneath the mucosa. The sublingual gland is in relation to the mandible laterally and to the duct of the submaxillary gland medially. It is also in relation to the mylohyoid, hyoglossus, and genioglossus muscles. Its secretion is canalized by a thin duct opening in the floor of the mouth next to, and sometimes into, the submaxillary duct.

Lymphatics. The salivary glands have a large interlobular network of lymphatics anastomosing in the form of plexuses and following the direction of the blood vessels and ducts. The lymphatics of the *parotid gland* end in the lymph nodes found within the substance of the gland and frequently also a collecting trunk of lymphatics follows a downward and forward direction and empties into one of the retrovascular submaxillary lymph nodes.

The lymphatics of the *submaxillary gland* gather into one or two trunks that are drained by one of the prevascular submaxillary lymph nodes. Some of the deep lymphatics of the submaxillary gland gather into a collecting trunk that follows the facial artery and ends in one of the subdigastric nodes of the anterior jugular chain.

The lymphatics of the *sublingual gland* are divided into those that are drained by submaxillary lymph nodes and those that follow in a posterior direction, have a long trajectory, and finally end in the deep nodes of the internal jugular chain between the digastric and the omohyoid muscles. Very rarely, the lymphatics of the sublingual gland may be emptied by submental lymph nodes (Rouvière[59]).

Epidemiology

Tumors of the major salivary glands are rare. In the states of New York and Connecticut, they constitute only 0.4% of all malignant tumors diagnosed. In the 1947 United States survey, the age-adjusted incidence rates per 100,000 population were 2.1 and 2.0 for male and female whites, with a 1.1 male:female ratio, and 2.5 and 2.6 for male and female nonwhites, with a 1.0 male:female ratio. One in four salivary gland tumors occurred in patients under 40 years of age. There seems to be an equal proportion of malignant tumors in both sexes, but there is a preponderance of women with mixed tumors. Of twenty-four salivary gland tumors found in children, seventeen were benign mixed tumors (Byars et al.[12]). It has often been claimed that these tumors are more frequent among the Africans and Asians (Marsden[44]) of tropical climates, but serious statistical studies have found no evidence for this claim (Edington and Sheiham[18]). The relative frequency of these, in relation to other tumors, has been found to be higher in Malays (Loke[41]) and in Eskimos (Wallace et al.[69]). In Egypt there seems to be a much higher ratio, 10:1, of parotid to submaxillary tumors, with a predominance in males (Gazayerli and Abdel-Aziz[28]), whereas in Uganda a higher than usual proportion of submaxillary tumors is found (Davies et al.[14]). The proportion of malignant tumors among all salivary gland tumors increases from the parotid to the submaxillary and sublingual; the total number of reported malignant tumors of the sublingual gland is thirty-seven (Rankow and Mignogna[53a]).

Pathology
Gross pathology

The major mucous and salivary gland tumors are, for the most part, found in salivary glands. They are also found in many other locations such as the buccal mucosa, base of the tongue, hard palate, soft palate, alveolar ridge, floor of the mouth, pharynx, sinuses, trachea, lip, and bronchi. Mixed tumors can arise from these areas that do not differ from those arising in the parotid or the submaxillary gland.

In a series of 573 tumors of the salivary glands observed at Washington University School of Medicine in St. Louis, there were 478 arising from the parotid gland, fifty-six from the submaxillary gland, and thirty-nine from other locations. There was a slightly higher proportion of benign tumors than malignant tumors in the parotid gland, whereas the opposite was true in the sub-maxillary gland (Table 42). In other reported series, these proportions vary because of obvious, although involuntary, preselection of material. The proportion of malignant tumors among those arising from the minor salivary glands has been found to be of the order of 50% to 85% (Bardwil et al.[8]).

The typical benign mixed tumor varies in size depending upon the duration of the disease. In exceptional cases, it may reach huge dimensions. It is firm, resilient, and at times cystic. Differences in consistency are due to connective tissue and cartilage content. On section, it has a definite connective tissue capsule, and the surface of the tumor not infrequently presents a variegated appearance. There may be myxoid areas, zones suggesting cartilage, cystic changes (Fig. 419, *B*), and gray zones of connective tissue proliferation. Small burgeoning nodules may extend out from the capsule, but they, too, are surrounded by a definite capsule. The tumor is usually attached to, and intimately associated with, the gland but portions of normal gland invariably remain for identification.

The malignant salivary gland tumor is usually much smaller than the benign variant. Its consistency depends on its cellularity and the amount of connective tissue. The tumors that are predominantly made up of connective tissue cut with increased

Table 42. Incidence of benign and malignant tumors of major salivary glands*†

Parotid gland		
Mixed tumors		322
Primary benign	254	
Recurrent benign (persistent)	49	
Malignant	19	
Carcinoma		82
Epidermoid	30	
Acinic cell adenocarcinoma	2	
Undifferentiated	25	
Mucoepidermoid	25	
Adenocarcinoma		35
Simple	12	
Papillary	3	
Adenoid cystic	20	
Papillary cystadenoma lymphomatosum (Warthin's tumor)		34
Unilateral	30	
Bilateral	4	
Oxyphil adenoma		4
Lipoma		1
Total in parotid gland		478
Submandibular gland		
Mixed tumors		31
Primary benign	25	
Recurrent benign (persistent)	5	
Malignant	1	
Carcinoma		12
Epidermoid	4	
Undifferentiated	6	
Mucoepidermoid	2	
Adenocarcinoma		12
Simple	1	
Adenoid cystic	11	
Papillary cystadenoma lymphomatosum (Warthin's tumor)		1
Total in submandibular gland		56
Other locations		
Mixed tumors		19
Primary benign	17	
Malignant	2	
Carcinoma		7
Undifferentiated	2	
Acinic cell adenocarcinoma	1	
Mucoepidermoid	4	
Adenocarcinoma		13
Simple	1	
Adenoid cystic	12	
Total in other locations		39
Grand total		573

*Surgical Pathology Laboratory, Washington University School of Medicine, St. Louis, Mo.
†From Ackerman, L. V.: Surgical pathology, ed. 4, St. Louis, 1968, The C. V. Mosby Co.

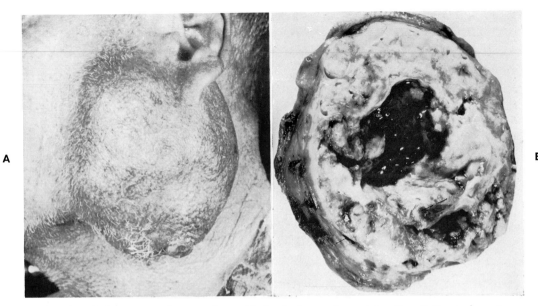

Fig. 419. A, Benign mixed tumor of parotid gland of several years' duration. **B,** Surgical specimen of same tumor presenting large area of central cystic degeneration. Note that tumor is enclosed in fairly well-defined capsule.

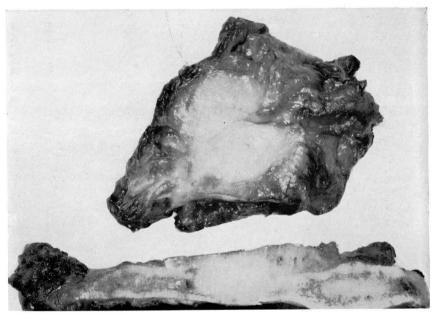

Fig. 420. Adenoid cystic carcinoma (cylindromatous type) of submaxillary gland of seven years' duration and with direct extension into mandible.

resistance and obliterate the normal architecture of the gland. They grow into the skin and insinuate themselves in the interstices of the surrounding tissue, where they speedily become fixed to bone. Those in the submaxillary area may invade the man-

dible and grow into the surrounding muscles (Fig. 420). Malignant tumors of the parotid gland may cause thrombosis of the external jugular vein and compression of the external carotid artery. The more cellular tumor is softer and cystic and may exist

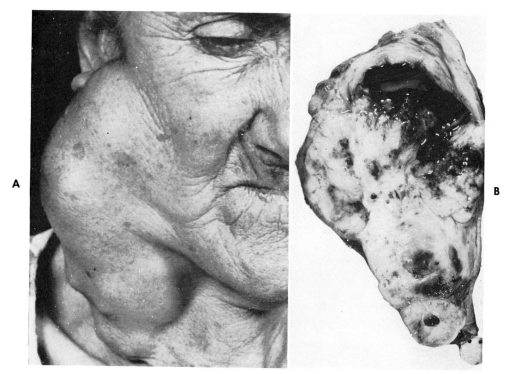

Fig. 421. A, Malignant mucoepidermoid type of tumor of parotid gland. Patient died with recurrence one year after operation. **B,** Grayish white and fairly homogeneous appearance showing mucinous changes in cross section of same tumor.

for a time within the substance of the parotid gland, but with increased growth it will ulcerate through the skin and form a voluminous mass that is ulcerating, vegetating, and foul smelling. It is prone to hemorrhage and spontaneous necrosis. It speedily invades the sternocleidomastoid, masseter, temporal, and pterygoid muscles. It is not infrequent for the temporomaxillary articulation to be invaded early. The superficial cervical plexus on the external surface of the sternocleidomastoid muscle can be surrounded and compressed. The malignant submaxillary gland tumors extend first to the soft tissue and the neighboring muscles, including the digastric, the mylohyoid, and even the sternocleidomastoid. The hypoglossal nerve and the superior branches of the superior cervical plexus may be surrounded. Extension along the internal prolongation of the submaxillary gland to the sublingual gland can occur.

The lowermost portion of the parotid gland lies anteriorly in contact with the posterosuperior aspect of the submaxillary gland. Because of this intimate relationship, the actual origin of some salivary gland tumors may remain in doubt. Tumors may also arise from separate glandular masses in the intramural and buccinator portions of the parotid duct (Eneroth et al.[19]). The mucoepidermoid carcinoma (Fig. 421), the adenocarcinoma, and the papillary carcinoma may all secrete mucin and, therefore, have a mucoid appearance. The rare primary lymphosarcomas are gray in color and highly cellular. When metastatic carcinoma is present in the lymph nodes of the parotid gland, often it is possible to diagnose its metastatic nature through identification of lymph node remnants.

Microscopic pathology

The classification of salivary gland tumors is confusing. The usual neoplasm of the salivary gland is a tumor in which the benign variant is less benign than the usual benign tumor and the malignant variant is less malignant than the usual malignant tumor. There are also numerous appellations appended to the same type of tumor, which makes the classification difficult even for a pathologist. It is therefore thought worthwhile to attempt a simple tentative classification of the salivary gland tumors:

1 Benign tumors
    a Hemangioma
    b Lipoma
    c Neurilemoma
    d Oxyphil adenoma (oncocytoma)
    e Papillary cystadenoma lymphomatosum (Warthin's tumor)
2 Mixed tumor (pleomorphic adenoma)
    a Malignant change in mixed tumors
3 Malignant tumors
    a Mucoepidermoid carcinoma
    b Adenoid cystic carcinoma (cylindroma type)
    c Papillary adenocarcinoma
    d Epidermoid carcinoma
    e Carcinoma—acinic cell
    f Carcinoma—unclassified
    g Malignant lymphoma
    h Metastatic carcinoma

Benign tumors. The *hemangioma* is found most frequently in the parotid region, probably rarely arises from the salivary gland itself, and undoubtedly comes from subcutaneous blood vessels. It is the most common tumor found in infants (Kauffman and Stout[35]). The *lymphangioma* is rarely observed.

Lipomas arise from fatty tissue in the region of the parotid gland and do not differ from lipomas found elsewhere. *Neurilemomas* arising from the facial nerve may form small encapsulated tumors within the parotid gland (Roos et al.[58]).

Oxyphil adenomas (oncocytomas) are rare. They seem to develop from the epithelium of the excretory ducts and also from the acini (Meza-Chávez[45]). They are histogenetically related to the *cystadenoma lymphomatosum* (Warthin's tumor), which rarely arises from the submaxillary gland. Thompson and Bryant[68] believe that these tumors arise from parotid duct epithelium and that the accumulation of lymphoid tissue is a secondary phenomenon. Microscopically, cystadenomas have a characteristic appearance that can be recognized easily. They are composed of two elements, lymphoid and epithelial, intimately asso-

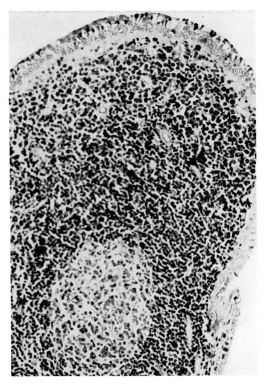

Fig. 422. Papillary cystadenoma lymphomatosum demonstrating intimate association of lymphoid and epithelial elements. (Low-power enlargement.)

ciated (Fig. 422). These papillary epithelial structures are embedded in lymphoid stroma that may contain germinal centers. The projections are lined by tall, nonciliated, eosinophilic epithelium. The epithelium may be exactly like that seen in the oxyphil adenoma. An extremely rare benign neoplasm that we have designated sebaceous lymphadenoma may occur. This tumor may be confused microscopically with mucoepidermoid carcinoma (McGavran et al.[43]).

Mixed tumors. The true mixed tumors are complex in nature, but majority opinion holds that they are entirely epithelial in origin. Favata[23] was able to grow these tumors in tissue culture. His findings support the theory of their epithelial origin. Ahlbom[2] believed that they arose from the epithelium of adult excretory ducts and acini and perhaps also from detached embryonal epithelial anlage. The typical mixed tumors are the most common tumors of the salivary glands, and names given to them have depended often upon

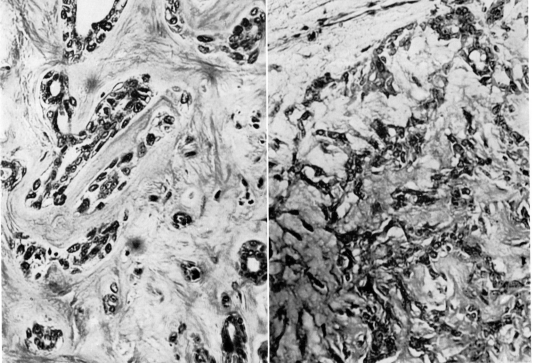

the predominant tissue, so that designations such as chondroma, fibroepithelioma, fibromyxoma, etc. have been used. Duct-like structures, stroma, and cartilage-like material are usually present, but true hyaline cartilage is infrequently found (Figs. 423 to 425), and rarely is bone formation encountered. Epithelium in the ducts may be mucin-secreting, but more frequently there is mucoid degeneration of the stroma. Mixed tumors contain two types of mucus, an epithelial type in the glandular structures and a mesenchymal type in the myxomatous areas, which can be identified by different staining reactions (Grishman[32]; Azzopardi and Smith[4]). The presence of cartilage indicates slow growth. It is rarely found in malignant tumors (Ahlbom[2]).

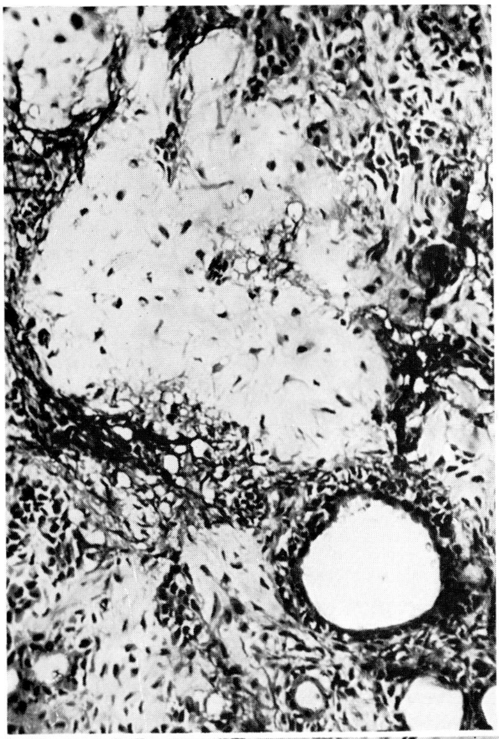

Fig. 423. Typical mixed tumor of salivary glands presenting cartilage, loose fibrous tissue, and glands. (Moderate enlargement.)

424

425

Fig. 424. Typical mixed tumor with well-differentiated glands in dense hyalinized stroma. (Moderate enlargement.)

Fig. 425. Recurrent typical mixed tumor. This resembled primary tumor exactly. (Moderate enlargement.)

These tumors frequently show small nests of cells within the capsule, and frequently also form satellite nodules in the periphery of the main mass.

Malignant tumors. *Mucoepidermoid carcinomas* described by Foote and Becker[24] make up about 25% of the malignant tumors. They are reported to constitute a majority of salivary gland tumors encountered in Jamaica (Gore et al.[30]). They are found most frequently in the parotid gland and next in the palate (Bhasker and Bernier[10]). They arise from duct epithelium and are composed of two elements, squamous cells and mucin-producing cells (Fig. 426) (Gray et al.[31]). The mucin causes cystic areas to develop, and the release of keratin into the interstitial tissue causes fibrosis and chronic inflammation. Usually this neoplasm does not grow to a large size. Microscopically it may show variations from an apparently benign to a highly malignant tumor. It is probably dangerous to underestimate its potentiality to invade, metastasize, and recur.

The *adenoid cystic carcinoma*, often designated as *cylindroma* or *basal cell carcinoma*, makes up for another 25% of the malignant salivary gland tumors. It has glandlike structures superficially resembling the cystic type of basal cell carcinoma and often containing small amounts of mucus within its center (Fig. 427). It is often associated with hyaline stroma but never with cartilage. There is frequent neural space involvement (Quattlebaum et al.[53]) that probably accounts for the high proportion of facial paralyses that occurs (Fig. 428). This tumor is much more malignant than is generally suspected. We believe that, regardless of uniform cellularity which suggests benignity, this neoplasm is always malignant and capable of producing distant metastases (Hertig[33]).

The other malignant epithelial neoplasms of the salivary glands constitute a poorly understood group. There are relatively rare

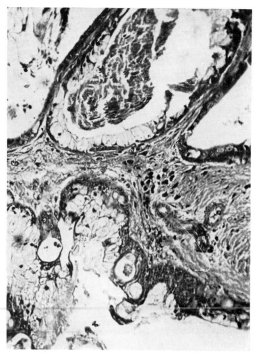

Fig. 426. Malignant mucoepidermoid tumor of salivary gland presenting squamous elements and cells producing mucin. (Moderate enlargement.)

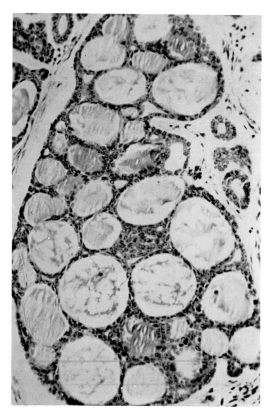

Fig. 427. Adenoid cystic carcinoma (cylindromatous type) of salivary gland with overproduction of mucin. Note resemblance to cystic type basal cell carcinoma.

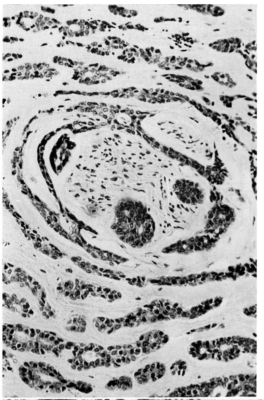

papillary adenocarcinomas that may produce mucin, often grow to rather large size, and have a slow rate of growth. The *epidermoid carcinoma* arising from duct epithelium is usually a highly malignant neoplasm (Fig. 429). Perhaps in some instances it represents, in fact, an overgrowth of squamous carcinoma in a mucoepidermoid carcinoma. In other instances, these tumors represent metastatic carcinoma. *Acinic cell carcinoma* is a rare, slowly growing neoplasm occurring almost exclusively in the parotid gland (Abrams et al.[1]). It usually appears in patients in the fourth to sixth decade and may metastasize to regional lymph nodes (Godwin et al.[29]). This tumor arises from acinar cells (Echevarria[17]) (Fig. 431).

Fig. 428. Perineural space invasion by adenocarcinoma (cylindromatous type) of salivary gland. (Moderate enlargement.)

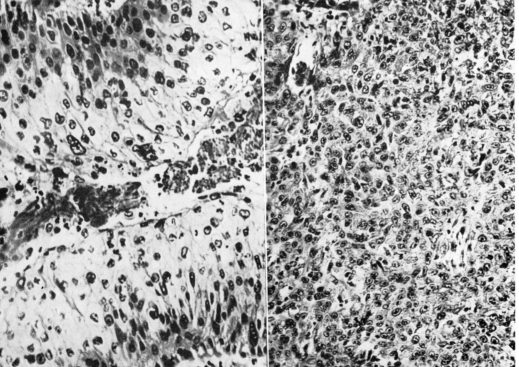

429

430

Fig. 429. Relatively undifferentiated epidermoid carcinoma of salivary gland. (High-power enlargement.)

Fig. 430. Very undifferentiated carcinoma of salivary gland. This tumor could easily be mistaken for sarcoma. (High-power enlargement.)

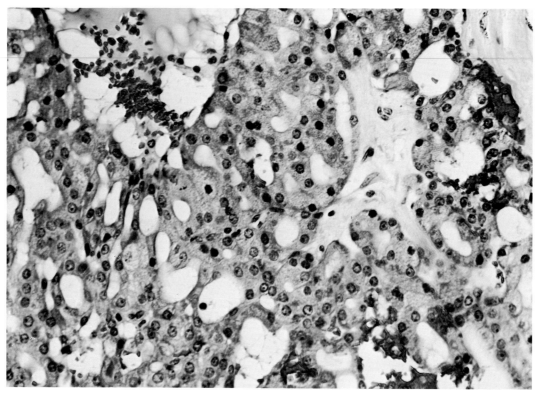

Fig. 431. Classic pattern of well-differentiated acinic cell cancer. This was recurrent after surgery several years previously. (×300; WU neg. 68-141A.)

There remains a group of highly undifferentiated *unclassifiable carcinomas* that metastasize rapidly. We have seen a few apparent primary *lymphosarcomas* arising from the parotid gland. They grow slowly, and their microscopic diagnosis may be difficult. Sarcomas of the parotid gland are extremely infrequent. Most reported sarcomas of the salivary glands are actually highly malignant tumors of epithelial origin (Fig. 430).

Metastatic spread

Metastases from malignant tumors of the salivary glands occur more frequently than is generally believed. The incidence of reported metastases depends on the adequacy of the initial treatment and the length of the follow-up. Of eighty-two patients with malignant tumors reported by Ahlbom,[2] sixteen (20%) had metastases on admission, but the proportion of metastases rose later to 33%. Of forty-four patients who were followed from initial symptom to necropsy, twenty-four (50%) had lymph node metastases. Metastases usually occur in the lymph nodes of the parotid, the submaxillary, the cervical, and the supraclavicular regions and sometimes in the mediastinum. The mucoepidermoid carcinomas, the adenocarcinomas, and the very undifferentiated carcinomas are, in general, prone to the production of metastases.

Metastases to the lungs occur with a certain number of malignant tumors of the salivary glands. They are found in extensive and terminal undifferentiated malignant tumors, and they are a rather common occurrence in the group of tumors usually diagnosed as cylindromas and pseudoadenomatous basal cell carcinomas (Lampe and Zatzkin[38]). Bone metastases have also been found, particularly in the skull, mandible, ribs, vertebrae, and pelvis (Wilner[71]). A mixed tumor that metastasized to the lungs and preserved its benign microscopic appearance in the metastatic lesions has been reported (Foote and Frazell[25]).

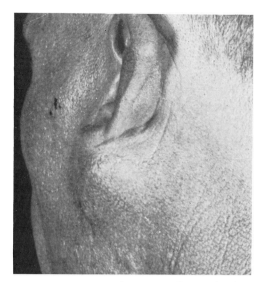

Fig. 432. Typical small benign salivary gland tumor of parotid gland with eversion of lobule of ear.

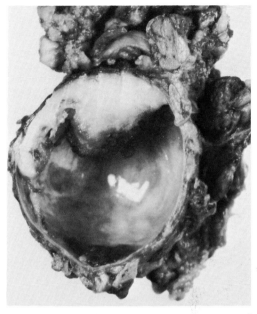

Fig. 433. Cystic benign mixed tumor of parotid gland. (WU neg. 67-7613.)

Clinical evolution

The benign mixed tumors of the salivary glands show variable speeds of growth, but their usual duration before diagnosis is invariably long (average, seven years). The first symptom in practically all patients is a small, *painless* lump that almost imperceptibly increases in size. If it is in the region of the submaxillary gland, it is often dismissed as an inflammatory lesion of a regional lymph node. However, with increase in size, there are unsightly facial asymmetry and pain. Tumors of the region of the parotid gland usually extend downward and appear as lobulated masses on the lateral surface of the neck. If there is retroauricular involvement of the parotid gland by tumor (Fig. 432), there may be eversion of the lobe of the ear. The tumor may become cystic (Fig. 433).

The benign mixed tumor, whether it arises from the parotid or the submaxillary gland, is only rarely the cause of death. The huge tumors of the parotid region with pharyngeal extension cause difficulty in mastication and deglutition. Benign mixed tumors treated inadequately, either by irradiation or by surgery, have been reported to become malignant after numerous recurrences. Such a history, however, may hide an initially malignant tumor that was not morphologically recognized.

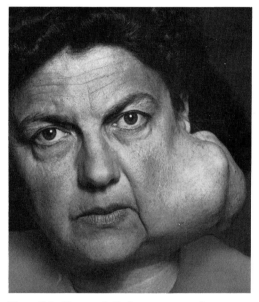

Fig. 434. Tumor had been present for twenty years and had grown slowly until three months prior to patient's admission to hospital. After that, growth was rapid. On histologic study, undifferentiated carcinoma was superimposed on mixed tumor. Treatment was total parotidectomy. Patient died fifteen months later of widespread metastases. (From Beahrs, O. H., et al.: Carcinomatous transformation of mixed tumors of the parotid gland, Arch. Surg. [Chicago] **75:**605-614, 1957.)

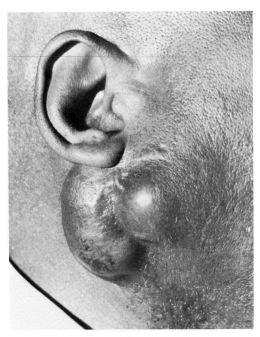

Fig. 435. Large adenoid cystic carcinoma incorrectly diagnosed pathologically, treated inadequately by surgery, and then irradiated. This evolution occurred over ten-year period and patient died from brain and pulmonary metastases shortly after this photograph was taken.

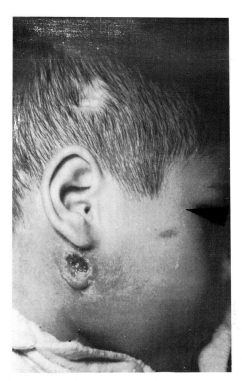

Fig. 436. Child with mucoepidermoid carcinoma treated by radical surgical excision. (Courtesy Dr. Humberto Torloni, São Paulo, Brazil.)

The malignant tumor of the salivary gland grows much more rapidly than the benign tumor (Fig. 434). However, the adenoid cystic carcinoma may also evolve over a number of years (Fig. 435). Evolution before examination is usually measured in months rather than in years. The first sign of carcinoma of the parotid gland may be the presence of a small nodule or a zone of irregular induration located just in front of the tragus or slightly below or above the angle of the mandible (Fig. 436). The skin becomes adherent to the subjacent tumor and becomes depressed. With involvement of deep structures and fixation, *pain* appears. Rarely, the tumors in the region of the parotid gland may invade the base of the skull to cause intractable pain and paralyses of various cranial nerves. The tumor producing large amounts of connective tissue quickly causes retraction of the skin and fixation of deep structures with increasing pain, and it seldom ulcerates. Infiltration of the skin often forms a veritable "collar of iron" that may immobilize the head in an attitude of torticollis. The softer tumors grow even more rapidly, tend to cause facial paralysis earlier, and are frequently accompanied by severe pain. They may erupt quickly through the skin, ulcerate, hemorrhage, and produce foul discharge.

If a malignant tumor of the parotid gland arises from the masseteric prolongation, the tumor may present itself as a lesion of the cheek, and if it infiltrates the masseter or the pterygoid muscles or involves the articulation of the temporomaxillary region, trismus may appear. It also may extend from this location in a retrograde fashion to involve the facial nerve and to be associated with facial paralysis and typical metastatic adenopathy. The tumor may also arise in the pharyngeal prolongation, and thus the tumor will bulge into the pharynx. The first symptom may be profound pain radiating to the neck and ear, and often dysphagia, dysphonia, and dyspnea occur.

The presence or absence of partial or complete *paralysis* of the facial nerve is an important factor that must be noted carefully in all tumors of the parotid gland. We have not seen a benign mixed tumor cause paralysis by compression of the nerve. It is present in about one-third of the patients with malignant tumors but may not occur in those with carcinomas originating deep within the gland or in its inferior pole. The paralysis is peripheral in type. Early paralysis may be localized to only one of the two branches (temporocervical and cervicofacial), but as the tumor grows, the paralysis becomes complete. It is usually due to perineural space involvement, but in certain instances, compression alone may cause these changes. If a malignant tumor of the parotid gland arises in the retroparotidian space, a syndrome characterized by paralyses of the ninth, tenth, eleventh, twelfth, and sympathetic nerves may appear. The symptoms and signs due to this involvement in the retroparotidian space have been dealt with in the discussion on cancer of the nasopharynx. It is also not rare to find cutaneous anesthesia in the juxtaparotid region due to the destruction of superficial cutaneous nerve filaments. Malignant submaxillary gland tumors can invade the periosteum or break into the cavity of the mandible, where they may compress or invade the dental nerve and cause pain referred along the jaw to the region of the ear and temple.

The malignant tumor of the salivary gland, in its rapid growth and extension, may metastasize to the regional lymph nodes and infrequently to lungs, bones, and other distant organs. Not infrequently, bronchopneumonia may occur as a terminal event. The extensive pulmonary metastases of adenoid cystic carcinomas, or so-called cylindromas, may develop silently for a number of years without affecting the apparent well-being of the patient (Lampe and Zatzkin[38]). Usually, however, death is caused by a number of factors. The tumor may ulcerate through the surface and become infected. This, in turn, results in secondary anemia, sepsis, and subsequent loss of weight. If the tumor arises in the region of the parotid gland, it may ulcerate through the external jugular vein and, on rare occasions, may even ulcerate into the external carotid artery and cause hemorrhages.

Diagnosis
Clinical examination

The clinical diagnosis of *benign salivary gland tumors* is not difficult. They are of variable consistency but usually firm, somewhat resilient and bosselated, not attached to the skin or underlying structures, and nontender to palpation.

At times, it may be difficult to determine whether the tumor arises within the anteroinferior portion of the parotid gland or in the submaxillary gland. This is of practical importance, for it may determine whether operation will necessitate excision of portions of the facial nerve. If this differentiation is kept in mind, the point of origin is usually resolved at the time of operation. Bimanual palpation with one finger in the mouth and the free hand on the external surface of the tumor also may be helpful in establishing the point of origin. The buccal prolongation of the parotid gland is behind and above the orifice of the parotid duct, and, by buccal palpation, association with the anterior border of the parotid gland can easily be demonstrated. Parotid tumors may present in the cervical region and be mistaken for adenopathy. Bimanual palpation is also helpful with tumors of the submaxillary gland to determine whether or not there is extension toward the duct and oral cavity.

Malignant salivary gland tumors may vary considerably in their clinical manifestations, which makes the diagnosis difficult. A small, soft, inconspicuous malignant tumor of the parotid gland may have its clinical onset with facial paralysis. The first sign of the tumor may be a cervical adenopathy. The tumor may cause the impression of a chronic inflammatory lesion of the gland or of a lymph node. Later in its development, the diagnosis may become evident.

It is often obvious that a primary tumor of the salivary glands exists, but it may be difficult to determine whether it is a benign or a malignant tumor. This determination is extremely important, particularly when the tumor arises in the parotid gland, for the treatment of a benign tumor is much more conservative than that of a malignant tumor. Some of the main differences between benign and malignant tumors are indicated in Table 43. It is true

Table 43. Differentiation between benign and malignant salivary gland tumors

	Benign	*Malignant*
Clinical history		
Rate of growth	Slow (years)	Rapid (months)
Sex	More frequent in females	No essential difference
Age	Peak before 40 years	Peak about 50 years
Pain	Usually absent	Invariably present
Physical examination		
Fixation	Freely movable	Often fixed to skin, deep structures, bone
Facial nerve paralysis (parotid tumors)	Practically never	Common (about 33%)
Consistency	Firm, cystic, nodular	May be stony hard
Gross pathology	Well-circumscribed capsule; often shows cartilage	No capsule; invasion of bone and contiguous tissue
Metastases	Never	Rather frequent (lymph nodes, lungs, bone)

that there are some cases in which it is impossible to differentiate, and the decision must rely on a biopsy.

A benign mixed tumor may become malignant, infiltrate, and metastasize. The patient with a malignant mixed tumor is, on the average, ten years older than the one with a benign lesion (Beahrs et al.[9]). The patients usually have had a slow-growing tumor for years which suddenly grows very rapidly and causes pain and facial paralysis. In a group of 353 mixed tumors studied at Washington University, twenty apparently underwent malignant transformation. Thomas and Coppola[67] collected forty-three cases with metastases, some of them to bone.

Roentgenologic examination

If the tumor is large and there is any suspicion of involvement of contiguous bony structures, the roentgenologic examination may reveal destructive processes in the base of the skull, zygoma, or mandible. Sialography may be useful as a roentgenologic procedure to demonstrate the presence or absence of distortion or involvement of the parotid salivary gland. After injection of the opaque material in the salivary duct, the roentgenograms usually show a well-demarcated and uniform glandular shadow with normal or limited visualization of ducts but no irregularities. In other instances, there is no definite demarcation between the tumor and the glandular shadow and the ducts are irregular in contour (Kimm et al.[36]). These

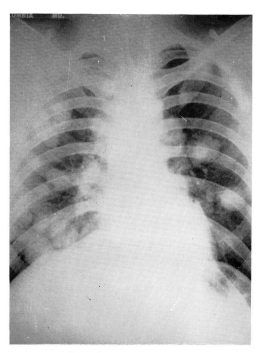

Fig. 437. Bilateral extensive spherical pulmonary metastasis from adenoid cystic carcinoma (cylindromatous type) of parotid gland. There were no symptoms of lung involvement.

findings must be interpreted in the light of clinical manifestations of the tumor.

A routine roentgenogram of the chest should be taken in all patients with salivary gland tumors. The pulmonary metastases of the adenoid cystic carcinomas are characteristically spherical and numerous. They may develop slowly and symptomlessly for years (Fig. 437). Bone metastases are usually osteolytic.

Biopsy

In well-delimited lesions of the salivary glands, it is best to attempt a surgical excision rather than a biopsy. Frozen sections may help in deciding on the radicality of the surgical procedure. In other instances, an incisional biopsy may be justified as a preliminary step to the therapeutic decision. Needle biopsies are not recommended for operable cases, for they may lead to erroneous diagnoses. However, needle biopsies are justified in the presence of advanced tumors and their metastatic adenopathies prior to the institution of radiotherapy.

Differential diagnosis

Acute inflammations of the parotid gland can be mistaken for tumor. However, in the presence of inflammation, the gland usually is diffusely involved and tender, and there is frequently tenderness of the other parotid salivary gland. The submaxillary gland may also be involved by inflammatory processes, and it is not too infrequent to find either gland presenting secondary changes due to the presence of *stones* within its main ducts. With these calculi there are increase in size and considerable induration of the entire gland. Frequently, there are paroxysms of pain that coincide with eating. These painful crises are usually accompanied by very rapid swelling of the gland and tend to recur at shorter and shorter time intervals. Between meals, the pain ceases. The calculus can often be felt by careful bimanual examination, or it may be seen on roentgenographic examination. It may be impossible to canalize the excretory salivary canal.

When an inflammatory process of the salivary glands is suspected, pressure along the duct may force the drainage of mucopurulent fluid through the duct opening. Chronic inflammation involving particularly the parotid salivary gland, with the formation of microliths and obstruction of the ducts, can result in secondary squamous metaplasia and may be incorrectly diagnosed microscopically as mucoepidermoid carcinoma.

Actinomycosis is an extreme rarity that can be diagnosed either by examination of the secretion in the ulceration or by biopsy. There is no facial paralysis, the lymph nodes are not often enlarged, and there may be some trismus. If fistulas exist, they exude yellowish pus. In both the fistulas and the ulcerations, typical sulfur granules may be observed on the smear.

Mikulicz's disease is a poorly understood entity in which there is symmetrical bilateral swelling with frequent simultaneous involvement of the parotid, submaxillary, and sublingual glands and, in addition, of the palatine, labial, and lacrimal glands. The disease progresses slowly and does not produce facial paralysis. It is certainly related to Sjögren's syndrome. In Sjögren's syndrome there are enlargement of salivary glands and conjunctivitis associated, at times, with rheumatoid arthritis (Bloch et al.[11]). The glands show increased lymphoid tissue and intraductal proliferation of epithelial and myoepithelial elements (Morgan and Raven[48]). Mikulicz's disease may be confused with papillary cystadenoma lymphomatosum.

Boeck's sarcoid may involve the parotid gland, but usually the involvement is bilateral, and there may be other signs of the disease. *Hypertrophy of the masseter muscle* may be taken for a parotid tumor.

Epidermoid *inclusion cysts* and *branchial cleft cysts* have been confused with tumors of the parotid gland. Advanced *carcinomas of the skin* with ulceration into the region of the parotid may be taken for malignant tumors of the gland.

Metastatic lesions in the lymph nodes in and around the salivary glands may offer difficulties in differential diagnosis. Carcinomas arising in the skin (Ridenhour and Spratt[57]) of the face and scalp, melanomas of the skin in these areas or from the oral cavity, pharynx, and orbit, and other tumors arising in distant organs may metastasize to nodes within the parotid gland or to lymph nodes in the close neighborhood of the parotid or submaxillary glands. In such instances, a thorough physical examination and a careful search in the probable areas of primary development are the most valuable assets in defining the diagnosis.

Treatment
Surgery

The treatment of choice for the majority of salivary gland tumors is surgical excision. Radical surgical removal of submaxillary tumors implies no important mutilation and is usually carried out without difficulty (Simons et al.[61]). Surgery of parotid tumors is influenced by the presence of the facial nerve, which is intimately associated with the gland. The anatomic concept of the parotid gland as a bilobed structure has facilitated the adaptation of surgical techniques by which the facial nerve may be totally or partially preserved (Davis et al.[15]). This anatomic viewpoint is not supported by many surgeons.

An unquestionably *benign tumor* of the parotid gland should be removed extracapsularly with a minimal amount of surrounding normal parotid tissue. Because of this, Bailey[6] believes that in some instances a superficial lobectomy can be done. Other surgeons have proposed a total parotidectomy, with preservation of the facial nerve, in the treatment of mixed tumors. This is a difficult procedure that is not always successful and is followed by facial paralysis or Frey's syndrome (flushing and perspiration during or after meals) which has occurred in as many as one-fourth of the patients in whom the operation is done (Patey and Thackray[51]). We believe that an adequately wide excision is sufficient and justified in these cases. The facial nerve should be preserved by exposing it at its emergence from the stylomastoid foramen and dissecting it forward. After operation, there is sometimes development of a facial paralysis due to edema. However, this promptly subsides.

In definitely *malignant tumors*, a total parotidectomy should be carried out with sacrifice of the facial nerve when necessary. Preservation of the nerve, however, is occasionally possible (Bailey[7]). Infrequently, a facial paresis may be due to compression, not invasion. Conley[13] has shown the value of nerve grafting and masseter muscle transplantation whenever it becomes necessary to transect the nerve. Tumors presenting a retromandibular or pharyngeal extension may present difficulties (Morfit[46]), but a pharyngeal approach is not necessary (Patey and Thackray[50]). In the presence of cervical metastases, the resection should be done in continuity with a radical neck dissection (Roux-Berger and Moyse[60]; Kirklin et al.[37]). Changes occurring in a submaxillary gland after a course of radio-

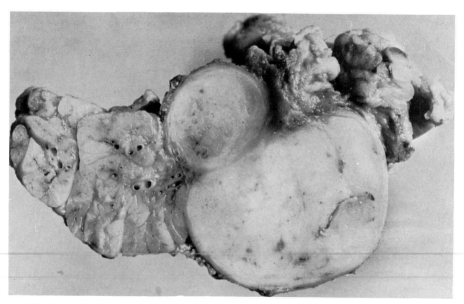

Fig. 438. Large benign recurrent mixed tumor of submaxillary gland. Tumor had been removed in 1946. It recurred in 1953, and this was the second recurrence in 1955. There has been no recurrence for the past five years. (WU neg. 55-4562.)

therapy may give the false impression of metastases (Staley et al.[65]). In our opinion, a prophylactic neck dissection (i.e., one that would be carried out in the absence of clinically ostensible metastases) is not indicated. MacComb and Fletcher[42] reported on thirty-two such dissections, with only one patient showing metastases. Others still advocate its use (Eneroth et al.[20]).

Postoperative recurrences

The recurrence of mixed tumors following surgery is one of their most common and disconcerting characteristics (Fig. 438). If the tumors are always removed with a margin of normal salivary gland, however, the recurrence rate is negligible. But if the tumor is only enucleated, remaining tumor foci result in subsequent recurrence. Sometimes, also, the surgeon may implant tiny nodules along the line of the incision. Redon[56] believes that these tumors have no true capsule. Delarue[16] stated that by careful sectioning of the surgical specimens, multiple foci of origin may be demonstrated. We have not been able to demonstrate them. In the absence of obvious signs that the tumor has been incompletely removed, it is not possible to predict, by simple microscopic examination of the tu-mor, whether or not it will recur. The adequacy of the surgical excision is a more reliable measure than the microscopic pattern. The recurrence usually mimics the original tumor very closely, but in some instances it may be difficult to note morphologically the malignant character of a recurrent tumor. There seems to be no doubt that some benign mixed tumors may become malignant (Fig. 434), with the chance being of the order of 2% according to Rawson et al.[55] In order to prove such transformation, one should demonstrate microscopic evidence of transition from typical benign mixed tumor areas to malignant ones.

Radiotherapy

The classical surgical literature makes repetitious remarks as to the palliative effects of radiations in salivary gland tumors. In practice, radiotherapy is seldom called upon except for the treatment of obviously inoperable or postoperative recurrent tumors. Thus, any comparison of results of surgery and radiotherapy alone in the treatment of these tumors is not possible. Yet, in the past thirty-five years, a number of serious workers have testified to the value of radiotherapy as a curative proce-

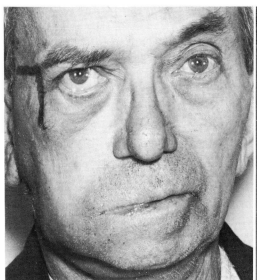
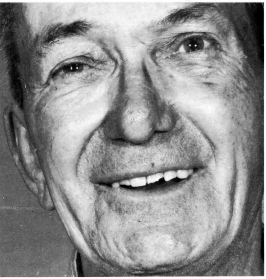

A **B**

Fig. 439. A, Patient, 72 years of age, seen in November, 1956, with anaplastic carcinoma of right parotid gland with complete right facial paralysis. **B,** Same patient in May, 1962, after irradiation and recovery of most of facial function. (From Mustard, R. A., and Anderson, W.: Malignant tumors of the parotid, Ann. Surg. **159:**291-304, 1964.)

dure either alone or as a routine postoperative measure. Ahlbom,[2] Baclesse,[5] Smiddy,[62] Watson,[70] Stewart et al.,[66] and Eneroth et al.[20] have published evidence of the radiocurability of all malignant varieties of these tumors (Fig. 439). We have verified these facts on a succession of postoperative recurrences from various malignant tumors. The slowly accumulated evidence has resulted in greater utilization of radiotherapy in recent years. Present evidence points to the indication of skillful radiotherapy with an aim to cure in the presence of any postoperative recurrence or histopathologic evidence of incomplete removal of a malignant salivary gland tumor. There is, moreover, some indication that routine postoperative irradiation of benign as well as malignant tumors may prove beneficial to any surgical series (Alaniz and Fletcher[3]).

Radiotherapy is best administered taking advantage of fractionation in order to avoid untoward effects on the bone and other adjacent structures that may be involved. Cobalt[60] teletherapy and supervoltage roentgentherapy facilitate meeting the requirements and permit a higher average daily dose throughout the entire area of potential involvement and a sufficiently high total dose without heavy reactions or untoward effects.

Prognosis

The prognosis of salivary gland tumors depends on their histopathology, their extent, their location, and the adequacy of the treatment. Recurrences are rare after excision of cystadenomas and other *benign tumors*. A great number of failures are due to lack of histopathologic recognition of the malignant potential of some apparently innocent tumors (Patey et al.[52]). Recurrences from benign *mixed tumors* are primarily dependent on the inadequacy of their excision rather than on multicentricity of their origin. Significantly, the rate of recurrence from benign mixed tumors of the submaxillary gland is much lower than for those in the parotid gland. Recurrences reach their peak one year after operation (Rawson et al.[55]).

Patients with *mucoepidermoid tumors* seem to do rather well after surgery, Gray et al.[31] reported on a series of thirty-five patients, twenty of whom lived from five to twenty years without evidence of recurrence following surgical treatment. Patients with *adenoid cystic carcinomas* (cylindromas) must be followed for a long time for evidence of recurrence or metastases. In a series of twenty-three patients in whom resections were done for cylindromas of the sublingual, submaxillary, and parotid glands, Smith et al.[64] reported six patients living from seven to fourteen years after surgery. Ten recurrences took place within three years, but six others occurred from five to eight years after treatment. *Acinic cell adenocarcinomas* arising mostly from the parotid gland are highly curable. Abrams et al.[1] reported on a series of seventy-two patients treated by conservative surgery, with only six local recurrences and five cases of metastases.

Patey et al.[52] reported on a series of ninety-five cases of malignant tumors of the *parotid gland* treated surgically. The results were excellent in mucoepidermoid, cylindromatous, and acinic cell tumors, but most of the forty-seven patients with tumors classified as carcinomas had died. Another series of 129 malignant tumors of the parotid gland was reviewed by Freeman et al.[27] The rate of recurrence was 27% and 35% for the tumors classified as low to moderate and high degree of malignancy, respectively, and the five-year survival rates were 92% and 60%, respectively. In a report of fifty-one patients with malignant tumors of the *submaxillary gland*, there were eighteen (36%) known recurrences and twenty-three (46%) five-year survivals (Simons et al.[61]). Rankow and Mignogna[53a] reported seven patients with malignant tumor of the sublingual gland treated surgically, with four patients apparently well and surviving from three to thirteen years.

The reported rate of recurrences of surgically treated benign mixed tumors varies from 20% to 30%. In seventy-five cases given routine postoperative irradiation, Watson[70] reported only five recurrences, all of which were surgically controlled. In several cases of postoperative recurrence, radiotherapy alone was able to control the tumors. Watson[70] believes that the case for postoperative radiotherapy is even stronger for malignant tumors: twelve of seventeen patients with malignant mixed tumors, nine of fourteen with adenocarcinomas, four of five with mucoepidermoid tumors, and six of six with carcinomas survived five years. Stewart et al.[66] reported on the results of radical radiotherapy in a series of nineteen patients with inoperable carcinomas of the parotid gland, with three living and well six to 10 years and 6 others dying without evidence of local recrudescence of the disease. In a small series irradiated at the Penrose Cancer Hospital, the curability of postoperative recurrences has been verified for all varieties of salivary gland tumors. The primary lesion was controlled in two patients with repeated recurrent malignant mixed tumors, one of whom had proved cervical metastases, with one dying of pulmonary metastases and the other remaining well for over ten years. Of two patients with recurrent adenoid cystic cancer, one survived twelve years and one died from metastases without local recurrence. Of three patients with recurrent mucoepidermoid tumors, two survived five and six years, respectively, and one died from metastases. Of four patients with carcinomas, two survived seven and ten years, respectively, one died from metastasis, and one died from intercurrent disease.

REFERENCES

1 Abrams, A. M., Cornyn, J., Scofield, H. H., and Hansen, L. S.: Acinic cell adenocarcinoma of the major salivary glands, Cancer **15**:1145-1162, 1965.
2 Ahlbom, H. E.: Mucous- and salivary-gland tumours, Acta Radiol. (Stockholm) (suppl. 23), pp. 1-452, 1935.
3 Alaniz, F., and Fletcher, G. H.: Place and technics of radiation therapy in the management of malignant tumors of the major salivary glands, Radiology **84**:412-419, 1965.
4 Azzopardi, J. G., and Smith, O. D.: Salivary gland tumours and their mucins, J. Path. Bact. **77**:131-140, 1959.
5 Baclesse, F.: Les métastases et la radio-sensibilité des cylindromas et des tumeurs mixtes des glandes salivaires, Rev. Stomat. (Paris) **47**:469-474, 1946.
6 Bailey, H.: Parotidectomy; indications and results, Brit. Med. J. **1**:404-407, 1947.
7 Bailey, H.: The surgical anatomy of the parotid gland, Brit. Med. J. **2**:245-248, 1948.
8 Bardwil, J. M., Reynolds, C. T., Ibanez, M. L., and Luna, M. A.: Report of one hundred tumors of the minor salivary glands, Amer. J. Surg. **112**:493-497, 1966.
9 Beahrs, O. H., Woolner, L. B., Kirklin, J. W., and Devine, K. D.: Carcinomatous transformation of mixed tumors of the parotid gland, Arch. Surg. (Chicago) **75**:605-614, 1957.
10 Bhaskar, S. N., and Bernier, J. L.: Mucoepidermoid tumors of the major and minor salivary glands, Cancer **15**:801-817, 1962.
11 Bloch, K. J., Buchanan, W. W., Wohl, M. J., and Bunim, J. J.: Sjogren's syndrome, Medicine (Balt.) **44**:187-231, 1965 (extensive bibliography).
12 Byars, L. T., Ackerman, L. V., and Peacock, E.: Tumors of salivary gland origin in children; a clinical pathologic appraisal of 24 cases, Ann. Surg. **146**:40-51, 1957.
13 Conley, J. J.: Facial nerve grafting in treatment of parotid gland tumors, Arch. Surg. (Chicago) **70**:359-366, 1955.
14 Davies, J. N. P., Dodge, O. G., and Burkitt, D. P.: Salivary-gland tumors in Uganda, Cancer **17**:1310-1322, 1964.
15 Davis, R. A., Anson, B. J., Budinger, J. M., and Kurth, L. E.: Surgical anatomy of the facial nerve and parotid gland based upon a study of 350 cervicofacial halves, Surg. Gynec. Obstet. **102**:385-412, 1956.
16 Delarue, J.: Les "tumeurs mixtes" plurifocales de la glande parotide, Ann. Anat. Path. (Paris) **1**:34-58, 1956.
17 Echevarria, R.: Ultrastructure of the acinic cell carcinoma and clear cell carcinoma of the parotid gland, Cancer **20**:563-571, 1967.
18 Edington, G. M., and Sheiham, A.: Salivary gland tumours and tumours of the oral cavity in Western Nigeria, Brit. J. Cancer **20**:425-433, 1966.
19 Eneroth, C. M., Fluur, E., and Moberger, G.: Unusual localization of mixed tumours of the parotid region, Pract. Otorhinolaryng. (Basel) **28**:108-116, 1966.
20 Eneroth, C. M., Hamberger, C. A., and Jakobsson, P. A.: Malignancy of acinic cell carcinoma, Ann. Otol. **75**:1-13, 1966.
21 Eneroth, C. M., and Zajicek, J.: Aspiration biopsy of salivary gland tumors. III. Morphologic studies on smears and histologic sections from 368 mixed tumors, Acta Cytol. (Balt.) **10**:440-454, 1966.
22 Evans, J. C.: Radiation therapy of salivary gland tumors, Radiol. Clin. (Basel) **35**:153-191, 1966.
23 Favata, B. V.: Characteristics of mixed tumors of the parotid gland growing in vitro, Surg. Gynec. Obstet. **86**:659-662, 1948.
24 Foote, F. W., and Becker, W. F.: Mucoepidermoid tumors of the salivary glands, Ann. Surg. **122**:820-844, 1945.
25 Foote, F. W., Jr., and Frazell, E. L.: Tumors of the major salivary glands. In Atlas of tumor pathology, Sect. IV, Fasc. II, Washington, D. C., 1954, Armed Forces Institute of Pathology.
26 Frazell, E. L.: Clinical aspects of tumors of the major salivary glands, Cancer **7**:637-659, 1954.
27 Freeman, F. J., Beahrs, O. H., and Woolner, L. B.: Surgical treatment of malignant tumors of the parotid gland, Amer. J. Surg. **110**:527-533, 1965.
28 Gazayerli, M. M., and Abdel-Aziz, A. S.:

Salivary gland tumors in Egypt and non-Western countries, Brit. J. Cancer 18:649-654, 1964.

29 Godwin, J. T., Foote, F. W., Jr., and Frazell, E. L.: Acinic cell adenocarcinoma of the parotid gland; report of twenty-seven cases, Amer. J. Path. 30:465-477, 1954.

30 Gore, D. O., Annamunthodo, H., and Harland, A.: Tumors of salivary gland origin, Surg. Gynec. Obstet. 119:1290-1296, 1964.

31 Gray, J. M., Hendrix, R. C., and French, J.: Mucoepidermoid tumors of salivary glands, Cancer 16:183-194, 1963.

32 Grishman, E.: Histochemical analysis of muco-polysaccharides occurring in mucus-producing tumors; mixed tumors of the parotid gland, colloid carcinomas of the breast and myxomas, Cancer 5:700-707, 1952.

33 Hertig, P.: Histology and prognosis of the cylindromas, Oncologia (Basel) 10:91-107, 1957.

34 Hintze, A.: Gutartige und bösartige Parotis-geschwülste und ihre Heilungsmöglichkeiten, Arch. Klin. Chir. 180:606-636, 1934.

35 Kauffman, S. L., and Stout, A. P.: Tumors of the major salivary glands in children, Cancer 16:1317-1331, 1963.

36 Kimm, H. T., Spies, J. W., and Wolfe, J. J.: Sialography, with particular reference to neo-plastic diseases, Amer. J. Roentgen. 34:289-296, 1935.

37 Kirklin, J. W., McDonald, J. R., Harrington, S. W., and New, G. B.: Parotid tumor; histo-pathology, clinical behavior, and end results, Surg. Gynec. Obstet. 92:721-727, 1951.

38 Lampe, I., and Zatzkin, H.: Pulmonary metas-tases of pseudoadenomatous basal-cell carci-noma (mucous and salivary gland tumor), Radiology 53:379-385, 1949.

39 Lathrop, F. D.: Carcinoma of salivary gland origin; a follow-up survey, Laryngoscope 70:580-594, 1960.

40 Lederman, M.: Mucous and salivary gland tumors, Brit. J. Radiol. 14:329-375, 1941.

41 Loke, Y. W.: Salivary gland tumours in Ma-laya, Brit. J. Cancer 21:665-674, 1967.

42 MacComb, W. S., and Fletcher, G. H.: Can-cer of the head and neck, Baltimore, 1967, The Williams & Wilkins Co.

43 McGavran, M. H., Bauer, W. C., and Acker-man, L. V.: Sebaceous lymphadenoma of the parotid salivary gland, Cancer 13:1185-1187, 1960.

44 Marsden, A. T. H.: The distinctive features of the tumours of the salivary glands in Malaya, Brit. J. Cancer 5:375-381, 1951.

45 Meza-Chávez, L.: Oxyphilic granular cell adenoma of the parotid gland (oncocytoma), Amer. J. Path. 25:523-547, 1949.

46 Morfit, H. M.: Retromandibular parotid tu-mors, Arch. Surg. (Chicago) 70:906-913, 1955.

47 Morgan, W. S., and Castleman, B.: A clinico-pathologic study of "Mikulicz's disease," Amer. J. Path. 29:471-503, 1953.

48 Morgan, A. D., and Raven, R. W.: Sjogren's

syndrome; a general disease, Brit. J. Surg. 40:154-162, 1952.

49 Mustard, R. A., and Anderson, W.: Malignant tumors of the parotid, Ann. Surg. 159:291-304, 1964.

50 Patey, D. H., and Thackray, A. C.: The pathological anatomy and treatment of parotid tumours with retropharyngeal extension (dumb-bell tumours), Brit. J. Surg. 44:352-358, 1957.

51 Patey, D. H., and Thackray, A. C.: The treat-ment of parotid tumours in the light of a pathologic study of parotidectomy material, Brit. J. Surg. 45:477-487, 1958.

52 Patey, D. H., Thackray, A. C., and Keeling, D. H.: Malignant disease of the parotid, Brit. J. Cancer 19:712-737, 1965.

53 Quattlebaum, F. W., Dockerty, M. B., and Mayo, C. W.: Adenocarcinoma, cylindroma type, of the parotid gland, Surg. Gynec. Obstet. 82:342-347, 1946.

53a Rankow, R. M., and Mignogna, F.: Cancer of the sublingual salivary gland, Amer. J. Surg. 118:790-795, 1969.

54 Rawson, A. J., and Horn, R. C., Jr.: Sebaceous glands and sebaceous gland-containing tumors of the parotid salivary gland, Surgery 27:93-101, 1950.

55 Rawson, A. J., Howard, J. M., Royster, H. P., and Horn, R. C., Jr.: Tumors of the salivary glands; a clinicopathological study of 160 cases, Cancer 3:445-458, 1950.

56 Redon, H.: Traitement des épitheliomas re-namés de la parotide, Rev. Stomat. (Paris) 57:757-762, 1956.

57 Ridenhour, C. E., and Spratt, J. S., Jr.: Epi-dermoid carcinoma of the skin involving the parotid gland, Amer. J. Surg. 112:504-507, 1966.

58 Roos, D. B., Byars, L. T., and Ackerman, L. V.: Neurilemomas of the facial nerve present-ing as parotid gland tumors, Ann. Surg. 144:258-262, 1956.

59 Rouvière, H.: Anatomie des lymphatiques de l'homme, Paris, 1933, Masson et Cie.

60 Roux-Berger, J. L., and Moyse, P.: Les parot-idectomies totales élargies, Mem. Acad. Chir. (Paris) 75:279-284, 1949.

61 Simons, J. N., Beahrs, O. H., and Woolner, L. B.: Tumors of the submaxillary gland, Amer. J. Surg. 108:485-494, 1964.

62 Smiddy, F. G.: Treatment of mixed parotid tumours, Brit. Med. J. 1:322-325, 1956.

63 Smith, M. J., and Stenstrom, K. W.: Parotid tumors; a review of ninety-three cases, Radiol-ogy 52:655-661, 1949.

64 Smith, L. C., Lane, N., and Rankow, R. M.: Cylindroma (adenoid cystic carcinoma), Amer. J. Surg. 110:519-526, 1965.

65 Staley, C. J., Kaupp, H. A., Jr., and Fischer, E.: The submandibular salivary gland in radical neck dissection specimens, Amer. J. Surg. 106:831-834, 1963.

66 Stewart, M. A., Jackson, A. W., and Chew, M. K.: The role of radiotherapy in the man-agement of malignant tumors of the salivary glands, Amer. J. Roentgen. 102:100-108, 1968.

67 Thomas, W. H., and Coppola, E. D.: Distant

metastases from mixed tumors of the salivary glands, Amer. J. Surg. **109:**724-730, 1965.

68 Thompson, A. S., and Bryant, H. C., Jr.: Histogenesis of papillary cystadenoma lymphomatosum (Warthin's tumor) of the parotid salivary gland, Amer. J. Path. **26:**806-849, 1950.

69 Wallace, A. C., MacDougall, J. T., Hildes, J. A., and Lederman, J. M.: Salivary gland tumors in Canadian Eskimos, Cancer **16:**1338-1353, 1963.

70 Watson, T. A.: Irradiation in the management of tumours of the head and neck, Amer. J. Surg. **110:**542-548, 1965.

71 Wilner, D.: A roentgen study of skeletal and intrathoracic metastases from salivary gland cancer, Radiology **55:**801-806, 1950.

72 Woolner, L. B., Pettet, J. R., and Kirklin, J. W.: Mucoepidermoid tumors of major salivary glands, Amer. J. Clin. Path. **24:**1350-1362, 1954.

Pancreas

Anatomy

The pancreas is a gland that extends from the second portion of the duodenum to the spleen, following an almost transverse direction at about the height of the first two lumbar vertebrae (Fig. 440). It measures 15 cm to 20 cm in length, 4 cm to 5 cm in height, and about 2 cm to 3 cm in thickness and has an irregular surface. It is usually divided into a head, body, and tail. The head is framed within the first three portions of the duodenum. The body and the tail run in line with the head and occupy a position slightly above and behind it. Pancreatic secretions empty into the duodenum.

The anterior surface of the head of the pancreas is covered by the peritoneum and crossed by the line of attachment of the transverse mesocolon. The supramesocolic area is in contact with the stomach, and the inframesocolic area is in contact with loops of the small intestine. The posterior surface of the head is in direct relation with numerous vessels of the portal and caval systems. The posterior surface is covered by the ligament of Treitz. The body is in direct relation with the stomach anteriorly and with the aorta, splenic veins, left kidney, and suprarenal gland posteriorly. The tail has very variable relations, but it is usually in direct contact with the spleen. The uncinate process of the pan-

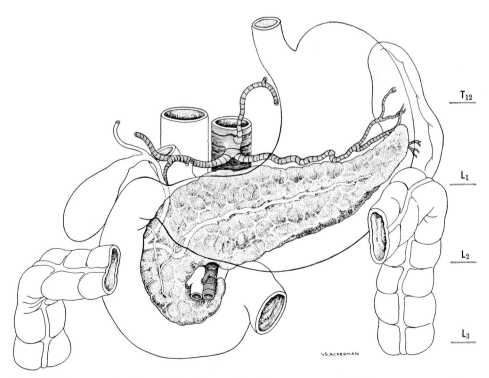

Fig. 440. Pancreas showing relationships to first three portions of duodenum, common duct, stomach, spleen, and transverse colon. Note its projection in reference to vertebrae.

creas extends downward from the lower left lateral border of the head and may actually encircle the portal vein.

The pancreas is a racemose gland similar to the salivary glands and is formed by secreting acini, each one of which constitutes a pancreas in miniature. The secretion of these acini is canalized toward the canal of Wirsung, which extends from the tail toward the head of the gland. In addition, in most instances there is an accessory canal, the canal of Santorini, which is 5 cm to 6 cm long, is found in the upper half of the head of the pancreas, and ends independently in the duodenum. The main pancreatic duct enters into the duodenum in conjunction with the common bile duct to form a common termination (ampulla) in about 55% of the instances. In the remainder, there are various other anatomic arrangements. At the point at which the

main duct empties, there is a smooth muscle sphincter.

The blood supply to the pancreas is derived from the superior pancreaticoduodenal, inferior pancreaticoduodenal, and splenic arteries. The principal veins accompany these arterial branches. The anterior and inferior surfaces of the tail and body are covered only by peritoneum, the anterior surface facing the lesser peritoneal sac and the inferior surface facing the general peritoneal cavity.

Lymphatics. The lymphatics of the pancreas are very rich, having numerous communications with those of the duodenum. They follow the interlobular spaces and come to the surface of the gland, where they follow the direction of the vessels and are drained by the following trunks (Bartels[3]):

1 The *trunks of the left side* empty into

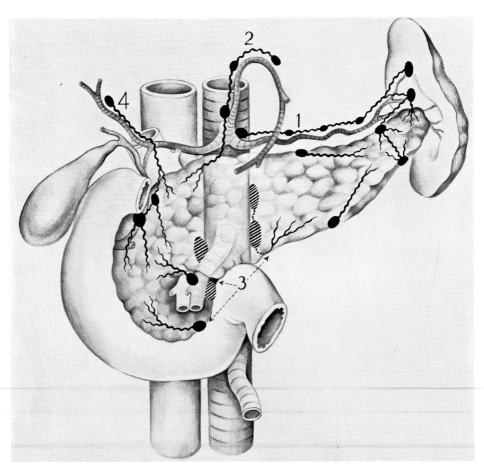

Fig. 441. Lymphatics of pancreas drained by trunks of left side, **1**; superior trunks, **2**; inferior trunks, **3**; trunks of right side, **4**.

the nodes of the hilum of the spleen, the nodes of the pancreatic or splenic ligament, and those nodes found in the superior and inferior border of the tail of the pancreas.

2 The *superior trunks* for the most part drain the body of the pancreas. They follow an upward direction and end in the superior pancreatic lymph nodes.

3 The *inferior trunks* also drain the body of the pancreas and empty into the inferior pancreatic, mesenteric, and left lateroaortic lymph nodes.

4 The *trunks of the right side* are divided into two groups:

  a The anterior lymphatics, which follow the anterior surface of the head, some toward the infrapyloric lymph nodes and the others downward toward pancreaticoduodenal and mesenteric lymph nodes

  b The posterior lymphatics, which are emptied by the posterior pancreaticoduodenal lymph nodes and the lateroaortic lymph nodes on the right side (Fig. 441)

Epidemiology

Carcinoma of the pancreas is a relatively rare neoplasm, making up only 1% to 2% of all forms of cancer. In the 1947 United States survey, the age-sex adjusted incidence rate was 9.51 and 5.57 for males and females, respectively, per 100,000 population. It occurs mainly between the ages of 30 and 70 years and is practically never found in patients under 25 years of age. A relatively high proportion of cases of cancer of the pancreas has been observed among natives of Uganda, Africa, and has been attributed to dietetic factors (Gillman et al.[36]). In a series of eighty-four cases of carcinoma of the pancreas collected from three hospitals of Israel, the majority were found in European Jews and rarely in Jews of oriental origin (Birnbaum and Kleeberg[10]).

It is difficult to obtain an idea of the occurrence of carcinoma in the different parts of the gland, for carcinoma of the head of the pancreas occurs most frequently in clinical material, but carcinoma of the body and tail predominates in autopsy material (Duff[24]). Also, many cases

diagnosed as carcinoma of the head of the pancreas undoubtedly arise within the bile ducts. Carcinoma of the *head* makes up approximately two-thirds and carcinoma of the *body* probably makes up about one-fourth of all the carcinomas of the pancreas. The reported ratio of cases of carcinoma of the body to those of the head of the pancreas is somewhat determined by the stage of the disease, because carcinoma of the body terminally may have extension to the head.

The *islet cell tumors* of the pancreas make up a small but distinctive group of neoplasms. In a review of the literature, Howard and Rhoads[44] found 398 cases of islet cell tumors, thirty-seven (10%) of which were carcinomas. In 9000 consecutive autopsies at the Presbyterian Hospital in New York, twenty-four adenomas were found (Frantz[32]).

Pathology
Gross pathology

In *carcinoma of the head* of the pancreas, the primary tumor is hard, and the head is deformed by a nodular mass. On cut section, the pancreas is replaced by homogeneous tumor obliterating the normal lobulated pancreatic tissue. The canal of Wirsung and the common bile duct are often obstructed and, at times, are invaded by neoplastic masses. The obstruction of the common bile duct is often associated with carcinoma in the lymph nodes along the biliary tract. This neoplastic lymph node involvement results in invasion of the duct wall (Kaplan and Angrist[47]) which, in turn, fixes the duct and permits its compression instead of mere displacement. Because of the complete obstruction of the common bile duct, the gallbladder is usually distended, and the liver, too, is invariably enlarged, its color ranging from dark green to olive yellow. The longer the biliary obstruction is present, however, the smaller the size of the liver and the greater its connective tissue content. The bile ducts within the liver are always found to be dilated, and there is increased interlobular and intralobular connective tissue. In the early stages of biliary obstruction, the bile is thick and inspissated, only later becoming pale and thin. Dilatation of the main pancreatic duct occurs at the head of the pancreas but usually does not occur in inflammatory disease.

Cancer of the head of the pancreas tends to remain fairly well localized, for spread is blocked by the duodenum on three sides, by the proximal transverse colon, and by the posterior wall of the abdomen. Spread to the peritoneal cavity is restricted because the head is in contact with the peritoneum in only one small area near the lower margin of its anterior surface.

With spread of the tumor, the head of the pancreas becomes fixed by inflammation or neoplastic connective tissue. These adhesions firmly anchor the carcinoma to the stomach, duodenum, transverse colon, and diaphragm. The carcinoma also invariably becomes adherent to the retropancreatic tissue and the vertebral column. The lesser omental cavity becomes smaller. The adhesions may even cause a partial pyloric obstruction. With further advance of the disease, the carcinoma infiltrates the musculature of the duodenum, the stomach, or the transverse colon, and this may result in mucosal edema and ulceration. It can even penetrate through the diaphragm to implant on the pleural and pericardial surfaces. The tumor often surrounds or even invades the portal vein, at times causing thrombosis followed by ascites.

Carcinoma of the *body* and *tail* of the pancreas presents a large nodular mass that readily becomes fixed to the vertebral column and promptly involves the retropancreatic tissues. It may cause thrombosis of the splenic vein and infarction of the spleen. Posteriorly, spread may extend to the diaphragm, left suprarenal gland, kidney, and spleen. The involvement of nerve trunks is also common in carcinoma of the body of the pancreas because the nerves of the celiac plexus are in intimate relation to the body. Involvement of nerves also occurs in cancer of the tail and head of the pancreas but not so frequently.

Carcinomas of the body and tail are commonly associated with *venous thrombosis* (Sproul[87]). In an extensive review of the literature and a careful study of a large group of cases, Sproul[87] noted that 56% of the patients with carcinoma of the body or tail had at least one thrombus, and 31% had multiple venous thrombi. On the contrary, if the carcinoma arose in the head, venous thrombi occurred in only about 10% of the patients. Kenney[48] found that carcinomas accompanied by multiple venous thrombi were of the mucinous type.

Mikal and Campbell[63] found twenty-eight cases of thrombophlebitis in 100 cases of carcinoma of the pancreas, with 18% of the tumors of the head and 48% of those of the body and tail presenting this complication. Other authors do not agree that this is a peculiar feature of carcinoma of the pancreas (Anlyan et al.[1]), and although it is the most frequent type, it may also be seen rather commonly with carcinoma of the lung or of the female reproductive tract. This thrombophlebitis in association with carcinoma of the pancreas may be recurrent or migratory but resistant to anticoagulants and may show an increased risk of pulmonary embolism (Lieberman et al.[53]):

The *islet cell tumors* are usually situated in the body or the tail and may be within the substance of the gland or located on its surface. About one-fourth of them appear at the head of the pancreas or at the junction of the body and the tail. Islet cell tumors are well circumscribed and usually rather small, varying from a little over 1 mm up to 5 cm in diameter. They have a reddish gray color that contrasts sharply with the lobulated yellow of the pancreas. They may exhibit considerable fibrosis and calcification during their evolution because of regressive changes. When these tumors become malignant, which is rare, they break through their capsule and invade the surrounding tissue. Multiple adenomas occur in about 10% of the patients.

Microscopic pathology

Carcinomas of the pancreas can be divided into three types: those arising from ducts, those arising from acini, and those arising from islet tissue.

The carcinomas arising from the ducts are by far the most common (Fig. 442). They are often accompanied by very prominent connective tissue reaction, and the picture is easily confused by blockage of the main ducts. The cells of the acini are fragile and tend to be effaced by the process developing within the ducts. If the neoplastic process blocks the ducts for any length of

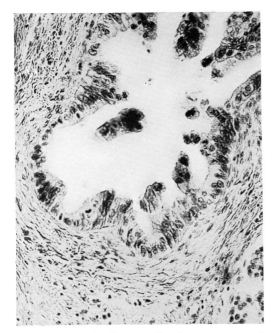

Fig. 442. Well-differentiated adenocarcinoma of duct origin, with fibrosis and persisting islet tissue. (Low-power enlargement.)

time, the acinar cells disappear completely. On the other hand, the cells of the islands are very resistant and capable of proliferating and conserving their structural characteristics. There may be considerable dilatation of the ducts, which can be cystic in nature, and there may be papillary enfoldings of the epithelium. At times, there may be focal areas of squamous metaplasia which can also be mistaken for carcinomas arising from acini, but if enough sections are taken, their duct origin becomes apparent. The tumors that arise from acini are much fewer in number and resemble acini. Areas of transition between the tumor and the glandular acinar tissue can be observed.

The rare so-called *cystadenoma* arising from the ducts of the pancreas appears most frequently in the tail. These tumors typically show a multilocular cyst, the cavity of which is lined by papillomatous vegetations. They strikingly resemble the serous cystadenomas of the ovary. Rarely they do become malignant, but it may be difficult to determine microscopically whether they are benign or malignant. They are usually large. These true tumors have to

be distinguished from the pseudocysts that may occur following trauma or infection. With blockage of the ducts, retention cysts appear and occasionally may result from defective development or be associated with polycystic disease of the kidney.

Histologically, *islet cell tumors* arise from the cells of the islets. They usually have a definite capsule and compress the adjacent pancreatic parenchyma. At times, their fibrous encapsulation is incomplete, and they are usually well vascularized. Special fixatives and stains are necessary to bring out the histologic details, and electron microscopy can identify the specific pattern of the secreting granules of the different types of cells (McGavran et al.[57]). In Ellison and Wilson's review[27] of 260 cases with the Zollinger-Ellison syndrome, the male:female ratio was 6:4. This syndrome occurred most commonly in the third through the fifth decades of life, but twelve of the patients were children under 15 years of age. Metastases may become manifest years after removal of the primary tumor (Frantz[33]). We believe that tumor cells lying free within veins have no significance. However, if true tumor thrombi are present within veins, this is significant. For instance, we had an islet cell tumor in which the only evidence of malignant change was true tumor thrombi. The patient developed liver metastases eight years following removal of the primary neoplasm. Heterotopic pancreatic tissue may give rise to hyperfunctioning, insulin-producing, benign or malignant neoplastic tissue (de Castro Barbosa et al.[15]).

Metastatic spread

Metastases from carcinoma of the pancreas most frequently involve the regional lymph nodes. Involved nodes in the region of the head of the pancreas become fused with the gland by direct extension. Large metastatic nodes may form in the hilum of the liver, and mesenteric, para-aortic, and posterior mediastinal nodes may also be involved. Blood-borne liver metastases are usually multiple but small. Metastases to lungs and bone are not unusual. Lisa et al.[54] found that carcinomas of the tail of the pancreas have a greater tendency to metastasize to the lungs and thoracic lymph nodes than do those of the head or body.

Carcinomas of the *head* of the pancreas have a relative tendency to remain localized, whereas those of the *body* and *tail* metastasize widely. *Islet cell carcinomas* metastasize first to regional lymph nodes and liver.

Clinical evolution
Carcinoma of head of pancreas (jaundice predominating)

The rich symptomatology of cancer of the pancreas is, above all else, a function of the extension of the tumor, and symptoms are due to compression or invasion of neighboring organs. Therefore, the clinical picture varies according to the site of origin of the tumor. The onset of cancer of the head of the pancreas is *insidious*. Often there is a preliminary period of *weight loss*, asthenia, slow or vague indigestion, gaseous distention, and nausea. In some rare instances, the appearance of tenacious anorexia introduces the illness. These phenomena, however, are not too alarming. It takes the appearance of *jaundice* or the sudden manifestation of a painful *crisis* to provoke a realization of actual illness.

The jaundice that accompanies cancer of the pancreas has a distinctive evolution. It may be preceded by an acute digestive episode associated with vomiting or diarrhea, but more often it develops slowly and is consequently unobserved even by the patient. It appears first on the mucous membranes and the palms of the hands but gradually becomes generalized, reaching a maximum intensity after a period of several weeks. The yellow color of the skin deepens little by little, passing from a light yellow to a dark saffron, and, in certain instances, to a greenish or olive color. Very rarely, a veritable black jaundice occurs. Whatever its intensity, the jaundice predominates generally on the face, the region of the genital organs, and the linea alba. The jaundice is characterized by its persistence. It does not regress. With jaundice, *pruritus* is usually severe. The patient often notes deepening of the color of the urine and the clay color of the stools. There is obstruction of the biliary tree with dilatation of the extrahepatic and intrahepatic ducts. With these changes, there may be

an apparent enlargement of the right lobe of the liver, and the gallbladder may become palpable (50% to 65% of the patients).

Pain accompanies carcinoma of the pancreas in a fairly high percentage of patients, but it seldom precedes the appearance of jaundice. It is often continuous and tends to radiate to the right upper quadrant (Gullick[39]). At times, the pain has a colicky nature, even in the absence of concomitant gallstones (about 20% of the patients have associated gallstones).

Emaciation is a constant finding. The patient may lose twenty or thirty pounds in a few weeks. The muscles rapidly become atrophic, and there are profound metabolic disturbances initiated by prolonged cholemia and extensive liver damage. This results in a natural tendency to hemorrhage, and, terminally, biliary infection is common.

Carcinoma of body of pancreas (pain predominating)

Tumors of the body of the pancreas grow silently. They tend to metastasize early because of their extensive close relation to the peritoneal cavity and because of this often present a mass in the epigastrium. This mass is made up mainly of metastatic nodes in the region of the primary carcinoma. With further development of the tumor, infringement on the abundant nerve plexus in the region of the body causes *pain* (Chauffard[17]). Morgagni[68] reported a case in which the intense pain was described by the patient as comparable to dogs tearing away the superior portion of the abdomen.

Crises of pain occur in cancer of the body of the pancreas without apparent reason, often taking place three or four hours after eating. This pain is relieved by sitting up and leaning forward or by lying on the right side with the legs drawn up and bending forward at the hips. It is increased by a recumbent position, probably because the solar plexus anterior to the vertebral column is placed under tension. Usually these pains are of short duration (fifteen minutes) but may occur more than once in a twenty-four-hour period. They can be regular or irregular. The pain is usually more severe at night and makes sleep impossible. Ultimately, these crises may either take on a paroxysmal character or be angioid in character, complicated by vomiting. In these instances, the patient rests immobile, the arms inert and the face pale, and shows marked anxiety and fear of imminent death. The pain often extends through to the back and radiates to the scapula, but its most permanent location is the epigastrium. At times, nerve involvement is accompanied by pigmentation of the skin, suggesting melanosis. Psychiatric problems, such as depression, agitation, and intractable insomnia, may develop in patients with carcinoma of the body and tail of the pancreas. Of eighty-seven cases reported by Ulett and Parsons,[89] nine had important psychiatric problems.

Weight loss is often rapid and occurs in nearly every patient. Obstinate constipation is frequent. It is not too unusual to find an enlarged liver. In eleven of sixteen patients, the liver was enlarged (Duff[24]). The spleen may also be enlarged due to infarction. Jaundice is practically never present except terminally.

Carcinoma of tail of pancreas

Cancer of the tail of the pancreas has the most insidious development of all the pancreatic carcinomas. Usually emaciation, asthenia, vague indigestion, and anorexia prevail. Gripping upper abdominal pain, splenomegaly, and upper gastrointestinal bleeding may be among the early manifestations; arterial embolism and the auscultation of a local bruit may lead to the diagnosis (Arlen and Brockunier[2a]). The initial symptoms are frequently caused by metastases to the peritoneum, lungs, bones, and other organs. Pain, although not nearly so common as in carcinoma of the body of the pancreas, radiates invariably to the left hypochondrium and left side of the chest. Jaundice almost never occurs. An abdominal tumor is one of the most common findings.

Islet cell tumors

The symptoms that occur with beta islet cell tumors are those due to the overproduction of insulin. However, practically all the patients in the lower age groups who have been reported on had symptoms of hypoglycemia. The size of the tumor bears no relation to the degree of hyperinsulinism. These symptoms are protean in nature, derive mainly from nervous system disturbances, and can be divided into three stages (Wauchope[93]). In the first stage, there is slight hypoglycemia characterized by fatigue, lassitude, indefinite restlessness, and malaise. In the second stage, symptoms suggesting compensatory secretion of epinephrine occur: pallor, clammy perspiration, palpitation, tremor of the fingers, fear, sensation of hunger, lowered temperature, increased pulse rate, and elevated blood pressure. The third stage resembles alcoholic intoxication with clouded sensorium, double vision, staggering, violence, and hysteria. These advanced symptoms are easily confused with epilepsy or alcoholism (Fonkalsrud et al.[30]). Blood sugar level may be low during an attack. Excessive weight gain can occur (Fig. 443). Brain changes similar to those described in pa-

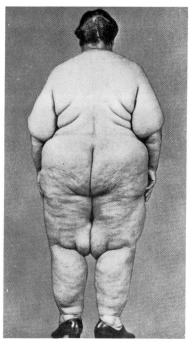

Fig. 443. Patient, 64-year-old woman, had had attacks of hypoglycemia for eight years. Her weight was 276 pounds. She had gained this weight because of 2.5 cm functioning benign islet cell tumor of head of pancreas. (From Frantz, V. K.: Tumors of the pancreas. In Atlas of tumor pathology, Sect. VII, Fascs. 27 and 28, Washington, D. C., 1959, Armed Forces Institute of Pathology.)

tients receiving overdosages of insulin have been reported (Malamud and Grosh[59]). If the tumor recurs after surgical removal of a carcinoma of islet cell origin, then hypoglycemic symptoms may appear with the recurrence. Benign islet cell tumors infrequently cause death. In islet cell carcinomas, death is caused by a combination of hypoglycemic reactions and wide dissemination of the neoplasm.

Zollinger and Ellison[100] reported a fulminating peptic ulcer diathesis, frequently fatal, associated with noninsulin-producing islet cell tumors of the pancreas. The syndrome is accompanied by extreme gastric hypersecretion. Multiple jejunal ulcers may be seen in the roentgenograms (Christoforidis and Nelson[18]). Moore et al.[67] used a bioassay of the serum, gastric juice and urine, for gastric acid secretagogue activity which is not present in patients with pure peptic ulcers. Ellison and Wilson[27] reviewed 260 patients with the Zollinger-Ellison syndrome. In 61% of the patients, the tumors were malignant. Pain was a predominant symptom and was related to ulcerations. Diarrhea and vomiting were common, and intestinal hemorrhage occurred in 22%. In fifty-six of the 260 patients, there were associated lesions of other endocrine organs (pituitary tumors, functioning parathyroid tumors, adrenal cortical tumors). Zollinger and Grant[101] pointed out that only a total gastrectomy is effective against the gastric hypersecretion in this syndrome. McGavran et al.[57] reported on a glucagon-secreting alpha-cell carcinoma of the pancreas. The primary neoplasm contained large amounts of glucagon, the hyperglycemic-glycogenolitic hormone of the alpha cells.

Diagnosis
Clinical examination

Carcinomas of the *head* of the pancreas are usually easily diagnosed by the progressive, obstinate, unrelenting jaundice that is generally accompanied by pain and profound weight loss. The laboratory findings all give evidence of complete biliary obstruction with acholia, a rising icterus index, and large amounts of bilirubin in the urine. The liver is frequently palpable and rather smooth. The gallbladder is enlarged in a high percentage of patients.

No mass is felt in the region of the pancreas. When obstructive jaundice and pain, digestive disturbances, and rapid weight loss occur in a male about 60 years of age, carcinoma of the head of the pancreas should be strongly suspected.

Carcinomas of the *body* and *tail* of the pancreas are rarely diagnosed before surgical exploration or necropsy. In Duff's group[24] of nineteen cases, none was diagnosed. Jaundice is practically never present in carcinoma of the body of the pancreas except terminally. In about one-half of the patients, a palpable tumor mass is present in the subumbilical region or in the region of the left hypochondrium. It is hard, is quite sharply limited, and gives an impression of resistance. If it is fixed to the vertebral column, it may be adherent to large vessels and may therefore pulsate. In carcinoma of both the body and the tail, excruciating pain is often present. Occasionally, pain is provoked by abdominal palpation. Careful questioning concerning the type of pain may give information that will suggest involvement of the celiac plexus. Thrombophlebitis may suggest the diagnosis. In eight of twenty-one patients with carcinoma of the body and carcinoma of the body and tail of the pancreas, a definite bruit was heard in the left hypochondrium that was caused by compression of the splenic artery by tumor (Serebro[83]).

Carcinoma of the body or tail of the pancreas should be suspected in men between 40 and 60 years of age with a palpable tumor mass in the epigastrium, extreme weight loss, pain, and peripheral venous thrombi. Persistent diarrhea with abdominal pain is also suggestive of pancreatic neoplasm (Dashiell and Palmer[22]).

Roentgenologic examination

To determine the presence of a neoplasm of the head and body of the pancreas, an upper gastrointestinal tract barium study is the most rewarding single approach (Mani et al.[60]). The most important changes are those observed *radioscopically* in the stomach and duodenum (Fig. 444) during the passage of barium. In most instances, these changes may be recorded radiographically after careful choice of position, compression, etc. Some

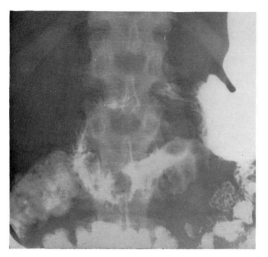

Fig. 444. Widening of loop of duodenum with extensive mucosal destruction and irregularity of third portion of duodenum due to invasion by carcinoma of pancreas.

authors advocate a routine examination of the opacified stomach in six different orientations (Beranbaum[8]). Retroperitoneal insufflation combined with tomography (Fig. 445) has been advocated (Frimann-Dahl[34]). Exact localization of the pancreatic tumor may be possible through arteriographic studies (Lunderquist[56]). The arteriogram may reveal displacement or invasion of vessels or the presence of tumor vessels (Fig. 446). Selective celiac and superior mesenteric arteriography may be useful in identifying carcinoma (Meaney et al.[61]). However, a negative angiogram does not exclude the possibility of carcinoma (Ranniger and Saldino[78]).

Beeler[6] reported on a study of seventy cases of carcinoma of the pancreas that were diagnosed roentgenologically. The most frequent changes observed were deformity, narrowing, obstruction, ulceration,

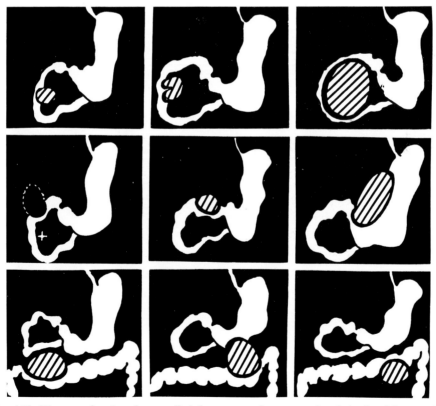

Fig. 445. Diagram showing that small defects occur first on inside of duodenal loop and in pyloric region. These defects caused by cancer can probably be diagnosed before patient develops jaundice. Larger indentations of stomach and colon represent tumors of body and can be cancer (usually inoperable), cyst, or pseudocyst. (From Frimann-Dahl, J.: Radiology in tumours of the pancreas, Clin. Radiol. **12:**73-79, 1961.)

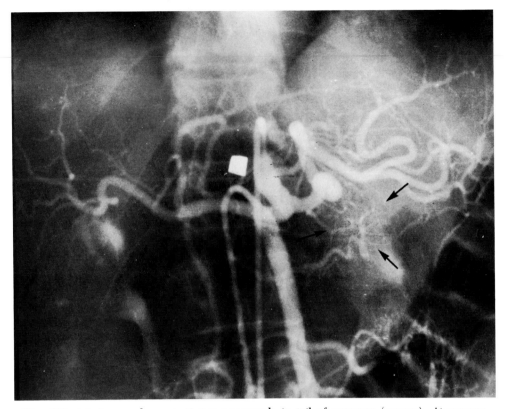

Fig. 446. Arteriogram demonstrating tumor vessels in tail of pancreas (arrows). At surgery, carcinoma 2.5 cm in diameter was found. (From Ranniger, K., and Saldino, R. M.: Arteriographic diagnosis of pancreatic lesions, Radiology **86:**470-474, 1966.)

and filling defect of the duodenum. Less frequently, gastric deformities, filling defects, and dilatation were noted. The pancreatic tumor may become sufficiently large to cause obvious widening of the duodenal loop, or it may become palpable, but many of the earlier signs can be elicited or discovered only through astute observation during radioscopy and special maneuvers:

1 The *"padding sign" of the stomach* may be observed under gentle pressure, in horizontal position, betraying a mass behind the stomach.

2 *Flattening of the duodenal folds* in the medial aspect of the descending portion of the duodenum results from distention and infiltration of the bowel wall.

3 An *"inverted three sign"* is sometimes observed due to enlargement of the pancreas around the ampulla of Vater.

4 A *compression of the duodenum,* caused by the dilatation of the common duct, may also be visible.

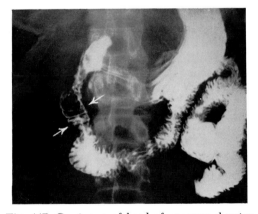

Fig. 447. Carcinoma of head of pancreas showing "pad" effect on stomach (arrows). (Courtesy Dr. Philip J. Hodes, Philadelphia, Pa.)

5 Direct or indirect signs of *duodenal obstruction* may be observed.

6 Direct or indirect signs of *gastric compression* may be visible (Fig. 447).

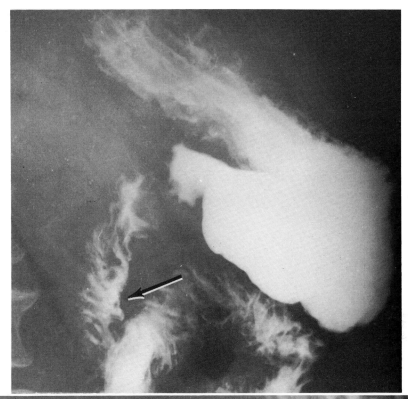

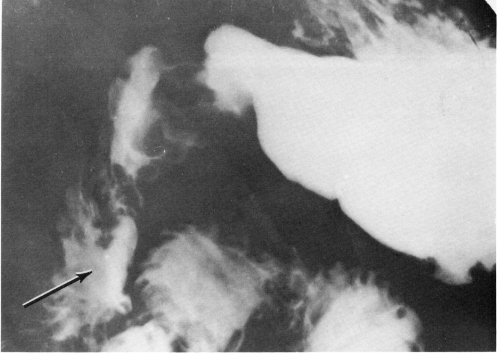

Fig. 448. Disruption of mucosa with several areas of ulceration in second portion of duodenum (arrows). Specimen showed large carcinoma of pancreas invading duodenum and ampulla of Vater, with ulceration of duodenum. (From Perez, C. A., et al.: Roentgenologic-pathologic correlation of resectable carcinoma of the pancreatico-duodenal region, Amer. J. Roentgen. **94**: 438-448, 1965; WU negs. 57-4306 and 57-4035.)

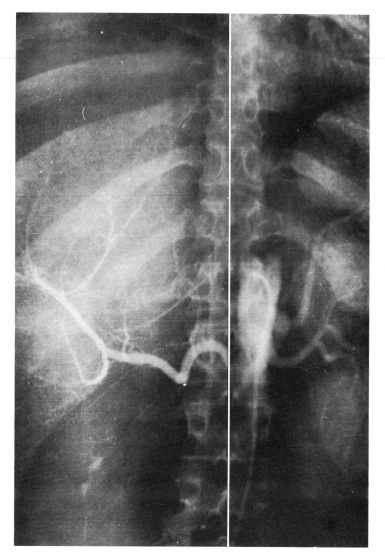

Fig. 449. Celiac arteriogram showing distortion of branches of hepatic artery about tumor masses in right lobe of liver. In later phase of arteriogram, tumor stain is seen in tail of pancreas. The tumor is fed chiefly by splenic and gastric arteries. (From McGavran, M. H., et al.: A glucagon-secreting alpha-cell carcinoma of the pancreas, New Eng. J. Med. **274:** 1408-1413, 1966; WU negs. 65-8582 and 65-8583.)

Ulceration of the duodenal mucosa and intraluminal mass is most often seen in carcinoma of the papilla of Vater (Perez et al.[74]) (Fig. 448).

Unless ulceration of the duodenum is demonstrated, the radiographic diagnosis of carcinoma of the head of the pancreas is uncertain. Pancreatic calcification is common in cases of alcoholism and of pancreatitis. In 677 patients with pancreatic calcification, twenty-four had coexisting pancreatic carcinoma (Johnson and Zintel[45]). Pancreatic cystadenomas may be suspected roentgenologically because of the calcification (Haukohl and Melamed[42]). In Swanson's case,[88] the angiographic findings localized the tumor and displayed its extremely vascular nature. In the islet cell carcinoma described by McGavran et al.,[57] selective arteriography localized the

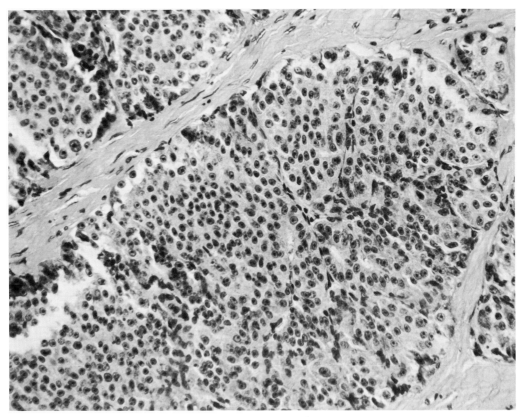

Fig. 450. Primary islet cell carcinoma showing lobular and acinar arrangement of uniform cells with large oval nuclei and prominent nucleoli. Well-vascularized connective tissue stroma surrounds nests of cells. (Hematoxylin and eosin stain; ×300; from McGavran, M. H., et al.: A glucagon-secreting alpha-cell carcinoma of the pancreas, New Eng. J. Med. **274:**1408-1413, 1966; WU neg. 65-8440A.)

neoplasm (Figs. 449 and 450). Madsen[58] has summarized angiography in pancreatic tumors of islet cell origin.

Laboratory examination

The laboratory findings in carcinoma of the *head* of the pancreas all give evidence of complete biliary obstruction. The icterus index constantly increases. Bile is prominent in the urine but absent in the stools. Urobilinogen is absent in the urine. At times, there may be blood in the stool from ulceration of some part of the gastrointestinal tract. There may be increased tendency to intestinal hemorrhage because of liver damage. The tests of external pancreatic function are important and should include a determination of pancreatic ferment activity (amylase, protease, and lipase) and a quantitative estimation of fat

absorption (Bauman[4]). Johnson reported on thirty patients, sixteen of whom showed elevation of the serum lipase. Hyperglycemia developing during the course of carcinoma of the pancreas occurs in from 13% to 25% of patients (Gullick[39]).

True diabetes, when present, develops in patients with tumors of the pancreatic tail in which islets are most prominent. Exfoliative cytology studies can be done, and a diagnosis of malignant cells can be obtained in some instances. Raskin et al.[80] recovered malignant cells in twenty-eight of forty-three cases of pancreatic, biliary, and duodenal carcinoma. The procedure is aided by the intravenous injection of secretin (Wenger and Raskin[95]).

In *islet cell tumors*, the evidence of origin can be substantiated by a positive assay for insulin in either the primary tumor or its metastasis. Of the twenty-one cases reported by Hanno and Banks,[41] in only three instances was the assay successful. Wilder et al.[98] made the first report. Plasma insulin immunoassay is valuable in islet cell tumors since, with prolonged fasting, there should be practically no measurable serum insulin except in the presence of an islet cell tumor (Williams et al.[98a]). The fasting blood sugar level must be 50 mg/100 ml or less during an attack, and the symptoms should be promptly alleviated by the administration of glucose by vein or mouth. The blood sugar level after a fast of twelve to fifteen hours is more reliable than the glucose tolerance curve, which is more a liver function than a pancreatic function test (Whipple[96]). Disorders of the suprarenal glands, anterior lobe of the pituitary gland, liver, thyroid gland, and thalamus, in which hypoglycemia may also occur, must be ruled out. The islet cells of the pancreas elaborate several hormones (Demling and Ollenjann[23]) and can certainly produce secretin (Zollinger et al.[103]), glucagon (McGavran et al.[57]), serotonin (van der Veer et al.[90]), and gastrin (Gregory et al.[38]).

The diagnosis of carcinoma of the pancreas is often difficult at the time of exploratory laparotomy. Chronic pancreatitis fixes the lobules, and palpation reveals a hard mass that can easily be mistaken for carcinoma. It must be remembered that the operative mortality for the radical operation for carcinoma of the head of the pancreas is high (25% to 40%), and there are few patients cured of carcinoma of the head of the pancreas. It is granted that a few surgeons can do this procedure with a much lower mortality.

In view of the high operative mortality and the difficulty of cure, we feel that the surgeon must have a positive histologic diagnosis before doing this radical procedure. There are many pitfalls for the pathologist, for chronic pancreatitis may greatly distort pancreatic lobules, and excretory ducts running through the wall of the duodenum may be mistaken for cancer. The surgeon may not take the biopsy from the right area, and no cancer will be identified. We do frozen section diagnosis on all lesions in which one-stage Whipple procedure is contemplated, and the operation is not done without positive biopsy. Our

accuracy rate is 91% (Spjut and Ramos[86]) with all of our errors on the false negative side. We have also utilized needle biopsy with frozen section to make a diagnosis. This type of procedure will reduce the chance of implantation (Coté et al.[19]).

Differential diagnosis

The differential diagnosis of carcinoma of the pancreas often concerns *common duct obstruction due to stone, chronic pancreatitis,* or other *carcinomas of the periampullary region.*

The assessment of certain laboratory findings may be of very great differential value. It is of particular importance to determine whether the obstruction is complete. This can be determined by repeated examinations of the stools for the presence of bile and repeated examinations of the urine for the presence of urobilin. If urobilin and bile are constantly absent, then the obstruction must be complete. The duodenal contents should be aspirated and assayed for the presence of bile pigment and pancreatic ferments. Some of the information that can be gained by laboratory examinations of the duodenal contents is summarized in Table 44. In numerous instances, however, in spite of the most careful clinical and roentgenologic examination, differentiation may be resolved only by a prompt exploration. *Common duct lithiasis* may exactly mimic carcinoma of the head of the pancreas. Usually, however, the patients are younger and have a previous history of attacks of acute colicky pain, the biliary obstruction is not complete, and weight loss and weakness are not so pronounced as in carcinoma of the pancreas.

Further points of differentiation have been shown by Zollinger and Kevorkian[102] (Table 45). Dilatation of the gallbladder is present in a high percentage of patients with carcinoma, whereas the gallbladder is practically never dilated in the presence of a biliary lithiasis, even when the common bile duct is obstructed by a calculus. Courvoisier[20] explains this by recalling that in cases of lithiasis, obstruction is invariably preceded by an inflammatory process which scleroses the vicinity of the biliary tract and renders it less distensible. Dila-

Table 44. Differential diagnosis of carcinoma of pancreas and other conditions

	Carcinoma of head of pancreas	*Carcinoma of ampulla*	*Carcinoma of common bile duct*	*Obstruction of common bile duct due to stone*
Bile in duodenal contents	Usually absent	Intermittently present	Usually absent	Intermittently present
Blood	Invariably absent	Frequently present	Invariably absent	Usually absent
Pancreatic ferments	Invariably absent	Invariably absent or greatly diminished	Invariably present	Invariably present
Gallbladder	Usually enlarged	Usually enlarged	Usually enlarged	Usually normal size
Roentgenologic examination	Occasional displacement of stomach and invasion of duodenum, widening of its loop	May show filling defect	No useful findings	15% of stones radiopaque

Table 45. Differential characteristics of common duct stone and carcinoma of head of pancreas*

Symptom or finding	*Common duct stone in 75 cases (%)*	*Carcinoma of head of pancreas in 49 cases (%)*
Males	13	69
Females	87	31
Past history suggesting gallbladder disease	100	18
Colicky pain	91	16
Referred to dorsal region	67	18
Weight loss	25	86
Jaundice	81	86
Intermittent	35	12
Vomiting	77	37
Chills	33	8
Enlarged gallbladder	12	55
Enlarged liver	25	80

*From Zollinger, R., and Kevorkian, A. Y.: Surgical aspects of obstructive jaundice, New Eng. J. Med. **221:**486-488, 1939.

tation of the gallbladder is not present in about 15% of the patients with carcinoma of the head of the pancreas because of concomitant gallstones. Conversely, in relatively rare instances the gallbladder may be dilated when cystic duct obstruction from stone also compresses the common duct (Brunschwig[13]).

Chronic pancreatitis is a disease entity in which the clinical symptoms and laboratory examination may strongly suggest a carcinoma of the head of the pancreas. This similarity may not be resolved even at the time of surgical exploration, for the firmness of the pancreas due to inflammation may be easily mistaken for carcinoma. If the region is biopsied and frozen section done, this may show chronic inflammation. Conversely, a negative biopsy of the pan-

creas does not always rule out the presence of carcinoma. There have been numerous cases reported in which the short-circuiting operations performed for a supposed carcinoma of the head of the pancreas have resulted in complete and permanent disappearance of symptoms.

Usually intrinsic liver disease, particularly differential *viral hepatitis*, which occurs in younger individuals, is not a difficult differential diagnosis. Biliary obstruction is intermittent, and the patients tend to improve spontaneously. Other *carcinomas of the periampullary region* can produce almost all the findings that are present in carcinoma of the head of the pancreas. Their differentiation will be detailed in discussions on carcinoma of the gallbladder and extrahepatic ducts later in this chapter. However, exact differentiation is only of academic interest, for surgical treatment is the same in both lesions.

The extreme pain that is present in carcinoma of the body of the pancreas is often confused with that of other painful lesions such as *intercostal neuralgia, diaphragmatic pleurisy,* and *renal calculus* (Levy and Lichtman[52]). It may even suggest a tabetic crisis. If, however, profound weight loss with peripheral venous thrombi is present together with a palpable epigastric mass, this should strongly suggest carcinoma of the pancreas. We have seen a case in which secondary implantation had occurred on the serosal surface of the large bowel and signs suggesting a primary large bowel tumor were present.

Metastases to the pancreas from primary lesions elsewhere are relatively infrequent. They occur in about 5% of carcinomas of the lung and in widely disseminating tumors such as the malignant melanoma.

Neoplastic cysts of the pancreas are extremely rare. Becker et al.[5] collected 115 cases of cystadenoma of the pancreas, a rare, benign, slow-growing tumor arising usually in the body or tail. It occurs usually in young or middle-aged women. Diabetes is present in about three of five patients with such cysts (Bowers et al.[12]), and there is quite frequently a history of disease of the biliary tract. Examination usually shows a rounded mass in the upper portion of the abdomen. Roentgenograms may reveal displacement of the colon downward with displacement of the stomach medially (Bowers et al.[12]) (Fig. 451). At times, intravenous pyelograms may reveal poor function of the left kidney because of pressure by the cyst on the renal veins or artery.

Pseudocysts, or collections of fluid in the peripancreatic tissues of the lesser omental sac, may cause displacements of neighboring organs which in the roentgenogram may suggest a pancreatic tumor or cyst. They are not accompanied by glycosuria (Meyer et al.[62]).

The most difficult problem in the differential diagnosis of islet cell tumors of the pancreas is that offered by spontaneous hypoglycemia. A blood sugar level under 50 mg/100 ml on prolonged fasting is,

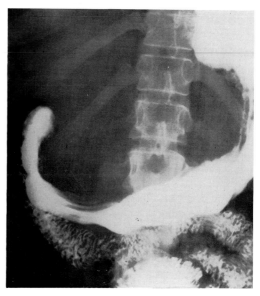

Fig. 451. Displacement of wall of stomach by enormous benign cyst of pancreas. Defect in wall of stomach has smooth margins. There is also displacement of duodenum and colon.

however, strong evidence in favor of tumor (Perkins et al.[75]).

Treatment
Surgery

Surgical resection for carcinoma of the head of the pancreas has been perfected during the past two decades. This formidable procedure requires meticulous preoperative and postoperative care and a surgeon of outstanding ability. Unfortunately, the patients are often extremely poor operative risks.

We agree with Porter[76] that before doing one-stage Whipple procedures a careful search must be made for disease outside the zone of proposed resection, and appropriate material must be submitted for frozen section. *It is unfortunate that the number of patients suitable for this radical operation remains small.* Practically all patients when first seen are inoperable because of extension of carcinoma or because liver damage and other metabolic changes have become irreversible, making operative risk prohibitive. Because of the sparsity of cures of carcinoma of the pancreas and the high operative mortality, it has even been proposed by some surgeons that this operation be abandoned (Crile[20a]). However, in spite of the meager yield, this operation should continue to be used by the experienced surgeon, for occasional cures are now being reported. It should be stressed that the patient with a questionable carcinoma of the head of the pancreas should not be observed over a long period of time while the diagnosis is being modified but rather should be explored promptly while the lesion may still be resectable. At the present time the one-stage Whipple operation seems to be most popular and logical. It eliminates the dangers of two anesthesias and two major procedures.

Almost none of the patients with carcinoma of the *body* of the pancreas are operable because when diagnosed, extensive metastases invariably are present. The mass is made up mainly of metastatic lymph nodes. Brunschwig[14] reported on six patients in whom he resected the body of the pancreas with splenectomy. There are only isolated reports of cures of carcinoma of the body and tail of the pancreas.

In *islet cell tumors*, exploration is indicated. If an adenoma is found, it should be resected. Very careful exploration may not reveal an adenoma, and the surgeon convinced of the clinical syndrome may do a subtotal removal of the pancreas. At the subsequent careful pathologic examination of the specimen, tumor may be found, hyperplasia of the islet cells may exist, or the pancreas may be normal. It should be remembered that symptoms may continue after removal of an adenoma because adenomas tend to be multiple, and reexploration may be necessary. At times, symptoms may be due to adenomatosis of islet cells (Frantz[32]). It is remotely possible that hypoglycemic symptoms may be caused by pathologic alterations in an aberrant pancreas. In the patient with the Zollinger-Ellison syndrome, there is about a 60% chance that the tumor is malignant. *Scintograms* may be done preoperatively if it is thought that liver metastases are present. If the tumor, at operation, is resectable and there is no evidence of distant disease, then only surgical resection is indicated. However, if the tumor is unresectable or if there are metastases beyond the possibility of removal, then resection must be combined with total gastric resection in order to rid the patient of gastric

hypersecretion. This radical approach is well indicated because a malignant islet cell tumor may have an extremely long clinical evolution even in the presence of metastases (Kernen et al.[49]). Furthermore, patients with the Zollinger-Ellison syndrome have to be followed because of the possibility of pluriglandular involvement of other organs. This would include the pituitary, parathyroid, and adrenal glands. Moreover, this syndrome may be familial.

The operative mortality of pancreatoduodenectomies is relatively high. Waugh[94] reported a mortality rate of 21%. Cattell and Pyrtek[16] reported on a reduction of mortality from 18.5% to 7.3% in two series of cases. It must be remembered that the operative mortalities quoted are by the surgeons experienced in pancreatic surgery. The well-trained surgeon who has done few radical pancreatoduodenectomies will have an operative mortality that may be double or triple that quoted.

Radiotherapy

Billingsley et al.[9] reported on a series of thirteen cases of carcinoma of the pancreas that were irradiated with cobalt[60] and concluded that the patients received no appreciable palliative benefit. In another series of ninety-one patients, all of whom had been explored prior to irradiation, the average survival was 6.6 months. In 10% of the patients, the palliative results were considered excellent, mostly through relief of pain and decrease of jaundice (Miller and Fuller[65]).

Prognosis

In 1965, there were in the United States 16,002 deaths from carcinoma of the pancreas, a crude death rate of 8.3 per 100,000 population. There seems to have been an increase in death rate in the past two decades. About 90% of the untreated patients die within a year. Among those resected, few survive (Newton[71]). Glenn and Thorbjarnarson[37] emphasized that the surgical treatment of *carcinoma of the pancreas* is, in most instances, only palliative. Surgical procedures for relief of the obstruction of the common duct, duodenum, and pancreatic duct alleviate symptoms but do not prolong life. In a total of 564 cases of proved carcinoma of the pancreas

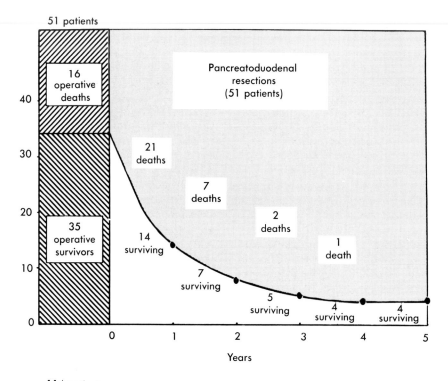

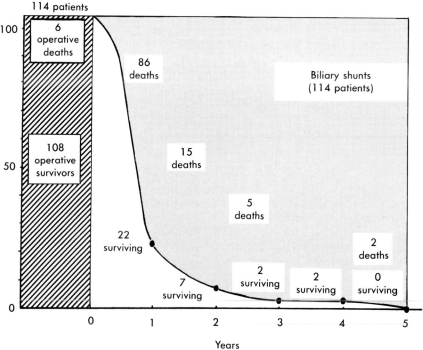

Fig. 452. Carcinoma of head of pancreas. Comparative survival curves in fifty-one patients undergoing pancreatoduodenectomy and 114 patients undergoing biliary shunts only. (From Bowden, L., et al.: Carcinoma of the head of the pancreas, Amer. J. Surg. 109:578-582, 1965.)

seen over a ten-year period at several hospitals in Portland, Oregon, only 5% of the patients underwent a resection with an aim to cure and only two patients survived resection and lived five years without evidence of tumor (Neilson et al.[70]). Klintrup[50] reviewed 1556 cases. Radical operation could be performed in only 2%, and only one patient survived five years. Bowden et al.[11] reviewed 190 patients with carcinoma of the head of the pancreas studied at the Memorial Hospital in New York: 114 of the patients had biliary shunts and none lived five years, and fifty-one underwent a pancreatodudenal resection and four survived five years (Fig. 452). Mongé et al.[66] reviewed 119 patients of carcinoma of the head of the pancreas seen at the Mayo Clinic. Four of sixty-four patients who had pancreatoduodenectomy survived five years. In a series of 134 patients with pancreatic carcinoma seen at the M. D. Anderson Hospital, three survived over five years—two had islet cell carcinomas and the other one died of cancer after six years (Gallitano et al.[35]). Morris and Nardi[69] recorded 121 patients with carcinomas of the head of the pancreas, twenty-six of whom had surgical resections, with fifteen surviving the operation and two surviving over eight years. Contrary to these gloomy results, the infrequent bulky *cystadenocarcinoma* of the pancreas can be treated with a hope of cure. Cullen et al.[21] reported seven patients surviving out of eleven operated upon. Warren and Hardy[91] reported on seventeen patients with cystadenocarcinoma, seven of whom had a resection with good results.

Carcinomas of the pancreas often extend along the ducts and involve contiguous structures and lymph nodes. Frequently, even though the margin appears adequate at the operation, a recurrence follows because of microscopic extension beyond the line of transection. Tumor may be present in the nerve sheaths, in the resected end of the common duct, or in invading vessels. Even though resection appears adequate, a high percentage of the patients have metastases beyond the scope of the operation, within the liver or lungs. Patients surviving the operation are capable of maintaining a satisfactory nutritional status with the help of special diets.

Patients with benign islet cell adenomas do well following excision, although diabetes may persist. Islet cell carcinomas may have a slow course. Whipple[97] reported an instance of five-year survival, but the patient developed a nodular liver in the sixth year (Parson[73]). The cure rates in patients with the Zollinger-Ellison syndrome depend upon whether the tumor is benign or malignant. In the group with malignant tumors, there is an appreciable five-year survival (over 50%), but this, of course, does not mean cure.

REFERENCES

1 Anlyan, W. G., Shingleton, W. W., and DeLaughter, G. D., Jr.: Significance of idiopathic venous thrombosis and hidden cancer, J.A.M.A. **161**:964-966, 1956.

2 Arkin, A., and Weisberg, S. W.: Carcinoma of the pancreas; a clinical and pathologic study of seventy-five cases, Gastroenterology **13**:118-126, 1949.

2a Arlen, M., and Brockunier, A.: Clinical manifestations of carcinoma of the tail of the pancreas, Cancer **20**:1920-1923, 1967.

3 Bartels, P.: Ueber die Lymphgefässe des Pankreas. II. Das feinere Verhalten der lymphatischen Verbindungen zwischen Pankreas und Duodenum, Arch. Anat. Entwcklngsgesch. pp. 250-287, 1906.

4 Bauman, L.: Tests of the external pancreatic function. In Nelson Loose-leaf medicine, New York, 1945, Thomas Nelson & Sons, chap. XXVI-A, pp. 547-553.

5 Becker, W. F., Welsh, R. A., and Pratt, H. S.: Cystadenoma and cystadenocarcinoma of the pancreas, Ann. Surg. **161**:845-863, 1965.

6 Beeler, J. W.: Roentgenologic findings accompanying carcinoma of the pancreas, Amer. J. Roentgen. **67**:576-584, 1952.

7 Bell, E. T.: Carcinoma of the pancreas. I. A clinical and pathologic study of 609 necropsied cases. II. The relation of carcinoma of the pancreas to diabetes mellitus, Amer. J. Path. **33**:499-523, 1957.

8 Beranbaum, S. L.: Carcinoma of the pancreas: a bi-directional roentgen approach, Amer. J. Roentgen. **96**:447-467, 1966.

9 Billingsley, J. S., Bartholomew, L. G., and Childs, D. S., Jr.: A study of radiation therapy in carcinoma of the pancreas, Proc. Staff Meet. Mayo Clin. **33**:426-430, 1958.

10 Birnbaum, D., and Kleeberg, J.: Carcinoma of the pancreas; a clinical study based on 84 cases, Ann. Intern. Med. **48**:1171-1184, 1958.

11 Bowden, L., McNeer, G., and Pack, G. T.: Carcinoma of the head of the pancreas, Amer. J. Surg. **109**:578-582, 1965.

12 Bowers, R. F., Lord, J. W., and McSwain, Barton: Cystadenoma of the pancreas; re-

port of five cases, Arch. Surg. (Chicago) **45**:111-122, 1942.

13 Brunschwig, A.: The surgery of pancreatic tumors, St. Louis, 1942, The C. V. Mosby Co.

14 Brunschwig, A.: Results of pancreatoduodenectomy, Cancer **2**:763-766, 1949.

15 de Castro Barbosa, J. J., Dockerty, M. B., and Waugh, J. M.: Pancreatic heterotopia, Surg. Gynec. Obstet. **82**:527-542, 1946.

16 Cattell, R. B., and Pyrtek, L. J.: An appraisal of pancreatoduodenal resection; a follow-up study of 61 cases, Ann. Surg. **129**:840-849, 1940.

17 Chauffard, A.: Le cancer du corps du pancreas, Bull. Acad. Med. (Paris) **60**:242-255, 1908.

18 Christoforidis, A. J., and Nelson, S. W.: Radiological manifestations of ulcerogenic tumors of the pancreas, J.A.M.A. **198**:511-516, 1966.

19 Coté, J., Dockerty, M. B., and Priestley, J. T.: An evaluation of pancreatic biopsy with the Vim-Silverman needle, Arch. Surg. (Chicago) **79**:588-596, 1959.

20 Courvoisier; quoted by Oberling, C., and Guerin, M.: Cancer du pancreas, Paris, 1931, Gaston Doin.

20a Crile, G., Jr.: The advantages of bypass operations over radical pancreatoduodenectomy in the treatment of pancreatic carcinoma, Surg. Gynec. Obstet. **130**:1049-1053, 1970.

21 Cullen, P. K., Jr., ReMine, W. H., and Dahlin, D. C.: A clinicopathological study of cystadenocarcinoma of the pancreas, Surg. Gynec. Obstet. **117**:189-195, 1963.

22 Dashiell, G. F., and Palmer, W. L.: Carcinoma of the pancreas, Arch. Intern. Med. (Chicago) **81**:173-183, 1948.

23 Demling, L., and Ottenjann, R.: Non-insulin producing tumors of the pancreas, Stuttgart, 1969, Georg Thieme (excellent review monograph).

24 Duff, G. L.: The clinical and pathological features of carcinoma of the body and tail of the pancreas, Bull. Hopkins Hosp. **65**:69-100, 1939.

25 Duff, G. L.: The pathology of islet cell tumors of pancreas, Amer. J. Med. Sci. **203**:437-451, 1942.

26 Ellison, E. H.: The ulcerogenic tumor of the pancreas, Surgery **40**:147-170, 1956.

27 Ellison, E. H., and Wilson, S. D.: The Zollinger-Ellison syndrome; re-appraisal and evaluation of 260 registered cases, Ann. Surg. **160**:512-530, 1964 (extensive bibliography).

28 Engel, A., and Lysholm, E.: A new roentgenological method of pancreas examination and its practical results, Acta Radiol. (Stockholm) **15**:635-651, 1934.

29 Evans, B. P., and Ochsner, A.: The gross anatomy of the lymphatics of the human pancreas, Surgery **36**:177-191, 1954.

30 Fonkalsrud, E. W., Dilley, R. B., and Longmire, W. P.: Insulin secreting tumors of the pancreas, Ann. Surg. **159**:730-736, 1964.

31 Frantz, V. K.: Tumors of islet cells with hyperinsulinism, benign, malignant, and questionable, Ann. Surg. **112**:161-176, 1940.

32 Frantz, V. K.: Adenomatosis of islet cells, with hyperinsulinism, Ann. Surg. **119**:824-844, 1944.

33 Franz, V. K.: Tumors of the pancreas. In Atlas of tumor pathology, Sect. VII, Fascs. 27 and 28, Washington, D. C., 1959, Armed Forces Institute of Pathology.

34 Frimann-Dahl, J.: Radiology in tumours of the pancreas, Clin. Radiol. **12**:73-79, 1961.

35 Gallitano, A., Fransen, H., and Martin, R. G.: Carcinoma of the pancreas; results of treatment, Cancer **22**:939-944, 1968.

36 Gillman, T., Gillman, C., and Gilbert, C.: Observations on the etiology of cancer of the liver; symposium on geographical pathology and demography of cancer; published under the auspices of the World Health Organization, 1950.

37 Glenn, F., and Thorbjarnarson, B.: Carcinoma of the pancreas, Ann. Surg. **159**:945-958, 1964.

38 Gregory, R. A., Tracy, H. J., French, J. M., and Sircus, W.: Extraction of a gastrin-like substance from a pancreatic tumour in a case of Zollinger-Ellison syndrome, Lancet **1**:1045-1048, 1960.

39 Gullick, H. D.: Carcinoma of the pancreas; a review and critical study of 100 cases, Medicine (Balt.) **38**:47-84, 1959 (extensive bibliography).

40 Hallwright, G. P., North, K. A. K., and Reid, J. D.: Pigmentation and Cushing's syndrome due to malignant tumor of the pancreas, J. Clin. Endocr. **24**:496-500, 1964.

41 Hanno, H. A., and Banks, R. W.: Islet cell carcinoma of pancreas, with metastasis, Ann. Surg. **117**:437-449, 1943.

42 Haukohl, R. S., and Melamed, A.: Cystadenoma of pancreas, Amer. J. Roentgen. **63**:334-345, 1952.

43 Holm, O. F.: Ueber den Wert der Röntgenuntersuchung des Pankreas, Acta Radiol. (Stockholm) **22**:620-642, 1941.

44 Howard, J. M., and Rhoads, J. E.: Hyperinsulinism and islet-cell tumors of the pancreas, Int. Abstr. Surg. **90**:417-455, 1950 (extensive bibliography).

45 Johnson, J. R., and Zintel, H. A.: Pancreatic calcification and cancer of the pancreas, Surg. Gynec. Obstet. **117**:585-588, 1963.

46 Jordan, G. L.: Surgical management of carcinoma of the pancreas and periampullary region, Amer. J. Surg. **107**:313-316, 1964.

47 Kaplan, N., and Angrist, A.: The mechanism of jaundice in cancer of the pancreas, Surg. Gynec. Obstet. **77**:199-204, 1943.

48 Kenney, W. E.: The association of carcinoma in the body and tail of the pancreas with multiple venous thrombi, Surgery **14**:600-609, 1943.

49 Kernen, J. A., Scofield, G., Koucky, C., Benitez, R. E., and Ackerman, L. V.: Long survival with islet cell carcinoma of the pancreas, Amer. J. Clin. Path. **39**:137-141, 1963.

50 Klintrup, H. E.: Carcinoma of the pancreas;

a statistical, clinical and pathological study, Acta Chir. Scand. 362(suppl.):1-96, 1966.

51 Leven, N. L.: Primary carcinoma of the pancreas, Amer. J. Cancer 18:852-874, 1933.

52 Levy, H., and Lichtman, S. S.: Clinical characterization of primary carcinoma of the body and tail of the pancreas, Arch. Intern. Med. (Chicago) 65:607-626, 1940.

53 Lieberman, J. S., Borrero, J., Urdaneta, E., and Wright, I. S.: Thrombophlebitis and cancer, J.A.M.A. 177:542-545, 1961.

54 Lisa, J. R., Trinidad, S., and Rosenblatt, M. B.: Pulmonary manifestations of carcinoma of the pancreas, Cancer 17:395-401, 1964.

55 Lopez-Kruger, R., and Dockerty, M. B.: Tumors of the islets of Langerhans, Surg. Gynec. Obstet. 85:495-511, 1947.

56 Lunderquist, A.: Angiography in carcinoma of the pancreas, Acta Radiol. [Diagn.] (Stockholm) 235(suppl.):1-143, 1965.

57 McGavran, M. H., Unger, R. H., Recant, L., Polk, H. C., Kilo, C., and Levin, M. E.: A glucagon-secreting alpha-cell carcinoma of the pancreas, New Eng. J. Med. 274:1408-1413, 1966.

58 Madsen, B.: Demonstration of pancreatic insulomas by angiography, Brit. J. Radiol. 39:488-493, 1966.

59 Malamud, N., and Grosh, L.: Hyperinsulinism and cerebral changes, Arch. Intern. Med. (Chicago) 61:579-599, 1938.

60 Mani, J. R., Zboralske, F. F., and Margulis, A. R.: Carcinoma of the body and tail of the pancreas, Amer. J. Roentgen. 96:429-446, 1966.

61 Meaney, T. F., Winkelman, E. I., Sullivan, B. H., and Brown, C. H.: Selective splanchnic arteriography in the diagnosis of pancreatic tumors, Cleveland Clin. Quart. 30:193-197, 1963.

62 Meyer, K. A., Sheridan, A. I., and Murphy, R. F.: Pseudocysts of the pancreas; report of 31 cases, Surg. Gynec. Obstet. 88:219-229, 1949.

63 Mikal, S., and Campbell, A. J. A.: Carcinoma of the pancreas; diagnostic and operative criteria based on one hundred consecutive autopsies, Surgery 28:963-969, 1950.

64 Miller, J. R., Baggenstoss, A. H., and Comfort, M. W.: Carcinoma of the pancreas; effect of histological type and grade of malignancy on its behavior, Cancer 4:233-241, 1951.

65 Miller, T. R., and Fuller, L. M.: Radiation therapy of carcinoma of the pancreas, Amer. J. Roentgen. 80:787-792, 1958.

66 Mongé, J. J., Judd, E. S., and Gage, R. P.: Radical pancreatoduodenectomy; a 22-year experience with the complications, mortality rate and survival rate, Ann. Surg. 160:711-722, 1964.

67 Moore, F. T., Murat, J. E., Endahl, G. L., Baker, J. L., and Zollinger, R. M.: Diagnosis of ulcerogenic tumor of the pancreas by bioassay, Amer. J. Surg. 113:735-737, 1967.

68 Morgagni; quoted by Oberling, C., and

Querin, M.: Cancer du pancreas, Paris, 1931, Gaston Doin.

69 Morris, P. J., and Nardi, G. L.: Pancreaticoduodenal cancer; experience from 1951 to 1960 with a look ahead and behind, Arch. Surg. (Chicago) 92:834-837, 1966.

70 Neilson, R. O., Grout, J. G., Groshong, L. E., Remer, W. C., Marcum, R. W., Dennis, D. L., and Foster, J. H.: A ten-year experience with carcinoma of the pancreas, Arch. Surg. (Chicago) 94:322-325, 1967.

71 Newton, W. T.: Mortality and morbidity associated with resection of pancreaticoduodenal cancers, Amer. Surg. 27:74-79, 1961.

72 Oberling, C., and Guerin, M.: Cancer du pancreas, Paris, 1931, Gaston Doin.

73 Parson, W. B.: Radical operations on the head of the pancreas, Surg. Clin. N. Amer. 27:356-359, 1950.

74 Perez, C. A., Powers, W. E., Holtz, S., and Spjut, H. J.: Roentgenologic-pathologic correlation of resectable carcinoma of the pancreatico-duodenal region, Amer. J. Roentgen. 94:438-448, 1965.

75 Perkins, H. A., Desforges, J. F., and Guttas, C. G.: Adenoma of the islands of Langerhans; its differentiation from functional hypoglycemia, New Eng. J. Med. 243:281-285, 1950.

76 Porter, M. R.: Carcinoma of the pancreaticoduodenal area; operability and choice of procedure, Ann. Surg. 148:711-723, 1958.

77 Priestley, J. T., Comfort, M. W., and Sprague, R. G.: Total pancreatectomy for hyperinsulinism due to islet-cell adenoma; follow-up report five and one-half years after operation including metabolic studies, Ann. Surg. 130:211-217, 1949.

78 Ranniger, K., and Saldino, R. M.: Arteriographic diagnosis of pancreatic lesions, Radiology 86:470-474, 1966.

79 Ransom, H. K.: Carcinoma of the body and tail of the pancreas, Arch. Surg. (Chicago) 30:584-606, 1935.

80 Raskin, H. F., Wenger, J., Sklar, M., Pleticka, S., and Yarema, W.: The diagnosis of cancer of the pancreas, biliary tract, and duodenum by combined cytologic and secretory methods, Gastroenterology 34:996-1008, 1958.

81 Sallick, M. A., and Garlock, J. H.: Obstructive jaundice due to carcinoma of the pancreas; the choice of operative procedure, Ann. Surg. 115:25-31, 1942.

82 Sanders, R. L., and Porter, C. H.: Palliative operations for carcinoma of the pancreas, Southern Surg. 15:383-392, 1949.

83 Serebro, H.: A diagnostic sign of carcinoma of the body of the pancreas, Lancet 1:85-86, 1965.

84 Soloway, H. B.: Constitutional abnormalities associated with pancreatic cystadenomas, Cancer 18:1297-1300, 1965.

85 Soloway, H. B., and Sommers, S. C.: Endocrinopathy associated with pancreatic carcinomas; review of host factors including hyperplasia and gonadotropic activity, Ann. Surg. 164:300-304, 1966.

86 Spjut, H. J., and Ramos, A. J.: An evaluation of biopsy-frozen section of the ampullary region and pancreas; a report of 68 consecutive patients, Ann. Surg. **146:**923-930, 1957.

87 Sproul, E. E.: Carcinoma and venous thrombosis; the frequency of association of the carcinoma in the body or tail of the pancreas with multiple venous thrombosis, Amer. J. Cancer **34:**566-585, 1938.

88 Swanson, G. E.: A case of cystadenoma of the pancreas studied by selective angiography, Radiology **81:**592-595, 1963.

89 Ulett, G., and Parsons, E. H.: Psychiatric aspects of carcinoma of the pancreas, J. Missouri Med. Ass. **45:**490-493, 1948.

90 van der Veer, J. S., Choufoer, J. C., Zuerido, A., van der Heul, R. O., Hollander, C. F., and van Rijssel, T. G.: Metastasizing islet cell tumor of the pancreas associated with hypoglycemia and carcinoid syndrome, Lancet **1:**1416-1419, 1964.

91 Warren, K. W., and Hardy, K. J.: Cystadenocarcinoma of the pancreas, Surg. Gynec. Obstet. **127:**734-736, 1968.

92 Warren, S.: Adenomas of the islands of Langerhans, Amer. J. Path. **2:**335-340, 1926.

93 Wauchope, G. M.: Critical review; hypoglycaemia, Quart. J. Med. **2:**117-156, 1933.

94 Waugh, J. M.: Personal communication, 1951.

95 Wenger, J., and Raskin, H. F.: The diagnosis of cancer of the pancreas, biliary tract and duodenum by combined cytologic and secretory methods, Gastroenterology **34:**1009-1017.

96 Whipple, A. O.: Present-day surgery of the pancreas, New Eng. J. Med. **226:**513-526, 1942.

97 Whipple, A. O.: Pancreaticoduodenectomy for islet carcinoma, Ann. Surg. **121:**847-852, 1945.

98 Wilder, R. M., Allan, F. N., Power, M. H., and Robertson, H. E.: Carcinoma of the islands of the pancreas, J.A.M.A. **89:**348-355, 1927.

98a Williams, C., Jr., Bryson, G. H., and Hume, D. M.: Islet cell tumors and hypoglycemia, Ann. Surg. **169:**757-773, 1969.

99 Young, E. L., Jr.: Pancreatic cyst, New Eng. J. Med. **216:**334-339, 1937.

100 Zollinger, R. M., and Ellison, E. H.: Primary peptic ulcerations of the jejunum associated with islet cell tumors of the pancreas, Ann. Surg. **142:**709-728, 1955.

101 Zollinger, R. M., and Grant, G. N.: Ulcerogenic tumor of the pancreas, J.A.M.A. **190:**181-184, 1964.

102 Zollinger, R., and Kevorkian, A. Y.: Surgical aspects of obstructive jaundice, New Eng. J. Med. **221:**486-488, 1939.

103 Zollinger, R. M., Tompkins, R. K., Amerson, J. R., Endahl, G. L., Kraft, A. R., and Moore, F. T.: Identification of the diarrheogenic hormone associated with non-beta islet cell tumors of the pancreas, Ann. Surg. **168:**502-521, 1968.

Liver

Anatomy

The liver occupies an extraperitoneal and subdiaphragmatic position on the right side of the upper abdomen. It is divided into a right and a left lobe. The caudate lobes are subdivisions of the right main lobe. The right kidney, right suprarenal gland, right colic flexure, and proximal duodenum all bear a close relationship to the inferior surface of the liver. The biliary secretion is transmitted from the left and caudate lobes to the left hepatic duct and from the right and quadrate lobes to the right hepatic duct.

Lymphatics. The *superficial* lymphatics of the liver arise from the superficial lobules and go directly to the periphery and travel beneath the peritoneum. Some of them enter the suspensory coronary and triangular ligaments, pass through the diaphragm, and end in the pericardial nodes and those of the posterior mediastinum. Others follow the direction of the esophagus and descend to end in the nodes of the coronary chain. Still others follow the lower aspect of the liver to end in the nodes of the hepatic pedicle and the inferior vena cava (Fig. 453). The *deep* lymphatics arise from deep lobules and follow the trajectory of the portal and suprahepatic veins, or they may pass through the diaphragm to end in the supradiaphragmatic nodes. Others follow the course of the portal vein branches, receive the lymphatics of the biliary tree, and end in the nodes of the hepatic pedicle, hepatic artery, or coronary chain. A few of the deep lymphatics may end in the juxta-aortic nodes neighboring the renal arteries (Rouvière[58]).

Epidemiology

Primary carcinoma of the liver is rare in the United States. In the 1947 cancer survey, the total sex-age adjusted incidence (including biliary passages) was 8.34 per 100,000 population. The incidence in the United States is lower for blacks than for whites (Dorn[15]). The actual age-adjusted 1947 incidence for whites was 7.2 and 8.6 for males and females, whereas it was 6.7 and 4.7 for male and female non-whites per 100,000. In Los Angeles, the

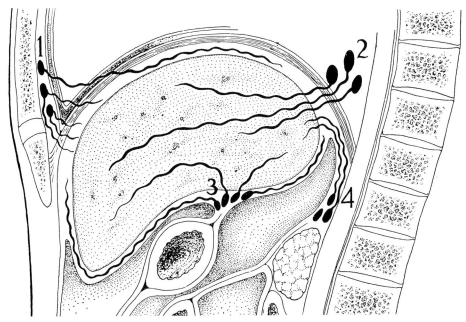

Fig. 453. Superficial and deep lymphatics of liver leading to pericardial nodes, **1**; juxtaphrenic nodes of posterior mediastinum, **2**; nodes of hepatic pedicle, inferior vena cava, and hepatic artery, **3**; nodes of coronary chain and renal arteries, **4**.

occurrence of cancer of the liver is higher among Japanese and Filipinos than among whites (Edmondson and Steiner[16]). The incidence increases to reach its maximum in the eighth and ninth decades of life. The incidence appears to be low in Latin America (Lopez-Corella et al.[42]).

Berman[9] observed a high occurrence of primary cancer of the liver among Bantus of South Africa. In male Bantus under 45 years of age, half of all cancer arises in the liver (Oettlé[54]). The highest incidence of primary carcinoma of the liver occurs in Portuguese East Africa (Torres[72]). Bergeret[8] reported 135 cases of primary cancer of the liver observed at the Hôpital Central Indigène of Dakar between 1939 and 1945, while only ninety-nine other cases of cancer were observed during the same period. The incidence of cancer of the liver in some Asian countries seems to be also in disproportion with that observed in Western Europe and the American continent. Snijders and Straub[65] found that almost one of every five cases of cancer among natives of Java was hepatic carcinoma. The occurrence is higher among Chinese who live in Java (Kouwenaar[37]).

The occurrence is higher also among immigrant than among indigenous Chinese in Singapore (Shanmugaratnam[63]).

Primary carcinomas of the liver are commonly associated with cirrhosis, and this relationship has been long debated. It seems now certain that carcinoma is associated with the postnecrotic and posthepatitic types of cirrhosis but not with the nutritional type (Sagebiel et al.[59]). If cirrhosis is present with carcinoma in the Bantu, it is of the postnecrotic type (Higginson[28]; Steiner and Davies[69]). In the United States, it is also associated with postnecrotic cirrhosis (MacDonald[43]; Gall[20]; Miyai and Ruebner[47]). However, autopsies done on 167 Bantu patients, revealed that 47% had no cirrhosis (Geddes and Falkson[21]).

Carcinomas of the bile duct cell type are only infrequently associated with cirrhosis and rarely arise on the basis of congenital cysts (Willis[74]). However, following longstanding inflammation, fibrosis, cholelithiasis, etc., carcinoma may develop. According to Steiner,[67] the occurrence of cholangiocellular carcinomas (bile duct carcinomas) is the same throughout the world, except where it is increased by liver flukes. Hou[30] theorized that 15% of all primary carcinomas observed in Hong Kong are caused by *Clonorchis sinensis.* Thorotrast, used for diagnostic purposes, may result in cancer of the liver after considerable time (Batzenschlager et al.[5]). The types of tumors observed following its use include malignant vascular neoplasms as well as hepatomas (Kuisk et al.[38]).

Isaacson[33] noted how rarely Bantu patients with postnecrotic cirrhosis gave a history of previous jaundice. He was also impressed by a report of Miyake et al.[48] of a high frequency of toxic liver injuries and liver cirrhosis in mice and rats after long-term feeding with rice contaminated with *Penicillium islandicum.* This suggested that contamination of maize (a diet staple of the Bantu) by a mycotoxin might be a factor in the etiology of postnecrotic cirrhosis and hepatoma. Such toxins, particularly aflatoxin, have caused the deaths of turkeys, trout, and bears with liver necrosis and, at times, with hepatomas. The sequential morphologic changes produced by aflatoxin B_1 in the rat liver hepatoma have been described by Newberne and Wogan.[52] Oettlé[55] has demonstrated that there is major contamination of maize in Africa. He indicates that the hypothesis of mycotoxicosis fits the distribution of cancer of the liver—it would account for its rarity in the dry areas where mold spoilage is minimal. Alpert et al.[3] emphasize that the highest incidence of hepatoma appears in countries where there is poverty, food scarcity, or a tropical climate. All these factors tend to increase the amount of fungal contamination of food. If this theory is confirmed throughout the world, a substantial proportion of cancer of the liver may be prevented.

Pathology
Gross pathology

Tumors arising from the liver may form a large, single nodule (Fig. 454) but very frequently have satellite tumor nodules around them (Fig. 455). Another form presents a diffuse nodulation throughout the organ, usually with evidence of coexisting cirrhosis. There may be evidence of collateral circulation, portal obstruction with ascites, esophageal varices, and splenic enlargement. For the most part, the liver itself is enlarged. In fifty-one cases reported by Berman,[9] the average weight of the liver was around 4000 gm, and the right lobe was found to be most frequently invaded. Gross evidence of blood vessel invasion is seen frequently, and it is not unusual to find evidence of invasion of the vena cava. Tumor thrombosis of the inferior vena cava and of the right auricle may occur (Gregory[24]). Direct invasion of the diaphragm, gallbladder, and pleura sometimes occurs, and sometimes there is involvement of the mesentery and the peritoneum.

The liver is very often the site of metastatic disease. This is due, for the most part, to the abundant vascular supply to the liver from the widely ramifying portal system and from the hepatic artery. The portal system drains the pancreas, large bowel, and stomach and also has numerous anastomoses with the caval system. Tumors that develop in the lung, whether primary or metastatic, easily break into the branches of the pulmonary veins and from there to the heart, where they pass to the systemic circulation and eventually to the hepatic artery and liver. Other tumors, such as cancer of the breast, may reach the liver through the lymphatics, and still others, such as carcinoma of the stomach, may invade the liver directly. The liver also seems to be a very fertile soil for the growth of tumors of all types, which probably enhances the frequent finding of metastatic tumor there.

In metastatic carcinoma, the liver itself is tremendously enlarged. This is particularly true of a metastatic melanocarcinoma, which may weigh as much as 10 kg. It should be remembered, however, that the liver can be extensively seeded with metastases and yet weigh within normal limits. The metastatic nodules of the liver are usually spherical and are often seen bulging beneath a tense elevated capsule. These metastatic nodules will vary somewhat in appearance according to their vascularity and connective tissue content. Their size will vary from a few millimeters to that of an entire lobe. As they increase in size, secondary changes with hemorrhage and central necrosis occur, giving the nodulation a typical umbilicated ap-

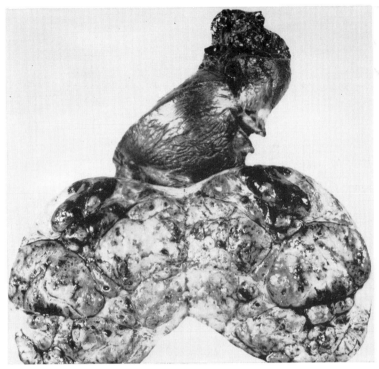

Fig. 454. Well-encapsulated and pedunculated adenoma of liver. Patient, 63-year-old woman, was well over ten years after operation.

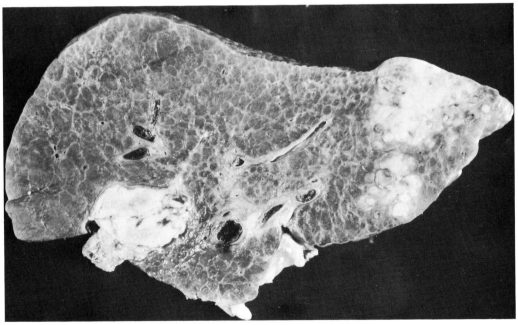

Fig. 455. Classic primary hepatoma of liver occurring in Bantu with portal vein thrombosis by tumor. (Courtesy Dr. J. Murray, Johannesburg, R.S.A.; SA neg. 5179.)

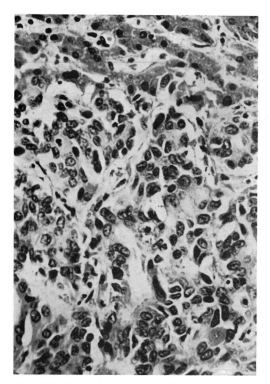

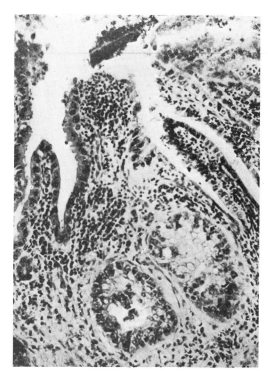

Fig. 456. Primary carcinoma of liver cell type. Note extreme anaplasia and bizarre forms. (Moderate enlargement.)

Fig. 457. Bile duct type of adenocarcinoma of liver. Note dilated duct with carcinoma originating from it. (From Sanes, S., and MacCallum, J. D.: Primary carcinoma of the liver; cholangioma in hepatolithiasis, Amer. J. Path. **18**:675-687, 1942.)

pearance. With the growth of the tumor, compression and destruction of contiguous liver parenchyma occur. Not infrequently, tumor will be found in the branches of the portal vein. Metastatic carcinoma of the liver is found more frequently than metastatic sarcoma of the liver. Sarcomas as a group are more cellular and softer and, therefore, more readily subjected to degenerative changes.

Microscopic pathology

Primary carcinomas of the liver are classified broadly as hepatocellular and cholangiocellular carcinomas. There is frequently great variation in the microscopic pathology of the tumors of the liver cell type (Fig. 456), whereas the bile duct cell type has a more uniform pattern (Loesch[41]) (Fig. 457). There is usually a well-developed capillary stroma in the liver cell type that is absent in the bile duct cell variety. The liver cell variety frequently

produces bile that may be present in the metastases as well as in the primary tumor (Steiner[67]). Bile secretion is not usually found in the bile duct carcinomas, but at times bile pigment is present within the lumina of the small bile ducts (Winternitz[75]).

The consensus is that primary carcinomas of the liver are unicentric rather than multicentric and that the reason for the apparent multiplicity of lesions is readily explained because of the early distribution of tumor through the blood vessels.

Metastatic spread

Because of the tendency of carcinoma of the liver to invade the hepatic and portal veins, the tumor easily migrates to the heart and thence to the lungs. There were pulmonary metastases in 89% of the cases of primary carcinoma of the liver reported by Berman.[9] Other sites of metastatic involvement are the hilar, portal, mesenteric, and retroperitoneal nodes, the heart, the brain, and the skeletal system (Berman[9]).

Clinical evolution

About two-thirds of all carcinomas of the liver have a clinical onset characterized by indefinite abdominal symptoms usually attributed to gastric disturbances (Berman[9]). Nausea and vomiting may be present with a sense of fullness and abdominal pressure in the epigastrium. Constipation occurs rather frequently. Pain is generally present in the form of a dull ache, frequently localized to the right hypochondrium. It becomes more severe as the disease progresses but bears no relation to digestion. The increase of pain is explained by the progressive distention of the liver capsule or invasion of the diaphragm. When jaundice is present, it is usually minimal. Anemia and esthenia are remarkably constant and alarmingly progressive. Weight loss is observed in most patients but may be obscured by the presence of ascites or edema. Dyspnea occurs as a late symptom and is usually related to ascites, anemia, and pulmonary metastases. Hematemesis due to esophageal varices or invasion of the stomach may also be observed in advanced disease.

The liver is invariably enlarged, particularly the right lobe, and occasionally the total growth may be outlined from week to week. There may be a dilatation of the superficial veins of the chest and the abdomen preceded by edema of the lower extremities. The dilatation probably occurs because hepatic invasion by tumor interferes with the portal circulation as an important collateral return (Gregory[24]).

About one-third of all carcinomas of the liver present an exceptional clinical onset, but they may be found only at autopsy. Berman[9] described an acute abdominal type characterized by intraperitoneal hemorrhage. In some of his patients there was a febrile onset that often suggested a liver abscess. Not infrequently, hypoglycemia may be observed (Imperato and Lipton[32]), at times leading to convulsions (Thompson and Hilferty[71]). A Cushing's syndrome may be present in patients with primary carcinoma of the liver. In a case reported by Burmeister et al.,[11] a biological assay of the tumor revealed the presence of ACTH. A number of other associated changes have been observed: precocious puberty with circulating gonadotropin (Hung et al.[31]), virilization (Behrle et al.[6]), and congenital defects (Fraumeni et al.[19]). Polycythemia has been found in association with carcinoma of the liver (Nakao et al.[50]). Four of the patients reported by Geddes and Falkson[21] had thrombocytopenic purpura.

Diagnosis

Because carcinoma of the liver is comparatively rare in this hemisphere, the clinician is often reluctant to diagnose it, and the disease may develop for several months before a diagnosis is established. In pediatric practice, the overwhelming majority of patients with primary carcinoma of the liver are under 2 years of age.

Examination invariably reveals an enlarged tender liver, and if there is coexisting cirrhosis, there may be ascites, edema, evidence of circulatory changes, and hematemesis. The ascitic fluid is quite frequently blood-tinged, and it is not too infrequent for carcinomas of the liver to produce fatal hemorrhage. Rarely, in the presence of evident thrombosis of the inferior vena cava, there is a sudden increase of edema of the extremities and in the size and tenderness of the liver, accompanied by orthopnea and increasing venous pressure. These changes should be interpreted as evidence of a tumor thrombosis of the right auricle (Gregory[24]).

Roentgenologic examination

A roentgenogram is of value in establishing evidence of deformity of the liver and invasion of the diaphragm. The radioscopic examination furnishes information as to the fixation of the right side of the diaphragm. In certain instances, due to tumor emboli, there may be extremely prominent vascular markings seen by roentgenographic examination of the chest. The heart, however, will be normal in size. Primary malignant tumors of the liver can be identified in infants and children by rather simple roentgen studies (Margulis et al.[45]).

Arteriography can be used to determine the extent of the primary tumor and to facilitate the planning of adequate surgery

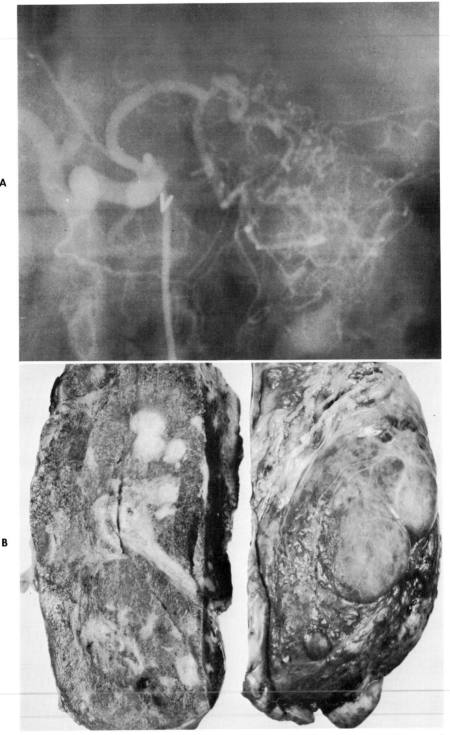

Fig. 458. A, Arteriogram of liver demonstrating numerous, large, anastomosing vessels in 63-year-old man. Nature of tumor could not be determined. **B,** Grossly, it proved to be large benign vascular tumor of left lobe measuring 15 cm × 10 cm × 4 cm. (**A,** WU neg. 68-8254; **B,** WU neg. 68-8099.)

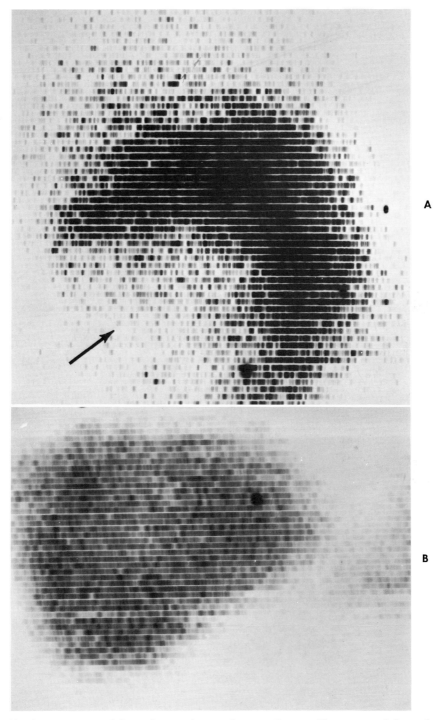

Fig. 459. A, Scintigram of liver showing large 15 cm × 18 cm cold area caused by malignant tumor. Right hepatic lobectomy was performed. **B,** Scintigram taken six months later shows almost complete regeneration of lobe. (From Dillard, B. M.: Experience with twenty-six hepatic lobectomies and extensive hepatic resections, Surg. Gynec. Obstet. **129:**249-257, 1969; by permission of Surgery, Gynecology & Obstetrics; **A,** WU neg. 68-5185; **B,** WU neg. 68-5183.)

(Yu[77]) (Fig. 458). Boijsen and Abrams[10] utilized the celiac axis and the **superior** mesenteric arteries. Arteriography may also be found helpful in the differential diagnosis of benign vascular tumors.

Photoscanning of the liver after injection of radioactive isotopes may prove helpful in the identification of primary or metastatic neoplasms of the liver (Fig. 459). Combined scanning utilizing iodine[131], rose bengal, and gold[198] provides useful information (Ariel[4]). A nonfunctioning mass within an enlarged liver may be due to a primary hepatic carcinoma but, in order to be so recognized, a mass must be larger than 2 cm (Zubovskiĭ[78]). Achaval et al.[1] found iodine[131] and rose bengal to be diagnostic in twenty-three of thirty-six cases.

Laboratory examination

An extensive replacement of the liver parenchyma has to occur before there is any significant measurable impairment of hepatic function, and for this reason most liver function tests are of little or no value in the diagnosis of primary carcinoma of the liver. The cephalin cholesterol test may be negative in patients with carcinoma of the liver without cirrhosis; this negative finding is of value in the differential diagnosis. In patients with primary carcinoma of the liver, the serum bilirubin is only slightly elevated, but there is high alkaline phosphatase activity together with an increase in the transaminase levels (Saragoça et al.[61]). The liver function tests reflect biliary tree obstruction with associated hepatocellular injury (San Jose et al.[60]). Alpha-feto-protein is present in the serum in about three-fourths of all patients with primary carcinoma of the liver. This protein has a striking tendency to change only slightly during the course of the disease. This test appears to be specific (Purves et al.[57]). False positives, for all practical purposes, do not occur. *Therefore, if the results are positive, the patient has a primary carcinoma of the liver.*

Biopsy

A needle biopsy, particularly when nodules are felt beneath the anterior abdominal wall, may be of definite value. When the procedure is successful, it easily solves the problem of diagnosis and treatment. When the pathologic process is localized, positive needle biopsy may be difficult to obtain.

Differential diagnosis

A *metastatic carcinoma* of the liver is considerably more frequently found than a primary tumor, and for this reason the first effort should always be to eliminate this probability. The liver is often the site of metastases from primary tumors of the stomach, bowel, endometrium, lung, and breast. Melanomas of the skin and eye also frequently metastasize to, and considerably enlarge, the liver. Particular attention consequently should be paid to the history of suspicious nevi or enucleations of the eye that might appear irrelevant in the history of the patient. At times, an exploration of the abdomen may be necessary to establish a definite diagnosis.

Cirrhosis of the liver may be mistaken for carcinoma, but the cirrhotic liver is usually small instead of large, and a long history of gastrointestinal difficulties is usually given. In *hemochromatosis,* the liver may be indurated and nodular, and, if sudden improvement of the diabetes (even hypoglycemic intervals), accompanied by fever, anemia, leukocytosis, and weight loss, occurs, the coexistence of a primary carcinoma of the liver should be strongly suspected. Benz and Baggenstoss[7] reported a number of cases of what he designated as *focal cirrhosis.* This lesion has been called by many names and probably represents a focal area of cirrhosis with evidence of regeneration. These lesions were all described at necropsy, but we have seen three cases at the time of surgery, all three of which were incorrectly identified by the surgeon as metastatic cancer.

If a tumor is localized to, and apparently primary in, the liver, it may be difficult to determine whether it is benign or malignant (Malt et al.[44a]). A single movable, nontender mass that causes vague gastrointestinal disturbances in a patient in good general condition is usually a benign lesion. However, if there are systemic symptoms, with anemia, weight loss, and hard, often multiple, tender masses, a malignant tumor probably is present. Roentgenologic study and an exploratory laparotomy may be necessary to establish a diagnosis.

Hydatid cysts of the liver may cause enlargement and suggest the possibility of a tumor. A good number of these cysts become calcified, and their diagnosis is thus simplified (Schlanger and Schlanger[62]). Small hemangiomas of the liver are usually discovered as incidental findings in the course of abdominal surgery. Henson et al.[27] reported thirty-five cases of hemangioma of the liver, twenty-four of which were incidental findings, and only one showed calcification. Eleven of the thirty-five cases presented as palpable masses. Ten of those were found in women. Large vascular benign tumors of the liver may be resected (Greville[25]). Hemangiomas of the liver rarely are associated with heart failure (Winters et al.[76]), probably because of vascular shunts. Mesenchymal hamartoma of the liver is a benign tumor seen in children under 2 years of age. It is made up of fibrous tissue and of multiple cysts probably of bile duct origin (Ishida et al.[34]).

Treatment and prognosis

Carcinoma of the liver can be cured only by a surgical excision, and this is possible only when the lesion is so localized that it can be removed (Flanagan and Foster[18]). The excision does not appreciably impair the functional capacity of the liver, which has a tremendous reserve. The regenerative capacity has been well demonstrated experimentally and clinically (Fig. 459). Ch'eng-en and Kuo-ts'ai[12] explored 336 patients with primary carcinoma of the liver and were able to resect 130 of the lesions with an operative mortality of 25%. Forty-three patients survived over six months and two for more than five years. Primary carcinoma of the liver in children is often a large neoplasm not associated with cirrhosis. It does not metastasize early and, therefore, can often be resected with a hope of cure (Nixon[53]). When carcinoma is associated with cirrhosis, however, failure of treatment is certain. A poor prognosis is also associated with a high gamma globulin

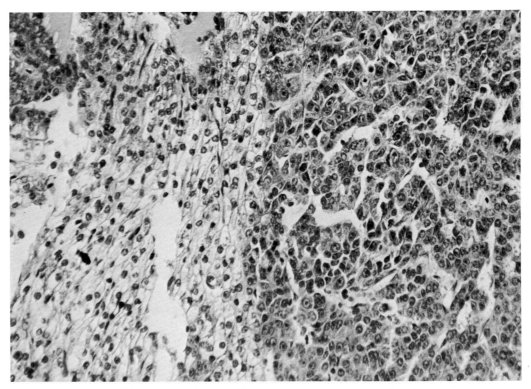

Fig. 460. Hepatoblastoma in 7-month-old infant. Tumor was resected and patient remains well three and one-half years later. (×300; courtesy Dr. Tien-Yu Lin, Taipei, Taiwan; WU neg. 68-10947.)

level and rising SGOT (serum glutamic ox-aloacetic transaminase) and SGPT (serum glutamic pyruvic transaminase) levels (Geddes and Falkson[21]). Fish and McCary[17] collected thirty-seven cases in which the patients survived the operation, with seven living over five years. Lin et al.[40] reported on twenty-one infants and children, six of whom were treated by lobectomy, with one surviving three and one-half years (Fig. 460). Modlin et al.[49] reported a postoperative survival rate of seventeen years. Children with hepatoblastoma have a better prognosis than those with hepatocellular carcinoma (Ishak and Glunz[35]).

Nelson et al.[51] employed 5-fluorouracil, Thio-TEPA, and other chemotherapeutic agents in twenty-one patients with some appreciable effect but no significant difference in results. Watkins and Khazei[73] utilized continuous infusion of antimetabolites in the treatment of advanced cancer of the liver, with temporary regressions and appreciable clinical benefit. In their therapeutic trial series, Geddes and Falkson[21] reported that intrahepatic artery infusion by methotrexate gives the best palliation.

In a series of cases of carcinoma of the liver reported by Gustafson,[26] the average course from the first symptom to death was 3.2 months, the average duration being longer in the bile duct cell type of tumor than in the liver cell type.

REFERENCES

1 Achaval, A., Tauxe, W. M., and Gambill, E. E.: Scintillation scanning of the liver, Mayo Clin. Proc. **40**:206-215, 1965.
2 Alagille, D., Borde, J., Le Tan Vinh, Gubler, J. P., Cochard, A. M., and Wucher, R.: Vascular tumors of the liver in babies; an anatomical-clinical classification based on 6 personal observations, Rev. Int. Hepat. **16**:71-125, 1966.
3 Alpert, M. E., Hutt, M. S. R., and Davidson, C. S.: Hepatoma in Uganda, Lancet **1**:1265-1267, 1968.
4 Ariel, I. M.: An aid for determining treatment of liver cancer by combined hepatic gamma-scanning, Surg. Gynec. Obstet. **121**:267-274, 1965.
5 Batzenschlager, A., Weill-Bousson, M., and Mandard, A. M.: Cancers hépatiques et biliaires par thorotrastose hépato-ganglionnaire, Arch. Anat. Path. (Paris) **15**:295-300, 1967.
6 Behrle, F. C., Mantz, F. A., Jr., Olson, R. L., and Trombold, J. C.: Virilization accompany-

ing hepatoblastoma, Pediatrics **32**:265-271, 1963.
7 Benz, E. J., and Baggenstoss, A. H.: Focal cirrhosis; its relation to the so-called hamartoma, Cancer **6**:743-755, 1953.
8 Bergeret, C.: Le cancer primitif du foie à l'Hôpital Central Indigène de Dakar, Bull. Med. Afr. Occid. Fr. **3**:9-11, 1946.
9 Berman, C.: Primary carcinoma of the liver; a study in incidence, clinical manifestations, pathology and etiology, London, 1951, H. K. Lewis & Co., Ltd.
10 Boijsen, E., and Abrams, H. L.: Roentgenologic diagnosis of primary carcinoma of the liver, Acta Radiol. [Diagn.] (Stockholm) **3**: 257-277, 1965.
11 Burmeister, P., Bianchi, L., Klietmann, W., and Torhorst, J.: Paraneoplastisches Cushing-Syndrom bei primärem Leberkarzinom, Deutsch. Med. Wschr. **93**:164-165, 1968.
12 Ch'eng-en, W., and Kuo-ts'ai, L.: Surgical treatment of primary carcinoma of liver, Chin. Med. J. (Peking) **82**:65-78, 1963.
13 Davies, J. N. P.: The pathology of carcinoma of the liver, Leech **27**:11-15, 1958.
14 Dillard, B. M.: Experience with twenty-six hepatic lobectomies and extensive hepatic resections, Surg. Gynec. Obstet. **129**:249-257, 1969.
15 Dorn, H. F.: Cancer of the liver, infectious hepatitis and cirrhosis of the liver in the United States, Acta Un. Int. Cancr. **13**:573-578, 1957.
16 Edmondson, H. A., and Steiner, P. E.: Primary carcinoma of the liver, Cancer **7**:462-503, 1954.
17 Fish, J. C., and McCary, R. G.: Primary cancer of the liver in childhood, Arch. Surg. (Chicago) **93**:355-359, 1966.
18 Flanagan, L., Jr., and Foster, J. H.: Hepatic resection for metastatic cancer, Amer. J. Surg. **113**:551-557, 1967.
19 Fraumeni, J. F., Jr., Miller, R. W., and Hill, J. A.: Primary carcinoma of the liver in childhood; an epidemiologic study, J. Nat. Cancer Inst. **40**:1087-1099, 1968.
20 Gall, E. A.: Primary and metastatic carcinoma of the liver; relationship to hepatic cirrhosis, Arch. Path. (Chicago) **70**:226-232, 1960.
21 Geddes, E. W., and Falkson, G.: Malignant hepatoma in the Bantu, Cancer **25**:1271-1278, 1970.
22 Gillman, J., and Payet, M.: Primary cancer of the liver, Acta Un. Int. Cancr. **13**:860-873, 1957.
23 Gillman, T., Gillman, C., and Gilbert, C.: Observations on the etiology of cancer of the liver; symposium on geographical pathology and demography of cancer; published under the auspices of the World Health Organization, 1950.
24 Gregory, R.: Primary carcinoma of the liver; tumor thrombosis of the inferior vena cava and right auricle, Arch. Intern. Med. (Chicago) **64**:566-578, 1939.
25 Greville, Y. A.: Large haemangioma of the liver, Brit. J. Surg. **51**:505-510, 1964.

26 Gustafson, E. G.: An analysis of 62 cases of primary carcinoma of the liver based on 24,000 necropsies at Bellevue Hospital, Ann. Intern. Med. 11:889-900, 1937.

27 Henson, S. W., Jr., Gray, H. K., and Dockerty, M. B.: Benign tumors of the liver. II. Hemangiomas, Surg. Gynec. Obstet. 103:3217-3231, 1956.

28 Higginson, J.: Primary carcinoma of the liver in Africa, Brit. J. Cancer 10:609-622, 1956.

29 Higginson, J.: Pathogenesis of liver cancer in the Johannesburg area (South Africa), Acta Un. Int. Cancr. 13:590-598, 1957.

30 Hou, P. C.: The relationship between primary carcinoma of the liver and infestation with Clonorchis Sinensis, J. Path. Bact. 72:239-246, 1956.

31 Hung, W., Blizzard, R. M., Migeon, C. J., Camacho, A. M., and Nyhan, W. L.: Precocious puberty in a boy with hepatoma and circulating gonadotropin, J. Pediat. 63:895-903, 1963.

32 Imperato, P. J., and Lipton, M. S.: Hypoglycemia in primary carcinoma of liver, New York J. Med. 65:2707-2710, 1965.

33 Isaacson, C.: The aetiology of cirrhosis and hepatoma in the Bantu—an appraisal, S. Afr. Med. J. 40:11-13, 1966.

34 Ishida, M., Tsuchida, Y., Saito, S., and Sawaguchi, S.: Mesenchymal hamartoma of the liver, Ann. Surg. 164:175-182, 1966.

35 Ishak, K. G., and Glunz, P. R.: Hepatoblastoma and hepatocarcinoma in infancy and childhood, Cancer 20:396-422, 1967.

36 Johnson, P. M., and Grossman, F. M.: Radioisotope scanning in primary carcinoma of the liver, Radiology 84:868-872, 1965.

37 Kouwenaar, W.: On cancer incidence in Indonesia; symposium on geographical pathology and demography of cancer; published under the auspices of the World Health Organization, 1950.

38 Kuisk, H., Sanchez, J. S., and Mizuno, N. S.: Colloidal thorium dioxide (thorotrast) in radiology with emphasis on hepatic cancerogenesis, Amer. J. Roentgen. 99:463-475, 1967.

39 Lawrence, G. H., Gauman, D., Lasersohn, J., and Baker, J. W.: Primary carcinoma of the liver, Amer. J. Surg. 112:200-210, 1966.

40 Lin, T.-Y., Chen, C.-C., and Liu, W.-P.: Primary carcinoma of the liver in infancy and childhood, Surgery 60:1275-1281, 1966.

41 Loesch, J.: Primary carcinoma of the liver, Arch. Path. (Chicago) 28:223-235, 1939.

42 Lopez-Corella, E., Ridaura-Sanz, C., and Albores-Saavedra, J.: Primary carcinoma of the liver in Mexican adults, Cancer 22:678-685, 1968.

43 MacDonald, R. A.: Cirrhosis and primary carcinoma of the liver, New Eng. J. Med. 255:1179-1183, 1956.

44 McFadzean, A. J. S., Todd, David, and Tsang, K. C.: Polycythemia in primary carcinoma of the liver, Blood 8:427-435, 1958.

44a Malt, R. A., Hershberg, R. A., and Miller, W. L.: Experience with benign tumors of the liver, Surg. Gynec. Obstet. 130:285-291, 1970.

45 Margulis, A. R., Nice, C. M., Jr., and Rigler, L. G.: The roentgen findings in primary hepatoma in infants and children; an analysis of eleven cases, Radiology 66:809-816, 1956.

46 Misugi, K., Okajima, H., Misugi, N., and Newton, W. A., Jr.: Classification of primary malignant tumors of liver in infancy and childhood, Cancer 20:1760-1771, 1967.

47 Miyai, K., and Ruebner, B. H.: Acute yellow atrophy, cirrhosis, and hepatoma, Arch. Path. (Chicago) 75:609-617, 1963.

48 Miyake, M., Saito, M., Enomoto, M., Shikato, T., Ishiko, T., Uraguchi, K., Sakai, F., Tatsuno, T., Tsukioka, M., and Sakai, Y.: Toxic liver injuries and liver cirrhosis induced in mice and rats through long term feeding with Penicillium islandicum Sopp—growing rice, Acta Path. Jap. 10:75-123, 1966.

49 Modlin, J. J., Perez-Mesa, C. M., Johnson, R. E., and Yeager, H.: Long term survival in carcinoma of the liver; case report, Missouri Med. 64:985-987, 1967.

50 Nakao, K., Kimura, K., Miura Y., and Takaku, F.: Erythrocytosis associated with carcinoma of the liver (with erythropoietin assay of tumor extract), Amer. J. Med. Sci. 251:161-165, 1966.

51 Nelson, R. S., de Elizalde, R., and Howe, C. D.: Clinical aspects of primary carcinoma of the liver, Cancer 19:533-537, 1966.

52 Newberne, P. M., and Wogan, G. M.: Sequential morphologic changes in aflatoxin B carcinogenesis in the rat, Cancer Res. 28:770-781, 1968.

53 Nixon, H. H.: Hepatic tumours in childhood and their treatment by major hepatic resection, Arch. Dis. Child. 40:169-172, 1965.

54 Oettlé, A. G.: The incidence of primary carcinoma of the liver in the southern Bantu, I. Critical review of the literature, J. Nat. Cancer Inst. 17:249-287, 1956.

55 Oettlé, A. G.: The aetiology of primary carcinoma of the liver in Africa; a critical appraisal of previous ideas with an outline of the mycotoxin hypothesis, S. Afr. Med. J. 39:817-825, 1965.

56 Peden, J. C., Jr., and Blalock, W. N.: Right hepatic lobectomy for metastatic carcinoma of the large bowel, Cancer 16:1133-1140, 1963.

57 Purves, L. R., Bersohn, I., and Geddes, E. W.: Serum alpha-feto-protein and primary cancer of the liver in man, Cancer 25:1261-1270, 1970.

58 Rouvière, H.: Anatomie des lymphatiques de l'homme, Paris, 1932, Masson et Cie.

59 Sagebiel, R. W., McFarland, R. B., and Taft, E. B.: Primary carcinoma of the liver in relation to cirrhosis, Amer. J. Clin. Path. 40:516-520, 1963.

60 San Jose, D., Cady, A., West, M., Chomet, B., and Zimmerman, H. J.: Primary carcinoma of the liver, Amer. J. Dig. Dis. 10:657-674, 1965.

61 Saragoça, A., Barros, B., and Santos, S. C.: Primary neoplasms of the liver; the possibility of biochemical diagnosis, Amer. J. Dig. Dis. 9:337-344, 1964.

62 Schlanger, P. M., and Schlanger, H.: Hydatid

disease and its roentgen picture, Amer. J. Roentgen. **60**:331-347, 1948.

63 Shanmugaratnam, K.: Primary carcinomas of the liver and biliary tract, Brit. J. Cancer **10**: 232-246, 1956.

64 Sheldon, J. H.: Haemochromatosis, New York, 1935, Oxford University Press.

65 Snijders, E. P., and Straub, M.: Geneesk, T. Nederl. Indie **61**:625, 1921; also Trans. Fifth Biennial Congr. Far Eastern Ass. Trop. Med. (Singapore), p. 779, 1923.

66 Steiner, M. M.: Primary carcinoma of the liver in childhood, Amer. J. Dis. Child. **55**: 807-824, 1938.

67 Steiner, P. E.: Cancer of the liver and cirrhosis in Trans-Saharan Africa and the United States of America, Cancer **13**:1085-1166, 1960 (extensive bibliography).

68 Steiner, P. E., Camain, R., and Netik, J.: Observations on cirrhosis and liver cancer at Dakar, French West Africa, Cancer Res. **19**: 567-579, 1959.

69 Steiner, P. E., and Davies, J. N. P.: Cirrhosis and primary liver carcinoma in Uganda Africans, Brit. J. Cancer **11**:523-534, 1957.

70 Stewart, M. J.: Precancerous lesions of alimentary tract (Croonian lecture), Lancet **2**: 565, 617, 669, 1931.

71 Thompson, C. M., and Hilferty, D. J.: Primary carcinoma of the liver (cholangioma) with hypoglycemic convulsions, Gastroenterology **20**: 158-165, 1952.

72 Torres, F. D.: Personal communication, 1970.

73 Watkins, E., Jr., and Khazei, A. M.: Arterial infusion chemotherapy of liver cancer, Bull. Soc. Int. Chir. **25**:279-292, 1966.

74 Willis, R. A.: Carcinoma arising in congenital cysts of the liver, J. Path. Bact. **55**:492-495, 1943.

75 Winternitz, M. C.: Primary carcinoma of the liver, Johns Hopkins Hosp. Rep. **17**:143-184, 1916.

76 Winters, R. W., Robinson, S. J., and Bates, G.: Hemangioma of the liver with heart failure, Pediatrics **14**:117-121, 1954.

77 Yu, C.: Primary carcinoma of the liver (hepatoma); its diagnosis by selective celiac arteriography, Amer. J. Roentgen. **99**:142-149, 1967.

78 Zubovskiĭ, G. A.: Radioizotopnoe skennirovanie v diagnostike opukholeĭ pecheni, Vop. Onkol. **12**:12-18, 1966.

Gallbladder

Anatomy

The gallbladder is normally attached directly to the inferior surface of the right lobe of the liver by loose areolar tissue. This attachment separates the quadrate lobe from the remainder of the right lobe. The gallbladder has a deep, medially directed neck, a body, and a free distal fundus. Its arterial supply is derived di-

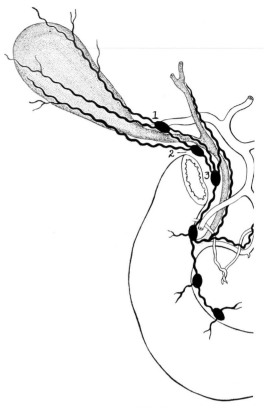

Fig. 461. Lymphatics of gallbladder showing pathways to cystic node, 1; node of anterior border of foramen of Winslow, 2; superior retropancreaticoduodenal node, 3.

rectly from the cystic artery, which lies between the gallbladder and the hepatic surface. The venous drainage goes directly into the hepatic divisions of the portal vein.

Lymphatics. The lymphatics of the gallbladder, arising from the mucosa, travel through the muscular wall to empty into a subserous lymphatic network. The trunks empty into lymph nodes of the anterior border of the foramen of Winslow, the lymph node of the neck of the gallbladder, and the hepatic lymph node (Fig. 461). These lymphatics have abundant anastomoses with the lymphatics of the liver.

Epidemiology

Of all malignant tumors of the accessory organs of digestion, carcinoma of the gallbladder is fifth in incidence. It is rarely observed before the age of 40 years, and over two-thirds of the cases are found in patients 50 to 70 years of age. It is encountered from two to four times more often in women than in men (Arminski[3]). It occurs more frequently in Mexican women and often at an earlier age (Steiner[28]). When vital statistics are recorded, the gallbladder and the extrahepatic ducts, including the ampulla of Vater, are combined under the heading of biliary passages.

Primary carcinoma of the gallbladder is found in approximately 1% of the patients operated upon for a clinically diagnosed cholecystitis. When gallstones are present, the incidence of carcinoma is between 4% and 5% (Jankelson[13]). If the patients under 60 years of age are excluded, the proportion of carcinomas found in association with cholelithiasis is much higher. In routine autopsies on adults, the incidence of cancer of the gallbladder is low, ranging between 0.25% and 0.33% (Bennett and Jepson[4]). In a collected group of 46,480 operations on the biliary system compiled by various hospitals, there were 569 carcinomas of the gallbladder, or 1.22% (Arminski[3]). Gallstones are present in a high proportion of patients with carcinoma of the gallbladder, the reported figures ranging from 65% to 100% (Janowski[14]). The views concerning this coexistence can be condensed in three viewpoints:

1 The gallstones may cause the carcinoma to develop.
2 The gallstones form because of the presence of carcinoma.
3 An initial inflammation causes both the carcinoma and the gallstones.

The type of stone usually associated with carcinoma is the solitary cholesterol or mixed type. It is possible that the chemical structure of some compounds naturally excreted in bile could be altered metabolically to produce carcinogenic hydrocarbons (Fortner[9]). Papillomas of the gallbladder rarely precede carcinoma (Phillips[24]).

There is little experimental proof that stones or foreign bodies could cause carcinoma of the gallbladder (Burrows[5]). Petrov and Krotkina,[23] however, produced unequivocal carcinoma of the gallbladder in guinea pigs following the introduction of sterile hard foreign bodies into the gallbladder, and distant metastases developed in four of the five carcinomas so produced.

Pathology
Gross and microscopic pathology

About 80% of the carcinomas of the gallbladder arise in the dome or neck and the other 20% in the lateral walls. These tumors are of two varieties, epidermoid and adenocarcinoma. The epidermoid carcinoma is rare, frequently exists with stones, and undoubtedly occurs because of metaplasia of the epithelium, which can be seen at times (Fig. 462). Of the three varieties of the adenocarcinoma, the scirrhous type is the most common (approximately 55%), is accompanied by considerable connective tissue, and invades contiguous structures rather quickly. The papillary type of adenocarcinoma (approximately 25%) has a papillary overgrowth that tends to grow within the lumen and to form a bulky, rather slowly growing tumor. It is frequently accompanied by necrosis and infection. The colloid or mucinous adenocarcinoma (15%) tends to form large, soft masses.

Carcinoma of the gallbladder invades the liver fairly early in its evolution and may also directly extend into the extra-

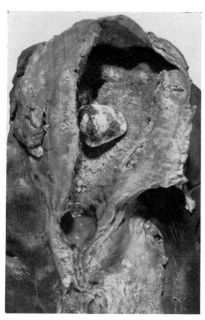

Fig. 462. Epidermoid carcinoma of gallbladder with local invasion of surrounding structures associated with single large gallstone.

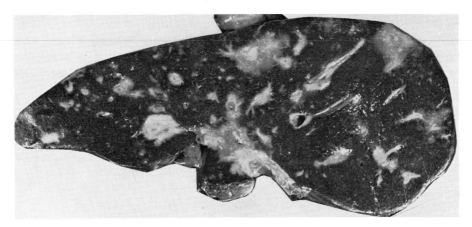

Fig. 463. Local spread of carcinoma of gallbladder by means of biliary duct system.

hepatic ducts (Fig. 463). Direct spread to the stomach and the duodenum with even complete pyloric obstruction can occur. Rarely, the disease implicates the hepatic flexure or transverse colon. Peritoneal involvement is quite common, the gelatinous type of carcinoma sometimes implanting on the peritoneal surface and causing secondary invasion of the bowel. Fistulous communication may develop between the gallbladder, stomach, duodenum, and colon.

When tumor is present within the gallbladder, infection often follows. This complication may cause empyema of the gallbladder, perforation, gangrene, generalized peritonitis, ascending suppurative cholangitis, and liver abscesses (Liebowitz[17]). Direct invasion of the gallbladder by carcinoma arising in the liver, bile ducts, stomach, or pancreas can occur, but metastatic lesions are rare.

Botryoid sarcoma of the common bile duct has been reported by Davis et al.[7] Carcinoid tumors can arise from the presence of argentaffin cells in the human gallbladder and account for the rare instances of this neoplasm (Christie[6]). We have seen a single case of a carcinoid tumor. This tumor was an incidental finding that presented as a slightly raised, sessile, yellowish nodule. Primary melanomas arising from the mucosa of the gallbladder have been reported (Raffensperger et al.[25]).

A benign neoplasm of the gallbladder is rare and is found in only about 1 of every 100 surgically removed gallbladders. It is usually a polyp, an adenomyoma, or a fibroma (Arbab and Brasfield[2]).

Metastatic spread

A carcinoma of the gallbladder most frequently spreads by the lymphatics to involve the cystic and periportal nodes, then the nodes about the head of the pancreas, and finally the retroperitoneal lymph nodes (incidence, about 50%). Metastases to the liver are frequently reported, but they are often the result of direct extension. Distant spread to the suprarenal glands, lungs, spleen, bones, and other distant organs have been observed (Arminski[3]), but they are not the rule.

Clinical evolution

Carcinoma of the gallbladder has an insidious onset, eludes early diagnosis, and is often recognized only at exploration or necropsy. The clinical picture depends, to a great extent, upon the location of the lesion, its extension and metastases, and upon associated conditions related to infection, stones, or pancreatitis. A typical case is a woman about 60 years of age with a history of biliary colic and complaint of pain, steady and severe, of one or two months' duration in the right upper quadrant. There may be nausea and vomiting also, and she may or may not be jaundiced. The liver and tumor may both be palpable.

About 70% of the patients with carcinoma of the gallbladder have a long history of repeated gallbladder attacks. These attacks eventually change in character insofar as they are followed by a short period of pain, vomiting epigastric distress, diarrhea, belching, progressive weakness, weight loss, and anorexia, all appearing within a six-month period (Mohardt[21]). Just as in other gallbladder disease, the pain caused by cancer radiates to the left upper or lower quadrants of the abdomen. As the tumor increases in size, the pain becomes more frequent and persistent, and jaundice appears in about 60% of the patients. This jaundice, obstructive in type, is caused by neoplastic involvement of the regional lymph nodes pressing on the extrahepatic ducts. Ascites may occur due to portal vein obstruction secondary to involved metastatic nodes.

With further progress of the disease, the tumor very frequently causes inflammatory complications that may result in cholangitis with high fever. At times, a liver abscess may form, and perforation of the gallbladder with terminal peritonitis is not unusual. The disease is terminated more frequently by these inflammatory complications than by a widespread metastatic process.

Diagnosis

The diagnosis of an early carcinoma of the gallbladder is practically impossible. In only seven of 105 patients reported by Warren et al.[32] was a preoperative diagnosis made. The frequent association of carcinoma and stones makes it imperative that any patient with stones (particularly a woman over 40 years of age) be examined carefully for evidence of carcinoma of the gallbladder. Usually, symptoms and signs of cholecystitis and cholelithiasis are present. When the disease become advanced, the gallbladder becomes palpable, firm, and, later in its evolution, fixed. Early jaundice is seldom present. Clinical signs of weight loss and anemia are not apparent until the end. A "dissociated" Courvoisier's syndrome has been described in association with carcinoma of the ampullary portion of the gallbladder (Ginzburg and Payson[10]). The distention of the gallbladder would be due to hydrops caused by obstruction of the cystic duct, and the jaundice would result from the neoplastic obstruction of the proximal portion of the common hepatic duct.

In a group of seventy-five patients reported by Lichtenstein and Tannenbaum,[16] fifty (67%) had pain in either the right upper quadrant or the epigastrium. In twenty-six (52% of those with pain), the pain was present fewer than six months, and in thirty-one (62% of those with pain), it was present for less than a year. Weight loss occurred in forty-three (or 57.3%) and jaundice in forty-one (or 54.7%). The combined symptoms of pain, weight loss, and jaundice were present in fifteen of the seventy-five patients. If the tumor originates in the fundus, it may not give rise to symptoms until after dissemination has taken place. On the other hand, if it arises in the neck, cystic duct obstruction may occur early. The inflammatory complications occurring near the end of the evolution are often confusing.

Roentgenologic examination

In some instances, a plain roentgenogram of the abdomen reveals the presence of a bulge between the liver edge and the colon. The presence of air in the center of the mass, due to a biliary fistula, may be observed. Barium enemas may be less satisfactory than a plain roentgenogram. The most valuable procedure seems to be the upper gastrointestinal barium study, for a distinct deformity of the stomach or duodenum caused by the tumor may be demonstrated. A cholecystogram is useless as a diagnostic measure, for if a carcinoma exists, the gallbladder does not fill with the dye. Kirklin[15] reviewed sixteen cases of carcinoma of the gallbladder in which cholecystographic examination had been done. Of these, fourteen showed no gallbladder shadow, but seven revealed stones. The fifteenth showed multiple stones and normal function, and the sixteenth showed function with no stones.

Asymptomatic localized mucosal lesions of the gallbladder may have a papillomatous character. They may represent a nonneoplastic inflammatory lesion, a true papilloma, or even carcinoma in situ occurring in a papillomatous lesion (Tabah and McNeer[30]). These lesions may be demonstrated radiographically (Loitman et al.[19]). Kirklin,[15] by means of cholecystograms, accurately diagnosed papillomas and adenomas of the gallbladder. Laboratory tests for liver function are usually non-contributory.

Differential diagnosis

Cholecystitis and *cholelithiasis* are invariably accompaniments of carcinoma of the gallbladder. In early carcinoma, it is impossible to be sure clinically that it coexists with these two conditions. Inflammatory complications with cholangitis or peritonitis may obscure the underlying neoplastic process. Carcinoma should be suspected, however, if previous signs and symptoms of cholelithiasis have been present or if there is a firm mass in the region of the gallbladder. A tumor of the gallbladder is not usually confused with the lesions of the periampullary region or with stone in the common bile duct, for these conditions (in contrast to carcinoma) produce an intense jaundice and present other laboratory or roentgenologic findings to help differentiate them.

Treatment

The only chance of curing a carcinoma of the gallbladder is by complete surgical removal. If the clinical diagnosis is obvious, usually the patient is inoperable. It is unfortunate that the symptoms of carcinoma confined to the gallbladder and chronic cholecystitis and cholelithiasis are the same. It is only when the tumor extends beyond the gallbladder that other signs and symptoms supervene, but at this time the disease unfortunately is incurable. In the past, Moynihan,[22] Graham,[11] and Finsterer[8] advised prophylactic removal of all gallbladders containing stones because of the risk of concomitant carcinoma. In a six-year period at Barnes Hospital, 2226 cholecystectomies were done. In this group, there were twenty carcinomas of the gallbladder, practically all were advanced cases. There was one cancer of the gallbladder for every 110 gallbladders removed, or less than 1%.

Lund[20] presented almost 100% complete five-year to twenty-year follow-up on 526 patients with gallstones who were not operated upon. One-third to one-half of these patients subsequently developed severe symptoms and/or complications from these stones. From this study, prophylactic removal of the gallbladder was certainly in-

dicated. The risk of cancer of the gallbladder, however, was no higher than the operative mortality in elected cholecystectomy.

Robertson and Dochat[26] demonstrated that the incidence of gallstones at postmortem examination was 22.3% for the age group 40 to 49 years and that it rose to 38.7% in the age group 60 to 69 years. It probably should not be inferred that this is the incidence of gallstones in the living population.

In an elderly female patient who is a good surgical risk, we would recommend cholecystectomy in the presence of signs and symptoms of cholecystitis and cholelithiasis. We would certainly recommend it because of the danger of complications from cholelithiasis, together with the hope that in removing such gallbladders an early cancer might be found, and therefore the patient might be cured. The only patients cured at Barnes Hospital from carcinoma of the gallbladder had superficial tumors found incidentally at an operation done for cholecystitis and cholelithiasis. Appleman et al.[1] believe that cancer of the gallbladder can be cured only when it is

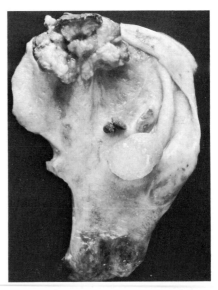

Fig. 464. Polypoid adenocarcinoma 2.5 cm in diameter in fundus and single cholesterol stone. Patient was well eight years after cholecystectomy. (From Appleman, R. M., et al.: Long term survival in carcinoma of the gallbladder, Surg. Gynec. Obstet. **117:**459-464, 1963; by permission of Surgery, Gynecology & Obstetrics.)

localized to that organ and that radical procedures offer nothing.

Postoperative irradiation may prove of value in some of these cases. At the Penrose Cancer Hospital, a case that presented invasion through and beyond the wall and blood vessels was given intensive postoperative cobalt[60] irradiation, and the patient remained well for five years.

Prognosis

The prognosis for carcinoma of the gallbladder is extremely poor. In most of the large reported series, only a very few patients live five years, the majority dying within a year after operation, and frequently the mortality rate is 100%. Strauch[29] reviewed 1061 cases of carcinoma of the gallbladder and found that only eleven patients lived five years or longer.

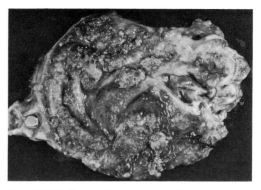

Fig. 465. Diffuse multicentric papillary carcinoma. Despite penetration of lesion through muscle in several areas, patient has survived five years after cholecystectomy. Note stone in cystic duct. (From Appleman, R. M., et al.: Long term survival in carcinoma of the gallbladder, Surg. Gynec. Obstet. 117:459-464, 1963; by permission of Surgery, Gynecology & Obstetrics.)

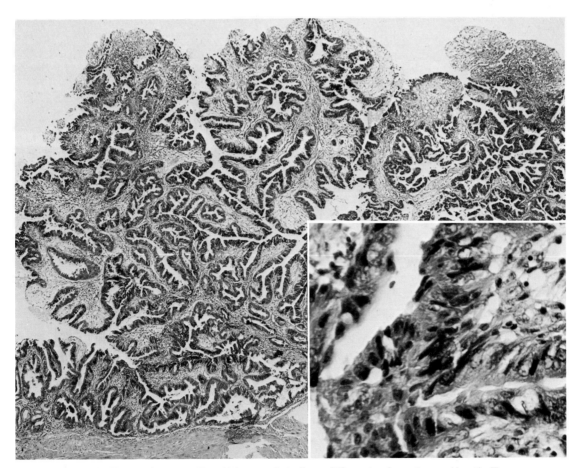

Fig. 466. Tumor shown in Fig. 464 was relatively undifferentiated carcinoma (**inset**). Tumor shown in Fig. 465 had a papillary character and was fairly well differentiated. (Slides contributed by Dr. D. C. Dahlin, Rochester, Minn.; WU neg. 69-3951.)

In fifty-four patients operated upon and reported by Vadheim et al.,[31] eight were alive at the end of five years, but the lesions in seven of these were well differentiated and limited to the mucosa and the submucosa. Appleman et al.[1] studied twenty-one patients who had survived five or more years from a group of 166 operated upon at the Mayo Clinic for cancer of the gallbladder, all of whom had been considered to have inflammatory gallbladder disease before surgery and all but one of whom had stones. There was invasive carcinoma in thirteen of these patients, and in ten the tumor had grown completely through the muscular wall but there was no involvement of the liver (Figs. 464 to 466). One of these patients died after nine years and another had a recurrence after twenty-six years. Only one of forty-one patients seen at the Akron City Hospital from 1958 to 1968 lived five years (Gradisar and Kelly[10a]).

REFERENCES

1 Appleman, R. M., Morlock, C. G., Dahlin, D. C., and Adson, M. A.: Long term survival in carcinoma of the gallbladder, Surg. Gynec. Obstet. 117:459-464, 1963.

2 Arbab, A. A., and Brasfield, R.: Benign tumors of the gallbladder, Surgery 61:535-540, 1967.

3 Arminski, T. C.: Primary carcinoma of the gallbladder; a collective review with the addition of twenty-five cases from the Grace Hospital, Detroit, Michigan, Cancer 2:379-398, 1949 (extensive bibliography).

4 Bennett, R. C., and Jepson, R. P.: Carcinoma of the gallbladder, Aust. New Zeal. J. Surg. 34:278-283, 1965.

5 Burrows, H.: An experimental inquiry into the association between gall-stones and primary cancer of the gall-bladder, Brit. J. Surg. 20:607-629, 1933.

6 Christie, A. C.: Three cases illustrating the presence of argentaffin (Kultschitzky) cells in the human gallbladder, Amer. J. Clin. Path. 7:318-321, 1954.

7 Davis, G. L., Kissane, J. M., and Ishak, K. G.: Embryonal rhabdomyosarcoma (sarcoma botryoides) of the biliary tree; report of five cases and a review of the literature, Cancer 24:333-342, 1969.

8 Finsterer, H.: Das Karzinom der Gallenblase, Med. Klin. 28:432-436, 1932.

9 Fortner, J. G.: An appraisal of the pathogenesis of primary carcinoma of the extrahepatic biliary tract, Surgery 43:563-571, 1958.

10 Ginzburg, L., and Payson, B. A.: A variant of the Courvoisier syndrome in carcinoma of the gall bladder, Ann. Surg. 146:976-982, 1957.

10a Gradisar, I. A., and Kelly, T. R.: Primary

11 Graham, E. A.: Prevention of carcinoma of the gall-bladder, Ann. Surg. 93:317-322, 1931.

12 Jaguttis, P.: Ueber das Schicksal der 1900-1914 in der Medizinischen Klinik zu Konigsberg in Pr. behandelten Gallensteinkranken, Mitt. Grenzgeb. Med. Chir. 39:255-269, 1926.

13 Jankelson, I. R.: Clinical aspects of primary carcinoma of the gall bladder, New Eng. J. Med. 217:85-88, 1937.

14 Janowski, W.: Ueber Veranderungen in der Gallenblase bei Vorhandensein von Gallensteinen, Beitr. Path. Anat. 10:499-480, 1891.

15 Kirklin, B. R.: Cholecystographic diagnosis of neoplasms of the gallbladder, Amer. J. Roentgen. 29:8-16, 1932.

16 Lichtenstein, C. M., and Tannenbaum, W.: Carcinoma of the gallbladder, Ann. Surg. 111:411-415, 1940.

17 Liebowitz, H. R.: Primary cancer of the gallbladder, Amer. J. Dig. Dis. 6:381-387, 1939.

18 Litwin, M. S.: Primary carcinoma of the gallbladder; a review of 78 patients, Arch. Surg. (Chicago) 95:236-240, 1967.

19 Loitman, B. S., Cassel, M. A., and Holtz, S.: Papillomas of the gallbladder, Amer. J. Roentgen. 88:783-791, 1962.

20 Lund, J.: Surgical indications in cholelithiasis; prophylactic cholecystectomy elucidated on the basis of long-term follow up on 526 nonoperated cases, Ann. Surg. 151:153-162, 1960.

21 Mohardt, J. H.: Carcinoma of the gallbladder, Int. Abstr. Surg. 69:440-451, 1939.

22 Moynihan, B. G. A.: Quoted by Finsterer, H.: Das Karzinom der Gallenblase, Med. Klin. 28:432-436, 1932.

23 Petrov, N. N., and Krotkina, N. A.: Experimental carcinoma of the gallbladder, Ann. Surg. 125:241-248, 1947.

24 Phillips, J. R.: Papilloma of the gall bladder, Amer. J. Surg. 21:38-42, 1933.

25 Raffensperger, E. C., Brason, F. W., and Triano, G.: Primary melanoma of the gallbladder, Amer. J. Dig. Dis. 8:356-363, 1963.

26 Robertson, H. E., and Dochat, G. R.: Pregnancy and gall stones; a collective review, Int. Abstr. Surg. 78:193-204, 1944.

27 Robertson, W. A., and Carlisle, B. B.: Primary carcinoma of the gallbladder; review of fifty-two cases, Amer. J. Surg. 113:738-742, 1967.

28 Steiner, P. E.: Cancer-producing agents from human sources; collective review, Int. Abstr. Surg. 76:105-112, 1943; in Surg. Gynec. Obstet., Feb. 1943.

29 Strauch, G. O.: Primary carcinoma of the gallbladder; presentation of 70 cases from the Rhode Island Hospital and a cumulative review of the last 10 years of the American literature, Surgery 47:368-383, 1960.

30 Tabah, E. J., and McNeer, G.: Papilloma of gall bladder with in situ carcinoma, Surgery 34:57-71, 1953.

31 Vadheim, J. L., Gray, H. K., and Dockerty, M. B.: Carcinoma of the gallbladder, Amer. J. Surg. 63:173-180, 1944.

32 Warren, K. W., Hardy, K. J., and O'Rourke, M. G. E.: Primary neoplasia of the gallbladder, Surg. Gynec. Obstet. **126**:1036-1040, 1968.

Extrahepatic ducts and periampullary region

Anatomy

The extrahepatic bile ducts vary considerably in length, structure, course, and relationship to one another, and it is difficult to distinguish the normal from the abnormal. The left and right hepatic ducts originate in the transverse fissure of the liver but unite at a 90° angle to form the common hepatic duct that courses backward, downward, and medially in the gastrohepatic ligament.

The common hepatic duct has an average length of 3.5 cm and crosses the branches of the hepatic artery and the portal vein. At the point at which the duct leaves the hilus, it overlies the anterolateral portion of the portal vein, and the hepatic artery passes to the left of the duct.

The cystic duct is a continuation of the neck of the gallbladder and averages 4 cm in length. The upper proximal portion has a redundant lining arranged in spiral folds to form Heister's valve. The distal portion extends downward to join the hepatic duct. This point of union may be of three types: the parallel type, usually deep behind the duodenum, present in 36% of the instances, the spiral type seen posteriorly to the left in 28%, and the angular type, usually on the right of the hepatic duct, present in 36% (Nuboer[29]).

The common bile duct averages 7 cm in length and can be divided into three portions: suprapancreatic, pancreatic, and ampullary. The suprapancreatic portion lies behind the duodenum and naturally varies in length according to the point of confluence between the cystic and the hepatic ducts. If this point of confluence is low, the suprapancreatic portion is absent. The duct descends to the right of the hepatic artery anterior to the portal vein and along the lesser omentum at its right margin. The second or pancreatic portion of the common bile duct is within a groove or tunnel in the posterior surface of the pancreas where it enters the descending duodenum. This portion is 3 cm to 5 cm in length and is separated from the vena cava by a thin segment of pancreas or by connective tissue. The third portion of the common bile duct is the ampulla. A true ampulla in the sense of a pouch lying within the papilla is present in only about one-third of the cases (Lettule and Nattan-Larrière[20]). Besides the true ampulla (type 1), there are three other variations: the pancreatic duct empties into the choledochus at some distance from the duodenal wall without formation of a true ampulla (type 2), the two ducts open side by side on the surface of the intestine without the formation of a papilla (type 3), or the two ducts form a prominent papilla in the duodenal lumen but remain separate (type 4) (Fig. 467).

Lymphatics. The lymphatics of the he-

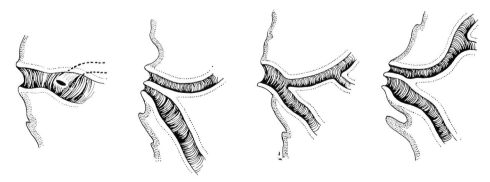

Fig. 467. Four anatomic types of ampulla of Vater (according to Lettule and Nattan-Larrière[20]).

patic, cystic, and common bile ducts arise from a mucous network that communicates directly with the network on the external surface of the ducts. The lymphatic collecting trunks of the cystic duct empty into the cystic node and into the node on the anterior border of the foramen of Winslow. The lymphatics of the hepatic duct empty into the node of the foramen of Winslow and into a superior retropancreaticoduodenal node. The collecting trunks of the common bile duct are drained by the lymph node of the foramen of Winslow and the posterior pancreaticoduodenal lymph nodes. The lymphatics of the ampulla of Vater anastomose with those of the duodenum and the main pancreatic duct and of necessity, therefore, with the lymphatics of the pancreas.

Epidemiology

Malignant tumors that develop in the extrahepatic ducts are relatively few in number. The ratio of carcinoma of the head of the pancreas to carcinoma of the extrahepatic ducts is about 4:1. In 109 verified cases reported by Ransom,[32] eighty-three arose from the pancreas and twenty-six from the extrahepatic ducts. Of these twenty-six, eighteen were from the ampullary region. The ratio of carcinoma of the extrahepatic duct to carcinoma of the gallbladder is about 1:3. In 312 cases of carcinoma of the gallbladder and extrahepatic ducts collected by Judd and Gray,[16] 100 arose from the extrahepatic biliary ducts. Cancer of the extrahepatic duct is found twice as frequently in males as in females. These tumors are associated with stones in approximately 40% of the patients. That cancer of the biliary tract may be caused by a specific carcinogen of the bile has been inferentially suggested (Fortner[10]).

Pathology

Gross pathology

Cancer of the extrahepatic ducts may be specifically located in the cystic duct, in the hepatic duct, in the confluence formed by the cystic and hepatic ducts, or in the common bile duct. In a series of 570 bile duct carcinomas collected by Sako et al.,[33] the distribution was as follows: hepatic ducts, 47; common hepatic duct, 79;

triple junction, 137; cystic duct, 34; common bile duct, 203; unclassified, 70. It should be noted that the highest proportion of these cases occurred at the lower end of the common bile duct and at the confluence of the cystic and hepatic ducts. Steward[38] critically analyzed all the cases of carcinoma of the extrahepatic ducts that had been reported and found thirty-five arising from the hepatic duct, forty-eight from the confluence of the extrahepatic duct, and twenty-one from the common bile duct. He pointed out that it was often very difficult to establish with certainty the site of origin of these tumors when the pathologic process was far advanced. He could not definitely discover a single primary carcinoma of the cystic duct, feeling that most of them represented direct invasion from a primary carcinoma of the gallbladder. He also found it difficult to establish the exact point of origin in the lower third of the common bile duct.

In the periampullary region, the tumor can arise from the common bile duct, duct of Wirsung, mucosa of the duodenum overlying the papilla, ampulla, or, very rarely, from aberrant pancreas or even Brunner's glands. The first three are by far the most common, but it should be remembered that carcinoma that arises from the head of the pancreas may simulate a primary tumor of the extrahepatic ducts. The number of tumors of the periampullary region in which the exact site of origin can be ascertained remains very small inasmuch as so very few cases have complete postmortem ex-

Table 46. Tumors of periampullary region*

Location	Cases
Primary carcinoma of ampulla	1
Primary carcinoma of terminal duct of Wirsung	3
Primary carcinoma of terminal common bile duct	7
Primary carcinoma of intestinal mucous membrane covering papilla of Vater	3
Primary carcinoma involving all structures detailed in first four groups	182
Primary carcinoma involving all structure comprising papilla of Vater except tumors arising from intestinal mucous membrane	33

*Data from Lieber, M. M., et al.: Carcinoma of the peripapillary portion of the duodenum, Ann. Surg. **109**:383-429, 1939.

aminations. Lieber et al.[22] analyzed all the reported tumors from the periampullary region but was forced to reject many of them because of inadequate data. They finally grouped them as shown in Table 46.

Carcinomas of the extrahepatic ducts may be either papillary or flat and ulcerated. They may be localized or diffuse. Stewart et al.[38] grouped their cases as shown in Table 47. The same is true of the tumors that arise in the periampullary region. All of these tumors spread to invade contiguous tissue. The carcinomas arising from the head of the pancreas or from the duct of Wirsung may invade the terminal third of the common bile duct, but the reverse does not often take place. In 117 tumors arising from the common bile duct, there was secondary invasion in only thirty-four (Lieber et al.[22]). The tumors arising from the hepatic ducts quickly invade the liver or extend farther down the ducts. Carcinoma of the bile ducts tends to spread in their walls and may transform the duct into a hard and rigid tube without becoming enlarged (Thorbjarnarson[41]). The carcinoma arising at or below the confluence blocks off ducts and causes dilatation of the common bile duct and gallbladder.

Confirmation of the slow growth of these tumors has been obtained from observations at exploratory operations and ultimate postmortem examination. Invariably, there is partial or complete obstruction of the common bile duct with consequent dilatation of the duct. When the duct is completely obstructed, it usually measures between 5 cm and 8 cm in diameter. This obstruction is due to neoplastic annular constriction (most common cause), pressure of the primary duodenal tumor, and secondary invasion of the pancreas after metastases to regional nodes or to concomitant biliary calculi.

Along with these changes, there may be inflammatory lesions which, particularly in the periampullary region, may be accompanied by pancreatitis, which in turn is sometimes associated with fat necroses. With obstruction of the duct of Wirsung, there may be cystic dilatation of all its ramifications, giving the pancreas a firm, indurated consistency and causing diminution of function. There also may be an ascending infection of the biliary tree with cholangitis or empyema of the gallbladder. The liver is usually enlarged and the surface smooth, but occasionally it may be finely or coarsely nodular. The cut surface is deeply bile-stained, and there may be considerable distention of the intrahepatic ducts.

Microscopic pathology

All tumors of the extrahepatic ducts and periampullary region are adenocarcinomas (Figs. 468 and 469). It would be very helpful if the primary origin could be identified by the histologic character of the cells. In fact, some workers have thought that they could distinguish tumors having primary origin from the duct of Wirsung or head of the pancreas from those arising from the terminal third of the common bile duct, but in our experience this cannot be done.

Two rare cases of botryoid sarcoma of the common bile duct in children have been reported (Farinacci et al.[9]). Clinically, the cases may be confused with infectious hepatitis.

Metastatic spread

Carcinomas of the extrahepatic ducts metastasize rather early to the regional lymph nodes (Neibling et al.[28]). Lieber et al.[22] reported metastases in 43% of 182 neoplasms involving the papilla of Vater. Carcinomas arising from the mucosa overlying the ampulla tend to metastasize late.

Table 47. Carcinoma of extrahepatic ducts; gross characteristics of neoplasms and frequency of metastasis*

Location	Cases	Form	Metastases
Hepatic duct	35	Local tumor 75%—diffuse 25%	48%
At confluence	48	Local growth 56%—diffuse 44%	46%
Common bile duct	21	Local growth 57%—diffuse 43%	52%

*Data from Stewart, H. L., et al.: Carcinoma of the extrahepatic bile ducts, Arch. Surg. (Chicago) 41:662-713, 1940.

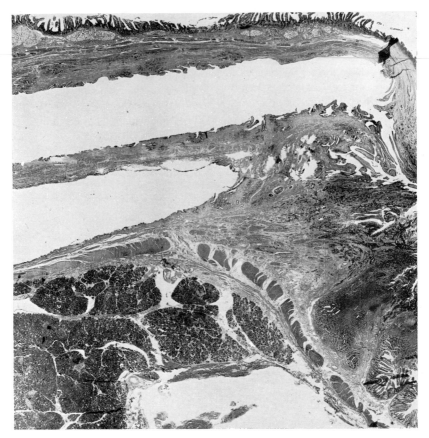

Fig. 468. Carcinoma of ampulla of Vater. (Low power; courtesy Dr. A. P. Stout, New York, N. Y.)

Clinical evolution

One of the first signs of a carcinoma of the common bile duct or of the ampulla of Vater is jaundice. It was the first symptom in 136 of 222 patients (Lieber et al.[22]) and was eventually present in all but four patients. The jaundice accompanying carcinoma of the ampulla, although slowly progressive, often fluctuates because of ulceration of the papilla. It is also true that ulceration of the duodenum may cause bleeding into the gastrointestinal tract.

Pain is frequently a symptom of the disease. The frequency of symptoms and signs found by Cooper[6] and Lieber et al.[22] is listed in Table 48. The longer the duration of obstructive jaundice, the greater the degree of liver damage which may lead to hemorrhage and cause death. Cholangitis and other local inflammatory conditions are often the cause of death, whereas widespread metastases are rarely the cause.

Diagnosis

Tumors of the extrahepatic ducts are seldom diagnosed because they are seldom even considered. Only thirty-nine of 222 cases were accurately diagnosed clinically, and the correct diagnosis was obtained in only eighty-three of the 122 patients in whom exploration was carried out (Lieber et al.[22]). In sixty-two cases, one or more diagnoses were made. The most common was carcinoma of the head of the pancreas (twenty-five), calculus choledochitis (fourteen), calculus cholecystitis (ten), and obstruction of the bile ducts (twelve).

Clinical examination

Jaundice is invariably present with tumors arising from the extrahepatic ducts and periampullary region. It is very frequently the first sign of a tumor of the ampulla, and it may wax and wane due to ulceration. In neoplastic obstruction of the

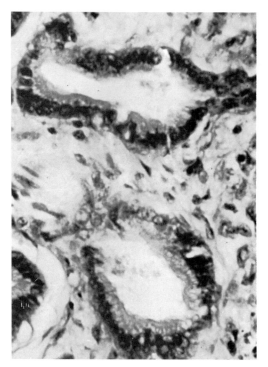

Fig. 469. Well-differentiated adenocarcinoma of terminal third of common bile duct. (Moderate enlargement.)

Table 48. Relative frequency of symptoms and signs in carcinoma of the extrahepatic ducts*

Symptom or sign	Cooper[6] (%)	Lieber et al.[22] (%)
Jaundice	95	98
Abdominal pain	86	59
Weight loss	78	
Anorexia	71	
Vomiting	36	58
Diarrhea	21	
Palpable gallbladder	50	50
Enlarged liver	86	78
Occult blood in stool	82	
Duodenal defect in gastro-intestinal series	80	32

*From Hyde, L., and Young, E. L.: Carcinoma of the ampulla of Vater, New Eng. J. Med. 223:96-99, 1940.

common bile duct, however, jaundice appears slowly and only gradually deepens to become intense. The gallbladder is frequently palpable, and the liver is often enlarged in all of the patients. The gallbladder may not be felt, however, if there is poor cooperation on the part of the patient, if the abdominal wall is very thick, or if the patient is obese.

Roentgenologic examination

Roentgenologic studies of the gallbladder and gastrointestinal tract may show failure of the gallbladder to fill and may, upon occasion, show a duodenal defect. A gastrointestinal series done on forty-nine patients revealed a lesion of the papilla in sixteen, recognizable by a continued duodenal deformity most often in the second portion (Lieber et al.[22]). Radiographically, Clemett[5] has shown that these tumors can be demonstrated by direct cholangiography and rarely shown by indirect methods (Fig. 470). Perez et al.[31] reviewed the roentgenographic changes in twenty-nine carcinomas of the pancreaticoduodenal

area and correlated these findings with the pathologic changes (Fig. 471). A correct diagnosis was made in about 70% of the cases. The following were the most common findings:

1 Smooth extrinsic pressure defect in the medial wall of the descending duodenum
2 Deformity of the postbulbar area relating to dilation of the common duct or infrequently to a distended gallbladder
3 Ulceration of the duodenal mucosa, a most important finding (Fig. 472)
4 An intraluminal mass, most frequently seen in carcinoma of the papilla of Vater

From the radiographic standpoint, benign tumors practically never occur within the major bile ducts, and primary sclerosing cholangitis shows diffuse thickening of the ducts. The latter is much rarer than primary bile duct carcinoma. Transcutaneous hepatic cholangiography can be useful in localizing carcinoma of the extrahepatic ducts (Shaldon et al.[35]) (Fig. 473).

Laboratory examination

Laboratory procedures (as detailed for carcinoma of the head of the pancreas, p. 565) are also indicated here. The investigations are directed to finding out whether or not complete biliary obstruction is present. Fecal urobilinogen tests were evaluated in fifty-eight patients with cancer involving the extrahepatic bile duct and head of the pancreas. Some reached the plateau after a few weeks of jaundice, and usually the obstruction was not complete (Wollaeger and Gross[43]).

Exfoliative cytology

The examination of duodenal sediment for cancer cells may facilitate a correct preoperative diagnosis. In fifty-eight cases

reported by Lemon and Byrnes,[19] the diagnosis was made in eleven patients. There were no false positive results.

Differential diagnosis

The patient with a carcinoma of the extrahepatic ducts or ampulla invariably has jaundice. Therefore, differentiation has to

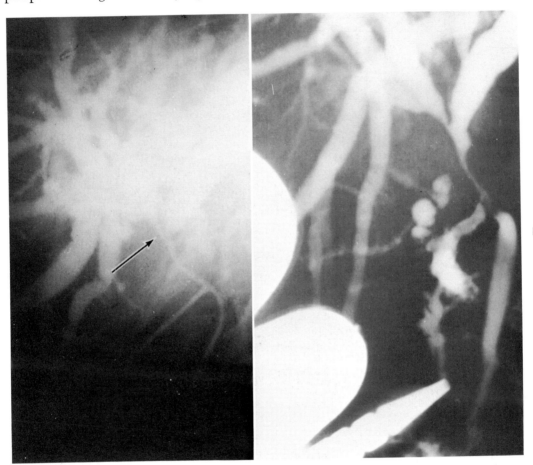

Fig. 470. A, Operative т-tube cholangiogram. Dilated intrahepatic ducts and nonfilling of common duct. Proximal margin of tumor extending to right hepatic duct is evident (arrow). **B,** Injection of biliary fistula. Fairly extensive (4 cm) stenosing tumor of common hepatic duct. (From Clemett, A. R.: Carcinoma of the major bile ducts, Radiology **84:**894-903, 1965.)

Fig. 471. A, Mass 2.5 cm in diameter in periampullary region without mucosal alteration. Extrinsic pressure defect is present in distal second portion of duodenum (arrows). **B,** Cholecystocholangiogram demonstrating filling defect producing complete obstruction in distal common duct (arrow). **C,** Polypoid tumor 2.7 cm in diameter replacing papilla of Vater and extending into head of pancreas and muscularis of duodenum (arrow). **D,** Open common duct demonstrating dilatation in ulcerating tumor at its distal portion (arrow). (From Perez, C. A., et al.: Roentgenologic-pathologic correlation of resectable carcinoma of the pancreatico-duodenal region, Amer. J. Roentgen. **94:**438-448, 1965; **A,** WU neg. 57-4292; **B,** WU neg. 57-4293; **C,** WU neg. 54-2207; **D,** WU neg. 54-2206.)

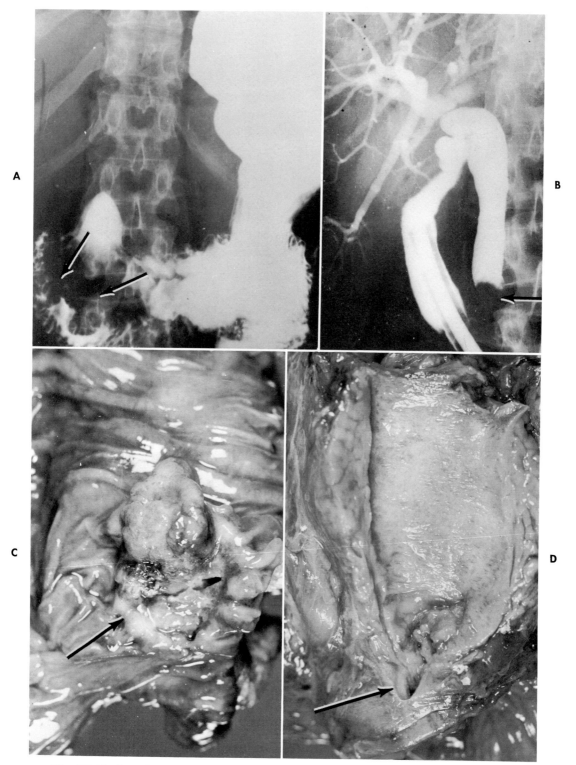

Fig. 471. For legend see opposite page.

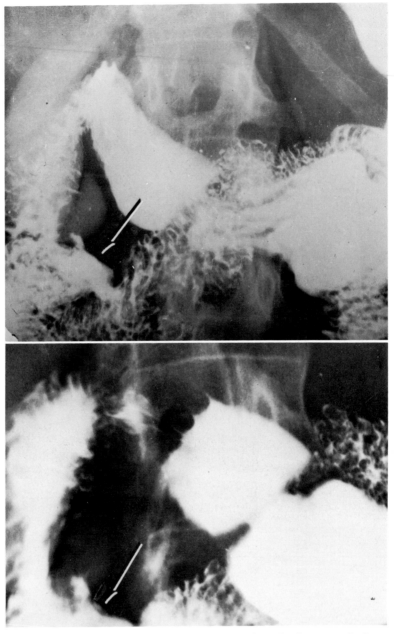

Fig. 472. Flat mass in concave border of distal descending duodenum with destruction of mucosal pattern and 2 cm ulcer crater (arrows). (From Perez, C. A., et al.: Roentgenologic-pathologic correlation of resectable carcinoma of the pancreatico-duodenal region, Amer. J. Roentgen **94:**438-448, 1965; WU negs. 57-4294 and 57-4295.)

be made from other conditions that give jaundice. In the first place, nonobstructive forms of jaundice have to be ruled out, but usually the cause is obvious. At times, *viral hepatitis* may be confusing and the obstruction temporarily complete. However, this inflammatory process generally ap-

pears in young individuals, the jaundice tends to clear, and, with adequate laboratory tests, the obstruction is proved incomplete.

Carter et al.[3] reported on a series of 3607 patients with disease of the liver and biliary tract admitted to the New York

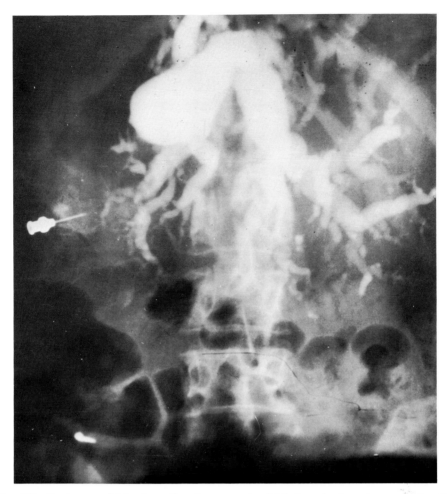

Fig. 473. Carcinoma of bile duct. Complete stenosis of left hepatic duct close to its junction with right hepatic duct, with gross distention of left hepatic duct and its branches proximal to site of obstruction. Left lobe of liver is enlarged, and there is no filling of right hepatic duct. (From Shaldon, S., et al.: Percutaneous transhepatic cholangiography; a modified technique, Gastroenterology **42:**371-379, 1962; © 1962, The Williams & Wilkins Co., Baltimore. Md., U.S.A.)

Postgraduate Hospital between 1916 and 1936 (Table 49). From the statistical standpoint, the chances are high that when obstructive jaundice occurs, it results from a benign cause such as a stone rather than from a malignant neoplasm.

Benign neoplasms of the extrahepatic ducts may cause obstruction and jaundice that may be interpreted to be due to carcinoma. Such benign tumors are extremely rare. It is certain that most of these are not true neoplasms. They form polypoid masses and have been designated as adenomas, adenomyomas, or papillomas. Because of their critical location, they can produce symptoms mimicking a carcinoma. Frozen section diagnosis would be critical, for they should be treated conservatively (Dowdy et al.[8]). A preoperative diagnosis had not been made in any of them.

Of the benign conditions, the most difficult one to differentiate is *common duct stone*. The associated symptoms are biliary colic, jaundice, chills, and fever; usually in that order. Dark urine and acholic stools usually follow the attack. Colic frequently indicates the passing of a stone from the cystic duct into the common duct. The jaundice that follows may wane as the stone passes into the duodenum or into a

Table 49. Comparative incidence of jaundice and age incidence of different obstructive biliary conditions*

	Operative cases	Cases with jaundice	Age (yr)
Cholelithiasis	1,346	296 (22%)	30 to 50
Acute cystitis cholelithiasis	356	103 (29%)	40 to 60
Cholelithiasis (stone in common duct)	105	65 (62%)	40 to 60
Carcinoma of pancreas	94	61 (65%)	50 to 60
Carcinoma of gallbladder	47	19 (41%)	60 to 70

*From Carter, R. F., et al.: Diagnosis and management of diseases of the biliary tract, Philadelphia, 1939, Lea & Febiger.

true ampulla. Only rarely is complete obstructive jaundice present. It is usually intermittent. In a series of 106 cases reported by Jordan and Weir,[15] all of the patients had symptoms of recurrent colic for variable periods of time, but fourteen (13%) never had any jaundice at all. About 80% of the patients with common duct stone have a contracted, atrophic, functionless gallbladder, and when evidence of intermittent block is also apparent, bile will be found in the stool and urobilinogen in the urine, particularly if frequent tests are made. There are a few patients in the older age group who give no history of pain suggesting calculi, and a preoperative diagnosis of carcinoma of the head of the pancreas is made.

Stones in the ampulla give approximately the same signs and symptoms as stones in the common bile duct. In 160 cases reviewed by Judd and Marshall,[17] 75% of the patients were between 40 and 60 years of age, and seventy-two of these had had one or more previous operations. The usual story was that of repeated attacks of paroxysms of pain followed by chills, fever, jaundice, and residual tenderness. Pain (mild or severe) was apparent in 155 of the 160 patients. In 73% of the patients, jaundice appeared for a few days or a few weeks (only thirty-seven escaped developing jaundice altogether). At times, the laboratory tests show absolute obstruction, but if these tests are repeated, evidence of intermittent obstruction will be found. Sepsis as manifested by chills and fever was present in 51% of the patients. In 110 patients, stones in the gallbladder were also present.

The presence or absence of a palpable gallbladder is very important in deciding whether the lesion is benign or malignant.

A high percentage of the malignant neoplasms of the periampullary region cause a dilated gallbladder, whereas conversely an extremely small proportion of benign obstructive lesions are accompanied by enlargement of the gallbladder. However, even a dilated gallbladder may not be felt if the patient is obese, if a large right lobe of the liver is overlying it, or if there is lack of cooperation on the part of the patient.

After there is no doubt that the lesion causing the jaundice is malignant, its origin must then be determined. Tumors of the extrahepatic ducts are relatively few compared with the number arising from the head of the pancreas and the gallbladder. In *carcinoma of the pancreas,* the weight loss, anemia, and other symptoms are usually followed by jaundice, whereas in carcinoma of the common bile duct or ampulla, jaundice is one of the first symptoms. The jaundice accompanying a pancreatic tumor is of a greater intensity than that associated with ampullary and bile duct tumors. It is also progressive and unrelenting. Because of the ulceration that may occur in carcinomas of the terminal third of the common bile duct, and particularly in those arising from the ampulla and from the intestinal epithelium overlying the ampulla, bleeding into the gastrointestinal tract can occur. This bleeding usually is minimal in amount, and gross hemorrhages do not occur. It is also possible, however, for carcinoma of the head of the pancreas to ulcerate the intestinal mucosa. Bile may be intermittently present in the feces of patients with carcinoma of the terminal third of the common bile duct and in those with carcinoma of the ampulla because of intermittent alleviation of the obstruction due to necrosis of the tumor.

Table 50. Differential character of benign and malignant lesions involving biliary tract, periampullary region, and head of pancreas

	Carcinoma of gallbladder	Carcinoma of periampullary region	Carcinoma of head of pancreas	Cholelithiasis	Stone in common bile duct
Age	50 to 70 yr (80% over 50)	50 yr (peak age)	60 yr (peak age)	30 to 50 yr	40 to 60 yr
Sex	Females 4:1	Males about 1.5:1	Males 3:1	Females 4:1	Females 2:1
Character of jaundice	Usually occurs late	Usually first symptom; tends to be incomplete	Other symptoms precede; progresses to high level; obstruction complete	Follows colic in high percentage; tends to be incomplete	Follows colic in high percentage; tends to be incomplete
Percentage with jaundice	About 50%	About 95%	About 75%	About 20%	About 70%
Percentage with pain	About 70%	About 65%	About 85%	High	About 75% have real colic; 20% have slight pain
Palpable gallbladder	About 50%	Common bile duct invariably dilated	About 65%	Less than 5%	Less than 5%
Blood in stools	Practically never	About 80%	Less than 5%	Practically never	Less than 5%
Roentgenologic findings	Nonvisualization	Ulceration; continued duodenal deformity	Widening of duodenal curve; invasion of duodenum; invasion of stomach	Failure to visualize; stones seen in 15%	Failure to visualize

By contrast, the carcinoma of the head of the pancreas never produces any bile in the feces. Pancreatic enzymes are invariably absent in carcinoma of the head of the pancreas, but they may be present in carcinoma of the terminal third of the common bile duct or ampulla (Table 50).

The differential diagnosis of obstruction is always difficult (Moynihan[27]). Problems arise from coincident phenomena such as secondary hepatitis in patients with prolonged obstruction (Steigmann and Popper[37]).

Treatment

Surgery is the only form of treatment that can be offered to patients with cancer of the extrahepatic biliary ducts, but surgical treatment is fraught with difficulties due to the proximity of the biliary tree to the blood supply of the liver and to the extension of the tumor through the ducts to the adjacent tissues. Usually, palliative procedures such as local resection for distal duct lesions are the most satisfactory (Glenn and Hill[11]). Various types of biliary by-pass procedures have been reported by Buckwalter et al.[2] It is best to employ the common duct rather than the gallbladder. These procedures give palliation but practically no prolongation of life. Carcinoma may occur in the bifurcation of the hepatic duct within the porta hepatis. Frequently it is not recognized at the time of surgery. The lesion could be recognized if the duct is explored by probing and cholangiography. Palliative surgery to relieve this obstruction may give good results (Klatsin[18]).

Carcinomas of the periampullary region are more suitable for surgical treatment because they tend to remain localized (Siler and Zinninger[36]). At the time of exploration, the liver, head of the pancreas, and regional lymph nodes should be examined carefully. Tumors in the region of the ampulla may be difficult to diagnose at exploration, for they are often soft and difficult to palpate through the bowel wall. There should be no hesitation in opening the duodenum. Papillary tumors of the ampullary region are often well differentiated, and when biopsy is taken from a superficial area, the microscopic pattern may appear benign (Child[4]). In a large proportion of these, carcinoma will be found at the base. Accessory pancreatic ducts may be microscopically confused with carcinoma in the region of the papilla (Loquvam and Russell[23]). Proved metastatic lymph nodes or liver nodules militate against radical surgery.

If carcinoma is proved, a radical one-stage pancreatoduodenectomy rather than a local resection should be done. Of ninety-eight patients in whom local excision with transplantation of the common bile duct and pancreatic duct was done, there was an immediate 20% operative mortality (Hunt[12]). Only five patients were alive at the end of four years.

Prognosis

The prognosis of carcinoma of the extrahepatic ducts is dismal. The Mayo Clinic reported follow-up information on sixty-seven patients. Of 62 of the surgical cases, only one patient was living at thirty-seven months (Van Heerden et al.[42]). However, Braasch et al.[1] reported 173 cases of cancer of the extrahepatic bile ducts. Of the entire group, only twenty-five patients have survived one year or longer. The only patients with long-term survival had lesions in the region of the distal duct. There were sixty-two patients in this group, twenty-seven of whom were treated by pancreatoduodenal resection. There were seven postoperative deaths and six patients survived without disease for four, six, six, nine, nine, and fifteen years, respectively.

Prognosis of the ampulla of Vater and the periampullary portion of the duodenum is much better. Moody and Thorbjarnarson[26] reported thirty-seven cases of carcinoma of the ampulla of Vater. Thirty-one patients were explored, but only twenty-four could have radical pancreaticoduodenectomy. Six patients were alive and free of disease two and one-half to seventeen year later. Salmon[34] reported thirty-five pancreatoduodenectomies for cancer of the ampulla of Vater. Fifteen patients died within three years. Ten of these had recurrent cancer, and seven of this group had negative lymph nodes at operation. Of fourteen patients

who lived for a prolonged period of time, eleven lived for more than five years. Of eighty-six cases of carcinoma of the ampulla of Vater and periampullary portion of the duodenum, thirty-six of the patients were living and well, but only ten had survived three years or longer. Of the twenty-six who were known to have died of disease, sixteen died within the first year, and only two showed evidence of recurrence after thirty months.

In forty-seven untreated patients reported by Outerbridge,[30] the average time from onset of symptoms to death was a little over seven months, and in 50% of the patients the duration of life was less than six months. In 100 inadequately treated patients, ninety-seven survived for an average of six months from the onset of the disease (Lieber et al.[22]).

REFERENCES

1 Braasch, J. W., Warren, K. W., and Kune, G. A.: Malignant neoplasms of the bile ducts, Surg. Clin. N. Amer. **47**:627-637, 1967.
2 Buckwalter, J. A., Lawston, R. L., and Tidrick, R. T.: Bypass operations for neoplastic biliary tract obstruction, Amer. J. Surg. **109**:100-106, 1965.
3 Carter, R. F., Greene, C. H., and Twiss, J. R.: Diagnosis and management of diseases of the biliary tract, Philadelphia, 1939, Lea & Febiger.
4 Child, C. G., III: Pancreaticojejunostomy and other problems associated with the surgical management of carcinoma involving the head of the pancreas, Ann. Surg. **119**:845-855, 1944.
5 Clemett, A. R.: Carcinoma of the major bile ducts, Radiology **84**:894-903, 1965.
6 Cooper, W. A.: Carcinoma of the ampulla of Vater, Ann. Surg. **106**:1009-1034, 1937.
7 Den Besten, L., and Liechty, R. D.: Cancer of the biliary tree, Amer. J. Surg. **109**:587-589, 1965.
8 Dowdy, G. S., Jr., Olin, W. G., Jr., Shelton, E. L., Jr., and Waldron, G. W.: Benign tumors of the extrahepatic bile ducts; report of three cases and review of the literature, Arch. Surg. (Chicago) **84**:503-513, 1962 (extensive bibliography).
9 Farinacci, C. J., Fairshild, J. P., Sulak, M. H., and Gilpatrick, C. W.: Sarcoma botryoids (a form of embryonal rhabdomyosarcoma) of the common bile duct, Cancer **9**:408-417, 1956.
10 Fortner, J. G.: An appraisal of the pathogenesis of primary carcinoma of the extrahepatic biliary tract, Surgery **43**:563-571, 1958.
11 Glenn, F., and Hill, M. R., Jr.: Extrahepatic biliary tract cancer, Cancer **8**:1218-1225, 1955.
12 Hunt, V. C.: Surgical management of carcinoma of the ampulla of Vater and of the periampullary portion of the duodenum, Ann. Surg. **114**:570-602, 1941.

13 Hunt, V. C., and Budd, J. W.: Transduodenal resection of the ampulla of Vater for carcinoma of the distal end of the common duct, Surg. Gynec. Obstet. **61**:651-661, 1935.

14 Hyde, L., and Young, E. L.: Carcinoma of the ampulla of Vater, New Eng. J. Med. **223**: 96-99, 1940.

15 Jordan, F. M., and Weir, J. F.: Stone in the common bile duct, Med. Clin. N. Amer. **15**: 1529-1544, 1932.

16 Judd, E. S., and Gray, H. K.: Carcinoma of the gall bladder and bile ducts, Surg. Gynec. Obstet. **55**:308-315, 1932.

17 Judd, E. S., and Marshall, J. M.: Gallstones in the ampulla of Vater, J.A.M.A. **95**:1061-1064, 1930.

18 Klatsin, G.: Adenocarcinoma of the hepatic duct at its bifurcation within the porta hepatis; an unusual tumor with distinctive clinical and pathological features, Amer. J. Med. **38**:241-256, 1965.

19 Lemon, H. M., and Byrnes, W. W.: Cancer of the biliary tract and pancreas diagnosed from cytology of duodenal aspirations, J.A.M.A. **141**:254-257, 1949.

20 Lettule, M., and Nattan-Larriére, L.: Region vaterienne du duodenum et l'ampoule de Vater, Bull. Soc. Anat. Paris **78**:491-506, 1898.

21 Lieber, M. M., Stewart, H. L., and Lund, H.: Carcinoma of the infrapapillary portion of the duodenum, Arch. Surg. (Chicago) **35**:268-289, 1937.

22 Lieber, M. M., Stewart, H. L., and Lund, H.: Carcinoma of the peripapillary portion of the duodenum, Ann. Surg. **109**:219-245, 383-429, 1939.

23 Loquvam, G. S., and Russell, W. O.: Accessory pancreatic ducts of the major duodenal papilla, Amer. J. Clin. Path. **20**:305-313, 1950.

24 Meyerowitz, B. R., and Aird, I.: Carcinoma of the hepatic ducts within the liver, Brit. J. Surg. **50**:178-184, 1962.

25 Miller, E. M., Dockerty, M. B., Wollaeger, E. E., and Waugh, J. M.: Carcinoma in the region of the papilla of Vater, Surg. Gynec. Obstet. **92**:172-182, 1951.

26 Moody, F., and Thorbjarnarson, B.: Carcinoma of the ampulla of Vater, Amer. J. Surg. **107**: 572-579, 1964.

27 Moynihan, B. G. A.: Gall-stones and their surgical treatment, Philadelphia, 1905, W. B. Saunders Co., p. 236.

28 Neibling, H. A., Dockerty, M. B., and Waugh, J. M.: Carcinoma of the extrahepatic bile ducts, Surg. Gynec. Obstet. **89**:429-438, 1949.

29 Nuboer, J. F.: Studien über das extrahepatische Gallenwegssystem, Frankfurt. Z. Path. **41**:198-249, 1931.

30 Outerbridge, G. W.: Carcinoma of the papilla of Vater, Ann. Surg. **57**:402-426, 1913.

31 Perez, C. A., Powers, W. E., Holtz, S., and Spjut, H. J.: Roentgenologic-pathologic correlation of resectable carcinoma of the pancreatico-duodenal region, Amer. J. Roentgen. **94**:438-448, 1965.

32 Ransom, H. K.: Carcinoma of the pancreas and extrahepatic bile ducts, Amer. J. Surg. **40**:264-281, 1938.

33 Sako, K., Seitzinger, G. L., and Garside, E.: Carcinoma of the extrahepataic bile ducts, Surgery **41**:416-437, 1957 (extensive bibliography).

34 Salmon, P. A.: Carcinoma of the pancreas and extrahepatic biliary systems, Surgery **60**:554-565, 1966.

35 Shaldon, S., Barber, K. M., and Young, W. B.: Percutaneous transhepatic cholangiography; a modified technique, Gastroenterology **42**:371-379, 1962.

36 Siler, V. E., and Zinninger, M. M.: Surgical treatment of carcinoma of the ampulla of Vater and the extrahepatic bile ducts, Arch. Surg. (Chicago) **56**:199-223, 1948.

37 Steigmann, F., and Popper, H.: Pitfalls in the diagnosis of the jaundiced patient; intrahepatic arrest of bile flow, Rev. Gastroent. **15**:367-380, 1948.

38 Stewart, H. L., Lieber, M. M., and Morgan, D. R.: Carcinoma of the extrahepatic bile ducts, Arch. Surg. (Chicago) **41**:662-713, 1940.

39 Strohl, E. L., Reed, W. H., Diffenbaugh, W. G., and Anderson, R. E.: Carcinoma of the bile ducts, Arch. Surg. (Chicago) **87**:567-577, 1963.

40 Thorbjarnarson, B.: Carcinoma of the intrahepatic bile ducts, Arch. Surg. (Chicago) **77**: 908-917, 1958.

41 Thorbjarnarson, B.: Carcinoma of the bile ducts, Cancer **12**:708-713, 1959.

42 Van Heerden, J. A., Judd, E. S., and Dockerty, M. B.: Carcinoma of the extrahepatic bile ducts; a clinicopathologic study, Amer. J. Surg. **113**:49-56, 1967.

43 Wollaeger, E. E., and Gross, J. B.: Complete obstruction of the extrahepatic biliary tract due to carcinoma as determine by the fecal urobilinogen test: incidence and effect on serum bilirubin concentrations, Medicine (Balt.) **45**:529-536, 1966.

Chapter 11

Cancer of the genitourinary tract

Kidney
Urinary bladder

Kidney

Anatomy

The kidneys are paired organs situated on both sides of the midline in the posterior portion of the abdomen at a level between the eleventh rib and the third lumbar transverse process. The right kidney is usually situated 2 cm lower. The kidneys assume a slightly oblique position and present an anterolateral and a posteromedial surface. Anteriorly, they are in direct relationship with the suprarenal gland at their superior pole. The right kidney is in relation to the descending portion of the duodenum, peritoneal cavity, hepatic flexure of the colon, and right lobe of the liver. Anteriorly, the left kidney is in relation to the tail of the pancreas and with the posterior wall of the stomach through the omental bursa. The posterior relationships are fairly constant on both sides, formed by the psoas major, quadratus lumborum, diaphragm, and the transversus abdominis muscles with the overlying twelfth dorsal, ileohypogastric, and ileoinguinal nerves.

The kidney in its fibrous capsule and the perinephric fat are enveloped by Gerota's fascia, which arises from the transversalis fascia and divides into a posterior layer (fascia of Zuckerkandl), attached medially to the vertebral bodies, and a thinner anterior layer (fascia of Toldt), which extends beyond the midline to the opposite side.

Lymphatics. The lymphatics of the kidney parenchyma and those of the fibrous capsule are continuous, but they do not communicate with those of the adipose tissue. In the parenchyma, two separate systems of channels have been demonstrated (Rawson[69]). One begins close to the Bowman's capsule and enlarges to form nets about the cortical blood vessels that accompany the interlobular vessels, wind around the arcuate and interlobar vessels, and leave the kidney at the hilus. Another system of lymphatic vessels begins beneath the mucosa of the papillae, ascends through the medulla parallel to the blood vessels, and enlarges to form the lymphatic channels that surround the arcuate arteries and veins. No lymphatics are demonstrable in the glomeruli, about the afferent or efferent arterioles, or about the intertubular capillaries (Rawson[69]). At the pedicle, the lymphatic channels of the kidney divide into three main trunks (Rouvière[76]), anterior, middle, and posterior, which are located in front, between, and behind the renal vessels (Fig. 474):

1 The *anterior trunks* drain the anterior half of the kidney and terminate in the lateroaortic nodes between the renal and inferior mesenteric arteries. On the left side, the highest trunks may empty into a node situated at the junction of the left renal and suprarenal veins and into a node located at the point at which the left spermatic vein drains into the renal vein. At times, they may also drain into a node lying below the termination of the renal vein and into a precaval lymph node.

2 The *middle trunks* of the right kidney usually terminate in the right latero-

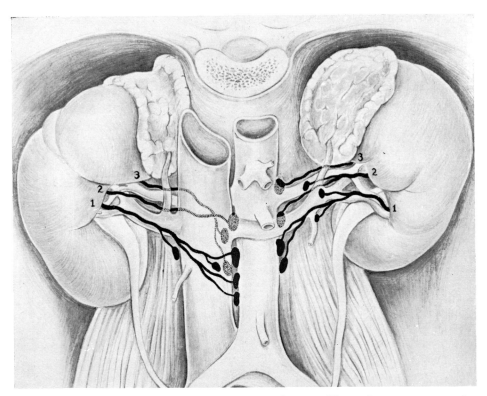

Fig. 474. Lymphatics of kidneys showing anterior trunks, **1**; middle trunks, **2**; posterior trunks, **3**. (After Rouvière, H.: Anatomie des lymphatiques de l'homme, Paris, 1933, Masson et Cie.)

aortic node. On the left side, they end in a node that is near the junction of the suprarenal and renal veins or in a lateroaortic node.

3 The *posterior trunks* originating from the posterior half of the kidney terminate in the right side in nodes that are located behind the inferior vena cava along the right border of the aorta, between the renal artery and the inferior mesenteric artery. On the left side the posterior trunks empty into the lateroaortic nodes near the origin of the renal artery.

The lymphatics of the *renal pelvis* are drained by the lateroaortic nodes that lie near the origin of the corresponding renal artery and the termination of the aorta and also by common iliac, hypogastric, and external iliac nodes.

Epidemiology

Kidney tumors constitute about 2% of all malignant tumors of the adult and 20% of those occurring in children. In the 1947 cancer survey in the United States, the age-adjusted incidence rates were 5.6 and 3.1 for white males and females per 100,000 population, whereas they were 4.3 and 3.0, respectively, for nonwhites. A comparison of the 1945-1949 and 1960-1962 surveys in the state of Connecticut revealed an increase in the incidence rate for males from 5.2 to 7.0, or 35%, whereas the rates for females remained the same. The comparison of the 1949-1951 and 1958-1960 surveys of the state of New York revealed an increase of 32% in the male rate and of 25% in the female rate. The incidence rates rise from around 1.0 in patients 35 to 39 years of age to around 35.0 in patients in the eighth decade of life.

Adenocarcinomas constitute about 80% of all malignant renal tumors and occur more frequently in men than in women and are rarely seen in children (Aron and Gross[4]). *Epidermoid carcinomas* of the kidney pelvis make up only about 10% of all renal tumors and are mostly found in persons in the fifth and sixth decades of life (Gahagan and Reed[31]). *Wilms' tumors*

constitute only about 6% of all renal neoplasms and are found predominantly in
children, mostly under 4 years of age. A
collected series of 1106 cases of Wilms'
tumor included forty-nine cases in adults
(Klapproth[49]).

A history of retrograde pyelography
with Thorotrast has been reported in some
patients with renal carcinomas (Dunant
and Rutishauser[23]). Production of stilbes-
trol-induced renal tumors in hamsters led
Bloom et al.[12, 13] to the interesting observation that the kidney, not an endocrine or
secondary sex organ, may nevertheless be
the site of hormone-dependent tumors subject to regression by the administration of
sex hormones. Renal adenocarcinomas have
been observed in association with hypercalcemia and containing a parathyroid
hormonelike substance (Goldberg et al.[38]).
A great number of carcinomas of the renal pelvis are associated with calculi and
renal infections (Gahagan and Reed[31]).
The development of bilateral Wilms' tumors (Snyder et al.[84]) and their occurrence
in identical twins (Gaulin[34]) would seem
to attest to possible genetic factors.

Pathology

Gross and microscopic pathology

Adenocarcinomas of the kidney are often
found unexpectedly at necropsy, usually
in kidneys that show evidence of previous
disease. Mintz and Gaul[58] collected sixty-
one kidneys containing sixty-nine circumscribed lesions, the majority of which were
less than 5 cm in diameter. There were
only eleven without evidence of pre-existing renal disease. Seven were so-called
fetal adenomas, forty-seven were papillary
cystadenomas, and seven were adrenal
rests. These small circumscribed cortical
lesions were well delineated, were often
homogeneously light yellow in color, and
created a slight bulge in the overlying capsule of the kidney. The differentiation of
adenoma and carcinoma cannot be made
grossly.

The *adenocarcinomas* vary in size but,
as a general rule, do not reach the huge
size of the Wilms tumor. These tumors
have been designated as hypernephromas,
a name that specifies neither origin nor
structure. Rarely, they are bilateral. The
infiltrating type without enlargement of

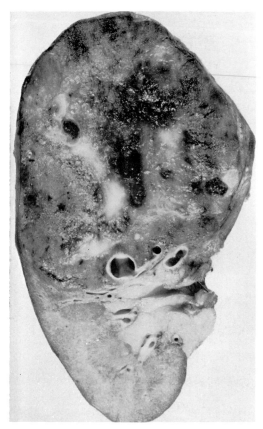

Fig. 475. Well-delineated adenocarcinoma of superior pole of kidney with areas of hemorrhage.

the kidney is rare. Adenocarcinomas are
well circumscribed even when large and
tend to grow toward the medullary portion
of the kidney and its pelvis. On section,
they are usually bright yellow in color,
and hemorrhage and necrosis are common
(Fig. 475). Heslin et al.[41] reported two instances in which a renal cell carcinoma implanted in the lower urinary tract. We
have not seen this type of spread.

Microscopically, it may sometimes be
impossible to determine if a tumor is an
adenoma or an adenocarcinoma, for encapsulation is often present in both, and individual acini are regular in appearance.
Frequently, the papillary cell type of adenocarcinoma with granular cytoplasm is replaced in a few areas by large cells with
foamy cytoplasm (Fig. 476). These tumors
can be divided into three microscopic variants designated as papillary diffuse, granular cell, or clear cell types. Multiple or
large sections frequently reveal transi-

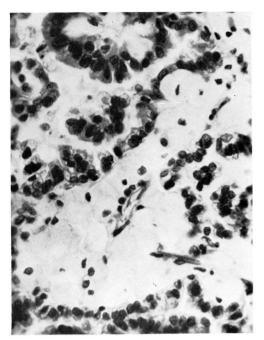

Fig. 476. Adenocarcinoma of kidney showing small areas in which tumor cells have foamy cytoplasm. (High-power enlargement.)

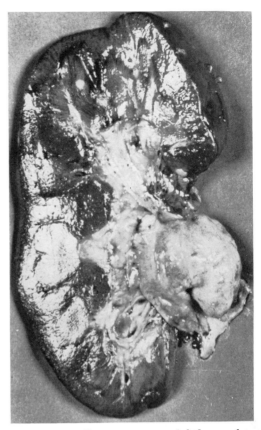

Fig. 477. Papillary carcinoma of kidney pelvis. First symptom was profuse hematuria.

tions and variations of all forms in the same tumor, and it is therefore logical to designate them all simply as adenocarcinomas of the kidney. They undoubtedly arise from renal tubules and, like renal tubules, may show hyaline droplets and a tendency to phagocytosis of broken-down blood pigment. They have been shown by electron microscopy to arise from the cells of the convoluted tubules (Oberling et al.[63]).

The transition point between *benign papilloma* and *papillary carcinoma* of the kidney pelvis is indefinite. Papillary carcinomas of the kidney pelvis form soft red or gray mammilated masses with smooth, glistening surfaces, as if covered by mucus. The tumor is made up of arborescent ramifying papillary masses and sometimes resembles small pedunculated polyps with irregular surfaces (Fig. 477). Surrounding the main tumor are often smaller masses that may represent direct invasion of the ureter by the papillomatous neoplasm. Tumor is also frequently present in the upper and lower thirds of the ureter, but the midportion may be free of disease. These papillary tumors are not associated with leukoplakia, stones, or infection. Local re-

currences after excision are frequent, but distant metastases are relatively uncommon.

Carcinomas of the kidney pelvis have the notorious quality of being accompanied by satellite lesions in the ureter and also in the opposite kidney pelvis or ureter. It is debatable whether this multiplicity on the same side is due to implantation or is merely a reflection of an increased tendency of the mucous membrane of the genitourinary tract to form this type of tumor. We feel that it is probably caused by a malignant tendency of the epithelium similar to the tendency of the mucosa of the large bowel to produce multiple polyps and adenocarcinomas. Further supportive evidence lies in the fact that solitary papillary tumors of the ureters are rare. Kimball and Ferris[47] reported seventy-four kidney tumors involving more than one portion of the urinary tract. Very few cases of

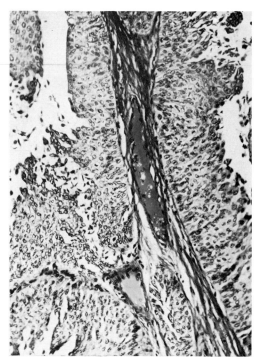

Fig. 478. Malignant papillary tumor of kidney pelvis. (Moderate enlargement.)

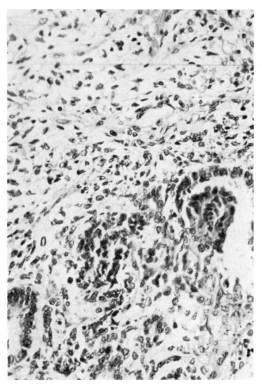

Fig. 479. Wilms' tumor showing adenomatoid and sarcomatous elements. (Moderate enlargement.)

adenocarcinoma of the kidney pelvis have been recorded (Ashley and Hickey[5]).

Microscopic examination shows the central portion of the tumor made up of a connective tissue axis continuous with the submucosal tissue of the pelvis (Fig. 478) or ureter, and there may be small strands of smooth muscle at the base. The epithelium is transitional in type, and the cellular characteristics are similar to those of papillary carcinomas of the bladder. Kidney tumors, unlike the ulcerating squamous carcinomas of the pelvis, are usually not associated with infection. The firm, flat, *ulcerating epidermoid carcinoma* arising from the pelvis of the kidney is a rare tumor commonly associated with nephrolithiasis and concomitant pyelonephritis.

The *Wilms tumor* (or embryoma) probably arises from embryonic nephrogenic tissue and represents a neoplastic exaggeration of the normal developmental process occurring in the growth zones of the renal cortex in late fetal life or the first few months after birth. The tumor is usually well delineated, globular, and large (over 250 gm). It has a definite connective tissue capsule which is continuous with that of the kidney. Because of this capsule, the tumor tends to remain confined, often reaching a large size before breaking through. As the neoplasm distends the capsule, its surface becomes bosselated and tense. The cross section of the tumor usually shows a gray or grayish white substance, but hemorrhage and necrosis may alter this color. The consistency varies with the amount of cartilage and connective tissue present. The remaining kidney substance is often atrophied because of pressure.

At necropsy, Wilms' tumors are often huge and attached to the contiguous organs by inflammatory or neoplastic adhesions. They spread by continuity toward the pelvis, with invasion of the renal veins and, rarely, the vena cava. When the tumor has penetrated the capsule, it may cause rupture and perineal extension. Adrenal invasion is most common in Wilms' tumors that arise in the superior portion of the kidney. Infrequently, the

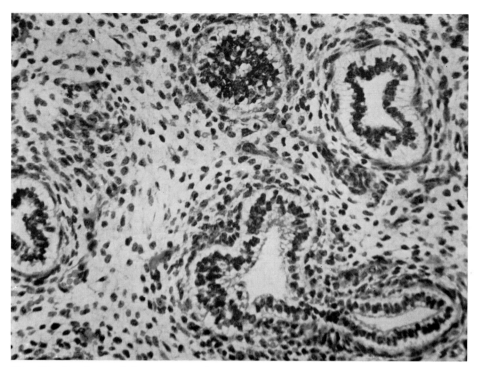

Fig. 480. Developing kidney in 3 cm fetus. Note resemblance to Wilms' tumor. (WU neg. 60-2529.)

tumor may directly invade the small bowel, large bowel, liver, or vertebrae.

Wilms' tumors with a pure almost sarcomatous appearance may show cells of both epithelial and connective tissue origin. Smooth muscle and sometimes bone and cartilage may be found. Striated muscle is present in about 40% of the cases. Adenomatous areas and occasional glomeruli are often also found (Fig. 479). This complex constitution is the cause of the variegated nomenclature given this neoplasm. The pattern of the tumor shows a close resemblance to fetal kidney (Fig. 480). Fetal hamartoma of the kidney is a benign symptomatic congenital tumor often mistaken for Wilms' tumor. It may be partially responsible for the statement that Wilms' tumor in the extremely young patient has an unexpectedly good prognosis (Wigger[92]).

Metastatic spread

Adenocarcinomas of the kidney frequently metastasize to the lymph nodes of the renal pedicle and the immediately adjacent para-aortic lymph nodes. Lymphatic spread may also be found in the mediastinum, in the hilar, carinal, and paratracheal lymph nodes, and, beyond these, in the supraclavicular lymph nodes. Frequently, also, early renal vein and vena cava involvement results in blood-borne metastases that are often found in the lung in the form of typically large spherical nodules. Finally, adenocarcinomas do involve also the paravertebral vein plexus and spread to the bones of the axial skeleton in particular. *Squamous carcinomas* of the kidney pelvis are often found to have metastasized to the regional lymph nodes. *Wilms' tumors* spread to the regional lymph nodes but, also favoring vein involvement, do metastasize to the lungs, liver, and brain.

Clinical evolution

Renal cell carcinomas may be the unsuspected primary lesion of a variety of metastatic manifestations. Since metastases may occur early and involve any tissue of the body, the symptoms and signs produced may mimic and suggest a diversity of clinical disorders not evoking the presence of a silent primary kidney tumor (Rusche[79]). Aside from the not infrequent asymptomatic primary tumor, hematuria is the most common presenting symptom in patients with adenocarcinomas of the kidney. It is the first clinical manifestation in between 45% and 60% of the patients, and between 70% and 80% eventually present it. Pain is the first symptom in about one-third of the patients and eventually appears in the majority. The presence of a palpable mass completes the triad of symptoms and signs most frequently observed in these tumors. These symptoms and signs may not coincide chronologically but the more advanced the stage of development, the more frequently the association.

Blood clots may form, causing severe spasmodic pain as they pass down the ureter. As the tumor disseminates, anemia, cough, and pleural pain may occur. Fever and anemia are commonly found and not necessarily related to local necrosis nor to the presence of metastases (Clarke and Goade[17]). Metastases to the brain are not unusual in the terminal stages. Low-grade fever may accompany the tumor, disappear with its surgical removal, and reappear with a recurrence. It is not unreasonable to presume that certain carcinomas of the kidney remain latent or grow at a slow rate for a number of years and then suddenly accelerate their growth, disseminate, and cause death. In the series reported by Albarrán and Imbert,[2] the mean duration of carcinoma of the kidney was 4.5 years.

Several unusual manifestations have been found associated with renal cell carcinomas (Table 51). *Polycythemia* has been reported in some twenty cases (Damon et al.[21]). It usually antedates the discovery of the tumor. It has been suggested that these renal tumors may put in circulation an erythropoietic factor (Jacobson et al.[43]). After removal of the tumor, the blood may return to normal, only to rise again in the presence of metastases (Giger[37]). In nonmetastatic renal cell carcinoma, *hypercalcemia* and metabolic *alkalosis* can occur. In the patient reported by O'Grady et al.,[65] a substance immunochemically similar to parathyroid hormone was found in the urine. The hypercalcemia may be severe enough to cause lassitude and even

psychosis. *Hypertension* may be associated with a renal cell carcinoma because of associated arteriovenous fistula within the tumor and will disappear after removal of the neoplasm (Bosniak[14]). Weidmann et al.[89] also reported hypertension associated with tumors adjacent to the renal arteries. In addition, a *salt-losing syndrome* has been reported (Lassen and Sagild[51]).

Carcinomas of the kidney pelvis manifest themselves initially in almost all of the patients by painless but profuse bleeding, and this naturally leads to a certain degree of anemia. These symptoms may be present over a relatively long period of time, and hematuria may wax and wane. Often, there are multiple tumors. Kimball and Ferris[47] reported that 33% of seventy-four patients had tumors in the ureter and bladder as well as in the kidney at the time they were first seen by a urologist. *Epidermoid carcinomas* often have a long previous history of symptoms suggesting renal lithiasis. They are often accompanied by evidence of kidney infection with recurring bouts of fever, tenderness in the region of the kidney, and rather marked painless hematuria. The clinical course is quite rapid not only because of the presence of infection, but also because squamous carcinomas metastasize early. Death, however, is predominantly due to kidney infection.

The *Wilms tumor* develops insidiously and painlessly and is invariably large when first discovered (Fig. 481). Over three-fourths of these tumors are found in children under 7 years of age. As the tumor grows to involve the capsule or nerves in

Table 51. Renal cell carcinoma—clinical presentation*

"Surgical"	"Medical"
Triad	Pyrexia of unknown origin
Hematuria	Polycythemia
Pain	Hypercalcemia
Mass	Hypertension
	Leukemoid reaction
	Salt-losing syndrome
	Arteriovenous fistulae
	Anemia
	Abnormalities of liver function
	Lindau–von Hipple disease
	Cushing's syndrome

*From Gregg, D.: Tumours of the kidneys and suprarenals. II. Renal and suprarenal tumours in adults, Brit. J. Radiol. **37:**128-141, 1964.

the immediate area, pain becomes apparent. Anemia is common. In the advanced stages of the disease, anorexia and weight loss appear. *In contrast to other kidney tumors, hematuria is infrequently* found as a single symptom throughout the course of the disease. The first symptoms or signs of a Wilms tumor are listed in Table 52. In spite of the fact that lung metastases are often massive (Fig. 482), dyspnea is seldom present. The symptoms and signs of brain metastases appear only terminally. George and Harley[35] reported on four patients with bilateral aniridia and genital abnormalities. If a boy under 3 years of age has aniridia without a family history of this disorder and genital abnormalities

and/or mental retardation, Wilms' tumor must be considered.

Diagnosis

Hematuria is frequently present in patients with kidney tumors, but its presence does not necessarily indicate invasion of the kidney pelvis. The tumors that arise within the pelvis naturally bleed much more readily than those arising from the cortical area, but hematuria may be caused simply by congestion or invasion of vessels contiguous with the tumor. There may be a considerable variation in the amount of bleeding. Hematuria is very infrequent in the Wilms tumor, is found more often in carcinoma of the kidney and papillary carcinomas of the pelvis, but is very frequent in papillomas. The epidermoid carcinoma, because of hornification and relative avascularity, does not have such a marked tendency to bleed. Because the patients have a long history of infection and kidney stones, epidermoid carcinomas are usually

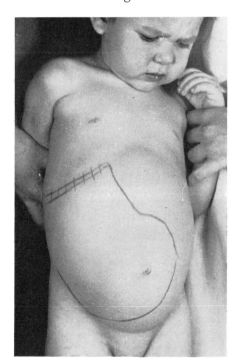

Fig. 481. Wilms' tumor in 3-year-old child. Outline indicates extent of palpable tumor. Note excellent general condition of patient.

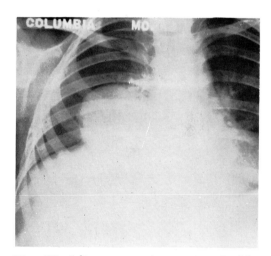

Fig. 482. Solitary metastatic mass in right hilar region from Wilms' tumor one year following operation.

Table 52. Symptoms in Wilms' tumor of kidney*

	Cases studied	Symptoms and signs		
		Tumor (%)	Pain (%)	Hematuria (%)
First symptom	98	71	20	5
During entire illness	140	96	18	16
With two symptoms	140	80		—

*From Albarrán, J., and Imbert, L.: Les tumeurs du rein, Paris, 1903, Masson & Cie.

not diagnosed until postmortem examination or at the time of operation.

Hematuria may occur at any time during the illness. At times, there is a hemorrhage every few days. The bleeding may be regular, with variation only in intensity, or it may disappear abruptly, only to reappear with the same suddenness. This uncertain characteristic is striking when the urine specimens are kept separately, for although the color of the urine remains uniform through each micturition, it may vary from bright red to normal. This variation is one of the most common signs of renal neoplasm. *Pain* and *costovertebral tenderness* occur when a blood clot passing down the ureter causes contraction or when the pelvis is considerably distended by a clot. The pain can radiate either to the groin or toward the chest and may suggest kidney stone if severe and colicky.

Clinical examination

Palpation of the kidneys is not always possible even in normal individuals, and only a careful bimanual palpation may succeed in revealing the presence of a tumor. The patient should assume a dorsal decubitus position and be relaxed. The examiner should stand on the side of the kidney to be palpated. With one hand placed in the angle formed by the last rib and the sacrolumbar muscles, the other hand depresses deeply the anterior abdominal wall just below the costal margin. Thus the kidney may be held down between the two hands, and its volume, form, and consistency may be appreciated. Tumors developing in the upper pole of the kidney usually cannot be palpated, whereas those that grow on the lower pole are more accessible and consequently more easily detected. When a tumor arises in a ptotic kidney, it may be apprehended in any early stage of its evolution. It is better detected on the right side because the liver forms a natural barrier to its growth. On the left side, a kidney tumor may enlarge upward without interference from other organs.

On percussion of kidney tumors, dullness is found as a rule, but a tympanic column may be found crossing the tumor area. This only indicates that the tumor is retroperitoneal. A tympanic column may

also be found on percussion of many other tumors.

An *adenocarcinoma* of the kidney may be so small that it cannot be palpated, but if the kidney is enlarged, the lesion can usually be outlined by bimanual palpation. It does not move on respiration. The first sign of an adenocarcinoma may be bone or soft tissue metastases. Voluminous and easily palpable metastatic bone lesions may *pulsate* due to abundant vascularization. These bone and soft tissue metastases are often confused with primary osteogenic or soft tissue sarcomas. They usually occur in the region of the nutrient arteries, particularly of the femur. They are most difficult to diagnose when the primary tumor is occult and hematuria is absent. Biopsy may suggest carcinoma of the kidney, and pyelography may then reveal kidney alterations. A varicocele sometimes accompanies the kidney tumor, most frequently on the left side (Albarrán and Imbert[2]), and may be complicated by a hydrocele, but a tumor or its adenopathy must attain a fair size before the spermatic vein is compressed and occluded. Infrequently, the varicocele is caused by simple thrombosis of the spermatic vein, but this is usually a sign of far-advanced development.

Physical examination for papillary carcinomas of the kidney pelvis is usually negative. If the kidney is palpable, it is usually due to a coexisting hydronephrosis. If infection occurs with any of these tumors, costovertebral tenderness and fever may be present. Cystoscopic examination of patients with these neoplasms frequently reveals blood coming from one ureteral orifice, and retrograde pyelograms demonstrate a filling defect.

In a *Wilms tumor*, the mass is usually large, the overlying skin is tense and shiny, and often there is a network of enlarged veins in which the blood flows from the abdomen toward the chest. On bimanual palpation, the tumor is fairly firm and has an irregular surface, variable consistency, and great depth. It may pulsate. If the Wilms tumor arises on the right side and is attached to the liver, a false impression of its true size may result because of lack of definition. It may displace the transverse and ascending colon so that the large bowel extends in a diagonal line from the cecum to the anchored splenic flexure. This displacement of the bowel may be suspected because of resonance, which can be outlined by percussion. If the Wilms tumor arises on the left side, it may extend upward and displace the diaphragm. There may also be an area of sonority on the left between the tumor and the liver. Ascites is infrequent.

Exfoliative cytology and biopsy

It has been hoped that exfoliative cytology might give definitive information in patients with suspected renal neoplasms in whom urographic examination reveals inconclusive but suggestive findings. Exfoliative cytology has proved most valuable in tumors of the pelvis and ureter. Undifferentiated transitional cell carcinoma and squamous carcinoma can usually be identified without too much difficulty. The well-differentiated tumors, however, are impossible to identify. Unfortunately, in carcinomas arising from the cortex the percentage of false negative results is high, and false positive results are also encoun-

tered. Focal hyperplasia of renal tubules may result in exfoliation of cells impossible to differentiate from carcinoma arising from these tubules.

Needle biopsy may be used to establish a histologic diagnosis of soft tissue extensions of renal tumors or of their metastases. However, needle biopsy of lesions confined to the kidney may prove to be detrimental due to implantation along the unresectable needle tract.

Roentgenologic examination

The roentgenologic exploration of the kidneys is an important complement of other examinations and may, in many instances, demonstrate an asymptomatic or unsuspected lesion. A complete study requires a preliminary "scout" roentgenogram (flat film), excretory urography, and retrograde urography. In recent years, renal angiography and nephrotomography have proved to be valuable diagnostic resources (Fig. 483). An arteriogram of a pararenal abscess may demonstrate pooling and abnormal vessels which can be diag-

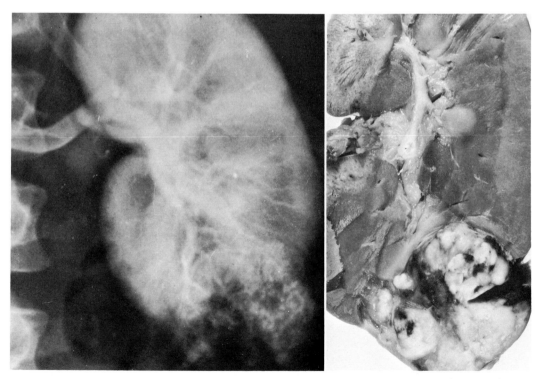

Fig. 483. Classic well-delineated adenocarcinoma of kidney. (WU negs. 68-3019 and 68-3535.)

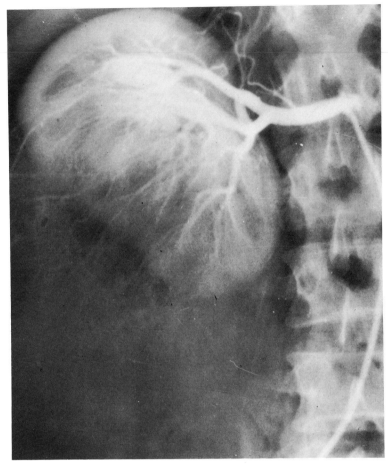

Fig. 484. Pooling and abnormal vessels diagnosed as possible carcinoma. Lesion proved to be perirenal abscess. (WU neg. 68-3609.)

nosed incorrectly as carcinoma (Fig. 484). We have seen rarely a solitary cyst incorrectly diagnosed as tumor (Fig. 485), and a rare lesion diagnosed as cholesteatoma may actually simulate a neoplasm (Fig. 486) (Osius et al.[66]). Other procedures such as pneumopyelography and perirenal insufflation are not without some risks and are seldom resorted to.

The "scout" roentgenogram may give information as to the size, position, and outline of the kidneys. Calcifications may be observed in association with tumors but are more often found with other renal and pararenal conditions. The presence of calculi does not exclude the possibility of a carcinoma of the renal pelvis. Excretory urography (intravenous pyelography) may give leading information of value toward the diagnosis. Failure of the kidney to ex-

crete the dye may be due to thrombosis or compression of the renal vein by tumor. In sixteen patients with adenocarcinoma with renal vein involvement, eight failed to excrete the dye (Beer[8]), but a nonfunctioning kidney may be related to other causes. Irregularities may be demonstrated by excretory urography, for the pelvis is elongated by the development of a neighboring tumor. A diagnosis can seldom be established on this basis alone, and, whether negative or suggestive, the procedure is to be followed by retrograde urography. Preliminary cytoscopy permits detection of unilateral bleeding, but often it is best to carry out bilateral catheterization and urography. In some cases, the routine roentgenograms should be complemented by lateral views. This procedure may put clearly in evidence the distortion or elongation of the calices produced by a parenchymal tumor or filling defects of the pelvis. Bleeding lesions may be accompanied by clots and consequent filling defects.

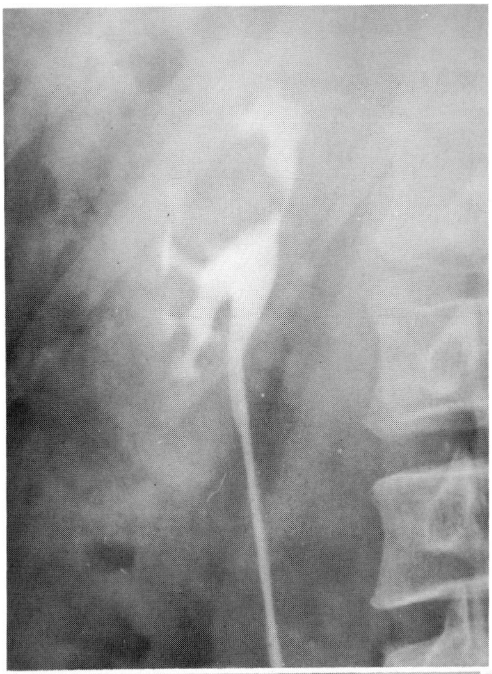

Renal angiography may reveal very small carcinomas of the kidney not demonstrable by other means (Löfgren[53]). Sophisticated techniques of angiography adapted to the study of renal carcinomas have been reviewed by Kahn et al.[46]—selective renal arteriography after epinephrine hydrochloride injection, selective phlebography of the renal veins, selective catheterization of small

Fig. 485. Well-delimited mass in superior portion of right kidney. This defect was considered to be cancer of kidney but proved to be solitary cyst. (WU neg. 68-8035.)

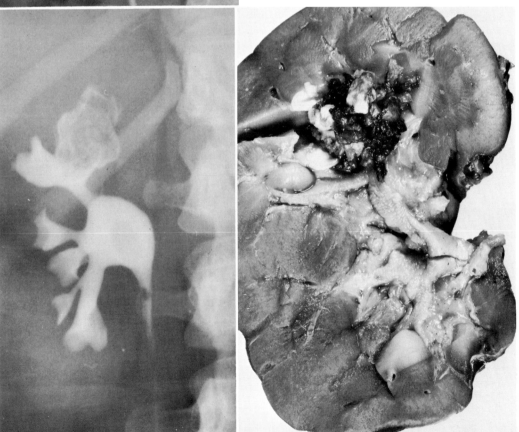

A   B

Fig. 486. **A,** Persistent filling defect of upper calyx of right kidney in 38-year-old white woman. Nephrectomy was performed. **B,** Lesion proved to be cholesteatoma—a rare lesion. (**A,** WU neg. 68-10648; **B,** WU neg. 68-10381.)

retroperitoneal arteries, etc. They concluded that any one or all of these procedures may be of additional value in the preoperative evaluation of a case. The preoperative demonstration of anomalous blood supply may become a useful forewarning to the surgeon of the preliminary steps to be taken. Fontaine et al.[30] have reported that some renal carcinomas are not hypervascularized, having, on the contrary, a reduced or practically absent blood circulation. *Nephrotomoangiography* is a combination of body section roentgenography and renal angiography (Evans[24]). The accuracy of this procedure approaches 100% in the differentiation of tumors from cysts (Tables 53 and 54). Angiography often reveals a rich vascularization with fine

vessels in cases of Wilms' tumor (Farah and Lofstrom[25]).

The diagnosis of kidney tumors by means of *scanning* following administration of a radioactive isotope has been studied (Morris et al.[59]; Rosenthall[75]). The procedure is innocuous and expeditious and may help but does not preclude or surpass the thorough radioangiographic studies.

Differential diagnosis

There are several lesions of the kidney that may suggest adenocarcinoma because of hematuria and pyelographic alterations. A single *renal cyst* is one of the most difficult differentiating lesions. It usually presents a well-defined homogeneous pyelographic shadow in the lower pole. If calcification is present, it is usually in the wall and is curvilinear in shape. Angiography may be of distinct value in the differential diagnosis of renal cysts. Unless the patient is a poor operative risk, he should be explored. If needle aspiration of the exposed cystic lesion reveals a bloody fluid, the chance that the lesion is malignant is 1 in 3. In a series of nephrotomographic examinations reported by Witten et al.,[94] 147 lesions were diagnosed as cysts. Only two of these proved to be carcinoma, whereas of thirty-eight thought to be neoplasms, only four proved to be cysts.

In Wilms' tumors, the radiographic findings are usually a nonfunctioning kidney displaced by a large mass. These radiographic findings are diagnostic in a high proportion of patients. When the mass arises in the upper pole, it may be impossible to differentiate it from a *neuroblastoma* of the suprarenal gland. A review of cases seen at Barnes Hospital in St.

Table 53. Nephrotomographic criteria for renal cysts and neoplasms*

Cyst	Neoplasm
Arterial phase 　Mass avascular Nephrotomogram 　Mass homogeneously 　　radiolucent 　　throughout 　Well-defined, thin 　　walls 　Sharp demarcation 　　from normal 　　functioning 　　parenchyma 　Acute sharp angle 　　formed at junc- 　　tion of cyst wall 　　and cortex	Pathologic vessels, pooling or laking of contrast media in vessels within mass Arteriovenous aneurysms Mass equal or greater density than surrounding parenchyma Necrosis will result in blotchy, irregular, poorly defined zones of radiolucency within mass Thick or irregular wall

*Based on data in Chynn, K. Y., and Evans, J. A.: Nephrotomography in the differentiation of renal cyst from neoplasm: a review of 500 cases, J. Urol. 83:21-24, 1960; from Evans, J.: The accuracy of diagnostic radiology, J.A.M.A. 204:223-226, 1968.

Table 54. Accuracy of nephrotomographic diagnosis*

Diagnosis	Patients		Error proved by operation or autopsy	Percentage of error
Normal	127		5	4
Renal cysts	203 }	240 cases	13	5
Polycystic	37 }			
Renal carcinoma	77		5	6
Miscellaneous including pyelonephritis, anomalies, extrarenal mass, renal abscess, etc.	56		2	4

*Compiled from data in Chynn, K. Y., and Evans, J. A.: Nephrotomography in the differentiation of renal cyst from neoplasm: a review of 500 cases, J. Urol. 83:21-24, 1960, and data in Southwood, W. F., and Marshall, V. F.: A clinical evaluation of nephrotomography, Brit. J. Urol. 30:127-141, 1958; from Evans, J.: The accuracy of diagnostic radiology, J.A.M.A. 204:223-226, 1968.

Louis revealed eight instances of erroneous preoperative diagnosis of Wilms' tumor. The resected kidneys revealed two cases of hydronephrosis, one case of pyelonephritis with perinephric abscess, one renal vein thrombosis with infarction, one renal malrotation, one unilocular cyst, one multilocular cyst, and one renal dysplasia. In only two cases was salvageable renal parenchyma present (Black and Ragsdale[11]).

Hydatid cysts of the kidney often give a typical pyelographic image. *Hemangiomas* of the kidney are seldom diagnosed preoperatively (Waller et al.[88]). They usually produce profuse hematuria without renal colic and may be bilateral. *Necrotizing renal papillitis,* usually found in diabetic patients, may simulate a tumor in the pyelogram, for it may have unilateral manifestations.

Pyelitis may produce clots within the pelvis that may necessitate repeated urograms to eliminate a diagnosis of tumor. Diffuse *lipomatous replacement* of the kidney can cause pyelographic anomalies and also be confused with a tumor (Hamm and De Veer[40]). A *carcinoma of the cecum or of the ascending colon* may simulate a kidney tumor of the right side, but this tumor is movable from side to side, and barium enema reveals a typical filling defect. Tumors of the tail of the pancreas, adrenal tumors, retroperitoneal sarcomas, abdominal aneurysms, and several other rare conditions may have to be differentiated from tumors of the kidney.

Splenomegaly, caused by numerous conditions, may have to be differentiated from a kidney tumor of the left side. This usually offers little difficulty since the spleen is superficial and may present a palpable notch. *Primary tumors of the spleen* are rare (Krumbhaar[50]). Lymphosarcomas are the most common primary malignant tumor of the spleen and often grow to a large size and generalize frequently. Hemangiomas (Pines and Rabinovitch[68]) and hemangioendotheliomas can also cause extreme enlargement of the spleen. Epidermal cysts of the spleen may become large (Bostick[15]), and they occur in young individuals (Shawan[82]). Dermoid cysts, epithelial cysts, and mesothelial inclusion cysts have also been reported. Infarction of the spleen with sudden pain may occur in both benign and malignant tumors. The roentgenologic examination may be of value in the differentiation of all large splenic tumors. Calcifications, displacement of the left kidney, encroachment in the greater curvature of the stomach, and obliteration of the psoas muscle may be demonstrated.

It is impossible to differentiate *renal tuberculosis* from a primary carcinoma of the kidney when there is hematuria and the kidney is slightly enlarged but there are no symptoms of pulmonary tuberculosis and the bladder appears normal. Coexistence of renal tuberculosis and cancer is rare (Neibling and Walters[61]). *Kidney stones* can be more easily differentiated, for pain is often increased by urination or activity and is relieved by repose. The pain in kidney tumor is not influenced by urination, rest, or movement. The kidney with stone is also sensitive to pressure, and the urine is frequently infected. *Renal lithiasis, tuberculosis,* and *pyelitis* (Fig. 487) have to be differentiated from carcinomas of the pelvis. *Leukoplakia* of the kidney pelvis is seldom diagnosed preoperatively. Most cases are associated with infections and chronic inflammation and present a history of pollakiuria, pyuria, etc., but the passage of flaky debris or gritty flakes becomes diagnostic (Thompson[87]). Pyelograms of patients with leukoplakia reveal an overall moth-eaten appearance and lacy striations of the kidney pelvis.

Primary tumors of the ureter are extremely rare. Lazarus and Marks[52] were able to collect only 183 cases, and they occurred in the male in a ratio of 2:1, with the highest frequency in the sixth and seventh decades. These rare tumors can arise either from the lining mucosal epithelium or from the wall of the ureter. By far the greatest number arise from the epithelium and can be classified as papillary or nonpapillary carcinomas (Fig. 488). These tumors are comparable to those arising from the renal pelvis. The true epidermoid carcinomas, few in number, are often associated with calculi. In their growth, these tumors naturally cause obstruction of the ureter with secondary hydronephrosis and, at times, pyelonephritis. Metastases to regional and peritoneal lymph nodes oc-

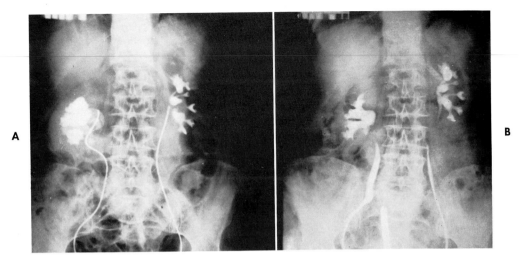

Fig. 487. A, Filling defect of right kidney that was thought to be due to carcinoma. **B,** Complete clearing of defect forty-eight hours later. Primary cause was pyelitis plus blood clot.

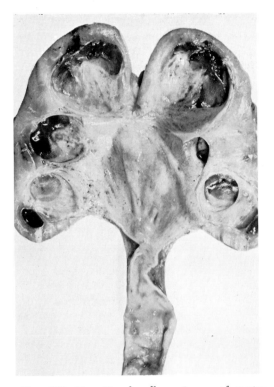

Fig. 488. Transitional cell carcinoma of ureter producing complete block with extreme hydronephrosis.

curred in 29% of a large group collected by Lazarus and Marks.[52] Distant metastases to liver and lungs also occurred. The first symptom of carcinoma of the ureter is hematuria. It is usually profuse, in-

termittent, and painless, but colic is frequently present due to the formation of blood clots. This bleeding naturally causes anemia. Hematuria occurred as the outstanding symptom in 70% of the reported cases (Lazarus and Marks[52]). With ureteral block, renal infection is also common, and this causes symptoms of pyelonephritis, from which death usually occurs. In patients with carcinoma of the ureter, the retrograde pyelogram shows either a complete obstruction or an irregular filling defect of the ureteral lumen (Savignac[80]). By cystoscopy, the tumor may sometimes be seen protruding from the ureteral meatus. Obstruction is usually encountered at the site of tumor, and manipulation of the catheter produces bleeding.

A *neuroblastoma* of the suprarenal gland may have to be differentiated from a Wilms tumor, but it seldom attains a large size and before it becomes palpable has usually metastasized to bone, liver, lungs, or regional lymph nodes. Wilms' tumors rarely metastasize to bone, whereas neuroblastomas have bone metastases in a large percentage of cases. Retroperitoneal *lymphosarcoma*, if present, is usually accompanied by peripheral lymphadenopathy. A *splenomegaly*, which in a child is usually due to some blood dyscrasia, must be differentiated from Wilms' tumor. The enlarged spleen moves on respiration. Hematologic findings and pyelograms will also usually serve to distinguish the conditions. A massive hydronephrosis may be confused easily with a Wilms tumor because of its size or failure of the kidney to be visualized by pyelography. It will not diminish in size under radiotherapy, and the diagnosis may be made only at exploration. *Ovarian tumors, omental cysts,* and *new growths of the liver* have all been confused with Wilms' tumor, but these conditions are extremely rare and usually have other identifiable characteristics that are sufficient for differentiation.

Treatment

Surgery

The treatment of choice of *adenocarcinomas* of the kidney is a radical nephrectomy, which implies removal of the kidney and a good length of the ureter, the perinephric fat, Gerota's fascia, the adrenal gland, and the paracaval and adjacent para-aortic lymph nodes. An early preliminary ligation of the vascular pedicle is advisable, but this is not always possible with large tumors (Riches[72]). A lumbar approach is satisfactory for the excision of small renal tumors. A thoracoabdominal approach is widely preferred, for it affords a wider exposure of the kidney, facilitating handling of the renal pedicle. In the presence of a definite preoperative diagnosis of tumor, and particularly for large ones, this approach is indicated. Others prefer a flank approach with an extensive incision along the tenth rib, removal of the twelfth rib, and division of the diaphragm (Nalle and Kennedy[60]). This permits a wide preliminary exploration of the kidney and retroperitoneal space and, if necessary, withdrawal, with a minimum of trauma. The presence of retroperitoneal involvement, liver involvement, or distant lymph node metastases may contraindicate the completion of the radical surgical procedure. The presence of dilated and tortuous veins in the fatty capsule often means that a tumor thrombus occludes the main trunk of the renal vein (Ahlberg et al.[1]). Perirenal fixation may mean extracapsular spread of the tumor but may be caused also by perinephritis.

In a patient with a solitary kidney with a small carcinoma, it may be possible to do a partial resection with resulting cure

(Zinman and Dowd[96]). In the presence of evident pulmonary metastases, a nephrectomy has been reported to have caused their disappearance (Beer[8]). In one case, the regression persisted nine years after the removal of the kidney (Mann[56]). Rarely, an adenocarcinoma of the kidney may be accompanied by a single pulmonary metastasis. In such instances, a nephrectomy followed by lobectomy may result in long-standing survival (Barney[7]). However, nephrectomy does not result in prolonged survival of patients with numerous distant metastases (Middleton[57]).

Epidermoid carcinomas of the kidney pelvis are best treated by a nephroureterectomy. The entire ureter, including its intramural portion in the bladder wall, must be removed to eliminate the high risk of recurrence. A transperitoneal approach seems to be preferred in the performance of nephrectomies for *Wilms' tumors.*

Radiotherapy

The variable radiosensitivity of renal *adenocarcinomas* has long favored the palliative irradiation of inoperable residual, recurrent, or metastatic lesions. In recent years, slowly accumulating evidence has opened new opportunities for radiotherapy as a surgical adjuvant in renal cell carcinomas. Riches[74] has repeatedly called attention to the fact that perinephric spread, vein invasion, and para-aortic lymph node metastases often thwart the surgical efforts. For years, he has subjected a number of these patients to postoperative radiotherapy and has been gratified by the improved results, as compared with those obtained in nonirradiated patients. A similar experience has subsequently been reported by other observers (Bixler et al.[10]; Flocks and Kadesky[29]; Reboul et al.[70]). As in all instances in which postoperative radiotherapy seems to be of value, it is likely that preoperative irradiation may be of still greater value. Both these propositions call for a seriously planned prospective clinical trial (Bratherton[16]; Regato and Kagan[71]).

Preoperative irradiation of adenocarcinomas need not be carried out to doses needed for curative purposes. Nevertheless, it should encompass all of the potential primary involvement and the adjacent nodes, it should administer a sufficiently high dose of radiations throughout the entire tumor area, and it should be done over a period of four to five weeks. Following preoperative irradiation, the nephrectomy should be carried out after an interval of no less than three weeks.

Postoperative irradiation of adenocarcinomas should be administered in all instances in which the surgeon's exploration or the histopathologic examination of the specimen reveals evidence of residual tumor in the kidney bed, vein invasion, or para-aortic lymphatic involvement. The doses of radiations to be administered should make it possible to control the remaining tumor—the higher the dose, the greater the chance of control. Thus, the postoperative irradiation requires longer time and care. The concern should be to minimize the irradiation of the spinal cord and avoid the irradiation of the remaining kidney (Regato and Kagan[71]).

Radiotherapy has shown little usefulness in the treatment of *epidermoid carcinomas* of the kidney pelvis. We have observed one instance, however, of radiotherapeutic control of a postoperative recurrence in the path of the ureter.

Radiotherapy has been long advocated postoperatively in the treatment of *Wilms' tumors*, but although it has controlled inoperable tumors, postoperative recurrences, and metastases, it is often called to correct the irremediable (Schweisguth et al.[81]). If postoperative irradiation is of any value, preoperative irradiation is likely to be much more useful. Again, if the irradiation is to be administered preoperatively, a reasonably smaller amount of radiations would be required than when it is administered postoperatively. In both instances, however, precautions should be taken to avoid or minimize the untoward effects of irradiation. Since patients with Wilms' tumor are usually young children, intensive unilateral irradiation may result in subsequent scoliosis (Rubin et al.[78]). The best safeguard against such effects is a long fractionation of the treatment over several weeks (six to eight weeks). In addition, radiations should be distributed as homogeneously as possible, and irradiation of the spinal cord and opposite kidney should be minimized or avoided. When administering postoperative radiotherapy, one must keep in mind that subsequent recrudescences cannot be reirradiated nor are they controllable by surgery. Thus, a reasonable risk of scoliosis, etc. may be justifiable. Radiotherapy may be found useful in the treatment of metastases in Wilms' tumors, even when in the lung, or in the treatment of a second Wilms' tumor in the remaining kidney (Stein and Goodwin[85]).

Hormonotherapy and chemotherapy

Bloom et al.[12, 13] have succeeded in producing marked regressions of renal tumors in the experimental animal and in patients with advanced *adenocarcinomas* by means of progestational drugs and also testosterone. The matter does require further study, but it opens interesting opportunities. No chemotherapeutic agent has been found which offers any help in the management of hopeless renal carcinomas. Woodruff et al.[95] obtained only twenty-seven objective responses in 260 patients in a trial of thirty-six different drugs. Among the various compounds that have been tried in the treatment of *Wilms' tumors*, dactinomycin has proved most effective (Farber[26]). With this drug, it is possible to produce complete regressions of primary or metastatic manifestations of Wilms' tumor. Farber et al.[27] have observed advantages in the simultaneous administration of dactinomycin and radiotherapy. It is claimed that its routine administration at the time of nephrectomy followed by radiotherapy prevents the development of metastases. That dactinomycin is a true radiosensitizer (D'Angio et al.[22]) is open to question, but there may be advantages to gain in exploiting the additivity of the effects of both forms of treatment. If the combined treatment results in lesser dosage from radiotherapy, it has an unquestionable value in the treatment of pulmonary metastases from Wilms' tumors. Dactinomycin is a very toxic drug; it requires sustained observation and control. When administered jointly with radiotherapy, it brings the disadvantage that its toxic effects may force an undesirable interruption or discontinuation of irradiations. Maier and Harshaw[54] did not find any advantage in regard to cure of Wilms' tumors with the use of dactinomycin combined with radiotherapy as compared with adequate irradiation alone. Vincristine has also been tried with some degree of success. In four children with inoperable Wilms' tumors, it was given preoperatively, resulting in dramatic regression of the tumor. After nephrectomy, the drug was continued, and the tumor bed and the entire chest were irradiated. All four of the children were well five to twenty-one months later (Sullivan et al.[86]).

Prognosis

In 1965, there were in the United States 5634 deaths from kidney tumors or a rate of 2.9 per 100,000 population. From 1930 to 1960, the mortality rates have doubled for white and nonwhite males and for nonwhite females, whereas the rates for white females have shown only a very slight increase. In Denmark, a comparison of surveys of 1943-1947 and 1953-1957 reveals an increase of 40% for both males and females. In the United States, cancer of the kidney accounts for about 10% of all deaths in children under 5 years of age.

Adenocarcinoma

The smaller the tumor the less the chance of distant metastases. Therefore, the best prognosis may be given to those patients in whom the tumors are diagnosed early. The patients with a doubtful preoperative diagnosis or in whom the tumor is small at the time of operation have a good prognosis. On the other hand, large tumors may be present for many years without metastasizing, and small tumors may show wide dissemination.

The survival of patients operated upon for renal carcinomas can be correlated also with differentiation of the tumor and the presence or absence of vein invasion. In Riches' series[73] of cases, there were thirty-six patients with differentiated carcinomas and no evidence of vein invasion, twenty-seven (75%) of whom survived five years. By contrast, of twenty other patients with undifferentiated carcinomas and vein invasion, only four survived five years. The prognosis of tumors which remain circumscribed and do not involve the kidney pelvis is definitely better (Arner et al.[3]). Riches' experience[74] suggests that postoperative irradiation improves the prognosis of cases with vein invasion and para-aortic lymph node involvement.

Mintz and Gaul[58] operated upon sixty-two patients (1900-1923), seven of whom lived five years, but three of these had recurrences, leaving only four survivors at ten years. They operated upon another group of sixty-five patients (1924-1935) with ten survivors at five years and five at ten years. In total, Mintz and Gaul[58] had nine patients (7%) surviving ten years out of 127 operated upon.

Papillary and epidermoid carcinomas of kidney pelvis

The prognosis of tumors of the kidney pelvis is conditioned largely by the type of operation done. Kimball and Ferris[47] reported on forty patients treated by nephrectomy. There were thirty recurrences and twenty-one second recurrences, mostly in the ureteral stump, with 33% operative mortality. Culp[20] reported on eighty-nine patients with tumors of the kidney pelvis treated by nephroureterectomy, yet thirty-eight of these (43%) developed subsequent similar tumors of the bladder.

The prognosis of the epidermoid carcinoma of the kidney pelvis is invariably very poor. In a series of 15 cases treated at the Roswell Park Memorial Institute there were no 5-year survivals (Oberkircher et al.[62]). Gahagan and Reed[31] could find no 5-year survivals in a collected series of 106 cases of epidermoid carcinoma. With nephroureterectomy the prognosis for the superficial papillary *carcinoma of the ureter* is good. For the nonpapillary infiltrating carcinoma the prognosis is extremely poor (Whitlock et al.[91]).

Wilms' tumors

The best results in the treatment of Wilms' tumors are obtained when the patients are treated in the first two years of life (Garcia et al.[32]; Westra et al.[90]), and particularly when the tumors are localized and are removed intact. The worst results are observed in patients with hematuria or with large tumors or in those in whom the tumor is broken into during surgery. Postoperative radiotherapy is widely credited with improving on the

Table 55. Results of various methods of treatment of Wilms' tumor*

Type of treatment	Cases	Cures	%
Nephrectomy alone	282	59	20.9
Preoperative irradiation and nephrectomy	103	28	27.2
Nephrectomy and post-operative irradiation	423	111	26.2
Preoperative irradiation, nephrectomy, post-operative irradiation	145	35	24.1

*From Klapproth, H. J.: Wilms tumor: a report of 45 cases and an analysis of 1,351 cases reported in the world literature from 1940 to 1958, J. Urol. 81:633-648, 1959.

Table 56. Series of 384 cases of Wilms' tumor collected at Baylor University*†

	Patients	%
Developed recurrence or died within period of risk	240	71.9
Alive and well beyond period of risk without recurrence	92	27.5
Survived beyond period of risk but developed later recurrence	2	0.6
	334	100.0

*From Collins, V. P.: Data presented at the A.M.A. meeting in San Francisco, June, 1958.
†Of the 384 patients, fifty still at risk.

results of surgery alone (Baert et al.[6]; Schweisguth et al.[81]), but no large series of cases or randomized study has been produced. Preoperative radiotherapy has not been given the trial it deserves. If nothing else, it diminishes considerably the risk of spillage at operation. Klapproth[49] reviewed 1351 cases and the results of various combinations of surgery and radiotherapy (Table 55). Dactinomycin has been credited with adding further to the combination of surgery and radiotherapy, the main claim being that it diminishes the proportion of metastases that appear after operation (Farber et al.[27]; Fernbach and Martyn[28]), but it is also administered for the treatment of metastases after they have appeared (Schweisguth et al.[81]). Farber[26] reported on fifty-three patients with no demonstrable metastases who were treated by a combination of dactinomycin, surgery, and radiotherapy, with forty-seven (89%) alive and well from two to nine years after treatment. Sixteen of these patients subsequently presented metastases

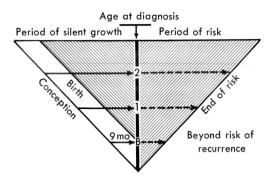

Fig. 489. Growth of Wilms' tumor proceeds from left to right. Diagnosis is preceded by period of silent growth that as a maximum is equal to nine months' gestation plus age of child at diagnosis. Diagnosis is followed by period of risk equal to maximum period of silent growth. If patient lives beyond period of risk without recurrence, he should be beyond risk of recurrence. (From Collins, V. P.: The treatment of Wilms's tumor, Cancer 11:89-94, 1958.)

and were given additional chemotherapy and radiotherapy, with ten apparently well at least two years afterward. Local excision of recurrences is sometimes successful (Garrett et al.[33]).

Collins et al.[18] studied 384 patients with Wilms' tumors. All recurrences in this group fell within a postoperative period equal to the patients' age at the time of diagnosis plus nine months. Collins et al.[18] concluded that the prognosis varies with age and that it is possible to predict the period of greatest risk (Table 56) (Fig. 489). For instance, a 1-year-old child could be considered cured if he lives twenty-one months after surgery without evidence of disease, whereas a 5-year-old child would have to survive sixty-nine months before he can be considered cured. We feel that this method of determining cure has definite merits.

Rarely, patients with Wilms' tumors have been reported cured by radiotherapy alone. Johnson and Marshall[45] reported a patient who survived eight years. Bilateral Wilms' tumors have been successfully treated by judicious combination of surgery and radiotherapy (Snyder et al.[84]; Stein and Goodwin[85]).

REFERENCES

1 Ahlberg, N. E., Bartley, O., Chidekel, N., and Wahlquist, L.: An anatomic and roentgenographic study of the communications of the

renal vein in patients with and without renal carcinoma, Scand. J. Urol. Nephrol. 1:43-51, 1967.

2 Albarrán, J., and Imbert, L.: Les tumeurs du rein, Paris, 1903, Masson et Cie.

3 Arner, O., Blanck, C., and von Schreeb, T.: Renal adenocarcinoma, Acta Chir. Scand. **346:** 11-50, 1965.

4 Aron, B. S., and Gross, M.: Renal adenocarcinoma in infancy and childhood; evaluation of therapy and prognosis, J. Urol. **102:**497-503, 1969.

5 Ashley, D. J. B., and Hickey, B. B.: Adenocarcinoma of the renal pelvis, Brit. J. Urol. 36:309-312, 1964.

6 Baert, L., Verduyn, H., and Vereecken, R.: Wilms' tumors (nephroblastomas); report of 57 histologically proved cases, J. Urol. **96:** 871-874, 1966.

7 Barney, J. D.: A twelve year cure following nephrectomy for adenocarcinoma and lobectomy for solitary metastasis, J. Urol. 52:406-407, 1944.

8 Beer, E.: Some aspects of malignant tumors of the kidney (B. A. Thomas Oration), Surg. Gynec. Obstet. 65:433-446, 1937.

9 Bennington, J. L., and Kradjian, R. M.: Renal carcinoma, Philadelphia, 1967, W. B. Saunders Co.

10 Bixler, L. C., Stenstrom, K. W., and Creevy, C. D.: Malignant tumors of the kidney; review of 117 cases, Radiology 42:329, 1944.

11 Black, W. C., and Ragsdale, E. F.: Wilms' tumor, Amer. J. Roentgen. 103:53-60, 1968.

12 Bloom, H. J. G., Baker, W. H., Dukes, C. E., and Mitchley, B. C. V.: Hormone-dependent tumours of the kidney. II. Effect of endocrine ablation procedures on the transplanted oestrogen-induced renal tumour of the Syrian hamster, Brit. J. Cancer 17:646-656, 1964.

13 Bloom, H. J. G., Dukes, C. E., and Mitchley, B. C. V.: Hormone-dependent tumours of the kidney. I. The oestrogen-induced renal tumour of the Syrian hamster; hormone treatment and possible relationship to carcinoma of the kidney in man, Brit. J. Cancer 17:611-645, 1964.

14 Bosniak, M. A.: Radiographic manifestations of massive arteriovenous fistula in renal carcinoma, Radiology 85:454-459, 1965.

15 Bostick, W. L.: Primary splenic neoplasms, Amer. J. Path. 21:1143-1165, 1945.

16 Bratherton, D. G., III: The place of radiotherapy in the treatment of hypernephroma, Brit. J. Radiol. 37:141-146, 1964.

17 Clarke, B. G., and Goade, W. J., Jr.: Fever and anemia in renal cancer, New Eng. J. Med. 254:107-110, 1956.

18 Collins, V. P., Loeffler, R. K., and Tivey, H.: Observations on growth rates of human tumors, Amer. J. Roentgen. 76:988-1000, 1956.

19 Cornell, S. H., and Dolan, K. D.: Angiographic findings in renal carcinoma, J. Urol. 98:71-76, 1967.

20 Culp, O. S.: Treatment of tumors of the renal pelvis and ureter, Trans. Amer. Ass. Genitourin. Surg. 47:101-112, 1955.

21 Damon, A., Holub, D. A., Melicow, M. M., and Uson, A. C.: Polycythemia and renal carcinoma; report of ten new cases, two with long hematologic remission following nephrectomy, Amer. J. Med. 25:182-197, 1958.

22 D'Angio, G. J., Farber, S., and Maddock, C. L.: Potentiation of x-ray effects by actinomycin D, Radiology 73:175-177, 1959.

23 Dunant, J. H., and Rutishauser, G.: Thorotrast tumors of the kidney, Schweiz. Med. Wschr. 96:1156-1160, 1966.

24 Evans, J.: The accuracy of diagnostic radiology, J.A.M.A. 204:223-226, 1968.

25 Farah, J., and Lofstrom, J. E.: Angiography of Wilms's tumor, Radiology 90:775-777, 1968.

26 Farber, S.: Chemotherapy in the treatment of leukemia and Wilms' tumor, J.A.M.A. 198: 826-836, 1966.

27 Farber, S., D'Angio, G., Evans, A., and Mitus, A.: Clinical studies of actinomycin D with special reference to Wilms' tumor in children. Part III. Clinical significance, Ann. N. Y. Acad. Sci. 89:421-425, 1960.

28 Fernbach, D. J., and Martyn, D. T.: Role of dactinomycin in the improved survival of children with Wilms' tumor, J.A.M.A. 195: 1005-1009, 1966.

29 Flocks, R. H., and Kadesky, M. C.: Malignant neoplasms of the kidney; an analysis of 353 patients followed five years or more, Trans. Amer. Ass. Genitourin. Surg. 49:105-110, 1957.

30 Fontaine, R., Kiény, R., Suhler, A., and Rieffel, R.: L'artériographie rénale sélective dans les cancers et kystes du rein (a propos de 25 cas), J. Radiol. Electr. 47:391-402, 1966.

31 Gahagan, H. Q., and Reed, W. K.: Squamous cell carcinoma of the renal pelvis, J. Urol. 62:139-151, 1949.

32 Garcia, M., Douglass, C., and Schlosser, J. V.: Classification and prognosis in Wilms's tumor, Radiology 80:574-580, 1963.

33 Garrett, R. A., Donohue, J. P., and Arnold, T. L.: Metastatic renal embryoma; survival following therapy, J. Urol. 98:444-449, 1967.

34 Gaulin, E.: Simultaneous Wilms' tumors in identical twins, J. Urol. 66:547-550, 1951.

35 George, A. M., and Harley, R. D.: The association of aniridia, Wilms' tumor and genital abnormalities, Arch. Ophthal. (Chicago) 75: 796-798, 1966.

36 Gerota, D.: Beiträge zur Kenntnis des Befestigungsapparates der Niere, Arch. Anat. Entwcklngsgesch., pp. 265-282, 1895.

37 Giger, K.: Sekundäre Polyglobulie bei Nierentumoren, Schweiz. Med. Wschr. 97:1067-1070, 1967.

38 Goldberg, M. F., Tashjian, A. H., Jr., Order, S. E., and Dammin, G. J.: Renal adenocarcinoma containing a parathyroid hormone-like substance and associated with marked hypercalcemia, Amer. J. Med. 36:805-814, 1964.

39 Gregg, D.: Tumours of the kidneys and suprarenals. II. Renal and suprarenal tumours in adults, Brit. J. Radiol. 37:128-141, 1964.

40 Hamm, F. C., and DeVeer, J. A.: Fatty replacement following renal atrophy or destruction, J. Urol. 41:850-866, 1939.

41 Heslin, J. E., Milner, W. A., and Garlick, W. B.: Lower urinary tract implants or metastases from clear cell carcinoma of the kidney, J. Urol. 73:39-46, 1955.

42 Holmes, R. B.: Primary tumors of the ureter; their roentgen diagnostic features, Radiology 56:520-527, 1951.

43 Jacobson, L. O., Goldwasser, E., Fried, W., and Plzak, L.: Role of kidney in erythropoiesis, Nature (London) 179:633, 1957.

44 Jenkins, G. D.: Regression of pulmonary metastasis following nephrectomy for hypernephroma; eight year followup, J. Urol. 82:37-40, 1959.

45 Johnson, S. H., III, and Marshall, M., Jr.: Primary kidney tumors of childhood, J. Urol. 74: 707-720, 1955.

46 Kahn, P. C., Wise, H. M., Jr., and Robbins, A. H.: Complete angiographic evaluation of renal cancer, J.A.M.A. 204:753-757, 1968.

47 Kimball, F. N., and Ferris, H. W.: Papillomatous tumors of pelvis associated with similar tumors of ureter and bladder; review of literature and report of two cases, J. Urol. 31: 257-304, 1934.

48 King, J. S., Jr., editor: Renal neoplasia, Boston, 1967, Little, Brown and Co.

49 Klapproth, H. J.: Wilms' tumor: a report of 45 cases and an analysis of 1,351 cases reported in the world literature from 1940 to 1958, J. Urol. 81:633-648, 1959 (extensive bibliography).

50 Krumbhaar, E. B.: The incidence and nature of splenic neoplasms, Ann. Clin. Med. 5:833-860, 1927.

51 Lassen, U. V., and Sagild, U.: Salt-losing syndrome due to unilateral renal disease (hypernephroma), Acta Med. Scand. 168:65-70, 1960.

52 Lazarus, J. A., and Marks, M. S.: Primary carcinoma of ureter with special reference to hydronephrosis, J. Urol. 54:140-157, 1945.

53 Löfgren, F. O.: Renal tumour not demonstrable by urography but shown by renal angiography, Acta Radiol. (Stockholm) 42:300-304, 1954.

54 Maier, J. G., and Harshaw, W. G.: Treatment and prognosis in Wilms' tumor; a study of 51 cases with special reference to the role of actinomycin D, Cancer 20:96-102, 1967.

55 Mann, L. T.: Spontaneous disappearance of pulmonary metastases after nephrectomy for hypernephroma; four year follow-up, J. Urol. 59:564-566, 1948.

56 Mann, L. T.: Personal communication, 1953.

57 Middleton, R. G.: Surgery for metastatic renal cell carcinoma, J. Urol. 97:973-977, 1967.

58 Mintz, E. R., and Gaul, E. A.: Kidney tumors; some causes of poor end results, New York J. Med. 39:1405-1411, 1939.

59 Morris, J. G., Coorey, G. J., Dick, R., Evans, W. A., Smitananda, N., Pearson, B. S., Loewenthal, J. I., Blackburn, C. R. B., and McRae, J.: The diagnosis of renal tumors by radioisotope scanning, J. Urol. 97:40-54, 1967.

60 Nalle, B. C., and Kennedy, L. J.: Renal-cell carcinoma with capsular calcification, Cancer Seminar 2:2-5, 1956.

61 Neibling, H. A., and Walters, W.: Adenocarcinoma and tuberculosis of the same kidney; review of the literature and report of seven cases, J. Urol. 59:1022-1035, 1948.

62 Oberkircher, O. J., Staubitz, W. J., and Blick, M. S.: Squamous cell carcinoma of the renal pelvis, J. Urol. 66:551-560, 1951.

63 Oberling, C., Rivière, M., and Haguenau, F.: Ultrastructure des épithéliomas à cellules claires du rein (hypernephromes ou tumeurs de Grawitz) et son implication pour l'histogénèse de ces tumeurs, Bull. Ass. Franc. Cancer 46:356-381, 1959.

64 Ochsner, M. G.: Renal cell carcinoma; five-year follow-up study of 70 cases, J. Urol. 93: 361-363, 1965.

65 O'Grady, A. S., Morse, L. J., and Lee, J. B.: Parathyroid hormone-secreting renal carcinoma associated with hypercalcemia and metabolic alkalosis, Ann. Intern. Med. 63:858-868, 1965 (excellent review).

66 Osius, T. G., Harrod, C. S., and Smith, D. R.: Cholesteatoma of the renal pelvis, J. Urol. 87: 774-778, 1962.

67 Peterson, C. A.: Personal communication, January, 1960.

68 Pines, B., and Rabinovitch, J.: Hemangioma of the spleen, Arch. Path. (Chicago) 33:487-503, 1942.

69 Rawson, A. J.: Distribution of the lymphatics of the human kidney as shown in a case of carcinomatous permeation, Arch. Path. (Chicago) 47:283-292, 1949.

70 Reboul, J., Ballanger, F., Delorme, G., Tavernier, J., and Geindre, M.: Association radiothérapie préopératoire et chirurgie dans le traitement du cancer primitif du rein de l'adulte, Ann. Radiol. (Paris) 5:283-288, 1962.

71 del Regato, J. A., and Kagan, A. R.: Basic considerations in radiotherapy of renal carcinomas. In King, J. S., Jr., editor: Renal neoplasia, Boston, 1967, Little, Brown and Co., chap. 22, pp. 547-557.

72 Riches, E.: On carcinoma of the kidney, Ann. Roy. Coll. Surg. Eng. 32:201-218, 1963.

73 Riches, E. W.: Analysis of patients with adenocarcinoma in a personal series. In Riches, E. W., editor: Tumors of the kidney and ureter, London, 1964, E. & S. Livingstone, Ltd., pp. 357-368.

74 Riches, E.: The place of radiotherapy in the management of parenchymal carcinoma of the kidney, Trans. Amer. Ass. Genitourin. Surg. 57:120-124, 1965.

75 Rosenthall, L.: Radionuclide diagnosis of malignant tumors of the kidney, Amer. J. Roentgen. 101:662-668, 1967.

76 Rouvière, H.: Anatomie des lymphatiques de l'homme, Paris, 1933, Masson et Cie.

77 Royce, R. K., and Tormey, A. R., Jr.: Malignant tumors of the renal parenchyma in adults, J. Urol. 74:23-35, 1955.

78 Rubin, P., Duthie, R. B., and Young, L. W.: The significance of scoliosis in postirradiated Wilms' tumor and neuroblastoma, Radiology 79:539-559, 1962.

79 Rusche, C. F.: Silent adenocarcinoma of the kidney with solitary metastases occurring in brothers, J. Urol. 70:146-151, 1953.

80 Savignac, E. M.: Primary carcinoma of the ureter, Amer. J. Roentgen. **74**:628-634, 1955.

81 Schweisguth, O., Guy, E., and Sentenac, J. P.: La place de la radiothérapie dans le traitement du néphroblastome de l'enfant, J. Radiol. Electr. **46**:376-380, 1965.

82 Shawan, H. K.: Epidermoid cysts of the spleen, Arch. Surg. (Chicago) **27**:63-74, 1933.

83 Sherman, R. S., and Pearson, T. A.: The roentgenographic appearance of renal cancer metastasis in bone, Cancer **1**:276-285, 1948.

84 Snyder, H. E., Brockman, S. K., Grant, B. P., and Foster, J. H.: Bilateral Wilms' tumor, Amer. J. Surg. **110**:492-494, 1965.

85 Stein, J. J., and Goodwin, W. E.: Bilateral Wilms' tumor, including report of a patient surviving ten years after treatment, Amer. J. Roentgen. **96**:626-634, 1966.

86 Sullivan, M. P., Sutow, W. W., Cangir, A., and Taylor, G.: Vincristine sulphate in management of Wilms' tumor; replacement of preoperative irradiation by chemotherapy, J.A.M.A. **202**:381-384, 1967.

87 Thompson, R. F.: Leukoplakia of the renal pelvis, Trans. South Centr. Sect. Amer. Urol. Ass., pp. 64-69, 1954.

88 Waller, J. I., Throckmorton, M. A., and Barbosa, E.: Renal hemangioma, J. Urol. **74**:186-190, 1955.

89 Weidmann, P., Siegenthaler, W., Ziegler, W., and Sulser, H., Endres, P., and Werning, C.: Hypertension associated with tumors adjacent to renal arteries, Amer. J. Med. **47**:528-533, 1969.

90 Westra, P., Kieffere, S. A., and Mosser, D. G.: A summary of 25 years of experience before actinomycin-D, Amer. J. Roentgen. **100**:214-221, 1967.

91 Whitlock, G. F., McDonald, J. R., and Cook, E. N.: Primary carcinoma of the ureter; a pathologic and prognostic study, J. Urol. **73**:245-253, 1955.

92 Wigger, H. J.: Fetal hamartoma of kidney, Amer. J. Clin. Path. **51**:323-337, 1969.

93 Wilms, M.: Die Mischgeschwulste der Niere, Leipzig, 1899, Arthur Georgi, pp. 1-90.

94 Witten, D. M., Greene, L. F., and Emmett, J. L.: An evaluation of nephrotomography in urologic diagnosis, Amer. J. Roentgen. **90**:115-123, 1963.

95 Woodruff, M. W., Salman, D. G., and Jones, R., Jr.: The current status of chemotherapy for advanced renal carcinoma. In King, J. S., Jr., editor: Renal neoplasia, Boston, 1967, Little, Brown and Co., chap. 24, pp. 573-592.

96 Zinman, L., and Dowd, J. B.: Partial nephrectomy in renal cell carcinoma, Surg. Clin. N. Amer. **47**:685-693, 1967.

Urinary bladder

Anatomy

The urinary bladder is a muscular membranous sac occupying the anterior part of the pelvis and the lower abdomen. It has the form of a tetrahedron with a postero-inferior triangular base, the trigone, extending from the origin of the urethra to the ureteral orifices. Its posterosuperior wall extends from the urachus to the ureteral orifices, and the anterolateral walls join it to complete the tetrahedron and end in an anterosuperior summit at the point of fixation of the urachus.

The inferolateral surfaces are related to the endopelvic fascia covering the levator ani muscles and extending upward to the level of the arcus tendineus. With distention, the obturator nerve and vessels, umbilical artery, and ductus deferens are brought into relationship with this surface. The fundus, with a more fixed position, is directly related to the seminal vesicles in the male, portions of the vas deferens, and the ampullary portion of the rectum. In the female, it is related to the anterior surface of the vaginal wall and the corpus uteri. In the male, the inferior angle of the bladder at the urethral orifice rests directly on the base of the prostate, from which it gains support through the puboprostatic ligaments of the endopelvic fascia. In the female, this point is attached to the transverse sphincter urethra muscle with a similar fascial support. The superior angle continues onto the anterior abdominal wall as the median umbilical ligament. The arterial supply to the bladder is derived from the superior and inferior vesical branches of the hypogastric artery. The venous drainage forms a plexus in the lower fundic area that empties into the hypogastric veins.

Lymphatics. The mucosa and the muscular layers of the bladder possess rich intercommunicating networks of lymphatics (Albarrán[3]). According to Rouvière,[118] they give rise to the following:

1 The *collecting trunks of the trigone* emerge from points medial to the ureters or to the deferent ducts. They follow the uterine or the deferent artery and terminate in the medial and middle group of external iliac nodes.

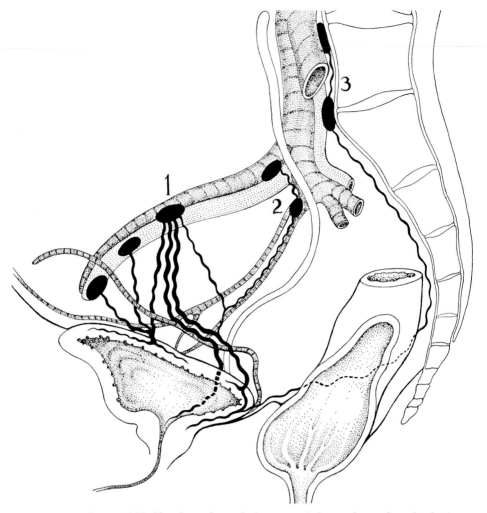

Fig. 490. Lymphatics of bladder drained mainly by external iliac nodes, **1**, but also by hypogastric nodes, **2**, and common iliac nodes, **3**.

2 The *collecting trunks of the posterior wall* may empty into the collecting trunks of the trigone or reach the posterolateral angle of the bladder, cross the umbilical artery, and terminate (a) in one of the medial or middle external iliac nodes, (b) less frequently, in the retrofemoral nodes, and (c) in the hypogastric or the lateral nodes of the external iliac chain.

3 The *collecting trunks of the anterior wall* converge toward the middle third of the lateral border of the bladder, descend toward the origins of the middle vesicle artery and of the umbilical artery, meet and merge with the collecting trunks of the posterior wall, and terminate in the nodes of the external iliac chain.

In summary, the lymphatics of the bladder are drained particularly by the medial and middle groups of nodes of the external iliac chain but occasionally also by the hypogastric and the common iliac nodes (Fig. 490).

Epidemiology

In the 1947 cancer survey in the United States, the age-adjusted incidence rates of cancer of the bladder were found to be 17.3 and 8.1 for male and female whites and 4.9 and 5.6 for male and female nonwhites per 100,000 population. The rate for males 35 to 39 years of age is about 3, but it rises steadily to around 155 per 100,000 in men 75 to 79 years old. The comparisons of the Connecticut surveys of 1945-1949 and 1960-1962 and the New York surveys of 1949-1951 and 1958-1960 show an increase in the incidence rate of about 25% in both states. The highest reported male rate is from South Africa and the lowest from Japan (Clemmesen et al.[24]).

It has been known for a long time that chronic industrial exposure to certain dye intermediates implies a high risk of carcinoma of the bladder (about thirty times greater than that of the general population). Cases of vesical cancer among aniline dye workers were first reported in Germany (Rehn[115]), and as such industry developed in other countries, cases were reported in Switzerland, England, France (Billiard-Duchesne[9]), Russia, Italy, and the United States. Hueper[68] collected about 200 cases of cancer of the bladder over a period of twenty years in persons connected with dye industries in the United States. The length of necessary exposure varies considerably and may be as long as forty years (Oppenheimer[105]). The most frequently recognized and incriminated agent is beta-naphthylamine, but alpha-naphthylamine, 4-aminodiphenyl, benzidine, and auramine are also suspect. These agents are not carcinogenic to other tissues. The common denominator seems to be an aromatic amine that can be excreted as an orthohydroxylated urinary metabolite (Bonser et al.[11]).

Holsti and Ermala[66] observed that the oral application of tobacco tars in mice was followed in 75% of the animals by the development of bladder papillomas that failed to develop in any of the controls. A high degree of association of long-standing smoking habits and cancer of the bladder in men has been reported from several sources (Lockwood,[87] Denoix and Schwartz[35]). Clemmesen et al.[23] showed a parallel increase of cases of papilloma of the bladder in men and tobacco consumption in Copenhagen. Cobb and Ansell[26] have suggested that a combination of acid urine, some degree of urinary obstruction, and heavy cigarette smoking may increase the risk of cancer of the bladder.

Patients with cancer of the bladder ex-crete excessive quantities of tryptophan metabolites. This is also true of lower animals with spontaneous cancer of the bladder. Kerr et al.[77] have observed a rise of tryptophan metabolites in smokers and, therefore, believe that smoking may contribute to the cause of vesical cancer by inhibiting the metabolism of tryptophan.

There is a definite association between leukoplakia and epidermoid carcinoma of the urinary tract. Leukoplakia results from metaplasia of the transitional epithelium of the bladder. It can exist independently and can precede or accompany an epidermoid carcinoma. The metaplasia is initiated by long-standing chronic inflammation or mechanical irritation plus unknown factors. In 124 cases of leukoplakia of the urinary bladder collected by Rabson,[113] eighteen were associated with carcinoma (thirteen epidermoid) and one with sarcoma. Patch[108] found thirteen cases of leukoplakia of the bladder, seven coexistent with epidermoid carcinoma in the bladder and one with simultaneous epidermoid carcinoma of the bladder and the left kidney pelvis. Under the influence of infection, metaplasia can progress to the formation of glandular epithelium (cystitis glandularis). These changes may progress to adenocarcinoma (Stirling and Ash[132]; Patch[109]). Davis[32] described two cases of carcinoma of the bladder that showed spontaneous regression following ureterosigmoidostomy. Microscopic examination revealed evidence of residual tumor. deGironcoli[34] collected thirteen cases of tumors of the bladder that regressed following supravesical diversion of the urinary stream.

Cancer of the bladder may develop in patients with bilharziasis, a parasitic infection that is associated with cancer of the bladder. Parallelism does not exist between the frequency of bilharzial infection and the frequency of bladder carcinoma. There are undoubtedly other factors associated with this infection that may have a bearing on the frequency of carcinoma. Abdel-Tawab et al.[2] indicated that the etiology could be related to excretion of tryptophan metabolites and beta-glucuronidases in the urine. Furthermore, Fripp[58] believes that *Schistosoma haematobium* infestation may precipitate tumor development by increasing the excretion of beta-glucuronidase, which could hydrolyze any inactivated carcinogenic glucuronide excreted in the urine. Bilharziasis occurs almost always in men, and cancer associated with it makes its appearance at an early age (between 30 and 40 years). It is estimated that from 70% to 90% of the population of Egypt is infected with *Schistosoma haematobium* (bilharziasis). The tumors vary in their microscopic pattern and are often asso-ciated with metaplastic epithelial changes. In ninety cases reported by Dimmette et al.,[39] fifty were squamous, thirty-three were transitional, six were adenocarcinoma, and one was mixed in type.

Pathology
Gross pathology

The well-differentiated *papilloma* of the bladder is best designated as Grade I *transitional cell carcinoma.* The tumors can be implanted and often recur. They have been grown in the eyes of guinea pigs (Hovenanian and Deming[67]).

Grade I transitional cell carcinoma (papilloma) arises on the paler mucous membrane of the bladder and has a large base that hides the point of implantation like a mushroom hides its base. It is pink or red in color and friable and soft. Only under some tension does it become evident that this tumor is attached by an often flat and very soft pedicle formed, for the most part, by the mucous membrane itself. At times, the bladder can be entirely replaced by these well-differentiated neoplasms (Fig. 491). If multiple tumors are present, they may show varying degrees of differentia-

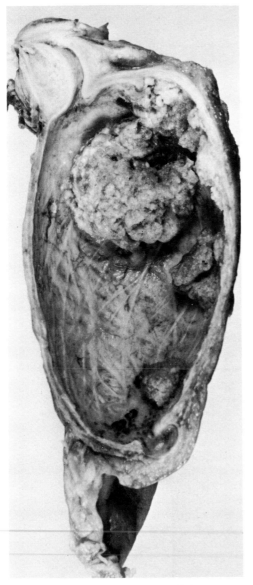

Fig. 491. Cystectomy specimen including prostate and seminal vesicles. There are multiple papillary transitional cell carcinomas and direct extension into left ureter. (WU neg. 68-5455.)

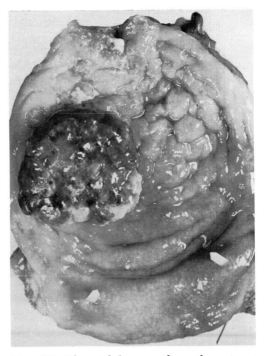

Fig. 492. Ulcerated large epidermoid carcinoma of bladder that was treated by cystectomy.

tion. Grossly, the well-differentiated neoplasms are usually pedunculated. As these tumors become undifferentiated, the proportion of papillary ones among them decreases. Infrequently, the highly malignant carcinomas are papillary in character. In the poorly differentiated tumors, ulceration, infection, and fixation are common. When a papillary tumor shows poor differentiation, it tends to invade the base and become fixed. Later, it ulcerates and becomes infected, but the majority of transitional cell carcinomas develop as a papillary mass. *Epidermoid carcinomas* (only a small percentage of the total number of carcinomas) are usually firm, deeply ulcerated, and heavily infected and often involve the musculature of the bladder (Fig. 492).

In a large series of single bladder tumors of the transitional cell type collected by the Carcinoma Registry of the American Urological Society, the points of origin were as shown in Table 57 (Mostofi[101]). In 243 cases reported by Barringer,[5] 195 (80%) were around the bladder base near or involving the internal urethra or one or both ureters. In another series reported

by the Registry, there were 643 single and 250 multiple bladder carcinomas, 45% of which were more than 5 cm in diameter.

In the group collected by the Registry, only 34% were limited to a single area. This figure contrasts with that of the vesical adenocarcinomas, of which 63% were in a single area, with 57% of them located in the dome (Mostofi[101]).

Carcinoma of the bladder gradually extends through the wall, the speed of its extension being related to the degree of differentiation (Jewett[72]). Intramural spread

Table 57. Points of origin of single bladder tumors*

Region	%
Trigone	21
Lateral walls	47
Posterior wall	18
Dome	6
Anterior wall	8
Total	100

*Data from Mostofi, F. K.: A study of 2678 patients with initial carcinoma of the bladder. I. Survival rates, J. Urol. 75:480-491, 1956.

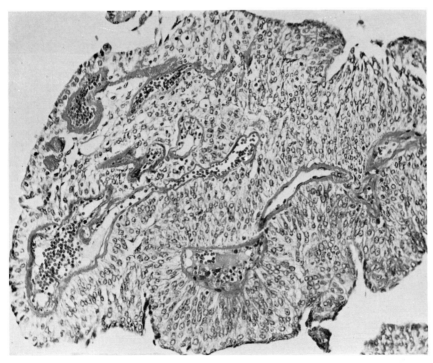

Fig. 493. Grade I transitional cell carcinoma of bladder. Note uniformity of cells. (Moderate enlargement.)

beyond the apparent boundary of the tumor is not unusual. In poorly differentiated tumors growing close to the prostatic urethra, invasion of the prostate may take place. Invasion of the seminal vesicles, urethra, and ureters is rare. In some rare instances, the large bowel has been found invaded.

Microscopic pathology

For the most part, tumors of the bladder arise from the transitional epithelium, and when they form well-differentiated tumors, they are supported by an abundantly vascularized connective tissue stroma. The connective tissue in Grade I *transitional cell carcinoma* (papilloma) is in the center of and forms the framework for lobules (Fig. 493). As the tumor becomes more malignant, it invades these lobules, and connective tissue is often seen about the periphery (Fig. 494). Some of these tumors may contain nerves and small collections of smooth muscle cells. The location of recurrent Grade I *transitional cell carcinoma* (papilloma) corresponds exactly to the opposing points of the mucosa.

Multiple foci of origin can also occur. The most malignant zones in a papillary tumor are found not only in the base, but also frequently in the peripheral portions accessible to biopsy. These changes may be localized so that one area of a neoplasm may be more malignant than another.

With the frankly ulcerating *transitional cell carcinoma,* the origin from transitional epithelium is still apparent. As the tumor becomes more undifferentiated, it shows a tendency to infiltrate diffusely, and destruction and permeation of the bladder musculature by masses of tumor cells within the lymphatics are seen quite frequently. When a carcinoma is far advanced and quite undifferentiated, it may be difficult to tell whether it originated in the prostate or the bladder. Primary adenocarcinoma of the bladder often coexists with cystitis cystica and cystitis glandularis, suggesting origin from such lesions (Wheeler and Hill[141]).

Sarcoma botryoides, a rare form of malignant bladder tumor, usually occurs in young children. It has myxomatous tissue in which striated tumor cells can often be seen (Batsakis[7]).

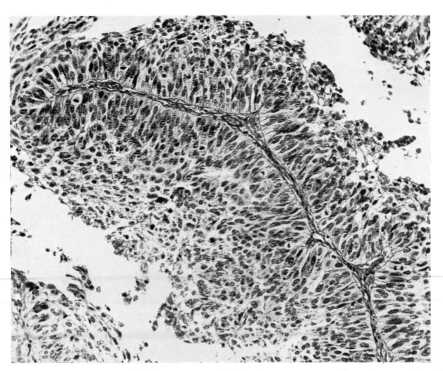

Fig. 494. Grade II transitional cell carcinoma of bladder. Note increased prominence of nuclei and variation in cell size. (Moderate enlargement.)

Metastatic spread

Autopsy studies of metastases in carcinoma of the bladder reveal a variable proportion of lymph node involvement (Fetter et al.[49]). Many patients die because of concomitant infection and pyelonephritis or of postoperative complications before the tumor has had an opportunity to metastasize. Spooner[129] found metastases in only forty-nine (29%) of 167 cases seen at autopsy, whereas Colston and Leadbetter[28] found metastases in fifty-nine (61%) of ninety-eight cases seen at autopsy. Jewett and Eversole[73] studied a group of eighty-nine patients with extravesical direct invasion by the tumor, fifty-two of whom presented metastases. Thirty-three had regional lymph node involvement, twenty-six had liver implants, eighteen had lung involvement, and eleven had bone involvement. One-third of the patients with metastases had no regional node involvement. The most frequent node involvement is found at the bifurcation of the iliac artery. It has been suggested that direct involvement of the prostate or parametria may increase the chances of metastases (Saphir[123]). Skin metastases may be observed but rarely (Bischoff and Fishkin[10]).

Clinical evolution

Hematuria is the most common presenting symptom of carcinoma of the bladder (Table 58). In 163 patients reported by Smith and Mintz,[128] 125 had hematuria. Hematuria often appears abruptly without pain and is not relieved by repose or motion. Its persistence and repetition are the most important characteristics of the evolution of the disease. There is often disproportion between the amount of bleeding and the amount of disease present. One micturition may be bloody, whereas the next is entirely clear or the urine may change slowly to a normal color over a period of days. In some instances, the amount of bleeding may be marked, and if clots appear, they may be followed by enormous enlargement of the bladder and by painful spasms of the bladder musculature. With removal of the clots, the pain ceases. Hematuria is often most prominent in the terminal stages of a carcinoma of the bladder (Albarrán[3]) but may be severe even in benign papillomas. In carcinomas

Table 58. Tabulation of initial symptom and later symptoms and their incidence in 902 cases of carcinoma of bladder*

	Cases
Initial symptom	
Hematuria	573
Frequency of urination (pollakiuria)	176
Dysuria (painful micturition)	40
Pain unrelated to urination	16
Difficulty in urination	16
Acute retention	7
Total	828
Later symptoms	
Intermittent hematuria	704
Constant hematuria	122
Frequency of urination (pollakiuria)	644
Dysuria (painful micturition)	375
Pain unrelated to micturition	312
Retention of urine	113
Urinary incontinence	19
Passage of fragments of tumor	32

*Data from Committee on Carcinoma Registry: Cancer of the bladder, J. Urol. 31:423-472, 1934.

with a low degree of malignancy, there is excessive hematuria in the symptomatology, whereas in the more malignant varieties, probably because of invasion of the bladder wall, there is a preponderance of pain and pollakiuria (Royce and Ackerman[119]).

The removal of Grade I transitional cell carcinomas (papillomas) does not necessarily imply cure, for they are likely to recur within a period of months. There may be intermittent hematuria during a period of years until, for no apparent reason, the tumor becomes more malignant and takes an aggressive character. Unfortunately, if a papillary tumor of the bladder is controlled locally by conservative therapy, it is impossible to predict whether the patient will develop further tumors or whether he will develop an invasive cancer. It is obvious that once a patient has developed a papillary tumor, follow-up is mandatory (Pyrah et al.[111]). New tumors may actually represent evidence of multiple foci of origin. Eventually, pollakiuria, nycturia, and pain become preponderant.

Carcinoma of the bladder varies in the speed of its evolution. Wallace and Harris[140] emphasize that some bladder tumors remain confined to the bladder mucosa for months or years, whereas others spread rapidly to lymph nodes in the pelvic wall within weeks or months. The papillary type of carcinoma tends to grow more slowly than the deeply ulcerating variety. The poorly differentiated carcinomas usually have a relatively rapid growth. Since a high percentage of the tumors grow in close relation to the ureters, urinary infection is common. It produces fever, weight loss, and costovertebral tenderness. The patient with untreated carcinoma of the bladder usually dies of urinary infection associated with unilateral or bilateral pyelonephritis. It is most uncommon for extensive generalized metastases to be the cause of death.

Cutaneous metastases from carcinoma of the bladder have been rarely observed (Higgins and Hausfeld[64]; McDonald et al.[90]). These skin manifestations usually appear in terminal stages. Osteolytic bone metastases are infrequently observed in the course of the disease.

Diagnosis
Clinical examination

A tumor of the bladder can be felt best by rectal or vaginal palpation further supported by pressure on the hypogastrium and with the patient under spinal anesthesia. At times, the tumor can be felt suprapubically. The bladder should, of course, be empty. Perivesical extension may be detected by palpation. This examination may be unsatisfactory if the prostate is enlarged. Jewett and Eversole[73] have long insisted that this examination can easily reveal whether or not the bladder wall is invaded, thus facilitating the establishment of a prognosis.

Cystoscopy

Cystoscopic examination of all bladder tumors is essential. The typical Grade I transitional cell carcinoma (papilloma) is attached by a delicate pedicle usually to the lower lateral or posterior part of the bladder wall. Its grayish pink branches float in the irrigating fluid, giving the appearance of seaweed. With infection, the tips of this fernlike growth become edematous and necrotic. It is not always possible on cystoscopy to determine how malignant a given tumor may be. In early papillary carcinoma, the base is infiltrated. In the deeply ulcerating tumors, the sur-

rounding mucosa is often thrown up into folds. With carcinomas, secondary infection may be present that also contributes to the rigidity of the wall. Bullous edema, in the untreated case, usually indicates submucosal growth of the tumor (Franksson[52]). The capacity of the bladder is often reduced. It may be difficult to differentiate this type of carcinoma from chronic inflammatory lesions and encrusted phosphatic cystitis. In a few instances, mainly when carcinoma develops on the anterior wall, the tumor may not be seen on cystoscopy.

Staging

The following clinical classification has been suggested by Edsmyr et al.[41]; bimanual palpation and a positive biopsy are assumed in every case.

Stage I

Tumor freely movable within the bladder and soft to palpation; no biopsy evidence of muscular infiltration

Stage II

Induration of the bladder wall as revealed by palpation and/or biopsy evidence of muscular infiltration

Stage III

Hard nodular tumor but movable in all directions and/or biopsy evidence of deep muscular infiltration

Stage IV

Tumor fixed or invading adjoining areas (vagina; prostate)

Biopsy

Biopsy through a cystoscope may be difficult because of the secondary infection present. A negative biopsy in the presence of an apparent carcinoma should always be repeated. Transurethral biopsy has been found practicable. Microscopic examination of cystoscopic biopsies often reveals a lower grade of malignancy than the deeper portions of the tumor examined after surgery (Dean[33]). A diagnosis of carcinoma of the bladder may be made through recognition of exfoliated malignant cells in the urine or bladder washings. Schmidlapp and Marshall[125] found malignant cells in forty-nine of sixty-seven cases of proved malignant tumors, but this method of diagnosis is rarely of practical value. There are unusual instances in which a bladder tumor may be concealed within a diverticulum, and the recognition of malignant cells will make an unexpectetd diagnosis (Papanicolaou[107]).

Roentgenologic examination

"Scout" roentgenograms of the pelvis may reveal the presence of a suspicious soft tissue mass. Excretory urography is helpful in revealing kidney damage or concomitant ureteral tumors. Retrograde urography may be preferable, but often the presence of an infected bladder tumor interferes with its performance. In 229 urographic examinations in bladder tumors, Franksson and Lindblom[53] found fifty-eight cases of dilatation of one or both ureters. The majority of these were found to be infiltrating tumors. The presence of ureteral block plus thickening of the bladder wall and a sloping contour of the tumor suggest cancer (Franksson[52]). Increasingly, cystography is used to determine the extent of a bladder carcinoma (Fig. 495). Wise and Fainsinger[144] used angiography to define the limits of the tumor. Lang et al.[83] found arteriography

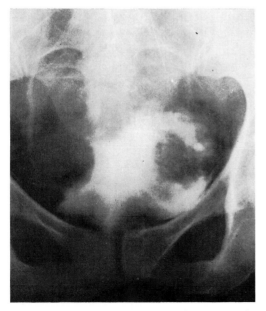

Fig. 495. Cystogram showing multiple irregular filling defects due to multiple papillomatosis.

of value in staging, with an overall accuracy of over 90%.

Differential diagnosis

Because a very high percentage of carcinomas of the bladder produce hematuria, other lesions presenting this symptom have to be ruled out. In 860 cases of hematuria studied by Kretschmer,[80a] there were 126 lesions of the prostate and fifty-four lesions of the ureter. The bleeding was caused by renal lesions in 331 patients and by bladder lesions in 307. Bladder bleeding was caused by carcinoma in 163 patients, by papillomas in seventy-two, by lithiasis in thirty-one, by tuberculosis in fourteen, and by cystitis in six. Radiographic examination may be sufficient to diagnose the clearly benign or obviously malignant lesions of the bladder.

Tuberculosis may be mistaken for tumor. Fairly often, however, there is evidence of tuberculosis in the epididymis or seminal vesicles, or pyelograms may show a primary lesion in the kidney. Practically all cases of tuberculosis of the genitourinary tract are secondary to primary lung lesions. Biopsies may show tuberculosis, and guinea pig inoculation or culture, if positive, is unequivocal proof of the presence of acid-fast infection. The hematuria that is present in tuberculosis is usually not so frequent or so painful as in carcinoma of the bladder.

Carcinoma of the female urethra is rarely observed. It is usually an undifferentiated epidermoid carcinoma. Occasionally transitional cell carcinomas occur, and rarely adenocarcinomas arise from paraurethral ducts and glands (Walker and Huffman[139]). McCrea[89] was able to collect 546 cases of urethral carcinomas. These tumors occur most frequently in women after the menopause. There is no evidence that urethral caruncle or leukoplakia has any etiologic significance in their development. The proximal half of the urethra is most commonly affected, but the tumor may invade the vaginal wall and the vulva. Inguinal lymph node metastases are most common, but metastases may also be found in the external iliac, hypogastric, retrofemoral, and sacral nodes. Interstitial irradiation has been successful in the treatment of carcinomas of the female urethra (Staubitz et al.[130]). Buschke and Cantril[19] reported successful external roentgentherapy for carcinoma of the female urethra in four patients. Hultberg[70] reported on the results of combined roentgentherapy and interstitial radium therapy. Seven of eleven patients treated by this method were free from symptoms after a minimum of four years. Others have preferred a combination of surgery and radiotherapy (Fagan and Hertig[48]; Brack and Dickson[14]). The best results are obtained in patients with carcinomas limited to the anterior urethra (Monaco et al.[97]). The frequency of metastases requires a bilateral inguinal dissection in some cases. Fricke and McMillan[55] reported fifteen five-year survivals in a series of thirty-five patients treated at the Mayo Clinic.

Kidney tumors are not difficult to differentiate, for on cystoscopy blood is often seen coming from the ureteral orifice of the involved kidney. The presence of a mass in the kidney region is confirmatory evidence.

Simple *chronic interstitial cystitis* may be difficult to differentiate because the induration and infection so strongly suggest bladder carcinoma. Repeated biopsies and cystoscopic examinations may be necessary to rule out tumor. A stone which accompanies cystitis also produces an induration around the bladder and may cause an erroneous diagnosis of cancer. Tumor may coexist with cystitis, and this may give a false impression of a tumor much larger than that which is present. Lesions of the prostate may cause hematuria, but again rectal and cystoscopic examinations usually suffice to differentiate them.

Direct invasion of the bladder by *tumors of other organs* is quite common, particularly the prostate, cervix, and rectum. The primary source of these tumors can usually be determined by careful pelvic and rectal examination or by biopsy.

Primary carcinomas and papillomas of the bladder apex are relatively rare, but they have to be distinguished from the mucinous adenocarcinoma arising from the epithelium of the urachal canal. Begg[8] collected thirty-four cases of *adenocarcinoma of the urachus* showing areas of circumscribed ulceration. Elimination of mucus and necrotic material in the urine is often observed. Few cases have been diagnosed before the tumor perforated the vesical mucosa.

Rare benign tumors of the bladder are *neurofibromas* (Thompson and McDonald[135]), *fibromyxomas* (Higgins[63]), *hemangiomas* (Segal and Fink[126]), and *leiomyomas* (Kretschmer and Doerhing[81]). *Adenomatoid tumors* of the bladder reproducing renal structures (nephrogenic adenomas) have been observed and studied (Friedman and Kuhlenbeck[57]). Pheochromocytoma of the bladder may be associated with hypertension provoked by urination (Bourne and Beltaos[12]). *Lymphosarcoma* has been reported by Jacobs and Symington.[71] *Leiomyosarcomas* may arise (Kretschmer and Doerhing[81]). Mostofi and Morse[102] reported ten cases of polypoid *rhabdomyosarcoma* (botryoid sarcoma) in infants. Hanbury[62] reported a similar group in the bladder and prostate. These tumors caused death by local infiltration rather than by distant metastases. Rare bony and cartilaginous tumors of the bladder may occur (Pang[106]). Malacoplakia predominates in female patients and is characterized, at times, by submucosal plaques suggesting a neoplasm (Smith[127]).

Treatment
Prevention

Prevention of occupational tumors is possible, for the carcinogenic agent doubtless enters the respiratory tract, and protection can and should be utilized. Workers admitted into industrial plants that use aromatic amines should be healthy and between 20 and 45 years of age and should not have had any previous history of occupational exposure to those agents that are known to cause carcinoma of the bladder. Employment should be limited to a maximum of three years, and frequent routine cystoscopic examinations should be done. If, at any time, there is evidence of any changes in the bladder suggestive of beginning neoplasm, the worker should immediately be taken out of his occupational environment (Hueper[69]). Effective control of cancer hazards related to work with beta-naphthylamine has proved to be so difficult that certain English, Swiss, and German manufacturers have discontinued its production. Crabbe et al.[29] have used cytology as an effective method in discovering cancer of the bladder in patients working in dangerous industries. Koss et al.[79] studied by cytology the bladder sediment of workers exposed to para-aminodiphenyl over a number of years. They found that the time necessary to develop invasive cancer was long and that there was a period of years in which abnormal cytology progressed from carcinoma in situ to invasive carcinoma, without detectable clinical abnormalities. Clemmesen et al.[23] have suggested that patients with bladder papillomas abstain from smoking because of the correlation between smoking and bladder cancer.

Surgery

For single, superficial, well-delimited Grade I transitional cell carcinomas (so-called papillomas), biopsy followed by *fulguration* may be the treatment of choice (Royce and Spjut[120]), but casual attention to follow-up of these cases may result in considerable harm. There is no doubt that carcinoma of the bladder is often multicentric and that local treatment may offer temporary results only. By delaying more radical procedures, this approach may also be harmful.

Cases suitable for *segmental resection* make up a small percentage of all bladder tumors. They should be single, sharply defined, and preferably situated high up in the bladder. Masina[94] emphasizes that papillary tumors of a low grade are not suitable, and there must be an abrupt change from the tumor to normal mucosa.

Cystectomy is most successful in the treatment of extensive well-differentiated and superficial lesions, but this radical procedure is not indicated when the tumors have penetrated through the wall, in very undifferentiated tumors, or in the presence of lymph node metastases (Whitmore and Marshall[143]). Thus, before cystectomy is decided upon, the size, location, and histologic features of the tumor or tumors should be known, as well as the extent of infiltration and the presence or absence of lymph node involvement. The general condition of the patient and, in particular, the cardiovascular and renal reserves should be evaluated (Dean[33]). The operative mortality of cystectomies has been reduced. Total cystectomy and ileal diversion were performed in 146 patients with seven operative mortalities (Bowles and Cordonnier[13]). Resection of the prostate and seminal vesicles seems to reduce complications (Romanus[117]). Leadbetter and Cooper[85] devised an operative procedure that provides for en bloc dissection of lymphatic channels and draining nodes, but it is unlikely that any surgical procedure will be successful in the presence of lymph node metastases except in rare instances. Riches' indications[116] for total cystectomy extend much beyond the limits accepted by others. Long et al.[87a] have devised a radical abdominoperineal cystectomy with urethrectomy in continuity. This procedure is particularly effective in the advanced cancers for, as might be expected, it reduces the incidence of local recrudescence.

The success of a cystectomy depends on the effectual transplantation of the ureters. They may be transplanted into the sigmoid, perineum, rectum, urethra, vagina, skin near the incision, or surgical wound or near the anterosuperior iliac spine (Hinman[65]). Nephrostomy and lumbar ureterostomy may be done. The nephrostomy and the skin transplantation seem to have the lowest operative mortality, but the necessity of taking care of the urine through the use of an artificial bladder makes this operation undesirable. Transplantations into the vagina and urethra carry a high operative mortality. Transplantation into the rectum often causes death from kidney infection. The diversion of the urinary flow into an isolated segment of the ileum, as devised by Bricker,[16] is the most satisfactory method to deal with this problem.

Radiotherapy

Interstitial implantation of radon seeds through a suprapubic cystostomy enjoyed acceptance for some time as a procedure of choice for the irradiation of tumors of the urinary bladder (Barringer[6]), but a reappraisal of this method has been disappointing (Marshall[92]). The irradiation of the tumor in this manner is seldom sufficiently homogeneous—hence, the great possibility of necrosis or recurrence or both. Interstitial irradiation with radium element needles has proved successful in papillary lesions (Darget[31]). More recently, nylon thread containing cobalt[60] pellets has been used for the same purpose (Vermooten[138]). The intracavitary instillation of a soluble radioactive material has also been tried in the treatment of very superficial lesions. The elements used are mostly emitters of soft, little-penetrating beta radiations: sodium[24], bromine[82], yttrium[90], and gold[198] (Ellis and Oliver[47]; Einhorn et al.[44]; Touvinen and Kettunen[136]; Cuccia[30]). The lesions suitable for this approach constitute an extreme minority. Radioactive gold has received greater use in a distensible latex bag placed within the bladder (Dickson and Lang[38]; Dyche and McKay[40]). Even papillary lesions may be relatively thick and thus unevenly irradiated by the soft radiations of the radioactive gold. The lesion to be irradiated is not usually evenly distributed around the bag, and the possibility of infiltration of the wall always remains unsuspected. Friedman and Lewis[56] introduced a technique of intracavitary irradiation by means of a radium source within a distensible balloon placed in the bladder and connected to a urethral catheter. The use of radium as an intracavitary source of radiations offers the advantage of greater penetration of gamma radiations, but it has limited applicability and success.

External pelvic irradiation by means of conventional roentgentherapy of 250 kv seldom succeeded in destroying completely carcinomas of the bladder. The relatively low quality of radiations produced by these units resulted in marked systemic and superficial reactions, insufficient penetration, inhomogeneous distribution of radiations, and invariable underdosage. The skillful application of cobalt[60] and supervoltage roentgentherapy has brought radiotherapy to a key position in the management of cancer of the bladder. Buschke and Cantril[18] first reported worthy results. The dedicated efforts of many others have now demonstrated the great value of radiotherapy as a curative method (Morrison and Deeley[98]; Regato and Chahbazian[114]; Miller et al.[96]; Sagerman et al.[122]). Modalities of treatment and results vary, but radiotherapy has been progressively accepted by urologic surgeons who, only a few years ago, were fearful of the procedure. Naturally, radiotherapy has been sought as a surgical adjuvant by many who would still hold to a surgical procedure as the method of choice.

The use of *preoperative radiotherapy* has made many converts, for it has proved not only beneficial but at times curative in itself (Whitmore et al.[142]; DeWeerd and Colby[37]; Edsmyr et al.[41]; Galleher et al.[59]; Wizenberg et al.[145]). In a cooperative study by the Urological Group of the Royal Marsden Hospital of London, twenty-four patients had radical surgery following preoperative irradiation without a single operative death; four of the surgical specimens showed no residual carcinoma, and there was a surprisingly low proportion of verifiable metastatic nodes (Bloom[10a]). An American study carried out by urologists and radiotherapists under a cooperative protocol has also found instances of no residual tumor after relatively moderate preoperative irradiation (Prout[110a]). An adequate comparison of series of patients receiving or not receiving preoperative irradiation is hampered by the fact that staging of irradiated cases must be strictly based on clinical findings and biopsy evidence, whereas purely surgical cases can yield more detailed histopathologic evidence of the extent of disease at the time of treatment. Irradiation of advanced cases for palliation has proved surprisingly rewarding (Brizel and Scott[17]), and the irradiation of postoperative recurrences has proved effective (Morrison and Deeley[99]).

Successful radiotherapy depends on the homogeneous distribution of a rather high dosage of radiations throughout the potential area of direct or metastatic involvement. Fractionation over a period of six to eight weeks is the best safeguard against untoward effects. Bladder and rectal symptoms that accompany the treatments can be medically palliated and tolerated without interruption of irradiations except in rare cases (Finney[50]). A surprising proportion of patients recover a normal or nearly normal bladder capacity (Buschke and Jack[21]; Regato and Chahbazian[114]). Depending on the amount of destruction of the bladder wall by the tumor, there may be subsequent breakdown of avascular areas or bursting of telangiectases with consequent hematuria—conservative management is usually rewarding. When carcinoma recurs, it is usually within the first two years after treatment. The multicentric character of the tumor or its appearance de novo is always a possibility, but recurrences may be due to inadequate or insufficient irradiation (Goodman and Balfour[60]). The most important complication is the possibility of small bowel injury (Edwards[43]). If suspected early, this complication is easily resolved by surgical intervention and resection of the terminal ileum.

Chemotherapy

Some drugs have been found that are capable of producing regression of bladder tumors, either by systemic administration or intracavitary instillation, but these agents are not sufficient in themselves to cause a complete regression (Morrow[100]; Deren and Wilson[36]). Thio-TEPA and 5-fluorouracil have been sought as surgical or radiotherapeutic adjuvants with unsatisfactory results (Stein and Kaufman[131]). The hopes and support once placed on chemotherapy have now turned to radiotherapy.

Prognosis

In 1965, there were 8110 deaths in the United States from cancer of the bladder or a crude mortality rate of 4.2 per 100,000 population. The death rates were 6.1 and 2.7 for male and female whites and 3.4 and 2.3 for male and female nonwhites. In spite of increased incidence, the mortality rates have remained stable for over thirty years. The mortality risks are higher for nonwhites than for whites among young persons, but the reverse is true of older individuals (King and Bailar[78]).

The average duration of life from onset of symptoms to death in patients with untreated carcinoma of the bladder is 13.2 months (Sauer et al.[124]). The duration of life is shorter for patients with infiltrating tumors. Papillary lesions, first diagnosed as benign but capable of later following a malignant course, are not included in such appraisal of survivals. If they were included, the average life expectancy would be considerably longer. All forms of treatment claim better results in the papillary tumors and admit poor results in the infiltrating variety. Under these circumstances,

the overall results of any form of treatment are highly influenced by the proportions of these varieties included in the group reported. Pathologists classify papillomas separately or include them as Grade I carcinomas. These facts may also influence the reported results.

Mostofi[101] collected 2678 cases of carcinoma of the bladder treated in various fashions. He found that Grade I papillary carcinoma was cured in 96% of the patients after one year, in 85% after five years, and in 67% after ten years. By contrast, Grade II or Grade III infiltrating carcinomas were cured in 50% after one year, in 20% after five years, and in 12% after ten years. The survival rates for females with infiltrating cancer were better than for males.

Lund and Lundwall[88] followed a group of 183 patients with so-called papillomas (Grade I transitional cell carcinoma). When there were multiple tumors, 73% recurred, and in 18% the tumors became obviously malignant microscopically. When there were solitary tumors, 28% recurred and 5% became malignant microscopically.

Buschke and Jack[21] reported nine patients living ten years (13%) in a series of sixty-six patients treated by supervoltage roentgentherapy. Regato and Chahbazian[114] treated with cobalt[60] thirty consecutive patients who were ineligible for surgical treatment. The disease was considered advanced in two-thirds, and several of the biopsies showed muscle invasion. Fourteen patients (48%) survived three years and twelve patients (40%) survived five years without evidence of recurrence or metastases. Six additional patients died without residual disease in the bladder, bringing the total of healed bladders in this series to 60%. Collins[27] reported that previous surgery lessens the chance of cure by radical radiotherapy. Goodman and Balfour[61] reported on forty-nine patients treated with cobalt[60], twenty-eight of whom were alive and well and with good bladder function after two years. A cystectomy was performed in four of the survivors following radiotherapy, and none showed residual disease in the bladder or lymph nodes.

The results of radiation therapy have tremendously improved during the last few years. This improvement has been due to the use of megavoltage, and it has been shown that it is possible to cure patients with superficial or deep involvement of the muscle. Furthermore, even when tumor extends beyond the bladder wall or involves regional lymph nodes in the immediate vicinity, radiation therapy can, at times, effect a cure. It is recognized that adequate irradiation may result in cure of patients who are not eligible for such benefit following the most radical surgery. Depending on the extent and location of the tumor, as well as on its intensity, the bladder capacity has been reported to be reduced (Bloom[10a]) or very largely recovered (Regato and Chahbazian[114]).

Mackenzie et al.[91] feel that preliminary irradiation followed by cystectomy in the earlier infiltrative stages of the disease offers the greatest hope to patients with carcinoma of the bladder (Table 59).

Segmental resection of bladder carcinoma is successful when the lesion is well defined and small enough so that a 2 cm margin of normal vesical wall can encompass the lesion. In the region of the trigone, resection naturally is more difficult, and recurrences appear more frequently. Survival is directly related to the depth of infiltration (Jewett et al.[74]) (Table 60).

Total cystectomy has been widely applied in recent years. The operative mortality, initially high, has decreased to negligible levels in experienced hands. Late mortality from pyelonephritis is relatively more important. Bowles and Cordonnier[13] reported on seventy-three selected patients who were operated upon, thirty of whom were well five or more years. They have emphasized that if the carcinoma of the bladder extends outside the bladder, a pelvic evisceration and radical iliac node dissection are not indicated, for this procedure results only in high operative mortality and morbidity with few patients salvaged.

The curability of bladder tumors is greatly influenced by the degree of infiltration of the bladder wall (Jewett[72]) (Figs. 496 and 497). If lymph node metastases are present at the time of cystectomy or pelvic exenteration, the prognosis is practically hopeless. Sarcoma botryoides may be cured by cystectomy (Cleveland and Forsythe[25]).

Because such a high percentage of these tumors (approximately 80%) are located in close proximity to the trigone, infection of the genitourinary tract is common. The presence or absence of this infection and the amount of functioning kidney tissue present are very frequently the sole determining factors of whether a patient lives or not. In some instances, it is true that the infection can be controlled or stabilized so that cure of a local condition can still be effected. If, however, when the patient is first seen there has been irreparable profound kidney damage, hope of cure is im-

Table 59. Two-year and three-year survival following treatment of bladder cancer*

| Clinical stage | Preoperative irradiation and radical cystectomy (onset 1959) | |
	2 yr	3 yr
O, A, B₁	8/13 (61%)	7/13 (54%)
B₂, C	8/19 (42%)	8/19 (42%)
D	0/1 (0%)	0/1 (0%)

*From Mackenzie, A. R., et al: Supervoltage x-ray therapy of bladder cancer, Cancer 18:1255-1260, 1965.

Table 60. Segmental resection (133 cases)—relation of survivorship to depth of infiltration*

| Stage | Lived 5 yr or longer without cancer | Died with cancer | Died within 5 yr | |
			Late complications	Unrelated cause
A	15/26 (58%)	8/26 (31%)	1/26 (4%)	2/26 (7%)
B₁	7/12 (58%)	5/12 (42%)	0	0
B₂	4/25 (16%)	21/25 (84%)	0	0
C	11/70 (16%)	55/70 (78%)	4/70 (6%)	0
Total	37/133	89/133	5/133	2/133

*From Jewett, H. J., et al.: A study of 365 cases of infiltrating bladder cancer; relation of certain pathological characteristics to prognosis after extirpation, J. Urol. 92:668-678, 1964; © 1964, The Williams & Wilkins Co., Baltimore, Md., U.S.A.

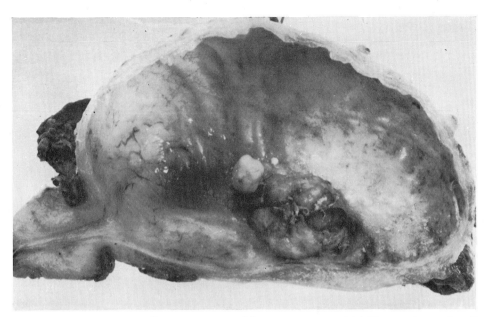

Fig. 496. Patient, 45-year-old man, was treated by cystectomy in 1945. He was alive and well without evidence of disease in 1961. Tumor was undifferentiated transitional cell carcinoma with squamous metaplasia that invaded muscle. (Courtesy Sir Eric Riches, London, England.)

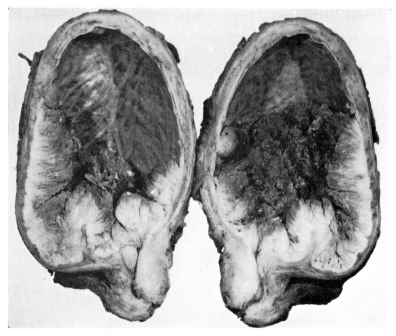

Fig. 497. Patient, 50-year-old man, was treated by cystectomy in 1958. Tumor was well-differentiated transitional cell carcinoma invading muscle and left ureter. In 1959, it was growing in apex of urethra, and pulmonary metastases were observed in 1961. (Courtesy Sir Eric Riches, London, England.)

possible, and death results from kidney insufficiency. Death from widespread dissemination of the disease is relatively infrequent. Since patients with carcinoma of the bladder are often elderly and subject to concomitant ailments, their life expectancy is naturally limited at best, and five-year and ten-year statistics must suffer from the toll of intercurrent diseases and fail to reflect the actual results. Kurohara et al.[82] have sought a better statistical method of reporting results.

REFERENCES

1 Abdel-Tawab, G. A., el-Zoghby, S. M., Abdel-Samie, Y. M., Zaki, A., and Saad, A. A.: Studies on the aetiology of bilharzial carcinoma of the urinary bladder. VI. Beta-glucuronidases in urine, Int. J. Cancer 1: 383-389, 1966.

2 Abdel-Tawab, G. A., Kelada, F. S., and Kelada, N. L.: Studies on the aetiology of bilharzial carcinoma of the urinary bladder. V. Excretion of tryptophan metabolites in urine, Int. J. Cancer 1:377-382, 1966.

3 Albarrán, J.: Les tumeurs de la vessie, Paris, 1891, G. Steinheil.

4 Austen, G., Jr., and Friedell, G. H.: Observations on local growth patterns of bladder cancer, Trans. Amer. Ass. Genitourin. Surg. 56:38-43, 1964.

5 Barringer, B. S.: Twenty-five years of radon treatment of cancer of the bladder, J.A.M.A. 135:616-618, 1947.

6 Barringer, B. S.: Five year control of bladder cancers by radon implants. J.A.M.A. 120: 909-911, 1942.

7 Batsakis, J. G.: Urogenital rhabdomyosarcoma; histogenesis and classification, J. Urol. 90:180-186, 1963.

8 Begg, R. C.: The colloid adenocarcinomata of the bladder vault arising from the epithelium of the urachal canal; with a critical survey of the tumours of the urachus, Brit. J. Surg. 18:422-466, 1931.

9 Billiard-Duchesne, J.-L.: Cas français de tumeurs professionnelles de la vessie. Statistiques; remarques, Bull. Ass. Franc. Cancer 45:376-380, 1958.

10 Bischoff, A. J., and Fishkin, B. G.: Carcinoma of the urinary bladder with cutaneous metastasis; report of 4 cases, J. Urol. 75:701-710, 1956.

10a Bloom, H. J. G.: Radiotherapy of carcinoma of the bladder, Tenth International Congress of Cancer, Main Panel no. 14, May, 1970, Houston, Texas.

11 Bonser, G. M., Clayson, D. B., Jull, J. W., and Pyrah, L. N.: The genesis of tumours of the bladder and other tissues with special reference to the industrial amines, Proc. Roy. Soc. Med. 51:965-970, 1958.

12 Bourne, R., and Beltaos, E.: Pheochromocytoma of the bladder; case report and summary of literature, J. Urol. 98:361-364, 1967.

13 Bowles, W. T., and Cordonnier, J. J.: Total cystectomy for carcinoma of the bladder, J. Urol. 90:731-735, 1963.

14 Brack, C. B., and Dickson, R. J.: Carcinoma of the female urethra, Amer. J. Roentgen. 79:472-478, 1958.

15 Brack, C. B., Nesbitt, R. E. L., Jr., and Everett, H. S.: Neoplasms of the female urinary bladder, J. Urol. 80:24-30, 1958.

16 Bricker, E. M.: Bladder substitution after pelvic evisceration, Surg. Clin. N. Amer. 30: 1511-1521, 1950.

17 Brizel, H. E., and Scott, R. M.: Palliative irradiation for bladder carcinoma, Amer. J. Roentgen. 100:909-915, 1967.

18 Buschke, F., and Cantril, S. T.: Roentgentherapy of carcinoma of the urinary bladder; an analysis of 52 patients treated with 800 k.v. roentgentherapy, J. Urol. 48:368-383, 1942.

19 Buschke, F., and Cantril, S. T.: Roentgen therapy of carcinoma of the female urethra and vulva, Radiology 51:155-165, 1948.

20 Buschke, F., Cantril, S. T., and Parker, H. M.: Supervoltage roentgentherapy, Springfield, Ill., 1950, Charles C Thomas, Publisher.

21 Buschke, F., and Jack, G.: Twenty-five years' experience with supervoltage therapy in the treatment of transitional cell carcinoma of the bladder, Amer. J. Roentgen. 99:387-392, 1967.

22 Clayton, S. G.: Carcinoma of the female urethra, J. Obstet. Gynaec. Brit. Emp. 52: 507-511, 1945.

23 Clemmesen, J., Lockwood, K., and Nielsen, A.: Smoking habits of patients with papilloma of urinary bladder, Danish Med. Bull. 5: 123-128, 1958.

24 Clemmesen, J., Nielsen, A., and Lockwood, K.: Mortality rates for cancer of urinary bladder in various countries, Brit. J. Cancer 11:1-7, 1957.

25 Cleveland, J. C., and Forsythe, W. E.: Sarcoma botryoides; report of three-year survival, J. Urol. 89:683-685, 1963.

26 Cobb, B. C., and Ansell, J. S.: Cigarette smoking and cancer of the bladder, J.A.M.A. 193:329-332, 1965.

27 Collins, C. D.: Influence of previous surgery on results of megavoltage radiotherapy in carcinoma of bladder, Lancet 2:988-990, 1964.

28 Colston, J. A. C., and Leadbetter, W. F.: Infiltrating carcinoma of the bladder, J. Urol. 36:669-683, 1936.

29 Crabbe, J. G. S., Cresdee, W. C., Scott, T. S., and Williams, M. H. C.: The cytological diagnosis of bladder tumours amongst dye-stuff workers, Brit. J. Indust. Med. 13:270-276, 1956.

30 Cuccia, C. A.: The radiotherapeutic approach to carcinoma of the bladder, J. Urol. 82:86-89, 1959.

31 Darget, R.: Tumeurs malignes de la vessie;

traitement par la radium thérapie à vessie ouverte, Paris, 1951, Masson et Cie.

32 Davis, E.: Disappearance of carcinomatous ulceration of bladder following ureterosigmoidostomy, J.A.M.A. **137**:450-453, 1948.

33 Dean, A. L.: Comparison of the malignancy of the bladder tumors as shown by the cystoscopic biopsy and subsequent examination of the entire excised organ, J. Urol. **59**: 193-194, 1948.

34 deGironcoli, F.: Intorno alla scomparsa di alcuni tumori vescicali in seguito alla derivazione sopravescicale dell'urina, Urologia **19**:1-10, 1952.

35 Denoix, P. F., and Schwartz, D.: Tabac et cancer de la vessie, Bull. Ass. Franc. Cancer **43**:387-393, 1956.

36 Deren, T. L., and Wilson, W. L.: Use of 5-fluorouracil in treatment of bladder carcinomas, J. Urol. **83**:390-393, 1960.

37 DeWeerd, J. H., and Colby, M. Y.: Bladder carcinoma—combined radiotherapy and surgical treatment, J.A.M.A. **199**:109-111, 1967.

38 Dickson, R. J., and Lang, E. K.: Treatment of papillomata of the bladder with radioactive colloidal gold (AU[198]), Amer. J. Roentgen. **83**:116-122, 1960.

39 Dimmette, R. M., Sproat, H. F., and Sayegh, E. S.: The classification of carcinoma of the urinary bladder, associated with schistosomiasis and metaplasia, J. Urol. **75**:680-686, 1956.

40 Dyche, G. M., and Mackay, N. R.: The intracavitary treatment of the bladder with radioactive colloidal gold, Brit. J. Radiol. **32**:757-763, 1959.

41 Edsmyr, F., Jacobsson, F., Dahl, O., Walstam, R., and Nilsson, A.: Teamwork in treatment of bladder carcinoma, Strahlentherapie **132**:19-23, 1967.

42 Edsmyr, F., Dahl, O., and Walstam, R.: Cobalt 60 teletherapy of carcinoma of the bladder, Acta Radiol. [Ther.] (Stockholm) **6**: 81-99, 1967.

43 Edwards, D. N., Complications following megavoltage radiation for carcinoma of the bladder, Clin. Radiol. **16**:27-33, 1965.

44 Einhorn, J., Larsson, L. G., and Ragnhult, I.: Radioactive yttrium (Y[90]) as possible adjunct to the treatment of papillomatosis of the urinary bladder, Acta Radiol. (Stockholm) **43**:298-304, 1955.

45 Elliott, G. B.: and Freigang, B.: Observations on the nature of mucin secreting urachal cystadenoma, Ann. Surg. **157**:613-617, 1963.

46 Ellis, F.: Bladder neoplasms—the challenge to the radiotherapist, Clin. Radiol. **14**:1-16, 1963.

47 Ellis, F., and Oliver, R.: Treatment of papilloma of the bladder with radioactive colloidal gold (AU[198]), Brit. Med. J. **1**:136-139, 1955.

48 Fagan, G. E., and Hertig, A. T.: Carcinoma of the female urethra. Review of the literature; report of eight cases, Obstet. Gynec. **6**: 1-11, 1955.

49 Fetter, T. R., Bogaev, J. H., McCuskey, B., and Seres, J. L.: Carcinoma of the bladder; incidence and sites of metastases, J. Urol. **81**:746-748, 1959.

50 Finney, R.: The treatment of carcinoma of the bladder with megavoltage irradiation—a clinical trial, Clin. Radiol. **16**:324-327, 1965.

51 Flocks, R. H.: Treatment of patients with carcinoma of the bladder, J.A.M.A. **145**:292-301, 1951.

52 Franksson, C.: Tumours of the urinary bladder, Acta Chir. Scand. **151**(suppl.):1-203, 1950.

53 Franksson, C., and Lindblom, K.: Roentgenographic signs of tumor infiltration of the wall of the urinary bladder, Acta Radiol. (Stockholm) **37**:1-7, 1952.

54 Franksson, C., Lindbolm, K., and Whitehouse, W.: The reliability of roentgen signs of varying degrees of malignancy of bladder tumors, Acta Radiol. (Stockholm) **45**:266-272, 1956.

55 Fricke, R. E., and McMillan, J. T.: Radium therapy in carcinoma of the female urethra, Radiology **52**:533-540, 1949.

56 Friedman, M., and Lewis, L. C.: Irradiation of carcinoma of the bladder by a central intracavitary radium of cobalt[60] source (The Walter Reed Technique), Amer. J. Roentgen. **79**:6-31, 1958.

57 Friedman, N. B., and Kuhlenbeck, H.: Adenomatoid tumors of the bladder reproducing renal structures (nephrogenic adenomas), J. Urol. **64**:657-670, 1950.

58 Fripp, P.-J.: Bilharziasis and bladder cancer, Brit. J. Cancer **19**:292-296, 1965.

59 Galleher, E. P., Jr., Young, J. D., Jr., Beyer, O. C., Bloedorn, F. G., and Dow, J.: Supravoltage irradiation followed by cystectomy for bladder cancer, J. Urol. **93**:598-603, 1965.

60 Goodman, G. B., and Balfour, J.: Local recurrence of bladder cancer after supervoltage irradiation, J. Canad. Ass. Radiol. **15**:92-98, 1964.

61 Goodman, G. B., and Balfour, J.: Carcinoma of bladder; cobalt therapy, J. Urol. **92**:30-36, 1964.

62 Hanbury, W. J.: Rhabdomyomatous tumours of the urinary bladder and prostate, J. Path. Bact. **64**:763-773, 1952.

63 Higgins, C. C.: Benign tumors of the bladder, Ann. Surg. **93**:886-890, 1931.

64 Higgins, C. C., and Hausfeld, K. F.: Cutaneous metastases from carcinoma of the urinary bladder; report of 2 cases, J. Urol. **59**:879-886, 1948.

65 Hinman, F.: The technic and late results of uretero-intestinal implantation and cystectomy for cancer of the bladder. In reports of Seventh Congress of the International Society of Urology, pp. 464-555, 1939.

66 Holsti, L. R., and Ermala, P.: Papillary carcinoma of the bladder in mice, obtained after peroral administration of tobacco tar, Cancer **8**:679-682, 1955.

67 Hovenanian, M. S., and Deming, C. L.: Heterologous transplantation of uroepithelial

tumors. Part II. Transplantation of bladder tumors, Yale J. Biol. Med. 19:149-153, 1946.

68 Hueper, W. C.: "Aniline tumors" of the bladder, Arch. Path. (Chicago) 25:856-899, 1938.

69 Hueper, W. C.: Environment and cancer, J.A.M.A. 157:679-685, 1955.

70 Hultberg, S.: Kombinierte Roentgen- und Radiumbehandlung bei Urethra-Carcinom, Strahlentherapie 99:171-184, 1956.

71 Jacobs, A., and Symington, T.: Primary lymphosarcoma of urinary bladder, Brit. J. Urol. 25:119-126, 1953.

72 Jewett, H. J.: Carcinoma of the bladder; influence of depth of infiltration on the 5-year results following complete extirpation of the primary growth, J. Urol. 67:672-676, 1952.

73 Jewett, H. J., and Eversole, S. L., Jr.: Carcinoma of the bladder; characteristic modes of local invasion, J. Urol. 83:383-389, 1960.

74 Jewett, H. J., King, L. R., and Shelley, W. M.: A study of 365 cases of infiltrating bladder cancer; relation of certain pathological characteristics to prognosis after extirpation, J. Urol. 92:668-678, 1964.

75 Joshi, D. P., Wessely, Z., Seery, W. H., and Neier, C. R.: Rhabdomyosarcoma of the bladder in an adult; case report and review of the literature, J. Urol. 96:214-217, 1966.

76 Kaplan, G. W., Bulkley, G. J., and Grayhack, J. T.: Carcinoma of the male urethra, J. Urol. 98:365-371, 1967.

77 Kerr, W. K., Barkin, M., Levers, P. E., Woo, S. K. C., and Menczyk, Z.: The effects of cigarette smoking on bladder carcinogens in man, Canad. Med. Ass. J. 93:1-7, 1965.

78 King, H., and Bailar, J. C., III.: Epidemiology of urinary bladder cancer, J. Chronic Dis. 19:735-772, 1966.

79 Koss, L. G., Melamed, M. R., Ricci, A., Melick, W. F., and Kelly, R. E.: Carcinogenesis in the human urinary bladder, New Eng. J. Med. 272:767-770, 1965.

80 Kretschmer, H. L.: Haematuria; a clinical study based on 933 consecutive cases, Surg. Gynec. Obstet. 40:683-686, 1925.

81 Kretschmer, H. L., and Doerhing, P.: Leiomyosarcoma of the urinary bladder, Arch. Surg. (Chicago) 38:274-286, 1939.

82 Kurohara, S. S., Rubin, P., and Silon, N.: Analysis in depth of bladder cancer treated by supervoltage therapy, Amer. J. Roentgen. 95:458-467, 1965.

83 Laign, A. H., and Dickinson, K. M.: Carcinoma of bladder treated by supervoltage irradiation, Clin. Radiol. 16:154-164, 1965.

84 Lang, E. K., Nourse, M. H., Wishard, W. N., Jr., and Mertz, J. H. P.: The accuracy of preoperative staging of bladder tumors by arteriography, J. Urol. 95:363-367, 1966.

85 Leadbetter, W. F., and Copper, J. F.: Regional gland dissection for carcinoma of the bladder, J. Urol. 63:242-260, 1950.

86 Lee, D. A., Cockett, A. T. K., Caplan, B. M., and Chiamori, N.: Urinary lactic acid dehydrogenase activity in the diagnosis of urologic neoplasms, J. Urol. 95:77-78, 1966.

87 Lockwood, K.: On the etiology of bladder tumors in Kobenhavn-Frederiksberg; an inquiry of 369 patients and 369 controls, Acta Path. Microbiol. Scand. 51:1-166, 1961.

87a Long, R. T. L., Grummon, R. A., and Spratt, J. S.: Survival after radical abdomino-perineal cystourethrectomy (with topical intravesical chemotherapy) for carcinoma of the urinary bladder; a comparison with radical abdominal, simple, and paritial cystectomy (to be published).

88 Lund, F., and Lundwall, F.: Epithelial tumours of the urinary tract; follow-up and appraisal of the treatment in 480 cases, Danish Med. Bull. 6:59-63, 1959.

89 McCrea, L. E.: Malignancy of the female urethra, Urol. Survey 2:85-149, 1952 (extensive bibliography).

90 McDonald, J. H., Heckel, N. J., and Kretschmer, H. L.: Cutaneous metastases secondary to carcinoma of urinary bladder; report of two cases and review of the literature, Arch. Derm. Syph. (Chicago) 61:276-284, 1950.

91 Mackenzie, A. R., Whitmore, W. J., Jr., and Nickson, J. J.: Supervoltage x-ray therapy of bladder cancer, Cancer 18:1255-1260, 1965.

92 Marshall, V. F.: Results of radiation therapy of bladder cancer, New York J. Med. 48:875-876, 1948.

93 Marshall, V. F., and Whitmore, W. F., Jr.: Simple cystectomy for cancer of the urinary bladder; one hundred consecutive cases: two years later, J. Urol. 63:232-241, 1950.

94 Masina, F. S.: Segmental resection for tumours of the urinary bladder; ten year follow-up, Brit. J. Surg. 52:279-283, 1965.

95 Melamed, M. R., Voutsa, N. G., and Grabstald, H.: Natural history and clinical behavior of in situ carcinoma of the human urinary bladder, Cancer 17:1533-1545, 1964.

96 Miller, L. S., Crigler, C. M., and Guinn, G. A.: Supervoltage irradiation for carcinoma of the urinary bladder, Radiology 82:778-785, 1964.

97 Monaco, A. P., Murphy, G. B., and Dowling, W.: Primary cancer of the female urethra, Cancer 11:1215-1221, 1958.

98 Morrison, R., and Deeley, T. J.: The treatment of carcinoma of the bladder by supervoltage x-rays, Brit. J. Radiol. 38:449-458, 1965.

99 Morrison, R., and Deeley, T. J.: The treatment of recurrent carcinoma of the bladder by supervoltage radiotherapy, Brit. J. Urol. 38:319-322, 1966.

100 Morrow, J. W.: Chemotherapy of carcinoma of the bladder; preliminary report of forty-four cases treated with citral, Brit. J. Urol. 32:69-78, 1960.

101 Mostofi, F. K.: A study of 2678 patients with initial carcinoma of the bladder. I. Survival rates, J. Urol. 75:480-491, 1956.

102 Mostofi, F. K., and Morse, W. H.: Polypoid rhabdomyosarcoma (sarcoma botryoides) of

bladder in children, J. Urol. **67**:681-687, 1952.

103 Mostofi, F. K., Thomson, R. V., and Dean, A. L., Jr.: Mucous adenocarcinoma of the urinary bladder, Cancer **8**:741-758, 1955.

104 Munro, A. I.: The results of using radioactive gold grains in the treatment of bladder growths, Brit. J. Urol. **36**:541-548, 1964.

105 Oppenheimer, R.: Ueber die bei Arbeitern chemischer Betriebe beobachteten Erkrankungen des Harnapparates, Z. Urol. Chir. **21**: 336-370, 1927.

106 Pang, L. S. C.: Bony and cartilaginous tumours of the urinary bladder, J. Path. Bact. **76**:357-377, 1958.

107 Papanicolaou, G. N.: Cytology of the urine sediment in neoplasms of the urinary tract, J. Urol. **57**:375-379, 1947.

108 Patch, F. S.: The association between leukoplakia and squamous-cell carcinoma in the upper urinary tract, New Eng. J. Med. **200**: 423-437, 1929.

109 Patch, F. S.: Epithelial metaplasia of the urinary tract, J.A.M.A. **136**:824-827, 1948.

110 Pontius, E. E., Nourse, M. H., Paz, L., and McCallum, D. C.: Primary malignant lymphomas of the bladder, J. Urol. **90**:58-61, 1963.

110a Prout, G. R., Jr.: Personal communication, 1970.

111 Pyrah, L. N., Raper, F. P., and Thomas, G. M.: Report of a follow-up of papillary tumours of the bladder, Brit. J. Urol. **36**:14-25, 1964.

112 Rabkova, L. M., and Shraer, D. P.: Clinical and bacteriological parallels in patients with urogenital tumours, Vop. Onkol. **9**:55-60, 1963.

113 Rabson, S. M.: Leukoplakia and carcinoma of the urinary bladder, J. Urol. **35**:321-341, 1936.

114 del Regato, J. A., and Chahbazian, C. M.: Radiotherapy for transitional-cell carcinoma of the urinary bladder with cobalt⁶⁰, Radiology **87**:1053-1057, 1966.

115 Rehn, L.: Ueber Blasenerkrankungen bei Anilinarbeitern, Verh. Deutsch. Ges. Chir. **35**: 313-314, 1906.

116 Riches, E.: Tumours of the kidney and ureter, Edinburgh/London, 1964, E. & S. Livingstone, Ltd.

117 Romanus, R.: Cystectomy in the male, the significance of the combined prostato-seminal vesiculo-cystectomy with special reference to the sexual function, Acta Chir. Scand. **97**: 389-409, 1949.

118 Rouvière, H.: Anatomie des lymphatiques de l'homme, Paris, 1932, Masson et Cie.

119 Royce, R. K., and Ackerman, L. V.: Carcinoma of the bladder; study of clinical, therapeutic, and pathologic aspects of 135 cases, J. Urol. **65**:66-86, 1951.

120 Royce, R. K., and Spjut, H. J.: Transitional cell carcinoma of the bladder; Grade I (socalled papilloma), J. Urol. **82**:486-489, 1959.

121 Rubin, P.: Cancer of the urogenital tract; bladder cancer, incidence, frequency, etiological factors, J.A.M.A. **206**:1761-1776, 1968.

122 Sagerman, R. H., Bagshaw, M. A., and Kaplan, H. S.: Linear accelerator supervoltage radiation therapy; carcinoma of the bladder, Amer. J. Roentgen. **93**:122-127, 1965.

123 Saphir, O.: Certain aspects of primary carcinoma of the urinary bladder, Urol. Cutan. Rev. **48**:552-554, 1944.

124 Sauer, H. R., Blick, M. S., and Meehan, D. J.: A study of untreated bladder cancers, J. Urol. **63**:124-127, 1950.

125 Schmidlapp, C. J., and Marshall, V. F.: The detection of cancer cells in the urine; a clinical appraisal of the Papanicolaou method, J. Urol. **59**:599-603, 1948.

126 Segal, A. D., and Fink, H.: Cavernous hemangioma of the bladder, J. Urol. **47**:453-460, 1942.

127 Smith, B. H.: Malacoplakia of the urinary tract, Amer. J. Clin. Path. **43**:409-417, 1965.

128 Smith, G. G., and Mintz, E. R.: Bladder tumor; observations on one hundred and fifty cases, Amer. J. Surg. **20**:54-63, 1933.

129 Spooner, A. D.: Metastasis in epithelioma of the urinary bladder, Trans. Amer. Ass. Genitourin. Surg. **27**:81-89, 1934.

130 Staubitz, W. J., Carden, L. M., Oberkircher, O. J., Lent, M. H., and Murphy, W. T.: Management of urethral carcinoma in the female, J. Urol. **73**:1045-1053, 1955.

131 Stein, J. J., and Kaufman, J. J.: The treatment of carcinoma of the bladder with special reference to the use of preoperative radiation therapy combined with 5-fluorouracil, Amer. J. Roentgen. **102**:519-529, 1968.

132 Stirling, W. C., and Ash, J. E.: Tumors of the bladder, J.A.M.A. **141**:1036-1039, 1949.

133 Swinney, J.: Treatment of bladder cancer by megavoltage therapy, Brit. J. Urol. **29**:241-243, 1957.

134 Thiede, T., Chievitz, E., and Christensen, B. C.: Chlornaphazine as a bladder carcinogen, Acta Med. Scand. **175**:721-725, 1964.

135 Thompson, G. J., and McDonald, J. R.: Benign tumors of the urinary bladder; report of a case of neurofibroma, J. Urol. **43**:831-835, 1940.

136 Touvinen, P. I., and Kettunen, K.: Superficial malignant lesions of bladder treated by radioactive colloidal gold (AU¹⁹⁸), Brit. Med. J. **1**:1090-1092, 1957.

137 Van der Werf-Messing, B.: Treatment of carcinoma of the bladder with radium, Clin. Radiol. **16**:16-26, 1965.

138 Vermooten, V.: Use of radioactive cobalt (Co⁶⁰) in treatment of bladder tumors, J. Urol. **74**:85-92, 1955.

139 Walker, L. M., and Huffman, J. W.: Adenocarcinoma of the female urethra; a review, Quart. Bull. Northwestern Univ. Med. School **21**:115-125, 1947.

140 Wallace, D. M., and Harris, D. L.: Delay in treating bladder tumours, Lancet **2**:332-334, 1965.

141 Wheeler, J. L., and Hill, W. T.: Adenocar-

cinoma involving the urinary bladder, Cancer **7**:119-135, 1954.

142 Whitmore, W. F., Jr., Grabstald, H., Mackenzie, A. R., Iswariah, J., and Phillips, R.: Preoperative irradiation with cystectomy in the management of bladder cancer, Amer. J. Roentgen. **102**:570-576, 1968.

143 Whitmore, W. F., Jr., and Marshall, V. F.: Radical surgery for carcinoma of the urinary bladder, Cancer **9**:596-608, 1956.

144 Wise, H. M., Jr., and Fainsinger, M. H.: Angiography in the evaluation of carcinoma of the bladder, J.A.M.A. **192**:1027-1034, 1965.

145 Wizenberg, M. J., Bloedorn, F. G., Young, J. D., Jr., and Galleher, E. P., Jr.: Radiation therapy and surgery in the treatment of carcinoma of the bladder, Amer. J. Roentgen. **96**:113-118, 1966.

146 Wynder, E. L., Onderdonk, J., and Mantel, N.: An epidemiological investigation of cancer of the bladder, Cancer **16**:1388-1407, 1963.

Chapter 12

Cancer of the male genital organs

Prostate
Testis
Penis

Prostate

Anatomy

The prostate gland lies at the base of the bladder just anterior to the rectum, above the levator ani, and around the initial portion of the urethra. Physiologically, it is part of the male genital system. The ejaculatory ducts pass down and forward through the posterior portion of the gland to end in the urethra. The *anterior lobe* forms the roof of the urethra, the *median lobe* consists of a narrow strip of tissue that lies between the internal sphincter and the verumontanum and forms the floor of the urethra, the *posterior lobe* lies posterior to the plane that passes through the ejaculatory ducts, and the *lateral lobes* are the portions of the gland that lie between the anterior and posterior lobes. Functionally, the prostatic glands are divided into an inner and an outer group. The inner or periurethral short glands become increasingly prominent with age and may give rise to benign hyperplasia, whereas the outer group of larger submucosal glands undergoes atrophy of epithelium and stroma and may be the site of both hyperplasia and carcinoma (Franks[44]).

Just outside the prostatic capsule lies a venous plexus communicating with the deep dorsal vein of the penis and the vesical plexus and draining into the internal iliac veins. This plexus communicates also with the vertebral vein plexus. The arterial supply to the prostate comes from the inferior vesical and the middle hemorrhoidal branches of the hypogastric artery.

Within the immediate periprostatic area, there is an abundant network of nerves from the hypogastric plexus. The whole of the prostate and its plexuses is surrounded by the prostatic fascia, the posterior portion of which, the *fascia of Denonvilliers,* forms an effective barrier between the prostate and rectum (Fig. 498).

Lymphatics. The lymphatics of the prostate arise from the glandular acini. They run toward the capsule and there form a dense network that is most abundant on the posterior and superior surfaces. This network of lymphatics is drained by four major collecting trunks that follow the course of the prostatic arteries:

1 The *external iliac pedicle* arises from the base of the prostate and from the upper part of its posterior surface. It follows the seminal vesicle and then passes above the terminal segment of the ureter to terminate in one of the middle nodes of the external iliac chain.

2 The *hypogastric pedicle* arises from the inferior aspect of the prostate, travels toward the posterior surface of the gland, and then turns along the prostatic artery to terminate in one of the hypogastric nodes.

3 The *posterior pedicle* arises from the posterior surface of the prostate and follows an anteroposterior direction to end in lymph nodes located on the medial side of the second sacral foramen or in other nodes in the region of the promontory of the sacrum.

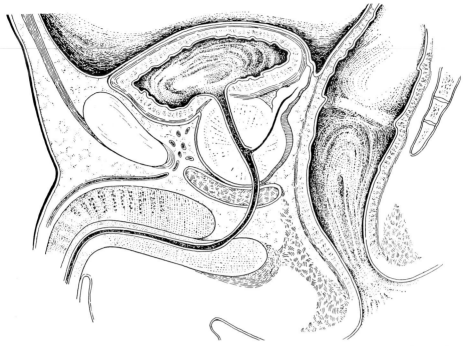

Fig. 498. Sagittal section of male pelvis showing relationship of prostate to urethra and its separation from rectum by Denonvilliers' fascia.

4 The *inferior pedicle,* usually formed by a single trunk, follows a downward direction on the anterior surface of the prostate until it reaches the perineal floor. It follows the internal pudendal artery to terminate in one of the hypogastric nodes near its origin.

The lymphatics of the prostate anastomose with those of the bladder fundus, seminal vesicles, ampulla of the ductus deferens, and rectum. There are also intercalating lymph nodes between the prostate and the rectum, but the lymphatics of the prostate, for the most part, are drained by the external iliac, hypogastric, and sacral lymph nodes (Fig. 499).

Epidemiology

Carcinoma of the prostate is uncommon in Asia, Africa (Houston[64]), and Latin America in that relative order, but it is not entirely absent (Dodge[31]). The highest incidence for this form of cancer is found in the United States. In the 1947 survey, the age-adjusted rate per 100,000 population was 34.8 for white and 49.9 for nonwhite males. Considering only males over 35 years of age, the incidence rate is 127 per 100,000. For individuals 40 to 44 years of age, the incidence rate is 0.4, but it rises steadily to about 747.7 per 100,000 individuals 80 to 84 years old. (Connecticut, 1960-1962). The age-adjusted incidence rate for the state of Connecticut increased from 29 to 39 per 100,000 from 1945-1949 to 1960-1962. An increase has also been reported in Denmark. The low incidence rate in Japanese rises appreciably for Japanese Americans (King et al.[75]).

There seems to be no relationship between prostatic hypertrophy and carcinoma of the prostate. A hormonal cause for the latter has been variously suggested. In patients with cirrhosis of the liver, there seems to be a lowered occurrence of carcinoma of the prostate (Glantz[51]). Apt's observation[1] that prostatic carcinoma is less frequent in circumcised men needs confirmation.

Sarcomas of the prostate are very rare (Melicow et al.[86]). Leiomyosarcomas (Prince and Vest[95]) and rhabdomyosarcomas occur mostly in the first two decades of life.

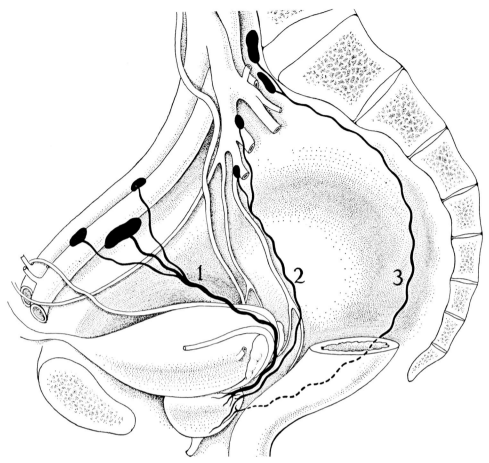

Fig. 499. Lymphatics of prostate showing external iliac pedicle, **1**; hypogastric pedicle, **2**; posterior pedicle, **3**. Inferior pedicle, which follows downward direction and ends in hypogastric nodes, is not illustrated here.

Pathology

Gross pathology

Carcinoma of the prostate most frequently arises from the posterior lobe but rarely involves the median lobe. Gaynor[49] plotted the location of these tumors and found that the overwhelming majority arose in the posterior lobe. Over 95% were located in the subcapsular areas (Fig. 500).

The recognition of early cancer of the prostate is the most difficult when it is small and closely resembles normal prostatic tissue. A normal prostate is usually gray tinged with light yellow and on cross section is not homogeneous, often showing a clear alveolar network. An early carcinoma often reveals a brighter color, ranging from sulfur to butter yellow. In ninety early macroscopically diagnosed carci-

nomas, Gaynor[49] found that fifty-three presented this yellow appearance. Most of the carcinomas measuring 0.5 cm or more were diagnosed grossly. They were fairly firm but not stony hard. A few carcinomas may be very hard because of increased connective tissue content and on section are gray to bluish white in color. Only their more homogeneous character can serve to differentiate them from normal prostatic tissue. This variety is not usually recognized until it reaches almost 1 cm in diameter. Both types have irregular, poorly defined borders. Small carcinomas may be difficult to differentiate from areas of atrophy, hyperplastic tuberculosis, and small areas of infarction. The large carcinomas are of a grayish white color spotted with numerous yellow foci. At times, invasion of the capsule can be observed grossly. Multiple primary carcinomas are quite common within the prostate.

The tumors that arise in the anterior lobe tend to remain localized longer and invade more reluctantly (Gaynor[49]). When tumor arises in the subcapsular area (Fig. 500), involvement of the capsule and the perineural space occurs early and is fre-

quently seen in latent carcinomas (Moore[89]) (Fig. 501). In 204 of 232 carcinomas found by Gaynor,[49] there was capsular invasion. Of 195 cases, 91% showed similar involvement of the capsule (Kahler[73]). The outer capsular layer, made up of connective and elastic tissue as well as muscle, prevents further spread. This barrier is particularly efficient in the posterior lobe in the region of Denonvilliers' fascia, which was infiltrated in only seventy-nine of Gaynor's 232 cases.[49] The spread of tumor to the rectum is also blocked by Denovilliers' fascia. In 800 patients with carcinoma of the prostate, Young[116] found the rectal mucosa to be involved in only twelve instances. Local vessel and nerve space invasion is common because of the location of the plexus between the capsule and the fascia. As the tumor continues to spread, it involves the seminal vesicles but seldom affects the urethra. Invasion of the bladder is a late phenomenon, but if present, partial or complete block of both ureters with secondary hydronephrosis and pyelonephritis can occur. Prostatic stones may or may not be associated with carcinoma. About 50% of the patients with carcinoma have coincident benign prostatic hypertrophy. In thirty-eight autopsies reported by Graves and Militzer,[52] genitourinary

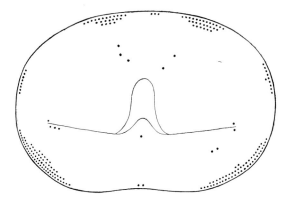

Fig. 500. Schematic representation of 203 prostatic carcinomas on frontal section that passes through verumontanum. Note that almost all tumors are subcapsular. All but three of those apparently arising in center are also subcapsular in location. (From Gaynor, E. P.: Zur Frage des Prostatakrebses, Virchow Arch. Path. Anat. **301:** 602-652, 1938.)

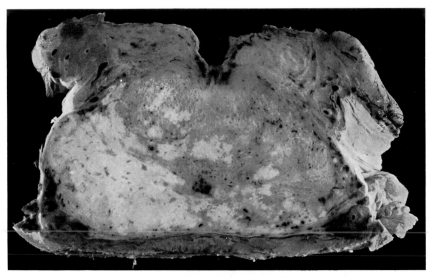

Fig. 501. Carcinoma arising in posterior lobe of prostate and growing in immediate proximity to capsule. (Material reported by Moore[89]; from Dixon, F. J., and Moore, R. A. Tumors of the male sex organs. In Atlas of tumor pathology, Sect. 8, Fascs. 31B and 32, Washington, D. C., 1952, Armed Forces Institute of Pathology.)

complications were prominent. There was unilateral obstruction of the ureters in twenty-six instances and bladder invasion in sixteen. A significant degree of pyelonephritis was present in twenty-eight, and it was the most common immediate cause of death.

Microscopic pathology

Carcinomas of the prostate are adenocarcinomas that vary considerably in appearance. The most common type is the small cell variety, but the cells may be larger with brightly staining eosinophilic cytoplasm and columnar epithelium (Fig. 502). In certain instances, the tumor can closely resemble normal prostatic tissue. Moore[89] stressed the fact that prostatic acini are surrounded by a collagenous band of connective tissue and that with the onset of carcinoma this limiting zone is lost. But in the well-differentiated carcinomas it is not rare for the basement membrane to persist (Fig. 503). Perineural space involvement, which is extremely common (Fig. 504), may be a means of definitely identifying a well-differentiated carcinoma when the microscopic diagnosis is in doubt.

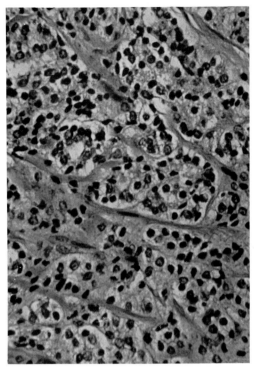

Fig. 502. Undifferentiated carcinoma of prostate. (×370; WU neg. 60-790.)

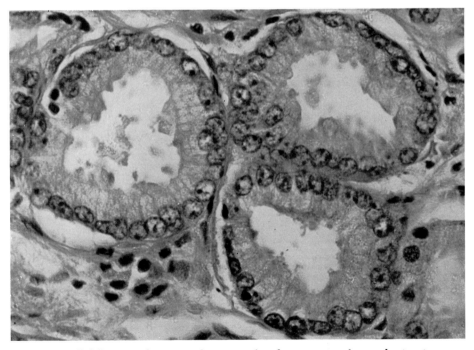

Fig. 503. Well-differentiated cancer of prostate found at margin of enucleation in suprapubic prostatectomy. Patient was treated with estrogens and died six years later with metastases. (High power; WU neg. 58-6123.)

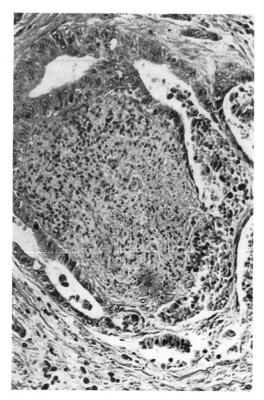

Fig. 504. Perineural space involvement by adeno-carcinoma of prostate. (Low-power enlargement.)

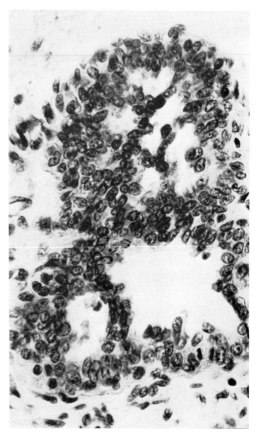

Fig. 505. Intraductal hyperplasia of breast following stilbestrol therapy in elderly man. (Moderate enlargement.)

There are no perineural lymphatics—only spaces into which carcinoma invades (Smith[105]; Larson et al.[78]; Rodin et al.[101]). The involvement of these spaces indicates that the lesion is a carcinoma, but such involvement has no prognostic significance (Pennington et al.[93]). The small cell type of carcinoma tends to invade and metastasize more quickly than the well-differentiated type. Fat is commonly present, but Gaynor[49] believes this is not a degenerative process, for it lies within the lumen of the carcinomatous alveoli and at times is seen as droplets within the cytoplasm. Mucin-producing carcinoma of the prostate is relatively infrequent but does occur (Edgar[32]; Sika and Buckley[104]; Franks et al.[47]). Islands of metaplastic epithelium, particularly when associated with infarction of the prostate, can be confused with carcinoma (Baird et al.[10]).

Carcinoma of the prostate and its metastatic lymph nodes change their microscopic appearance after orchiectomy or after administration of estrogens. The tu-mor often becomes smaller, and individual tumor cells show shrinkage with diminution of cell cytoplasm and sometimes rupture. Pyknosis of nuclei and loss of nuclear details occur. Rarely, nuclear vacuolation as well as cytoplasmic vacuolation occurs. This response is often patchy rather than uniform. With the passage of time, the tumor cells frequently lose their sensitivity to estrogens, but the normal cells do not (Fergusson and Franks[38]). Skin metastases may completely regress under therapy. The breasts become enlarged and their stroma somewhat edematous, and the ducts, which previous to stilbestrol therapy were atrophic, may show intraductal hyperplasia (Fig. 505). With stilbestrol, there may be excessive squamous metaplasia within the prostate that can be confusing (Bain-borough[9]). It was thought by Huggins and Scott[68] at one time that the poorly differentiated carcinomas did not respond clinically, but Nesbit and Cummings[91] could not substantiate this finding. The few reported cases of *sarcoma* of the prostate are primarily leiomyosarcomas, rhabdomyosarcomas, and lymphosarcomas.

Metastatic spread

Pelvic lymph node metastases in cancer of the prostate are found in decreasing order of frequency in hypogastric, obturator, and iliac nodes (Flocks et al.[41]). Invasion of the seminal vesicles by the tumor magnifies the chances of lymph node metastases: Arduino and Glucksman[3] found pelvic lymph node metastases in seventeen patients with seminal vesicle involvement, whereas in fifty-four others in whom the vesicles were free, only four cases had lymph node metastases. At autopsy of patients *who die of prostatic carcinoma,* only 20% fail to show evidence of metastases (Arnheim[4]). Extrapelvic lymph node metastases are found in the para-aortic and mediastinal nodes and, rarely, in the axillary and cervical regions. Visceral metastases are most frequently found in the kidneys, adrenal glands, liver, and lungs. The overwhelming majority of cases which come to autopsy have osseous metastases along the distribution of the vertebral vein plexus (Franks[42])—pelvic bones, femora, lumbar spine (Fig. 506). By contrast, more than 80% of cases of carcinoma of the prostate *discovered at autopsy* do not present evidence of metastases. *Sarcomas* metastasize freely to lungs and liver.

Clinical evolution

In early carcinoma of the prostate restricted to single lobe (usually the posterior) and not associated with hypertrophy, there are usually no symptoms. The initial symptoms of a large group of patients examined over a quarter of a century ago and tabulated by Young[116] are given in Table 61. The pain, due probably to perineural space invasion, is referred to the bladder and urethra, rectum and perineum, sacrum and gluteal region, and legs. It often suggests sciatic pain and is eventually present in most patients. Dysuria may be due to encroachment on the urethra or extension to the wall of the bladder and ureters. Gross hematuria is infrequently observed. In some patients, there may be

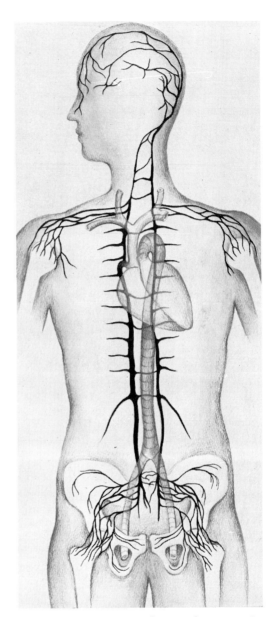

Fig. 506. Vertebral vein plexus with its extensive ramifications and communications with other venous systems. Note particularly distribution in pelvis, where it conforms to distribution of metastases so common in cancer of prostate.

rectal obstruction and also edema of the lower extremities. Lumbar and pelvic pain is frequently caused by the presence of metastases. Dorsolumbar pain may be caused by hydronephrosis and urinary infection. A syndrome of serious bleeding has been associated with metastatic carcinoma of the prostate. This is apparently

Table 61. Initial symptoms of carcinoma of prostate*

Symptoms	%
Frequency of urination (pollakiuria)	69
Difficult or painful urination	43
Pain	31
Complete urinary retention	3
Hematuria	3

*Data from Young, H. H.: The cure of cancer of the prostate by radical perineal prostatectomy (prostatoseminal vesiculectomy): history, literature and statistics of Young's operation, J. Urol. **53:**188-256, 1945.

due to fibrinolysis and consequent hypofibrinogenemia (Phillips et al.[94]). The patients with progressive carcinoma of the prostate develop severe anemia and become bedridden. The usual immediate cause of death is renal insufficiency complicated by infection. *Sarcomas* of the prostate become rapidly generalized and have a short clinical history.

Diagnosis
Clinical diagnosis

An early diagnosis of cancer of the prostate can only be expected from the routine rectal palpation of the prostate of symptomless individuals. The yield of such routine palpation is, of course, greater in elderly males, but the systematic rectal palpation of all males over 40 years of age will uncover a surprising proportion of asymptomatic nodules. The most satisfactory palpation of the prostate is done with the patient in knee-chest position. In contrast with the discrete raised nodule, a cellular carcinoma may be felt as an enlarged soft gland. The examiner should be aware of the fact that not all carcinomas are hard or well delineated. Palpation may establish whether or not the tumor is limited within the gland or has already reached the capsule and whether or not the tumor has already extended to the seminal vesicles and beyond.

The diagnosis of a prostatic tumor is rather obvious in the symptomatic or advanced stage. There may be pronounced dysuria and pain. The pain may be felt deep in the pelvic midline, in the perineum, or along a sciatic distribution. More extensive pain may be due to bony metastases. Inguinal and, more rarely, cervical and axillary metastases may be noted.

A diagnostic innovation was embodied in a report of occult carcinomas in men who had not sought medical advice (Hudson et al.[65]); an arbitrary perineal biopsy was done on the posterior lobe of the prostate of 100 random individuals: eighteen cases of occult carcinoma were found of which only seven had been suspected on clinical examination. There are no criteria to evaluate the biologic potential of these lesions as well as of *latent carcinomas* found at autopsy (Franks[44]).

Staging

The following clinical classification, adopted by the *Cooperative Study of Radiotherapy for Carcinoma of the Prostate* (Regato[99]) is recommended:

Stage I
a Occult carcinoma (microscopic foci found on specimens of TUR done for a benign condition)
b Latent carcinoma (microscopic foci discovered at autopsy)

Stage II
Carcinomas confined within the prostatic capsule without elevation of serum acid phosphatase

Stage III
a Carcinomas apparently confined within the capsule that are accompanied by an elevated serum acid phosphatase
b Carcinomas that are no longer confined within the capsule and those that have extended to extracapsular structures (seminal vesicles, urethra, bladder, etc.) with or without elevation of serum acid phosphatase

Stage IV
Carcinomas with demonstrable bony or any extrapelvic involvement.

Biopsy

Patients with a localized nodule can be biopsied adequately by means of a Silverman needle. Larger lesions offer less difficulty. For these purposes, either the transrectal or perineal approach may be utilized with little risk (Guillemin and Guillemin[55]). Rarely, carcinoma of the prostate may be implanted in the surface of a percutaneous needle biopsy (Burkholder and Kaufman[21]). The material obtained by a needle biopsy

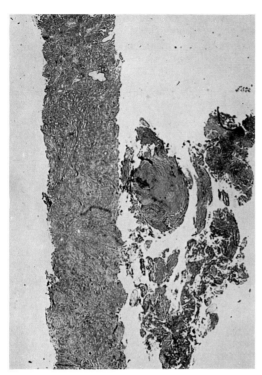

Fig. 507. Transrectal needle biopsy of prostate. Note adequacy of biopsy. (Low power; WU neg. 60-794.)

is often abundant (Fig. 507), but the procedure is of value only if a positive diagnosis is established. In some instances, frozen section diagnosis may be required on a needle biopsy. This is simple if the tumor is undifferentiated but difficult with well-differentiated carcinomas. Histopathologic evidence of nerve space involvement, however, is evidence of cancer (Culp and McDonald[27]).

A special *thin needle* has been devised (Franzén et al.[48]), with a guide placed on the examining finger, to be used as a simplified means of transrectal biopsy. The small aspirated fragments may permit a histologic or *cytologic* diagnosis (Esposti[36]). The diagnosis of carcinoma of the prostate by microscopic study of *exfoliated cells* remains a difficult problem (Mason[84]). Positive diagnosis may be obtained after massage of advanced lesions (Jönsson and Fajers[72]), but the method is not fruitful in the diagnosis of discrete nodules (Mason[85]). False positive diagnoses are caused by cells from the seminal vesicles or by the presence of infection. Diagnosis by ex-

foliative cytology is impractical and costly as a screening procedure (Boyer[18]). A *bone marrow biopsy* is indicated in most, if not all, cases of carcinoma of the prostate. Particularly in the presence of anemia, the bone marrow is likely to show general involvement (Chua et al.[23]).

In carcinomas of the prostate which cause urethral obstruction a transurethral approach may produce abundant material for histopathologic diagnosis; usually, but not always, carcinomas so diagnosed are relatively advanced. Conversely, in transurethral resections done for benign prostatic hypertrophy, microscopic foci of *occult carcinoma* may be found.

Cytoscopy

Cytoscopic examination may be of value in facilitating identification of a carcinoma of the prostate. There may be puckering of the bladder wall at the level of the trigone, or nodules may be visible. There may be obstruction of one or both ureters in advanced cases or in cases of unsuspected spread.

Roentgenologic examination

The roentgenologic examination of the prostate can be done only by indirect methods such as urethrography. Edling[34] reported that a large proportion of cases of carcinoma of the prostate present an elongation of the prostatic urethra and a bulging into the base of the bladder that is appreciable in urethrocystography. These changes are never sufficient in themselves for a diagnosis, and cases of definite cancer may not present any apparent changes.

It is important to recognize that carcinoma of the prostate may cause an annular constriction of the rectum (Davis[29]) and present as acute obstruction (Davies[28]). On radiographic examination, a prostatic origin should be suspected when the mucosa is not affected (Becker[15]).

A rather frequent roentgenologic finding is the presence of bone metastases (Table 62). Of 539 patients examined by Bumpus,[20] 123 showed involvement of the pelvic bones, and 107 showed involvement of the vertebrae. Bone metastases from carcinoma of the prostate are most frequently osteoplastic, seldom osteolytic, but sometimes mixed. Most of the metastases are osteo-

Table 62. Distribution of metastasis from carcinoma of prostate as determined by roentgenographic examination*

Bones or organs involved	Cases	%
Pelvic bones and sacrum	69	85
Lumbar vertebrae	48	59
Dorsal vertebrae	19	23
Cervical vertebrae	3	4
Femora	28	35
Ribs	18	22
Shoulder girdles	11	14
Humeri	4	5
Skull	1	1
Lungs	7	9

*From Graves, R. C., and Militzer, R. E.: Carcinoma of the prostate with metastases, J. Urol. 33:235-251, 1935.

blastic (Figs. 508 to 510) and often follow the distribution of the vertebral vein plexus. Metastatic disease may be demonstrated, prior to its radiographic demonstration, by means of *strontium*[85] photoscans (Williams and Blahd[112]). Seminal *vesiculography* is a difficult technical procedure. Its use as a means of demonstrating involvement of seminal vesicles is not worthwhile.

Laboratory examination

The most significant laboratory examination is the *acid and alkaline phosphatase* determination. Present in the normal prostate of man, the enzyme does not appear in any quantity until sexual maturity. Prostatic carcinomatous tissues, their soft tissue extensions, and their bony metastases continue to be able to secrete acid phosphatase (Gutman[57]). Unfortunately, the serum acid phosphatase level is not elevated until tumor has extended beyond the prostatic capsule. Gutman et al.[58] found an elevation of the serum acid phosphatase level in 85% of 177 patients with pathologically verified metastatic carcinoma of the prostate. In patients with infarction of the prostate, the acid phosphatase level may be extremely elevated (Stewart et al.[106]). The same may be true of any condition that disturbs the barriers normally present between the prostate and its blood vessels (Woodard[114]). The acid phosphatase level may be found elevated after massage of benign prostates (Still and Warwick[107]; Marberger et al.[83]) or in the presence of urinary retention (Wray[115]). The test should be employed in all patients with suspected carcinoma of the prostate. Prostatic cancer produces acid phosphatase but usually in reduced amounts proportional to the degree of dedifferentiation. The vast majority produces no aminopeptidase activity (Kirchheim et al.[76]).

Measurement of serum "prostatic" acid phosphatase does show some advantages (Fishman et al.[40])—it is a more effective indicator of metastatic carcinoma of the prostate than the measure of total serum acid phosphatase. Cook et al.[26] reported the results of over 2000 determinations of "prostatic" acid phosphatase. No positive tests occurred in patients with localized cancer, and it was elevated in 47% of patients with locally invasive carcinoma, in 87% of those with bony metastases, and in 100% of those with soft tissue metastases.

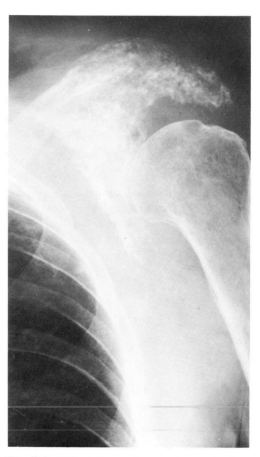

Fig. 508. Metastatic carcinoma of scapula from adenocarcinoma of prostate after partial calcification following palliative radiotherapy. (PCH 68-601.)

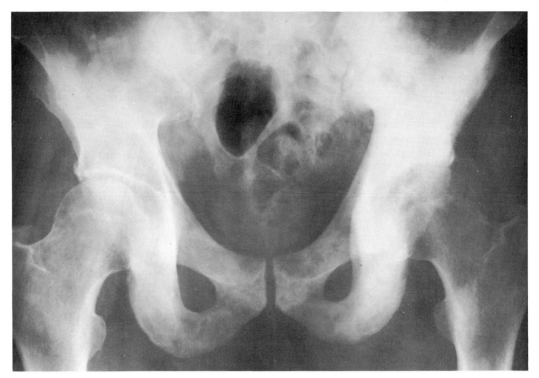

Fig. 509. Metastatic carcinoma of prostate in 64-year-old patient with intense marbleized appearance (eburnation) and peculiar unilaterality. (PCH 68-604.)

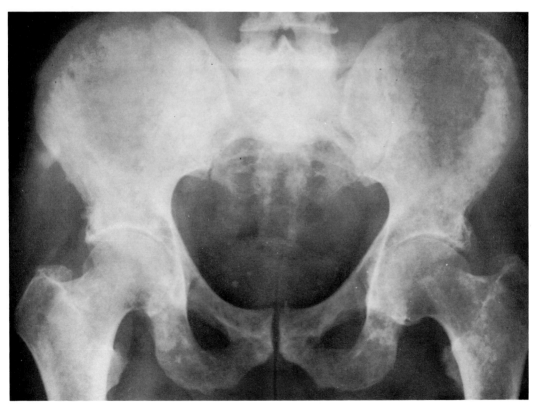

Fig. 510. Typical extensive osteoblastic metastasis of pelvic bones in 74-year-old patient with carcinoma of prostate that had been diagnosed only eight months previously. (PCH 68-1010.)

The *alkaline phosphatase level* is also frequently elevated when metastases to bone are present. However, increase of alkaline phosphatase represents a nonspecific response to bone injury, bone growth, or attempts at bone repair, and consequently osteoblastic metastases cause elevation, but the serum alkaline phosphatase level may be normal with osteolytic metastases. It is elevated with Paget's disease.

The acid phosphatase level falls precipitously within twenty-four to forty-eight hours after orchiectomy, whereas the alkaline phosphatase may rise over a period of several months because of new bone formation. The same changes may be observed after administration of stilbestrol, but they are slower in their evolution. In patients undergoing orchiectomy, the changes in alkaline phosphatase may reflect the clinical course rather closely (Woodard[114]). As metastatic areas heal, the alkaline phosphatase drops to normal; as new bony metastases develop, the alkaline phosphatase rises again. Administration of androgens may cause further rise of acid phosphatase (Huggins[67]) but, in general, the results are unpredictable (Prout and Brewer[96]).

Differential diagnosis

The differential diagnosis between *benign prostatic hypertrophy* and carcinoma may be difficult, for both entities may present the same symptoms. A palpable indurated nodule within the prostate may be due to a localized area of hypertrophy or to an *infarct*. Prostatic *calculi* may be large and on palpation may be confused with carcinoma, but they are invariably radiopaque. In 211 palpable nodules, Jewett[70] found that only one-half were due to cancer. Seven nodules in the median furrow were all benign. Carcinoma of the prostate may encircle and invade the rectum. A diagnosis of the true origin of the carcinoma is important because of the frequent response of carcinoma of the prostate to palliative therapy.

The most important differential roentgenologic diagnostic problem is that of *Paget's disease*. If the skull shows the typical changes of Paget's disease, then the other bone lesions are probably due to the same process. In Paget's disease, there is a bowing of the long bones without cortical thickening and without reduction of marrow spaces. Rib lesions are usually due to metastatic carcinoma. It is also possible for the two conditions to coexist. In osteoblastic metastases and in Paget's disease, the alkaline phosphatase level is elevated. If the acid phosphatase level is also elevated, then the bone changes must be due, at least in part, to metastatic carcinoma from the prostate. In a relatively few instances, roentgenologic examination may not suffice to make the diagnosis (de-Vries[30]). Primary *adenocarcinomas of Cowper's gland* are extremely rare and are confused with carcinoma of the prostate. This rare carcinoma is associated with pain and swelling of the perineal scrotal area, fistula, and ulceration but does not cause urinary or rectal distress.

Primary *carcinoma of the seminal vesicles* is extremely rare (McNally and Cochens[82]). It is usually accompanied by pelvic pain, hematuria, and urinary obstruction. Rectal examination usually reveals a large, firm mass in the region of the seminal vesicles, but since the vesicles are frequently secondarily invaded by cancer (Lazarus[79]), proof of their primary involvement is unusual. The findings must be differentiated from a rectal shelf due to metastatic carcinoma. Leiomyosarcomas have been reported originating in the prostate (Barone and Joelson[13]).

Treatment
Surgery

The *radical perineal prostatectomy*, advocated by Young[116] in the beginning of the century, implies removal of the prostatic capsule, the fascia of Denonvillier, the vesical neck, much of the trigone, the seminal vesicles, and the ampulla of the vas deferens. The operation is followed by impotence in practically all cases. Perineal leakage and difficulties in urinary control may also follow. The operation can be performed now with minimal operative mortality. The *retropubic prostatectomy* is advocated by few (Hand and Sullivan[60]; Millin[88]), but it has been adopted by many urologists. Arduino and Glucksman[3] emphasize that this extravesical removal of the gland permits also the extirpation of regional lymph nodes. There is no information, however, as to the questionable advantages of this extension of the procedure.

In responsible and competent hands, prostatectomy has been reserved for a minority of patients (Whitmore[111]), mostly because very few carcinomas of the prostate are diagnosed in an operable stage (i.e., when still confined within the capsule). Inoperability is often due also to advanced age or to the pathologic stage of the individual patient. Approximately 5% of all patients with carcinoma of the prostate diagnosed at present are eligible for a radical prostatectomy. At the Massachusetts General Hospital, there were only 196 such patients in the twenty-five years between 1932 and 1956 (Vickery and Kerr[110]). A few of the relatively younger patients refuse the operation because of consequent impotence. Others who apparently should not be concerned also refuse to accept the consequences.

Androgen control

Under this designation are placed both the elimination of the testicular androgens by *orchiectomy* and their neutralization through the administration of *estrogens*.

The work of Huggins and Scott[68] demonstrated the frequent hormone dependence of carcinomas of the prostate and, as a consequence, the value of orchiectomy and the administration of estrogens in the *palliative treatment* of incurable patients with advanced carcinoma of the prostate.

The immediate response of symptomatic patients to androgen control may be spectacular (Figs. 511 and 512). Relief of pain may often occur within twenty-four to forty-eight hours following orchiectomy. With stilbestrol therapy, the response may be variably delayed. Patients recover their appetite, gain weight, and often return to their normal activities. In many cases, there is gradual softening and regression of the tumor, and it may be difficult to find any palpable evidence of the neoplasm. The most striking regressions are those of the soft tissue extensions and lymph node metastases, but osseous metastases may regress also (Middleton[87]). Regressive changes of the primary lesion and of its bony metastases have been histologically verified. In patients who first respond to orchiectomy and then show a recrudescence of symptoms, bilateral adrenalectomies have been

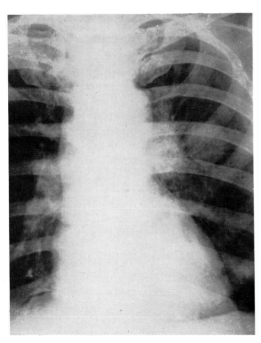

Fig. 511. Roentgenogram showing spherical metastasis close to hilum and overlying left third rib anteriorly.

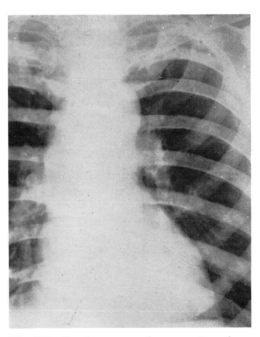

Fig. 512. Roentgenogram of same patient shown in Fig. 511 three months following bilateral orchiectomy. Metastatic lesion of lung has completely disappeared.

done with disappointing results, and the same is true of hypophysectomies. Destruction of the pituitary gland by means of yttrium[90] is a simpler procedure which affords some worthwhile relief of pain (Straffon et al.[108]).

The administration of estrogens results in unpleasant side effects such as nausea, vomiting, gynecomastia, and accumulation of fat in a feminine distribution. Retention of sodium and water may precipitate congestive heart failure. Arduino[2] has presented evidence that the use of preoperative estrogen therapy in patients with possible operable cancer of the prostate is associated with a high operative risk as compared to patients who do not receive preoperative estrogen therapy.

The palliative success of androgen control has motivated a decreasing performance of prostatectomies (Whitmore[111]) and an almost universal application of orchiectomy or administration of estrogens, or both, to patients with operable or inoperable carcinoma of the prostate. The assumptions have been that these measures would retard the development of metastases and prolong life. Unfortunately, because of the uncertainty and frustration resulting from these palliative procedures, the patient has difficulty adjusting mentally to the realization of the incurability of his cancer.

The Veterans Administration Co-Operative Urological Research Group[109] has reported on the results of a study of androgen control measures in over 2300 patients with previously untreated carcinomas of the prostate. *Operable* patients (those with Stage I or Stage II lesions) were submitted to prostatectomy and were randomized to receive also either estrogens or a placebo. The survival of those receiving placebos was significantly better. *Inoperable* patients without evidence of distant metastases (those with Stage III lesions) were randomized to receive (1) orchiectomy alone, (2) orchiectomy plus estrogens, (3) estrogens alone, or (4) supportive measures only plus a placebo. The study revealed no statistical differences in the observed results in various parameters, including delay in the occurrence of metastases and symptoms, loss of weight, performance, and five-year survival

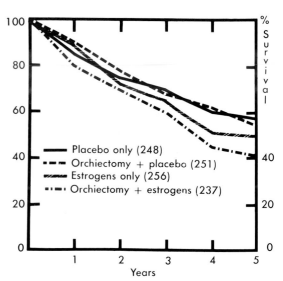

Fig. 513. Survival rates in 992 patients with carcinoma of prostate no longer confined within prostatic capsule but without elevation of acid phosphatase level or evidence of distant metastases (Stage III) who were randomized in four different groups. (Courtesy Veterans Administration Co-Operative Urological Research Group; from del Regato, J. A.: Radiotherapy in the conservative treatment of operable and locally inoperable carcinoma of the prostate, Radiology **88**:761-766, 1967.)

(Fig. 513). Patients with *distant metastases* (those with Stage IV lesions) were also randomized among the four groups mentioned, and the study revealed a relative advantage in these patients for the orchiectomy. The outstanding finding of this worthy study has been to show that estrogens, at a dosage of 5 mg daily, resulted in a considerably and statistically significantly greater number of deaths from cardiovascular accidents in operable as well as in inoperable patients. Reduction of this dosage level is indicated (Bailar and Byar[7a]).

In our opinion, androgen control measures should be judiciously reserved for the palliation of patients in whom all other means of treatment have failed. These measures should not be applied to the asymptomatic patient, regardless of the extent of the disease. Patients in good health and good general condition may live for years without treatment. An orchiectomy and its physical, social, and emotional consequences, even in elderly individuals, is not as innocuous as it is often assumed (Pennington et al.[93]).

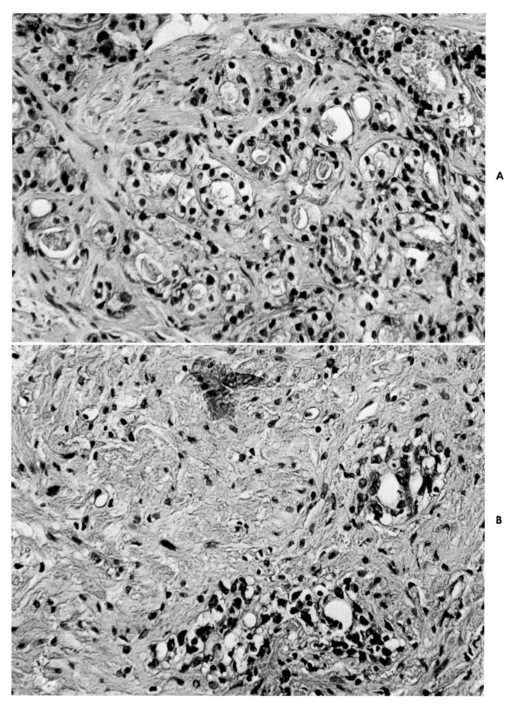

Fig. 514. A, Typical adenocarcinoma of prostate. Patient was given full course of cobalt[60] tele-therapy with a total dose of about 6500 R in five weeks at center of prostate. **B,** Six months later showing extensive fibrosis but no evidence of tumor. (**A,** ×340; PCH 67-1194; WU neg. 68-10948; **B,** ×340; WU neg. 68-10949.)

Radiotherapy

Irradiation of bony metastases has been long utilized for palliative purposes, but irradiation of the primary prostatic lesion has been tried only sporadically. The fact that adenocarcinomas often respond slowly to irradiation has been misinterpreted as "radioresistance" of these tumors. *Radium applications* in various ways have failed because of limited and uneven irradiation (Calais[22]). Flocks et al.[41] have made a sustained effort to treat primary carcinomas of the prostate by means of localized injection of *radioactive gold* through various approaches (Kerr et al.[74]; Elkins et al.[35]). The procedure, not without complications, fails often because of its inability to irradiate homogeneously the potential area of tumor involvement. However, Flocks et al.[41] have indisputably shown that these tumors are radiocurable.

External pelvic irradiation by means of conventional roentgentherapy was never sufficient to irradiate these deep-seated tumors. But, surprisingly, the advent of supervoltage roentgentherapy in the 1930's did not invite serious attempts at curative irradiation of carcinomas of the prostate. In the previous edition of this book (1962), it was stated that there was ". . . evidence that adequate utilization of supervoltage equipment and cobalt[60] units may permit very adequate irradiation of moderately advanced carcinomas of the prostate . . . the approach may be most suitable for most inoperable cases." Subsequent experience now permits the assertion that adequate external irradiation may prove to be the treatment of choice for the majority of these patients (Fig. 514). Irradiation of carcinoma in the prostate, and of its extracapsular extensions and metastases, has been sought in various ways with supervoltage roentgentherapy and cobalt[60] teletherapy (Budhraja and Anderson[19]; Reboul et al.[97]). Rotation therapy aims at a high differential irradiation of the prostate and surrounding structures (Bagshaw et al.[7]), but carcinoma of the prostate is often not limited to the anatomic site of the gland. It spreads eccentrically to the bladder wall and ureters and metastasizes to obturator, hypogastric, and iliac nodes. A rather homogeneous irradiation of the entire pelvic contents can be achieved by two (anterior and posterior) portals of entry (George et al.[50]). An excellent approach is the additional utilization of a perineal field (Regato[98]). External irradiation is accompanied by mild and temporary dysuria and diarrhea. Late sequelae may be limited to urethral narrowing necessitating periodic dilatations, particularly in patients who had been subject to repeated transurethral resections before irradiation.

Prognosis

In 1965, there were 15,911 deaths from cancer of the prostate in the United States. The mortality rates were 16.5 and 18.7 for white and nonwhite men, respectively, with 94% of the deaths occurring in those over 60 years of age. The mortality rates have remained rather constant in the state of Connecticut since 1949. The prevalence of carcinoma of the prostate found at autopsy is far in excess of that diagnosed clinically (Ashley[5]). In a postmortem study of 292 individuals over 50 years of age, forty-one cases (14%) of carcinoma of the prostate were found, only fourteen of which had been diagnosed clinically (Rich[100]). The proportion of cases found rises with the age groups—41% for individuals 70 to 79 years of age (Halpert and Schmalhorst[59]) and more than 70% for those over 90 years of age (Franks[44]). In another series reported by Schmalhorst and Halpert,[102] carcinoma was found at autopsy in thirty-three of fifty-eight patients over the age of 80 years. Most cases found at autopsy are localized to the prostate (Table 63).

In a series of 485 untreated patients with prostatic carcinoma reviewed by Bumpus,[20]

Table 63. Increasing occurrence of carcinoma of prostate found in postmortem studies*

Age (yr)	Cases studied	Carcinomas found	
		Cases	%
20-29	15	0	0.0
30-39	25	1	4.0
40-49	122	6	4.9
50-59	241	25	10.4
60-69	312	54	17.8
70-79	237	67	28.3
80-89	93	36	38.7
90+	5	2	40.0
Total	1050	191	18.4

*From Gaynor, E. P.: Zur Frage des Prostatakrebses, Virchow Arch. Path. Anat. **301:**602-652, 1938.

the average length of life from onset of symptoms to death was thirty-one months. Two-thirds of those who presented metastases when first seen died within nine months. Griswold[54] reported on another series of 544 untreated patients, only thirty-eight (7%) of whom survived.

In carcinomas found after prostatectomy for an assumed benign hypertrophy, the five-year and ten-year survival rates were 75% and 47%, respectively, for the *differentiated* tumors. This survival compares with that reported by Vickery and Kerr[110] after radical perineal prostatectomy—79% and 49% five-year and ten-year survival rates, respectively. One would expect a similarly good survival for the Bowery patients operated upon by Hudson et al.[65] for latent symptomless carcinomas. It is regrettable that Hudson's cases were not randomized between radical prostatectomy and abstention.

The results of radical perineal prostatectomy in small nodules limited within the capsule are excellent. Jewett[69] reported on eighty-six patients with such limited lesions, twenty-eight of whom lived over fifteen years free of disease. Several of the tumors were so small that they had been removed completely by the incisional biopsy. On the other hand, no patient with *undifferentiated* carcinoma or with carcinomas *extending beyond the capsule* survived.

Bailar et al.[8] have attempted to develop a numerical formula that would serve to establish a prognosis. The factors considered for this purpose are the stage of the disease (range 1 to 4), the primary or predominant pattern of histologic differentiation (range 1 to 5), and the secondary pattern (range 1 to 5). Thus, the numerical prognostic formula itself ranges from 3, the most favorable, to 14, the most unfavorable. This combination of the extent of the disease and the histologic character in the appreciation of prognosis does have definite merits.

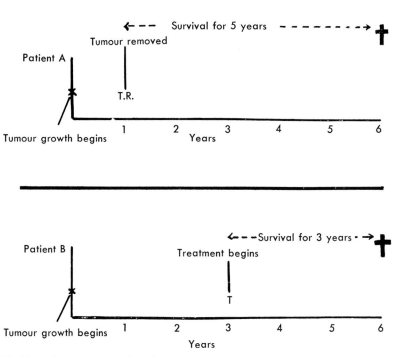

Fig. 515. Chart demonstrating that if two patients each has tumor with same expected duration, efficacy of given type of treatment will seem superior if Patient A is treated earlier in evolution of disease than is Patient B. Patient A survived for five years after removal of tumor, whereas Patient B survived for only three years after beginning of treatment. Unfortunately, total duration of life of both patients with their tumors was exactly same. (From Franks, L. M.: Some comments on the long-term results of endocrine treatment of prostatic cancer, Brit. J. Urol. **30**:383-388, 1958.)

As indicated, the degree of extension and the degree of differentiation of the tumor are important factors in the prognosis. But Franks[45] points out that the results simply depend on the time in its chronologic evolution when treatment is instituted (Fig. 515). The study of the Veterans Administration Co-Operative Urological Research Group[109] revealed the following results: for the operable patients (Stage I and Stage II), the five-year survival rate after prostatectomy was about 70% for all patients; the inoperable patients without distant metastases (Stage III) who received various palliative procedures had a five-year survival of about 50%, and the patients who had bony or distant metastases before receiving palliative measures (Stage IV) had a five-year survival of about 25%.

The results of curative radiotherapy for the operable as well as for the locally advanced cases cannot be adequately assessed at this time. Regato[98] reported on four inoperable patients who had been irradiated and who were living and well five to eight years after radiotherapy at the time of the report. Bagshaw[6] reported a group of fifty-nine patients followed for more than five years, with twenty-five living apparently free of disease. Ten of the latter patients had also received endocrine therapy. George et al.[50] made a report on their experience in the irradiation of nine patients and their early response. Bennett[16] also reported a series of eleven patients treated with cobalt[60].

Scott[103] reported on thirty-one selected patients with advanced carcinoma of the prostate treated by endocrine therapy plus radical perineal prostatectomy. Sixteen (51%) survived ten years or more without evidence of cancer. Cook and Watson[25] analyzed retrospectively records of 367 men with carcinoma of the prostate treated palliatively at the Ellis Fischel State Cancer Hospital. They contended that carcinoma of the prostate that metastasizes to bone has a different natural history from that which metastasizes to lungs. The mean age of patients in the former group was less than that of the latter.

REFERENCES

1 Apt, A.: Circumcision and prostatic cancer, Acta Med. Scand. **178**:493-504, 1965.

2 Arduino, L. J.: Personal communication, 1968.

3 Arduino, L. J., and Glucksman, M. A.: Lymph node metastases in early carcinoma of the prostate, J. Urol. **88**:91-93, 1962.

4 Arnheim, F. K.: Carcinoma of the prostate, J. Urol. **60**:599-603, 1948.

5 Ashley, D. J. B.: On the incidence of carcinoma of the prostate, J. Path. Bact. **90**:217-224, 1965.

6 Bagshaw, M. A.: Definitive radiotherapy in carcinoma of the prostate, J.A.M.A. **210**:326-327, 1969.

7 Bagshaw, M. A., Kaplan, H. S., and Sagerman, R. H.: Linear accelerator supervoltage radiotherapy. VII. Carcinoma of the prostate, Radiology **85**:121-129, 1965.

7a Bailar, J. C., III, and Byar, D. P.: Estrogen treatment for cancer of the prostate, Cancer **26**:257-261, 1970.

8 Bailar, J. C., III, Mellinger, G. T., and Gleason, D. F.: Survival rates of patients with prostatic cancer, tumor stage, and differentiation—preliminary report, Cancer Chemother. Rep. **50**:129-136, 1966.

9 Bainborough, A. R.: Squamous metaplasia of prostate following estrogen therapy, J. Urol. **68**:329-336, 1952.

10 Baird, H. H., McKay, H. W., and Kimmelstiel, P.: Ischemic infarction of the prostate gland, Southern Med. J. **43**:234-240, 1950.

11 Baird, S. S., and Hare, D. M.: Metastasis of prostatic carcinoma to the testicle, J. Urol. **59**:1208-1211, 1948.

12 Barnes, R. W.: Personal communication; cited by Jewett et al.[71]

13 Barone, A. M., and Joelson, J. J.: Leiomyosarcoma of the prostate; report of a case, J. Urol. **63**:533-538, 1950.

14 Bauer, W. C., McGavran, M. H., and Carlin, M. R.: Unsuspected carcinoma of the prostate in suprapubic prostatectomy specimens, Cancer **13**:370-378, 1960.

15 Becker, J. A.: Prostatic carcinoma involving the rectum and sigmoid colon, Amer. J. Roentgen. **94**:421-428, 1965.

16 Bennett, J. E.: Treatment of carcinoma of the prostate by cobalt-beam therapy, Radiology **90**:532-535, 1968.

17 Blennerhasset, J. B., Cohen, R. B., and Vickery, A. L.: Carcinoma of the prostate; enzyme histochemistry, Cancer **20**:2133-2138, 1967.

18 Boyer, W. F.: Carcinoma of the prostate; a cytological study, J. Urol. **63**:334-345, 1950.

19 Budhraja, S. N., and Anderson, J. C.: An assessment of the value of radiotherapy in the management of carcinoma of the prostate, Brit. J. Urol. **36**:535-540, 1964.

20 Bumpus, H. C., Jr.: Carcinoma of the prostate, Surg. Gynec. Obstet. **43**:150-155, 1926.

21 Burkholder, G. V., and Kaufman, J. J.: Local implantations of carcinoma of the prostate with percutaneous needle biopsy, J. Urol. **95**:801-804, 1966.

22 Calais, A.: Contribution à l'étude du traitement du cancer de la prostate par la radium-

thérapie, Thèse, Faculté de Médecine, Bordeaux, France, 1954.

23 Chua, Domingo T., Ackermann, Wolfgang, and Veenema, Ralph J.: Bone marrow biopsy in patients with carcinoma of the prostate, J. Urol. 102:602-606, 1969.

24 Colby, F. H.: Carcinoma of the prostate, results of total prostatectomy, J. Urol. 69: 797-812, 1953.

25 Cook, G. B., and Watson, F. R.: Events in the natural history of prostate cancer; using salvage curves, mean age distributions and contingency coefficients, J. Urol. 99:87-96, 1968.

26 Cook, W. B., Fishman, W. H., and Clarke, B. G.: Serum acid phosphatase of prostatic origin in the diagnosis of prostatic cancer; clinical evaluation of 2408 tests by the Fishman-Lerner method, J. Urol. 88:281-287, 1962.

27 Culp, O. S., and McDonald, J. R.: Importance of frozen section in evaluating prostatic nodules, Trans. Amer. Ass. Genitourin. Surg. 45:180-186, 1953.

28 Davies, A. L.: Prostatic carcinoma presenting as acute obstruction of large bowel, Cancer 20:1035-1037, 1967.

29 Davis, J. M.: Carcinoma of the prostate presenting as disease of the rectum, Brit. J. Urol. 32:197-203, 1960.

30 deVries, J. K.: The differential diagnosis of carcinoma of the prostate with skeletal metastases and osteitis deformans (Paget's disease of bone), J. Urol. 46:981-996, 1941.

31 Dodge, O. G.: Carcinoma of the prostate in Uganda Africans, Cancer 16:1264-1268, 1963.

32 Edgar, W. M.: Mucin-secreting carcinoma of the prostate, Brit. J. Urol. 30:213-216, 1958.

33 Edling, N. P. C.: On the roentgen aspect of prostatic cancer by urethrocystography, Acta Radiol. (Stockholm) 29:461-474, 1948.

34 Ekman, H., Hedberg, K., and Persson, P. S.: Cytological versus histological examination of needle biopsy specimens in the diagnosis of prostatic cancer, Brit. J. Urol. 39:544-548, 1967.

35 Elkins, H. B., Flocks, R. H., and Culp, D. A.: Evaluation of the use of colloidal radioactive gold in the treatment of prostatic carcinoma, Radiology 70:386-389, 1958.

36 Esposti, P.-L.: Cytologic diagnosis of prostatic tumors with the aid of transrectal aspiration biopsy; a critical review of 1,110 cases and a report of morphologic and cytochemical study, Acta Cytol. (Balt.) 10:182-186, 1966.

37 Fergusson, J. D.: Endocrine control therapy in prostatic cancer, Brit. J. Urol. 30:397-406, 1958.

38 Fergusson, J. D., and Franks, L. M.: The response of prostatic carcinoma to estrogen treatment, Brit. J. Surg. 40:422-428, 1953.

39 Fetter, T. R., Yunen, J. R., Greening, R. R., and Benjamin, A.: Seminal vesiculography; diagnostic aid in prostatic carcinoma, J. Urol. 87:718-725, 1962.

40 Fishman, W. H., Bonner, C. D., and Hom-berger, F.: Serum "prostatic" acid phosphatase and cancer of the prostate, New Eng. J. Med. 255:925-933, 1950.

41 Flocks, R. H., Culp, D. A., and Porto, R.: Lymphatic spread from prostatic cancer, J. Urol. 81:194-196, 1959.

42 Franks, L. M.: The spread of prostatic carcinoma to the bones, J. Path. Bact. 66:91-93, 1953.

43 Franks, L. M.: Latent carcinoma of the prostate, J. Path. Bact. 68:603-616, 1954.

44 Franks, L. M.: Latency and progression in tumours; the natural history of prostatic cancer, Lancet 2:1037-1039, 1956.

45 Franks, L. M.: Some comments on the long-term results of endocrine treatment of prostatic cancer, Brit. J. Urol. 30:383-388, 1958.

46 Franks, L. M.: An assessment of factors influencing survival in prostatic cancer; the absence of reliable prognostic features, Brit. J. Cancer 12:321-326, 1958.

47 Franks, L. M., O'Shea, J. D., and Thomson, A. E. R.: Mucin in the prostate; a histochemical study in normal glands, latent, clinical and colloid cancers, Cancer 17:983-991, 1964.

48 Franzén, S., Giertz, G., and Zajicek, J.: Cytological diagnosis of prostatic tumours by transrectal aspiration biopsy; a preliminary report, Brit. J. Urol. 32:193-196, 1960.

49 Gaynor, E. P.: Zur Frage des Prostatakrebses, Virchow Arch. Path. Anat. 301:602-652, 1938.

50 George, F. W., Carlton, C. E., Dykhuizen, R. F., and Dillon, J. R.: Cobalt-60 telecurie-therapy in the definitive treatment of carcinoma of the prostate; a preliminary report, J. Urol. 93:102-109, 1965.

51 Glantz, S. M.: Cirrhosis and carcinoma of the prostate gland, J. Urol. 91:291-293, 1964.

52 Graves, R. C., and Militzer, R. E.: Carcinoma of the prostate with metastases, J. Urol. 33:235-251, 1935.

53 Greene, L. F., and Simon, H. B.: Occult carcinoma of the prostate; clinical and therapeutic study of eighty-three cases, J.A.M.A. 158:1494-1498, 1955.

54 Griswold, M. H.: Cancer of the prostate in Connecticut, Connecticut Med. J. 10:106-109, 1946.

55 Guillemin, A., and Guillemin, P.: Ponction-biopsie de la prostate par voie trans-rectale (300 cas), J. Urol. (Paris) 62:496-500, 1956.

56 Gutman, A. B.: Serum "acid" phosphatase in patients with carcinoma of the prostate gland, J.A.M.A. 120:1112-1116, 1942.

57 Gutman, A. B.: The development of the acid phosphatase test for prostatic carcinoma, Bull. N. Y. Acad. Med. 44:63-76, 1968.

58 Gutman, A. B., Gutman, E. B., and Robinson, J. M.: Determination of serum "acid" phosphatase activity in differentiating skeletal metastases secondary to prostatic carcinoma from Paget's disease of bone, Amer. J. Cancer 38:103-108, 1950.

59 Halpert, B., and Schmalhorst, W. R.: Carci-

noma of the prostate in patients 70 to 79 years old, Cancer 19:695-698, 1966.

60 Hand, J. R., and Sullivan, A. W.: Retropubic prostatectomy; analysis of one hundred cases, J.A.M.A. 145:1313-1321, 1323-1324, 1951.

61 Herbut, P. A.: Cytologic diagnosis of carcinoma of the prostate, Amer. J. Clin. Path. 19:315-319, 1949.

62 Hinman, F.: The early diagnosis and radical treatment of prostatic carcinoma, Calif. Med. 68:338-343, 1948.

63 Hinman, F., Jr., and Hinman, F.: Occult prostatic carcinoma diagnosed upon transurethral resection, J. Urol. 62:723-729, 1949.

64 Houston, W.: Prostatic cancer in Bantu, J. Roy. Coll. Surg. Edinb. 4:1-3, 1968.

65 Hudson, P. B., Finkle, A. L., Hopkins, J. A., Sproul, E. E., and Stout, A. P.: Prostatic cancer. XI. Early prostatic cancer diagnosed by arbitrary open perineal biopsy among 300 unselected patients, Cancer 7:690-703, 1954.

66 Hudson, P. B., Finkle, A. L., Trifilio, A., Jost, H. M., Sproul, E. E., and Stout, A. P.: Prostatic cancer. VIII. Detection of unsuspected adenocarcinoma in the aging male population, J.A.M.A. 155:426-429, 1954.

67 Huggins, C.: Prostatic cancer treated by orchiectomy; the five year results, J.A.M.A. 131:576-581, 1946.

68 Huggins, C., and Scott, W. W.: Bilateral adrenalectomy in prostatic cancer; clinical features and urinary excretion of 17-ketosteroids and estrogen, Ann. Surg. 122:1031-1041, 1945.

69 Jewett, H. J.: Radical perineal prostatectomy for cancer of the prostate; an analysis of 190 cases, J. Urol. 61:277-280, 1949.

70 Jewett, H. J.: Significance of the palpable prostatic nodule, J.A.M.A. 160:838-839, 1956.

71 Jewett, H. J., Bridge, R. W., Gray, G. F., and Shelley, W. M.: The palpable nodule, of prostatic cancer; results 15 years after radical excision, J.A.M.A. 203:115-119, 1968.

72 Jönsson, G., and Fajers, C. M.: Cancer cells in prostatic secretion, Acta Chir. Scand. 99: 545-559, 1950.

73 Kahler, J. E.: Carcinoma of the prostate gland; a pathologic study, J. Urol. 41:557-574, 1939.

74 Kerr, H. D., Flocks, R. H., Elkins, H. B., and Culp, D. A.: Follow-up study of one hundred cases of carcinoma of the prostate treated with radioactive gold, Radiology 64:637-641, 1955.

75 King, H., Diamond, E., and Lilienfeld, A. M.: Some epidemiological aspects of cancer of the prostate, J. Chronic Dis. 16:117-153, 1963.

76 Kirchheim, D., Niles, N. R., Frankus, E., and Hodges, C. V.: Correlative histochemical and histological studies on thirty radical prostatectomy specimens, Cancer 19:1683-1969, 1966.

77 Kristianstad, A. A.: Circumcision and prostatic cancer, Acta Med. Scand. 178:493-504, 1965.

78 Larson, D. L., Rodin, A. E., Roberts, D. K.,

O'Steen, W. K., Rapperport, A. S., and Lewis, S. R.: Perineural lymphatics; myth or fact, Amer. J. Surg. 112:488-492, 1966.

79 Lazarus, J. A.: Primary malignant tumors of the retrovesical region with special reference to malignant tumors of the seminal vesicles; report of a case of retrovesicle sarcoma, J. Urol. 55:190-205, 1946.

80 McCrea, L. E.: Primary carcinoma of the seminal vesicles, J.A.M.A. 136:679-682, 1948.

81 McGavran, H. G.: Giant prostate without symptoms; neurofibroma, J. Urol. 60:254-259, 1948.

82 McNally, A., and Cochens, F. M.: Primary carcinoma of the seminal vesicles, J. Urol. 36:532-537, 1936.

83 Marberger, H., Segal, S. J., and Flocks, R. H.: Changes in serum acid phosphatase levels consequent to prostatic manipulation or surgery, J. Urol. 78:287-293, 1957.

84 Mason, M. K.: Cytology of the prostate, J. Clin. Path. 17:581-590, 1964.

85 Mason, M. K.: The cytological diagnosis of carcinoma of the prostate, Acta Cytol. (Balt.) 11:68-71, 1967.

86 Melicow, M. M., Pelton, T. H., and Fish, G. W.: Sarcoma of the prostate gland: review of literature; table of classification; report of four cases, J. Urol. 49:675-707, 1943.

87 Middleton, A. W.: Union of pathologic fracture of femur following castrations for carcinoma of the prostate, Amer. J. Surg. 64: 144-146, 1944.

88 Millin, T.: Retropubic prostatectomy; a new extravesical technique; report of 20 cases, Lancet 2:693-696, 1945.

89 Moore, R. A.: The morphology of small prostatic carcinoma, J. Urol. 33:224-234, 1935.

90 Nesbit, R. M., and Baum, W.-C.: Endocrine control of prostate carcinoma, J.A.M.A. 143: 1317-1320, 1950.

91 Nesbit, R. M., and Cummings, R. H.: Prostatic carcinoma treated by orchiectomy, J.A.M.A. 120:1109-1111, 1942.

92 Okada, K.: Ultrastructural changes in prostatic cancer cells following castration, Jap. J. Urol. 57:803-821, 1966.

93 Pennington, J. W., Prentiss, R. J., and Howe, G.: Radical prostatectomy for cancer; significance of perineural lymphatic invasion, J. Urol. 97:1075-1077, 1967.

94 Phillips, L. L., Skrodells, V., and Furey, C. A.: The fibrinolytic enzyme in prostatic cancer, Cancer 12:721-730, 1959.

95 Prince, C. L., and Vest, S. A.: Leiomyosarcoma of the prostate, J. Urol. 46:1129-1143, 1941.

96 Prout, G. R., Jr., and Brewer, W. R.: Response of men with advanced prostatic carcinoma to exogenous administration of testosterone, Cancer 20:1871-1878, 1967.

97 Reboul, J., Ballanger, F., Delorme, G., and Tessier, J. P.: La radiothérapie dans le cancer de la prostate, Ann. Radiol. (Paris) 8: 353-358, 1965.

98 del Regato, J. A.: Radiotherapy in the conservative treatment of operable and locally

inoperable carcinoma of the prostate, Radiology **88**:761-766, 1967.

99 del Regato, J. A. (chairman): Radiotherapy for cancer of the prostate. Protocol and experimental design for a Cooperative Study of Radiotherapy for Carcinoma of the Prostate Stage C, Colorado Springs, pp. 1-40, 1967.

100 Rich, A. R.: On the frequency of occurrence of occult carcinoma of the prostate, J. Urol. **33**:215-223, 1935.

101 Rodin, A. E., Larson, D. L., and Roberts, D. K.: Nature of the perineural space invaded by prostatic carcinoma, Cancer **20**:1772-1779, 1967.

102 Schmalhorst, W. R., and Halpert, B.: Carcinoma of the prostate gland in patients more than 80 years old, Amer. J. Clin. Path. **42**:170-173, 1964.

103 Scott, W. W.: An evaluation of endocrine therapy plus radical perineal prostatectomy in the treatment of advanced carcinoma of the prostate, J. Urol. **91**:97-102, 1964.

104 Sika, J. V., and Buckley, J. J.: Mucus-forming adenocarcinoma of the prostate, Cancer **17**:949-952, 1964.

105 Smith, M. J. V.: The lymphatics of the prostate, Invest. Urol. **3**:439-444, 1966.

106 Stewart, C. B., Sweetser, T. H., and Delory, G. E.: A case of benign prostatic hypertrophy with recent infarcts and associated high serum acid phosphatase, J. Urol. **63**:128-131, 1950.

107 Still, B. M., and Warwick, R. T.: Prostatic massage and the plasma acid phosphatase level, Brit. J. Urol. **38**:279-282, 1966.

108 Straffon, R. A., Kiser, W. S., Robitaille, M.,

and Dohn, D. F.: 90-yttrium hypophysectomy in the management of metastatic carcinoma of the prostate gland in 13 patients, J. Urol. **99**:102-105, 1968.

109 Veterans Administration Co-Operative Urological Research Group: Treatment and survival of patients with cancer of the prostate, Surg. Gynec. Obstet. **124**:1011-1017, 1967.

110 Vickery, A. L., and Kerr, W. S., Jr.: Carcinoma of the prostate treated by radical prostatectomy; a clinicopathological survey of 187 cases followed for 5 years and 148 cases followed for 10 years, Cancer **16**:1598-1608, 1963.

111 Whitmore, W. F., Jr.: The rationale and results of ablative surgery for prostatic cancer, Cancer **16**:1119-1132, 1963.

112 Williams, D. F., and Blahd, W. H.: The diagnostic and prognostic value of strontium-85 photoscanning in carcinoma of the prostate, J. Urol. **97**:1070-1074, 1967.

113 Winter, C. C.: The problem of rectal involvement by prostatic cancer, Surg. Gynec. Obstet. **105**:136-140, 1957.

114 Woodard, H. Q.: The interpretation of phosphatase findings in carcinoma of the prostate, New York J. Med. **47**:379-381, 1947 (classic).

115 Wray, S.: The significance of the blood acid and alkaline phosphatase values in cancer of the prostate, J. Clin. Path. **9**:341-346, 1956.

116 Young, H. H.: The cure of cancer of the prostate by radical perineal prostatectomy (prostato-seminal vesiculectomy): history, literature and statistics of Young's operation, J. Urol. **53**:188-256, 1945 (classic).

Testis

Anatomy

The testis is formed by glandular tissue and convoluted tubules surrounded by connective tissue containing the interstitial cells of internal secretion. It is completely invested in a dense membrane, the tunica albuginea, which sends radiating septa into the gland. The tubules converge at the hilum, known as the *rete testis*, from which point a single convoluted tubule further extends to form the epididymis (Fig. 516).

In the process of its descent from the abdomen into the scrotum, the testis develops several coats of tissue, the most significant of which is the tunica vaginalis, which nearly surrounds the organ except at the point at which the epididymis is attached. Surrounding the vaginalis successively are the fibrous, muscular, and cellular layers, all of which are included in the tunica dartos and the scrotum (**Fig. 517**). There is a virtual cavity between the visceral and the parietal layers of the vaginalis.

Lymphatics. The lymphatic channels of each testis, numbering four to eight, place themselves on the surface of the spermatic vessels, the course of which they follow. They curve medially across the ureter and end on the lateral para-aortic lymph nodes that extend from the renal vein to the bifurcation of the aorta. Some of the lymphatics end on the medial preaortic nodes, and some may cross the midline. On the right side, some lymphatics occasionally end in a node placed in the angle formed by the vena cava and the renal vein. On both sides, some of the channels abandon the spermatic vessels after they reach the

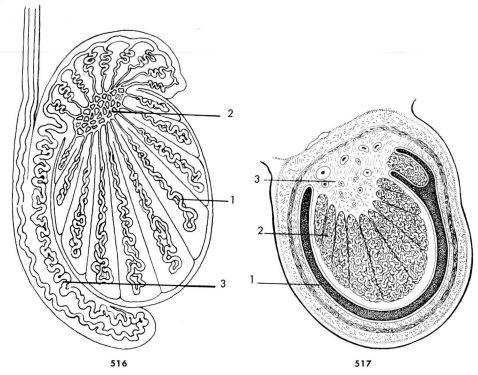

516   **517**

Fig. 516. Section of normal adult testis showing convoluted tubules, **1**; rete testis, **2**; epididymis, **3**.

Fig. 517. Section of normal adult testis showing tunica vaginalis, **1**; convoluted tubules, **2**; rete testis, **3**.

vesical peritoneum, turning laterally to end on nodes lying on the external iliac vein (Fig. 518). The lymphatics of the epididymis follow this latter course.

Lymphographic studies have shown that in the male adult the draining para-aortic lymph nodes are situated from the eleventh thoracic to the fourth lumbar vertebrae (Busch and Sayegh[9]). Those studies suggest also that there is a principal node area or testicular lymphatic center, laterally situated about the level of the first to second lumbar vertebrae, from which spread to other nodes takes place (Chiappa et al.[13]).

Epidemiology

Testicular tumors constitute fewer than 1% of all malignant tumors, but they are about the most common malignant tumor found in men 30 to 34 years of age. The majority occur in individuals 20 to 40 years of age. *Seminomas* do not occur in children (Phelan et al.[70]). Their frequency rises after the age of 15 years to reach a maximum between 40 and 45 years of age. The frequency of *teratocarcinomas* is about the same in the first six decades of life. Testicular tumors are rare in Negroes (Kaplan et al.[49]; Koehler et al.[50]). They are also extremely rare in the Bantu and infrequent in the Cape colored (Tiltman[90]). In childhood, the distinctive tumor (Teoh et al.[89]) is an *adenocarcinoma* (sometimes designated as *orchioblastoma*), which is probably neither a teratoma nor a seminoma (Huntington et al.[47]), but the most common testicular tumor is the *embryonal carcinoma* (Tefft et al.[88]). *Lymphosarcomas* occur mostly in elderly persons.

The occurrence of tumors in cases of *cryptorchidism* is notable. About 1 in 80 inguinal testes and 1 in 20 abdominal testes may be expected to develop neoplasms (Campbell[11]). It has also been suggested that the congenital imperfection of the testis, rather than its abnormal

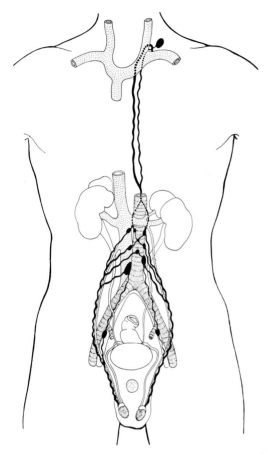

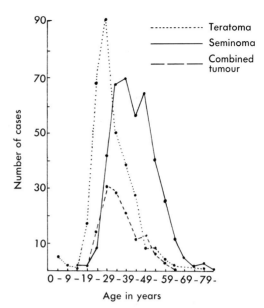

Fig. 519. Age distribution of patients at time of orchiectomy: 400 cases of seminoma, 322 cases of teratoma, and 136 cases of combined tumor. Note how peak age of combined tumors occupies intermediate position between peaks for seminoma and teratoma. (From Collins, D. H., and Pugh, R. C. B., editors: The pathology of testicular tumours; classification and frequency of testicular tumours, Brit. J. Urol. 36[suppl.]:1-11, 1964; WU neg. 69-6396.)

Fig. 518. Lymphatics of testis showing main drainage in para-aortic lymphatics and further lymphatic extension by way of thoracic duct. Left supraclavicular node is fairly frequently involved. Lymphatics of epididymis drain into external iliac lymph nodes.

location, is the predisposing factor (Sohval[82]). The presence of undescended testes may be related to hormonal influences. In lower animals, bilateral cryptorchidism is characterized by an excessive secretion of gonadotropins (Hamilton and Leonard[39]). Sumner[85] collected sixty-five cases in which a tumor had developed years after orchiopexy and suggested that the operation be done early. Hand[40] prefers an orchiectomy if the testis has not descended spontaneously at puberty or cannot be brought down surgically. *Trauma* is often claimed as an initial factor in the history, being reported in as large a proportion as 10% of patients (Fergusson[26]). However, the importance of this factor is difficult to assess. In many instances, trauma may simply call attention to the presence of a tumor, or the presence of the tumor makes the trauma more possible. Giertsen[33] reported five cases occurring between the ages of 6 and 26 months following *orchitis* due to mumps. He questioned whether or not the atrophy combined with hormonal imbalance could cause the development of tumor.

The relatively frequent occurrence of successive bilateral testicular tumors may also point to a hormonal cause (Hamilton and Gilbert[38]). Peirson[69] collected forty-six cases of teratoma in which another tumor occurred in the other testis. Six of the patients suffered from cryptorchidism, a proportion far in excess of the expected occurrence.

Pathology
Gross pathology

Ewing[24] believed that all tumors of the testis are teratomas arising from the totipotent sex cells in the neighborhood of the

Table 64. Classification and frequency of primary germinal tumors*†

	Cases	%
Total	894	100.0
Pure tumor types	536	60.0
Mixed tumor types	358	40.0
Pure tumor types	536	100.0
Mature teratomas	34	6.3
Immature teratomas	15	2.8
Embryonal carcinomas	135	25.2
Choriocarcinomas	7	1.3
Seminomas	345	64.4

*From Dixon, F. J., and Moore, R. A.: Tumors of the male sex organs. In Atlas of tumor pathology, Sect. 8, Fascs. 31B and 32, Washington, D. C., 1952, Armed Forces Institute of Pathology.
†Excludes 46 cases classified as germinal on basis of type in metastasis; no slides for primary tumor available.

rete. The classification of Dixon and Moore[19] has been widely used in the United States. Of 976 testicular tumors studied by them, 940 were considered to be germinal in origin, and only 60% were considered pure tumor types (Table 64). A new classification by Collins and Pugh[15] divides all testicular tumors into two main types: seminomas and teratomas. Certainly, these two types have to be separated in considering the results of treatment. Seminomas and various types of teratomas may appear in the same testicular tumor. Azzopardi and Hoffbrand[3] insist that a seminoma of the testis can never give rise to metastases of the choriocarcinoma or embryonal carcinoma type. There may be regression of the teratoma in the involved testis, and if this teratoma is not identified by careful pathologic study, it may be suggested erroneously that the metastasis came from a seminoma.

Chevassu[12] considered seminomas a specific entity arising from the epithelium of the seminal tubules. In these tumors, prominent intratubular growth is often observed (Dixon and Moore[20]). In dogs, seminoma is one of the most common malignant tumors, and often spermatic epithelium is strongly suggested (Scully and Coffin[79]). Dixon and Moore's hypothesis[20] of maturation of testicular tumors is supported by instances in which the primary lesion showed only adult structures, whereas the metastases contained undifferentiated elements. These findings do not support a separation of adult teratomas from teratocarcinomas (Symeonidis[86]).

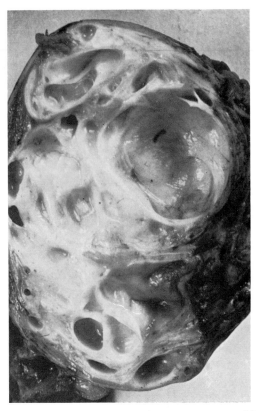

Fig. 520. Cystic teratoma of testis in 19-year-old youth. All elements were well differentiated, yet on retroperitoneal lymph node dissection several nodes were also found to be involved by well-differentiated teratomatous elements. (Courtesy Dr. George Scofield, Fort Leonard Wood, Mo.)

Testicular tumors vary greatly in size. They may enlarge the organ to ten times the normal dimensions or may be occult in a normal-sized testis. The tumor itself is usually fairly firm, depending upon cellularity, bone, cartilage, and connective tissue content. A cross section of the adult teratoma shows cystic spaces, mucinous areas, cartilage, and bone formation (Fig. 520). However, if these tumors are less differentiated, they are softer and often develop areas of hemorrhage and necrosis. Seminomas are usually homogeneous and may show areas of necrosis. It is not rare for a mixture of seminoma and some other form of testicular tumor to occur together. Halley[37] did careful sectioning of testicular tumors and found that coincident seminoma and teratoma are present in a much higher percentage than had previously been reported. He also emphasized that these

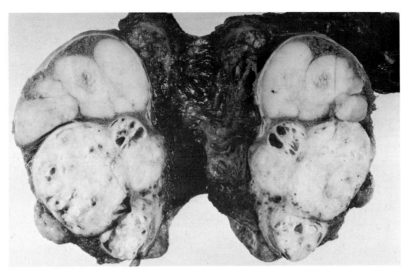

Fig. 521. Coincident but discrete seminoma and teratoma. Seminoma occupies upper half of testis. (From Halley, J. B. W.: Pathology and survival in testicular neoplasia, Cancer **16:** 1269-1280, 1963.)

two tumors are separate and dissimilar (Fig. 521).

The choriocarcinoma is usually small, hemorrhagic, and soft. Rarely, there may be widespread metastases from choriocarcinoma without a palpable tumor in the testis. Step sections of the testis may reveal a small tumor, or there may even be complete regression of the primary neoplasm. Study of the scar may show only fibrosis and hemosiderin pigmentation (Laipply and Shipley[51]) (Fig. 522).

Rather et al.[74] collected eighteen cases of testicular tumors showing various degrees of maturation and presenting regressions of the primary tumor in the face of florid growth of metastases and added six of their own cases. Of these twenty-four cases, seven testes presented scar tissue only, and nine showed seminomatous tissue in addition to fibrosis. In the remaining eight cases, there were cysts and tubular structures lying in zones of fibrosis, with a few instances of foci of calcification and depositions of hemosiderin. Azzopardi et al.[4] observed somewhat similar findings. In thirteen of their seventeen cases, peculiar amorphous hematoxylin-staining deposits were observed in dilated seminiferous tubules. The seminoma is customarily homogeneous noncystic pinkish yellow, only occasionally showing areas of hemorrhage and necrosis (Fig. 523).

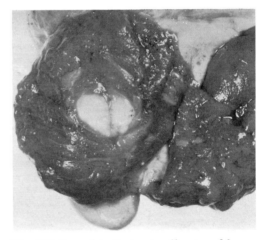

Fig. 522. Scar of testis showing fibrosis and hemosiderin pigmentation. This was only evidence of primary choriocarcinoma. Patient had extensive metastases. (Courtesy Dr. David Rosenbaum, Indianapolis, Ind.)

Paratesticular tumors of connective tissue and muscle occur infrequently. Gowing and Morgan[35] collected twenty-seven, eleven of which were rhabdomyosarcoma and embryonic sarcoma. Rarely, seminomas may be primary in the retroperitoneal area (Abell et al.[1]). Interstitial cell tumors of the testis are usually yellow-brown and are well delineated.

The direct extension of testicular tumors is limited somewhat by the tunica albu-

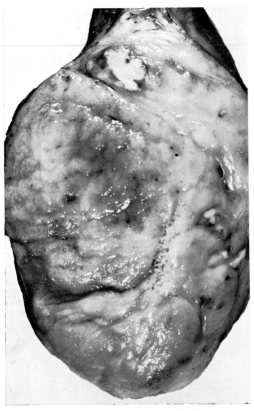

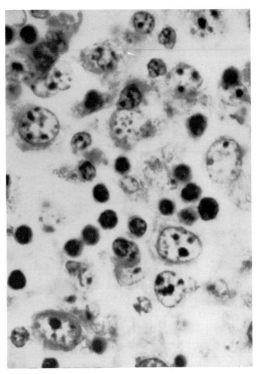

Fig. 524. Seminoma showing characteristic large cells with clear cytoplasm, well-defined nuclei, and rather prominent nucleoli. Lymphoid stroma is present. (High-power enlargement.)

Fig. 523. Seminoma of testis with characteristic zones of necrosis. Note homogeneous appearance with small foci of necrosis.

ginea, which, if encroached upon, may show surface nodules. Further extension beyond the tunica albuginea is rare, but tumors may involve and even ulcerate the skin of the scrotum.

Microscopic pathology

Microscopically, the adult teratoma shows all types of tissue with elements traceable to mesoderm, ectoderm, and entoderm. In subserial sections of an adult teratoma, it is not uncommon to find zones of poorly differentiated neoplasm. The anaplastic teratocarcinomas (embryonal carcinomas) can be distinguished from seminomas by their cellular anaplasia, variations in cell size, and large, irregular nuclei. Early trophoblastic differentiation may be seen. By contrast, seminomas have rather uniform cells with clear cytoplasm, well-defined nuclei, and usually a single prominent nucleolus (Fig. 524). Their lymphoid stroma is variable. Seminomas

may show intratubular growth and may have fibrous or even granulomatous stromal background. Choriocarcinomas are easily recognized through the presence of cyto-forming and somatic trophoblast-forming villuslike structures. Sharp differentiation into these various types does not always occur, and mixtures result. In a group of 358 tumors, 40% showed some mixture (Table 65). The term "embryonal carcinoma" as used by Ewing[24] and by Dixon and Moore[19] is confusing, and it is more rational to think of this type of tumor as an anaplastic teratocarcinoma.

Most tumors developing in ectopic testes are seminomas. Dixon and Moore[20] had twenty cases (twelve inguinal, eight abdominal), fifteen of which were seminomas.

There are two errors that pathologists make that obscure the prognosis. Seminomas are incorrectly diagnosed as embryonal carcinomas, and embryonal carcinomas are incorrectly called seminomas (Schnyder[78]). These pseudoseminomas are hormonally active and may cause a positive

Table 65. Frequency of combinations of tumor types*

	Cases	%
All mixed tumors	358	100.0
Embryonal carcinoma + seminoma	43	12.0
Embryonal carcinoma + immature teratoma	142	39.6
Embryonal carcinoma + seminoma + immature teratoma	40	11.2
Embryonal carcinoma + immature teratoma + mature teratoma	39	10.9
All other mixed types	94	26.2

*From Dixon, F. J., and Moore, R. A.: Unpublished data.

Aschheim-Zondek test, and careful sectioning may show teratoid elements. Eckert and Smith[21] found thirty-five cases among 665 patients with testicular tumors. Five of the patients had other simultaneous manifestations. We have seen lymphosarcoma of the testis. Tumor cells in this neoplasm grow between the tubules instead of arising within them. This is a helpful point in differentiating this tumor from a seminoma. Spermatocytic seminoma is a rare distinctive lesion often confused with seminoma (Rosai et al.[75a]).

Metastatic spread

Early lymphatic metastases to the para-aortic nodes are found in most testicular tumors. Involvement of the ipsilateral iliac nodes is not uncommon, particularly when the epididymis is invaded. The para-aortic node involvement is frequently bilateral, but not the iliac extension, which is always confined to the same side. When invasion of the albuginea has occurred, inguinal metastases may be expected. Inguinal metastases have also been observed after orchiopexy or orchiectomy for tumors in inguinal testes (Witus et al.[95]). Spread may also take place through the spermatic veins, either to the renal vein on the left or the vena cava on the right. Choriocarcinomas may metastasize exclusively by the veins without presenting lymphatic spread. Intracardiac metastases causing obstruction of the right auricle have been observed (Watts[92]). Rare cases of tridermal metastases have been reported (Adams[2]). Reporting on thirty-seven autopsy cases, Barringer and Earl[6] found lymph node involvement in 60%. In 27% of the cases, there was lymphatic involvement from the bifurcation of the aorta up to the supraclavicular region all along the course of the thoracic duct. Lung metastases were found in 78% of the cases, and in three-fourths of these the liver was also affected.

Clinical evolution

Tumors of the testes develop slowly and insidiously. An early symptom may be simply a sensation of discomfort due to the weight of the tumor. Testicular sensitivity may also decrease. These symptoms may give place to a *dull ache* or *pain* (Milner and Gilbert[65]). *Lumbar pain* may result from the development of retroperitoneal metastases which, in some cases, may be the first recognizable manifestation of the disease. The lumbar pain may radiate down to the thigh. Symptoms of *urinary obstruction*, with dysuria, anorexia, and vomiting may result from the compression of the renal pedicle. *Gynecomastia* and pigmentation of the nipples have been observed in patients with choriocarcinoma.

Primary lymphosarcomas of the testes are an accepted entity (Gowing[34]). It is not always possible to decide whether or not such tumors are metastatic. Eckert and Smith[21] reported on thirty cases, twenty of which had resulted in generalization and death within eighteen months, and half of the patients had bilateral testicular lymphoid tumors. This suggests that the testicular manifestation was probably, in many cases, secondary to a generalized process.

Testicular tumors may spread rapidly and result in death within six to eight months of diagnosis (Table 66). Lung metastases may be unsuspected or, on the contrary, cause considerable symptomatology. In extensive disease, brain metastases are not uncommon.

Interstitial cell tumors are most commonly observed in patients 5 to 10 and 30 to 35 years of age (Dalgaard and Hesselberg[17]). In children, they may result in precocious sexual and body development (Jungck et al.[48]) (Fig. 525). In adults, there may be virilization, feminization (gynecomastia), sexual indifference, loss of libido, (Reiners and Horn[75]), or no clinical symptoms at all. Few interstitial cell tumors are actually malignant in spite of histopathologic pleomorphism. Three

Table 66. Relation of symptoms to lesions due to metastatic spread of testicular tumors

Symptom	Lesion
Involved inguinal nodes	Tumor growing through tunica albuginea or tumor growing in operative scar
Lumbar pain Constipation Pain in sciatic distribution	Involvement of retroperitoneal nodes
Costovertebral tenderness Lumbar pain Pyuria Dysuria	Partial ureteral or renal pedicle obstruction by involved nodes
Vomiting Headache Drowsiness	Impending renal failure due to block of ureters or renal pedicle by involved nodes
Cough Dyspnea (may suggest tuberculosis)	Involvement of lung and mediastinal nodes
Hemoptysis	Involved bronchial or tracheal nodes eroding tracheobronchial tree
Cerebral symptoms	Brain metastases
Swelling of lower extremity	Inferior vena caval obstruction by lymph node metastases

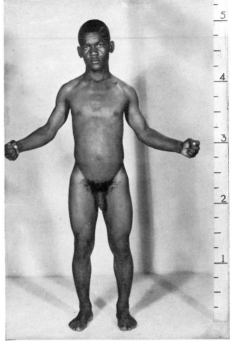

Fig. 525. Patient, 8-year-old boy, with adult genitalia and unusual muscular development. Benign interstitial cell tumor was removed. (From Jungck, E. C., et al.: Sexual precocity due to interstitial-cell tumor of the testis: report of two cases, J. Clin. Endocr. 17:291-295, 1957.)

cases of bilateral interstitial cell tumors have been recorded (Flynn and Severance[27]).

Diagnosis
Clinical examination

Dean[18] found that in two-thirds of patients, the average delay between first symptom and examination was four months, but an additional six and one half months lapsed before institution of treatment. Upon palpation of the testis, the examiner should detect changes in size, shape, and consistency. A normal testis may attain a rather large size, particularly when its mate has become atrophic, but it conserves its peculiar consistency and sensitivity. And yet a tumor may be present and even produce metastases without affecting the size of the testis. A testis enlarged by tumor is firm and painless. Usually, the epididymis is flattened on the posterior surface, although it is seldom involved. In rare instances, the testicular tumor has an inflammatory component (Whittle[94]). Rarely, testicular tumors may be bilateral. There may be a hydrocele with or without a tumor. To facilitate palpation, the fluid should be removed. Transillumination may be of assistance. Solid structures, such as tumors, gummas, and calcified hematomas, do not transilluminate.

The abdomen should be examined carefully for retroperitoneal lymph node metastases. The examination can be made best with the patient lying on his back with the legs slightly flexed on the abdomen and the arms at the sides and breathing through the mouth. Palpation must be fairly deep, since the metastatic nodes usually lie at the level of, or slightly caudal to, the umbilicus. The left supraclavicular node area should also be investigated. Metastases within the lung are scarcely ever detected on physical examination un-

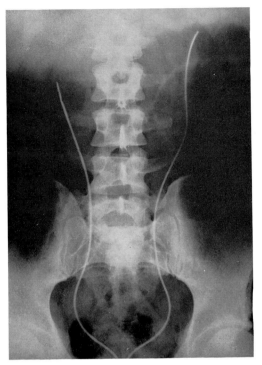

Fig. 526. Roentgenogram after catheterization of ureters showing lateral deviation of left ureter by para-aortic adenopathy.

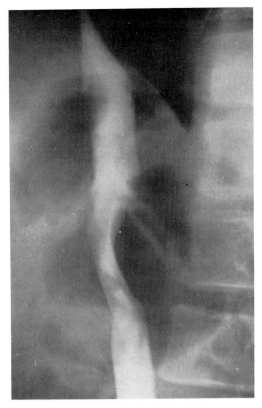

Fig. 527. Note smooth indentation of vena cava due to metastases in lymph node by seminoma. (Courtesy Department of Radiology, Mallinckrodt Institute of Radiology, Washington University School of Medicine, St. Louis, Mo.)

less they are very large, approach the pleura, or compress or invade the bronchi. Infrequently, rectal examination may reveal involvement of periprostatic lymph nodes (Barringer[5]).

Roentgenologic examination

Metastatic para-aortic lymph nodes may displace the ureter laterally (Fig. 526) and cause its partial or complete obstruction. To demonstrate the presence of metastatic nodes, a retrograde (rather than intravenous) *pyeloureterogram* is useful. The roentgenograms may reveal a rounding of the psoas muscle, as though it were contracted, with a convexity of the lumbar spine toward the affected side. *Phlebograms* may also be useful in demonstrating objectively the presence of metastatic lymph nodes (Fig. 527). In men 20 to 40 years of age, the fortuitous discovery of *pulmonary metastases* points frequently to a primary malignant tumor of the testis.

Lymphangiography has become a very useful part of the examination of patients with testicular tumors, providing valuable information as to the abdominal and pelvic lymph node involvement (Chiappa et al.[14]), and it is said to be more accurate than pyeloureterography or caval phlebograms (Markovits et al.[63]). The procedure, however, is not without errors (Cook et al.[16]). Lymphangiography may help in radiotherapeutic planning (Picard[71]). If done before surgery, it helps in determining the adequacy of retroperitoneal lymphadenectomy.

Hormone studies

The measurement of chronic gonadotropin may be helpful in establishing a diagnosis and in estimating the prognosis. Patients with choriocarcinoma have an extremely high titer, whereas those with seminomas and teratomas should have a low titer. It is important that the measurements be very carefully made by an accurate method. When a high titer remains after treatment of a choriocarcinoma, this indicates the presence of residual tumor. Similarly, a drop of the titer after treatment and a subsequent rise indicate the development of metastases. A high titer in patients with a tumor diagnosed as seminoma would indicate that the tumor has not been thoroughly examined and that areas of teratocarcinoma are present within it (Hobson[44]). In a tumor excreting large amounts of chronic gonadotropin, the uninvolved testis may show interstitial cell hyperplasia (Laqueur[52]; Mark and Hedinger[62]).

Differential diagnosis

Tuberculosis, which is invariably primary in the epididymis, results in nodularity and may cause "beading" of the vas deferens. Only in the late stages, however, does extension into the testis take place. With tuberculous involvement of the testis, other portions of the genitourinary tract and lungs may be affected, but this can usually be demonstrated by clinical and roentgenologic examination. Roentgenograms of the testis showing calcification in the region of the epididymis are presumptive evidence of tuberculosis. Further aid in diagnosis can be gained from roentgenograms of the lung, which will show any tuberculosis present, or from palpation of the prostate, which may reveal evidence of nodular caseous tuberculosis.

Syphilitic gumma of the testis is practically never observed today. It may be extremely difficult to differentiate from a tumor of the testis, because it is sharply circumscribed and fairly firm. The serology, however, will be positive, and other stigmas of syphilis may be present. These findings should not rule out the possibility of coexisting syphilis and tumor.

Spontaneous hemorrhage into the testis can occur, and because *hematoceles* do not transilluminate, they may easily be mistaken for tumor. In addition, the hematocele may be very firm if organization of the clot has taken place. Trauma often precedes a hematocele. Simple *orchitis* is seldom confused with a testicular tumor because of its evident elements of acute inflammation.

Granulomatous orchitis is a relatively rare condition that may be confused clinically with a testicular tumor because it presents as a firm mass. At times, there is a history of trauma. Grossly, the lesion also suggests a tumor. Microscopically, because it is highly cellular, it may be misdiagnosed as a seminoma or a reticulum cell sarcoma (Spjut and Thorpe[83]).

Metastatic carcinoma of the testis is rare and is usually observed in elderly patients (Price and Mostofi[72]). *Spermatic cord* tumors may be benign (Hinman and Gibson[42]) or malignant (Gray and Biorn[36]; Satter et al.[77]). If on careful palpation the tumor can be separated from the testis and appears just below the internal ring, a diagnosis of tumor of the spermatic cord should be entertained (Arlen et al.[2a]). A rare benign *tumor of the epididymis* of mesothelial origin has been reported (Fajers[25]). *Tumors of the tunica albuginea* are also seldom seen. *Malacoplakia* has been reported in the testis (Brown and Smith[8]). Symptomatic plasmacytomas of the testis are usually malignant (Levin and Mostofi[55]).

Treatment
Surgery

Orchiectomy is indicated for all tumors of the testis. Even if the clinical diagnosis of malignant tumor is not certain, no biologic loss is sustained by the surgical removal of the testis because benign tumors and syphilitic gummas may also displace and destroy the organ as they grow within it. The surgical removal of the testis also submits the entire specimen for pathologic study. At operation, the spermatic cord should be exposed and clamped at the external inguinal ring before the testis is removed. Palpation of the testis during this procedure should be avoided because of the possibility of spread of tumor resulting from this manipulation.

In the treatment of malignant tumors of the testis, however, an orchiectomy alone yields rather poor results. Tanner[87] reported only 6% four-year survivals following orchiectomy alone. The retroperitoneal node dissection is not a very adequate procedure for curative purposes, but the reduced operative mortality has encouraged its use in the treatment of embryonal carcinomas and teratomas (Staubitz et al.[83a, 84]; Leadbetter[54]; Patton and Mallis[68]). Mallis and Patton[61] reported a method for transperitoneal bilateral lymphadenectomy. The operation has the advantage of establishing the presence or absence of abdominal spread, depending of course on the adequacy of the intervention and of the histopathologic study of the specimen. It would obviate the need for postoperative irradiation when no metastatic nodes are found. However, the dissection may leave behind a considerable number of nodes as shown by lymphangiography. Moreover, the operation increases the risk of subsequent irradiation, and there is no evidence that it improves the results of abdominal irradiation of metastatic seminomas.

Radiotherapy

The administration of *preoperative radiotherapy* to the testicular tumor has not been shown to be of value. In addition, it usually modifies the architecture of the tumor and interferes with its proper pathologic study. Since a knowledge of the pathologic entity is so vital to the future welfare of the patient, we believe that roentgentherapy should never be administered before orchiectomy.

Irradiation of the potential areas of metastatic involvement, on the same side of the pelvis and on both sides of the abdominal midline, even when such involvement has not been proved, has definitely improved on the results of simple orchiectomy. This is particularly true of seminomas (Staubitz et al.[84]) and may be true also of other tumors. Seminomas are the most radiosensitive and radiocurable, but there is some evidence that benefit is also derived from irradiation of embryonal carcinomas (Friedman and Di Rienzo[92]) and of teratocarcinomas (Parker and Holyoke[67]).

Caldwell[10] believes that megavoltage radiotherapy is a more rational treatment of retroperitoneal node metastasis of non-seminomatous testicular tumors than surgical dissection. Following orchiectomy, he advises a lymphangiogram, preferably by injection of lymphatics of the spermatic cord, unilaterally, in order to decide the extent of the fields to be irradiated. If the lymphangiogram is negative in patients with nonseminomatous tumors, he advises postoperative radiotherapy to the potential area of metastasis in the ipsilateral pelvis and retroperitoneal space. When the lymphangiogram shows the presence of lymph node involvement, he advocates preoperative radiotherapy followed by retroperitoneal dissection or radiotherapy alone. He admits that only a well-conducted clinical study may definitely solve this dilemma.

There is no evidence that patients with choriocarcinoma are helped by abdominal irradiation. With the use of cobalt[60] and supervoltage roentgentherapy, it has become possible to administer, with ease, a satisfactory amount of radiations over the areas of possible metastatic involvement. Under these favorable circumstances, there is no need to irradiate intensively provided a reasonable total amount of radiations is distributed throughout the sites of potential metastases. Short intensive courses of radiotherapy only increase the chances of untoward effects on bowel and spinal cord (Lewis[57]). The kidneys should and, as a rule, can be shielded without detriment. Reports of radiation injury to the kidney (Notter and Ranudd[66]; Shepherd[80]) usually imply irradiation through posterior fields or irradiation of large masses. An anterior midline field extending only over the medial third of the kidney permits sufficient irradiation of the nodes without irradiation of the kidneys. Extension of the irradiated area, to include the mediastinum and neck, is justified in the presence of radiographic or histologic evidence of high para-aortic involvement, for in half of such instances the mediastinum is involved.

Friedman and Purkayastha[30] demonstrated the value of radiotherapy in the management of recurrent metastases or of metastases outside the area of immediate involvement. Parker and Holyoke[67] also have demonstrated control of pulmonary metastases by means of adequate irradiation.

Chemotherapy

Various drugs have shown capability to cause regression of metastatic testicular tumors, among them actinomycin D, methotrexate, chlorambucil, and vinblastine. However, responses are often obtained at the price of drug toxicity and may be short

Table 67. Embryonal carcinomas*

Authors	Year	Patients treated	Well 5 yr or longer	% 5-yr survivals
Cabot and Berkson	1939	41	12	30
Pelot and Hébrard	1951	42	11	26
Dixon and Moore	1953	517	242	45
Lewis	1953	62	22	35.5
Cox	1954	32	11	34
Trial, Rescanière and Hébrard	1958	75	16	20
Cibert, Papillon, and Dargent	1959	20	8	40
Host and Stokke	1959	134	60	44
Patton, Hewitt, and Mallis	1959	244	98	40
Hope-Stone, Blandy, and Dayan	1961	60	20	33
Friedman and Di Rienzo	1963	83	25	30
Notter and Ranudd	1964	110	24	22
Ennuyer and Gricouroff	1965	37	5	13
		1457	554	38

*From Ennuyer, A.: Radiothérapie des métastases des tumeurs germinales du testicule, Bull. Cancer (Paris) **53:** 307-328, 1966.

Table 68. Seminomas*

Authors	Year	Patients treated	Well 5 yr or longer	% 5-yr survivals
Cabot and Berkson	1939	64	42	68
Nash and Leddy	1943	103	70	68
Ahlbom	1947	65	42	65
Sauer and Burke	1949	94	56	60
Pelot and Hébrard	1951	68	43	63
Dixon and Moore	1953	315	282	89.5
Lewis	1953	49	41	84
Trial, Rescanière, Hébrard, and Bertojo	1958	101	60	60
Cibert, Papillon, and Dargent	1959	47	26	55
Host and Stokke	1959	176	124	70
Patton, Hewitt, and Mallis	1959	138	103	74
Hope-Stone, Blandy, and Dayan	1961	75	50	66
Notter and Ranudd	1964	173	120	69
Ennuyer and Gricouroff	1965	67	62	77
		1536	1111	72

*From Ennuyer, A.: Radiothérapie des métastases des tumeurs germinales du testicule, Bull. Cancer (Paris) **53:** 307-328, 1966.

lived. Retroperitoneal lymph node metastases seem relatively less responsive (Whitmore[93]). Drugs also have been tried in advanced cases (Li et al.[58]), with some instances of excellent palliation. In Mackenzie's experience,[60] actinomycin D is most effective in metastatic embryonal carcinoma, teratocarcinoma, and choriocarcinoma, whereas chlorambucil shows the best effects in seminomas. Samuels and Howe[76] used vinblastine alone and in combination with melphalan for patients with metastatic testicular tumors with good palliation.

Prognosis

There has been an undeniable improvement in the results of treatment of testic-ular tumors. Improvement has been due to more accurate histopathology, the development of lymphangiography (MacKay and Sellers[59]), and better understanding and better utilization of skillful radiotherapy (Smithers and Wallace[81]). Assuming proper treatment, the best prognosis occurs in seminomas, with embryonal carcinomas, teratocarcinomas, and lymphosarcomas following in that order. Patients with choriocarcinomas have a poor outlook at best. Ennuyer[22] collected the results of several institutions in the treatment of seminomas and embryonal carcinomas (Tables 67 and 68). The overall five-year survival for patients with seminomas varied from 55% to 89.5%, with an average of

Table 69. Testicular tumors treated by orchiectomy and lymphadenectomy*†

Type of tumor	Cases	Alive 5 yr	Dead			Alive or dead without tumor	
			Total	From tumor	Other cause	Total	%
Seminoma	100	83	17	4	13	96	96.0
Embryonal carcinoma	65	43	22	18	4	47	72.3
Teratocarcinoma	66	36	30	26	4	40	60.6
Miscellaneous	12	10	2	2	0	10	83.3
Total	243	172	71	50	21	193	79.4

*From Patton, J. F., and Mallis, N.: Tumors of the testis, J. Urol. 81:457-461, 1959.
†Of 243 patients followed, all but 16 were treated by irradiation.

72%. For those with embryonal carcinomas, the results varied from 13% to 45%, with an average five-year survival of 32%. MacKay and Sellers[59] reported their overall net five-year survival to be 64.9%. The survival for patients with seminomas and embryomas combined was 71%, and that for those with teratocarcinomas was 52%. MacKay and Sellers' results[59] of orchiectomy and radiotherapy compared favorably with the contemporaneous series of Patton and Mallis,[68] which also utilized lymphadenectomy (Table 69).

The best prognosis belongs to patients with seminomas confined to the testis (Halley[37]). Spermatocytic seminoma has an excellent prognosis (Rosai et al.[75a]). The advantage of routine postoperative irradiation of potential areas of metastatic involvement, within the abdomen and pelvis, is generally accepted for patients with *seminomas*. There is no clear evidence that a retroperitoneal node dissection is of any value in this group (Vechinski et al.[91]). There is some evidence that node dissection may hinder, in some cases, the subsequent performance of radiotherapy.

In the management of *embryonal carcinomas* and *teratomas*, the evidence in favor of abdominal and pelvic irradiation is promising (Parker and Holyoke[67]; Hope-Stone et al.[45]). A greater number of authors favor a retroperitoneal node dissection in these cases, but some favor subsequent irradiation also. Staubitz et al.[83a] treated twenty-six patients with embryonal carcinoma and teratocarcinoma with orchiectomy followed by retroperitoneal lymph node resection. Eight of the patients with embryonal carcinoma had involved lymph nodes, and seven are living and well over three years.

Seminomas arising in undescended testes have a good prognosis, but survivals from any other tumor complicating cryptorchidism are rare. Distinctive adenocarcinomas (orchioblastomas) of the infant testis have a good prognosis (Teoh et al.[89]; Brown[7]). The larger the primary tumor when first seen, the poorer the prognosis. Vascular invasion and penetration of the tunica and epididymis are ominous signs (Pugh[73]). Patients excreting a high level of chorionic gonadotropins have a bad prognosis unaffected by treatment.

REFERENCES

1 Abell, M. R., Fayos, J. V., and Lampe, I.: Retroperitoneal germinomas (seminomas) without evidence of testicular involvement, Cancer 18:273-290, 1965.

2 Adams, J. E.: A study of malignant testicular tumors including case reports of chorionepithelioma accompanied by hypertension and teratoma testis with single tridermal metastases, J. Urol. 47:491-507, 1942.

2a Arlen, M., Grabstald, H., and Whitmore, W. F., Jr.: Malignant tumors of the spermatic cord, Cancer 23:525-532, 1969.

3 Azzopardi, J. G., and Hoffbrand, A. V.: Retrogression in testicular seminoma with viable metastases, J. Clin. Path. 18:135-141, 1965.

4 Azzopardi, J. G., Mostofi, F. K., and Theiss, E. A.: Lesions of testes observed in certain patients with widespread choriocarcinoma and related tumors, Amer. J. Path. 38:207-219, 1961.

5 Barringer, B. S.: Prognosis in teratoma testis, J. Urol. 52:578-585, 1944.

6 Barringer, B. S., and Earl, D.: Teratoma testis; survey of thirty-seven autopsy records, Surg. Gynec. Obstet. 72:591-600, 1941.

7 Brown, J. J.: The pathology of testicular tumors; miscellaneous tumours of mainly epithelial type, Brit. J. Urol. 36(suppl.):70-77, 1964.

8 Brown, R. C., and Smith, B. H.: Malacoplakia of the testis, Amer. J. Clin. Path. 47:135-147, 1967.

9 Busch, F. M., and Sayegh, E. S.: Roentgenographic visualization of human testicular lymphatics; a preliminary report, J. Urol. **89:** 106-110, 1963.

10 Caldwell, W. L.: Why retroperitoneal lymphadenectomy for testicular tumors? Southern Med. J. **62:**1232-1236, 1969.

11 Campbell, H. E.: Incidence of malignant growth of the undescended testicle, Arch. Surg. (Chicago) 44:353-369, 1942.

12 Chevassu, M.: Les tumeurs du testicule, Thesis, no. 193, Paris, 1906.

13 Chiappa, S., Uslenghi, C., Bonadonna, G., Marano, P., and Ravasi, G.: Combined testicular and foot lymphangiography in testicular carcinomas, Surg. Gynec. Obstet. **123:**10-14, 1966.

14 Chiappa, S., Uslenghi, C. and Galli, C.: Lymphangiography and endolymphatic radiotherapy in testicular tumours, Brit. J. Radiol. 39:498-512, 1966.

15 Collins, D. H., and Pugh, R. C. B., editors: The pathology of testicular tumours; classification and frequency of testicular tumours, Brit. J. Urol. 36(suppl.):1-11, 1964.

16 Cook, F. E., Jr., Lawrence, D. D., Smith, J. R., and Gritti, E. J.: Testicular carcinoma and lymphangiography, Radiology 84:420-427, 1965.

17 Dalgaard, J. B., and Hesselberg, F.: Interstitial cell tumours of the testis, Acta Path. Microbiol. Scand. 41:219-234, 1957.

18 Dean, A. L., Jr.: Teratoid tumors of the testis, J.A.M.A. 105:1965-1971, 1935.

19 Dixon, F. J., and Moore, R. A.: Tumors of the male sex organs. In Atlas to tumor pathology, Sect. 8, Fascs. 31B and 32, Washington, D. C., 1952, Armed Forces Institute of Pathology.

20 Dixon, F. J., and Moore, R. A.: Testicular tumors, Cancer 6:427-454, 1953.

21 Eckert, H., and Smith, J. P.: Malignant lymphoma of the testis, Brit. Med. J. 2:891-894, 1963.

22 Ennuyer, A.: Radiothérapie des métastases des tumeurs germinales du testicule, Bull. Cancer (Paris) **53:**307-328, 1966.

23 Ennuyer, A., Gricouroff, G., and Thivet, M.: Les lymphoréticulocarcomes primitifs et secondaires du testicule, Bull. Cancer (Paris) **47:** 355-372, 1960.

24 Ewing, J.: Teratoma testis and its derivatives, Surg. Gynec. Obstet. **12:**230-261, 1911.

25 Fajers, C. M.: Mesotheliomas of the genital tract; a report of five new cases and a survey of the literature, Acta Path. Microbiol. Scand. 26:1-23, 1949.

26 Fergusson, J. D.: Tumours of the testis, Brit. J. Urol. 34:407-421, 1962.

27 Flynn, P. T., and Severance, A. O.: Bilateral interstitial-cell tumors of the testis, Cancer 4: 817-822, 1951.

28 Friedman, M.: Tumors of the testis and their treatment. In Portmann, U. V.: Clinical therapeutic radiology, New York, 1950, Thomas Nelson & Sons.

29 Friedman, M., and Di Rienzo, A. J.: Treatment of trophocarcinoma (embryonal carcinoma) of the testis, Radiology 80:550-565, 1963.

30 Friedman, M., and Purkayastha, M. C.: Recurrent seminoma; the management of late metastasis, recurrence, or a second primary tumor, Amer. J. Roentgen. 83:25-42, 1960.

31 Friedman, N. B.: The comparative morphogenesis of extragenital and gonadal teratoid tumors, Cancer 4:265-276, 1951.

32 Friedman, N. B., and Moore, R. A.: Tumors of testis; report on 922 cases, Milit. Surg. **99:** 573-593, 1946.

33 Giersten, J. C.: Malignant testicular tumours following mumps, Acta Path. Microbiol. Scand. 42:7-14, 1957.

34 Gowing, N. F. C.: The pathology of testicular tumours; malignant lymphoma of the testis Brit. J. Urol. 36(suppl.):85-94, 1964.

35 Gowing, N. F. C., and Morgan, A. D.: The pathology of testicular tumours; paratesticular tumours of connective tissue and muscle, Brit. J. Urol. 36(suppl.):78-84, 1964.

36 Gray, C. P., and Biorn, C. L.: Rhabdomyosarcoma of the spermatic cord, J. Urol. **74:** 402-406, 1955.

37 Halley, J. B. W.: Pathology and survival in testicular neoplasia, Cancer 16:1269-1280, 1963.

38 Hamilton, J. B., and Gilbert, J. B.: Studies in malignant tumors of the testis, Cancer Res. 2:125-129, 1942.

39 Hamilton, J. B., and Leonard, S. L.: The effect of male hormone substance upon the testes and upon spermatogenesis, Anat. Rec. **71:**105-117, 1938.

40 Hand, J. R.: Undescended testes; report of 153 cases with evaluation of clinical findings, treatment, and results on followup up to thirty-three years, Trans. Amer. Ass. Genitourin. Surg. 47:9-50, 1955 (extensive bibliography).

41 Hinman, F.: Principles and practice of urology, Philadelphia, 1935, W. B. Saunders Co.

42 Hinman, F., and Gibson, T. E.: Tumors of the epididymis, spermatic cord and testicular tunics, Arch. Surg. (Chicago) 8:100-137, 1924.

43 Hinman, F., Gibson, T. E., and Kutzmann, A. A.: The radical operation for teratoma testis, Surg. Gynec. Obstet. 37:429-451, 1923.

44 Hobson, B. M.: The excretion of chorionic gonadotrophin by men with testicular tumours, Acta Endocr. (Kobenhavn) 49:337-348, 1965.

45 Hope-Stone, H. F., Blandy, J. P., and Dayan, A. D.: Treatment of tumours of the testis; 282 testicular tumours seen at the London Hospital during 1926-61, Brit. Med. J. 1:984-989, 1963.

46 Host, H., and Stokke, T.: The treatment of malignant testicular tumors at the Norwegian Radium Hospital, Cancer 12:323-329, 1959.

47 Huntington, R. W., Jr., Morgenstern, L. N., Sargent, J. A., Giem, R. N., Richards, A., and Hanford, K. C.: Germinal tumors exhibiting the endodermal sinus pattern of Teilum in young children, Cancer 16:34-47, 1963.

48 Jungck, E. C., Thrash, A. M., Ohlmacher, A. P., Knight, A. M., Jr., and Dyrenforth, L. Y.: Sexual precocity due to interstitial-cell

tumor of the testis: report of two cases, J. Clin. Endocr. **17**:291-295, 1957.

49 Kaplan, G., Cohen, B. B., and Roswit, B.: Malignant testicular tumors; clinical and therapeutic evaluation of 158 cases, Amer. J. Roentgen. **66**:405-419, 1951.

50 Koehler, P. R., Fabrikant, J. I., and Dickson, R. J.: Observations on the behavior of testicular tumors with comments on racial incidence, J. Urol. **87**:577-579, 1962.

51 Laipply, T. C., and Shipley, R. A.: Extragenital choriocarcinoma in the male, Amer. J. Path. **21**:921-933, 1945.

52 Laqueur, G. L.: Testicular tumors and gonadotropic hormones, Stanford Med. Bull. **4**:67-77, 1946.

53 Leadbetter, W. F.: Treatment of testis tumors based on their pathological behavior, J.A.M.A. **151**:275-280, 1953.

54 Leadbetter, W. F.: Diagnosis and treatment tumors of the testis, Amer. J. Surg. **95**:341-352, 1958.

55 Levin, H. S., and Mostofi, F. K.: Symptomatic plasmacytoma of the testis, Cancer **25**:1193-1203, 1970.

56 Lewis, L. G.: Testis tumors; report of 250 cases, J. Urol. **59**:763-772, 1948.

57 Lewis, L. G.: Radioresistant testis tumors: results of 133 cases, five-year follow-up, J. Urol. **69**:841-844, 1953.

58 Li, M. C., Whitmore, W. F., Jr., Golbey, R., and Grabstald, H.: Effects of combined drug therapy on metastatic cancer of the testis, J.A.M.A. **174**:1291-1299, 1960.

59 MacKay, E. N., and Sellers, A. H.: A statistical review of malignant testicular tumors based on the experience of the Ontario Cancer Foundation, Canad. Med. Ass. J. **94**:889-899, 1966.

60 Mackenzie, R. A.: Chemotherapy of metastatic testis cancer, Cancer **19**:1369-1376, 1966.

61 Mallis, N., and Patton, J. F.: Transperitoneal bilateral lymphadenectomy in testis tumor, J. Urol. **80**:501-503, 1958.

62 Mark, G. J., and Hedinger, C.: Changes in remaining tumor-free testicular tissue in cases of seminoma and teratoma, Virchow Arch. Path. Anat. **340**:84-92, 1965.

63 Markovits, P., Gasquet, C., Grellet, J., Grosdemange, M., Vacant, J., and Lasserre, O.: La place de la lymphographie dans les tumeurs du testicule, Ann. Radiol. (Paris) **9**:355-366, 1966.

64 Martelli, A., Zaffagnini, V., and Platania, A.: Valeur pratique de la lymphographie associée à la cavographie dans l'étude de la diffusion lymphatique des tumeurs malignes du testicule, J. Urol. Nephrol. (Paris) **71**:127-139, 1965.

65 Milner, W. A., and Gilbert, J. B.: Painful malignant tumor of testis with and without hemorrhage, J. Urol. **64**:697-704, 1950.

66 Notter, G., and Ranudd, N. E.: Treatment of malignant testicular tumours; a report on 355 patients, Acta Radiol. [Ther.] (Stockholm) **2**:273-301, 1964.

67 Parker, R. G., and Holyoke, J. B.: Tumors of the testis, Amer. J. Roentgen. **83**:43-65, 1960.

68 Patton, J. F., and Mallis, N.: Tumors of the testis, J. Urol. **81**:457-461, 1959.

69 Peirson, E. L., Jr.: A case of bilateral tumors of the testicle with some notes on the effect of castration of the adult male, J. Urol. **28**:353-363, 1932.

70 Phelan, J. T., Woolner, L. B., and Hayles, A. B.: Testicular tumors in infants and children, Surg. Gynec. Obstet. **105**:569-596, 1957.

71 Picard, J. D.: Practical indication of lymphography in neoplasms and the outlook for the future, J. Belg. Radiol. **47**:231-242, 1964.

72 Price, E. B., Jr., and Mostofi, F. K.: Secondary carcinoma of the testis, Cancer **10**:592-595, 1957.

73 Pugh, R. C. B.: Tumours of the testis—some pathological considerations, Brit. J. Urol. **34**:393-406, 1962.

74 Rather, L. J., Gardener, W. R., and Frerichs, J. B.: Regression and maturation of primary testicular tumors with progressive growth of metastases, Stanford Med. Bull. **12**:12-25, 1954.

75 Reiners, O. R., Jr., and Horn, R. C., Jr.: Interstitial cell tumor of the testis; report of two cases, Amer. J. Clin. Path. **19**:1039-1047, 1949.

75a Rosai, J., Silber, I., and Khodadoust, K.: Spermatocytic seminoma, Cancer **24**:92-116, 1969.

76 Samuels, M. L., and Howe, C. D.: Vinblastine in the management of testicular cancer, Cancer **25**:1009-1017, 1970.

77 Satter, E. J., Heidner, F. C., II, and Wear, J. B.: Primary sarcoma of the spermatic cord and epididymis, J. Urol. **82**:148-154, 1959.

78 Schnyder, U.: Zur Frage der Seminome und Pseudoseminome des Hodens, Schweiz. Z. Allg. Path. **15**:331-353, 1952.

79 Scully, R. E., and Coffin, D. L.: Canine testicular tumors with reference to their histogenesis, comparative morphology, and endocrinology, Cancer **5**:592-605, 1952.

80 Shepherd, R. T. H.: Germ cell tumours of the testis, Clin. Radiol. **17**:280-288, 1966.

81 Smithers, D. W., and Wallace, E. N. K.: Radiotherapy in the treatment of patients with seminomas and teratomas of the testicle, Brit. J. Urol. **34**:422-435, 1962.

82 Sohval, A. R.: Testicular dysgenesis in relation to neoplasm of the testicle, J. Urol. **75**:285-291, 1956.

83 Spjut, H. J., and Thorpe, J. D.: Granulomatous orchitis, Amer. J. Clin. Path. **26**:136-145, 1956.

83a Staubitz, W. J., Magoss, I. V., Grace, J. T., and Schenk, W. G., III: Surgical management of testis tumors, J. Urol. **101**:350-355, 1969.

84 Staubitz, W. J., Magoss, I. V., Oberkircher, O. J., Lent, M. H., Mitchell, F. D., and Murphy, W. T.: Management of testicular tumors, J.A.M.A. **166**:751-758, 1958.

85 Sumner, W. A.: Malignant tumor of testis occurring 29 years after orchiopexy, J. Urol. **81**:150-152, 1959.

86 Symeonidis, A.: A process of regression and

scar formation in a testicular teratoma with widespread malignant metastases, Virchow Arch. Path. Anat. 321:623-636, 1952.

87 Tanner, C. O.: Tumors of the testicle with analysis of 100 original cases, Surg. Gynec. Obstet. 35:565-572, 1922.

88 Tefft, M., Vawter, G. F., and Mitus, A.: Radiotherapeutic management of testicular neoplasms in children, Radiology 88:457-465, 1967.

89 Teoh, T. B., Steward, J. K., and Willis, R. A.: The distinctive adenocarcinoma of the infant's testis; an account of 15 cases, J. Path. Bact. 80:147-156, 1960.

90 Tiltman, A. J.: The racial incidence of testicular tumours, S. Afr. Med. J. 43:97-98, 1969.

91 Vechinski, T. O., Jaeschke, W. H., and Ver-

mund, H.: Testicular tumors; an analysis of 112 consecutive cases, Amer. J. Roentgen. 95: 494-514, 1965.

92 Watts, R. W. E.: Testicular teratoma with extensive intracardiac metastases, Brit. Heart J. 9:175-180, 1947.

93 Whitmore, W. F., Jr.: Some experiences with retroperitoneal lymph node dissection and chemotherapy in the management of testis neoplasms, Brit. J. Urol. 34:436-447, 1962.

94 Whittle, R. J. M.: Tumours of the testicle, Brit. J. Radiol. 30:7-12, 1957.

95 Witus, W. S., Sloss, J. H., and Valk, W. L.: Inguinal node metastases from testicular tumors developing after orchiopexy, J. Urol. 81: 669-671, 1959.

Penis

Anatomy

The penis is a cylindrical organ formed by three tubes of fibrous tissue. Two of these tubes, the corpora cavernosa, are symmetrical and are next to each other on the anterior midline. The third, the corpus spongiosum, contains the urethra and runs posteriorly in a groove between the two corpora cavernosa. The corpus spongiosum ends anteriorly on a coniform expansion, the glans, at the summit of which is found the external urethral orifice. The base of the glans is marked by a prominent margin, the corona, above which is the retroglandular sulcus. Each one of the three cavernous bodies is encased in a fibrous sheath, the tunica albuginea, and the three are all enclosed in a common fascia that is surrounded by the subcutaneous tissue and the skin. Anteriorly, the skin and the subcutaneous tissue have a prolongation, the prepuce, which normally covers the glans. A small midline fold, the frenulum, passes from a point immediately behind the external urethral orifice to the deep surface of the prepuce.

The skin that covers the penis is remarkable for its thinness and elasticity. Sebaceous glands are found throughout. The dermis is entirely lacking in smooth muscle fibers and contains only connective and elastic tissue fibers. Deep in the preputial sac, the skin of the penis changes to a mucous membrane which, reflecting beyond itself, covers the glans. Numerous glands

of the sebaceous type, Tyson's glands, are found in the prepuce and in the mucosa of the penis.

Lymphatics. The lymphatics of the *prepuce* spring from a network that covers

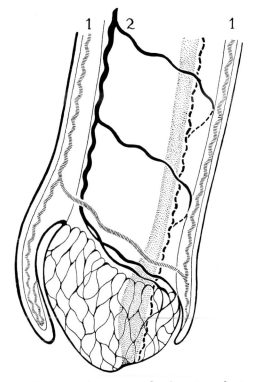

Fig. 528. Lymphatic network of penis gathering in subcutaneous trunks, **1**, and those of glans drained by subfascial trunk, **2**.

both its internal and external surfaces. They converge toward the dorsal aspect, join with the lymphatics coming from the skin of the shaft, and form several trunks that run toward the pubis, ending in the upper inner group of superficial inguinal lymphatics (Fig. 528).

The lymphatics of the *glans* form a very rich network that runs toward the frenulum. There they communicate with the lymphatics of the urethra and form several collecting trunks which follow the retroglandular sulcus, forming a collar of lymphatics that entirely surrounds the corona and finally forms one, two, or three trunks which run along the dorsal surface of the penis under the penile fascia together with the deep dorsal vein. Arriving at the suspensor ligament, these trunks form a presymphyseal plexus with multiple anasto-

moses and occasional nodules. From here, the lymphatic trunks are divided into two groups, those that follow the *femoral canal* and end in the superficial inguinal nodes, in the node of Cloquet, and in the retrofemoral nodes and those that follow the *inguinal canal* which, running under the spermatic cord, end in the external retrofemoral lymph nodes (Cunéo and Marcille[6]) (Fig. 529). It should be emphasized that the left and right inguinal lymph nodes have a rich communication with each other through the subcutaneous lymphatics.

The lymphatics of the *corpora cavernosa* end in the superficial upper and inner group of inguinal lymph nodes and sometimes also in the deep inguinal nodes and retrofemoral nodes. The lymphatics of the *urethra* and of the corpora cavernosa usually end in the deep inguinal lymph nodes.

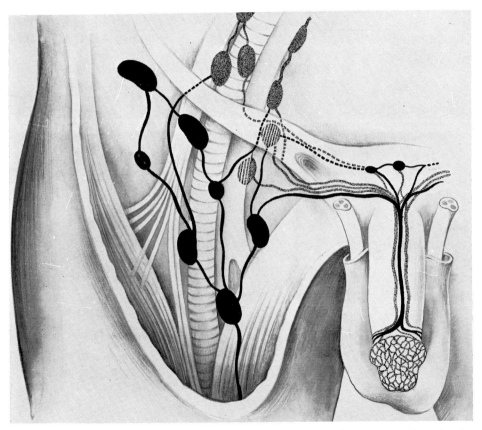

Fig. 529. Lymphatics of penis. Rich network of lymphatics gathers in several trunks that run toward symphysis, where they form presymphysial plexus. From there, lymphatic trunks divide into two groups: those following femoral canal which terminate in superficial lymph nodes (solid black) and those following inguinal canal which terminate in deep lymph nodes (shaded).

Epidemiology

In the United States, the reported incidence of carcinoma of the penis is 1.3 per 100,000 white males and 2.9 for nonwhites. A substantial proportion of cases diagnosed in the United States are found in foreign-born patients (Lenowitz and Graham[22]). In Puerto Rico, the incidence for the total male population varied from 3.9 to 4.9 from 1956 to 1960. In the same years, the age-adjusted incidence varied from 8.5 to 13.4 per 100,000 (Marcial et al.[25]). A high incidence of cancer of the penis is observed in Asia (Ngai[29]), particularly among the Chinese and Javanese (Kouwenaar[20]) but also among the Vietnamese (Nguyen Xuan Chu and Pham Bieu Tam[30]). In Uganda, carcinoma of the penis is the commonest cancer in the male population, accounting for more that 7% of all cases of cancer (Dodge and Linsell[10]). In the United States, six of ten patients with carcinoma of the penis are 60 years of age or over. Early occurrences are reported from Asia (Nguyen Xuan Chu and Pham Bieu Tam[30]), Paraguay (Riveros and Lebrón[34]), Uganda (Dodge[9]), and Puerto Rico (Marcial et al.[25]).

Cancer of the penis only rarely occurs in a circumcised Jew. There have been only five such cases reported (Melmed and Pyne[26]). This observation has led to considerable study and speculation in respect to the prophylactic role of circumcision (Wolbarst[43]; Kennaway[17]). Cancer of the penis occurs in other peoples, such as Moslems, who also practice ritual circumcision. Khanolkar[18] reported eighty-six cases of carcinoma of the penis in Hindus and only two cases in Moslems admitted to the Tata Memorial Hospital of Bombay, although Moslems and Hindus were in the proportion of 1:3 in the admissions. The occurrence of carcinoma of the penis in circumcised individuals other than Jews has been attributed to the fact that circumcision is done ritually by the Moslems between 3 and 14 years of age and for medical reasons in adults of other persuasions. Great emphasis is placed on the early circumcision as practiced by the Jews. Shabad[37] showed that late circumcision diminishes but does not prevent the occurrence of penile cancer. In Kenya, the occurrence of carcinoma of the penis is relatively low. Circumcision is practiced by all but two tribes, in which the majority of carcinomas of the penis are seen (Dodge and Linsell[10]). Admittedly, circumcision may favor better penile hygiene and decreases the smegna bacillus, phimosis, and other possible inflammatory complications which *could* predispose to carcinoma. But admittedly, too, circumcision does not, per se, assure penile hygiene. In all countries, this form of cancer is found in men of the lowest economic level with sordid living conditions and habits. In the eyes of many workers, early circumcision plays an important role in the prevention of this form of cancer. But it is possible that a certain racial immunity, similar to that observed in Jewish women for carcinoma of the cervix, may explain the low incidence in the Jew.

Syphilis and other venereal diseases have been incriminated as possible causative factors. Staubitz et al.[40] reported on 204 patients, forty of whom had a history of veneral disease or a positive Wassermann test. Erythroplasia of Queyrat,[32] a rare disease of the glans, has been thought to be a precancerous lesion. The changes in this lesion are those of carcinoma in situ that may become invasive carcinoma (Savatard[35]).

Pathology

Gross and microscopic pathology

Carcinoma of the penis may arise on the glans, retroglandular sulcus, and prepuce and, rarely, from the skin of the shaft. It is most common on the glans.

The gross appearance of the lesion may be either proliferative or ulcerative. The *proliferative type* first appears as a small wart, followed by the appearance of other nodules that coalesce to form numerous papillary projections. Sometimes, this tumor reaches a huge size, completely replacing the entire penis (Fig. 530). These exophytic tumors rarely invade the corpora cavernosa or the urethra but are usually accompanied by considerable secondary infection.

The infiltrative or *ulcerative type* is more common than the proliferative type and grows inwardly, destroying the glans and the prepuce (Figs. 531 and 532). Not infrequently, it invades the corpora cavernosa and the urethra, and contact lesions in the form of satellite nodules may grow on the prepuce and the glans at the same time.

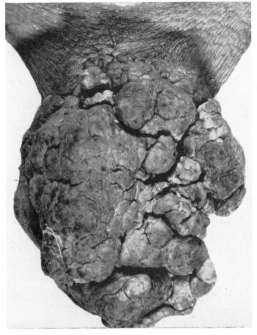

Fig. 530. Advanced, extensive, well-differentiated verrucous carcinoma of penis. There were no metastases.

The microscopic appearance is that of a squamous carcinoma which, in the proliferative type, often is very well differentiated (Fig. 533). The ulcerative infiltrative type tends to be more undifferentiated. In the microscopic examination of surgical specimens, particular attention should be paid to gross evidence of involvement of the urethra and the corpora cavernosa and to microscopic evidence of perineural extension. Sections should be taken at the limits of the excision in order to determine if the excision has been adequate. Carcinoma in situ has a reddish blue, slightly elevated, granular appearance, and often the clinical diagnosis is that of some inflammatory process. Microscopically, the changes are those of carcinoma in situ.

Metastatic spread

Inguinal metastases are rarely found in the proliferative type of lesion. The ulcerative type metastasizes more readily. Ekstrom and Edsmyr[11] found no correlations between the size and duration of the primary lesion and the presence of metastases, but carcinomas arising from the glans metastasize more frequently than preputial lesions, younger patients present metastases more frequently than elderly ones, and the proportion of metastases was found to be greater in patients with undifferentiated carcinomas. The vertebral vein plexus may

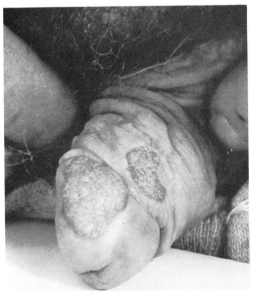

Fig. 531. Superficial carcinoma of glans with contact lesion of prepuce. (Courtesy Dr. R. E. Fricke, Rochester, Minn.)

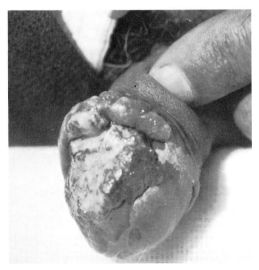

Fig. 532. Deeply ulcerating lesion of corona invading prepuce. (Courtesy Dr. R. E. Fricke, Rochester, Minn.)

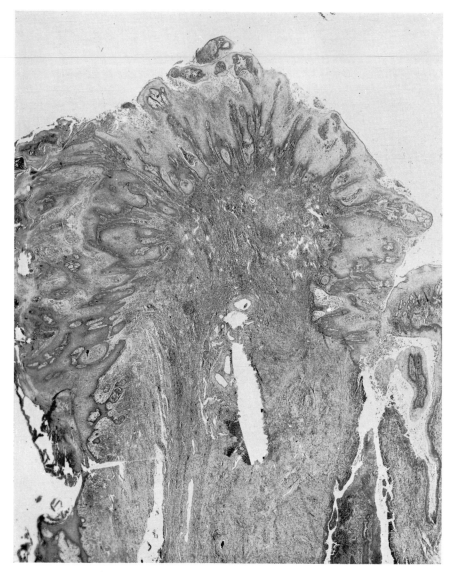

Fig. 533. Large, well-differentiated, proliferating epidermoid carcinoma (verrucous type) of penis. (Low power.)

rarely serve as a means of metastases. Distant metastases to abdominal nodes, liver, and lungs can occur.

Clinical evolution

Very often, the first symptom of carcinoma of the penis is a small nodule, warty growth, vesicle, or superficial ulceration, often painless, growing under an unretracted prepuce and consequently overlooked until it reaches considerable size. Rarely, the first symptom is a metastatic inguinal lymph node. As the lesion progresses, there is usually spontaneous bleeding, and secondary infection usually adds an offending odor. In as many as half of all cases, the carcinoma is found in patients with phimosis (Ekstrom and Edsmyr[11]).

When there is coexisting phimosis, edema of the glans and of the prepuce may rapidly increase. Rarely is there any dysuria. It is only after metastases have developed that any constitutional symptoms are evident. About 30% of the patients present inguinal metastases at the time of the first clinical observation (Tailhefer and

Courtial[41]). In late cases, the metastases to inguinal nodes will become fixed and infected and can even ulcerate through the skin. Infrequently, the large underlying vessels may be eroded, and profound hemorrhages can occur. At times, widespread metastases will contribute to the cause of death. Terminal infections such as bronchopneumonia are common in this group because of age and general debility.

Diagnosis

For a thorough examination of the glans, a surgical division of the prepuce may be warranted. This may facilitate the examination and biopsy of an early carcinoma hidden within the preputial sac (Buddington et al.[5]). The diagnosis of a typical proliferative or ulcerative growth presents no difficulties. There should be no hesitation in removing a specimen from the borders of the lesion for a pathologic diagnosis. It is often difficult to ascertain whether or not the inguinal nodes are involved, for they are frequently enlarged by inflammation, but when the nodes are more than 3 cm in diameter, they are usually metastatic. A needle biopsy may be indicated, but it is only of value when positive.

Murrell and Williams[28] staged their cases of cancer of the penis as follows:

Stage I

Tumor localized to the penis and without demonstrable lymph node metastases

Stage II

Tumor localized to the penis and with clinically positive operable lymph node metestases

Stage III

Tumor localized to the penis and with inoperable lymph node metastases

Stage IV

Direct spread of tumor from the penis to the perineum or distant metastases

Prospectively, this clinical classification has the disadvantage that a large proportion of the adenopathies observed are found to be due to inflammation (Frew et al.[13]). Thus, the classification is often used retrospectively.

Differential diagnosis

Benign *papillomas* may resemble an early carcinoma of the glans, but although they have a tendency to grow together, they may present relatively wide normal spaces between them. *Condyloma acuminatum* may also be confused with carcinoma, but it has a characteristic appearance and a long clinical history and, microscopically, does not show any tendency to infiltrate.

There is no difficulty in differential diagnosis with a *syphilitic chancre*, but it should not be forgotten that a carcinoma may coincide with a primary syphilitic lesion and that in a suspicious lesion the demonstration of spirochetes does not preclude the taking of a biopsy. *Soft chancres* are usually tender and are accompanied by voluminous, painful inguinal adenopathy. Infected *sebaceous cysts* of the prepuce may occur and should be considered in the differential diagnosis.

Peyronie's disease, a plastic induration of the penis, can be confused with carcinoma because of its firmness. This condition is accompanied by pain and distortion with erection and consequent interference with sexual intercourse. The condition may be found in patients with a tendency to keloid formations, Dupuytren's contracture of the palmar fasciae, diabetes, etc. Ossification of the plastic induration may take place (Smith[38]). Surgery has been advocated in the treatment of Peyronie's disease (Schourup[36]), but a trial of conservative treatment by means of radiotherapy is indicated first. Radiotherapy is often successful, but the results may not be noticed for several months.

Erythroplasia of the glans is characterized by its well-circumscribed, velvety, deep red appearance. Histologically, erythroplasia presents hyperplasia of the epithelium, thickening of the rete, and single or multiple ulcers that are surrounded by scaly dermatitis.

Primary carcinoma of the urethra is rare and seldom presents anteriorly. Mandler and Pool[24] reviewed thirty-seven cases. Kaplan et al.[16] collected 232 cases from the medical literature.

Metastatic carcinoma can involve the penis. Over seventy cases have been reported (McCrea and Tobias[23]), with the prostate, bladder, and rectum being the most common sites of primary lesions. A retrograde venous or lymphatic transport is believed to be the common route (Paquin and Roland[31]). *Malignant melanoma* of the penis has been rarely observed (Reid[33]). Ashley and Edwards[1] were able to collect fifty-four cases of various types of *sarcoma* of the penis. Dehner and Smith[7a] studied forty-six cases of soft tissue tumors of the penis. Most benign tumors were located on the glans, and the penile shaft was the common site for malignant types.

Treatment

Routine circumcision is advocated as a prophylactic measure to prevent carcinoma of the penis (Kennaway[17]). There are two main considerations in the treatment of carcinoma of the penis: treatment of the primary lesion, which in general offers no difficulty, and treatment of the inguinal metastases, which often requires judgment (Desaive and Ramioul[8]).

Primary lesion
Surgery

A partial or total penectomy is successful in the treatment of penile carcinomas. The operation is naturally shunned by the younger patients and lesser surgical procedures lead to failure. An adequate surgical excision requires a good margin of safety of no less than 1.5 cm. Surgical treatment of the penile lesion expedites the care of adenopathies (Bassett[3]). It is particularly well indicated in older patients and in those with large and infiltrating lesions that have already destroyed a great deal of the glans and corpora cavernosa (Murrell and Williams[28]). It is also the only way to deal with postirradiation recurrences (Lederman[21]; Jackson[15]).

Radiotherapy

Early approaches in the radiotherapy of carcinoma of the penis such as interstitial implantation and surface applications of radium, have been abandoned. Intensive irradiation results in considerable untoward effects and undesirable sequelae. Fractionated irradiation yields much better results, and this is best managed with roentgentherapy. The aim should be to destroy the tumor with a minimum of radiation effects. Total destruction of the tumor is possible, with a minimum loss of substance, provided a sufficient amount of radiations is administered to the entire area of involvement. With radiotherapy, the margin of safety can be extended farther than with surgery. Roentgentherapy results in a mucocutaneous reaction that requires careful attention to avoid secondary infection and necrosis. Epithelization of the denuded area may take considerable time, during which local dressings and antibiotics may be necessary to preserve the integrity of the remaining tissues. In many instances, close observation may indicate the need of surgical treatment for residual tumor (Knudsen and Brennhovd[19]; Jackson[15]).

Metastatic adenopathy

A *therapeutic inguinal dissection* is, of course, indicated in all patients in whom there is certainty of an inguinal metastasis. In general, all enlarged nodes more than 3 cm in diameter may be assumed to be metastatic. Clinical appraisal of the presence or absence of lymph node involvement is extremely difficult, and the only positive proof of metastases is a pathologic diagnosis. The dissection should be bilateral because of the subcutaneous lymphatic communications. Obviously, an inguinal dissection will not be indicated in patients with distant metastases nor in those in whom the lymph nodes have become definitely fixed.

A radical surgical excision of the penis, dorsal lymphatics, and inguinal and femoral lymph nodes as devised by Young[44] was practiced by the Brady Urological Institute for many years (Hudson et al.[14]). It is doubtful whether the continuity excision of the dorsal lymphatics is indicated. Bassett[3] pointed out that after amputation for a carcinoma of the penis, local recurrence along the pathway of these dorsal lymphatics practically never occurs. It is recommended, however, that if a lymph node dissection is done, the iliac lymph nodes be included.

A *prophylactic inguinal dissection* is seldom indicated in our opinion. In eighty-eight cases which Beggs and Spratt[4] considered free from metastases, they proved to be wrong in ten. Only two of these patients were considered to have died because of their inguinal metastases. In the absence of palpable adenopathy, a close follow-up is satisfactory, since it eliminates operative mortality and morbidity that would affect a number of patients without metastases.

Roentgentherapy of metastatic inguinal lymph nodes is justified only as a palliative measure when surgery is not indicated. External irradiation of these areas with a curative purpose requires administration of large amounts of radiations.

Prognosis

The prognosis of patients with carcinoma of the penis is very favorable when metastatic lymph nodes are not present. Ekstrom and Edsmyr[11] reported on 112 patients with carcinomas of the penis without inguinal metastases, 101 (90%) of whom were well after five years. Late recurrences are infrequent. Of twenty-six recurrences reported by Barney,[2] only four appeared after the fifth year. After surgical excision of the primary lesion, the more undifferentiated tumors and those that involve the corpora cavernosa and the urethra or show perineural space involvement have a worse prognosis because of their tendency for deep lymph node metastases. The prognosis for these patients is directly related to the existence of involved regional lymph nodes and to the therapeutic procedure employed and the time of its institution. In a total of sixty-five patients with metastases treated at the Radiumhemmet of Stockholm, twenty-one (32%) remained well five years (Ekstrom and Edsmyr[11]). Of forty-nine patients with carcinoma of the penis treated at the Fondation Curie, fifteen had inguinal metastases. The local lesions were treated with radium, and the metastases were surgically excised. The overall result was 23% five-year survival (Tailhefer and Courtial[41]). Of fifty-seven patients treated at the Norwegian Radium Hospital primarily by radiotherapy, and with conservative use of surgery, thirty-eight (67%) appeared well after five years (Engelstad[12]). Staubitz et al.[40] reported on twenty-seven patients with proved inguinal metastases treated at the Roswell Park Memorial Institute. Eleven were irradiated, with five cured. Sixteen had an inguinal

dissection, with eight cured. Patients with local recurrences have a poor prognosis but are far from hopeless (Engelstad[12]). Marcial et al.[25] reported six of eleven patients surviving five years after radiotherapy for postoperative recurrence. In advanced cases, radiotherapy may be followed by unavoidable loss of substance. In general, adequate irradiation results in minimal defect or dysfunction: in a case on record, the prurient beneficiary enjoyed his restoration until caught and killed by his wife in a flagrant act of adultery (Wildermuth[42]). In Lederman's series[21] of forty-four patients treated by radiations, amputation became necessary in seventeen. Twenty-four of his patients remained well five years, thirteen of whom had had radiotherapy only. Murrell and Williams[28] treated 108 patients with carcinoma of the penis with radiotherapy, with a five-year crude survival rate of 40%.

REFERENCES

1 Ashley, D. J. B., and Edwards, E. C.: Sarcoma of the penis, Brit. J. Surg. **45**:170-179, 1957.

2 Barney, J. D.: Epithelioma of the penis, Ann. Surg. **46**:890-914, 1907.

3 Bassett, J. W.: Carcinoma of the penis, Cancer **5**:530-538, 1952.

4 Beggs, J. H., and Spratt, J. S.: Epidermoid carcinoma of the penis, J. Urol. **91**:166-172, 1964.

5 Buddington, W. T., Kickham, C. J. E., and Smith, W. E.: An assessment of malignant disease of the penis, J. Urol. **89**:442-449, 1963.

6 Cunéo and Marcille, M.: Note sur les lymphatiques du gland, Bull. Soc. Anat. Paris **76**:671-674, 1901.

7 Dargent, M.: Positions respectives de la chirurgie et de la radiothérapie dans le traitement du cancer de la verge, J. Urol. (Paris) **53**:234-244, 1946-1947.

7a Dehner, L. P., and Smith, B. H.: Soft tissue tumors of the penis; a clinicopathologic study of 46 cases, Cancer **25**:1431-1447, 1970.

8 Desaive, P., and Ramioul, H.: Le cancer du pénis et son traitement actuel, Acta Chir. Belg. **49**:253-315, 1950.

9 Dodge, O. G.: Carcinoma of the penis in East Africans, Brit. J. Urol. **37**:223-226, 1965.

10 Dodge, O. G., and Linsell, C. A.: Carcinoma of the penis in Uganda and Kenya Africans, Cancer **16**:1255-1263, 1963.

11 Ekstrom, T., and Edsmyr, F.: Cancer of the penis; a clinical study of 229 cases, Acta Chir. Scand. **115**:25-45, 1958.

12 Engelstad, R. B.: Treatment of cancer of the penis at the Norwegian Radium Hospital, Amer. J. Roentgen. **60**:801-806, 1948.

13 Frew, I. D. O., Jefferies, J. D., and Swinney,

J.: Carcinoma of the penis, Brit. J. Urol. 39: 398-404, 1967.

14 Hudson, P. B., Hopkins, J. A., and Fish, G. W.: Carcinoma of the penis, Amer. J. Surg. 85:519-522, 1953.

15 Jackson, S. M.: The treatment of carcinoma of the penis, Brit. J. Surg. 53:33-35, 1966.

16 Kaplan, G. W., Bulkley, G. J., and Grayhack, J. T.: Carcinoma of the male urethra, J. Urol. 98:365-371, 1967.

17 Kennaway, E. L.: Cancer of the penis and circumcision in relation to the incubation period of cancer, Brit. J. Cancer 1:335-344, 1947.

18 Khanolkar, V. R.: Cancer in India in relation to race, nutrition and customs; symposium on geographic pathology and demography of cancer; published under the auspices of the World Health Organization, 1950.

19 Knudsen, O. S., and Brennhovd, I. O.: Radiotherapy in the treatment of the primary tumor in penile cancer, Acta Chir. Scand. 133:69-71, 1967.

20 Kouwenaar, W.: On cancer incidence in Indonesia; symposium on geographical pathology and demography of cancer; published under the auspices of the World Health Organization, 1950.

21 Lederman, M.: Radiotherapy of cancer of the penis, Brit. J. Urol. 25:224-232, 1953.

22 Lenowitz, H., and Graham, A. P.: Carcinoma of the penis, J. Urol. 56:458-484, 1946.

23 McCrea, L. E., and Tobias, G. L.: Metastatic disease of the penis, J. Urol. 80:489-500, 1958.

24 Mandler, J. I., and Pool, T.: Primary carcinoma of the male urethra, J. Urol. 96:67-72, 1966.

25 Marcial, V. A., Figureoa-Colón, J., Marcial-Rojas, R., and Colón, J. E.: Carcinoma of the penis, Radiology 79:209-220, 1962.

26 Melmed, E. P., and Pyne, J. R.: Carcinoma of the penis in a Jew circumcised in infancy, Brit. J. Surg. 54:729-731, 1967.

27 Mostofi, K.: Infantile testicular tumors, Bull. N. Y. Acad. Med. 28:684-687, 1952.

28 Murrell, D. S., and Williams, J. L.: Radiotherapy in the treatment of carcinoma of the penis, Brit. J. Urol. 37:211-222, 1965.

29 Ngai, S. K.: The etiological and pathological aspects of squamous-cell carcinoma of the penis among the Chinese, Amer. J. Cancer 19:259-284, 1933.

30 Nguyen Xuan Chu and Pham Bieu Tam: Le cancer de la verge chez le Vietnamiens, Presse Med. 62:125-126, 1954.

31 Paquin, A. J., Jr., and Roland, S. I.: Secondary carcinoma of the penis; a review of the literature and a report of nine new cases, Cancer 9:84-90, 1956.

32 Queyrat, M.: Erythroplasie du gland, Bull. Soc. Franc. Derm. Syph. 22:378-382, 1911.

33 Reid, J. D.: Melanocarcinoma of the penis, Cancer 10:359-362, 1957.

34 Riveros, M., and Lebrón, R. F.: Geographical pathology of cancer of the penis, Cancer 16:798-811, 1963.

35 Savatard, L.: Psoriasiform carcinoma of the penis, Brit. J. Derm. 52:87-93, 1940.

36 Schourup, K.: Plastic induration of the penis, Acta Radiol. (Stockholm) 26:313-323, 1945.

37 Shabad, A. L.: Some aspects of etiology and prevention of penile cancer, J. Urol. 92:696-702, 1964.

38 Smith, B. H.: Peyronie's disease, Amer. J. Clin. Path. 45:670-678, 1966.

39 Soiland, A.: Peyronie's disease or plastic induration of the penis, Radiology 42:183-185, 1944.

40 Staubitz, W. J., Melbourne, H. L., and Oberkircher, O. J.: Carcinoma of the penis, Cancer 8:371-378, 1955.

41 Tailhefer, A., and Courtial, J.: Le traitement des cancers primitifs de la peau et des orifices cutaneo-muqueux à la Fondation Curie, Bull. Ass. Franc. Cancer 31:85-115, 1943.

42 Wildermuth, O.: Personal communication, 1970.

43 Wolbarst, A. L.: Circumcision and penile cancer, Lancet 1:150-153, 1932.

44 Young, H. H.: A radical operation for the cure of cancer of the penis, J. Urol. 26:285-294, 1931.

Chapter 13

Tumors of the suprarenal gland

Anatomy

The suprarenal glands, crescentic in shape, rest on the upper pole and medial border of the kidneys. The right suprarenal gland lies against the diaphragm posteriorly, its anterior surface is molded by the liver and the inferior vena cava, and it reaches the duodenum inferiorly. The left suprarenal gland is separated from the stomach by the omental bursa, and inferiorly it is crossed by the splenic artery and the upper border of the pancreas. The right suprarenal vein drains into the inferior vena cava. The left suprarenal vein descends to the left renal vein. Their arterial blood supply is abundant, with branches from the inferior phrenic artery and the aorta. The very numerous nerve fibers that innervate the suprarenal glands arise from the greater splanchnic and postganglionic vagal fibers from the celiac plexus.

Accessory suprarenal cortex is frequently found in the kidneys and in the perirenal and retroperitoneal fascia. It may also be found in the broad ligament of the uterus, attached to the pedicle of the ovary, or associated with testicular tissue.

The suprarenal gland is divided into two portions, the cortex and the medulla, each of which has separate embryologic origins and is actually almost like two distinct organs. The cortex develops from the celomic mesoderm and the brownish medullary central portion arises from the ectoderm, which gives rise to the sympathetic nervous system.

Lymphatics. The lymphatics of the suprarenal gland arise from the cortex and the medulla and collect into several trunks that follow the direction of the vessels. The collecting trunks that accompany the superior suprarenal artery end in lymph nodes situated near the origin of the celiac artery and the inferior vena cava. The collecting trunks that accompany the middle suprarenal artery end in the lateroaortic nodes placed above the renal pedicle. Those that accompany the suprarenal vein are divided into anterior and posterior trunks, ending also in lateroaortic nodes (Fig. 534). In addition to these main trunks, some of the lymphatics of the suprarenal glands may pass through the diaphragm, following the splanchnic nerves, and terminate in a retroaortic node in the posterior mediastinum. Some of the lymphatics of the right suprarenal gland may penetrate into the liver (Rouvière[113]).

Epidemiology

Tumors of the suprarenal gland are not observed frequently, for they make up only a relatively small percentage of all tumors. Cortical *adenomas* are commonly found at autopsy. Functional tumors, benign or malignant, are rare. Rapaport et al.[109] collected all published cases from 1930 to 1949, and Heinbecker et al.[63] collected those from 1950 to 1955, a total of 285 cases. Approximately 80% were found in female patients. Three-fourths of the patients with Cushing's syndrome were over 12 years old, and one-half of all cases of virilization syndrome appeared before the age of 12 years.

Benign tumors of the medulla are pathologic rarities. McFarland[85] found only ninety-three reported cases of *ganglioneuroma* of the suprarenal gland or accessory suprarenal tissue in a review of the literature from 1905 to 1931. They are observed in children and young adults.

Neuroblastomas are the most common malignant tumors of the suprarenal gland. Farber[37] found forty neuroblastomas among 300 malignant tumors in children. Many are present at birth, and about one-third

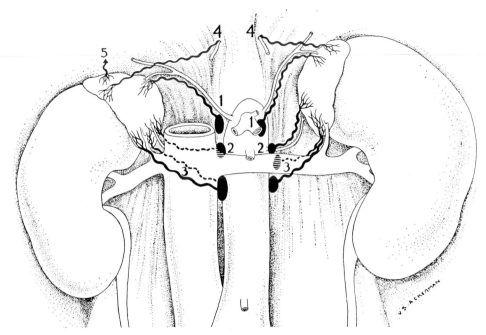

Fig. 534. Lymphatics of suprarenal glands illustrating their termination in lateroaortic nodes. Trunks accompanying superior suprarenal artery, **1**; collecting trunks accompanying middle suprarenal artery, **2**; collecting anterior and posterior trunks accompanying suprarenal vein, **3**; lymphatics perforating diaphragm and ending in posterior mediastinal nodes, **4**; lymphatics leading directly to liver, **5**.

are diagnosed during the first year and four-fifths within the first five years of life (Wittenborg[136]). In an epidemiologic approach, Miller et al.[92] found an increased frequency of congenital defects beyond normal expectation in patients with neuroblastoma, although there is little to suggest a genetic influence. They concluded that one cannot reject the possibility that some neuroblastomas may result from dominant lethal mutations.

Pheochromocytomas have been observed in patients in every decade of life. A review of over 200 cases with associated hypertension showed that 75% of the patients were between 20 and 49 years of age and more than 10% under 20 years of age (Graham[52]). Farquhar[38] was able to find fifty-seven cases of pheochromocytomas in children. Familial cases have been reported (Greenberg and Gardner[53]). These are often bilateral (Kelsall and Ross[68]). The question has been raised as to the possibility that pheochromocytomas are a definitely inherited abnormality (Carman and Brashear[20]; Smits and Huizinga[123]).

Pathology
Gross and microscopic pathology

Tumors that develop from the adrenal cortex have an epithelial character, whereas those that develop from the medulla are nervous system tumors. In order to facilitate their discussion, the following classification is adopted:

1 Tumors arising from cortex
  A Adenoma
    (1) Functioning
    (2) Nonfunctioning
  B Adenocarcinoma
2 Tumors arising from medulla
  A Ganglioneuroma
  B Pheochromocytoma
  C Neuroblastoma
  D Mixed type (ganglioneuroblastoma)

Tumors arising from cortex. Heterotopic cortical tumors also can occur in many locations, including the region of the adrenal glands, in the kidney substance, and along the course of the spermatic and ovarian veins (Nelson[95]). Although the origin of the cortical tissue is mesoblastic, the cells of the cortex acquire an epithelial character. The adrenal cortex is divided

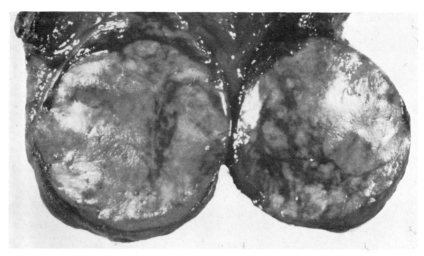

Fig. 535. Typical encapsulated homogeneous cortical adenoma of suprarenal gland.

into three zones. It is clear now that the zona glomerulosa is the site of aldosterone production. The zona fasciculata and zona reticularis are a functional unit. With ACTH stimulation, both of these zones produce increased amounts of cortical sterone, cortisone, and cortisol. There is increased enzymatic activity in the cells of the fascicular-reticular border. Most of the tumors originating in the cortex are benign.

The cortical *adenoma* is often bilateral and frequently found at postmortem examination. As a rule, the adenomas are small, measuring from a few millimeters to several centimeters in diameter. They are well delimited and somewhat spherical in shape, showing a rather deep brown, homogeneous appearance (Fig. 535). On microscopic examination, the capsule of the tumor is found to be formed of usually well-vascularized connective tissue, and the individual cells resemble those of the normal cortex.

Aldosterone-secreting tumors are invariably benign and are small, averaging 1.5 cm in diameter (Neville and Symington[96]). In a functioning tumor of this type, the uninvolved zona glomerulosa atrophies due to suppression of the renin-angiotensin-aldosterone system because of the high level of secretion of aldosterone by the tumor (Fig. 536). If renal biopsy shows hypertrophy and prominent granulation of the cells of the juxtaglomerular apparatus, this indicates secondary aldosteronism. If there is decreased granulation of the juxtaglomerular cells, this indicates decreased renin secretion and points to primary aldosteronism (Cohen et al.[21]). Hyalinized basophils (Crooke's cells) in the adenohypophysis are pathognomonic of hyperadrenocorticism (Heinbecker et al.[63]).

Adenocarcinomas that arise from the cortex may also appear to be encapsulated but are usually larger than the benign tumors (4 cm to 15 cm in diameter and often over 500 gm in weight). These tumors usually show zones of hemorrhage and necrosis. They seem to occur more frequently on the left than on the right. The tumor may break through the capsule and invade the surrounding tissues. On the right, tumor usually spreads directly to the liver but seldom invades the major veins. On microscopic examination, the tumor is often undifferentiated, and individual cells show striking variation in size and shape. There are numerous mitotic figures. The benign cortical tumor may have extremely atypical and giant nuclei, but such changes are not evidence that the tumor is malignant (Fig. 537). The size, necrosis, mitotic figures, and true vein invasion represent reliable evidence that the tumor is a carcinoma.

Areas may be found in which various layers of the cortex can be recognized. The adenocarcinoma may be difficult to differentiate microscopically from a malignant pheochromocytoma (rare). However, the presence of fat vacuoles within

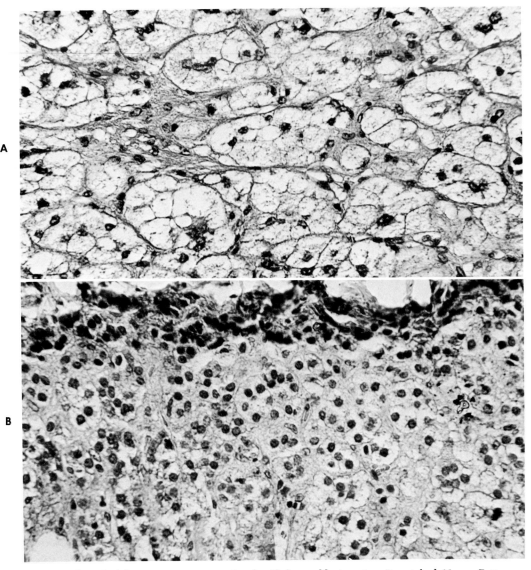

Fig. 536. **A,** Adenoma or tumor associated with hyperaldosteronism. It weighed 11 gm. Pattern of cells suggests zona fasciculata. **B,** Adrenal gland associated with this tumor. There is some atrophy of zona glomerulosa, and zona fasciculata has disturbed pattern. (**A,** ×300; WU neg. 68-11135; **B,** ×350; WU neg. 68-11136.)

cells and the absence of brown pigment after fixation in chromate solutions or other oxidizing agents are signs in favor of cortical origin, whereas, conversely, the absence of fat and the presence of pigment after chromate fixation are signs of a medullary origin (LeCompte[78]). In a study of the adrenal cortex in eighty-one patients with Cushing's syndrome, Neville and Symington[97] found bilateral adrenocortical hyperplasia in sixty-nine patients and neoplasms, seven of which were carcinoma,

in twelve patients. The contralateral adrenal glands showed cortical atrophy in the patients with neoplasms.

Tumors arising from medulla. Tumors that arise from the medulla are of nerve origin. The *ganglioneuroma* arises from, and is almost entirely made up of, mature ganglion cells. This tumor is usually found only by chance in the region of the suprarenal gland. The *pheochromocytoma* arises from the chromaffin cells or pheochromocytes and is composed of medul-

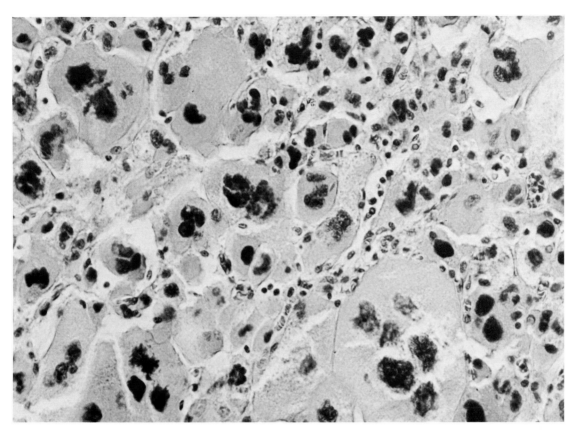

Fig. 537. Adrenal cortical tumor of large size but without necrosis or vein invasion. Nuclei are extremely atypical, but there are no mitotic figures. This should be classified as adenoma. (×350; slide contributed by Dr. R. E. Lovett, Springfield, Mo.; WU neg. 68-11133.)

lary tissue. It tends to be encapsulated and may reach a diameter of 12 cm. The tumor is usually of brownish color, showing cystic changes, hemorrhage, and necrosis. It shows rather large cells that have an affinity for chrome salts. It seldom shows evidence of fat by special stains.

Pheochromocytomas can vary tremendously in size, but their average weight is approximately 100 gm. Their microscopic pattern and their frequent invasion of the capsule are not evidence of malignant change. In the 107 cases reviewed by Sherwin,[119] there were only three malignant tumors, and they had a predominantly spindle cell pattern. In his group, a positive Henle chromoreaction was the most valuable aid in establishing the microscopic diagnosis. Pheochromocytomas, of course, may be multiple, and errors have been made in thinking that a second independent tumor was a metastasis. They are

bilateral in about 20% of the patients (Cahill[16]). About 20% of pheochromocytomas are found in unusual locations, and two or more tumors are present in about 30% of the patients. Fries and Chamberlin[41] collected 205 extra-adrenal pheochromocytomas (Table 70). Neurofibromatosis is sometimes associated with pheochromocytomas (Kirshbaum and Balkin[71]). Bilateral pheochromocytoma, medullary carcinoma of the thyroid gland, and parathyroid adenoma may be familial (Sarosi and Doe[115]).

The most important group of tumors arising from the suprarenal medulla are the *neuroblastomas* that derive from the primitive neuroblasts. These malignant tumors are usually small but may reach a size of 10 cm in diameter. As a rule, they are encapsulated and soft, invariably showing zones of hemorrhage and necrosis (Fig. 538, *A*). They are sharply delimited, but

Table 70. Distribution of extra-adrenal tumors*

Site	Tumors
Neck	5
Intrathoracic	24
Superior para-aortic	88
Inferior para-aortic	58
Urinary bladder	20
Sacrococcygeal	1
Anal	1
Vaginal	2
Extra-adrenal (site unspecified)	6
	205

*Compiled from various sources; from Fries, J. G. and Chamberlin, J. A.: Extra-adrenal pheochromocytoma: literature review and report of a cervical pheochromocytoma, Surgery 63:268-279, 1968.

as they increase in size, they erode through the capsule, grow luxuriantly in the surrounding tissue, and invade veins but do not encroach upon the substance of the kidney. On microscopic examination, the neuroblastoma is made up of large numbers of cells with narrow rims of cytoplasm that resemble, but are slightly larger than, normal lymphocytes. Neuroblastomas could easily be confused with sarcomas, but they can be differentiated because of the presence of rosettes (Fig. 538, *B*), which are formed by a concentric arrangement of the nuclei at the periphery of an indefinite mass of cytoplasm. The earliest stage of development of the rosettes is the formation of ball-like areas, the sympathoblasts forming more perfect rosettes than the sympathogonia (Blacklock[10]). Although rosettes are often present in the primary tumor, they are not often seen in the peripheral metastases.

Mixed tumors, presenting all transitions from neuroblasts to adult ganglion cells, are also observed. All of these transitions may be present in the same tumor, and there have even been cases reported in which there have been several tumors in different locations with different degrees of maturation (Wahl and Craig[131]; Dunn[35]).

Benign and malignant tumors showing the same character as those developing from the suprarenal medulla may arise from accessory suprarenal tissue found elsewhere. These tumors have been found arising from the paraganglionic tissue in immediate proximity to the suprarenal gland, in the celiac plexus, in the organ

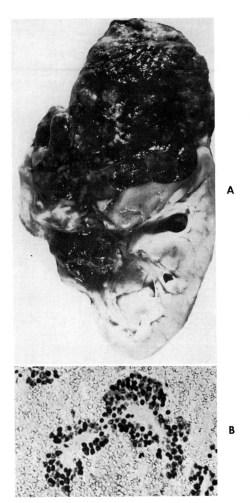

Fig. 538. **A,** Typical neuroblastoma of suprarenal gland—well delimited, hemorrhagic, and with extension into renal pelvis. **B,** Typical rosettes are visible.

of Zuckerkandl near the bifurcation of the iliac vessels, in the root of the lung, and in the superior cervical ganglion. Philips[106] found eleven pheochromocytomas outside of the suprarenal gland, nine of which arose from the organ of Zuckerkandl.

Metastatic spread

Malignant tumors of the suprarenal gland sometimes present markedly different forms of metastatic spread. The *adenocarcinomas* of the cortex metastasize predominantly to the liver, lungs, brain, and regional nodes. Bone metastases are rarely observed.

Some *neuroblastomas* are characterized by a massive involvement of the liver and mesenteric lymph nodes without producing bone metastases (Pepper type). Another type of neuroblastoma is characterized by the frequency of early metastases to the bones of the skull (Hutchison type). It must be emphasized that these two clinical types are not clear-cut. Frew[40] confirmed the presence of metastases to the skull in forty-seven of fifty-one neuroblastomas of the Hutchison type. It is probable that these metastases are related to the vertebral vein system. In addition to the skull metastases, metastatic implants are found in the sternum, vertebrae, ribs, and long bones. On microscopic examination, the vertebrae reveal a preserved architectural pattern, and the bone marrow appears in excessive amounts. In the long bones, subperiosteal extension with bone formation at right angles to the long axis is sometimes seen. In the skull, punched-out areas with complete destruction of the bone are often observed, together with soft tissue masses invading and distending the orbital tissues. The metastases in the liver tend to be very diffuse, enlarging and almost completely replacing it. Davis et al.[30] reported functioning metastases in a pheochromocytoma.

Clinical evolution

Tumors arising from cortex. The overwhelming majority of *adenomas* of the cortex do not produce clinical symptoms and are found only at autopsy. A small group of these tumors are characterized by their variable hormonal changes, the most common of which cause virilizing alterations in females. These changes usually occur after puberty and before the menopause. Amenorrhea is often noted, the body becomes masculine, the hair distribution acquires the characteristics of the male (Fig. 539), and the voice may change. Rarely, a feminizing tendency may be observed in the male, with changes in body type, painful enlargement of breasts, increased pigmentation of the nipples, and diminution in size of the testes (Gabrilone et al.[42]).

Tumors and hyperplasia of the adrenal cortex may be associated with Cushing's syndrome. Cushing's syndrome is characterized by hirsutism, sexual dystrophy (amenorrhea in females; impotence in males), facial plethora, truncal obesity,

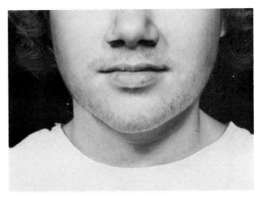

Fig. 539. Beard growth in 20-year-old woman with benign adrenal cortical tumor (17-ketosteroid excretion, 100 mg/24 hr). After excision of tumor, 17-ketosteroid excretion dropped to 6 mg. Patient became pregnant one month after operation. (WU neg. 61-7692.)

asthenia, acne, striae, and often hypertension. There may be prominent osteoporosis accompanied by rib fractures. This syndrome is associated with a high incidence of a great variety of tumors, many of which secrete corticotropic substance (Table 71) (O'Neal[99]). In twelve children with hyperadrenocorticism reported by Hayles et al.,[60] the most common clinical picture was a mixture of adrenogenital syndrome and Cushing's syndrome.

Simple hirsutism and increased skeletal musculature without other manifestations may be observed (Kinsell and Lisser[70]). There is a variety of possible vague manifestations. Cases of prolonged asthenia, peculiar weakness of the lower extremities, and craving for proteins (Goldberg et al[48]) have led to impressions of psychoneurosis until the diagnosis of suprarenal tumor was established. In some instances, the tumor may enlarge considerably and become palpable.

Aldosterone-producing tumors were described by Conn et al.[23] with a syndrome of hypokalemia and hypertension. It is not known how often hypertension is associated with aldosterone-producing tumor. The test for the identification of aldosterone and the renin determinations are available in only a small number of laboratories. The patients have numerous complaints (Table 72). All of the symptoms disappear following successful surgical removal.

Occasionally, *adenocarcinomas* of the

Table 71. Neoplasms in Cushing's syndrome*

	Cases	Adrenal adenoma	Adrenal carcinoma	Cortical hyperplasia; pituitary tumor	Cortical hyperplasia; other tumor	Cortical hyperplasia; no tumor anywhere	Cortical hyperplasia; pituitary status not known; no other tumor
Barnes Hospital	46	3 (6.5%)	9 (19.5%)	10 (21.7%)	7 (15.2%)	2 (4.3%)	15 (32.6%)
Literature 1940-1962	178	18 (10.1%)	32 (18.0%)	29 (16.3%)	26 (14.6%)	6 (3.4%)	67 (37.6%)
Total	224	21 (9.4%)	41 (18.3%)	39 (17.4%)	33 (14.7%)	8 (3.6%)	82 (36.6%)

*From O'Neal, L. W.: Pathologic anatomy in Cushing's syndrome, Ann. Surg. **160:**860-869, 1964.

Table 72. Presenting complaints in primary aldosteronism*

Complaint	%
Muscle weakness	73
Polyuria or nocturia	72
Headache	51
Polydipsia	46
Paresthesias	24
Visual disturbance	21
Intermittent paralysis	21
Tetany	21
Fatigue	19
Muscle discomfort	16
No symptoms	6

*From Conn, J. W., et al.: Clinical characteristics of primary aldosteronism from an analysis of 145 cases, Amer. J. Surg. **107:**159-172, 1964.

cortex are the cause of hormonal alterations, and these changes can be as variable as in the adenomas (McGavack[86]). Wood et al.[137] collected 35 cases of nonfunctioning carcinomas published over a period of thirty-four years. The patients often had pain in the loin and the hypochondrium and presented a low-grade fever and asthenia. A palpable mass was present in about one-third. The diagnosis is usually made late, when operation is not possible or metastases have occurred (Birke et al.[8]).

Tumors arising from medulla. The evolution of the *ganglioneuroma* is slow, and the tumor seldom produces any symptoms other than those due to its increased size.

The clinical evolution of the *pheochromocytoma* may be most dramatic and, once seen, it is never forgotten. The tumor causes paroxysmal attacks due to intermittent flooding of the bloodstream with pressor substances. Sweating, weakness, facial pallor (circumoral), and tachycardia occur. Dyspnea, shock, nervousness, nausea, vomiting, giddiness, blanching, pallor of the extremities, precordial pain, and a sense of constriction of the chest may occur. These paroxysms may occur for many years, and the physiologic changes can be extremely alarming. The attacks may vary in frequency from ten to twenty-five times per day or may occur only every two or three months (Kvale et al.[74]). Thomas et al.[127] believe that the clinical signs and symptoms of pheochromocytoma can be confused with intracranial tumors, vasodilating headache, focal arterial brain disease, a state of anxiety, hypertensive encephalopathy, and diencephalic-autonomic epilepsy (Table 73). In exceptional instances, the vascular changes produced by the hypertension lead to severe involvement of the vessels of the retina, heart, brain, and kidney (Thorn et al.[128]) and in some instances may cause death. The attacks may occur following exertion, change in position, deep breathing, massage of the suprarenal area, or palpation of the tumor mass, or they may be produced simply by emotion. If pheochromocytoma coincides with pregnancy, abortion may result (Cannon[19]). An active fetus may traumatize the tumor and provoke an attack (Dean[31]) (Fig. 540).

Whereas the hypertension is often paroxysmal, it may also be sustained (Cahill[16]) or may even be entirely absent. Excessive perspiration is found in patients with paroxysmal hypertension as well as in those who do not present that important manifestation. The perspiration may be a compensatory cooling mechanism when the metabolic rate is increased and vasoconstriction occurs to interfere with heat loss (Farquhar[38]). Elevation of tempera-

Table 73. Symptoms in 100 patients with pheochromocytoma*

Symptom	Patients (No. or %)
Headache	80
Perspiration	71
Palpitation (with or without tachycardia)	64
Pallor	42
Nausea (with or without vomiting)	42
Tremor or trembling	31
Weakness or exhaustion	28
Nervousness or anxiety	22
Epigastric pain	22
Chest pain	19
Dyspnea	19
Flushing or warmth	18
Numbness or paresthesia	11
Blurring of vision	11
Tightness in throat	8
Dizziness or faintness	8
Convulsions	5
Neck-shoulder pain	5
Extremity pain	4
Flank pain	4
Tinnitus	3
Dysarthria	3
Gagging	3
Bradycardia (noted by patient)	3
Back pain	3
Coughing	1
Yawning	1
Syncope	1
Unsteadiness	1
Hunger	1

*From Thomas, J. E., et al.: The neurologist's experience with pheochromocytoma, J.A.M.A. **197**:754-758, 1966.

ture may be observed (Smithwick[122]). Anxiety may predominate (Doust[34]). Pheochromocytomas may be associated with neurofibromatosis (Healey and Mekelatos[62]), may be accompanied by intestinal lesions that disturb motility and cause bleeding (Brown and Borowsky[12]), and also may have characteristic ocular manifestations (Gaines[43]). In fifteen cases of pheochromocytoma seen at autopsy, five patients had died of shock in the course of incidental operations (Minno et al.[93]).

Neuroblastomas occurring in utero have been the cause of fetal dystocia (Weinberg and Radman[132]). In general, this tumor has a rapid clinical course and may be found only at autopsy. There are two classic clinical types of evolution of neuroblastomas of the suprarenal gland. These do not correspond to any pathologic differences but are merely variations in the clinical findings and course.

The Pepper type is characterized by a distention of the abdomen from enlargement of the liver, mesenteric lymph node metastases, rapid loss of weight and strength, and anemia. The tumor here is found in the right suprarenal gland, which explains the rapid involvement of the liver. Metastases to the bones of the skull are seldom observed, but the mesenteric nodes are always considerably enlarged.

The Hutchison type is characterized by

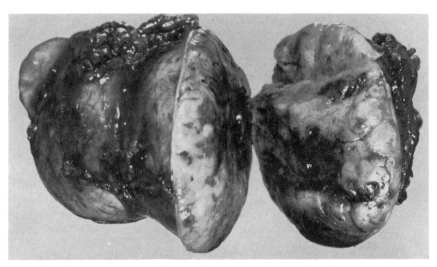

Fig. 540. Pheochromocytoma in 27-year-old pregnant woman. Catecholamines were elevated in urine. Patient had intermittent hypertension and abnormalities in carbohydrate metabolism. Tumor was removed and normal infant was delivered. (WU neg. 60-2493.)

the peculiar onset of ecchymosis of the eyelids, proptosis of the eye, and enlargement of the preauricular, submaxillary, and upper cervical lymph nodes on the same side (Fig. 541). These symptoms are caused by metastases in the bones of the skull, which have an unexplained predilection for the region of the orbit. Neuroblastomas that produce this clinical picture may be found in the left or the right suprarenal gland. It has been mistakenly thought that the Hutchison syndrome was produced by tumors arising in the left suprarenal gland, just as the Pepper syndrome was produced by those arising on the right side. Of the ten cases reported by Hutchison in his original publication,[64] only six arose from the left suprarenal gland. Frew[40] observed that when the tumor was on the right side, the metastasis to the orbit, the exophthalmos, and the ecchymosis also occurred on the right, and when the tumor was on the left, these changes developed first in the left orbit. The size of the primary tumor and the

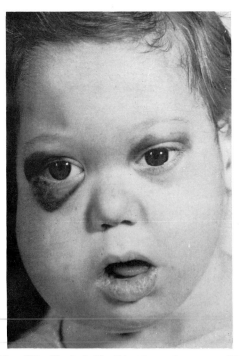

Fig. 541. Typical Hutchison's syndrome in 18-month-old child due to neuroblastoma of right suprarenal gland. Note ecchymosis, slight exophthalmos, and enlargement of right submaxillary and buccal lymph nodes.

enlargement of the mesenteric lymph nodes may be noticeable only in the later stages of the disease or may even be discovered at autopsy.

Diagnosis

The diagnosis of tumors of the suprarenal glands is often made because of the general symptoms produced or by the presence of metastases rather than by symptoms caused by the tumor in its local development. Symptoms of masculinization or premature sexual development, feminization, obesity, or hirsutism should encourage further investigation (Kinsell and Lisser[70]). The presence of an orbital ecchymosis, with exophthalmos and cervical adenopathy in children, is almost pathognomonic of metastatic neuroblastoma. Neuroblastoma is, next to Wilms' tumor, the second most common abdominal tumor in children. The actual diagnosis may be established only after surgical exploration has been done. *Epinephrine-producing* tumors in children usually cause a sustained hypertension with symptoms of adrenal intoxication. The illness appears to be more fulminating than in adults (Moore and Shumacker[94]).

Patients with paroxysmal hypertension should be observed carefully during the attack and the blood pressure charted closely. Exercise or postural changes or massage may be sufficient to bring about a paroxysmal attack. In one patient, massage of an abdominal mass caused an elevation of the systolic pressure to over 300. If the diagnosis can be established without precipitating the attack, such course is preferable. In functioning pheochromocytomas, the repeated basal metabolism rate may be helpful in the diagnosis, for a basal metabolic rate of over +20 is unusual in essential hypertension. Protein-bound radioactive iodine will not be taken up in large amounts by the thyroid gland. Examination of the eyegrounds may reveal vascular pathology which is often confused with that produced by essential hypertension (Bruce[13]) or optic neuritis (Gaines[43]).

Roentgenologic examination

A number of radiologic procedures may be utilized to demonstrate the presence of an adrenal neoplasm: scout abdominal roentgenograms, intravenous pyelography, nephrotomography, retroperitoneal pneumography, aortography, selective adrenal arteriography, and selective adrenal vein catheterization (Kahn[67]). O'Neal[99] is not enthusiastic about sophisticated procedures and relies primarily on intravenous pyelography, reasoning that, in any event, biochemical verification is more important than radiographic localization.

Scout roentgenograms of the abdomen may reveal the presence of suprarenal neoplasms because of their volume and kidney displacement. Rarely, calcifications are seen in pheochromocytomas and more frequently in neuroblastomas (Mandeville[87]). Visualization of an uninvolved apex in the presence of a mass within the remaining adrenal tissue is believed by Meyers[90] to be a specific finding for pheochromocytoma. Calcification often indicates that the tumor is malignant.

Pyelography is a useful procedure for the diagnosis of these tumors which depends, of course, on the size of the tumor. Neuroblastomas tend to displace the calyces and the renal pelvis downward. Tresidder[130] diagnosed an adrenal neoplasm by pyelography in twenty-seven patients, but the procedure failed to demonstrate

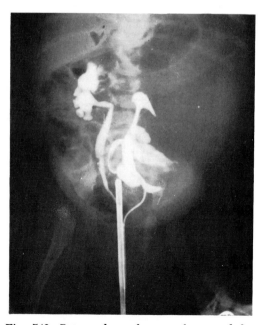

Fig. 542. Retrograde pyelogram of young baby girl with suprarenal neuroblastoma.

the presence in twenty-seven others (Fig. 542). A study by Greer et al.[55] showed that the tumors were not demonstrated in 70% of the patients (average weight of tumor, 48 gm), whereas the diagnosis was made in the remainder (average weight of tumor, 186 gm).

Nephrotomography is a combination of pyelography and planigraphy. With this procedure, Hartman et al.[59] identified thirty-one of thirty-nine proved tumors.

The vascular pattern revealed at *arteriography* may help both in localizing the tumor and indicating whether or not it is malignant (Rossi[112]), but the procedure is not without risk. Meaney and Buonocore[89] used *selective arteriography,* with constant monitoring of blood pressure, in fifteen patients suspected of having a pheochromocytoma. In some of the patients, it was necessary to discontinue the injection of contrast medium.

Because aldosterone-secreting tumors are usually small, selective adrenal *vein catheterization* has been utilized for their localization (Mikaelsson[91]). Eckström et al.[36] compared angiograms with microangiography and histologic studies of twenty-eight adrenal glands with varying patterns. In an intermediate group, the vascular pattern was not accurate for diagnosis.

For a suspected neuroblastoma, skeletal films should be taken. Metastases are usually generalized and in practically all bones proximal to the knee and elbow joints. If the long bones show bilateral symmetrical involvement, a neuroblastoma is probably present (Wyatt and Farber[139]). These changes will be present particularly in the diaphyseal portions of the humerus and the distal portions of the femur. Although they are usually osteolytic, they are not infrequently mixed in type. The bones of the pelvis and skull may show extensive replacement. Sherman and Leaming[118] pointed out that in the metastases of neuroblastoma, striking skull changes may occur, with separation of the sutures, enlargement of the head, perpendicular spiculation, and patchy productive and destructive changes within the vault. It is not rare for the metastases of a neuroblastoma to mimic the roentgenologic changes in Ewing's sarcoma, with elevation of the periosteum in the upper ends of long bones and with production of bone spicules at right angles to the shaft, due undoubtedly to tumor infiltration with separation of the periosteum. The skull very frequently shows massive osteolytic involvement with multiple areas of destruction (Doub[33]). In tumors of the cortex that give the clinical syndrome suggesting pituitary basophilism, roentgenograms of the skull are indicated. Generalized osteoporosis may also be present.

Laboratory examination

The diagnosis of tumors of neural crest origin is greatly aided by biochemical tests that measure increased urinary excretions of certain metabolites of catecholamines. These include norepinephrine (NE), epinephrine (E), dopamine (DM), and dopa (DA). Vanilmandelic acid (VMA) is the major terminal metabolite of norepinephrine and epinephrine, whereas homovanillic acid (HVA) represents the major terminal degradation product of endogenously and exogenously administered dopamine, the precursor of both norepinephrine and epinephrine. Patients with neuroblastoma, ganglioneuroblastoma, and ganglioneuroma excrete increased amounts of homovanillic acid and vanilmandelic acid in their urine (Williams and Greer[135]). Patients with pheochromocytoma excrete increased amounts of vanilmandelic acid but normal amounts of homovanillic acid. There is great variation in the synthesis and degradation of catechol metabolites in patients with neuroblastoma, but there is a well-defined metabolic pathway in those with pheochromocytoma (Greer et al.[55]). If a primary tumor of the sympathetic nervous system is removed, and previous to its removal there was an elevation of catecholamines, then these should fall to normal if all, or nearly all of the tumor is removed. If recurrence or metastases develop, then the catecholamines will again become elevated (Robinson et al.[111]). Tissue culture may be diagnostic in tumors of the sympathetic nervous system (Goldstein et al.[50]).

Cushing's syndrome may be caused by a benign or malignant tumor of the adrenal cortex or may be associated with bilateral hyperplasia (Scott et al.[117]). With hyperplasia of the cortex, stimulation with ACTH causes further elevation of plasma cortisol and 17-hydroxycorticosteroid levels. If the patient has a tumor, there is no increase or only an insignificant increase of these substances after stimulation with ACTH. Urinary 17-ketosteroids are usually elevated, particularly in patients with carcinoma of the cortex. High excretory levels of steroids may be present. Such elevation of hormone excretion will again appear following recrudescence of the neoplasm (Loutfi and Emerson[83]). Wotiz et al.[138] measured the urinary estrogens in a patient with a feminizing adrenal cortical tumor and found prominent elevations in the urinary titers, particularly of estriol. The diagnosis of an aldosterone-secreting tumor depends on the determination of aldosterone in plasma in urine as well as renin determinations. At the present moment, these determinations are expensive, technically difficult, and not widely available.

"The cells of the normal zona glomerulosa are responsible for the formation of aldosterone in animals and man,[4, 46, 120] and can form corticosterone but not cortisol. Since an 18-oxidase system is required for the biosynthesis of aldosterone and a 17α-hydroxylase system is needed for cortisol production, it follows that the cells of the normal zona glomerulosa possess the 18-oxidase system but lack the 17α-hydroxylase. By contrast, the clear cells of the normal zona fasciculata, which can form cortisol and corticosterone but not aldosterone, have the 17α-hydroxylase system but not the 18-oxidase system. Both enzyme systems must be present in tumors causing primary aldosteronism since they are capable of forming cortisol, corticosterone and aldosterone in vitro."[*4, 11, 29, 39, 82, 102]

All patients with tumors of the adrenal cortex, no matter what their clinical presentation, often secrete abnormal amounts of various steroid substances. These abnormal amounts will disappear with the removal of the tumor, only to reappear with recrudescence of the neoplasm. The urinary 17-ketosteroids in patients with adenocarcinoma of the cortex are often strikingly elevated (Schteingart et al.[116]). It

---

*From Neville, A. M., and Symington, T.: Pathology of primary aldosteronism, Cancer **19:** 1854-1868, 1966.

is unfortunate that not too many laboratories have the facilities to do these tests accurately. Pathology is totally inadequate in determining the pattern of hormone excretion. Furthermore, electron microscopy and radiochemical tests of various types are now being studied intensively. This type of study does not fall within the range of the usual diagnostic laboratory.

The bioassay with strips of rabbit's aorta is an accurate method. There are also fluorometric methods for quantitating epinephrine and norepinephrine in the blood and in the urine (Kvale et al.[74]). In patients with sustained hypertension, Regitine causes a profound fall in blood pressure, but this test may not be helpful in patients who have received heavy sedation or antihypertensive drugs.

Differential diagnosis

Cushing's syndrome produced by *pituitary basophilism* may be thought to be due to a tumor of the adrenal cortex. The most important differentiating point is the excretion of 17-ketosteroids, which is normal in patients with pituitary tumors (Crooke and Callow[25]). Cases of *female pseudohermaphroditism* may lead to the suspicion of a suprarenal tumor. They may result from

adrenal hypertrophy or from hormonal activity of the mother upon the fetus during gestation (Hain[57]). To complicate matters, pseudohermaphroditism and adrenal tumors are often found in members of the same family (Bentinck et al.[6]). Here, again, the androgen excretion may be of great value in differentiation, for although it may be found slightly elevated, it never attains the high levels observed in patients with adrenal tumors. *Arrhenoblastoma* of the ovary may also suggest an adrenal tumor because of its virilizing signs. The clinical examination will usually reveal lack of obesity and of hypertension that may accompany the adrenal tumors. The carbohydrate tolerance will be found normal, and the presence of an ovarian tumor may be ascertained on palpation or at laparotomy. *Tumors of the hypothalamus* may cause precocious puberty (Weinberger and Grant[133]), and *testicular tumors* may also cause sexual precocity (Rowland and Weber[114]).

Malignant hypertension may have to be differentiated from pheochromocytomas (Palmer and Castleman[100]). The administration of Regitine does not result in reduction of blood pressure, as it does in patients with sustained hypertension with

Table 74. Differential diagnosis of neuroblastoma of suprarenal gland

	Age (yr)	Abdominal mass	Orbit	Bone changes	Pyelograms	Bone marrow biopsy	Response to radiotherapy
Neuroblastoma	0 to 6	Often not felt	Proptosis of eye; ecchymosis of eyelids often present	Osteoplastic and osteoblastic; symmetrical changes in long bones and skull common	May reveal extrinsic tumor, distorting calyces	At times diagnostic	Immediate response
Wilms' tumor	0 to 9	Invariably large		Not present	Reveal intrinsic tumor of kidney	Normal	Delayed response
Chloroma (myelocytic leukemia) and acute leukemia	0 to 5	Not present but may have enlarged spleen and/or liver	Proptosis of eye; ecchymosis of eyelids may be present	Invariably osteolytic; very similar to neuroblastoma	Normal	May be diagnostic; white blood count invariably elevated	Immediate response
Ewing's sarcoma	5 to 25	Not present		Almost identical with neuroblastoma	Normal	May resemble neuroblastoma	Delayed response

pheochromocytomas mentioned previously. A basal metabolism rate that remains above +20 is not found in those with essential hypertension. *Hyperthyroidism* may also suggest a pheochromocytoma. The other signs of thyrotoxosis are usually present to help in the differentiation. The increased amount of pressor substance found in the blood at the height of a paroxysmal attack with pheochromocytomas is usually of great value in differentiation. In children, coarctation of the aorta, lead poisoning, and tumors of the hypothalamus may have to be considered in the differential diag-

nosis of pheochromocytomas (Snyder and Vick[124]). The symptoms and signs associated with *acute anxiety* and those produced by a renal cyst can be confused with the symptoms of pheochromocytomas.

A *Wilms* tumor may be mistaken for a neuroblastoma of the adrenal gland. In Wilms' tumor of the kidney, there is invariably a large abdominal mass, and the intravenous pyelogram reveals intrinsic deformity of the kidney in patients in good general condition. *Chloroma*, which produces ecchymosis of the eyelid, may suggest a Hutchison type of metastasizing

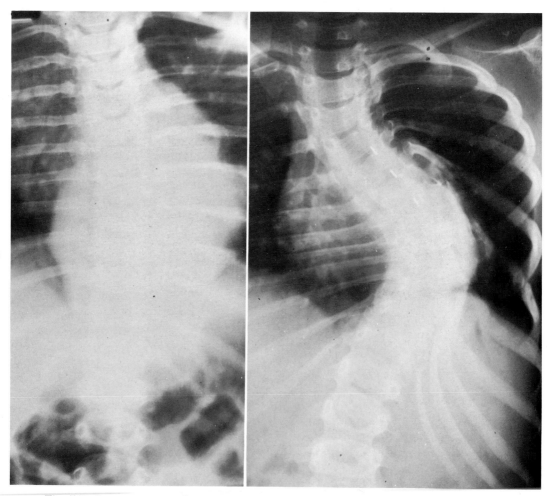

A

B

Fig. 543. Large mass in right posterior mediastinum with erosion of vertebral bodies in 11-month-old infant. **A,** Myelogram showing complete block at level of ninth thoracic vertebra due to tumor invasion. **B,** After surgical removal and administration of about 1200 rads to tumor area in a relatively short time, marked scoliosis developed, requiring casts and surgical correction. (From Perez, C. A., et al.: Tumors of the sympathetic nervous system in children; an appraisal of treatment and results, Radiology **88:**750-760, 1967; **A,** WU neg. 57-5527; **B,** WU neg. 59-7725.)

neuroblastoma (Olesen and Sjontoft[98]). In patients with chloroma, the spleen may be enlarged and may be taken for the primary abdominal lesion, but the peripheral blood count or the bone marrow biopsy should be decisive. Extensive cases of Ewing's tumor and generalized lymphosarcoma may suggest a widely metastasizing neuroblastoma. In such cases, a biopsy may not be sufficient to establish the differential diagnosis, and other factors may have to be taken into consideration (Table 74). Marin et al.[88] reported a patient with a *hematoma* in the region of the adrenal gland that simulated a tumor in a newborn infant. Adrenal cysts are rare lesions that are usually not diagnosed, for they may show calcification on the roentgenogram. They can be either a true cyst or a pseudocyst following hemorrhage (Abeshouse et al.[1]).

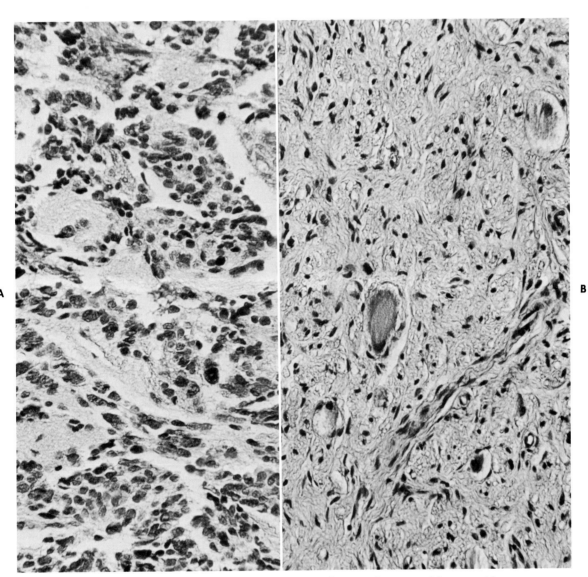

Fig. 544. Same tumor shown in Fig. 543. **A,** Removed tumor shows neuroblastoma with some cells forming pseudorosettes. **B,** Biopsy of small nodule found three years after initial treatment shows well-differentiated ganglioneuroma with numerous ganglion cells. (From Perez, C. A., et al.: Tumors of the sympathetic nervous system in children; an appraisal of treatment and results, Radiology **88:**750-760, 1967; **A,** WU neg. 66-4246; **B,** ×300; WU neg. 66-4247.)

It is well known that metastases from other primary tumors are frequently found in the suprarenal glands. In fact, in some autopsy series, the percentage of metastases to the suprarenal gland is more than 25% (Glomset[47]). In spite of this frequent occurrence, there is only rarely a question of differential diagnosis between these metastatic tumors and primary tumors of the suprarenal gland.

Treatment
Surgery

Tumors of the adrenal cortex are best approached through a transverse abdominal incision, for it facilitates the preliminary bilateral exploration that is indicated in all patients. The tumor may be bilateral, and the opposite adrenal gland may be atrophic or rarely absent (Lukens et al.[84]). If the tumor is situated anterior to the kidney, the abdominal approach facilitates its removal without simultaneous nephrectomy. In females with virilizing symptoms, an abdominal approach facilitates exploration of the ovaries. With enlarged palpable tumor, the thoracolumbar approach may facilitate more adequate exploration and removal of the neoplasm.

Before the advent of steroid hormones for substitution, operative mortality was high in patients with Cushing's syndrome. In the collected series of Rapaport et al.,[109] it was 56% between 1930 and 1949 and dropped to 20% between 1950 and 1955. In patients with virilism, it was about 30% between 1930 and 1949 and dropped to 6% between 1950 and 1955 (Heinbecker et al.[63]). Details concerning substitution therapy have been extensively reviewed by Thorn et al.[128] The differences in operative mortality between patients with Cushing's syndrome and the adrenogenital syndrome are probably due to the fact that in Cushing's syndrome the opposite adrenal gland is frequently atrophic, whereas such an atrophy in the adrenogenital syndrome is much less common (Labhart et al.[75]).

The surgical treatment of patients with pheochromocytomas is somewhat hazardous. Preoperative restoration of blood volume is important (Brunjes et al.[14]). Patients with sustained hypertension, particularly children (Moore and Shumacker[94]), should be given preoperative medication to reduce the blood pressure to reasonable levels. A thoracoabdominal approach is preferred by some (Lance et al.[76]). During operation, the tumor must be handled as little as possible. After removal, the patients often go into shock, and the blood pressure may have to be maintained with norepinephrine. If the blood pressure remains elevated, this may indicate the presence of a second neoplasm (Davis et al.[30]). Surgical removal should not be postponed because of pregnancy (Dean[31]). In the past, the operative mortality has been high, approximately 25% (Graham[52]), but better understanding of preoperative and postoperative care has greatly reduced it (Dahl-Iversen[27]). Cardiac arrhythmia should be promptly recognized by anesthetist and surgeon and the patient given appropriate protection (Riddell et al.[110]).

Neuroblastomas of the suprarenal gland are often recognized by their metastases in a stage in which few are eligible for curative treatment. Surgical removal of the primary lesion is capable of control if no metastases have occurred (Lehman[79]).

Radiotherapy

There is abundant evidence of the curative value of radiotherapy in poorly differentiated tumors of the sympathetic nervous system. Radiotherapy should be administered whenever a surgical intervention has been incomplete; radiotherapy should also be directed to the liver or to bony lesions that may be present, for it has been found surprisingly effective in these instances. A serious consideration should be entered as to the total dose administered and the duration of the course of treatments. Intensive short courses and very high doses are unnecessary and inadvisable. Since the patient is usually a growing child, the irradiation should be carried out with proper concern for the organs irradiated, such as the kidneys and the growing bones. Fractionated treatments, over several weeks, will minimize the effects and avoid scoliosis and kyphosis that result from intensive irradiation (Figs. 543 and 544). The risks of radiotherapy are outweighed by its excellent results. There seems to be no reason to administer postoperative radiotherapy in ganglioneuromas for these tumors are adequately controlled by surgery alone. There is no evidence that radiotherapy may be effective in pheochromocytomas (Graham[52]).

Chemotherapy

Various drugs have been tried in the palliative treatment of suprarenal tumors, and the trend is toward a combination of drugs. Cyclophosphamide has been found helpful in the management of disseminated *neuroblastomas.* Pinkel et al.[107] found the combination of cyclophosphamide and vincristine preferable to the administration of alkalating agents alone (Thurman and Donaldson[129]). Chemotherapy should not be resorted to in the treatment of localized tumors, whether alone or as a radiotherapeutic adjuvant. It has been suggested that such treatment could impair host resistance (Perez et al.[104]).

Bergenstal et al.[7] have reported the use of a drug that produces measurable response in inoperable patients with functioning and nonfunctioning adrenal carcinomas (Hutter and Kayhoe[65]). It is associated with considerable toxicity and should not be given unless other measures have been thoroughly exhausted.

Prognosis

Patients with benign tumors of the adrenal cortex who survive operation are subject to recurrences, but these may be permanently controlled (Goldberg et al.[48]). Obesity and secondary sexual changes may regress, but hirsutism and voice changes may remain. Isolated reports of long-standing control of suprarenal carcinomas have been made. Survival in spite of metastases may be long (Cottler[24]). In thirty-five patients with nonfunctioning adrenal cortical carcinomas reviewed by Wood et al.,[137] the prognosis was extremely poor, with only two patients surviving five years.

Patients with pheochromocytoma have a good prognosis following successful removal (Graham[52]). Results in children have been documented by Farquhar[38] (Fig. 545). Spontaneous hemorrhage into the tumor may give rise to a clinical picture of abdominal catastrophe (Jelliffe[66]) and may possibly result in spontaneous cure (Albers et al.[2]).

Patients with neuroblastomas adequately

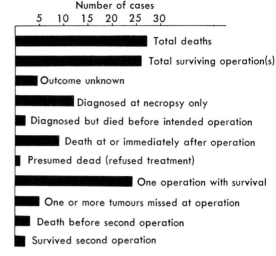

Fig. 545. Outcome of fifty-seven recorded cases of pheochromocytoma in children. (From Farquhar, J. W.: Phaeochromocytoma in childhood; case report and a brief review of 56 others recorded in the literature, J. Roy. Coll. Surg. Edinb. 3:301-310, 1958.)

treated by surgery or by irradiation may be cured in a fair percentage (Fig. 546). Wittenborg[136] reported on seventy-three cases of neuroblastoma seen at the Children's Hospital in Boston. Only forty-five of these patients were treated by surgery, radiotherapy, or a combination of both. Twenty-two patients (30%) survived three or more years, and some lived over twelve years. In this series, there were six patients with liver metastases, and all had survived at least three years after radiotherapy. Patients under 2 years of age do better than those over 2 years of age (Gross[56]). At least one case of remission resulted in recrudescence after eighteen years (Dargeon[28]). Stella et al.[125a] reported on 129 patients with neuroblastomas treated at the Gustave-Roussy Institute of Paris by a combination of radiotherapy and surgery and occasionally chemotherapy; ten additional patients received palliative treatment only and five received no treatment. Thirty-seven (21%) of the 129 patients treated remained well from thirty-two to sixty months. Patients with bone metastases usually do not survive, but we know of two patients who had spontaneous regression of the bone involvement and are cured. Maturation of the tumor can also occur with cure (Kissane and Ackerman[72]).

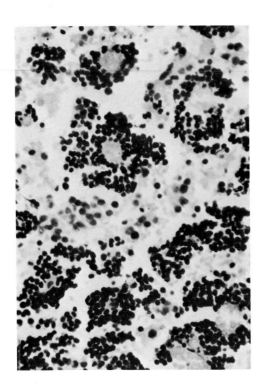

Spontaneous regression may occur without treatment or following biopsy.

In tumors of the sympathetic nervous system, there is a good correlation between microscopic pattern and outlook (Fig. 547). Patients with ganglioneuromas uniformly do well, and the percentage of cure in those with ganglioneuroblastomas is much higher than in those with neuroblastomas.

Fig. 546. Classic example of neuroblastoma with prominent rosettes. At the age of 7 weeks, patient had 4 cm tumor of right adrenal gland. Tumor, including kidney, was removed, and operation was followed by 3100 rads absorbed in region of tumor in three-week period. Patient is doing well fifteen years after therapy. Clinical and radiographic findings seven years after operation show severe lordotic deformity of lumbar spine without significant scoliosis. (×300; from Perez, C. A., et al.: Tumors of the sympathetic nervous system in children; an appraisal of treatment and results, Radiology 88:750-760, 1967; WU neg. 66-4248.)

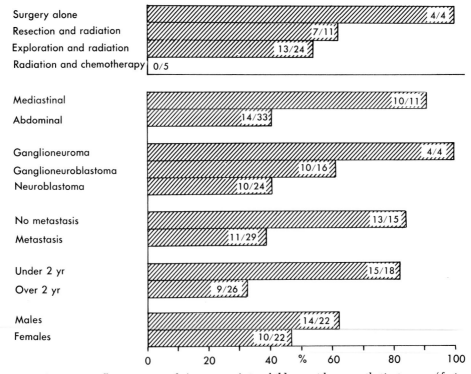

Fig. 547. Factors affecting survival (two years) in children with sympathetic tumors (forty-four patients). (Courtesy Dr. Carlos A. Perez, St. Louis, Mo.; collected material from Department of Radiotherapy, Mallinckrodt Institute of Radiology, Washington University School of Medicine, St. Louis, Mo.; WU neg. 67-1394.)

REFERENCES

1 Abeshouse, G. A., Goldstein, R. B., and Abeshouse, B. S.: Adrenal cysts; review of the literature and report of three cases, J. Urol. **81**:711-719, 1959.

2 Albers, D. D., Kalman, E. H., and Back, K. C.: Pheochromocytoma; report of five cases, one a spontaneous cure, J. Urol. **78**:301-308, 1957.

3 Allen, W. M., Hayward, S. J., and Pinto, A.: A color test for dehydroisoandrosterone and closely related steroid, of use in the diagnosis of adrenocortical tumors, J. Clin. Endocr. **10**:54-70, 1950.

4 Ayres, P. J., Barlow, J., Garrod, O., Kellie, A. E., Tait, S. A. A., Tait, J. F., and Walker, G.: Primary aldosteronism (Conn's syndrome). In An international symposium on aldosterone (A. F. Muller and C. M. O'Connor, editors), London, 1958, J. & A. Churchill, Ltd., pp. 143-154.

5 Bailey, R. E., Slade, C. I., Lieberman, A. H., and Luetscher, J. A., Jr.: Steroid production by human adrenal adenomata and nontumorous adrenal tissue in vitro, J. Clin. Endocr. **20**:457-465, 1960.

6 Bentinck, R. C., Hinman, F., Sr., Lisser, H., and Traut, H. F.: The familial congenital adrenal syndrome; report of two cases and review of the literature, Postgrad. Med. **11**:301-312, 1952.

7 Bergenstal, D. M., Hertz, R., Lipsett, M. B., and Moy, R. H.: Chemotherapy of adrenocortical cancer with o,p DDD, Ann. Intern. Med. **53**:672, 1960.

8 Birke, G., Franksson, C., Gemzell, C.-A., Moberger, G., and Plantin, L.-O.: Adrenal cortical tumours; a study with special reference to possibilities of correlating histologic appearance with hormonal activity, Acta Chir. Scand. **117**:233-246, 1959.

9 Biskind, G. R., Meyer, M. A., and Beadner, S. A.: Adrenal medullary tumor, J. Clin. Endocr. **1**:113-123, 1941.

10 Blacklock, J. W. S.: Neurogenic tumors of the sympathetic system in children, J. Path. Bact. **39**:27-48, 1934.

11 Brode, E., Grant, J. K., and Symington, T.: A biochemical and pathological investigation of adrenal tissues from patients with Conn's syndrome, Acta Endocr. (Kobenhavn) **41**:411-431, 1962.

12 Brown, R. B., and Borowsky, M.: Further observations on intestinal lesions associated with pheochromocytoma, Ann. Surg. **151**:683-692, 1960.

13 Bruce, G. M.: Changes in the ocular fundus associated with pheochromocytoma of the adrenal gland; report of 3 cases, Arch. Ophthal. (Chicago) **39**:707-730, 1948.

14 Brunjes, S., Johns, V. J., Jr., and Crane, M. C.: Pheochromocytoma; postoperative shock and blood volume, New Eng. J. Med. **262**:393-396, 1960.

15 Cahill, G. F.: Tumors of the adrenal and use of air insufflation in their diagnosis, Radiology **37**:533-544, 1941.

16 Cahill, G. F.: Pheochromocytomas, J.A.M.A. **138**:180-186, 1948.

17 Cahill, G. F., and Melicow, M. M.: Tumors of the adrenal gland, J. Urol. **64**:1-25, 1950.

18 Cahill, G. F., Melicow, M. M., and Darby, H. H.: Adrenal cortical tumors, Surg. Gynec. Obstet. **74**:281-305, 1942.

19 Cannon, J. F.: Pregnancy and pheochromocytoma, Obstet. Gynec. **2**:43-48, 1958.

20 Carman, C. T., and Brashear, R. E.: Pheochromocytoma as an inherited abnormality, New Eng. J. Med. **263**:419-423, 1960.

21 Cohen, E. L., Rovner, D. R., and Conn, J. W.: Postural augmentation of plasma renin activity; importance in diagnosis of renovascular hypertension, J.A.M.A. **197**:973-978, 1966.

22 Conn, J. W.: Primary aldosteronism; a new clinical syndrome, J. Lab. Clin. Med. **45**:661-664, 1955.

23 Conn, J. W., Knopf, R. F., and Nesbit, R. M.: Clinical characteristics of primary aldosteronism from an analysis of 145 cases, Amer. J. Surg. **107**:159-172, 1964.

24 Cottler, Z. R.: Nonhormonal adrenal cortical carcinoma; report of case with 5-year survival and relief of hypertension, J. Urol. **60**:363-370, 1948.

25 Crooke, A. C., and Callow, R. K.: The differential diagnosis of forms of basophilism (Cushing's syndrome) particularly by the estimation of urinary androgens, Quart. J. Med. **8**:233-249, 1939.

26 Cushing, H.: Basophil adenomas of the pituitary body and their clinical manifestations (pituitary basophilism), Bull. Hopkins Hosp. **50**:137-195, 1932.

27 Dahl-Iversen, E.: 18 phaeochromocytomas; clinical aspects and surgical results, Acta Chir. Scand. **116**:118-131, 1958.

28 Dargeon, H. W.: Problems in the prognosis of neuroblastoma, Amer. J. Roentgen. **83**:551-555, 1960.

29 Davignon, J., Tremblay, G., Nowaczynski, W., Koiw, E., and Genest, J.: Parallel biochemical and histochemical studies of an adrenocortical adenoma from a patient with primary aldosteronism, Acta Endocr. (Kobenhavn) **38**:207-219, 1961.

30 Davis, P., Peart, W. S., and van't Hoff, W.: Malignant phaeochromocytoma with functioning metastases, Lancet **2**:274-275, 1955.

31 Dean, R. E.: Pheochromocytoma and pregnancy, Obstet. Gynec. **11**:35-42, 1958.

32 Dorfman, R. I., Wilson, H. M., and Peters, J. P.: Differential diagnosis of basophilism and allied conditions, Endocrinology **27**:1-15, 1940.

33 Doub, H. P.: The roentgen aspect of sympathetic neuroblastoma, J.A.M.A. **109**:1188-1191, 1937.

34 Doust, B. C.: Anxiety as a manifestation of pheochromocytoma, Arch. Intern. Med. (Chicago) **102**:811-815, 1958.

35 Dunn, J. S.: Neuroblastoma and ganglioneuroma of the suprarenal body, J. Path. Bact. **19**:456-473, 1915.

36 Ekström, T., Ivemark, B., and Lagergren, C.: The vasculature of the adrenal gland in neoplasia and hyperplasia, Virchow Arch. Path. Anat. 343:189-196, 1968.

37 Farber, S.: American Pediatric Society Transactions, Amer. J. Dis. Child. 60:749-751, 1940.

38 Farquhar, J. W.: Phaeochromocytoma in childhood; case report and a brief review of 56 others recorded in the literature, J. Roy. Coll. Surg. Edinb. 3:301-310, 1958.

39 Fazekas, A. G., and Webb, J. L.: Personal communication, 1965.

40 Frew, R. S.: On carcinoma originating in the suprarenal medulla in children, Quart. J. Med. 4:123-140, 1910.

41 Fries, J. G., and Chamberlin, J. A.: Extra-adrenal pheochromocytoma: literature review and report of a cervical pheochromocytoma, Surgery 63:268-279, 1968.

42 Gabrilove, J. L., Sharma, D. C., Wotiz, H. H., and Dorfman, R. I.: Feminizing adrenocortical tumors in the male, Medicine (Balt.) 44:37-79, 1965.

43 Gaines, S. R.: Ocular changes in pheochromocytoma, Amer. J. Ophthal. 47:471-487, 1959.

44 Garrett, R. A.: Adrenal cortical carcinoma in children, J. Urol. 66:477-485, 1951.

45 Gilbert, J. W., Bell, N. H., and Bartter, F. C.: Primary aldosteronism; diagnosis and surgical treatment, Ann. Surg. 158:195-204, 1963.

46 Giroud, C. J., Stachenko, J., and Venning, E. H.: Secretion of aldosterone by the zona glomerulosa of rat adrenal glands incubated in vitro, Proc. Soc. Exp. Biol. Med. 92:154-158, 1956.

47 Glomset, D. A.: The incidence of metastasis of malignant tumors to the adrenals, Amer. J. Cancer 32:57-61, 1938.

48 Goldberg, M. B., Gordan, G. S., Deamer, W. C., and Hinman, F., Jr.: Mortality in surgically treated adrenocortical tumors. I. Report of three cases of Cushing's syndrome due to adrenocortical tumors, Postgrad. Med. 11:313-324, 1952.

49 Goldman, R. L., Winterling, A. N., and Wingerling, C. C.: Maturation of tumors of the sympathetic nervous system; report of long-term survival in 2 patients, one with disseminated osseous metastases and review of cases from the literature, Cancer 18:1510-1516, 1965.

50 Goldstein, M. N., Burdman, J. A., and Journey, L. J.: Long-term tissue culture of neuroblastoma. II. Morphologic evidence for differentiation and maturation, J. Nat. Cancer Inst. 32:165-199, 1964.

51 Goldzieher, M., and Koster, H.: Adrenal cortical hyperfunction, Amer. J. Surg. 27:93-106, 1935.

52 Graham, J. B.: Pheochromocytoma and hypertension; an analysis of 207 cases, Int. Abstr. Surg. 92:105-121, 1951; in Surg. Gynec. Obstet., Feb., 1951 (extensive bibliography).

53 Greenberg, R. E., and Gardner, L. K.: Pheochromocytoma in father and son; report of the eighth known affected kindred, J. Clin. Endocr. 19:351-362, 1959.

54 Greer, M., Anton, A. H., Williams, C. M., and Echevarria, R. A.: Tumors of neural crest origin, Arch. Neurol. (Chicago) 13:139-148, 1965.

55 Greer, W. E. R., Robertson, C. W., and Smithwick, R. H.: Pheochromocytoma; diagnosis, operative experiences, and clinical results, Amer. J. Surg. 107:192, 1964.

56 Gross, R. E.: The surgery of infancy and childhood, Philadelphia, 1953, W. B. Saunders Co.

57 Hain, A. M.: Adrenal tumours and pseudohermaphroditism; a hormone study of cases, J. Path. Bact. 59:267-292, 1947.

58 Hansman, C. F., and Girdany, B. R.: The roentgenographic findings associated with neuroblastoma, J. Pediat. 51:621-633, 1957.

59 Hartman, G. W., Witten, D. M., and Weeks, R. E.: The role of nephrotomography in the diagnosis of adrenal tumors, Radiology 86:1030-1034, 1966.

60 Hayles, A. B., Hahn, H. B., Jr., Sprague, R. G., Bahn, R. C., and Priestly J. T.: Hormone-secreting tumors of the adrenal cortex in children, Pediatrics 37:19-25, 1966.

61 Haymaker, W., and Anderson, E.: The syndrome arising from hyperfunction of the adrenal cortex; the adrenogenital and Cushing's syndromes—a review, Int. Clin. 4:244-299, 1938.

62 Healey, F. H., and Mekelatos, C. J.: Pheochromocytoma and neurofibromatosis, New Eng. J. Med. 258:540-543, 1958.

63 Heinbecker, P., O'Neal, L. W., and Ackerman, L. V.: Functioning and nonfunctioning adrenal cortical tumors, Surg. Gynec. Obstet. 105:21-33, 1957.

64 Hutchison, R.: On suprarenal sarcoma in children with metastasis in the skull, Quart. J. Med. 1:33-38, 1908.

65 Hutter, A. M., Jr., and Kayhoe, D. E.: Adrenal cortical carcinoma, Amer. J. Med. 41:572-580, 581-592, 1966.

66 Jelliffe, R. S.: Phaeochromocytoma presenting as a cardiac and abdominal catastrophe, Brit. Med. J. 2:76-77, 1952.

67 Kahn, P. C.: The radiologic identification of functioning adrenal tumors, Radiol. Clin. N. Amer. 5:221-230, 1967.

68 Kelsall, A. R., and Ross, E. J.: Bilateral pheochromocytoma in two sisters, Lancet 2:273-274, 1955.

69 Kerr, W. J., and Grodan, G. S.: Adrenal cortical carcinoma with excess androgen production in an adult man, Postgrad. Med. 11:278-283, 1952.

70 Kinsell, L. W., and Lisser, H.: Adrenal cortical tumor causing hirsutism without other evidence of virilization, J. Clin. Endocr. 12:50-54, 1952.

71 Kirschbaum, J. D., and Balkin, R. B.: Adrenalin producing pheochromocytoma of the adrenal associated with hypertension, Ann. Surg. 116:54-60, 1942.

72 Kissane, J. M., and Ackerman, L. V.: Maturation of tumours of the sympathetic nervous system, J. Fac. Radiol. 7:109-114, 1955.

73 Kolff, W. J., and Tjiook, K. B.: Hirsutism and virilism in a 5-year-old girl; remission following removal of adrenal carcinoma; recurrence after three and a half years, J. Clin. Endocr. 10:270-279, 1950.

74 Kvale, W. F., Bothe, C. M., Manger, W. M., and Priestley, J. T.: Present-day diagnosis and treatment of pheochromocytoma; a review of fifty cases, J.A.M.A. 164:854-861, 1957.

75 Labhart, A., Froesch, E. R., and Zieglaer, W.: Zur Diagnose und Therapie des Cushing-Syndroms, Schweiz. Med. Wschr. 89:44-52, 1959.

76 Lance, E. M., Cate, W. R., Liddle, G. W., and Scott, H. W.: Clinical experiences with pheochromocytoma, Surg. Gynec. Obstet. 106:25-37, 1958.

77 Lang, E. K.: The roentgenographic diagnosis of suprarenal masses, Radiology 87:35-45, 1966.

78 LeCompte, P. M.: Cushing's syndrome with possible pheochromocytoma, Amer. J. Path. 20:689-708, 1944.

79 Lehman, E. P.: Adrenal neuroblastoma in infancy—15-year survival, Amer. Surg. 95:473, 1932.

80 Lipsett, M. B., Hertz, R., and Ross, G. T.: Clinical and pathophysiologic aspects of adrenocortical carcinoma, Amer. J. Med. 35:374-383, 1963.

81 Lisser, H., and Player, L.: Follow-up report of a 5-year-old sexually precocious boy 20 years after removal of a malignant adrenal cortical tumor, Postgrad. Med. 11:267-271, 1952.

82 Louis, L. H., and Conn, J. W.: Primary aldosteronism—content of adrenocortical steroids in adrenal tissue, Recent Progr. Hormone Res. 17:415-436, 1961.

83 Loutfi, G. I., and Emerson, K., Jr.: Oestrogens in virilizing adrenal carcinoma, Acta Endocr. (Kobenhavn) 52:443-454, 1966.

84 Lukens, F. D. W., Flippin, H. F., and Thiguen, F. M.: Adrenal cortical adenoma with absence of opposite adrenal, Amer. J. Med. Sci. 193:812-820, 1937.

85 McFarland, J.: Ganglioneuroma of retroperitoneal origin, Arch. Path. (Chicago) 11:118-124, 1931.

86 McGavack, T. H.: Masculinizing and nonmasculinizing carcinomata of the cortex of the adrenal gland, Endocrinology 26:396-408, 1940.

87 Mandeville, F. B.: Calcification in sympathoblastoma (neuroblastoma), Radiology 53:403-405, 1949.

88 Marin, H. M., Graham, J. H., and Kickham, C. J. E.: Adrenal hematoma simulating tumor in newborn, Arch. Surg. (Chicago) 71:941-945, 1955.

89 Meaney, T. F., and Buonocore, E.: Selective arteriography as a localizing and provocative test in the diagnosis of pheochromocytoma, Radiology 87:309-314, 1966.

90 Meyers, M. A.: Characteristic radiographic shapes of pheochromocytomas and adrenocortical adenomas, Radiology 87:889-892, 1966.

91 Mikaelsson, C. G.: Retrograde phlebography of both adrenal veins, Acta Radiol. [Diagn.] (Stockholm) 6:348-354, 1967.

92 Miller, R. W., Fraumeni, J. F., and Hill, J. A.: Neuroblastoma; epidemiologic approach to its origin, Amer. J. Dis. Child. 115:253-261, 1968.

93 Minno, A. M., Bennett, W. A., and Kvale, W. F.: Pheochromocytoma; a study of 15 cases diagnosed at necropsy, New Eng. J. Med. 251:959-965, 1954.

94 Moore, T. C., and Shumacker, H. B., Jr.: Adrenalin producing tumors in childhood, Ann. Surg. 143:256-265, 1956.

95 Nelson, A. A.: Accessory adrenal cortical tissue, Arch. Path. (Chicago) 27:955-965, 1939.

96 Neville, A. M., and Symington, T.: Pathology of primary aldosteronism, Cancer 19:1854-1868, 1966.

97 Neville, A. M., and Symington, T.: The pathology of the adrenal gland in Cushing's syndrome, J. Path. Bact. 93:19-35, 1967.

98 Olesen, H., and Sjontoft, F.: Sympathicoblastomas with metastases to the orbit, Acta Ophthal. (Kobenhavn) 26:67-87, 1948.

99 O'Neal, L. W.: Pathologic anatomy in Cushing's syndrome, Ann. Surg. 160:860-869, 1964.

100 Palmer, R. S., and Castleman, B.: Paraganglioma (chromaffinoma, pheochromocytoma) of the adrenal gland simulating malignant hypertension, New Eng. J. Med. 219:793-796, 1938.

101 Pampari, D. and Lacerenzo, C.: Intrathoracic pheochromocytoma, J. Thorac. Surg. 36:174-181, 1958.

102 Pasqualini, J. R.: Conversion of tritiated-18-hydroxy-corticosterone to aldosterone by slices of human cortico-adrenal glands and adrenal tumour, Nature (London) 201:501, 1964.

103 Pepper, W.: A study of congenital sarcoma of the liver and suprarenal, Amer. J. Med. Sci. 121:287-299, 1901.

104 Perez, C. A., Vietti, T., Ackerman, L. V., Eagleton, M. D., and Powers, W. E.: Tumors of the sympathetic nervous system in children; an appraisal of treatment and results, Radiology 88:750-760, 1967.

105 Perez, C. A., Vietti, T. J., Ackerman, L. V., Kulapongs, P., and Powers, W. E.: Treatment of malignant sympathetic tumors in children; clinicopathological correlation, Pediatrics 41:452-462, 1968.

106 Philips, B.: Intrathoracic pheochromocytoma, Arch. Path. (Chicago) 30:916-921, 1940.

107 Pinkel, D., Pratt, C., Holton, C., James, D., Jr., Wrenn, E., Jr., and Hustu, O.: Survival of children with neuroblastoma treated with combination chemotherapy, J. Pediat. 73:928-931, 1968.

108 Rankin, F. W., and Wellbrook, W. L. A.: Tumors of the carotid body; report of 12 cases including one of bilateral tumor, Ann. Surg. 93:801-810, 1931.

109 Rapaport, E., Goldberg, M. B., Gordan, G. S., and Hinman, F., Jr.: Mortality in surgically treated adrenocortical tumors. II. Review of cases reported for the 20 year period 1930-1949, inclusive, Postgrad. Med. **11**:325-353, 1952.

110 Riddell, D. H., Schull, L. G., First, T. F., and Baker, T. D.: Experience with pheochromocytoma in 21 patients; use of Dichloroisoproterenol hydrochloride for cardiac arrhythmia, Ann. Surg. **157**:980-988, 1963.

111 Robinson, R., Smith, P., and Whittaker, S. R. F.: Secretion of catecholamines in malignant phaeochromocytoma, Brit. Med. J. **1**: 1422-1424, 1964.

112 Rossi, P.: Arteriography in adrenal tumors, Brit. J. Radiol. **41**:81-98, 1968.

113 Rouvière, H.: Anatomie des lymphatiques de l'homme, Paris, 1932, Masson et Cie.

114 Rowland, R. P., and Weber, P. F.: Growth of the left testicle with precocious sexual and bodily development (macro-genitosomia), Guy Hosp. Rep. **79**:401-408, 1929.

115 Sarosi, G., and Doe, R. P.: Familial occurrence of parathyroid adenomas, pheochromocytoma, and medullary carcinoma of the thyroid with amyloid stroma (Sipple's syndrome), Ann. Intern. Med. **68**:1305-1309, 1968.

116 Schteingart, D. E., Oberman, H. A., Friedman, B. A., and Conn, J. W.: Adrenal cortical neoplasms producing Cushing's syndrome; a clinicopathologic study, Cancer **22**:1005-1013, 1968.

117 Scott, H. W., Jr., Foster, J. H., Liddle, G., and Davidson, E. T.: Cushing's syndrome due to adrenocortical tumor, Ann. Surg. **162**: 505-516, 1965.

118 Sherman, R. S., and Leaming, R.: The roentgen findings in neuroblastoma, Radiology **60**: 837-849, 1953.

119 Sherwin, R. P.: Histopathology of pheochromocytoma, Cancer **12**:861-877, 1959 (extensive bibliography).

120 Siebenman, R. E.: Zur hokalisation der aldosteronbildung in der menschlichen nebennierenrinde, Schweiz. Med. Wschr. **89**:837-841, 1959.

121 Skanse, B., Moller, F., Gydell, K., Johansson, S., and Wulff, H. B.: Observations on primary aldosteronism, Acta Med. Scand. **158**: 181-194, 1957.

122 Smithwick, R. H., Greer, W. E. R., Robertson, C. W., and Wilkins, R. W.: Pheochromocytoma; a discussion of symptoms, signs and procedures of diagnostic value, New Eng. J. Med. **242**:252-257, 1950.

123 Smits, M., and Huizinga, J.: Familial occurrence of phaeochromocytoma, Acta Genet. (Basel) **11**:137-153, 1961.

124 Snyder, C. H., and Vick, E. H.: Hypertension in children caused by pheochromocytoma, Amer. J. Dis. Child. **73**:581-601, 1947.

125 Soffer, L. J.: Clinical manifestations of adrenal cortical hyperfunction, Bull. N. Y. Acad. Med. **23**:479-493, 1947.

125a Stella, J. G., Schweisguth, O., and Schlienger, M.: Neuroblastoma; a study of 144 cases treated in the Institut Gustave-Roussy over a period of 7 years, Amer. J. Roentgen. **108**: 324-332, 1970.

126 Talbot, N. B., Berman, R. A., MacLachlan, E. A., and Wolfe, J. K.: The colorimetric determination of neutral steroids (hormones) in a 24-hour sample of human urine (pregnanediol; total, alpha and beta alcoholic, and non-alcoholic 17-ketosteroids), J. Clin. Endocr. **1**:668-673, 1941.

127 Thomas, J. E., Rooke, E. D., and Kvale, W. F.: The neurologist's experience with pheochromocytoma, J.A.M.A. **197**:754-758, 1966.

128 Thorn, G. W., Forsham, P. H., and Emerson, K., Jr.: The diagnosis and treatment of adrenal insufficiency, ed. 2, pub. no. 29, American Lecture Series, monograph in American Lectures in Endocrinology, edited by Willard O. Thompson, Springfield, Ill., 1951, Charles C Thomas, Publisher.

129 Thurman, W. G., and Donaldson, M. H.: Cyclophosphamide (NSC-26271) therapy for children with neuroblastoma, Cancer Chemother. Rep. **51**:399-401, 1967.

130 Tresidder, G. C.: Tumors of the adrenal medulla, Brit. J. Urol. **35**:367, 1963.

131 Wahl, H. R., and Craig, P. E.: Multiple tumors of the sympathetic nervous system, Amer. J. Path. **14**:797-808, 1938.

132 Weinberg, T., and Radman, H. M.: Fetal dystocia due to neuroblastoma of the adrenals with metastases to the liver, Amer. J. Obstet. Gynec. **46**:440-444, 1943.

133 Weinberger, L. M., and Grant, F. C.: Precocious puberty and tumors of the hypothalamus, Arch. Intern. Med. (Chicago) **67**:762-792, 1941.

134 Wilkins, L.: A feminizing adrenal tumor causing gynecomastia in a boy of five years contrasted with a virilizing tumor in a five-year-old girl, J. Clin. Endocr. **8**:111-132, 1948.

135 Williams, C. M., and Greer, M.: Homovanillic acid and vanilmandelic acid in diagnosis of neuroblastoma, J.A.M.A. **183**:836-840, 1963.

136 Wittenborg, M. H.: Roentgen therapy in neuroblastoma; a review of seventy-three cases, Radiology **54**:679-688, 1950.

137 Wood, K. F., Lees, F., and Rosenthal, F. D.: Carcinoma of the adrenal cortex without endocrine effects, Brit. J. Surg. **45**:41-48, 1957.

138 Wotiz, H. H., Chattoraj, S. C., and Gabriloveo, J. L.: Urinary estrogen titers in a patient with feminizing adrenocortical carcinoma, J. Clin. Endocr. **28**:192-197, 1968.

139 Wyatt, G. M., and Farber, S.: Neuroblastoma sympatheticum, Amer. J. Roentgen. **46**:485-495, 1941.

Chapter 14

Cancer of the female genital organs

Ovary

Endometrium

Cervix (including cervical
stump and cervix and
pregnancy)

Vagina

Vulva

Ovary

Anatomy

The ovaries are situated on each side of the pelvis behind the broad ligament and the fallopian tubes and 1.5 cm to 2 cm in front of the sacroiliac symphysis. They have a somewhat flattened ovoid form and during genital life have a pink color and deep crevices. After the menopause, the ovaries have a tendency to become atrophied, sclerotic, and smooth. They are attached to the posterior aspect of the broad ligaments by the meso-ovarium and to the uterus medially by the utero-ovarian ligament, but the most important means of fixation is the suspensor ligament, which connects the ovary with the pelvic wall.

Lymphatics. The lymphatics of the ovary form a rich network that surrounds the graafian follicles. The collecting trunks follow an upward direction with the utero-ovarian vessels, cross the external iliac vessels, and reach the level of the lower pole of the kidney, where they turn medially, cross in front of the ureter, and terminate in the lumboaortic lymph nodes. Normally, the intersection with the ureter is found higher on the left than on the right. Also on the left side, the lymphatic trunks are more compact and terminate in a closely related group of nodes under the kidney pedicle. On the right side, the lymphatics become separated toward the end and diverge to terminate in precaval and

laterocaval nodes that may be found from the kidney pedicle down to the termination of the aorta (Rouvière[137]). In addition, another collecting trunk has been described (Marcille[95]) that is not constant (Fig. 548). This trunk follows a lateral direction in the broad ligaments to terminate in the nodes of the external iliac chain.

Epidemiology

In the 1947 cancer survey in the United States, the sex-age adjusted incidence of cancer of the ovary was 14.7 for white and 9.9 for nonwhite females per 100,000 population. The relative incidence in women 35 to 39 years old is under 10 per 100,000, rises with every decade to reach a height of over 50 per 100,000 in women 65 to 69 years old, and declines in the later decades. The surveys in both New York and Connecticut reveal an approximate 15% increase from the late 1940's to the early 1960's. The relative frequency increases with age, and most cases (50% to 60%) are found in patients 40 to 59 years of age (Allan and Hertig[4]).

There is one carcinoma for every five or six ovarian tumors (Taylor[162]). Allan and Hertig[4] found 265 carcinomas in a series of 1750 ovarian neoplasms, or an occurrence of 15%, whereas Randall[131] studied 897 ovarian neoplasms, 353 of which were malignant. Carcinomas of the ovary may be found in the second decade

713

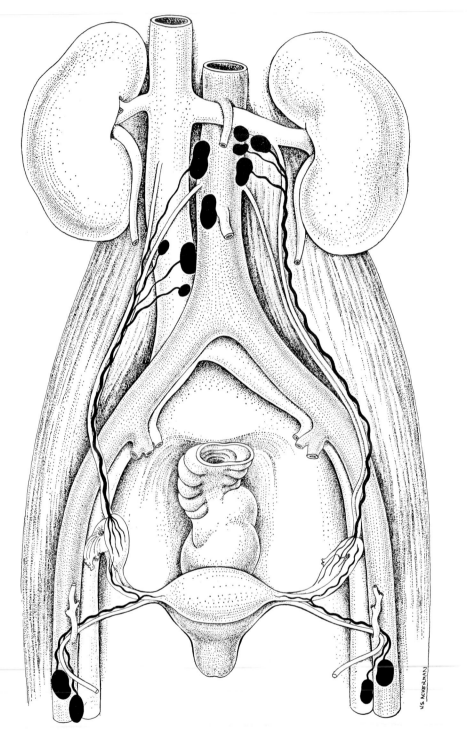

Fig. 548. Lymphatics of ovary showing drainage by para-aortic lymph nodes. On right, draining nodes extend from kidney pedicle to termination of aorta. There is also inconstant drainage toward external iliac nodes.

of life, but they are relatively rare before the age of 20 years. Dysgerminomas predominate in patients under 30 years of age, with over 6% found in the first decade of life, whereas thecomas are never seen before menarche. Rare instances of ovarian carcinomas in several members of the same family have been reported (Liber[79]).

Pathology
Gross and microscopic pathology

A knowledge of the embryology of the ovary is necessary for an understanding of the development of ovarian tumors. The following brief summary of the histogenesis of the ovary is based upon the excellent studies of Witschi,[182] Gillman,[45] and Pinkerton et al.[126]

The primordial germ cells are first seen in the thirteen-somite (3.5 mm) embryo in the yolk sac endoderm adjacent to the allantoic evagination (Witschi[182]). These cells move along the endoderm of the yolk sac into the gut, through the mesenteric mesenchyme, and into the mesonephric ridge by the eighth week. Although the mechanism of this migration is not entirely clear, the germ cells may be clearly recognized during this period both cytologically and by their characteristic histochemical staining for alkaline phosphatase and glycogen (Pinkerton et al.[126]). There is considerable mitotic proliferation from the eighth through the twentieth weeks, following which maturation begins, with gradual loss of histochemical activity. The coelomic mesoblasts overlying the developing gonad produce cordlike growths (or tubules) of mesenchymal cells that cluster about the enlarging germ cells and proliferate, forming a multilayered granulosa. There is no evidence that the surface epithelium ever produces germ cells. The stroma cells originate from the connective tissue that accompanies the blood vessels into the ovary during the twenty-eighth week. The theca cells develop from those stroma cells in contact with a growing follicle. When the developmental patterns of these cells are understood, many tumor variations such as granulosa cell tumors with tubular structures or the occurrence of granulosa and theca cells together in any proportion might well be anticipated (Gillman[45]).

Classification

The ovary is an extremely complex structure, having an intricate embryologic development with many details still imperfectly understood (Hertig and Gore[54]). Since there is no complete agreement on the histogenesis of many of the normally occurring structures in the ovary, it is not surprising that the histogenesis of the varied tumors arising from these structures should be controversial. We are in agreement with the concept that tumors with hormone production should be classified on a morphologic basis rather than according to their endocrine effects. These endocrine effects may vary within different lesions with the same appearance (Morris and Scully[105]) (Table 75). In some metastatic tumors of the ovary, endocrine function may be the result of ovarian stromal changes apparently unrelated to the type of tumor present (Scully and Richardson[149]).

The following classification* includes some recent concepts especially in the classification of gonadal stroma tumors (Morris and Scully[105]; Teilum[166]; Mostofi et al.[106]). It is not fundamentally different from classifications in recent monographs on this subject (Hertig and Gore[54]; Morris and Scully[105]; Abell[2]).

A Tumors of surface (müllerian) epithelial origin
  1 Serous cystomas and cystadenocarcinomas
  2 Mucinous cystomas and cystadenocarcinomas
  3 Endometrioid carcinomas and cystadenocarcinomas
  4 Brenner tumors
  5 Mesonephric tumors
B Tumors of germ cell origin
  1 Germinomas: dysgerminomas (and choriocarcinomas, endodermal sinus tumors, gonadoblastomas, embryonal carcinomas, etc.)
  2 Teratomas (cystic teratomas, solid teratomas, and teratocarcinomas)
C Tumors of ovarian stroma
  1 Granulosa–theca cell tumors
  2 Sertoli–Leydig cell tumors (arrhenoblastomas)

---

*Slightly modified from Ackerman, L. V. (in collaboration with Butcher, H. R., Jr.): Surgical pathology, ed. 4, St. Louis, 1968, The C. V. Mosby Co.

Table 75. Comparative data on ovarian tumors

Origin	Type of tumor		Endocrine effect	% all benign tumors	% all malignant tumors	% bilateral
Surface (müllerian) epithelium	Serous cystoma Serous cystadenocarcinoma	Benign 50% Malignant 50%	Rare	20	45	50
Surface (müllerian) epithelium	Mucinous cystoma Mucinous cystadenocarcinoma	Benign 90% Malignant 10%	Rare	25	10	5 20
Surface (müllerian) epithelium	Endometrioid carcinoma and adenoacanthoma (so-called)		Usually none	—	15	
Surface (müllerian) epithelium	Brenner tumor		Rare	1	—	5
Surface (müllerian) epithelium	Mesonephric clear cell carcinoma		Usually none	—	< 1	5*
Germ cell	Dysgerminoma (and choriocarcinoma, embryonal carcinoma, endodermal sinus tumor)		Uncommon	—	4	20
Germ cell	Gonadoblastoma		Usually masculinizing	?*	?*	?50*
Germ cell	Teratoma, cystic	Benign 97% Malignant 3%	Rare	15	1	12
Ovarian stroma	Granulosa cell tumor		Usually estrinism	?*	4-10	5
Ovarian stroma	Thecoma		Usually estrinism	3	< 1*	< 1
Ovarian stroma	Sertoli–Leydig cell tumors (androblastoma, Teilum; arrhenoblastoma, Meyer)		Usually masculinizing	< 1*	< 1*	< 5
Ovarian stroma	Lipid cell tumors (includes tumors of aberrant adrenal cortex as well as those Leydig cell and lutein cell tumors that may be morphologically indistinguishable from adrenal cortical cells)		Usually masculinizing	< 1*	< 1*	?*
Nonintrinsic stroma	Fibroma Fibrosarcoma		None	30 —	— < 1	30*
Undetermined	Carcinoma, unclassified		Usually none	—	5-10	> 50
Metastatic adenocarcinoma, especially stomach	Krukenberg tumor		Uncommon	—	< 2	100

*Insufficient data available for accurate figures.

3 Lipid cell tumors
4 Mixed and indeterminate types
D Nonintrinsic stromal tumors—fibromas
E Metastatic carcinoma
F Undifferentiated carcinoma

The percentage of all benign tumors in serous and mucinous neoplasms will be influenced by the pathologist's viewpoint. If he is conservative, then the percentage of all benign tumors must rise. On the other hand, if he calls all granulosa cell tumors malignant and interprets slight variations from the benign pattern in mucinous cystoma and serous cystoma as carcinoma, then the percentage of benign tumors must fall. How many carcinomas are unclassified depends upon the pathologist's knowledge of ovarian tumors, the thoroughness of the examination, and his ego.

To some extent, the *serous and mucinous tumors* are similar, and it is important to know the distinguishing gross characteristics (Table 76). The serous variety pre-

Table 76. Differential characteristics of serous and mucinous tumors of ovary

	Serous	*Mucinous*
Frequency	Benign varieties about equal in frequency; malignant types predominantly serous	
Bilateral	50%	5% in benign (20% in malignant)
Size	Moderate	Often huge
Character of fluid	Transudate	Slimy, viscid
Malignant	High percentage	Low percentage
Tendency to metastasize to regional and distant lymph nodes in malignant variant	High percentage	Low percentage
Tendency to implant	High percentage	Relatively frequent
Microscopic characteristics	Cuboidal	High columnar, basally situated nucleus
Cilia	Often present	Never present
Psammoma bodies	Frequent in well-differentiated types	Never present

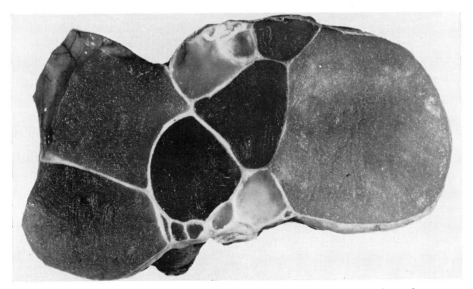

Fig. 549. Serous cystoma of ovary. Specimen frozen and then sectioned to demonstrate loculation.

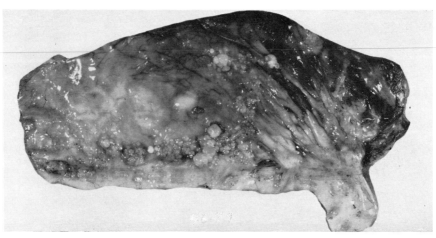

Fig. 550. Inner aspect of benign serous cystoma of ovary with typical small nodular growths.

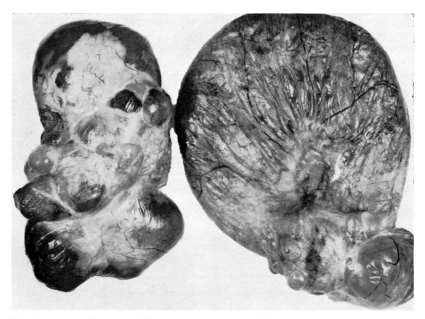

Fig. 551. Bilateral moderate-sized benign serous cystoma of ovaries.

sents characteristic loculations (Fig. 549) and papillary burgeoning outgrowths that are usually seen growing within the wall of the cyst (Fig. 550), on its surface, or on the peritoneum (Fig. 551). When the mucinous tumor grows in the peritoneum, it forms large masses of gelatinous tumor resembling frog spawn. The fluid of the serous tumor has the characteristics of a transudate, whereas that of the mucinous variety has a viscid, slimy quality. Both of these cystic tumors are moderate in size and freely movable and lie mostly out-

side of the pelvis (Fig. 552). Torsion of the pedicle occurs more frequently in the benign than in the malignant tumors of the ovary because the malignant variety quickly becomes fixed.

Microscopically, there are many variants of the serous cystoma (Taylor and Greeley[163]). The predominantly fibrous serous cystoma with very little epithelial element is invariably benign (Timonen and Purola[174]) (Fig. 553). This tumor tends to become more cellular, and since the acini show layering of the cells, it may be dif-

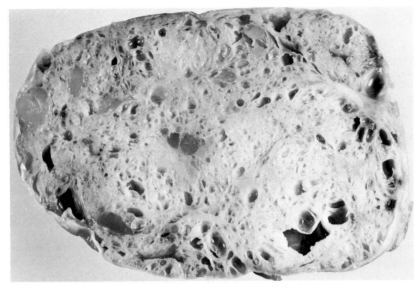

Fig. 552. Typical mucinous cystoma of ovary. (WU neg. 69-14.)

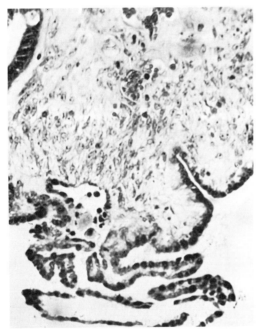

Fig. 553. Fibrous type of serous cystoma of ovary that is invariably benign. (Low-power enlargement.)

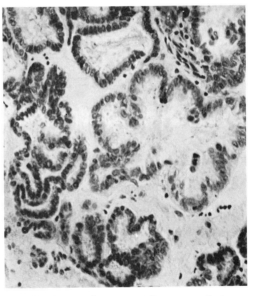

Fig. 554. Intermediate type of serous cystic tumor of ovary that usually behaves in benign fashion. (Moderate enlargement.)

ficult to determine whether it is benign or malignant (Fig. 554). Cilia are often seen in the serous variety, and psammoma bodies are plentiful in the more differentiated forms. This tumor is very frequently bilateral, but whether it arises spontane-ously in both ovaries or metastasizes from one to the other is hard to determine.

The mucinous tumor shows very tall, single-layer columnar cells with clear cyto-plasm and basally situated nuclei (Fig. 556). When it becomes malignant, the cells undergo stratification, there is variation in nuclear size and shape with many mitotic figures, and the tumor tends to invade the

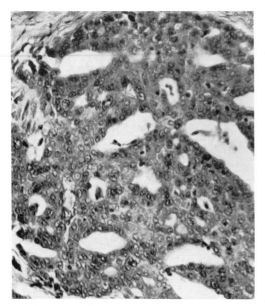

Fig. 555. Serous cystadenocarcinoma of ovary, obviously malignant. (Moderate enlargement.)

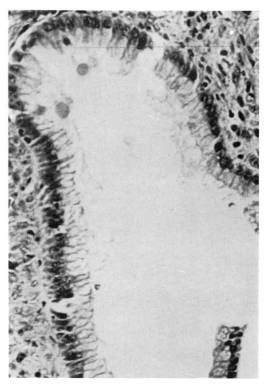

Fig. 556. Mucinous cystadenoma of ovary with tall columnar cells and basally situated nuclei. (Moderate enlargement.)

wall of the cyst. It does not form psammoma bodies or have cilia. The term pseudomucinous has always been used, but from the histochemical standpoint this name is incorrect. The correct term is mucinous cystadenoma (Fisher[39]). Both serous and mucinous neoplasms may present areas of necrosis, hemorrhage, infarction or torsion because of an excessively rapid growth.

Endometrioid carcinoma used to be considered a rare neoplasm, but Santesson[142] presented evidence in 1961 that this was a frequent ovarian tumor. In a review of 1274 primary malignant ovarian tumors, Santesson and Kottmeier[143a] reported 288 (22.5%) endometrioid carcinomas. Long and Taylor[83] found 17% in their series to be endometrioid. The gross pattern is nondiagnostic, but the microscopic pattern is that of primary carcinoma of the endometrium. There may be areas of squamous metaplasia (adenoacanthoma) (Fig. 557). According to Gricouroff,[48] primary ovarian tumors may arise from the epithelial or stromal manifestations of endometriosis, but, he feels that the histologic criteria are not sufficient to decide on the endometriotic origin. Gricouroff[48a] noted also that adenocarcinomas of the ovary have the same morphologic diversity as those arising from the endometrium. Scully and Barlow[147] have produced evidence that the ovarian "mesonephroma" is closely related to endometrioid tumors.

Brenner tumor, almost always unilateral and benign, may be very small or may grow slowly to weigh 15 pounds. However, Abell[1] reported three cases of malignant Brenner tumor and found nine other instances in the literature. The tumor is fairly firm and on cut section suggests a fibroma except for the yellowish tint to its surface. Gaines[43] observed small cavities (0.1 cm to 2 cm) containing opaque, viscid, yellow-brown fluid. At times, this tumor is solid and is situated in the wall of a cyst (usually pseudomucinous). Jondahl et al.[62] reported on thirty-one Brenner tumors. Nine of these were 1 cm or less in diameter, and five were found in the hilus of the ovaries. Meyer[100] and Reagan[132] believe that the Brenner tumors arise from the sexually indifferent cell inclusions described by Walthard, but Teoh[170] presented evidence that the Brenner tumors are of follic-

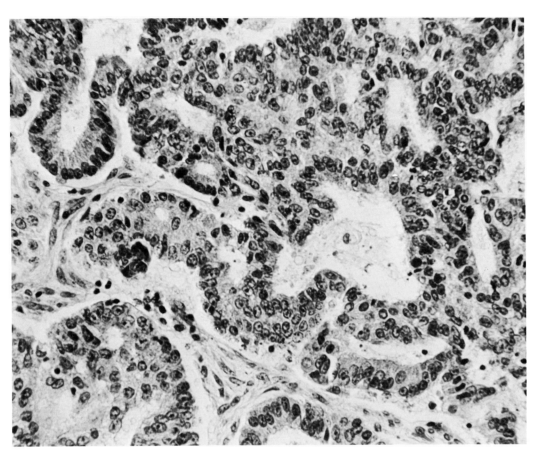

Fig. 557. Classic endometrioid carcinoma of ovary. Its pattern is that of endometrial carcinoma. (WU neg. 69-31.)

ular origin. Arey[8] serially sectioned and reconstructed two specimens of Brenner tumor and believed he demonstrated their origin from the so-called germinal epithelium of the ovarian surface. In the series reported by Jondahl et al.,[62] four tumors arose in the wall of a pseudomucinous cyst, two in the walls of a benign teratoma, and one in the wall of a malignant teratoma. The tumor is composed of abundant connective tissue with islands of compact polyhedral epithelial cells that have a characteristic longitudinal grooving or folding of their nuclei (Arey[7]) presenting no mitosis (Fig. 558). Novak and Jones[119] emphasized that this combination of epithelial cells and connective tissue framework must be present in order to make a diagnosis of Brenner tumor. There is some tendency to cystic degeneration of the epithelial nests, and the cells may take on a columnar appearance with a mucoid se-

cretion. Novak and Jones[119] and Meyer[100] believe that a small proportion of pseudomucinous cysts may originate in Brenner tumors. Brenner tumors contain no fat but do contain glycogen and invariably mucin. Granulosa cell tumors contain fat but no glycogen or mucin (Fox[41]).

Brenner tumors that show lipoid material in the stromal cells may produce estrogens (Kecskés and Szabó[65]). In a series of 402 Brenner tumors, thirty (7.5%) showed possible estrogen production arising from thecalike cells in the stroma (Farrar et al.[34]).

Germinomas are tumors of embryonal cells that resemble the immature germ cells of the developing gonad. Although the most common form is the dysgerminoma which resembles the testicular seminomas, rare tumors such as embryonal carcinoma, choriocarcinoma, and endodermal sinus tumor (Teilum[169]) have been

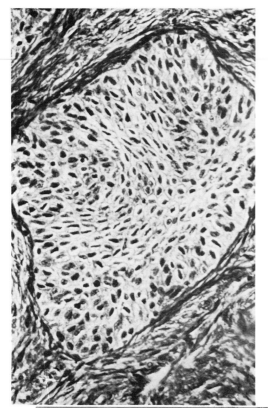

described. In addition, occasional tumors resembling dysgerminomas may contain elements of granulosa and theca cell origin also and have been designated gonadoblastomas (Scully[146]). Scully[146a] has reviewed seventy-four cases of gonadoblastoma; this tumor occurs always in sexually abnormal patients. Androgen production occurred in some tumors. Germinomas and occasionally other types of invasive germ cell tumors can develop from this neoplasm.

Dysgerminomas are often large, bilateral (about 25%), and apparently more common in the right ovary. Their surface is smooth and somewhat bosselated, and there is a resemblance to cerebral convolutions. They are soft and have a thin, smooth capsule (Fig. 559). On section, they are cellular and gray, and areas of hemorrhage and necrosis are common. Dysgerminomas probably arise from undiffer-

Fig. 558. Brenner tumor of ovary with typical well-delineated collection of epithelial cells. (Moderate enlargement.)

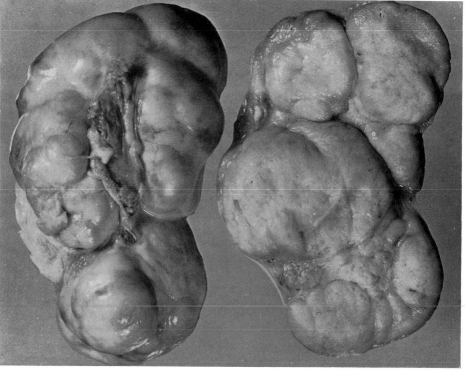

Fig. 559. Classic gross appearance of large dysgerminoma. External surface resembles convolutions of brain. (WU neg. 55-5537.)

entiated embryonic cells of the genital ridge (Meyer[100]). The individual cells are large with big nuclei, clear cytoplasm, and rather prominent nucleoli (Fig. 560). At times, a tuberculoid reaction of the stroma occurs and epithelioid and giant cells are seen, but this reaction is undoubtedly inflammatory and nonspecific (Heller[52]). Lymphoid infiltration of the stroma is prominent. It now appears that the dysgerminoma is a malignant neoplasm, and benign variants do not exist. The histologic appearance and behavior of dysgerminomas are somewhat similar to the seminoma. These tumors may be associated with gonadotropin excretion (Hobson and Baird[55]). They tend to recur, however, and it is certain that their malignancy is often underestimated because of short follow-up. A rare tumor with elements of both dysgerminoma and sex cord mesenchyme has been described by Scully.[146]

Fathalla et al.[37] studied the relationship between ovarian tumors and intersex states with special reference to dysgerminoma

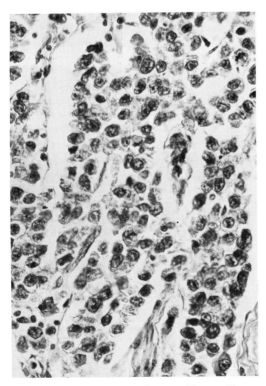

Fig. 560. Dysgerminoma of ovary. Note uniformity of cells and cordlike arrangement. (High power.)

and arrhenoblastoma. They found that two tumors originally reported as arrhenoblastomas were, in reality, testicular tubular adenomas replacing the undescended testes of genetic males with a testicular feminization syndrome. These patients also may have an increased risk of seminoma, perhaps because of the ectopic position of the testis. They concluded that no dysgerminoma arising in an intersex patient has been proved to arise in ovarian tissue. Gonadoblastomas occur in dysgenetic gonads of intersex patients who tend to look like masculinized females with primary amenorrhea. All of these tumors have been benign (Teter and Boczkonski[172]).

Teratomas may be cystic or solid. The *cystic teratoma* is sometimes designated as a dermoid cyst, but is more logically called a teratoma because it so frequently contains elements from all three embryologic layers. It has a smooth, shiny surface and, as a rule, does not attain a large size (average, 8 cm). Before surgical removal, the contents are fluid, but after removal the cyst wall becomes wrinkled and dry and the contents semisolid. On section, the cysts characteristically contain yellow, greasy material in which teeth may be found (Fig. 561). Hair is often present and may be of several colors in the same cyst. There is usually a white, shiny, unilocular protuberance in one part of the cyst. About 12% of these tumors are bilateral. Rarely, malignant transformation may be observed in a teratoma of the ovary, the most common form being squamous cell carcinoma. Alznauer[5] collected from the medical literature sixty-three acceptable cases of squamous cell carcinoma in teratomas. Peterson[125] found 147 carcinomas in a collected group of 8038 cystic teratomas (1.8%). Malignant change is twice as common in postmenopausal women (Malkasian et al.[90]). *Solid teratomas* of the ovary are rare, and 75% are malignant. Rarely, the elements within the tumor may appear to be completely benign (Thurlbeck and Scully[173]).

The origin of teratomas remains in doubt. Willis[181] believes that these are true neoplasms arising from foci of embryonic pluripotential tissue that escaped the primary organizer influence during early development. This escape would be in some

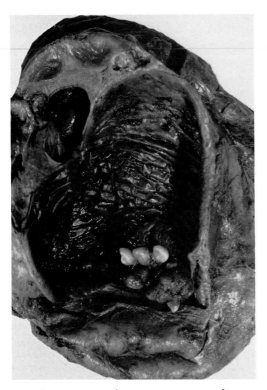

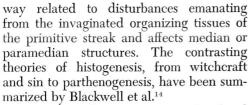

Fig. 561. Section of ovarian teratoma showing three teeth attached to rudimentary mandible.

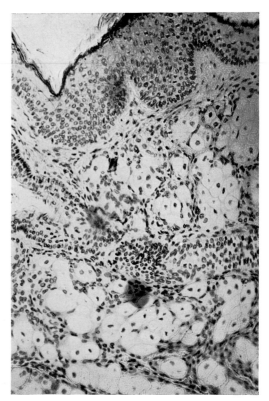

Fig. 562. Teratoma of ovary showing lining, squamous epithelium, hair follicles, and innumerable sebaceous glands. (Low-power enlargement.)

way related to disturbances emanating from the invaginated organizing tissues of the primitive streak and affects median or paramedian structures. The contrasting theories of histogenesis, from witchcraft and sin to parthenogenesis, have been summarized by Blackwell et al.[14]

Microscopically, teratomas are often lined throughout by stratified epithelium (resembling that of the skin) that very commonly contains sebaceous glands from which much of the greasy material emanates. Other skin appendages are commonly present (Fig. 562). All types of tissue can be found within a teratoma. In a large series of cases reported by Blackwell et al.,[14] 100% contained elements of ectoderm, 93% contained mesoderm, and 71% contained entoderm (Fig. 563). Plaut[127] studied three struma ovarii biologically and proved that they represented true functioning thyroid tissue. Struma ovarii may show the changes found in a nodular goiter, hyperplasia, or carcinoma (Emge[31]).

Teratomas may show an overgrowth of one element and become carcinoma, which is most frequently squamous in nature, but many types of malignant tumors arising from other elements have been reported. These rare malignant tumors include choriocarcinoma (Marrubini[97]), sweat gland carcinomas, malignant melanoma, and carcinoid tumors. Carcinoid tumors arising within the ovary in association with teratomas may have the dramatic carcinoid syndrome (increased production of serotonin, p. 472) (Ruckles and Stallkamp[139]). Eight cases have been reported (Nissen[113]).

Granulosa–theca cell tumors are discussed together because they have a common ancestry and because an increasing number of cases are being reported in which elements of both are found in the same tumor. The stromal cells of the ovary include the follicular granulosa cells, the surrounding theca cells, and large masses of unspecialized stromal cells that form the bulk of the tissue surrounding the ova

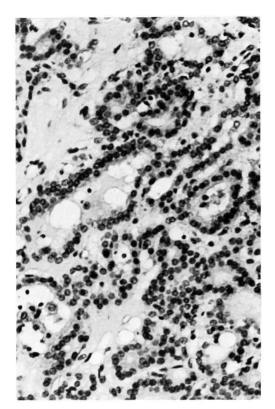

Fig. 563. Struma ovarii in teratoma of ovary. (Moderate enlargement.)

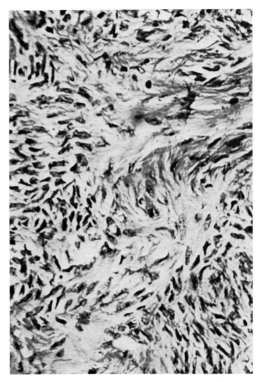

Fig. 564. Thecoma of ovary, with hyaline plaques and typical arrangement of cells. (Moderate enlargement.)

and follicles. Kempson[66] has shown that ovarian stroma is composed of two types of cells with ultrastructural characteristics similar to those found in Sertoli–Leydig cell, theca cell, and lipid cell tumors. A variety of tumors occurring in the ovary resemble the patterns produced by stroma during embryogenesis of both ovary and testis (Teilum[168]; Mostofi et al.[106]). Whether granulosa–theca cell tumors arise from the ovarian stroma or from the theca and granulosa cells that have differentiated from it is debatable.

The gross characteristics of granulosa and theca cell tumors are considerably different. The thecomas are usually benign and unilateral and do not reach a large size, measuring between 5 cm and 10 cm. These tumors are firm and on cut section the most important point in their differentiation from fibromas is the presence of small yellowish areas averaging 2 mm (Plate 3). The larger tumors tend to be edematous and cystic. Microscopic exami-

nation reveals large amounts of connective tissue with small, abundant hyaline plaques (Fig. 564), and if the tumor is stained by fat with sudan III, large amounts of intracellular, sudanophilic material are observed. Differential staining for various fat fractions has been shown by Wolfe and Neigus[183] to be of value. This fat represents an increase in cholesterol and cholesterol esters. Stromal hyperplasia is prominent in the nonneoplastic ovarian tissues. Sternberg and Gaskill[156] believe that this is the soil in which thecomas develop.

The granulosa cell tumor is a relatively common ovarian neoplasm. It is usually classified with malignant or solid ovarian tumors, and it is estimated to make up at least 10% of this group. Usually it is of moderate size, but very large granulosa cell tumors have been described.

Granulosa–theca cell tumors are bilateral in about 5% of the patients. On section, the tumor is cellular, and areas of hemorrhage and necrosis are frequent (Plate 3). Luteinization is not infrequent and gives the tumor a yellowish cast. Microscopically, a granulosa cell tumor may have a folliculoid, cylindroid, or sarcomatoid appearance. All these variants can coexist in the same tumor in different areas. Individual cells infrequently show mitotic figures.

Of fifty-one granulosa cell tumors reported by Nordén and Dahlberg,[115] twelve contained not only typical granulosa, but also tubular and cordlike structures such as those described as typical of arrhenoblastomas. These tumors are often divided into benign and malignant varieties, but the designation of malignant is often based on behavior rather than on microscopic pattern. It would seem more logical to consider them all as potentially malignant.

The theca cells are surrounded by reticulin, but no reticulin can be demonstrated surrounding granulosa and lutein cells. The granulosa cells contain argentaffin granules (Dockerty[27]). These differences may not always hold true (Knight[72]; Sternberg[155]). Special fat stains (Hoerr[56]) may reveal different types of fat. Traut et al.[175] believe that the hormone activity of these tumors is somewhat parallel to the phospholipid and free cholesterol content. McKay et al.[88] have done histochemical studies in granulosa cell tumors which indicate that the thecoma cell component of such tumors is the estrogen-secreting element rather than the granulosa cell. It is concluded that histochemical studies are capable of differentiating active thecomas from inactive ones and from fibromas. Luteinized stroma cells were demonstrated in the ovarian cortex of six of eighteen patients with thecoma (Nordén and Dahlberg[115]).

Both the granulosa cell and the theca cell tumors are associated with hyper-

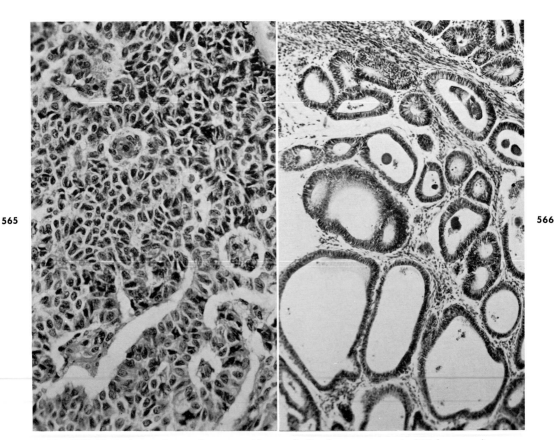

Fig. 565. Typical granulosa cell tumor with pseudoalveolar arrangement. (High power.)

Fig. 566. Cystic hyperplasia of endometrium occurring in conjunction with granulosa cell tumor.

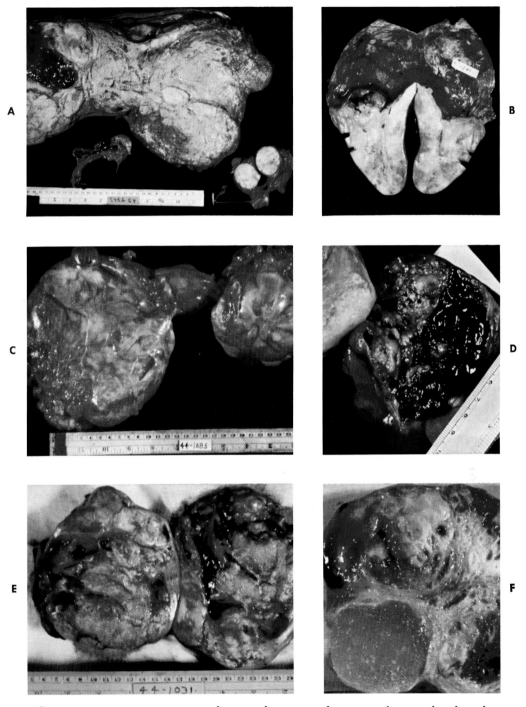

Plate 3. A, Leiomyosarcoma arising from intraligamentous leiomyoma that was thought to be carcinoma of ovary. **B,** Large thecoma of ovary with cystic changes and characteristic small, yellow areas. **C,** Bilateral serous cystadenocarcinomas of ovary with tumor growing on surface of largest cyst. **D,** Granulosa cell tumor with hemorrhage and yellowish zones. Myometrium shows hypertrophy. There was hyperplasia of endometrium. **E,** Bilateral undifferentiated carcinomas of ovary. **F,** Metastatic mucinous carcinoma in ovary from primary tumor of rectum.

estrogenism and myohypertrophy of the uterus, and endometrial hyperplasia is a frequent concomitant finding (Figs. 565 and 566). Endometrial carcinoma has been reported in conjunction with both of these tumors. Hyperplasia of the endometrium associated with these tumors is extremely difficult to differentiate from adenocarcinoma, and it is probable that a high percentage reported as carcinoma represent bizarre hyperplasia (Greene et al.[46]). Further evidence of this was reported by Stohr[157] who had a case diagnosed as endometrial adenocarcinoma before the removal of a granulosa cell tumor. Five weeks postoperatively repeat curettings of the endometrium showed normal early typical secretory epithelium coinciding with the menstrual cycle. In eighty-two granulosa cell tumors and sixteen thecomas studied by Kottmeier,[74] there were four carcinomas of the endometrium. In another nine, there were atypical changes in the endometrium. It has been our experience that these changes which simulate cancer invade the myometrium only superficially and metastases do not occur. Therefore, if a patient has a functioning tumor of the granulosa–theca cell type and endometrial curettings are diagnosed as carcinoma, this diagnosis may not be of any clinical significance. Fibroadenomas (McCartney[86]) and even mammary carcinoma (Finkler[38]) have also been concurrently reported.

Sertoli–Leydig cell tumors (arrhenoblastomas) are invariably unilateral, solid, and often hemorrhagic. Their color varies between yellow and reddish blue, and multicentric nodules are usually present. Javert and Finn[59] collected 122 cases from the medical literature, and twenty-seven were malignant.

Meyer[100] and Novak[118] believe that arrhenoblastomas arise from embryonic remnants of the seminiferous tubules in the region of the hilus of the ovary (Fig. 567). However, Kempson[66] has shown that the ultrastructural features of these tumors strongly support origin from ovarian stroma. Cells identical with Leydig cells of the testis are often found in the mesovarium and the hilus of the ovaries. Rarely, through hyperplasia or the formation of a true neoplasm, masculinizing signs may appear (Sternberg[155]). Microscopically, one

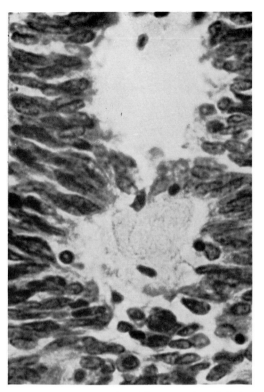

Fig. 567. Ovarian arrhenoblastoma of well-differentiated alveolar type. (Moderate enlargement.)

tumor can show all gradations from normal testis to abortive attempts at tubular formation of sarcoma-like tumor. These tumors were divided into three types by Meyer[100]:

1 The adenoma tubulare testiculare made up of tubules lined by large, orderly polygonal cells
2 A typical and an atypical tubular form, with solid cords or anastomosing strands
3 The solid form which may resemble a sarcoma but which, with careful study, is found to have cells containing lipoid suggesting interstitial cells or imperfect tubules

In the first group, which is the least common, masculinization or defeminization does not usually take place. The third group is most often associated with prominent hormonal alterations.

Gillman[45] demonstrated an embryologic homology between the ovarian theca and testicular interstitial cells and between the ovarian granulosa and the testicular Sertoli cells. He concluded that the former two cells are modified stromal cells of mesenchymal origin, whereas the latter two arise from the coelomic epithelium. This homology holds not only embryologically, but also functionally. The mesenchymally derived ovarian theca and testicular interstitial cells are the source of androgen (Shippel[150]), and the coelomically derived ovarian granulosa and testicular Sertoli cells are the source of estrogen. Potentially, therefore, either gonad is capable of giving rise to masculinizing and feminizing tumors. On the basis of this concept, it is now possible not only to explain the occurrence of a "feminizing androblastoma" in a male, as has been reported by Teilum,[164] but also to understand why masculinization in the female occurs so rarely in association with the highly differentiated arrhenoblastomas as compared with the less differentiated forms of these neoplasms. The new principle drawn from this is as follows:

"The more developed the coelomically derived granulosa or Sertoli cells are, the more likely is the estrogen to be the dominant hormone with the resultant persistence of the feminity in the female and the occurrence of feminization in the male; on the other hand, the more developed the gonadal mesenchymally derived theca or interstitial tissues are, the more likely is androgen to be the dominant hormone with the resultant persistence of masculinity in the male, and the occurrence of masculinization in the female."*

Teilum[168] prefers the term androblastoma to include the hormonally inactive group and believes that this lesion is identical to the testicular androblastoma. He reserves the term arrhenoblastoma for those androblastomas with masculinizing effects. The proper classification of these tumors is the subject of controversy (Mostofi et al.[106]). Morris and Scully[105] classified the variants of this tumor as Sertoli–Leydig cell tumors. Estrogen-producing tumors arising possibly from Sertoli cells have been described in the ovary (Teilum[165]) and are common in dogs (Scully and Cof-

*Translated from Wang, S. N.: Androblastoma tubulare lipoides (Sertoli cell tumor or testicular tubular adenoma) of ovary; report of case and review of literature, Chin. Med. J. (Peking) 73: 55-65, 1955.

fin[148]). Rarely, tumors producing both feminizing and virilizing signs may develop from the ovary and have been designated as gynandroblastomas (Mechler and Black[98]).

Fibromas of the ovary are usually firm, grayish white in color, and cystic. Calcification rarely occurs. The average size is 6 cm (Dockerty and Masson[28]). In 90% of the cases the tumor is unilateral. Fibromas probably arise from the ovarian stroma. They are made up of connective tissue that has a variable cellular quality, and intercellular edema is common. The mechanism of the hydrothorax in an ovarian fibroma as well as in the thecoma has been discussed at length. The fluid probably reaches the pleural cavity via the lymphatics, for it has been demonstrated that there are lymphatic vessels connecting the diaphragmatic peritoneum with subpleural lymph channels (Rubin et al.[138]).

Krukenberg tumors are metastatic neoplasms from primary lesions in the gastrointestinal tract and in particular from carcinomas of the stomach (Fig. 568). Primary tumors can also arise in the gallbladder, pancreas, and breast. It is doubtful if they are ever primary ovarian tumors. They are invariably bilateral, medium in size, and quite firm. The shape of the ovary is preserved. On section, small myxomatous areas are often observed. Microscopically, the stroma is usually quite pronounced, and a mucus-producing carcinoma is present with numerous signet-ring cells. In fifty-three instances of metastatic cancer of the ovary, there were three in which there was luteinization of the ovarian stroma cells, and Scully and Richardson[149] believe that such ovarian metastases may produce clinically significant quantities of steroid hormones.

Sarcomas make up a very small group of ovarian tumors. In the past, many of them were confused with other ovarian epithelial neoplasms that had sarcoma-like areas. They are bilateral in about 30% of instances, and the greater proportion of them are fibrosarcomas. They can arise from fibromas, and probably a few arise from teratomas.

An *unclassified* group of *carcinomas* is invariably found in textbooks on ovarian tumors. The more careful the study, how-

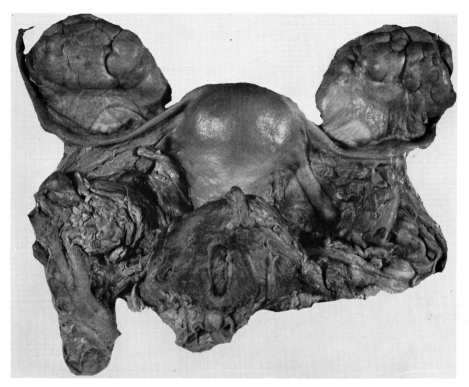

Fig. 568. Bilateral metastatic carcinoma in ovaries (Krukenberg tumor) from primary lesion in stomach.

ever, the fewer the number of tumors designated simply as carcinoma. Some of these lesions are probably dysgerminomas, arrhenoblastomas, and granulosa cell tumors, and undoubtedly a great many of them arise from previously existing serous cystomas. Various subdivisions have been given such as medullary, alveolar, and carcinoma simplex, but these divisions are artificial, for practically all of these tumors are very undifferentiated carcinomas tending to form acini. They are bilateral in about one-half of the instances, and most of them are solid. Some of the tumors designated as cystic are probably primarily solid, and secondary degenerative phenomena have caused cyst formation.

Metastatic spread

Serous and mucinous cystadenocarcinomas usually spread through the walls of the cyst and implant widely in the peritoneal surface. Implantation of innumerable gelatinous nodules on the surface of the peritoneum gives rise to pseudomyxoma peritonei; mucinous carcinomas seldom spread in other fashion than by direct implanta-tion. Metastases to the endometrium have been reported (Allan and Hertig[4]).

In serous cystadenocarcinomas, lymphatic metastases occur in the para-aortic nodes and in the inguinal regions. Node metastases may be observed in the cervical regions. Lung metastases are observed in fewer than 10% of cases (Burns et al.[19a]), metastases to the liver are less frequent, and bone metastases are rare except in dysgerminomas. Carcinomas that arise from cystic teratomas metastasize widely. Jew and Gross[61] reported the seventh known case of metastasizing thecoma. Sarcomas may metastasize widely.

Clinical evolution

In general, ovarian tumors grow insidiously and can reach a huge size before causing enough symptoms to bring the patient to the physician. Because of this, over one-half of the ovarian carcinomas are inoperable when first seen. There are general symptoms and signs that are common to all ovarian tumors (Table 77). A medium-sized tumor may cause abdominal discomfort accompanied by moderate low

Table 77. Symptoms and signs of ovarian tumors*

Symptoms and signs	Cases	% of cases
Symptoms		
Low abdominal pain	143	54
Abdominal enlargement	142	53
Gastrointestinal complaints	57	21
Genitourinary complaints	53	20
Abnormal vaginal bleeding	49	18
Pelvic pressure	46	17
Backache	36	13
Signs		
Pelvic mass	230	87
Abdominal mass	203	77
Ascites	82	31
Weight loss	75	28

*From Allan, M. S., and Hertig, A. T.: Carcinoma of the ovary, Amer. J. Obstet. Gynec. 58:640-653, 1949.

abdominal pain. As the tumor increases in size, however, pressure symptoms occur that result in dysuria from pressure on the bladder, constipation from pressure on the rectum, and swelling of the abdomen. Unfortunately, considerable expansion is possible within the pelvis without production of pressure symptoms. Butt[20] reported two cases of torsion cyst in infants and lutein cysts have been found in premature infants (Brune et al.[18]).

Torsion of a tumor pedicle may cause acute pain, fever, and leukocytosis. Ascites may develop with any of these tumors. It is frequently present in patients with serous cystadenocarcinoma (Taylor[162]), but its presence is not necessarily a sign of malignant tumor. Secondary abdominal masses and supraclavicular metastases may become palpable. Occasionally, a distant lymph node or skin metastasis may be the presenting symptom. Vaginal bleeding is seldom an early symptom in nonfeminizing tumors and, when present, is usually due to involvement of the uterus (Bayly and Greene[11]).

Brenner tumor seems to cause little pain and frequently is discovered accidentally (Jondahl et al.[62]). Ascites and hydrothorax (Meigs' syndrome) may be associated with ovarian fibromas but not exclusively (Rökaeus[135]). In 312 cases of fibroma reported by Dockerty and Masson,[28] ascites was present in fifty-one and hydrothorax in two. Ascites was present in seven of twenty-three patients with theca cell tumor reported by Rubin et al.[138] Granulosa and theca cell tumors may not cause clinically obvious enlargement of the ovary: such was the case in twenty-five of ninety-one patients reported by Fathalla.[36] Dysgerminomas are often accompanied by changes in the menstrual cycle or amenorrhea. Pseudohermaphroditism, hypogenitalism, and other forms of sexual maldevelopment are found associated with dysgerminoma (Santesson[142]).

There have been a number of instances of teratomas associated with autoimmune hemolytic anemia. Barry and Crosby[10] reported a case in a black woman with sickle cell trait, spherocytosis, and splenomegaly. Removal of the tumor resulted in disappearance of the spherocytosis and splenomegaly. Cystic teratomas make up about 20% of all ovarian tumors in adults. Malkasian et al.[90] reported 581 benign cystic teratomas with 415 in premenopausal and 160 in postmenopausal women. These neoplasms comprise about 50% of all ovarian tumors in children (Abell et al.[3]). Breen and Neubecker[16] reported that the malignant teratoma is one of the common malignant tumors in children.

In the prepubertal patient, granulosa cell tumors cause increase in size of the uterus and vaginal bleeding. The breasts increase in size, there may be secretion of colostrum, and the axillary and pubic hair and other secondary sex characteristics may appear. Sexual precocity was reported in a patient with a solid teratoma with choriocarcinoma (Pepus et al.[124]). In the adult, granulosa–theca cell tumors prolong the menstrual cycle or produce intermenstrual vaginal bleeding and mastalgia, but amenorrhea also may be observed. In the postmenopausal patient, cyclic bleeding may be reestablished, the uterus again undergoes hypertrophy, and the breasts enlarge. There is no relation between the size of the tumor and its endocrine function. Feminizing ovarian tumors are rarely observed in the course of pregnancy, and hirsutism is rarely seen (Diddle and O'Connor[25]).

Amenorrhea, gradual atrophy of the breasts, enlargement of the clitoris, and loss of feminine configuration may result from the development of an arrhenoblastoma. The hair takes a male distribution, with increased growth about the chin and loss on the scalp, and the voice may deepen. In some patients, there is menorrhagia before the development of amenorrhea. The libido is not affected, and pregnancy may take place if the uterus and opposite ovary are normal (Javert and Finn[59]), but infertility is more common (Nokes and Claiborne[114]).

Krukenberg tumors may arise like other ovarian tumors and often cause no symptoms suggestive of a primary lesion in the gastrointestinal tract. Ascites is frequently present. Rarely, patients with Krukenberg tumors have signs of masculinization (Bruno and Ober[19]). Turunen[176] reported evidence of estrogen secretion with this tumor. Almost any tumor of the ovary can have a functioning stroma (Scully and Richardson[149]).

The end stages of ovarian carcinomas are usually quite similar. Many of them develop peritoneal implants, causing increased ascites and progressive weight loss, with death usually brought about by some cause such as bronchopneumonia. Peritonitis commonly occurs in the mucinous group in which pseudomyxoma peritonei develops. After the masses become very bulky, invasion of the bladder or large bowel may occur. These changes result in death from infection or intestinal obstruction. The serous cystadenocarcinoma and the undifferentiated carcinomas often metastasize distantly, particularly to mediastinal lymph nodes, the evolution being quite rapid due to widespread dissemination. As a rule, the granulosa cell carcinomas and the dysgerminomas have a slow evolution, but death is still caused by generalized dissemination. Torsion of a pedicle or rupture of the tumor may result in hemorrhage and death.

Diagnosis

Clinical examination

Most ovarian tumors cause symptoms that recommend a thorough abdominal and pelvic examination. Large masses are easily palpated in the lower abdomen. Ascites (particularly with thecomas and fibromas) and metastatic masses in the omentum are also easily noticed. A bimanual pelvic examination may reveal the presence of a unilateral or bilateral unsuspected ovarian tumor. The examination requires considerable relaxation on the part of the patient, and consequently is better done under spinal anesthesia. Tumor implants in the peritoneal cul-de-sac may be felt by rectal palpation. Ovarian tumors can usually be differentiated from other pelvic masses in that they can usually be mobilized, but large tumors that become adherent to the wall may appear as metastatic pelvic masses. When torsion of the pedicle of a cyst has occurred, palpation is painful.

It should be stressed that small cystic lesions of the ovary are nonneoplastic in a high percentage of instances. In the series of 461 small ovarian cysts reported by Miller and Willson,[101] only 3% were neoplastic and only three cases were malignant. Most were simple cysts of the graafian follicle and corpus luteum (Fig. 569).

There are certain specific signs and symptoms that may identify various ovarian tumors. The cystic teratomas arise before the cessation of ovarian activity. If found after the menopause, they usually have a long previous history. Approximately 85% occur in patients between 16 and 55 years of age. They are probably the most common ovarian tumors prior to puberty and seldom become malignant before the patient reaches 40 years of age. They are somewhat more common in blacks. Although not usually attached to other or-

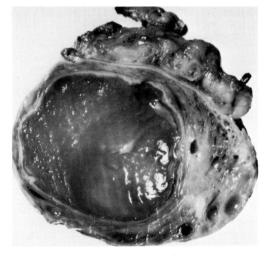

Fig. 569. Hemorrhagic corpus luteum cyst measuring 4.5 cm × 3.5 cm in diameter that had to be removed during course of abdominal surgery. (WU neg. 68-6255.)

gans, the cystic teratoma may become attached by inflammatory processes, and hair may be extruded through the rectum, bladder, or vagina. Struma ovarii arising in a cystic teratoma may cause signs of hyperthyroidism or even a malignant tumor (Nieminen et al.[102]). Rarely, a benign cystic teratoma may rupture, and the spillage of material within it may cause such a profound peritoneal reaction that the findings will be easily confused with advanced metastatic carcinoma (Auer et al.[9]).

Ovarian fibromas occur most commonly in the fourth, fifth, and sixth decades and practically never before puberty. Meigs and Cass[99] emphasized that they may be associated with ascites and pleural effusion. Because of hydrothorax there may be dyspnea, and an erroneous diagnosis of carcinoma of the ovary with metastases to the lungs may be made. Pleural effusion may also be associated with other tumors such as thecomas (Rubin et al.[138]), papillary cystadenocarcinomas (Schenck and Eis[144]), and mucinous cystomas (Millett and Shell[102]).

Brenner tumors do not appear before the age of 20 years, and the majority are found in patients 30 to 70 years of age, with two-thirds occurring after cessation of menses (McGoldrick and Lapp[87]).

In the estrogen-secreting group of tumors that produce signs and symptoms, it may be possible to make a definite clinical diagnosis. Granulosa cell tumors are fairly common, and their clinical signs and symptoms in the prepubertal and postmenopausal patient are pronounced because of the striking changes engendered. Such changes are not so apparent in patients who are still menstruating. In contrast to granulosa cell tumors, theca cell tumors are rarely observed before the age of 35 years, and signs of hyperestrogenism, while occurring, are not nearly so prominent as in the former. Estrogenic activity can occur in the cystadenoma of the ovary (Fox[40]).

Pregnancy luteomas are often multiple and occasionally bilateral; they result from hyperplastic overgrowth of theca-lutein cells in theca-lutein cysts and are not true neoplasms (Norris and Taylor[116]; Mandell et al.[93]).

Roentgenologic examination

The roentgenologic examination of the abdomen may reveal a large soft tissue tumor. This examination may be of value in differentiating ovarian tumors from partially calcified leiomyomas. Robins and White[134] pointed out that cystic teratomas invariably present a rounded or ovoid diminished area of density, banded and mottled in appearance. This area may be limited to the pelvis and is surrounded by a well-circumscribed ring of increased density sharply delineating it from the surrounding soft tissue. At times, teeth with fragments of a mandible may be observed. Of fifty-five proved cystic teratomas studied by Randall et al.,[130] twenty were not radiographically detected; the presence of teeth or abortive bone and the relative radiolucency of sebaceous contents facilitate the radiographic identification, but lesions under 5 cm in diameter are seldom visualized. In the serous cystomas or cystadenocarcinomas, psammoma bodies may present and characteristically cause multiple fine areas of calcification within the tumor (Dedick and Whelan[23]). A roentgenogram of the chest may reveal an insidious development of metastases. Pleural effusion may be found in association with thecomas and fibromas but should not be confused with pulmonary metastasis.

Laboratory examination

Watts and Adair[179] emphasized that fluids differ not only in different types of cysts but also in different cavities of the same tumor. But the examination of cystic fluid as a method of differentiation is not practical. There is some correlation with secretory activity: excessive amounts of estrogenic hormones may be present in granulosa cell tumors (Palmer[122]). Dysgerminomas may be associated with gonadotropin excretion (Hobson and Baird[55]). Plaut[127] proved that struma ovarii arising in cystic teratomas is biologically and chemically, as well as morphologically, true thyroid tissue: radioactive iodine may be used to evaluate thyroid function before and after surgical removal. Biosynthetic studies of endocrine tumors in vitro may help to determine histogenesis and to understand the patient's symptoms (Besch et al.[13]). Koudstaal et al.[76] studied ovarian tumors by histochemical methods.

Cytologic diagnosis

The examination of ascitic fluid may be helpful in making a diagnosis of malignant tumor of the ovary (Fig. 570). If the ascitic fluid is bloody, the probability is great that carcinoma is present. The fluid may be spun down and the sediment examined for morphologic evidence of tumor. Acini and papillary masses of cells are frequently observed. Malignant cells may be seen also in the vaginal smear in 10% to 20% of patients with advanced ovarian tumors (Koss and Durfee[73]). Psammoma bodies may be present. Cytologic examination of fluid aspirated from the cul-de-sac may be diagnostic (Grillo et al.[49]). In some instances, there may be an opportunity to make a morphologic diagnosis before laparotomy, as may be the case in metastatic adenopathies of the inguinal, cervical, or axillary regions or in metastatic

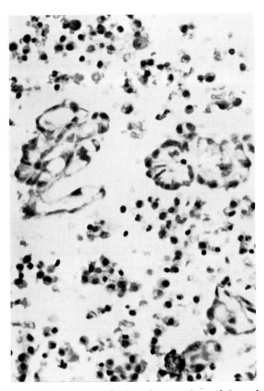

Fig. 570. Ascitic fluid sediment from bilateral serous cystadenocarcinomas of ovary with nests of tumor cells arranged in form of acini. (Moderate enlargement.)

skin or subcutaneous nodules. Rarely, positive diagnoses have been obtained from the rectum or from uterine curettages.

Differential diagnosis

In many patients the first symptoms and signs are due to a large mass that may be felt abdominally and pelvically. The most important differential diagnosis is to distinguish an ovarian tumor from a *uterine leiomyoma.* If the leiomyoma is intraligamentous or intimately associated with the uterus, it may be difficult, if not impossible, to differentiate it from an ovarian tumor before operation. Because of the characteristic calcification of leiomyomas, the roentgenologic examination may help to differentiate them from an ovarian tumor. Primary tumors of the broad ligaments are often, but not always, benign (Gardner et al.[44]). Their academic study is well justified, but a clinical differentiation is most often impossible and superfluous. True mesonephromas have rarely presented in this location (Teilum[167]).

It is sometimes difficult to decide at clinical examination whether the tumor is benign or malignant. It should be remembered that benign tumors such as fibromas, thecomas, mucinous cystomas, and some rather large serous cystomas may produce ascites probably because of mechanical reasons or partially because the tumor itself secretes fluid. The presence of such ascitic fluid does not, therefore, necessarily indicate malignant change.

In the granulosa–theca cell tumors, the diagnosis can be made if an ovarian mass, feminizing changes, and endometrial hyperplasia are present. Some very undifferentiated carcinomas of the ovary may cause cervical or vaginal ulceration. This occurs because of retrograde invasion of the endometrial canal, and the patient seeks advice because of vaginal bleeding. Not infrequently, these patients have an inguinal adenopathy. It is easy in such cases to be swayed by the appearance and to misdiagnose the case as a *carcinoma of the cervix* or *vagina.* Carcinoma of the ovary should be suspected if the microscopic examination shows secondary papillary branching and a configuration typical of ovarian carcinoma. There may also be a large mass in the region of the ovary.

Presacral meningoceles, chordomas, or neurofibromas and other rare tumors of the soft tissues or pelvic bones could suggest an ovarian tumor under certain circumstances. In children, retroperitoneal ganglioneuromas and gliomas could also be taken clinically for an ovarian tumor (Lovelady and Dockerty[84]). Rarely, tumors causing masculinization may arise from adrenal rests in the region of the ovaries (Nelson[111]; Kepler et al.[68]). Remission of the clinical picture with a lowering of 17-ketosteroid excretion following corticoid therapy indicates hyperplasia rather than neoplasia (Epstein et al.[33]). Masculinization is more often due to endocrine changes outside the ovary than to ovarian pathology. Carcinomas of the gastrointestinal tract and urinary tract have been mistaken clinically for ovarian cancer. Cavanagh et al.[21] point out that these cases can be discovered by proper preoperative radiographic studies before laparotomy.

Primary *carcinoma of the fallopian tube* is rare. Several series have been published over the past decade, bringing the total reported cases to over 800 (Hu et al.[58]; Jones[64]; Kneale and Atwood[71]; Ross et al.[136]). Most cases occur in patients 40 to 55 years of age, near the age of cessation of periods. Salpingitis and sterility may precede their development. Their most common symptoms are leukorrhea, often malodorous, and menorrhagia. Cramping pains in the lower abdomen and pelvis, often relieved by vaginal flow, may be present. On pelvic examination, the tumor may be palpable in the adnexal region in about 80% of the patients, but a diagnosis is seldom made before operation. Hysterosalpingography and culdoscopy are of little value in diagnosing the gross and radiographic appearance of carcinoma of the

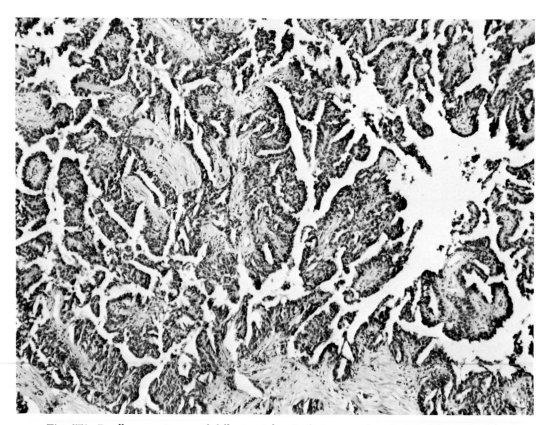

Fig. 571. Papillary carcinoma of fallopian tube. Such tumors often have solid or glandular areas as well as formed papillae. (×90; from Momtazee, S., and Kempson, R. L.: Primary adenocarcinoma of the fallopian tube, Obstet. Gynec. **32:**649-656, 1968; WU neg. 68-3486.)

fallopian tube, and the findings are frequently the same as those in chronic salpingitis and hydrosalpinx (Momtazee and Kempson[103]). The carcinoma starts usually in the fimbriated end of the tube. The occlusion of the os results in hydrosalpinx, hematosalpinx, or pyosalpinx, which may suggest an inflammatory disease. There are usually early adhesions to other organs. Metastases may be found in the ovaries, endometrium, and hypogastric, iliac, and inguinal lymph nodes. Microscopically, most of these tumors are adenocarcinomas, but a few are squamous cell carcinomas (Fig. 571). Rarely, tumor cells from carcinoma of the fallopian tube can be found in a vaginal smear. It may be difficult to ascertain whether or not the tumor originated in the ovary, uterus, or tube. Carcinoma of the fallopian tube should be treated surgically. In prognosis, the stage is more important than the differentiation of the tumor.

About twenty-five teratomas of the fallopian tube have been reported (Shirley et al.[152]).

Treatment
Prophylaxis

In a series of 10,000 pelvic examinations, Javert and Roscoe[60] estimated that only one symptomless case of malignant tumor of the ovary may be found. Thus, repeated routine pelvic examinations will detect very few cases. Moreover, in the presence of an enlarged ovary, an exploration often reveals a benign condition, so that surgeons are reluctant to operate except in the presence of more definite signs. Hence, few malignant tumors are operated upon in a curable stage. It becomes of the greatest importance to investigate carefully any patient with unexplained pelvic symptoms and to institute correct management of any pelvic masses found (Munnell et al.[109]). Unfortunately, however, no more than 2% of all ovarian tumors cause symptoms in their early stage.

About 8 of every 1000 American women over 40 years of age will develop a malignant ovarian tumor during the remainder of their life. Since about 15% of women over 40 years of age have had a laparotomy, a routine prophylactic oophorectomy done on that occasion would reduce their risk of having cancer of the ovary from 8 to 7 per 1000. This theoretical benefit would have to be balanced against the physical, emotional, and social consequences of an early artificial menopause in a large number of women (Randall[129]).

Exploration

An exploratory laparotomy is often necessary for the establishment of a diagnosis. In a high proportion of cases, it is known before exploration that the patient has an ovarian tumor, but in a few instances the exact nature is only strongly suspected (such as granulosa cell tumor or masculinizing arrhenoblastoma). Exploration should determine whether the tumor is unilateral or bilateral, solid or cystic, fixed or movable. Peritoneal implants in the immediate vicinity of the tumor, on the peritoneal surface, and in the cul-de-sac should be searched for. Approximately 80% of ovarian tumors are cystic, and a large proportion of these are benign. The other 20% are solid, and most of these are malignant.

Ovarian tumors may be first discovered at the time of pregnancy. If the tumor is more than 6 cm in diameter, it is probably a neoplasm rather than a cyst. In the ovarian tumors discovered during pregnancy, about 5% are malignant (Tawa and Baker[158]). If the tumor is discovered in the first trimester, exploratory laparotomy should be done at the time of the second trimester. If the tumor is discovered in the third trimester, treatment should be delayed until after delivery.

Treatment of the various types of ovarian tumors is often determined on the basis of the gross appearance. Frozen section histopathology may be helpful in the examination of implants or primary tumor; when the tumor appears confined to one ovary, frozen section of the removed ovary may be helpful in the decision as to the necessity of further surgery. Rupture of a tumor at the time of surgery usually raises questions as to the indicated procedure to follow. Grogan[50] reviewed 124 cases and found a 12.9% incidence of accidental rupture and intra-abdominal spillage: there was no demonstrated greater recurrence, seedling, metastases or compromise in life expectancy, especially in

Table 78. Indications for surgical treatment of ovarian tumors*

Tumor	Indication
Fibroma Brenner tumor Cystic teratoma Thecoma	Remove one ovary (at times, portions can be conserved)
Mucinous cystoma	Remove entire ovary
Solid teratoma Squamous carcinoma in a teratoma	Hysterectomy and bilateral salpingo-oophorectomy
Serous cystoma, apparently unilateral Serous cystoma, bilateral	Remove one ovary or remove both ovaries Remove both ovaries
Serous cysadenocarcinoma, apparently unilateral Serous cystadenocarcinoma, bilateral	Remove one ovary or do hysterectomy and bilateral salpingo-oophorectomy Hysterectomy and bilateral salpingo-oophorectomy
Carcinoma, either unilateral or bilateral Sarcoma, either unilateral or bilateral	Hysterectomy and bilateral salpingo-oophorectomy
Dysgerminoma Sertoli–Leydig tumor	Remove tumor or do hysterectomy and bilateral salpingo-oophorectomy
Granulosa cell tumor	Remove tumor or do hysterectomy and bilateral salpingo-oophorectomy

*Indications relative and mitigated by age of patient, operative risk, previous pregnancies, and other factors.

those with Stage I, Grade I lesions. Frequently, in these cases a hurried decision is made to instill radioactive gold or a chemotherapeutic agent: there is no proof of the effectiveness of these procedures. If postoperative radiotherapy is indicated, it should be possible to carry it out externally to a sufficiently high and homogeneously distributed dose throughout the area of potential residual disease without hindrance by internal inhomogeneous irradiation.

The question often arises as to whether to remove one ovary or both and whether to do a hysterectomy (Table 78). In a child or young patient with a tumor apparently confined to one ovary, the opposite ovary should be preserved. In the patient past childbearing age, there is little reason to preserve the ovary. In a follow-up on 345 patients with removal of an ovary for tumor, Randall et al.[130] found that twenty-four developed a second ovarian tumor, only four of which were malignant. On the basis of a study of forty-six patients treated for apparently unilateral cancer of the ovary with preservation of the normal-appearing ovary, Munnell[108] computed the risk of the presence of undetected cancer at 12%. In malignant, apparently unilateral serous tumors, it may be of value to biopsy the hilar region of the

opposite ovary for evidence of metastases. Roberts and Haines[133] showed that removal of a malignant cystic tumor within an ovary leaves the patient with an excellent chance of survival without removal of the opposite ovary. Terz et al.[171] reported fifty-five cases of ovarian carcinoma arising in the retained ovary. Thirty-four of the patients were over 50 years of age, and only two were cured; the assumption is easily made that all of the patients would have survived if the second ovary had been removed at the time of the first operation and if no consideration were given to physiology, parity, premature menopause, and emotional consequences. We favor the conservative attitude of Randall et al.[130] and Marchetti's summarization: two ovaries are better than one and one is better than none; save them when you can and remove them when you must.

The fibroma is most often unilateral, firm, and not very large and may be accompanied by ascites and pleural effusion. There are, however, no implants. The Brenner tumor, which occurs much less frequently, is also most often unilateral, fairly firm, and rarely associated with fluid. The thecoma, generally unilateral, may have the same gross appearance as the fibroma. It is firm and may also be associated with ascites and even pleural effusion. The cystic teratoma is usually unilateral (bilateral in about 15% of the cases), usually has a smooth surface, and its contents will be fluid.

The differentiation of the serous cystoma and the mucinous tumor is probably one of the most critical decisions in diagnosis. Mucinous tumors are usually unilateral and very large, whereas the serous variety is bilateral and of moderate size. The implants present with the serous and mucinous varieties are typical in appearance and easily recognized. If fluid is aspirated from a cystic ovarian tumor and if the tumor is of the serous type, the fluid will be a transudate. If the tumor is mucinous in nature, the fluid will be viscid and slimy. The dysgerminoma is a rare tumor, often large, brainlike, and rather soft. About 17% of dysgerminomas are bilateral (Santesson[142]). The Krukenberg tumors, invariably bilateral, retain the shape of the ovary, do not reach a large size, and are quite firm. In a woman under 45 years of age with bilateral ovarian tumors, a careful examination of the gastrointestinal tract, particularly the stomach, is indicated, but metastatic carcinomas of the uterus and breast may also present as an ovarian tumor (Wheelock and Putong[180]). At times, a unilateral ovarian tumor may be removed, immediately sectioned by the pathologist and a frozen section done in the operating room, and the decision as to further treatment made on the basis of the pathologic findings.

Surgery

Conservative surgical removal of one ovary is adequate treatment for a fibroma, thecoma, or Brenner tumor. Mucinous cystomas and cystic teratomas are benign tumors. However, bilateral involvement is frequent enough so that careful inspection of the opposite ovary or bisection of the ovary is indicated in premenopausal women. In dysgerminoma apparently confined to one ovary, the problem of not removing the opposite ovary occurs frequently because patients with this type of tumor are often young and desire children. At times, therefore, even with the risk of further trouble, conservatism is indicated. Furthermore, if this tumor occurs in a child, re-moval of both ovaries would not allow normal growth and development (Malkasian and Symmonds[92]). Obviously, malignant tumors such as serous cystadenocarcinoma and carcinomas and bilateral involvement by tumor demand hysterectomy and bilateral salpingo-oophorectomy. It is true that in spite of the clinical history and a careful examination plus all the other possible diagnostic procedures, it may be impossible to determine the type of tumor. In this instance, the surgical treatment depends on the training and judgment of the surgeon and the pathologist in attendance.

Radiotherapy

It is unfortunate that ovarian tumors, irrespective of histopathology, have often been reported together, thus not permitting an evaluation of radiotherapy either as a routine postoperative procedure or in the management of inoperable or recurrent tumors. The variety of approaches, sources of radiations, dosimetry, and reported results have often contributed to put the value of this procedure very much in question (Latour and Davis[77]). The experienced observer may review the available literature and draw favorable, though qualified, conclusions (Ellis[30]; Holme[57]).

Benign tumors such as thecomas, Brenner tumors, fibromas, cystic teratomas, and serous or mucinous adenomas, once surgically removed, need not be followed by radiotherapy. The *dysgerminoma* is definitely radiosensitive and radiocurable. Consequently, patients with this rare type of tumor should receive the benefit of postoperative radiotherapy unless the lesions are small and surgical removal is complete. Results obtained with postoperative irradiation of extensive *granulosa cell tumors* justify this procedure in most cases (Engle[32]). The results in the treatment of *serous* and *mucinous cystadenocarcinomas* seem better whenever routine postoperative irradiation is instituted. Moreover, radiotherapy decidedly palliates and prolongs life even when it fails to cure (Holme[57]). If, at exploration, a tumor is found impossible to remove completely, it is best to remove the ovaries for diagnosis and to proceed to administer postoperative radiotherapy. Endometrioid carcinomas are also radiosensitive, but mucinous cystadenocarcinomas are said to be less responsive (MacKay and Sellers[89]). In some instances, operation becomes possible after irradiation with chances of cure (Long et al.[82]). In any event, the overall survival of adequately irradiated inoperable patients is surprisingly satisfactory.

Vaeth and Buschke[177] have proposed a modus operandi that may permit proper evaluation of radiotherapy as an adjuvant to surgery in the treatment of ovarian tumors: at initial laparotomy, only a biopsy is to be performed; chemotherapy is to be administered in the presence of ascites or gross spread; radiotherapy is to be given to all; and, unless contraindicated, patients are to be operated upon about four weeks later (radical resection).

The aim of radiotherapy should be that of irradiating thoroughly and as homogeneously as possible the potential area of tumor involvement. External pelvic irradiation with supervoltages or cobalt[60] teletherapy would offer the best means of accomplishing this purpose. Some authors insist that the uterus be left in place to allow its use as a natural receptacle for radium sources and to complement thus the external irradiation (Kottmeier[74]; Ellis[30]). We fail to grasp the wisdom, the logic, and the physics of this approach, for it compromises the effectiveness of the surgical treatment for the sake of the use of radium placed in the uterus, which is neither indispensable nor the best vantage point for this purpose.

Injection of radioactive gold into the peritoneal cavity is advocated as a substitute for postoperative roentgentherapy. Such form of irradiation may result in sufficient dosage for the neoplastic cells immediately adjacent to the cavity, but it could not possibly irradiate sufficiently any remaining tumor outside the cavity. Radiations from Au^{198} have a very limited penetrability of a few millimeters. Thus, they cannot attain in fruitful amounts the neoplastic cells that are embedded in the tissues and nodes at a distance from the peritoneal cavity. In addition, the Au^{198} instilled into the peritoneum tends to become loculated so that radiations are poorly and unpredictably distributed. The value of intraperitoneal radioactive gold treatments as a routine postoperative procedure would be difficult to prove unless it is by a remarkable improvement of results that cannot be expected. The procedure is attended by definite hazards to the personnel and to the patient. We question that the cost and risk of this approach is justified by the results. There is no doubt that radioactive gold is valuable in controlling and reducing ascites caused by advanced ovarian cancer (Kligerman and Habif[70]; Moore and Langley[104]).

Chemotherapy

As in the case of other tumors, various drugs have been tried in patients with ovarian tumors with varied results (Kottmeier[75]): Thio-TEPA and methotrexate were tried by Greenspan[47] and endoxan and cyclophosphamide by Dvorak and Spirova[29] and Decker et al.[22] Rutledge and Burns[140] and Frick et al.[42] have reported relatively favorable results with no prolongation of life with L-phenylalanine mustard.

Prognosis

In 1965, there were 8933 deaths from ovarian cancer in the United States, a crude mortality rate of 9.5 for white and 5.5 for nonwhite females per 100,000 population. This accounts for 6.7% and 5%, respectively, of all reported deaths from cancer. The age-adjusted death rates in 1962-1963 were 1.69 in Japan and 11.02 in Denmark. In a comparison of mortality rates of Americans and Japanese-Americans, Wynder et al.[184] found suggestive differences in the background of premenopausal and postmenopausal patients with cancer of the ovary.

The survival statistics of patients with ovarian tumors are quite variable. In a series collected by Munnell et al.,[109] the five-year survival rates varied from 6% to 51%. These differences can be accounted for by the different extent and type of the tumors treated and by the liberality with which pathologists may decide on the malignancy of certain tumors.

It is obvious that the prognosis is excellent after surgical removal of Brenner tumors and thecomas. Excision of a fibroma quickly results in the disappearance of any ascitic or pleural fluid.

The cystic teratomas are, with a few exceptions, benign, and therefore their removal almost invariably results in an excellent prognosis. If the tumor is malignant when first seen, it is usually squamous carcinoma, and prognosis is always very poor, even with radical surgery. For instance, only four of sixty-three patients with squamous carcinoma in a teratoma are known to have survived for a period of five years or more (Alznauer[5]). Solid teratomas of the ovary in children have an extremely poor prognosis (London and Kazmers[81]).

The chances of curing a granulosa cell tumor are high if it is encapsulated and removed in its entirety. Even when it has extended beyond the capsule, surgical removal followed by postoperative irradiation gives a good prognosis. Kottmeier[75] reported on seventy patients, fifty-six of whom were well for five years. In a series of forty-four patients, twenty-nine were well after ten years. Norris and Taylor[117] recorded actuarial survival rates of 97% at five years and 93% at ten years in a group of ninety-seven patients with granulosa cell tumor. The sarcomatoid type of granulosa cell tumor appears to have a poor outlook. It has become increasingly apparent that granulosa cell tumors recur after long periods of time (Sommers et al.[153]). Long survivals have been obtained in some patients with advanced lesions with the use of postoperative roentgentherapy (Engle[32]).

In a group of 105 cases of dysgerminoma studied at the Armed Forces Institute of Pathology, Asadourian and Taylor[6] found an overall actuarial survival rate of 90% at five years and 83.5% at ten years. Although recurrence or metastasis occurred in twenty-three patients, additional treatment apparently cured ten. Of seventy-one patients with tumor confined to one ovary, the ten-year survival rate was the same in patients treated by unilateral oophorectomy (88%) as in those treated more extensively (83%). Local recurrences in some of the unilaterally treated patients responded to further treatment and did not affect survival rates. Successful pregnancy resulting in healthy children has proved possible in many patients (Brody[17]).

The original extent of disease is an important factor in evaluating prognosis. In Brody's series,[17] 95% of patients with encapsulated, unattached tumors and 78% with adhesions or rupture survived five years. Only 33% of patients with demonstrable metastases survived five years. The presence of immature or teratoid elements in a dysgerminoma may alter the prognosis for the worse (Morris and Scully[105]). Removal of arrhenoblastoma often permits development of pregnancy (Javert and Finn[59]). Endometrioid carcinoma has now been shown to be a frequent malignant ovarian tumor. Its separation into a distinctive type has demonstrated its favorable prognosis (Schueller and Kirol[145]). In Long and Taylor's series,[83] the survival curve for this neoplasm after two years was 80%.

Munnell et al.[109] reported on 148 patients treated from 1944 to 1951, two-thirds of whom had serous cystadenocarcinomas, with a total five-year survival rate of 29%. The best results were obtained in those with granulosa cell tumors and mucinous carcinomas, but there was no improvement over their previous series. Holme[57] reported on a series of 207 patients treated by surgery alone, with a 23% five-year survival, and he compared it with another series of 145 patients treated by surgery plus radiotherapy, which yielded a five-year survival rate of 39%. Henderson[53] reported a series of cases that excluded all equivocal cases and in which all patients received postoperative radiotherapy. In 110 patients in whom it was possible to remove the entire tumor, the five-year survival rate was 34%. In 349 patients with ovarian cancer reported by Kent and McKay,[67] the absolute five-year survival rate was 36.4%. The statistics should be dominated by the end results of the serous and mucinous tumors, which normally make up a large proportion of all ovarian neoplasms. The mucinous group, however, are fewer in number than the serous group, and their behavior from the standpoint of pathologic examination is more predictable. It is with the serous cystoma that the greatest discrepancy arises. Taylor and Greeley[163] reiterated and strongly emphasized that the interpretation of these tumors is difficult but that it has considerable influence on reported statistics. It is true that the serous cystomas that are predominantly fibrous behave in a benign fashion. It is also true that the very obviously malignant serous cystadenocarcinoma behaves in a malignant fashion. Taylor and Greeley[163] believe that tumors in the borderline group in time usually behave as malignant neoplasms.

Munnell and Taylor[110] summarized their five-year survival rate for papillary serous cystadenocarcinomas according to the degree of histologic malignancy. In the borderline group of twenty-eight cases, there was a 60% five-year survival; in the Grade I group of twenty-nine cases, a 48% five-year survival; in the Grade II group of nineteen cases, a 21% five-year survival; and in the Grade III group of forty-nine cases, a 6% five-year survival (Fig. 572). The absolute five-year survival in this group was 27.5%. A subsequent report by Munnell[107] in 1968 noted an improvement in the results of treatment of 235 patients treated in the 1952-1961 period, 40% of whom survived five years. This increase was attributed to the use of more aggressive and extensive surgery and to the more frequent and more precise use of postoperative radiotherapy.

Of 100 cases of ovarian tumors reported by Kerr and Einstein,[69] ninety-five were malignant and were treated by surgery and postoperative irradiation. There was a 40%

five-year survival. Forty-eight patients died within three years after irradiation, thirty-three of whom died in the first eighteen months. Nine died between three and five years after treatment. Kerr and Einstein[69] divided their cases into four groups. In Group I, in which the primary tumor could be removed, there were twenty-one patients, ten of whom survived over five years. In Group II, in which it was not possible to remove all of the tumor, there were forty-eight patients, with eighteen survivals. In Group III, there were eight cases representing recurrence of malignant tumor following operation or irradiation, and only one patient survived over five years. Group IV consisted of seventeen absolutely inoperable cases, and only three patients of this group survived five years. Delclos and Quinlan[24] reported on 161 patients with tumors of the ovary irradiated following surgical removal or exploration, thirty-nine of whom were living four or more years following irradiation by a large field, covering the abdomen and pelvis with a moving strip technique.

Some general statements can be made concerning a group of ovarian carcinomas. If the tumor is confined to the ovary or even confined to both ovaries, this is an important prognostic sign. These represent cases that are operable. In a group of patients reported by Javert and Roscoe,[60] twenty-two of thirty patients with operable tumors survived five years or more but only twenty of eighty patients with inoperable tumors survived five years or more. The most important prognostic finding is the extent of the tumor at the time of exploratory operation. If the cancer has disseminated into the upper abdomen, very few patients will be cured (Long et al.[82]).

The duration of symptoms bears little or no relation to the prognosis, although it is unquestionably related to the type of tumor. Low-grade malignancy confers a favorable prognosis. The best prognosis is that of borderline or low-grade papillary serous cystadenocarcinomas, the majority of papillary mucinous cystadenocarcinomas, and most granulosa cell neoplasms (Munnell et al.[109]). The undifferentiated carcinomas do poorly. If the tumor is solid or presents spread outside the capsule or is associated with ascites, the prognosis is un-

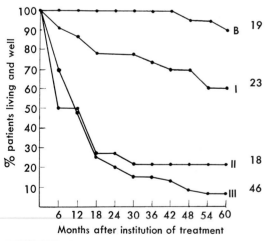

Fig. 572. Survival curves of patients with papillary serous cystadenocarcinoma of ovary according to degree of histologic malignancy. (From Munnell, E. W., and Taylor, H. C., Jr.: Ovarian carcinoma, Amer. J. Obstet. Gynec. **58:**943-955, 1949.)

favorably affected. About 60% of patients who die of carcinoma of the ovary do so within eighteen months. The remaining group may live for variable lengths of time (Munnell et al.[109]; Jones and TeLinde[63]).

REFERENCES

1 Abell, M. R.: Malignant Brenner tumors of ovary, Cancer 10:1263-1274, 1957.

2 Abell, M. R.: The nature and classification of ovarian neoplasms, Canad. Med. Ass. J. 94:1102-1124, 1966.

3 Abell, M. R., Johnson, V. J., and Holtz, F.: Ovarian neoplasms in childhood and adolescence. Part I. Tumors of germ cell origin, Amer. J. Obstet. Gynec. 92:1059-1081, 1965.

4 Allan, M. S., and Hertig, A. T.: Carcinoma of the ovary, Amer. J. Obstet. Gynec. 58:640-653, 1949.

5 Alznauer, R. L.: Squamous-cell carcinoma arising in benign cystic teratoma of the ovary; a report of three additional cases and review of the literature, Amer. J. Obstet. Gynec. 65:1238-1247, 1953.

6 Asadourian, L. A., and Taylor, H. B.: Dysgerminoma; an analysis of 105 cases, Obstet. Gynec. 33:370-379, 1969.

7 Arey, L. B.: The nature and significance of the grooved nuclei of Brenner tumors and Walthard cell islands, Amer. J. Obstet. Gynec. 45:614-624, 1943.

8 Arey, L. B.: The origin and form of the Brenner tumor, Amer. J. Obstet Gynec. 81:743-751, 1961.

9 Auer, E. A., Dockerty, M. B., and Mayo, C. W.: Ruptured dermoid cyst of the ovary simulating abdominal carcinomatosis, Proc. Staff Meet. Mayo Clin. 26:489-497, 1951.

10 Barry, K. G., and Crosby, W. H.: Autoimmune hemolytic anemia arrested by removal of an ovarian teratoma, Ann. Intern. Med. 41:1002-1007, 1957.

11 Bayly, M. A., and Greene, R. R.: Ovarian tumors and uterine bleeding, Amer. J. Obstet. Gynec. 57:984-988, 1949.

12 Bell, W. B.: So-called true hermaphroditism, with report of a case, Proc. Roy. Soc. Med. 8:77-94, 1915.

13 Besch, P. K., Watson, D. J., Vorys, N., Hamwi, G. J., Barry, R. D., and Barnett, E. B.: In vitro biosynthetic studies of endocrine tumors. VI. Malignant granulosa cell tumor, Amer. J. Obstet. Gynec. 96:466-477, 1966.

14 Blackwell, W. J., Dockerty, M. B., Masson, J. C., and Mussey, R. D.: Dermoid cysts of the ovary; their clinical and pathologic significance, Amer. J. Obstet. Gynec. 51:151-172, 1946.

15 Boivin, Y., and Richart, R. M.: Hilus cell tumors of the ovary, Cancer 18:231-240, 1965.

16 Breen, J. L., and Neubecker, R. D.: Ovarian malignancy in children, with special reference to the germ-cell tumors, Ann. N. Y. Acad. Sci. 142:658-674, 1967.

17 Brody, S.: Clinical aspects of dysgerminoma of the ovary, Acta Radiol. (Stockholm) 56:209-230, 1961.

18 Brune, W. H., Pulaski, E. J., and Shuey, H. E.: Giant ovarian cyst; report of a case in a premature infant, New Eng. J. Med. 257:876-878, 1957.

19 Bruno, M. S., and Ober, W. B.: Krukenberg tumor of the ovary, New York J. Med. 49:4001-4007, 1959.

19a Burns, B. C., Jr., Underwood, P. B., Jr., and Rutledge, F. N.: A review of carcinoma of the ovary at the University of Texas, M. D. Anderson Hospital and Tumor Institute at Houston. In Cancer of the uterus and ovary, Chicago, 1969, Year Book Medical Publishers, Inc.

20 Butt, J. A.: Ovarian tumors in children, Amer. J. Obstet. Gynec. 69:333-337, 1955.

21 Cavanagh, D., Egan, R. L., Dolan, P. A., and Tuledge, F.: Pelvic extragenital tumors in women; a study of 200 patients and a review of the literature, Obstet. Gynec. 20:70-108, 1965.

22 Decker, J. P., Hirsch, N. B., and Garnet, J. D.: Mixed mesodermal (mullerian) tumor of the ovary; report of two cases, Cancer 21:926-932, 1968.

23 Dedick, A. P., and Whelan, V. M.: Roentgen demonstration of psammoma bodies in cystadenocarcinoma of the ovaries; report of two cases, Radiology 64:353-356, 1955.

24 Delclos, L., and Quinlan, E. J.: Malignant tumors of the ovary managed with postoperative megavoltage irradiation, Radiology 93:659-663, 1969.

25 Diddle, A. W., and O'Connor, K. A.: Feminizing ovarian tumors and pregnancy, Amer. J. Obstet. Gynec. 62:1071-1078, 1951.

26 Diddle, A. W.: Granulosa- and theca-cell ovarian tumors; prognosis, Cancer 5:215-228, 1952.

27 Dockerty, M. B.: Theca cell tumors of the ovary; report of ten cases, Amer. J. Obstet. Gynec. 39:434-443, 1940.

28 Dockerty, M. B., and Masson, J. C.: Ovarian fibromas; a clinical pathologic study of 283 cases, Amer. J. Obstet. Gynec. 47:741-752, 1944.

29 Dvorak, O., and Spirova, M.: Report on the management of advanced ovarian cancer by medication with endoxan (ASTA) and cyclophosphamide, Zbl. Gynaek. 89:940-945, 1967.

30 Ellis, F.: Malignant disease of the ovary and radiotherapy; a survey of 168 cases with 10-year followup, J. Fac. Radiologists 7:1-10, 1955.

31 Emge, L. A.: Functional and growth characteristics of struma ovarii, Amer. J. Obstet. Gynec. 40:738-750, 1940.

32 Engle, R. B.: Roentgen treatment of granulosa cell carcinoma of the ovary, Amer. J. Roentgen. 80:793-798, 1958.

33 Epstein, J. A., Levinson, C. J., and Kupperman, H. S.: Ovarian adrenal rest tumor (masculinovoblastoma) simulating adrenal virilism, Amer. J. Obstet. Gynec. 74:982-988, 1957.

34 Farrar, H. K., Jr., Elesh, R., and Libretti, J.: Brenner tumors and estrogen production, Obstet. Gynec. Survey **15**:1-17, 1960.

35 Fathalla, M. F.: Malignant transformation in ovarian endometriosis, J. Obstet. Gynaec. Brit. Comm. **74**:85-92, 1967.

36 Fathalla, M. F.: The occurrence of granulosa and theca tumors in clinically normal ovaries; a study of 25 cases, J. Obstet. Gynaec. Brit. Comm. **74**:279-282, 1967.

37 Fathalla, M. F., Rashad, M. N., and Kerr, M. G.: The relationship between ovarian tumors and intersex states with special references to the disgerminoma and arrhenoblastoma, J. Obstet. Gynaec. Brit. Comm. **73**:812-820, 1966.

38 Finkler, R. S.: Granulosa cell tumor of ovary with carcinoma of breast, Amer. J. Obstet. Gynec. **36**:1064-1066, 1938.

39 Fisher, E. R.: Pseudomucinous cystadenoma; a misnomer? Obstet. Gynec. **4**:616-621, 1954.

40 Fox, H.: Estrogenic activity of the serous cystadenoma of the ovary, Cancer **18**:1041-1047, 1965.

41 Fox, R. A.: Brenner tumor of the ovary, Amer. J. Path. **18**:223-235, 1942.

42 Frick, H. C., Tretter, P., Tretter, W., and Hyman, G. A.: Disseminated carcinoma of the ovary treated by L-phenylalanine mustard, Cancer **21**:508-513, 1968.

43 Gaines, J. A.: Brenner tumors of the ovary, Amer. J. Obstet. Gynec. **32**:457-465, 1936.

44 Gardner, G. H., Greene, R. R., and Peckham, B.: Tumors of the broad ligament, Amer. J. Obstet. Gynec. **73**:536-555, 1967.

45 Gillman, J.: The development of the gonads in man, with a consideration of the role of fetal endocrines and the histogenesis of ovarian tumors, Contrib. Embryol. (nos. 207-212) **32**:83-131, 1948, Carnegie Institution of Washington.

46 Greene, R. R., Roddick, J. W., Jr., and Milligan, M.: Estrogens, endometrial hyperplasia and endometrial carcinoma, Ann. N. Y. Acad. Sci. **75**:586-600, 1959.

47 Greenspan, E. M.: Thio-tepa and methotrexate chemotherapy of advanced ovarian carcinoma, J. Mt. Sinai Hosp. **35**:52-67, 1968.

48 Gricouroff, G.: Endometrioid tumours of the ovary. In UICC Monograph Series—Vol. 11: Ovarian cancer (edited by F. Gentil and A. C. Junqueira), Berlin/Heidelberg/New York, 1968, Springer-Verlag, pp. 23-39.

48a Gricouroff, G.: Kystes dits "germinatifs," endometriose et tumeurs endometröides de l'ovaire, Bull. Cancer (Paris) **55**:343-352, 1968.

49 Grillo, D., Stienmier, R. H., and Lowell, D. M.: Early diagnosis of ovarian carcinoma by culdocentesis, Obstet. Gynec. **28**:346-350, 1966.

50 Grogan, R. H.: Accidental rupture of malignant ovarian cysts during surgical removal, Obstet. Gynec. **30**:716-720, 1967.

51 Harcourt, K. F., and Dennis, D. L.: Laparotomy for "ovarian tumors" in unsuspected carcinoma of the colon, Cancer **21**:1244-1246, 1968.

52 Heller, E. L.: Tuberculoid reaction in ovarian dysgerminoma, Arch. Path. (Chicago) **35**:674-680, 1943.

53 Henderson, D. N.: Granulosa and theca cell tumors of the ovary, Amer. J. Obstet. Gynec. **43**:194-210, 1942.

54 Hertig, A. T., and Gore, H.: Tumors of the female sex organs. Part 3—Tumors of the ovary and fallopian tube. In Atlas of tumor pathology, Sect. IX, Fasc. 33, Washington, D. C., 1961, Armed Forces Institute of Pathology.

55 Hobson, B. M., and Baird, D. T.: Dysgerminoma of the ovary and gonadotrophin excretion, J. Obstet. Gynaec. Brit. Comm. **73**:131-136, 1966.

56 Hoerr, N. L.: Histological studies in lipins, Anat. Rec. **66**:149-171, 317-342, 1936.

57 Holme, G. M.: Malignant ovarian tumours, J. Fac. Radiol. **8**:394-401, 1957.

58 Hu, C. Y., Taymor, M. L., and Hertig, A. T.: Primary carcinoma of the fallopian tube, Amer. J. Obstet. Gynec. **79**:24, 1960.

59 Javert, C. T., and Finn, W. F.: Arrhenoblastoma; the incidence of malignancy and the relation to pregnancy, to sterility, and to treatment, Cancer **4**:60-77, 1951 (extensive bibliography).

60 Javert, C. T., and Roscoe, R. R.: Serous cystadenocarcinoma of the ovary; a review of 127 cases, Surg. Clin. N. Amer. **33**:557-584, 1953.

61 Jew, E. W., Jr., and Gross, P.: Malignant thecoma with metastases, Amer. J. Obstet. Gynec. **69**:857-860, 1955.

62 Jondahl, W. H., Dockerty, M. B., and Randall, L. M.: Brenner tumors of the ovary; a clinicopathologic study of 31 cases, Amer. J. Obstet. Gynec. **60**:160-167, 1950.

63 Jones, G. E. S., and TeLinde, R. W.: The curability of granulosa-cell tumors, Amer. J. Obstet. Gynec. **50**:691-700, 1945.

64 Jones, V. O.: Primary carcinoma of the uterine tube, Obstet. Gynec. **26**:122, 1965.

65 Kecskés, L., and Szabó, E.: Menopausában vérzést okozó Brenner-daganat hormonalis hatása hüvelykenét vizsgálatokban, Magy. Noorv. Lap. **20**:182-186, 1957.

66 Kempson, R. L.: Ultrastructure of stromal tumors of the ovary; Sertoli-Leydig and adrenal rest tumor, Arch. Path. (Chicago) **86**:492-507, 1968.

67 Kent, S. W., and McKay, D. G.: Primary cancer of the ovary, Amer. J. Obstet. Gynec. **80**:430-438, 1960.

68 Kepler, E. J., Dockerty, M. B., and Priestly, J. T.: Adrenal-like ovarian tumor associated with Cushing's syndrome (so-called masculinovoblastoma, luteoma, hypernephroma, adrenal cortica carcinoma of the ovary), Amer. J. Obstet. Gynec. **47**:43-62, 1944.

69 Kerr, H. D., and Einstein, R. A. J.: Results of irradiation of ovarian tumors, Amer. J. Roentgen. **53**:376-384, 1945.

70 Kligerman, M. M., and Habif, D. F.: The use of radioactive gold in the treatment of effusion due to carcinomatosis of the pleura and peritoneum, Amer. J. Roentgen. **74**:651-656, 1955.

71 Kneale, B. L. G., and Atwood, H. D.: Primary carcinoma of the fallopian tube, Amer. J. Obstet. Gynec. **94**:840, 1966.

72 Knight, W. R., III: Theca-cell tumors of the ovary with a report of fifteen cases and a review of the literature, Amer. J. Obstet. Gynec. **56**:311-324, 1948.

73 Koss, L. G., and Durfee, G. R.: Diagnostic cytology and its histopathologic bases, Philadelphia, 1961, J. B. Lippincott Co.

74 Kottmeier, H. L.: The classification and treatment of ovarian tumours, Acta Obstet. Gynec. Scand. **31**:313-363, 1952.

75 Kottmeier, H. L.: Ovarian cancer; diagnosis and treatment, Med. Coll. Va. Quart. **3**: 47-53, 1967.

76 Koudstaal, J., Bossenbroek, B., and Hardonk, M. J.: Ovarian tumors investigated by histochemical and enzyme histochemical methods, Amer. J. Obstet. Gynec. **102**:1004-1017, 1968.

77 Latour, J. P. A., and Davis, B. A.: A critical assessment of the value of x-ray therapy in primary ovarian carcinoma, Amer. J. Obstet. Gynec. **74**:968-976, 1957.

78 Leddy, E. T.: Granulosa-cell tumor of the ovary with special reference to radiosensitivity, Amer. J. Roentgen. **59**:717-726, 1948.

79 Liber, A. F.: Ovarian cancer in mother and five daughters, Arch. Path. (Chicago) **49**: 280-290, 1950.

80 Lipschutz, A., Iglesias, R., Panasevich, V. I., and Salinas, S.: Granulosa-cell tumours induced in mice by progesterone, Brit. J. Cancer **21**:144-152, 1967.

81 London, J. L., and Kazmers, N.: Malignant solid teratoma of the ovary in children, Int. Surg. **46**:142-146, 1966.

82 Long, R. T. L., Johnson, R. E., and Sala, J. M.: Variations in survival among patients with carcinoma of the ovary, Cancer **20**: 1195-1202, 1967.

83 Long, M. E., and Taylor, H. C., Jr.: Endometrioid carcinoma of the ovary, Amer. J. Obstet. Gynec. **90**:936-950, 1964.

84 Lovelady, S. B., and Dockerty, M. B.: Extragenital pelvic tumors in women, Amer. J. Obstet. Gynec. **58**:215-234, 1949.

85 MacAulay, M. A., Weliky, I., and Schulz, R. A.: Ultrastructure of a biosynthetically active granulosa cell tumor, Lab. Invest. **17**: 562-570, 1967.

86 McCartney, J. S.: Malignant granulosa cell tumor of the ovary, Arch. Path. (Chicago) **29**:263-270, 1940.

87 McGoldrick, J. L., and Lapp, W. A.: Theca-cell tumors of the ovary, Amer. J. Obstet. Gynec. **48**:409-416, 1944.

88 McKay, D. G., Hertig, A. T., and Hickey, W. F.: The histogenesis of granulosa and theca cell tumors of the human ovary, Obstet. Gynec. **1**:125-136, 1953.

89 MacKay, E. N., and Sellers, A. H.: Ovarian cancer at the Ontario Cancer Foundation Clinics, 1938-1958, Canad. Med. Ass. J. **96**: 299-308, 1967.

90 Malkasian, G. D., Dockerty, M. B., and Symmonds, R. E.: Benign cystic teratomas, Obstet. Gynec. **29**:719-725, 1967.

91 Malkasian, G. D., Jr., Mussey, E., Decker, D. G., and Johnson, C. E.: Chemotherapy of gynecologic sarcomas, Cancer Chemother. Rep. **51**:507-516, 1967.

92 Malkasian, G. D., Jr., and Symmonds, R. E.: Treatment of the unilateral encapsulated ovarian dysgerminoma, Amer. J. Obstet. Gynec. **90**:379-382, 1964.

93 Mandell, G. H., Floyd, W. S., Cohn, S. L., and Goodman, P. A.: Luteoma of pregnancy, Amer. J. Clin. Path. **47**:148-153, 1967.

94 Marchetti, A. A.; quoted by Terz, J. J., Barber, H. R. K., and Brunschwig, A.: Incidence of carcinoma in the retained ovary, Amer. J. Surg. **113**:511-515, 1967.

95 Marcille, M.: Lympatiques et ganglions iliopelviennes, Thesis, Faculty of Medicine of Paris, 1902.

96 Marcus, C. C., and Marcus, S. L.: Struma ovarii, Amer. J. Obstet. Gynec. **81**:762-782, 1961 (extensive bibliography).

97 Marrubini, G.: Primary chorionepithelioma of the ovary; report of two cases, Acta Obst. Gynaec. Scand. **28**:251-284, 1949.

98 Mechler, E. A., and Black, W. C.: Gynandroblastoma of the ovary, Amer. J. Path. **19**: 633-654, 1943.

99 Meigs, J. V., and Cass, J. W.: Fibroma of the ovary with ascites and hydrothorax, Amer. J. Obstet. Gynec. **33**:249-267, 1937.

100 Meyer, R.: The pathology of some special ovarian tumors and their relation to sex characteristics, Amer. J. Obstet. Gynec. **22**:697-713, 1931.

101 Miller, N. F., and Willson, J. R.: Surgery of the ovary; the small ovarian cyst, New York J. Med. **42**:1851-1855, 1942.

102 Millett, J., and Shell, J.: Meigs' syndrome in a case of multilocular pseudomucinous cystadenoma of the ovary, Amer. J. Med. Sci. **209**:327-335, 1945.

103 Momtazee, S., and Kempson, R. L.: Primary adenocarcinoma of the fallopian tube, Obstet. Gynec. **32**:649-656, 1968.

104 Moore, D. W., and Langley, I. I.: Routine use of radiogold following operation for ovarian cancer, Amer. J. Obstet. Gynec. **98**: 624-630, 1967.

105 Morris, J. McL., and Scully, R. E.: Endocrine pathology of the ovary, St. Louis, 1958, The C. V. Mosby Co.

106 Mostofi, F. K., Theiss, E. A., and Ashley, D. J. B.: Tumors of specialized gonadal stroma in human male patients, Cancer **12**: 944-957, 1959.

107 Munnell, E. W.: The changing prognosis and treatment in cancer of the ovary, Amer. J. Obstet. Gynec. **100**:802-805, 1968.

108 Munnell, E. W.: Is conservative therapy ever

justified in Stage I (IA) cancer of the ovary? Amer. J. Obstet. Gynec. **103**:641-650, 1969.

109 Munnell, E. W., Jacox, H. W., and Taylor, H. C., Jr.: Treatment and prognosis in cancer of the ovary, Amer. J. Obstet. Gynec. **74**: 1187-1200, 1957.

110 Munnell, E. W., and Taylor, H. C., Jr.: Ovarian carcinoma, Amer. J. Obstet. Gynec. **58**:943-955, 1949.

111 Nelson, A. A.: Accessory adrenal cortical tissue, Arch. Path. (Chicago) **27**:955-965, 1939.

112 Nieminen, U., von Numers, C., and Widholm, O. I.: Struma ovarii, Acta Obstet. Gynec. Scand. **42**:399-424, 1963.

113 Nissen, E. D.: Consideration of the malignant carcinoid syndrome; primary argentaffin carcinomas arising in benign cystic teratomas of the ovary, Obstet. Gynec. **14**:459-488, 1959.

114 Nokes, J. M., and Claiborne, H. A., Jr.: A clinical evaluation of masculinizing tumors of the ovary, Ann. Surg. **143**:729-739, 1956.

115 Nordén, G., and Dahlberg, B.: On ovarian androblastoma, Lunds Universitets Arsskrift. Avd. 2, Bd. **52**:1-52, 1956.

116 Norris, H. J., and Taylor, H. B.: Nodular theca-lutein hyperplasia of pregnancy (so-called "pregnancy luteoma"), Amer. J. Clin. Path. **47**:557-566, 1967.

117 Norris, H. J., and Taylor, H. B.: Prognosis of granulosa-theca tumors of the ovary, Cancer **21**:255-263, 1968.

118 Novak, E.: Endocrine effects of certain dysontogenetic tumors of the ovary, Endocrinology **30**:953-958, 1942.

119 Novak, E., and Jones, H. W.: Brenner tumors of the ovary with report of 14 new cases, Amer. J. Obstet. Gynec. **38**:872-888, 1939.

120 Novak, E. R., and Woodruff, J. D.: Mesonephroma of the ovary, Amer. J. Obstet. Gynec. **77**:632-644, 1959.

121 O'Malley, B. W., Lipsett, M. B., and Jackson, M. A.: Steroid content and synthesis in a virilizing luteoma, J. Clin. Endocr. **27**: 311-319, 1967.

122 Palmer, A.: Estrogenic hormone in the urine and tumor of a patient with agranulosa cell tumor of the ovary, Amer. J. Obstet. Gynec. **37**:492-494, 1939.

123 Parker, T. M., Dockerty, M. B., and Randall, L. M.: Mesonephric clear cell carcinoma of the ovary; a clinical and pathologic study, Amer. J. Obstet. Gynec. **80**:417-425, 1960.

124 Pepus, M., Hutcheson, J. B., Ruffolo, E. H., and Smith, M. E.: Ovarian neoplasia and sexual precocity, Obstet. Gynec. **29**:828-833, 1967.

125 Peterson, W. F.: Malignant degeneration of benign cystic teratomas of the ovary—a collective review of the literature, Obstet. Gynec. Survey **12**:793-830, 1957.

126 Pinkerton, J. H. M., McKay, D. G., Adams, E. C., and Hertig, A. T.: Development of the human ovary; a study using histochemical technics, Obstet. Gynec. **18**:154-181, 1961.

127 Plaut, A.: Ovarian struma; a morphologic, pharmacologic and biologic examination, Amer. J. Obstet. Gynec. **25**:351-360, 1933.

128 Randall, C. L.: Postmenopausal ovarian function, Amer. J. Obstet. Gynec. **73**:1000, 1957.

129 Randall, C. L.: Ovarian carcinoma; risk of preserving the ovary, Obstet. Gynec. **3**:491-497, 1954.

130 Randall, C. L., Hall, D. W., and Armenia, C. S.: Pathology in the preserved ovary after unilateral oophorectomy, Amer. J. Obstet. Gynec. **84**:1233-1241, 1962.

131 Randall, J. H.: Treatment of ovarian carcinoma, Obstet. Gynec. **5**:445-451, 1955.

132 Reagan, J. W.: The ovarian Brenner tumor; its gross and microscopic pathology, Amer. J. Obstet. Gynec. **60**:1315-1323, 1950.

133 Roberts, D. W. T., and Haines, M.: Conserving ovarian tissue in treatment of ovarian neoplasms, Brit. Med. J. **2**:917-919, 1965.

134 Robins, S. A., and White, G.: Roentgen diagnosis of dermoid cysts of the ovary in the absence of calcification, Amer. J. Roentgen. **43**:30-34, 1940.

135 Rökaeus, S.: Fibroma of the ovary and two cases of Meigs' syndrome, Acta Obstet. Gynec. Scand. **28**:403-417, 1949.

136 Ross, W. M., Ward, C. V., and Lindsay, C. C.: Primary carcinoma of the fallopian tube, Amer. J. Obstet. Gynec. **83**:425-429, 1962.

137 Rouvière, H.: Anatomie des lymphatiques de l'homme, Paris, 1932, Masson et Cie.

138 Rubin, I. C., Novak, J., and Squire, J. J.: Ovarian fibromas and theca-cell tumors; report of 78 cases with special reference to production of ascites and hydrothorax (Meigs' syndrome), Amer. J. Obstet. Gynec. **48**:601-616, 1944.

139 Ruckes, J., and Stallkamp, B.: Morphology and genesis of primary ovarian carcinoids, Frankfurt. Z. Path. **76**:235-242, 1967.

140 Rutledge, F., and Burns, B. C.: Chemotherapy for advanced ovarian cancer, Amer. J. Obstet. Gynec. **96**:761-772, 1966.

141 Salm, R.: Pure and mixed hilus-cell tumours of ovary, Ann. Roy. Coll. Surg. Eng. **41**: 344-363, 1967.

142 Santesson, L.: Clinical and pathological survey of ovarian tumors treated at Radiumhemmet, Acta Radiol. (Stockholm) **28**:644-668, 1948.

143 Santesson, L.: Suggested classification of ovarian tumors; presented at meeting of The Cancer Committee of the International Federation of Gynecology and Obstetrics, Stockholm, Sweden, August 24-26, 1961.

143a Santesson, L., and Kottmeier, H. L.: General classification of ovarian tumors. In UICC Monograph Series—vol. 11: Ovarian cancer (edited by F. Gentil and A. C. Junqueira), Berlin/Heidelberg/New York, 1968, Springer-Verlag, pp. 1-8.

144 Schenck, S. B., and Eis, B. M.: Papillary cystadenocarcinoma of the ovary with hydro-

thorax, Amer. J. Obstet. Gynec. **38**:327-330, 1939.

145 Schueller, E. F., and Kirol, P. M.: Prognosis in endometrioid carcinoma of the ovary, Obstet. Gynec. **27**:850-858, 1966.

146 Scully, R. E.: Gonadoblastoma; a gonadal tumor related to the dysgerminoma (seminoma) and capable of sex-hormone production, Cancer **6**:455-463, 1953.

146a Scully, R. E.: Gonadoblastoma; a review of 74 cases, Cancer **24**:1340-1356, 1970.

147 Scully, R. E., and Barlow, J. F.: "Mesonephroma" of ovary; tumor of Müllerian nature related to the endometrioid carcinoma, Cancer **20**:1405-1417, 1967.

148 Scully, R. E., and Coffin, D. L.: Canine testicular tumors, with special reference to their histogenesis, comparative morphology and endocrinology, Cancer **5**:592-605, 1952.

149 Scully, R. E., and Richardson, G. S.: Luteinization of the stroma of metastatic cancer involving the ovary and its endocrine significance, Cancer **14**:827-840, 1961.

150 Shippel, S.: Ovarian theca cell; its function—critical review; variable endometrial responses to ovarian thecal function, J. Obstet. Gynaec. Brit. Emp. **57**:362-387, 1950.

151 Shippel, S.: Ovarian theca cell; unusual ovarian tumor, J. Obstet. Gynaec. Brit. Emp. **57**:557-565, 1950.

152 Shirley, W. C., Torpin, R., and Mullins, D. F., Jr.: Embryologic tumors of the uterine tube, Obstet. Gynec. **4**:194-196, 1954.

153 Sommers, S. C., Gates, O., and Goodof, I. I.: Late recurrences of granulosa cell tumors; report of two cases, Obstet. Gynec. **6**:395-398, 1955.

154 Spielman, F.: Tubular adenoma (arrhenoblastoma) of the ovary, Amer. J. Obstet. Gynec. **25**:517-521, 1933.

155 Sternberg, W. H.: The morphology, androgenic function, hyperplasia and tumors of the human ovarian hilus cells, Amer. J. Path. **25**:493-522, 1949.

156 Sternberg, W. H., and Gaskill, C. J.: Thecacell tumors, Amer. J. Obstet. Gynec. **59**:575-587, 1950.

157 Stohr, G.: Granulosa cell tumor of the ovary and coincident carcinoma of the uterus, Amer. J. Obstet. Gynec. **43**:586-599, 1942.

158 Tawa, K., and Baker, T. H.: Ovarian tumors in pregnancy, J. Int. Coll. Surg. **41**:60-74, 1964.

159 Taylor, C. W.: The pathology of malignant ovarian tumours, J. Obstet. Gynaec. Brit. Emp. **57**:328-334, 1950.

160 Taylor, H., Barter, R. H., and Jacobson, C. B.: Neoplasms of dysgenetic gonads, Amer. J. Obstet. Gynec. **96**:816-823, 1966.

161 Taylor, H. B., and Norris, H. J.: Lipid cell tumors of the ovary, Cancer **20**:1953-1962, 1967.

162 Taylor, H. C., Jr.: Malignant and semimalignant tumors of the ovary, Surg. Gynec. Obstet. **48**:204-230, 1929.

163 Taylor, H. C., Jr., and Greeley, A. V.: Factors influencing end-results in carcinoma of the ovary, Surg. Gynec. Obstet. **74**:928-934, 1942.

164 Teilum, G.: Feminizing tumor of testis, with same structures as arrhenoblastoma of ovary; studies on homologous tumors of ovary and testis, Nord. Med. **27**:1965-1967, 1945.

165 Teilum, G.: Estrogen-producing Sertoli tumors (androblastoma tubulare lipoides) of the human testis and ovary; homologus ovarian and testicular tumors, J. Clin. Endocr. **9**:301-318, 1949.

166 Teilum, G.: Classification of ovarian tumors, Acta Obstet. Gynec. Scand. **31**:292-312, 1952.

167 Teilum, G.: Histogenesis and classification of mesonephric tumors of the female and male genital system and relationship to benign so-called adenomatoid tumors (mesotheliomas); a comparative histological study, Acta Path. Microbiol. Scand. **34**:431-481, 1954.

168 Teilum, G.: Classification of testicular and ovarian androblastoma and Sertoli cell tumors; a survey of comparative studies with consideration of histogenesis, endocrinology and embryological theories, Cancer **11**:769-782, 1958.

169 Teilum, G.: Endodermal sinus tumors of the ovary and testis; comparative morphogenesis of the so-called mesonephroma ovarii (Schiller) and extraembryonic (yolk sac-allantoic) structures of the rat's placenta, Cancer **12**:1092-1105, 1959.

170 Teoh, T. B.: Further observations on the histogenesis of minute and small Brenner tumours, J. Path. Bact. **78**:145-150, 1959.

171 Terz, J. J., Barber, H. R. K., and Brunschwig, A.: Incidence of carcinoma in the retained ovary, Amer. J. Surg. **113**:511-515, 1967.

172 Teter, J., and Boczkowski, R.: Occurrence of tumors in dysgenetic gonads, Cancer **20**:1301-1310, 1967.

173 Thurlbeck, W. M., and Scully, R. E.: Solid teratoma of the ovary, Cancer **13**:804-811, 1960.

174 Timonen, S., and Purola, E.: Adenofibroma and cystadenofibroma of the ovary, Ann. Chir. Gynaec. Fenn. **56**(suppl. 154):1-33, 1967.

175 Traut, H. F., Kuder, A., and Cadden, J. F.: A study of the reticulum and luteinization in granulosa and theca cell tumors of the ovary, Amer. J. Obstet. Gynec. **38**:798-813, 1939.

176 Turunen, A.: Hormonal secretion of Krukenberg tumors, Acta Endocr. (Kobenhavn) **20**:50-56, 1955.

177 Vaeth, J. M., and Buschke, F. J.: The role of preoperative irradiation in the treatment of carcinoma of the ovary, Amer. J. Roentgen. **105**:614-617, 1969.

178 Wang, S. N.: Androblastoma tubulare lipoides (Sertoli cell tumor or testicular tubular adenoma) of ovary; report of case and review of literature, Chin. Med. J. (Peking) **73**:55-65, 1955.

179 Watts, R. M., and Adair, F. L.: On the chemistry of ovarian cysts, Amer. J. Obstet. Gynec. **48**:1-15, 1944.

180 Wheelock, M. C., and Putong, P.: Ovarian metastases from adenocarcinomas of colon and rectum, Obstet. Gynec. 14:291-295, 1959.

181 Willis, R. A.: The pathology of tumours, St. Louis, 1948, The C. V. Mosby Co., p. 980.

182 Witschi, E.: Migration of the germ cells of human embryos from the yolk sac to the primitive gonadal folds, Contrib. Embryol.

(nos. 207-212) 32:67-80, 1948, Carnegie Institution of Washington.

183 Wolfe, S. A., and Neigus, I.: Theca cell tumors of the ovary, Amer. J. Obstet. Gynec. 42:218-228, 1941.

184 Wynder, E. L., Dodo, H., and Barber, H. R. K.: Epidemiology of cancer of the ovary, Cancer 23:352-370, 1969.

Endometrium

Anatomy

The uterus is a pear-shaped muscular organ, slightly flattened anteroposteriorly, situated in the midline of the female pelvis between the bladder and the rectum. It is about 7.5 cm long and 5 cm wide. It is attached to the lateral walls of the pelvis by means of the broad ligaments, anteriorly by the round ligaments, and posteriorly by the uterosacral ligaments. Its walls are largely composed of thick layers of muscular fibers. Anteriorly, it is in almost direct relation to the bladder. Posteriorly, it is in close contact with portions of the small intestine and with the rectum. It may be divided into the *fundus* or superior portion, the *corpus* or intermediate section, and the *cervix* or lower portion.

The uterine cavity is a triangular space that extends from the cervical canal to the tubal orifices (cornua). It is lined by the *endometrium*, a mucous membrane of simple columnar epithelium containing numerous glands that extend deep into the thickness of the muscle. The endometrium is about 2 mm thick at the fundus, becoming thinner on the corpus and still thinner (0.5 mm) as it approaches the cervix. At the endocervical canal, it becomes smooth and more resistant. The endometrial mucous membrane undergoes physiologic hyperplasia and is periodically eliminated during menstruation.

Lymphatics. The uterus has several intercommunicating lymphatic networks that run in the mucosa, the muscularis, and the serous and subserous areas. The latter receive the lymph from the others, thereby becoming a point of origin for the collecting trunks. The collecting trunks originate in the lateral borders of the uterus and group themselves into three main pedicles (Fig. 573):

1 The *utero-ovarian pedicle* starts below the uterine tube and travels in the broad ligament until it reaches the hilus of the ovary. Here, there are wide anastomoses with the lymphatics of the tube and ovary, and they proceed to the preaortic and lateroaortic lymph nodes on the left and to the precaval and laterocaval lymph nodes on the right.

2 The *external iliac pedicle* contains a lesser number of trunks that follow a transverse direction outward and end in the lymph nodes of the external iliac group.

3 The *round ligament pedicle* is composed of a small number of trunks that follow the round ligament from its insertion in the uterine fundus to the inguinal canal and end in the superficial lymph nodes of the inguinal region.

Consequently, the lymphatic drainage of the body of the uterus may finally terminate in the para-aortic, paracaval, external iliac, and inguinal nodes (Testut and Latarjet[117]; Rouvière[95]).

Epidemiology

In the 1947 cancer survey in the United States, the sex-age adjusted incidence of carcinoma of the endometrium was 23.6 per 100,000 population. A comparison of the 1945-1949 and 1960-1962 surveys of the state of Connecticut did not show any change in incidence, and that of the New York state surveys of 1949-1951 and 1958-1960 showed a slight decrease. The incidence seems to be about the same for white and non-white women in the United States. In the South African Bantu, there is

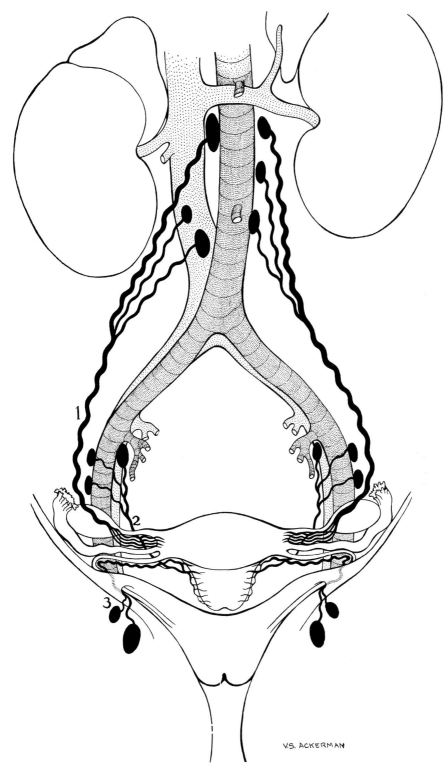

Fig. 573. Lymphatics of uterus showing utero-ovarian pedicle, **1**; external iliac pedicle, **2**; round ligament leading to inguinal lymph nodes, **3**.

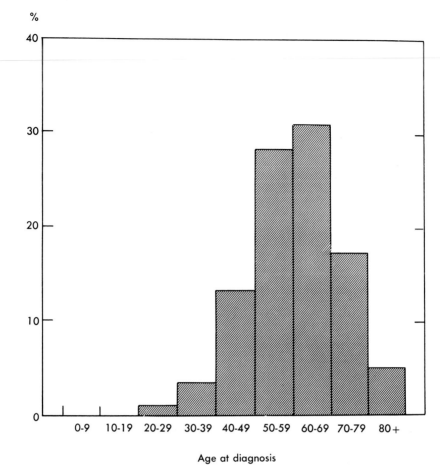

Fig. 574. Carcinoma of endometrium. Age distribution of patients diagnosed between 1955 and 1964. (From Cutler, S. J., et al.: End results in cancer, Report no. 3, United States Department of Health, Education, and Welfare, 1968.)

a low incidence of endometrial carcinoma; the ratio of carcinoma of the cervix to carcinoma of the endometrium is 8:1. The incidence rate is very low under the age of 35 years but rises steadily in the later decades of life (Fig. 574).

Carcinoma of the endometrium used to occur less frequently than carcinoma of the cervix. In a series of 1648 invasive carcinomas of the uterus reported by Christopherson et al.,[15] the overall ratio of cervical to endometrial carcinomas was 2.6:1. For women 30 to 39 years of age, the ratio was 24:1, whereas for those over 70 years of age it was 1.2:1. Clinical reports have emphasized a changing ratio in the occurrence of these two forms of cancer of the uterus. It is doubtful that the changing ratio is due to any true increase in occurrence of carcinoma of the endometrium.

Carcinoma of the endometrium has been found in patients who had been given previous radiotherapy for a benign condition, leading to the interpretation that radiations are a causative factor (Smith and Bowden[102]; Speert and Peightal[109]). However, these reports fail to emphasize that many of these patients were irradiated because of preexisting hyperplasia, in itself an indication of cancerous tendency (Hertig and Sommers[37]). Bernard and Hlasivec[8] have shown that such conclusions may be the result of false interpretation of the original histology. If radiations were the causative factor, carcinomas of the endometrium should be observed in women irradiated for and cured of carcinoma of the cervix—this has been rarely reported (Fernandez-Colmeiro[23]). The possibility that this form of cancer may develop after prolonged administration of estrogens also has been suggested (Vass[118]; Speert[107]). Speert[107] found four cases of cirrhosis among twelve patients who died of carcinoma of the endometrium and interpreted these findings as corroborative of the view that persistent estrogenic stimulation is a factor in the genesis of these tumors. Rosenblum and Hendricks[94] observed that the vaginal epithelium showed signs of estrogenation as frequently in the normal postmenopausal women as in those with carcinoma of the endometrium.

The overwhelming majority of carcinomas of the endometrium develop after the menopause, and the patients often have had a late menopause. Carcinoma of the endometrium, unlike carcinoma of the cervix, is frequently found in nulliparous women. In a special study, Moss[76] found a high proportion of diabetes, hypertension, and obesity among these patients. Fox and Sen[24a] also showed that endometrial adenocarcinoma was associated with hypertension, nulliparity, and a late menopause. An association between carcinoma of the endometrium and the Stein-Leventhal syndrome has been reported. The syndrome consists of menstrual irregularities, history of sterility, masculine hirsutism, obesity, and, in some patients, retarded development of the breasts (de Vere and Dempster[18]). Jackson and Dockerty[43] reported on forty-six patients with this syndrome, sixteen of whom had carcinoma of the endometrium.

Hyperplasia of the endometrium can coexist with endometrial carcinoma and, also, transitions between the two can be demonstrated (Goetchel[25]; Hall[30]). Te-Linde et al.[116] have pointed out that there are no absolute criteria for a diagnosis of hyperplasia and that the occurrence of hyperplasia decreases as that of carcinoma increases, after 50 years of age. However, the occurrence of hyperplasia is highest in the first five years after cessation of periods (McBride[64]). The coexistence of hyperplasia and carcinoma is five times more frequent in postmenopausal than premenopausal women (Payne[87]). Gray and Barnes[26] have verified the post menopausal association of both changes. Taylor[112] reported eighty-five cases of endometrial hyperplasia, two of which had apparently developed into carcinoma. In both instances, the apparent transformation was due to failure to detect carcinoma in the first examination. It seems obvious that only a small proportion of patients with a diagnosis of endometrial hyperplasia develop carcinoma. Hertig and Sommers[37] and Hertig et al.[38] studied thirty-two cases of carcinoma of the endometrium in which previous biopsies were available; seventeen patients had shown previous *cystic hyperplasia*, which the investigators[37, 38] concluded is a frequent important precursor of carcinoma.

Estrogen-secreting tumors may be accompanied by carcinoma of the endometrium. In patients over 50 years of age with granulosa–theca cell tumors, the coexistence of endometrial carcinoma may be found in one-fourth. McGoldrick and Lapp[66] collected forty-six cases of *theca cell tumors* of the ovary, thirty-six of which showed hyperplasia of the endometrium (thirty-two in postmenopausal patients) with five coexisting endometrial carcinomas. There is a case on record of a *granulosa cell tumor* of the ovary coexisting with a carcinoma of the endometrium that disappeared after surgical removal of the ovarian tumor (Stohr[111]). Naturally, questions have been raised as to the authenticity of these associated endometrial carcinomas. Hertig[36] has indicated that there is no endocrinologic proof, based on bioassay or on chemical tests, of this association.

Sarcomas of the uterus are rather infrequently observed, making up only about 4% of all malignant tumors of the uterus. They are found in patients 40 to 60 years of age. A large number of sarcomas of all types occur within the uterus. Leiomyosarcoma makes up the largest group. Ober[82] classified the remaining types of sarcomas. Mesodermal malignant *mixed tumors*, also rare, appear in women of *all* ages.

Pathology
Gross pathology

Endometrial carcinomas are usually flat, velvety lesions arising from the walls of the corpus, from the fundus, or in the region of the cornua. Sometimes they appear pedunculated. They are usually well circumscribed and grow toward the endo-

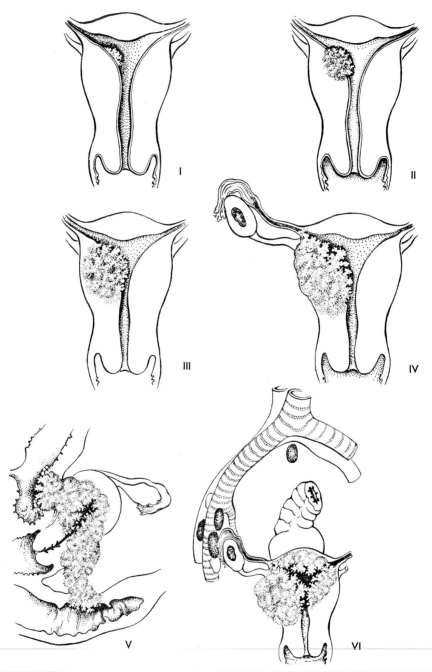

Fig. 575. Different stages of carcinoma of endometrium. **Stage I,** Early carcinoma without invasion of muscular layer. **Stage II,** Carcinoma with invasion of not more than half of muscular layer. **Stage III,** Carcinoma with invasion of entire muscular thickness. **Stage IV,** Carcinoma with invasion of serosa and with operable metastases to ovary. **Stage V,** Carcinoma with extension to bladder and rectum. **Stage VI,** Carcinoma with extension to external iliac nodes and nodes of promontory.

metrial cavity, but in some cases they are diffusely infiltrating. By direct invasion, the tumor may ulcerate the cervix and extend to the vaginal fornices. It may also invade the myometrium, increasing the size of the uterus and producing necrotic excavations. Invasion of the serosa, parametria, bladder, and small and large intestine may occur in patients with advanced lesions (Fig. 575).

Extension of the tumor to the region of the cornua and the fallopian tubes may result in direct invasion of these structures or in a tumor embolism leading to a separate growth (Lynch and Dockerty[63]). Höeg[40] demonstrated, through postoperative cytologic examination, that cells from carcinoma of the endometrium spread to the tubes and to the peritoneal cavity. It seems certain that the majority of these cells do not remain viable.

Carcinomas of the endometrium may be preceded by *endometrial polyps*. In the thirty-two patients with previous biopsies studied by Hertig and Sommers[37] and Hertig et al.,[38] ten had shown endometrial polyps. In 482 patients with endometrial polyps, seventeen developed carcinoma (Armenia[3]). In a study of 236 cases of postmenopausal uteri, Fahlund and Broders[22] found an incidence of endometrial polyps that was roughly eight times greater in the patients who had carcinoma than in those without disease. Polyps arise near the region of the cornua and are often observed after the menopause. They are usually well vascularized and may overlie a submucous leiomyoma.

It has been considered that leiomyosarcomas arise from preexisting leiomyomas, but this is difficult to prove, and probably most, if not all, leiomyosarcomas are malignant from their inception (Norris and Taylor[81]).

Microscopic pathology

Whether or not carcinomas of the endometrium arise from preexisting hyperplasia, the fact is that the two are often associated, and for this reason it is important to be able to differentiate them. In endometrial hyperplasia, there is marked glandular proliferation. The glands may be lined by several layers of cells, and there may even be some invasion of the muscle. The deeper glands may show cystic dilatation, which gives a typical appearance that has been called "Swiss cheese endometrium." Herrell and Broders[34] prefer the term cystic endometrium, and it is their opinion that sudden withdrawal or dysfunction of the ovarian tissue is usually accompanied by atrophy of the endometrium. However, many an endometrium removed after menopause histologically resembles that found in an active period of menstrual function. In 236 cases of postmenopausal uteri studied by Fahlund and Broders,[22] 41% of those that contained carcinoma of the endometrium presented an atrophic endometrium, whereas only 16% of those without carcinoma had an atrophic endometrium. Approximately 42% of the cases with carcinoma showed no cystic changes, whereas only 20% of those without carcinoma showed no cystic changes.

It used to be considered that the presence of mucin ruled out the possibility that an adenocarcinoma had originated in the endometrium. Meiser[72] studied 116 cases of adenocarcinoma, eighteen of which were assumed to have originated in the cervix due to positive mucin reaction. Microscopic study of the surgical specimens of these cases revealed that six of the eighteen had actually arisen from the endometrium. A detailed histochemical study has been made of the endometrium (McKay et al.[67]).

As a rule, pure endometrial hyperplasia is not difficult to differentiate from adenocarcinomas of the endometrium. The hyperplasia presents a velvety, thickened endometrium that may involve the entire cavity but stops abruptly at the internal os. Microscopically, unlike carcinoma it shows no areas of necrosis, and it reveals areas of hyperplasia of both the stroma and the glands with numerous cystic areas (Fig. 576).

Carcinoma in situ of the endometrium is characterized by few or many endometrial glands composed of large cells with abundant clear eosinophilic cytoplasm (Hertig and Sommers[37]; Hertig et al.[38]). The nuclei are pale with fine granular chromatin, and there is cellular disorientation and disparity in size, or stratification. Carcinoma in situ is often sharply demarcated. According to Hertig and Sommers[37] and Hertig

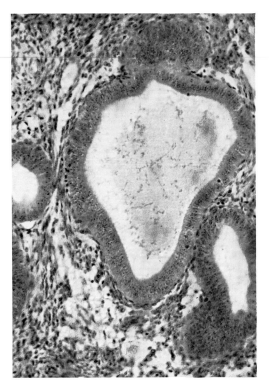

Fig. 576. Endometrial hyperplasia showing in detail large cystic glands and hyperplasia of stroma. (Moderate enlargement.)

et al.,[38] these changes are irreversible and would eventually progress to infiltrating carcinoma. The grading of carcinoma of the endometrium has some practical value. Well-differentiated adenocarcinoma may be present within a polyp in the endometrium. Most of the carcinomas are fairly well differentiated. A few are highly undifferentiated. The more undifferentiated tumors have a greater capacity for invasion. If an adenocarcinoma shows focal areas of squamous metaplasia, it is often designated as adenoacanthoma, a poor designation in our opinion. This has some practical value, but it is better designated adenocarcinoma with foci of squamous metaplasia. Kay[49] described a type of adenocarcinoma of the endometrium in which most of the cells have a rather clear appearance, and he feels this represents evidence of considerable endometrium glycogen secretion. This may be due to progesterone or progesterone-like stimulation. Bamforth[4] demonstrated that prominent secretory glandular activity is not rare in endometrial cancer.

The study of ovaries at the menopause shows a striking loss of follicular activity and a high incidence of stromal hyperplasia often accompanied by endometrial hyperplasia (Woll et al.[119]). Sommers and Meissner[106] found hyperplasia of the ovarian cortical stroma and of the adrenal cortex, as well as changes in the pituitary gland. Roddick and Greene[92] did not find any relationship between cortical stromal hyperplasia and endometrial carcinoma.

Metastatic spread

Lymph node involvement in *adenocarcinoma* of the endometrium usually does not appear until the disease is moderately advanced; it occurs in the external iliac chains (about 15%) (Lefèvre[58]), but also in the para-aortic chain and the inguinal region. In 4.7% of 251 cases reported by Heidler,[33] there were metastases to the tubes and ovaries. Retrograde permeation of lymphatics results in implants in the lower third of the vagina and vulva. Distant metastases to the liver, lungs, brain, and skeleton are observed mostly in advanced cases. *Sarcomas* metastasize widely through the bloodstream, most commonly to the liver and lungs. Spiro and McPeak[110] have recorded two additional instances of metastasis of histologically benign uterine leiomyoma. This is an extremely rare finding.

Clinical evolution

Early symptoms of carcinoma of the endometrium may not be unduly marked, but because they most commonly occur after the menopause, they cause immediate alarm. The most common early sign of disease is a slight *vaginal bleeding*, which may remain minimal but also may be shortly followed by a marked *hemorrhage*. *Watery discharge*, extremely malodorous, is at times present and is a very significant sign of the disease. In some instances, there may be spontaneous elimination of small fragments of friable tumor. Complaints of *menstrual pains* are often due to retention of blood or fluid and to the resulting uterine contractions. *Pain* is not an early symptom. When it appears, it is persistent and progressive, spreading from the lumbar region around the lower abdomen and radiating to the hips and thighs. *Urinary symptoms* are seldom present, and compression of the ureter and *anuresis* are less frequently observed than in carcinoma of the cervix. *Constipation* is caused by mechanical pressure over the rectosigmoid when the tumor become voluminous.

Most carcinomas of the endometrium develop slowly, and even though the disease may be considerably advanced, the patients may survive for years in a rather good general condition. *Anemia* may be present with markedly bleeding tumors. Death often occurs as a consequence of hemorrhage. In a study of 110 carcinomas of the endometrium, Gricouroff[27] found an unusually high percentage with metastases (about one-third of the cases). The majority of these were vaginal, vulvar, inguinal, and intra-abdominal metastases, but there were four cases of pulmonary metastases, two of intracranial metastases, and one of bone metastases.

Sarcomas develop slowly and cause discharge or bleeding after they invade the endometrium. Advanced cases are accompanied by severe pain. Generalization of the disease is more common than in carcinoma. Malignant mesodermal *mixed tumors* cause vaginal bleeding and frequently foul-smelling discharge.

Diagnosis

The overwhelming majority of carcinomas of the endometrium develop after the menopause. Patients complaining of postmenopausal uterine bleeding have a greater than even chance of having a malignant tumor of the gynecologic tract. In a study of a large series of cases of postmenopausal bleeding, TeLinde[115] found that 32% were due to carcinoma of the cervix, 15% to carcinoma of the endometrium, and 3% to malignant ovarian tumors, and that an additional 3% were made up of other rare malignant tumors of the vagina and uterus. The remaining cases presented benign lesions such as cervical ulcerations, prolapse of the uterus, vaginitis, rupture of vaginal adhesions, cervical polyps, endometrial polyps, endometritis, pyometra, leiomyomas, and benign ovarian tumors. In a very small group, no organic lesion was found to explain the bleeding. A similar study by Taylor and Millen[113] also emphasized the fruitfulness of the investigation of all cases of postmenopausal bleeding, for

over half of these may prove to be due to cancer (Fig. 577).

Hertig and Sommers[37] made a careful study of the history of patients with carcinoma of the endometrium. They found the following typical sequence: A 47-year-old patient has irregular vaginal bleeding preceding and following cessation of menstruation. Biopsy at this time may show adenomatous hyperplasia (Gusberg[28]). From the age of 49 to 57 years, bleeding continues. Biopsy now shows carcinoma in situ. Past 57 years of age, biopsy will probably show invasive adenocarcinoma. In other words, the mean age of patients with endometrial hyperplasia is 49 years and that of patients with carcinoma of the endometrium is 57 years, whereas the average duration of carcinoma in situ of the endometrium before its transformation into infiltrating carcinoma is six to eight years.

Miller[74] pointed out that carcinoma of the endometrium has not fully shared in the evident progress made in the diagnosis of carcinoma of the cervix. Indeed, an unfortunately large number of these patients are diagnosed in advanced stages due to delay by the patient (McCall[65]), to complacency in the investigation of postmenopausal bleeding, often assumed to be functional, and to the lack of a simple and sufficiently reliable early diagnostic procedure.

Clinical examination

Before an examination is started, a careful menstrual history should be recorded. The absence or presence of pain and its character, as well as other symptoms, should also be investigated. It should not be forgotten that obese multiparous patients with hypertension and a history of diabetes form a large proportion of those with adenocarcinoma of the endometrium (Moss[76]). Its association with feminizing ovarian tumors (p. 727), though not frequent, is greater than justified on the basis of chance alone (Ingram and Novak[42]; Dockerty and Mussey[19]). Gusberg and Kaplan[29] studied a group of patients with adenomatous hyperplasia of the endometrium, 12% of whom developed endometrial carcinoma. They believe that failure of ovulation, dysfunctional bleeding, and

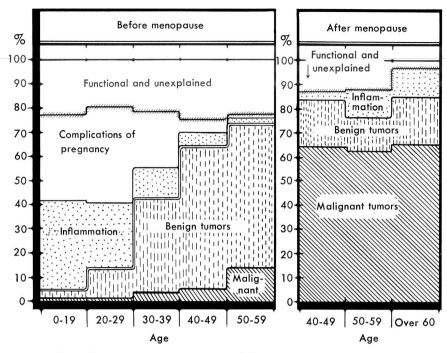

Fig. 577. Relative frequency of causes of vaginal bleeding in over 4000 cases. After menopause, vaginal bleeding is found to be due to cancer in more than half of cases. (Redrawn after Taylor, H. C., Jr., and Millen, R.: The causes of vaginal bleeding and the histology of the endometrium after the menopause, Amer. J. Obstet. Gynec. **36:**22-39, 1938.)

adenomatous hyperplasia is a triad that labels the patient as susceptible to carcinoma of the endometrium.

A thorough bimanual examination should be done in an attempt to establish the size of the uterus and its mobility. Because of obesity, pain, or lack of cooperation on the part of the patient, palpation may be handicapped and fail to reveal the actual size of the uterus. In such instances, an examination under anesthesia may be indicated. The examination, moreover, is useful to establish the differential diagnosis with ovarian tumors.

In the majority of patients with carcinoma of the endometrium, the cervix shows no involvement, but in some instances there may be an ulceration extending to the vaginal walls. Retrograde metastases of the vaginal wall, particularly around the urethra, may be detected. In general, the parametria will not be found invaded except in very advanced disease.

Biopsy

In most instances, a diagnosis is possible only after dilatation of the cervix and curettage of the uterine cavity. There should be no hesitation in carrying out this procedure in all patients with unexplained postmenopausal vaginal bleeding. It should be kept in mind, however, that this method carries some danger of perforating the uterus. A curettage of the uterus should secure tissue from the fundus, corpus, and endocervix, tissues that should be kept separately if possible.

It is important to demonstrate the presence or absence of cervical involvement. The pattern of spread to lymph nodes is different, and the vaginal recurrence rate will be high in those patients with cervical infiltration who do not receive radiation therapy (Rubin et al.[96]).

The microscopic diagnosis of carcinoma of the endometrium is not always obvious. Hertig et al.[38] described the changes of typical carcinoma in situ, and these are often focal. There are often atypical endometrial proliferations that are difficult to evaluate (Müller and Keller[77]). It is certain that some of these progress to carcinoma, but in the majority such development does not take place. Such atypical endometrial proliferation may be present with granulosa–theca cell tumors. Recently, with the use of various drugs, the problem has become even more complicated. Pseudo-malignant endometrial changes can be produced by synthetic progestins (Dockerty et al.[20]). Norethynodrel with added ethynyl estradial (Enovid) and norethindrone (Norlutin) can produce striking changes in the endometrium, particularly in the stroma, that even suggest a stromal sarcoma. Pseudodecidual reaction is produced. The most bizarre pathologic slide that we have seen was in a lesion of endometriosis of the large bowel that had been removed from a patient who had been treated with the progestin, Enovid. However, the endometrial glands are atrophic, the epithelium is low, and there is usually no difficulty in diagnosing the lesion as benign.

Exfoliative cytology is used in the diagnosis of carcinoma of the endometrium. Cytologic diagnosis of carcinoma of the endometrium is possible but requires acquaintance with the special features of exfoliated adenocarcinomatous cells (Berg and Durfee[6]). In Messelt's series,[73] only 64% of the patients with endometrial carcinoma had a positive cytologic examination. Hecht and Oppenheim[32] use endometrial aspiration smears in cytology, and they feel that such smears have increased their accuracy from 70% to 90%. In the follow-up of patients treated with radiotherapy alone, the examination of cervical smears may be of value in detecting persistent neoplasm.

Clinical classification

A clinical classification of carcinoma of the endometrium (comparable to the League of Nations' classification of carcinoma of the cervix) is desirable, but although several have been suggested, they are far from being as valuable in the prognosis as the one for carcinoma of the cervix. Healy and Cutler[31] pointed out that uterine enlargement in carcinomas of the endometrium has prognostic significance when radiotherapy alone is to be given. But the evaluation of the size of the uterus is a relative one, particularly in view of the fact that leiomyomas often accompany these tumors.

The International Federation of Obstetrics and Gynecology accepts the following classification:

Stage I

The carcinoma is confined to the corpus.

Stage II

The carcinoma has involved the corpus and the cervix.

Stage III

The carcinoma has extended outside the uterus but not outside the true pelvis.

Stage IV

The carcinoma has extended outside the true pelvis or has obviously involved the mucosa of the bladder or rectum.

In rare cases it may be difficult to decide whether the cancer actually is a carcinoma of the endocervix or a carcinoma of the endometrium involving the endocervix. If a clear decision cannot be made at the fractional curettage, an adenocarcinoma should be allotted to carcinoma of the corpus and an epidermoid carcinoma to the cervix (Kottmeier[56]).

In cases that are being curetted, it is of value to make note of the dimensions of the uterine cavity. This additional information may aid in the classification (Miller[74]).

Zsolnai and Nyire[121] have used hysterorography to help in the delimitation of the uterine cavity. It is particularly helpful after curettage and reveals a localization and extent of the process. If the size and shape of the uterus and the localization of the lesion are precisely outlined, radiotherapy can be carried out with more accuracy.

Differential diagnosis

Speculum examination easily reveals those cervical lesions that may cause vaginal bleeding (*carcinoma of the cervix and cervical polyps*). At times, carcinoma of the endometrium may invade the cervix and suggest a Stage I carcinoma of the cervix.

The most common sarcoma is a leiomyosarcoma. Other sarcomas include mixed mesodermal tumors, stromal sarcomas, and carcinosarcoma. These tumors arise from stromal cells that are multipotential. These tumor cells may differentiate into smooth

muscle, striated muscle, osteoblasts, cartilage, and glands. Origin of these tumors
from rests or primitive anlage is certainly
not true (Norris and Taylor[81]). The pathologic diagnosis of leiomyosarcomas is
difficult. Taylor and Norris[114] reported
sixty-three highly cellular uterine tumors
previously considered to be leiomyosarcomas. Lesions with fewer than ten mitoses
in ten high-powered fields proved benign
on follow-up, regardless of cytologic
atypism. If the tumor had ten or more
mitotic figures in ten high-powered fields,
there was recurrence or metastasis in thirty-one of thirty-six patients.

Most important in determining that a
smooth muscle tumor is malignant is evidence of infiltration and vascular invasion.
The incidence of leiomyosarcoma is low,
and at Indiana University there were only
5 leiomyosarcomas found out of a group
of 2,714 smooth muscle neoplasms, or
0.21% (Chang et al.[14]). Corscaden and
Singh[17] found a somewhat similar percentage. The incidence of lethal sarcomatous
change in a myoma was only 0.13% or 1
out of 800 cases.

Designations such as round cell, spindle
cell, or giant cell sarcoma are not justified
because they do not indicate histogenesis.
It is true that in many instances the extensive growth of the tumor has blotted
out any chance of determining histogenesis,
but the majority are leiomyosarcomas.
Rarely, sarcomas can arise from the lamina
propria of the endometrium or of a polyp
(Fienberg[24]). Curetted material from malignant *mesodermal mixed tumors* often
shows adenocarcinoma and sarcoma. Atypical cartilage and striated muscle are frequently present.

The malignant mesodermal tumor usually forms a polypoid mass with a broad
base and arises most frequently from the
posterior uterine wall in the region of the
fundus (Meikle[71]) (Fig. 578). The mesenchymal sarcomas of the uterus can be
traced to an origin "specifically that derived
from and surrounding the epithelium of
the Müllerian duct."[*]

Endometrial stromal sarcomas originate
either in the endometrium or from stroma-

like masses between myometrial muscle
bundles. Norris and Taylor[80] emphasized
the distinction between stromal nodules
(always benign), stromal sarcoma (malignant), and endolymphatic stromal myosis,
a characteristically intravascular growth of
intermediate aggressive tendency (Figs.
579 and 580).

A thorough bimanual palpation, particularly if carried out under anesthesia, can
reveal the presence of an *ovarian tumor*.
A dilatation of the cervix with curettage
of the endometrium facilitates the diagnosis of *endometritis*, pyometra, endometrial hyperplasia, and endometrial polyps.
Submucous leiomyomas may also be diagnosed by curettement. When *sarcomas*
have invaded the endometrium, they too
may be diagnosed from curettings. The
presence of leiomyomas that may be felt
on palpation does not eliminate an additional possibility of carcinoma of the endometrium. *Angiomas* of the uterus are very
rare (Marsh[68]).

Treatment
Prevention

From the studies of Hertig and Sommers[37] and Hertig et al.,[38] it appears that
patients who present endometrial polyps
and cystic or adenomatous hyperplasia may,

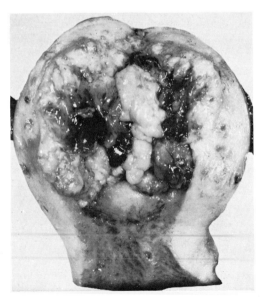

Fig. 578. Malignant mesodermal tumor of uterus.
Patient died with extensive metastases six months
after operation.

*[*]From Ober, W. B., and Tovell, H. M. M.:
Mesenchymal sarcomas of the uterus, Amer. J.
Obstet. Gynec. 77:246-268, 1959.

in a certain proportion of instances, develop endometrial carcinoma. It is imperative that those patients be followed closely and recuretted if symptoms continue. In

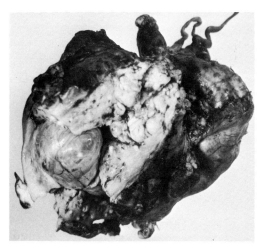

Fig. 579. Endometrial stromal sarcoma appearing in 59-year-old woman. Patient lived for six and one-half years in spite of extensive vascular invasion observed at time of initial surgery. (From Koss, L. G., et al.: Endometrial stromal sarcoma, Surg. Gynec. Obstet. **121:**531-537, 1965; by permission of Surgery, Gynecology & Obstetrics.)

patients with endometrial hyperplasia or carcinoma in situ, Kistner et al.[51] have pointed out that an effort should be made to secure ovulation. Carcinoma of the endometrium in association with Stein-Leventhal syndrome may respond to conservative treatment and require neither surgery nor radiotherapy; a wedge resection of the ovaries may be followed by ovulation, secretion of progesterone, and reversion of the hyperplastic process (Kaufman et al.[48]).

Radiotherapy

In the past, three important facts seem to have found wide assent in the treatment of carcinomas of the endometrium: (1) that the best results are obtained when a hysterectomy is practicable; (2) that the results are considerably improved by preoperative radiotherapy; and (3) that a large proportion of the inoperable cases can be cured by a skillful application of radiation therapy. Heyman[39] advocated radiumtherapy as the treatment of choice in all patients and advised hysterectomy only following radiotherapeutic failure. He supported this view with excellent results.

Intracavitary curietherapy of the uterus

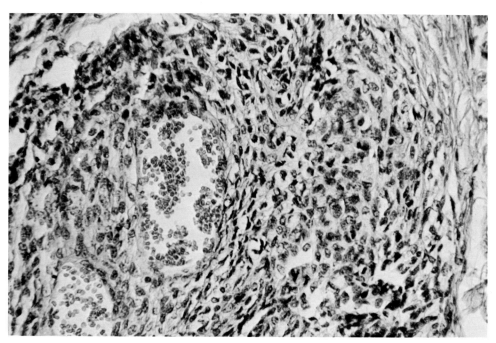

Fig. 580. Endometrial stromal sarcoma. Mass of tumor cells is lying within large blood vessel. Long duration and microscopic pattern suggest that this could be endometrial lymphatic stromal myosis. (×300; WU neg. 68-11031.)

affected by carcinoma of the endometrium offers unquestionable difficulties. In general, the uterine cavity is enlarged, and the "tandem" containing the radium needles or tubes may not occupy a desirable position in respect to the tumor. In addition, the development of tumor toward one side may greatly interfere with its homogeneous irradiation by internal sources of radiation. Numerous applicators for intrauterine radium have been devised, but they offer little advantage. Heyman's "packing method" appears most successful. A variable number of "irradiators" are placed within the cavity until it is filled, and these may be supplemented by a vaginal application of radium in a special holder. Nolan and Steele[78] made a study of distribution of radiations with the different applicators and concluded that Heyman's method shows unquestionable superiority.

Preoperative irradiation diminishes considerably the secondary infection and the volume of the tumor, facilitating its extirpation and, in all probability, diminishing the possibilities of postoperative recurrence and metastases.

The most widely used means of preoperative irradiation has been the intrauterine curietherapy (Fig. 581), but a thorough external pelvic irradiation may be equally valuable and may be used to advantage as an adjunct to intracavitary curietherapy.

Lampe[57] advocated external pelvic irradiation followed by hysterectomy after an interval of six weeks. In patients so treated, he reported complete destruction of the tumor in 88.6%. Supervoltage roentgentherapy and cobalt[60] teletherapy have rendered external pelvic irradiation, for these purposes, sufficient in itself to administer a rather large dose homogeneously throughout the area of tumor involvement. Unlike intracavitary radium application, external pelvic irradiation offers no complications of its own; it does not interfere nor does it increase the risk of the hysterectomy or its morbidity. Rutledge et al.[97] reported ninety-five patients treated by intrauterine and vaginal irradiation followed by hysterectomy. Only two developed vaginal metastases. In 127 patients treated by preoperative roentgentherapy followed by hysterectomy, there was not a single case

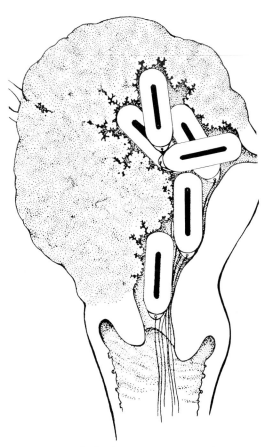

Fig. 581. Method of intracavitary curietherapy in advanced carcinoma of endometrium by means of Heyman's packed "irradiators."

of vaginal recurrence (Sala and Regato[98]). Whenever radiotherapy is not to be followed by surgery, external irradiation may be complemented by intracavitary curietherapy.

In judging the effect of preoperative irradiation, the pathologic examination of the surgical specimen is of great value, but the conclusions reported in the literature on the basis of this study are confusing. The fact that tumor is found remaining in the uterus following preoperative irradiation cannot be taken as a measure of the usefulness of this therapeutic step. On the other hand, the ability to find remaining persistent carcinoma depends on the thoroughness of the microscopic search. Obviously, a total disappearance of the tumor cannot be expected when surgery is done immediately after completion of the irradiation. All tumors, even the most radiosensitive, have a more or less prolonged period of latency before complete dissolution. On the other hand, a hysterectomy done several months after radiotherapy will show obvious evidence of recurrence if the amount of radiations has been insufficient to sterilize the tumor. In general, however, preoperative radiotherapy is given without intent of totally sterilizing the tumor, and to delay surgery is not justified. Sheehan and Schmitz[100] made a very thorough study of the effects of radiotherapy on carcinoma of the endometrium and found this sequence of events: simplification of glands, loss of glandular form, disintegration of glands, and inspissation of secretion with or without foriegn body giant cell reaction.

Surgical failures are usually due to vaginal recurrences or metastases. The treatment of such recurrences is necessarily variable according to the case. Interstitial curietherapy, especially in the form of implants of radium element needles, may be used to advantage in certain cases, for vaginal metastases are often the only manifestation of the recurrent disease, and their successful handling may save the life of the patient. In our experience, transvaginal roentgentherapy is an excellent method of treatment of these recurrences (Regato[91]).

Surgery

An abdominal hysterectomy with bilateral salpingo-oorphorectomy is preferable in the treatment of tumors of the endometrium. At operation, as large a vaginal cuff as is possible should also be removed. The operative mortality varies greatly but ranges between 5% and 15%. There are a few instances in which an operation without benefit of previous radiotherapy may be indicated. Patients with well-differentiated carcinoma of the endometrium in normal-sized uteri may be treated surgically without benefit of preoperative irradiation.

Carmichael and Bean[13] propose a total abdominal hysterectomy and bilateral salpingo-oophorectomy, without benefit of preoperative irradiation, in all patients with Stage I, group a, carcinomas of the endometrium. They propose postoperative radiotherapy in some patients on the basis of the surgical pathology findings such as invasion of the myometrium in the lower segment or gross myometrial involvement. Carmichael and Bean's objections[13] to preoperative irradiation are based on the use of intracavitary radium alone. Also, they overlook that postoperative radiotherapy, although capable of controlling some limited areas of residual tumor, is seldom as useful as preoperative irradiation.

A more extensive hysterectomy with wide parametrial excision and lymph node dissection has been advocated to diminish the proportion of recurrences, but whether more radical procedures would improve the results remains to be proved. The proportion of iliac and hypogastric lymph node metastases is relatively low (Javert and Hofammann[45]). In reality, undifferentiated tumors that give rise to early lymph node metastases are seldom controlled by any means. Parsons and Cesare[86] performed a Wertheim operation in fifty patients and found lymph node metastases in four. Only two of the four patients were living at the end of two years, and complications developed in 27% of the patients.

A fair number of patients with carcinoma of the endometrium (30% to 50%) are inoperable. The inoperability may be due to the extension of the tumor outside the uterus but is most often caused by vaginal extension or metastases. Very often, patients are judged inoperable on the basis of obesity, hypertension, or diabetes. Obesity in itself should not be considered a contraindication to surgery. Prem et al.[90] reported ninety-eight patients weighing over 200 pounds, eighty-eight of whom had surgery with only three operative deaths. Patients with locally inoperable carcinomas of the endometrium, without lymph node spread, may be eligible for a curative pelvic exenteration.

Sarcomas should be treated by a complete hysterectomy whenever possible, without previous irradiation.

Hormone control

Microscopic evidence of concomitant carcinoma of the endometrium may disappear following removal of granulosa–theca cell tumors. Wedge resection of the ovaries, curettage, or administration of progesterone may reestablish ovulation and cause disappearance of atypical endometrial

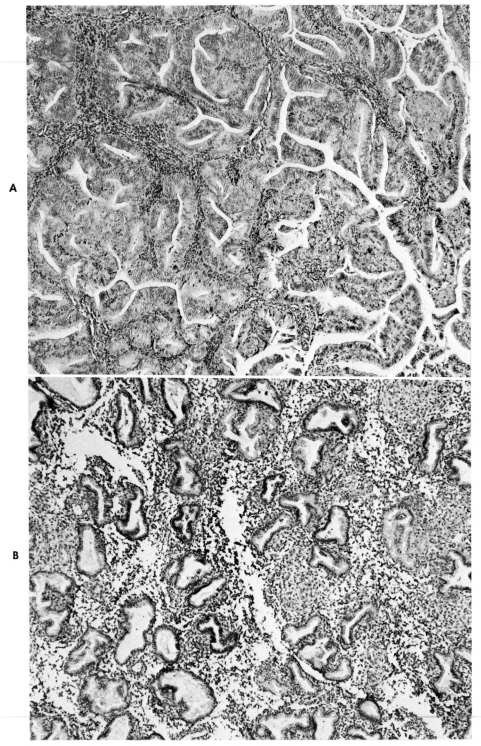

Fig. 582. A, On curettage, 27-year-old patient had this apparently well-differentiated adeno-carcinoma. Note glandular budding. **B,** Endometrium at repeat curettage three months later. Patient had ovulated and only secretory endometrium was present in specimen. Patient was well five years later. (From Kempson, R. L., and Pokorny, G. E.: Adenocarcinoma of the endometrium in women aged forty and younger, Cancer **21**:650-662, 1968; **A** and **B,** hema-toxylin and eosin; ×90; **A,** WU neg. 67-3363; **B,** WU neg. 67-3364.)

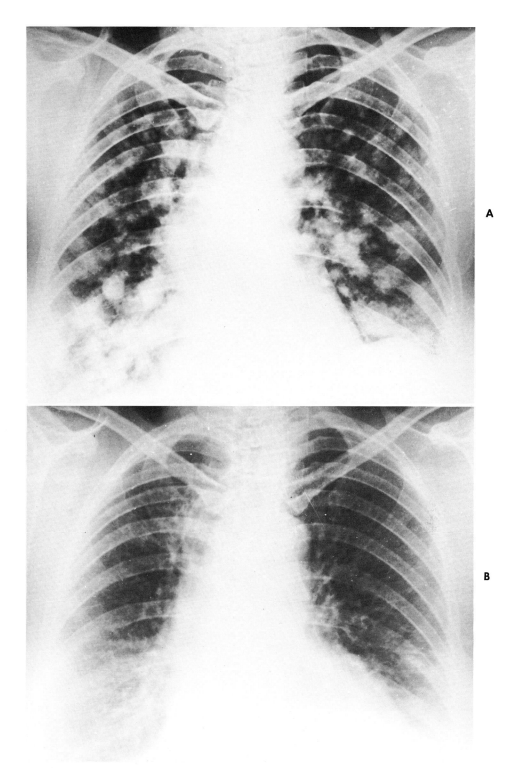

A

B

Fig. 583. **A,** Complete regression of extensive metastases from carcinoma of endometrium treated by medroxyprogesterone. **B,** Over two years later, metastases still in remission. (From Bonte, J., et al.: Traitement des adénocarcinomes du corps utérin par la medroxyprogestérone, Gynec. Obstet. [Paris] **65:**179-185, 1966.)

hyperplasia or carcinoma (Kaufman et al.[48]). This conservative approach may prove particularly fruitful in patients under 40 years of age, as shown by Kempson and Pokorny[50] (Fig. 582). Objective clinical and histopathologic regressions of distant metastases have been produced with the administration of relatively high doses of progesterone compounds. Andersen and Stephens[2] so treated twenty patients, with complete or partial regressions in eight. Bergsjø and Nilsen[7] observed regression of pulmonary metastases in four of thirteen patients. Others have reported observed regressions (Bonte et al.[10]; Smith et al.[104]; Phillips[88]) (Fig. 583). Progestational agents may be associated with radiotherapy as suggested by Kistner et al.,[52] but the usefulness of the combined approach remains to be proved (Lewis[59]; Lewis et al.[60]).

Prognosis

In 1965, there were 5785 deaths from carcinoma of the endometrium in the United States, a crude mortality of 5.9 per 100,000 population. There had been a slight progressive decline in the preceding fifteen years during which separate mortality records were kept for carcinoma of the cervix and endometrium.

The prognosis of carcinoma of the endometrium is relatively good, for the disease is curable in a goodly number of patients if adequate treatment is applied. Low histologic grade carcinomas and carcinomas arising in a polyp are often curable. The curability of others parallels their degree of differentiation (Roman et al.[93]). In patients under 40 years of age with carcinoma of the endometrium, the prognosis appears relatively more favorable than in older women (Kempson and Pokorny[50]). Patients with involvement of the cervix or vaginal infiltration have a poor outlook. The same is true for patients with parametrial spread (Long et al.[62]). A poor prognosis accompanies uterine perforation at curettage (Lindgren[61]), radiumtherapy, or hysterectomy. The lesser or greater depth of myometrial infiltration correlates rather well with the prognosis. Andersen and Stephens[2] reported twelve patients living five years out of twelve treated with no evidence of myometrial invasion, nineteen of twenty-two with infiltration of less than

half of the wall, nine of eleven with infiltration of more than half of the wall, and three of seven with complete invasion. Node involvement darkens the outlook, with only one patient surviving in a series of nine with lymph node metastases operated on by Javert and Douglas.[44]

In a properly selected series of early cases, *hysterectomy alone* may give a satisfactory result. At the Women's Clinic of the University of Helsinki, a selected series of 263 patients with carcinoma of the endometrium, constituting 61% of the total seen, were surgically treated, with a five-year survival rate of 72% (Ojanen et al.[84]).

The reported results of *preoperative radiotherapy and hysterectomy* are mostly based on a combination of radiumtherapy and surgery. Frequently, such series exclude the patients who have been selected for surgical treatment alone. Montgomery et al.[75] reported 104 (87%) five-year survivors in a series of 120 patients treated at the Jefferson Medical College by preoperative radiumtherapy and surgery. Johnson[47] reported 156 patients with carcinoma of the endometrium; in 121 patients treated by preoperative radium followed by surgery, there was a five-year survival of 81%. Utilizing a planned combination of preoperative radiumtherapy, surgery, and occasional postoperative radiotherapy, Bergsjø and Nilsen[7] obtained creditable overall results (Fig. 584). Of 173 patients with Stage I, group a lesions treated by preoperative irradiation (roentgentherapy and/or radiumtherapy) followed by hysterectomy, Lampe[57] reported that 145 (84%) were living and well at five years and eight had died of intercurrent disease without evidence of cancer; 28% of the surgical specimens showed no residual tumor. Lampe[57] believes the preoperative irradiation reduces the risk of local recurrence and remote dissemination. In 121 patients who received preoperative external pelvic irradiation only, the five-year survival rate was 90% In a consecutive series of patients treated at the Ellis Fischel State Cancer Hospital, Sala and Regato[98] found that the combination of external pelvic irradiation and surgery gave better results than that of radiumtherapy and surgery in operable lesions limited to the uterus. In a series of fifty-six consecutive

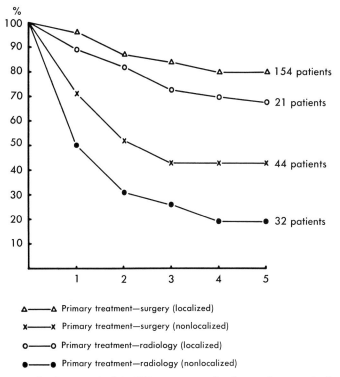

%

△——△ Primary treatment—surgery (localized)

✗——✗ Primary treatment—surgery (nonlocalized)

○——○ Primary treatment—radiology (localized)

●——● Primary treatment—radiology (nonlocalized)

Fig. 584. Five-year absolute survival in 251 patients with adequately treated adenocarcinoma of corpus uteri. (From Bergsjø, P., and Nilsen, P. A.: Carcinoma of the endometrium, Amer. J. Obstet. Gynec. **95:**496-507, 1966.)

patients treated by external irradiation followed by hysterectomy at the Penrose Cancer Hospital, there were forty-eight (86%) living and well five years or more after treatment: in twenty-eight cases (58%), no residual tumor was observed in the surgical specimen (only two of these patients died of cancer); a total of seven patients died of cancer, and two died of intercurrent diseases. There was no operative mortality and no morbidity or subsequent complications attributable to radiotherapy (Regato and Chahbazian[91a]).

If a thorough microscopic study of the surgical specimen reveals no evidence of residual carcinoma, the chances of permanent cure are excellent (90% plus). Of fifty-five patients reported by Schmitz et al.[99] in whom no tumor was found in the hysterectomy specimen, only two died of carcinoma.

The results of *radiotherapy alone* are good. Kottmeier[54] reported on the treatment of a series of 1433 consecutive patients with carcinoma of the endometrium

Table 79. Results of elective preoperative radiumtherapy, surgery, and postoperative radiumtherapy in treatment of carcinoma of endometrium*

	Patients	Well 5 yr
Stage I, group a	185	142 (77%)
Stage I, group b	40	22 (55%)
Stage II	31	6 (19%)
Total	256	170 (66%)

*From Bergsjø, P., and Nilsen, P. A.: Carcinoma of the endometrium, Amer. J. Obstet. Gynec. **95:**496-507, 1966.

at the Radiumhemmet in Stockholm. Radiumtherapy was the primary treatment used; 908 of the patients (63%) survived five years. Only 809 presented operable lesions confined to the uterus (Stage I, group I), and 638 of these (79%) survived five years (Kottmeier[56]). Sala and Regato[98] reported on a series of sixteen cases with posthysterectomy recurrences, nine of which were controlled by radiotherapy. Brown et al.[12] reported on thirty patients with vaginal recurrence treated at the Mayo Clinic, mostly by radiotherapy, with 50% surviving five years.

The *sarcomas* that arise in preexisting leiomyomas of the uterus have a variable prognosis depending upon their degree of differentiation (Aaro and Dockerty[1]; Evans[21]). Norris et al.[79] reported six patients cured in a series of thirty-one with *mixed mesodermal tumors.* Norris and Taylor[80] reviewed a series of fifty-three endometrial *stromal tumors* and found that those characterized as malignant (endometrioid sarcoma) yielded a 55% survival of five years. These tumors usually have a protracted course (Jensen et al.[46]). In a series of thirty-one patients with *carcinosarcoma,* none of those who survived had extrauterine extension.

REFERENCES

1 Aaro, L. A., and Dockerty, M. B.: Leiomyosarcoma of the uterus, Amer. J. Obstet. Gynec. **77**:1187-1198, 1959.

2 Andersen, J. LaC., and Stephens, S. R.: Survival in carcinoma of the endometrium following pelvic node dissection, Danish Med. Bull. **11**:1-13, 1964.

3 Armenia, C. S.: Sequential relationship between endometrial polyps and carcinoma of the endometrium, Obstet. Gynec. **30**:524-529, 1967.

4 Bamforth, J.: Carcinoma of the body of the uterus and its relationship to endometrial hyperplasia, J. Obstet. Gynaec. Brit. Emp. **63**:415-419, 1956.

5 Benjamin, F.: Glucose tolerance in dysfunctional uterine bleeding and in carcinoma of endometrium, Brit. Med. J. **5181**:1243-1246, 1960.

6 Berg, J. W., and Durfee, G. R.: The cytological presentation of endometrial carcinoma, Cancer **11**:158-172, 1958.

7 Bergsjø, P., and Nilsen, P. A.: Carcinoma of the endometrium, Amer. J. Obstet. Gynec. **95**:496-507, 1966.

8 Bernard, A., and Hlasivec, Z.: Intrauterine radium therapy in the treatment of climacteric and menopausal bleeding, Cesk. Gynek. **31**:164-168, 1966.

9 Beutler, H. K., Dockerty, M. B., and Randall, L. M.: Precancerous lesions of the endometrium, Amer. J. Obstet. Gynec. **86**:433-443, 1963.

10 Bonte, J., Drochmans, A., and Lassance, M.: Traitement des adénocarcinomes du corps utérin par la medroxyprogestérone, Gynec. Obstet. (Paris) **65**:179-185, 1966.

11 Brøbeck, O.: Heredity in cancer uteri; a genetical and clinical study of 200 patients with cancer of the cervix uteri and 90 patients with cancer of the corpus uteri, Doctor thesis, University of Copenhagen, Universitetsforlaget I Aarhus, 1949.

12 Brown, J. M., Dockerty, M. B., Symmonds, R. E., and Banner, E. A.: Vaginal recurrence of endometrial carcinoma, Amer. J. Obstet. Gynec. **100**:544-549, 1968.

13 Carmichael, J. A., and Bean, H. A.: Carcinoma of the endometrium in Saskatchewan, Amer. J. Obstet. Gynec. **97**:294-307, 1967.

14 Chang, H. Y., Melin, J. R., Vellios, F., Gastineau, D. C., and Huber, C. P.: Leiomyosarcoma of the uterus, Obstet. Gynec. **9**:212-218, 1957.

15 Christopherson, W. M., Mendez, W. M., Lundin, F. E., Jr., and Parker, J. E.: A ten-year study of endometrial carcinoma in Louisville, Kentucky, Cancer **18**:554-558, 1965.

16 Copenhaver, E. H., and Barsamian, M.: Management of adenocarcinoma of the endometrium, Surg. Clin. N. Amer. **47**:723-735, 1967.

17 Corscaden, J. A., and Singh, B. P.: Leiomyosarcoma of the uterus, Amer. J. Obstet. Gynec. **75**:149-155, 1958.

18 de Vere, R. D., and Dempster, K. R.: A case of the Stein-Leventhal syndrome associated with carcinoma of the endometrium, J. Obstet. Gynaec. Brit. Emp. **60**:865-867, 1953.

19 Dockerty, M. B., and Mussey, E.: Malignant lesions of the uterus associated with estrogen-producing ovarian tumors, Amer. J. Obstet. Gynec. **61**:147-153, 1951.

20 Dockerty, M. B., Smith, R. A., and Symmonds, R. E.: Pseudomalignant endometrial changes induced by administration of new synthetic progestins, Proc. Staff Meet. Mayo Clin. **34**:321-328, 1959.

21 Evans, N.: Malignant myomata and related tumors of the uterus, Surg. Gynec. Obstet. **30**:225-229, 1920.

22 Fahlund, G. T. R., and Broders, A. C.: Postmenopausal endometrium and its relation to adenocarcinoma of the corpus uteri, Amer. J. Obstet. Gynec. **51**:22-38, 1946.

23 Fernandez-Colmeiro, J.: Le cancer primitif de l'utérus après la guérison par radiothérapie d'un autre cancer du même organe, Presse Med. **57**:565-566, 1949.

24 Fienberg, R.: Endometrial sarcoma, Arch. Path. (Chicago) **29**:800-812, 1940.

24a Fox, H., and Sen, D. K.: A controlled study of constitutional stigmata of endometrial adenocarcinoma, Brit. J. Cancer **24**:30-36, 1970.

25 Goetchel, E.: Untersuchungen uber die bezeihungen der glandular-cystischen Hyperplasia zum corpuscarcinom des uterus, Gynaecologia (Basel) **160**:94-104, 1965.

26 Gray, L. A., and Barnes, M. L.: Carcinoma of the ovary—report of 106 cases. 2. Pathology, clinical course, treatment, Ann. Surg. **159**:279-290, 1964.

27 Gricouroff, G.: Répartition topographique et délai d'apparition des metastases extrapelviennes dans le cancer de l'utérus, Bull. Ass. Franc. Cancer **30**:90-117, 1942.

28 Gusberg, S. B.: Precursors of corpus carci-

noma estrogens and adenomatous hyperplasia, Amer. J. Obstet. Gynec. **54**:905-927, 1947.

29 Gusberg, S. B., and Kaplan, A. L.: Precursors of corpus cancer. IV. Adenomatous hyperplasia as stage 0 carcinoma of the endometrium, Amer. J. Obstet. Gynec. **87**:662-678, 1963.

30 Hall, K. V.: Irregular hyperplasia of the endometrium, Acta Obstet. Gynec. Scand. **36**:306-323, 1957.

31 Healy, W. P., and Cutler, M.: Radiation and surgical treatment of carcinoma of the body of the uterus, Amer. J. Obstet. Gynec. **19**:457-489, 1930.

32 Hecht, E. L., and Oppenheim, A.: The cytology of endometrial cancer, Surg. Gynec. Obstet. **122**:1025-1029, 1966.

33 Heidler, H.: Prinzipielles zur operativen Therapie des Carcinoma corporis uteri, Krebsarzt **9**:358-361, 1954.

34 Herrell, W. E., and Broders, A. C.: Histological studies of endometrium during various phases of menstrual cycle, Surg. Gynec. Obstet. **61**:751-764, 1935.

35 Hertig, A. T.: The aging ovary—a preliminary report, J. Clin. Endocr. **4**:581-582, 1944.

36 Hertig, A. T.: Endocrine ovarian-cancer relationships, Cancer **10**:838-841, 1957.

37 Hertig, A. T., and Sommers, S. C.: Genesis of endometrial carcinoma. I. Study of prior biopsies, Cancer **2**:946-956, 1949.

38 Hertig, A. T., Sommers, S. C., and Bengloff, H.: Genesis of endometrial carcinoma, III. Carcinoma in situ, Cancer **2**:964-971, 1949.

39 Heyman, J.: Improvement of results in the treatment of uterine cancer, J.A.M.A. **135**:412-416, 1947.

40 Höeg, K.: Superficial dissemination of cancer of the uterine body; cytological examination of smears from the tubes and the pouch of Douglas, J. Obstet. Gynaec. Brit. Emp. **63**:899-902, 1956.

41 Ingraham, C. B., Black, W. C., and Rutledge, E. K.: The relationship of granulosa cell tumors of the ovary to endometrial carcinoma, Amer. J. Obstet. Gynec.. **48**:760-773, 1944.

42 Ingram, J. M., Jr., and Novak, E.: Endometrial carcinoma associated with feminizing ovarian tumors, Amer. J. Obstet. Gynec. **61**:774-787, 1951.

43 Jackson, R. L., and Dockerty, M. B.: The Stein-Leventhal syndrome; analysis of 43 cases with special reference to association with endometrial carcinoma, Amer. J. Obstet. Gynec. **73**:161-173, 1957.

44 Javert, C. T., and Douglas, R. G.: Treatment of endometrial adenocarcinoma; a study of 381 cases at the New York Hospital; a preliminary report, Amer. J. Roentgen. **75**:508-514, 1956.

45 Javert, C. T., and Hofammann, K.: Observations on the surgical pathology, selective lymphadenectomy and classification of endometrial adenocarcinoma, Cancer **5**:485-498, 1952.

46 Jensen, P. A., Dockerty, M. B., Symmonds, R. E., and Wilson, R. B.: Endometrioid sarcoma ("stromal endometriosis"); report of 15 cases including 5 with metastases, Amer. J. Obstet. Gynec. **95**:79-90, 1966.

47 Johnson, F. L.: Adenocarcinoma of the endometrium, Obstet. Gynec. **27**:622-625, 1966.

48 Kaufman, R. H., Abbott, J. P., and Wall, J. A.: The endometrium before and after wedge resection of the ovaries in the Stein-Leventhal syndrome, Amer. J. Obstet. Gynec. **77**:1271-1285, 1959.

49 Kay, S.: Clear-cell carcinoma of the endometrium, Cancer **10**:124-130, 1957.

50 Kempson, R. L., and Pokorny, G. E.: Adenocarcinoma of the endometrium in women 40 years of age and younger, Cancer **21**:650-662, 1968.

51 Kistner, R. W., Gore, H., and Hertig, A. T.: Carcinoma of the endometrium—a preventable disease, Amer. J. Obstet. Gynec. **95**:1011-1024, 1966.

52 Kistner, R. W., Griffiths, C. T., and Craig, J. M.: Use of progestational agents in the management of endometrial cancer, Cancer **18**:1563-1579, 1965.

53 Koss, L. G., Spiro, R. H., and Brunschwig, A.: Endometrial stromal sarcoma, Surg. Gynec. Obstet. **121**:531-537, 1965.

54 Kottmeier, H. L.: The place of radiation therapy and surgery in the treatment of uterine cancer, J. Obstet. Gynaec. Brit. Emp. **62**:737-773, 1955.

55 Kottmeier, H. L., editor: Annual report, Treatment of carcinoma of the uterus, vol. 11, Stockholm, 1958, P. A. Norstedt & Söner.

56 Kottmeier, H. L., editor: Annual report on the results of treatment in carcinoma of the uterus and vagina, collated in 1968, vol. 14, Stockholm, 1968, P. A. Norstedt & Söner.

56a Kurohara, S. S., Badib, A. O., Beitia, A. A., and Webster, J. H.: Recurrent cancer of the corpus uteri, Acta Radiol. [Ther.] (Stockholm) **8**:373-389, 1969.

57 Lampe, I.: Endometrial carcinoma, Amer. J. Roentgen. **90**:1011-1015, 1963.

58 Lefèvre, H.: Node dissection in cancer of the endometrium, Surg. Gynec. Obstet. **192**:649-656, 1956.

59 Lewis, G. C., Jr.: Progestin therapy for cancer of the uterine corpus (presented at the Tenth International Cancer Congress, Houston, Texas, May, 1970).

60 Lewis, G. C., Jr., Nadler, S. H., Bross, I. D. J., and Slack, N. H.: Adjuvant chemotherapy for cancer of the corpus uteri; preliminary report, Obstet. Gynec. **29**:797-802, 1967.

61 Lindgren, L.: The prognosis of carcinoma of the endometrium in its different stages treated by surgery combined with post-operative radiotherapy, Acta Obstet. Gynec. Scand. **36**:426-438, 1957.

62 Long, R. T. L., Spratt, J. S., Jr., and Sala, J. M.: Problems in the management of advanced endometrium carcinoma; a report of 65 cases, Amer. J. Obstet. Gynec. **87**:942-947, 1963.

63 Lynch, R. C., and Dockerty, M. B.: The

spread of uterine and ovarian carcinoma with special reference to the role of the fallopian tube, Surg. Gynec. Obstet. **80**:60-65, 1945.

64 McBride, J. M.: The normal post-menopausal endometrium, J. Obstet. Gynaec. Brit. Emp. **61**:691-697, 1954.

65 McCall, M. L.: The causes and significance of delay in the management of adenocarcinoma of the endometrium; a review of 683 proven cases from the Philadelphia Pelvic Cancer Committee, South. Med. J. **50**:17-23, 1957.

66 McGoldrick, J. L., and Lapp, W. A.: Theca-cell tumors of the ovary, Amer. J. Obstet. Gynec. **48**:409-416, 1944.

67 McKay, D. G., Hertig, A. T., Barwahl, W., and Vilardo, J. T.: Histochemical observations in endometrium, Obstet. Gynec. **8**:140-156, 1956.

67a Marcial, V. A., Tome, J. M., and Ubinas, J.: The combination of external irradiation and curietherapy used preoperatively in adenocarcinoma of the endometrium, Amer. J. Roentgen. **105**:586-595, 1969.

68 Marsh, M. R.: Angioma of the uterus; a report of a case of submucous polypoid hemangioma of the uterus, Arch. Path. (Chicago) **49**:490-497, 1950.

69 Marrubini, G.: Doubtful malignant changes in the endometrial epithelium, Acta Radiol. (Stockholm) **31**:65-84, 1949.

70 Masson, J. C.: Sarcoma of the uterus, Amer. J. Obstet. Gynec. **5**:345-357, 1923.

71 Meikle, G. J.: Mesodermal mixed tumours of the uterus, J. Obstet. Gynaec. Brit. Emp. **43**:821-864, 1936.

72 Meiser, A.: Ueber Carcinoma cervicis uteri adenomatosum und seine histologische diagnostische Abgrenzung gegan das Schleimepithel enthaltende Carcinoma corporis uteri adenomatosum, Z. Geburtsh. Gynaek. **118**: 250-273, 1939.

73 Messelt, O. T.: Diagnosis of cancer in the female genital organs by smears, Acta Obstet. Gynec. Scand. **34**:345-365, 1955.

74 Miller, N. F.: Carcinoma of the endometrium, Obstet. Gynec. **15**:579-586, 1960.

75 Montgomery, J. B., Lang, W. R., Farell, D. M., and Hahn, G. A.: End results in adenocarcinoma of the endometrium managed by preoperative irradiation, Amer. J. Obstet. Gynec. **80**:972-983, 1960.

76 Moss, W. T.: Common peculiarities of patients with adenocarcinoma of the endometrium; with special reference to obesity, body build, diabetes and hypertension, Amer. J. Roentgen. **58**:203-210, 1947.

77 Müller, J. H., and Keller, M.: Atypische Proliferationserscheinungen des Endometriums und ihre Beziehung zum manifesten und latenten (Stad. 0) Corpus carcinom, Gynaecologica (Basel) **144**:31-39, 1957.

78 Nolan, J. F., and Steele, J. P.: Carcinoma of the endometrium; measurements of the radiation distribution around various multiple capsule applications of radium in irregular uteri, Radiology **51**:166-176, 1948.

79 Norris, H. J., Roth, E., and Taylor, H. B.: Mesenchymal tumors of the uterus. II. A clinical and pathologic study of 31 mixed mesodermal tumors, Obstet. Gynec. **28**:57-63, 1966.

80 Norris, H. J., and Taylor, H. B.: Mesenchymal tumors of the uterus. Part I. A clinical and pathological study of 53 endometrial stromal tumors, Cancer **19**:755-766, 1966.

81 Norris, H. J., and Taylor, H. B.: Mesenchymal tumors of the uterus. III. A clinical and pathologic study of 31 carcinosarcomas, Cancer **19**:1459-1465, 1966.

82 Ober, W. B.: Uterine sarcomas; histogenesis and taxonomy, Ann. N. Y. Acad. Sci. **75**: 568-585, 1959.

83 Ober, W. B., and Tovell, H. M. M.: Mesenchymal sarcomas of the uterus, Amer. J. Obstet. Gynec. **77**:246-268, 1959.

84 Ojanen, R., Turtola, V., and Olki, M.: Carcinoma of the corpus uteri; a study of 430 cases treated at the first and second Women's Clinics University of Helsinki from 1945 to 1954, Ann. Chir. Gynaec. Fenn. **50**(suppl. 100):1-27, 1961.

85 Papanicolaou, G. N., and Traut, H. F.: Diagnosis of uterine cancer by the vaginal smear, New York, 1943, The Commonwealth Fund.

86 Parsons, L., and Cesare, F.: Wertheim hysterectomy in the treatment of endometrial carcinoma, Surg. Gynec. Obstet. **108**:582-590, 1959.

87 Payne, F. L.: The clinical significance of endometrial hyperplasia, Amer. J. Obstet. Gynec. **34**:762-779, 1937.

88 Phillips, T. J.: Oral progesterones and adenocarcinoma of the uterus, J. Obstet. Gynaec. Brit. Comm. **73**:487-489, 1966.

89 Plotz, E. J., Stein, A. A., and Hahn, B. D.: Enzymatic activities related to steroidogenesis in postmenopausal ovaries of patients with and without endometrial carcinoma, Amer. J. Obstet. Gynec. **99**:182-197, 1967.

90 Prem, K. A., Mensheha, N. M., and McKelvey, J. L.: Operative treatment of adenocarcinoma of the endometrium in obese women, Amer. J. Obstet. Gynec. **92**:16-22, 1965.

91 del Regato, J. A.: Radiotherapy in the treatment of recurrences of carcinoma of the endometrium. In Lewis, G. C., Jr., Wentz, W. B., and Jaffe, R. M., editors: New concepts in gynecological oncology, Philadelphia, 1966, F. A. Davis Co.

91a del Regato, J. A., and Chahbazian, C. M.: External irradiation as a preoperative surgical adjuvant in the treatment of carcinoma of the endometrium (to be published).

92 Roddick, J. W., Jr., and Greene, R. R.: Relation of ovarian stromal hyperplasia to endometrial carcinoma, Amer. J. Obstet. Gynec. **73**:843-852, 1957.

93 Roman, T. N., Beck, R. P., and Latour, J. P. A.: Correlation of histologic grading with 5-year survival rates in endometrial carcinoma, Amer. J. Obstet. Gynec. **97**:117-119, 1967.

94 Rosenblum, J. M., and Hendricks, C. H.: Estrogenated vaginal epithelium; Relationship to the development of carcinoma of the endometrium, Obstet. Gynec. 3:535-545, 1954.

95 Rouvière, H.: Anatomie des lymphatiques de l'homme, Paris, 1932, Masson et Cie.

96 Rubin, P., Gerle, R. D., Quick, R. S., and Greenlow, R. H.: Significance of vaginal recurrence in endometrial carcinoma, Amer. J. Roentgen. 89:91-100, 1963.

97 Rutledge, F. N., Tan, S. K., and Fletcher, G. H.: Vaginal metastases from adenocarcinoma of the corpus uteri, Amer. J. Obstet. Gynec. 75:167-174, 1958.

98 Sala, J. M., and del Regato, J. A.: The treatment of carcinoma of the endometrium, Radiology 79:12-17, 1962.

99 Schmitz, H. E., Smith, C. J., and Fetherston, W. C.: Effects of preoperative irradiation on adenocarcinoma of the uterus, Amer. J. Obstet. Gynec. 78:1048-1059, 1959.

100 Sheehan, J. F., and Schmitz, H. E.: Histologic changes produced by radiation in adenocarcinomas of the uterus; comparison with changes produced in squamous cell carcinomas of cervix, Amer. J. Clin. Path. 20: 241-252, 1950.

101 Sherman, A. T., and Arneson, A. N.: Carcinoma of the endometrium, Amer. J. Med. Sci. 228:701-712, 1954.

102 Smith, F. R., and Bowden, L.: Cancer of the corpus uteri following radiation therapy for benign uterine lesions, Amer. J. Roentgen. 59:796-804, 1948.

103 Smith, G. Van S.: Quoted by Ingraham, C. B., Black, W. C., and Rutledge, F. K.: The relationship of granulosa cell tumors of the ovary to endometrial carcinoma, Amer. J. Obstet. Gynec. 48:760-773, 1944.

104 Smith, J. P., Rutledge, F., and Soffar, S. W.: Progestins in the treatment of patients with endometrial adenocarcinoma, Amer. J. Obstet. Gynec. 94:977-984, 1966.

105 Sommers, S. C., Hertig, A. T., and Bengloff, H.: Genesis of endometrial carcinoma. II. Cases 19 to 35 years old, Cancer 2:957-963, 1949.

106 Sommers, S. C., and Meissner, W. A.: Endocrine abnormalities accompanying human endometrial cancer, Cancer 10:516-521, 1957.

107 Speert, H.: Corpus cancer; clinical, pathological and etiological aspect, Cancer 1:584-603, 1948.

108 Speert, H.: Carcinoma of the endometrium in young women, Surg. Gynec. Obstet. 88: 332-336, 1949.

109 Speert, H., and Peightal, T. C.: Malignant tumors of the uterine fundus subsequent to irradiation for benign pelvic conditions, Amer. J. Obstet. Gynec. 57:261-273, 1949.

110 Spiro, R. H., and McPeak, C. J.: On the so-called metastasizing leiomyoma, Cancer 19:544-548, 1966.

111 Stohr, G.: Granulosa cell tumor of the ovary and coincident carcinoma of the uterus, Amer. J. Obstet. Gynec. 43:586-599, 1942.

112 Taylor, H. C., Jr.: Endometrial hyperplasia and carcinoma of the body of the uterus, Amer. J. Obstet. Gynec. 23:309-332, 1932.

113 Taylor, H. C., Jr., and Millen, R.: The causes of vaginal bleeding and the histology of the endometrium after the menopause, Amer. J. Obstet. Gynec. 36:22-39, 1938.

114 Taylor, H. B., and Norris, H. J.: Mesenchymal tumors of the uterus, Arch. Path. (Chicago) 82:40-44, 1966.

115 TeLinde, R. W.: Causes of postmenopausal bleeding, Amer. J. Surg. 48:289-293, 1940.

116 TeLinde, R. W., Jones, H. W., and Galvin, G. A.: What are the earliest endometrial changes to justify a diagnosis of endometrial cancer, Amer. J. Obstet. Gynec. 66:953-969, 1953.

117 Testut, L., and Latarjet, A.: Traité d'anatomie, humaine, ed. 8, vol. 5, Paris, 1931, Gaston Doin.

118 Vass, A.: Occurrence of uterine fundus carcinoma after prolonged estrogen therapy, Amer. J. Obstet. Gynec. 58:748-751, 1949.

119 Woll, E., Hertig, A. T., Smith, G. V. S., and Johnson, L. C.: The ovary in endometrial carcinoma, Amer. J. Obstet. Gynec. 56:617-633, 1948.

120 Wynder, E. L., Escher, G. C., and Mantel, N.: An epidemiological investigation of cancer of the endometrium, Cancer 19:489-520, 1966.

121 Zsolnai, B., and Hyirö, L.: Hysterography in corpus carcinoma, Zbl. Gynaek. 90:273-279, 1968.

Cervix (including cervical stump and cervix and pregnancy)

Anatomy

The cervix is a cylindrical structure that enters the vaginal canal pointing inferiorly and posteriorly. The vaginal wall forms a circular cul-de-sac around the cervix, which is arbitrarily divided into four *fornices*, one anterior, one posterior, and two lateral. The anterior fornix is represented by a shallow fold. The posterior fornix is the deepest. The cervix has a central orifice, the *external os,* which, in the normal adult multipara, is a transverse opening with an anterior and a posterior lip. It gives access to the cervical canal.

The cervix is covered by a squamous epithelium that is a continuation of the vaginal mucosa. At the external os, however, this mucosa changes abruptly into an arborescent, more rugous epithelium which is characteristic of the endometrium.

The cervix and the rest of the uterus are attached laterally to the pelvis by a thin elastic ligament, the broad ligament, which divides the pelvis into anterior (vesical) and posterior (rectal) compartments (Fig. 585). The broad ligament is formed by two layers of peritoneum which, descending on the anterior and posterior aspects of the uterus and tubes, come in almost immediate contact with each other. Arising from the posterior aspect of the broad ligament is a pedicle, the *meso-ovarium,* which supports the ovary. The portion of the broad ligament which lies above the meso-ovarium is the *mesosalpinx,* and that which lies below is the *mesometrium* or *parametrium* (Fig. 586). The parametrium contains a rich cobweblike adipose and connective tissue which is continuous with that surrounding the uterus and the one contained in the utero-sacral ligaments. It also contains the uterine artery, nerves, and numerous lymphatics. The ureters pass through the parametrium in a forward and inward direction and lie about 1.5 cm lateral to the cervix (Fig. 588). The *uterosacral ligaments* are of lesser importance. They are formed by secondary peritoneal folds that extend from the posterior surface of the cervix and isthmus, follow an anteroposterior direction on either side of the rectum, and end on both sides of the first sacral vertebra. The uterosacral ligaments contain some

alveolar tissue, which is continuous with the parametrium at its base, a few arteries and veins, and some lymphatic vessels. They are very elastic structures.

Anteriorly, the cervix is in close relation to the bladder, from which it is separated by only a few millimeters of celluloadipose

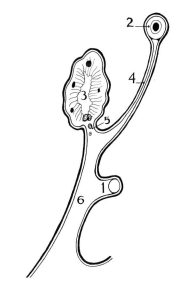

Fig. 586. Paramedian sagittal section of broad ligament illustrating round ligament, **1**; fallopian tube, **2**; ovary, **3**; mesosalpinx, **4**; meso-ovarium, **5**; mesometrium or parametrium, **6**.

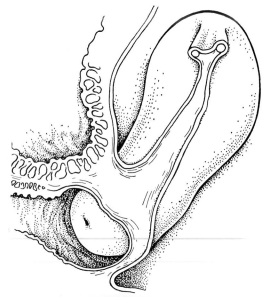

Fig. 587. Paramedian sagittal section of broad ligament at its insertion into lateral aspect of uterus.

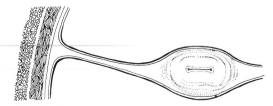

Fig. 585. Transverse section of parametrium and uterus showing division of pelvis into anterior (vesical) and posterior (rectal) compartments.

tissue (Fig. 589). Posteriorly, the cervix is separated from the rectal wall by only the posterior fornix.

Lymphatics. The lymphatics of the cervix form a rich plexus lateral to the cervix, presenting nodularities that have been interpreted as veritable lymph nodes (Lucas-Championnière[120]). From this plexus, the lymphatics gather into three main pedicles (Fig. 590):

1 The *preureteral pedicle* follows the direction of the uterine artery, passes in front of the ureters, crosses the umbilical artery and ends in the middle and internal groups of nodes of the external iliac chain. This pedicle is the *principal chain* of lymphatics of the cervix (Peiser[158]; Leveuf and Godard[114]).

2 The *retroureteral pedicle* follows the course of the uterine vein, passes behind the ureter, and ends in one of the hypogastric lymph nodes near the uterine artery.

3 The *posterior (uterosacral) pedicle,* less rich or constant than the other two, follows an anteroposterior direction on each side of the rectum and traces an upward curve to end in the laterosacral lymph nodes and sometimes in those of the promontory.

Epidemiology

Carcinoma of the cervix is the second most common form of cancer in American women. In the 1947 cancer survey, the sex-age adjusted incidence rate was 32.8 for white and 70.4 for nonwhite women per 100,000 population. The relative incidence rises after the age of 20 years, reaches its maximum for the group 65 to 69 years of age, and thereafter falls. In a survey among residents of Atlanta, Cutler[44] found that cancer of the cervix accounted for 14% of all cancer among white women and 31% among black women, with the difference being attributed to socioeconomic factors rather than to race (Christopherson and Parker[33]). Jewish women present a relatively low incidence of carcinoma in situ and invasive carcinoma (Ober and Reiner[151]; Kennaway[100]). This low incidence is confirmed in Israel (Hochman et al.[91]). A citywide study in the city of Cincinnati revealed an incidence of 26.4 for white, 49.4 for black, and 2.9 for Jewish women per 100,000 (Cole[38]). Cancer of the cervix is specially common in Latin America. In 1946-1950 Puerto Rico, it represented 40% of all recorded malignant tumors of the female. Several

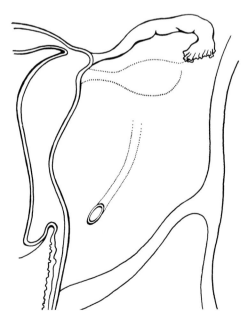

Fig. 588. Frontal section of pelvis showing approximate relationship of left ureter to cervix.

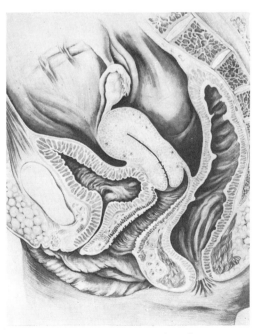

Fig. 589. Sagittal section of pelvis demonstrating close relationship of cervix to bladder and rectum.

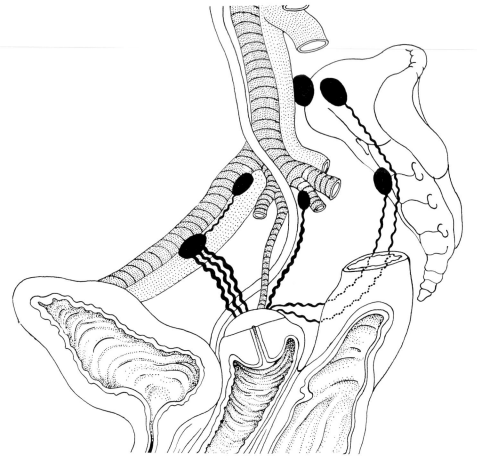

Fig. 590. Lymphatics of cervix showing preureteral, retroureteral, posterior, and uterosacral pedicles.

studies in Africa show that cancer of the cervix prevails among the Bantu women of Johannesburg (Oettlé[153]), Uganda (Davies et al.[45]), and other countries, whereas the incidence in Lourenço Marques is comparable to that of American whites (Prates and Torres[162]). An unusually large proportion of carcinomas of the cervix arising in prolapsed uteri has been reported by Díaz-Bazán[49] in El Salvador (Fig. 591). This is more likely to occur when the prolapse has been present for ten to fifteen years (Hesselberg[87]). Carcinoma of the cervix has been reported in identical twins (Stocking[201]).

In thoroughly screened communities, the prevalence rate of invasive carcinoma will decline (Marshall[129]). The yield of carcinoma in situ, in repeated surveys, will itself show a decline depending on the

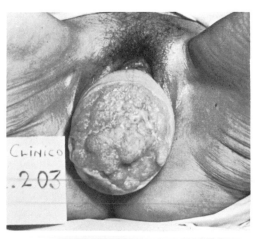

Fig. 591. Extensive fungating carcinoma of cervix occurring on prolapsed uterus. (Courtesy Dr. N. Díaz-Bazán, El Salvador.)

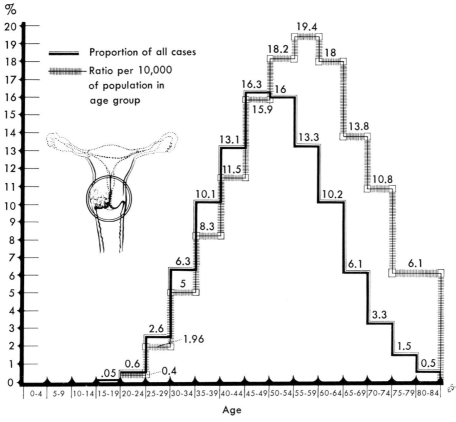

Fig. 592. Age distribution of patients with carcinoma of cervix in percentage of actual cases and in proportion to living female population in each age group. (Data from Sadugor, M. G., and Palmer, J. P.: Age, incidence, and distribution of 4,652 cases of carcinoma of the cervix, Amer. J. Obstet. Gynec. **56**:680-686, 1948.)

proportion of individuals examined and the stability of the population.

Carcinoma of the cervix is infrequently found in women under 20 years of age. In a review of 4652 patients admitted to the Roswell Park Memorial Institute, only one patient under that age was found (Sadugor and Palmer[187]) (Fig. 592). A few cases have been observed in girls under 12 years old (Speert[197]; Heckel[84]). The majority of cases recorded in young girls are adenocarcinomas, and in the absence of successful treatment or of autopsy, the authenticity of some of them can be disputed. The incidence of carcinoma of the cervix increases with age up to 65 years, when there is definite decrease at a faster rate than the decrease in the population of aged women (Maliphant[127]).

There is increasing circumstantial evidence favoring early coitus as a probable factor in the causation of cancer of the cervix (Terris et al.[206]; Higginson and Oettlé[89]; Schonberg et al.[190]). Early marriage has been invoked in Iran (Habibi[78]). It is a well known fact that this tumor occurs infrequently in unmarried women (Taylor et al.[203]). A study of 3280 nuns revealed 130 malignant tumors, including two of the endometrium, but not a single carcinoma of the cervix (Gagnon[63]). It has been indicated that women with cancer of the cervix often admit initiation to sexual activity in the second decade of life. Christopherson and Parker[35] noted that patients with carcinoma of the cervix declared twice as many marriages and more sexual mates than the controls (Moghissi and Mack[137]). The tumor arises more frequently in prostitutes than in other women (Røjel[174]). The low incidence rate observed in Ireland, second only to Israel, is due to late marriages, less frequent intercourse, and abundance of unmarried women (Magner and Bennett[125]). The relatively low incidence of cancer of the cervix among Amish women, in spite of high parity, has been attributed to the fact that they often have only one lifetime sexual partner (Cross et al.[41]). It is obvious that better epidemiologic research is needed (Rotkin [179, 180]) particularly in reference to early coitus, number of sexual partners, age at first pregnancy, etc. The low incidence among Jewish women has been attributed to the ritual circumcision of Jewish men, but it is more likely to be a genetic resistance. No difference in the occurrence of carcinoma of the cervix has been found among non-Jewish women whose husbands were circumcised (Stern and Dixon[200]). No difference was found in the circumcision status of the husbands of Christian and Moslem patients with carcinoma of the cervix and of control subjects (Abou-Daoud[1]). Nor can circumcision account for regional variations in incidence in the United States (Haenszel and Hillhouse[79]). Heredity plays no role (Rotkin[178]).

Sarcomas of the cervix are rare. Piquand[160] found only sixty-eight in a series of 325 sarcomas of the uterus. They are more frequently found in patients between 40 and 60 years of age, but the rare botryoid sarcoma arises predominantly in infancy.

Pathology
Gross pathology

In order of frequency, carcinomas of the cervix arise from the posterior lip, the cervical canal, and the anterior lip. There are three distinct gross types of tumor, ulcerating, exophytic, and nodular, but these differences are not related to histologic variations. The ulcerating tumor is characterized by its infiltration and by loss of substance. As the cavity enlarges to destroy the cervix and to deepen into the body of the uterus, the centrifugal spread of the ulceration involves the vaginal fornices (Figs. 602, *A*, and 604, *B*). The exophytic type may fill the entire upper half of the vagina without invading the fornices or the parametria. This so-called "cauliflower" growth is accompanied by considerable secondary infection and spontaneous necrosis (Figs. 602, *B*, and 603, *D*). The nodular variation usually arises in the endocervix, where the original ulceration is hidden. The tumor infiltrates through the submucosa, and the entire cervical structure is replaced by a granulating mass. The spread to the vaginal walls is accompanied by a hard, nodular elevation of the mucosa at the borders of the ulceration. Finally, there may be widespread ulceration (Figs. 604, *A*, and 605, *A*).

The clinical entity *verrucous carcinoma*, comparable to the one observed in the oral cavity (p. 222), is characterized by extensive superficial spread and infiltration. It occurs infrequently and does not metastasize.

In their relentless progress, carcinomas of the cervix spread in three distinct directions: (1) to the fornices and vaginal wall, (2) to the body of the uterus, and (3) to the parametria. Secondarily they invade the bladder, rectovaginal septum and rectum, vulva, and uterosacral ligaments. These events do not necessarily follow in chronologic sequence. A relatively early carcinoma of the anterior lip of the cervix may invade the bladder before infiltrating the parametria, and pelvic metastases may occur from early lesions still limited to the cervix, but this is rare.

The anterior fornix, much shallower than the others, is more easily but not so frequently invaded as are the lateral fornices. The posterior fornix is invaded by those tumors that have destroyed the posterior lip. Since this fornix is deep, its involvement is rarely an early occurrence. Once the vaginal wall is reached, the spread of tumor over it is accelerated. Besides invasion by contiguity, there may be retrograde permeation of the rich lymphatics of the vaginal mucosa. Isolated and sometimes pedunculated growths of the vaginal wall may be found at a distance from the primary tumor. From the anterior wall, the tumor rapidly reaches the introitus. The distance to the posterior wall is greater, and consequently this is usually the last region to be affected.

The thick uterine muscle is not often penetrated by carcinoma, but once the barrier of the isthmus has been passed, the tumor may spread into the uterine cavity and enlarge the whole organ. In these rare instances, the tumor remains for a long period of time within the muscular uterine frame, but it may eventually erode the serosa and even invade the neighboring intestine (Mitani et al.[136]).

Whether tumor breaks through the cervical muscle or whether it infiltrates out through lymphatic channels, once the surrounding areolar and subperitoneal tissue is reached, the tumor seems to develop easily and unhindered. This subperitoneal tissue is continuous with the one that fills the broad ligament, and it is toward the broad ligament that most carcinomas develop. The rich lymphatic network of the parametrium is perhaps responsible for this course. Within the parametrium, the tumor grows without restraint. It grows around the ureter, which traverses the parametrium behind the uterine artery and, in its course to the bladder, comes within 1.5 cm of the cervix. Rarely is the ureter invaded, but tumor may involve the periureteral lymphatics and compress and occlude the ureter 2.5 cm from the bladder. This results in hydroureters and hydronephrosis, which rarely may be bilateral (Fig. 593). The tumor may develop in a nodular fashion that imitates, but is not explained by, the presence of nodes in the parametrium. In reaching the lateral wall of the pelvis, the tumor finds its last barrier in the muscular fascia. Commonly, the parametrium becomes larger and harder before tumor finally invades the wall.

Inflammatory changes in the parame-

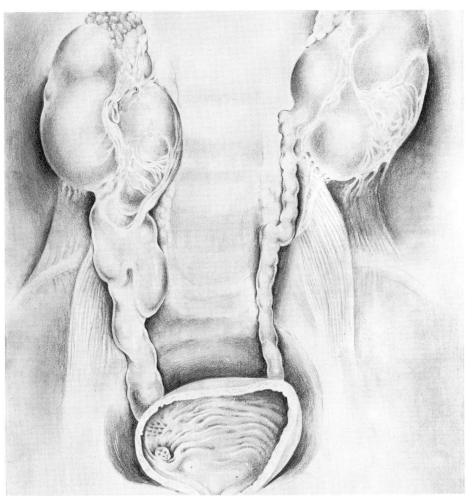

Fig. 593. Hydroureter and hydronephrosis due to compression of ureters in parametrium by carcinoma.

trium almost invariably accompany the neoplastic invasion, but in the majority of patients these changes are not remarkable. In some instances, however, the inflammation causes the parametrium to become diffusely indurated although not nodular.

When the anterior lip of the cervix is involved, the tumor passes rather easily into the lax tissue that separates it from the bladder. The same is true when cervical ulceration has extended into the anterior fornix and vaginal wall (Fig. 605, *D*). The bladder wall is at first displaced and distorted by the tumor and, because of this, the left ureter often may be first distended and its lumen obstructed. It takes time, however, for the tumor to pierce the thick bladder muscle and to ulcerate the mucosa. The invasion of the bladder wall is accompanied by edema. The ureteral orifices may be practically occluded. Moreover, the tumor may grow around the terminal portion of the ureter and contribute to this occlusion. Actual invasion and ulceration of the bladder mucosa are always accompanied by secondary infection and cystitis. With compression of the ureters and bladder invasion, there are often dilatations of the ureters and pyelonephritis resulting in kidney failure. Infection of the kidney may be retrograde or hematogenous.

When tumor has invaded the posterior fornix and extended over the posterior vaginal wall, it may remain static there for some time. There, little by little, tumor invades the muscular layer of the vagina and extends into the rectovaginal septum, which becomes enlarged and indurated. The rectal mucosa is actually ulcerated only in advanced cases (Fig. 605, *C*). The invasion of the lower third of the vaginal wall is sometimes accompanied by metastatic subcutaneous nodules in the thickness of the labia majora (Fig. 605, *A*). The ulceration itself, however, may extend to the introitus and also invade the urethra.

Once the tumor breaks through the muscular frame of the cervix, it spreads easily into the fatty subperitoneal tissue that extends into the lower half of the large ligament to form the parametrium and into the uterosacral ligament. The lymphatics of this ligament are not so rich as those of the parametrium, and for this reason it is not as often invaded. It is only in advanced disease that the uterosacral ligament becomes rigid on one or both sides of the rectum. As a result, there may be a constriction and, later, obstruction of the rectum (Pearson and Garcia[156]). The tumor may extend to the sacrum through this channel and directly invade that bone.

The autopsy findings in unsuccessfully treated patients differ somewhat in reference to treatment, with a greater proportion of cases with controlled primary lesions among those treated by radiations. Distant metastases are fairly widespread irrespective of therapy. Renal failure and sepsis are the leading causes of death (Badib et al.[8]).

Microscopic pathology

The overwhelming majority of carcinomas of the cervix are epidermoid, or squamous cell carcinomas. Even most of those that develop in the cervical canal, where the mucous membrane is columnar in type, are epidermoid carcinomas. The bulk of these tumors are moderately differentiated, falling in an intermediate group (Grade II) when a three-grade classification is used. Few are very anaplastic, and fewer yet are highly differentiated. Foraker and Denham[59] exhaustively studied squamous cancer of the cervix histochemically and found no reaction peculiar to cancer. Growing squamous cells, whether neoplastic or nonneoplastic, had essentially similar properties.

Epidermoid carcinoma in situ (intraepithelial or preinvasive carcinoma) is a definite entity (Fig. 594). It arises most frequently from the squamous-columnar junction. The location varies with the different ages of life. In young women, carcinoma in situ arises on the surface of the portio vaginalis, but in elderly women, it may arise in the endocervix (Hamperl and Kaufmann[82]). It may also be found, though rarely, in the vaginal fornices (Przybora and Plutowa[163]). Lesions now recognized as *basal cell hyperplasia, squamous metaplasia,* and *atypical epithelial proliferations* (Fig. 595) have been erroneously diagnosed as carcinoma in situ (Govan et al.[70]). The epithelial alterations of carcinoma in situ extend *through all layers.* Spread of these alterations to the glands does not

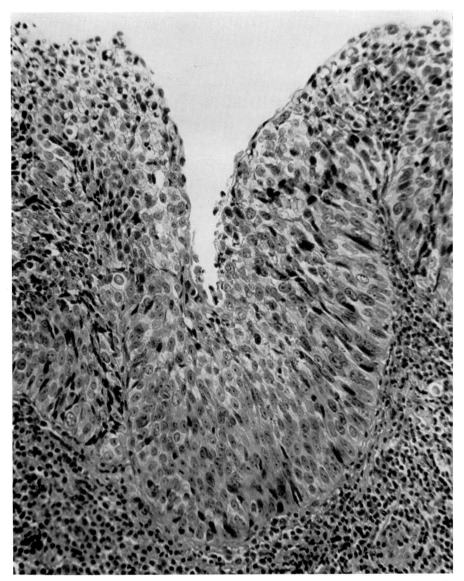

Fig. 594. Carcinoma in situ of cervix. There is complete disorganization of cells *throughout all layers*. Note extreme variation in size and shape of cells. (×275; WU neg. 57-4917.)

constitute invasiveness. The term *micro-invasion* has been coined to designate extension beyond the basement membrane, but this designation is confusing, for it is difficult to demonstrate even with the help of special stains. It seems certain that carcinoma in situ precedes the development of infiltrating carcinoma in a high proportion of instances. The retrospective study of cases with repeated biopsies supports this concept. Carter et al.[27] reported twenty-four patients with invasive carcinoma, seventeen of whom had had pre-

vious carcinoma in situ. The average age of patients with carcinoma in situ is ten years younger than that of patients with invasive carcinoma (38 and 48 years in the series of Carter et al.[27]). Changes diagnosed as carcinoma in situ in pregnant women have often been thought to be regressive. Spjut et al.[198] and Hamperl et al.,[83] independently, failed to confirm this concept. The sequence of dysplasia, carcinoma in situ, and invasive carcinoma occurs. The questions always arise concerning how often dysplasia progresses to car-

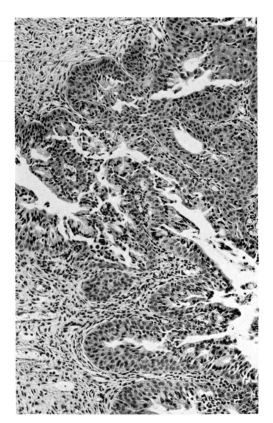

Fig. 595. Extensive papillary metaplasia of cervix which is often mistaken for cancer. There is uniformity of cells. (×125; WU neg. 61-168.)

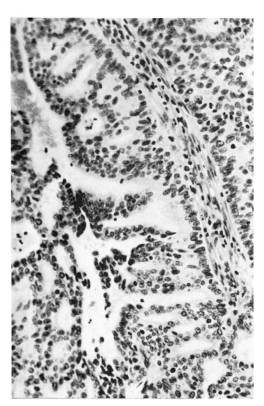

Fig. 596. Typical adenocarcinoma of cervix. Note resemblance to cervical glands.

cinoma in situ and whether all carcinomas in situ progress to invasive carcinoma. Naturally, this problem is complicated by therapy of such lesions by biopsy, and partial or complete excision. Dunn and Martin[51] charted the prevalence of rates of dysplasia, carcinoma in situ, and invasive cancer. There was an excess of dysplasia and carcinoma in situ. However, we tend to agree with Aitken-Swan and Baird[2] that there are two types of cervical cancer, the first rising in younger women and influenced by the factors that were indicated in the discussion of epidemiology. In this type, carcinoma in situ persists with development into invasive cancer. Carcinoma in situ is rare after the age of 60 years, and it is possible that the type of cancer of the cervix arising in elderly women is associated with advancing age and not related to other factors. It is possible that even in the early age group there are some carcinomas that do not pass

through the in situ stage or do it swiftly so that the preliminary stages are not recognized. Petersen[159a, 159b] followed the course of untreated cervical dysplasia and carcinoma in situ in a group of 127 women and reported that a progressive increase in the number with invasive cancer occurred. After twenty years, forty-four of the patients (34.7%) had developed invasive cancer (Sörensen et al.[195]).

In general, the grading of epidermoid carcinomas is of little prognostic value. The degree of extension of the disease as expressed by the clinical *stage* is more important, but within a given stage, the establishment of a relative prognosis may be helped by the histologic *grade*. Epidermoid carcinomas Grade III, although more radiosensitive, are more prone to produce early metastases to the lymph nodes in the upper abdomen. In a thorough histologic study of a large number of cases, Gricouroff[74] concluded that there was no histo-

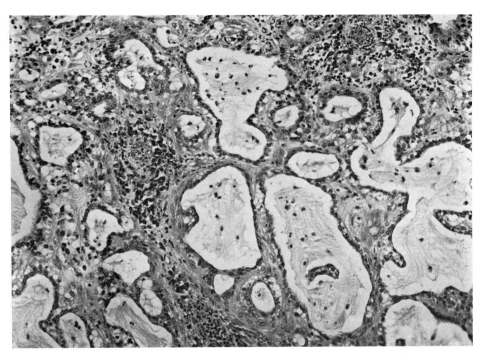

Fig. 597. Well-differentiated carcinoma of mesonephric origin occurring in cervix of 21-year-old woman. (×150; WU neg. 61-174.)

logic feature that could forewarn with certainty the possibility of metastases.

Adenocarcinoma of the cervix can, as a rule, be easily differentiated from epidermoid carcinoma. The typical adenocarcinoma of the cervix shows the characteristic tortuous cervical glands, and in many areas the resemblance to normal cervical epithelium can be recognized (Fig. 596). Carcinomas of the cervix of this type usually produce mucin which can be demonstrated by special stains. At times, carcinoma of the endometrium may be confused with adenocarcinoma of the cervix, but the glands resemble those of the endometrium and usually do not produce mucin. It must also be remembered that adenocarcinoma of the ovary may spread to involve the endometrial cavity and the cervix. This ovarian tumor can usually be recognized by the characteristic pattern, secondary branching of the glands, together with the clinical data. Cancer can rarely arise from remnants of the mesonephric duct, and such a tumor is often very well differentiated (Fig. 597). This type of adenocarcinoma is composed of clear cells that contain glycogen but not mucin. A relatively large proportion of cervical cancers of childhood and adolescence have this pattern (Fawcett et al.[53]). Sneeden[194] reported mesonephric duct remnants in 7.7% of cervices examined by bilateral longitudinal sections.

Metastatic spread

Through its copious lymphatic outlets, carcinoma of the cervix spreads to the lymph nodes of the external iliac and hypogastric groups and, less frequently, to the sacral nodes and the nodes of the promontory. Extension to the lumboaortic chain of nodes, mediastinum, and supraclavicular lymph nodes occurs by continued permeation of lymphatic channels, the cysterna chyli, and the thoracic duct.

Hematogenous spread may take place through the portal and caval vein systems and their anastomosis with the vaginal vein plexus (Javert[96]). Metastases to the liver, lungs, brain (Lipin and Davison[117]), and bones (Laborde and Kritter[112]) do occur but infrequently. Following treatment, the most common distant metastasis is found in the lung (Carlson et al.[26]). In the series of Cherry et al.,[31] the most frequently involved nodes were in the external iliac, obturator, common iliac, and the para-aortic chains, in that order. Henriksen,[85] in a meticulous autopsy study of untreated Stage I cancer, found lymph node metastases in nine of forty-nine cases; tumors with metastases exceeded 1 cm in diameter. In a study of 694 lymphadenectomy specimens for Stage Ib carcinoma, Kolstad[103] found lymph node metastases in 20%. Early lymphatic metastases take place only in the very undifferentiated carcinomas. Carcinomas measuring less than 1 cm in diameter are seldom accompanied by lymph node metastases: in 40 consecutive cases reported by Friedell and Graham[60] there was none with metastases. Carcinomas in situ, those showing microinvasion, and the verrucous type do not metastasize.

Clinical evolution

The onset of carcinomas of the cervix is seldom accompanied by alarming symptoms, as a result of which the disease progresses into a moderately advanced stage before it is deemed worthy of investigation. Early carcinomas of the cervix (Stage I) make up only about 10% of cases seen in the majority of clinics. In a goodly number of advanced cases, the absence of symptoms or the apparent benignity of those present is the main cause for the late diagnosis.

Early symptoms

The symptoms that could betray the existence of an early carcinoma of the cervix may give no concern to the patient during menstrual life. They are easily taken for inconsequential irregularities of a woman's physiologic burdens: *an elongation of the menstrual period* may be the only sign for months. Hypomenorrhea and even amenorrhea are rarely observed. *Watery discharge*, slight but continuous, may also be present for months before it becomes blood-stained. *Slight intermenstrual vaginal bleeding* may occur after coitus, exertion, or travel. Bleeding after coitus is usually startling enough to occasion an early examination. *Hemorrhage* is often the first symptom, but it is seldom associated with early lesions. In general, it accompanies rather advanced exophytic tumors that have developed rapidly and si-

lently. *Yellow vaginal discharge* is rarely a first symptom but occurs in the majority of patients with the later stages of the disease. *Pain* is seldom the first symptom unless it is in the form of a lumbar or lower abdominal ache, such as is sometimes present preceding menstrual periods. The first symptoms produced by the tumor after menopause are usually distressing enough to instigate quick consultation, for vaginal bleeding and discharge are then unexpected. It is also true, however, that when this occurs two or three years after cessation of menstrual life, the patients sometimes believe that they are menstruating again and delay a medical interview.

Late symptoms

In later stages of the disease, the symptoms acquire a different character, and other symptoms gradually become associated.

A *yellow vaginal discharge* is present in the majority of patients with advanced disease. It is characteristically foul smelling because of its high bacterial content. This discharge is very irritating to the vaginal and vulvar mucous membrane, and as a consequence a variable degree of vaginitis and vulvitis may ensue. Abundant watery discharge is seldom encountered. *Vaginal bleeding* may appear only after sexual intercourse or marked exertion. In the majority of cases there is always some degree of bleeding, but it is usually associated with large, rapidly growing exophytic growths. Profuse, continuous bleeding is exceptional. Death from hemorrhage may occur in these patients. Some patients have mild hemorrhages at intervals of weeks or months, usually found to originate from craterlike growths that bleed as they invade a major vessel.

Pain is almost invariably present with carcinoma of the cervix and is a guiding sign in the diagnosis. A vague lumbar ache accompanies a majority of gynecologic conditions, but in cancer of the cervix the pain is progressive, extending from the lumbar region to the hip, through the posterior or anterior aspect of the thigh, and stopping at the level of the knee. Later it extends to the ankle and toes. As a general rule, the greater the intensity and extension of the pain, the greater the pelvic involvement by the tumor. This pain is not easily explained. It is possibly a "reflex pain" resulting from a compression of the sympathetic nerves in the parametria. It may be unilateral or bilateral but is usually more intense and extensive on one side than on the other, according to the extension of the disease. A suprapubic pain is symptomatic of invasion of the anterior vaginal wall or bladder. Moderate tenderness is sometimes present in one or the other iliac fossa but is seldom acute.

Pain that extends high in the dorsolumbar region is usually due to compression of the ureters, hydroureter, and hydronephrosis. Epigastric pain is associated with involvement of the para-aortic nodes in patients in the terminal stage of disease. An intense sacrococcygeal pain usually accompanies the production of a rectovaginal fistula in those with advanced disease.

The *urinary symptoms* are variable and inconstant. An early tumor of the cervix may cause some pollakiuria and even nycturia without actual invasion of the bladder. These symptoms result either from neighboring inflammation and hyperemia of the mucosa with a diminution of the bladder capacity or from an irritation of the urethra by the vaginal discharge. There may be a sensation of heaviness and some pain immediately following micturition, but these signs are only the result of mechanical displacement of the bladder. In contrast, an advanced tumor that has invaded the wall of the bladder and has produced extensive bullous edema may give minimal urinary symptoms. Hence, the degree of bladder invasion cannot be appreciated by relying on these symptoms. As a general rule, however, there is some degree of pollakiuria and nycturia associated with the invasion of the bladder wall by tumor. When tumor has invaded the bladder and has perforated its mucosa, a *vesicovaginal fistula* may form. However, the passage of urine through the vagina may be small, and it may even pass unobserved or be considered merely as vaginal discharge. In other instances, the urine passes through the fistula in one impulse, lasting only a few seconds.

Constipation is present only in patients with advanced disease in whom compression and reduction of the lumen of the large bowel have occurred. It is progressive and becomes marked. *Diarrhea* may then develop as an automatic reaction of the bowel against a reduced bowel lumen. The passage of feces into the vagina through a *rectovaginal fistula* is rarely observed in spite of invasion of the rectal wall by tumor. The tumor growth usually obturates the area of destruction. However, when a slough of tumor does produce a fistula, the fecal material passes into the vaginal tube, causing both alarm and discomfort. As a general rule, however, a rectovaginal fistula forms only after treatment has melted the tumor.

Nausea and *vomiting* may be caused by upper abdominal metastases. *Vomiting, convulsions*, and finally *coma* may be due to uremia following compression of the ureters. *Anuresis* may be observed terminally.

Weight loss almost invariably accompanies cancer of the cervix. The appreciation of it and the period of time over which it occurs are important. Lack of appetite is common. Whether weight loss is the result of secondary infection, renal insufficiency, pain, or anorexia, the fact is that it may become prominent (ten to thirty pounds). Secondary *anemia* is more or less severe according to the duration of the disease but is more acute with the hemorrhagic type of tumor. Repeated transfusions may have to be given during the first weeks of treatment. In spite of the almost constant secondary infection of these tumors, *fever* is observed only rarely. With fever, however, there may be evidence of a pyometral or a urinary infection. All these symptoms combine to give the patient a grave appearance that is further aggravated by analgesics and hypnotics.

Patients not receiving treatment usually die of complications such as hemorrhage, toxemia, peritonitis, pyelonephritis, uremia, etc. Those in whom treatment has failed frequently meet with a similar end due to local recurrence. But with better therapeutic techniques, a greater number of patients have been presenting distant metastases after regional control of the disease. Gricouroff[74] reported 242 cases of distant metastases among 2186 patients with carcinoma of the cervix treated at the

Radium Institute of Paris. In 179 cases in which the approximate date of appearance was known, 130 occurred within three years, twenty in the fourth and fifth years, and only twenty-nine after five years. Of these cases, 113 presented no evidence of residual or recurrent carcinoma in the pelvis.

Sarcomas of the cervix develop very slowly. Sometimes they bleed profusely. Pain may become intense, but it is usually a late symptom. Blood-borne metastases to the liver and lungs are not uncommon.

Diagnosis
Screening and early detection

No other form of cancer offers the opportunity of early detection that is presented by carcinoma of the cervix. Adequate treatment and follow-up of patients with *carcinoma in situ* should decrease considerably the occurrence of infiltrating carcinoma and diminish the mortality from it. To some extent, this has been accomplished already. However, screening examinations have to be repeated periodically, vaginal smears obtained at intervals, and the cases detected properly handled. This is a time-consuming and costly task when it as applied to a large segment of the population. Accepting the finding of 2.5 cases of carcinoma in situ for every 10,000 smears examined, the cost of finding a case in the United States is approximately $2,400, considering only the salary of the special technologist and not that of the pathologist (Bryans et al.[24]); a lesser figure has been suggested (Constable and Truskett[39]). One would have to consider also the reduced cost of treating a lesser number of cases of invasive carcinoma. In 56,000 women examined, Macgregor[122] found no microinvasive carcinomas in situ in patients under 30 years of age and none in those over 65 years. The argument has been raised that in the screening of women with apparently healthy cervices, the vaginal smears need not be done annually. A practical procedure for self-obtained smears may simplify the screening procedure (Davis and Jones[46]). A pipette for self use has been utilized in mass screenings in Denmark for "irrigation smear" (Koch[102]): of 284 patients with suspicious cytology, tissue diagnosis was completed in 267, and seventy-six carcinomas in situ

and thirty-eight invasive carcinomas were found. Others prefer visualization of the cervix for direct scraping and for removal of material from the posterior fornix (Bryans et al.[24]). Jeffcoate[97] recommends repeated cytologic examination after six months as a protection against unsatisfactory specimens. Hammond et al.[81] recommend annual or biannual examination of patients showing Grade III smears. Others suggest as long an interval as five years between cytologic examinations (Macgregor[122]). An excellent opportunity for repeated cytologic examinations is afforded by young pregnant women attending gynecologic clinics. Roberts and Linkins[173] found an overall 85% accuracy in the cytologic diagnosis of 136 cases of cervical carcinoma.

Patients with carcinoma in situ are younger, on the average, than those with frank carcinoma. There seems to be an average interval of ten years between the two groups (Macgregor[122]). Patients with carcinoma in situ may be entirely asymptomatic or may have noted slight postcoitus bleeding. Physical examination may show no abnormality—hence the need to rely on vaginal smears. The occurrence of cases was found to be 2.4% in patients seen at the Strang Cancer Prevention Clinic in New York, 1% in those seen at the Women's Free Hospital of Boston, and 0.7% in those participating in a mass screening program in Aberdeen, Scotland. The latter study consisted of 56,000 married patients between 25 and 60 years of age (Macgregor[122]). A histologic study of 400 uteri removed for noncervical diseases revealed an occurrence of 3.5% carcinoma in situ (Howard et al.[92]). The effectiveness of cytologic screening in large populations has been demonstrated by a decrease in cases of invasive cervical cancer (Fidler et al.[55]). The invasive cancers found are detected at an earlier stage. Christopherson and Parker[36] found that the proportion of patients with Stage I cancer increased from 35% to 63% of the group of invasive lesions discovered in the population subjected to screening.

Clinical examination

Neither the extent of cancer of the cervix or its curability is necessarily indicated by the duration of symptoms or their intensity. Nor are the symptoms that accompany early carcinoma of the cervix pathognomonic of the disease, for they may be present in chronic cervicitis, uterine myomas, cervical polyps, and a number of other nonmalignant conditions. The early diagnosis depends mainly on a detailed history, careful examination, and intelligent evaluation of the findings.

A thorough and accurate recording of symptoms and their duration is an indispensable prerequisite to the examination of a patient suspected of having cancer of the cervix. Patients have a tendency to give the single complaint that appears most important to them, such as vaginal bleeding, whereas a careful questioning will reveal that there was vaginal discharge for months before the bleeding started, that there was lumbar pain that spread to the hip and later to the thigh on one side, or that micturition occurred several times in a night. All these details are of utmost importance.

The usual routine of gynecologic and obstetric examinations may not give enough information for a diagnosis, an evaluation of extension, and staging of cancer of the cervix. Certain details of examination are herewith emphasized which are most satisfactory and have found the sanction of experience.

Abdominal palpation. Before the gynecologic examination is started, a careful palpation of the abdomen must be done, for a voluminous, easily palpable lower abdominal mass can be missed. Palpation of the iliac fossae may disclose the presence of a metastatic mass that usually arises laterally from behind Poupart's ligament. If a mass is not present, this palpation may reveal tenderness on the side of greater extension of the tumor. This examination should also include the inguinal regions for detection of adenopathy.

Vaginal inspection. It is customary and safer to start a gynecologic examination by bimanual palpation, and most gynecologists insist that this be done before a speculum is introduced into the vagina. However, manipulation causes most tumors to bleed to such an extent that direct inspection through the speculum is hampered, and the investigation is, of necessity, hurried. It is therefore more convenient to start with the speculum examination following a mere exploration of the vagina with the gloved finger of one hand. In this way, the examiner may have a direct view of the tumor before it bleeds.

The *colposcope* of Henselmann has been recommended as a means of diagnosing early lesions of the cervix by direct examination. This instrument provides a magnified stereoscopic view of the cervix, thus a precise small biopsy can be obtained from a small lesion; it is also useful to determine whether or not such a lesion is entirely exocervical (Cartier[28]) and in identifying carcinoma in situ and invasive carcinoma (Coppleson[40]). Sakuraba[189] used the procedure in a large number of patients, including 465 with carcinoma of the cervix. By painting the cervix with an iodine solution (Gram's) the normal mucosa becomes brown, whereas areas of abnormal epithelium remain uncolored. This procedure *(Schiller's test)* is helpful in indicating the best place to take a biopsy in early cases of carcinoma, and it may also demonstrate local extent of carcinoma in situ onto the vaginal mucosa (Younge et al.[219]; Nyberg et al.[149]).

Vaginal palpation. With cancer of the cervix, vaginal palpation furnishes information as to the consistency of the cervix, the depth of all vaginal fornices, the size, position, and mobility of the uterus, and the possible extension of induration to the vaginal walls. This information cannot be accurately obtained unless the examiner, with gloves on both hands, does two bimanual examinations, one with the right hand in the vagina and the left hand above the symphysis pubis, and the other with the hands in a reverse position. The index and middle fingers of one hand must reach far into the lateral fornix in order to feel the induration of the mucosa or the diminution in depth of the fornix (Figs. 598 and 599). The same hand cannot reach equally deep into both fornices. The rotation of the hand is only an unsatisfactory maneuver that confuses the appreciation and comparison of the findings in the two sides.

When the tumor extends over the posterior fornix and wall, another type of bimanual examination is necessary. With the fingers of one hand placed in the vagina, palm facing down, and the index finger of the other hand introduced into the rectum, palm upward, the operator will be able to establish whether the invasion of the mucosa is superficial or if the tumor has invaded the rectovaginal septum.

Rectal palpation. Rectal examination establishes the extent of the parametrial infiltration, whereas vaginal palpation only gives a suspicion of it. The diminution in depth of a lateral fornix and loss of its elasticity and depressibility as felt via the vagina can be taken as signs that the tumor has broken out of the cervix and extended into the areolar tissue of the parametrium, but it cannot substantiate by itself how far out the tumor has spread.

Palpation via the rectum is limited to the use of either the index or the middle finger. With the right hand, the examiner can palpate the posterior surface of the right parametrium in its entire length to reach the pelvic wall on that side (Fig. 600). The use of the same finger of the right hand for exploration of the left parametrium is unsatisfactory. The left index or middle finger should be used to explore the left half of the pelvis (Fig. 601). The parametria are normally elastic and soft, but in some patients, particularly those with a history of pelvic inflammatory conditions, they may have become fibrotic and give a false impression of invasion by the tumor. These postinflammatory parametria are usually smooth, cordlike bands conserving some elasticity without increase in volume. Once a patient has received radiotherapy, the parametria may become entirely normal to palpation, but the appreciation of residual tumor in the parametria or the diagnosis of parametrial recurrence necessitates, in most cases, the support of symptoms such as pain and repeated follow-up examinations. Patients who have been heavily irradiated may have diffuse pelvic edema sometimes associated with minor postirradiation effect of the bowel. One should be cautious in diagnosing such bilateral indurations of the parametria as recurrences.

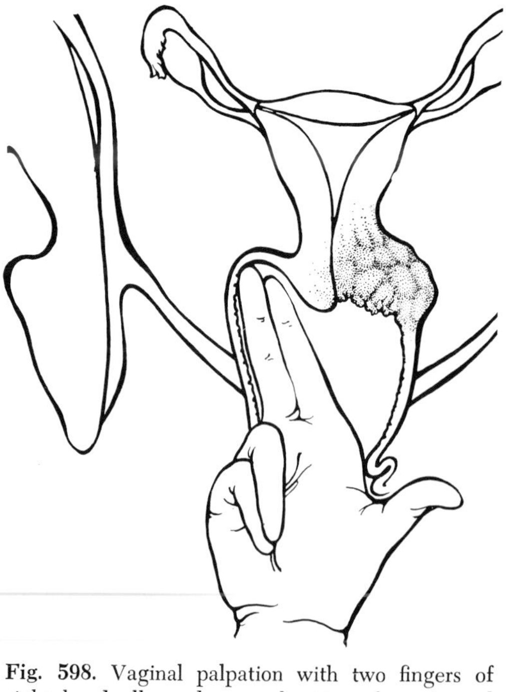

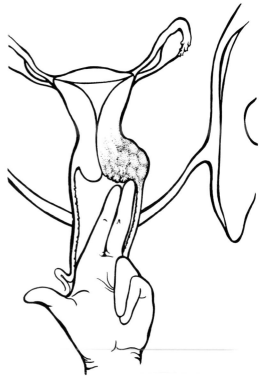

Fig. 598. Vaginal palpation with two fingers of right hand allows deep exploration of cervix and right fornix.

Fig. 599. Vaginal examination with left hand allows exploration of left side. Lack of elasticity suggests parametrial extension, but its limits cannot be definitely established by vaginal examination.

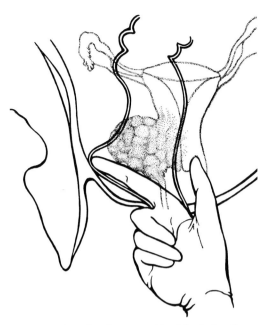

Fig. 600. Rectal palpation with right index finger allows complete exploration of right parametrium. When finger can be introduced between tumor mass and pelvic wall, parametrium is probably not totally invaded.

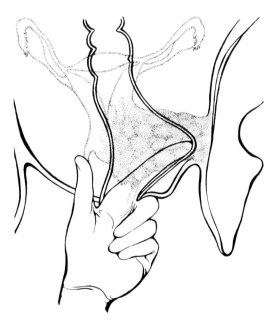

Fig. 601. Rectal palpation with left index finger allows complete exploration of left parametrium. When tumor mass is continuous with pelvic wall and there is no "notch" between tumor and pelvic wall, clinical assumption is that tumor has already invaded pelvic wall.

Clinical classification

The development of radiotherapeutic methods resulted in the necessity of a clinical classification not concerned with operability or inoperability. In 1929, the League of Nations Classification was first adopted. This clinical classification was revised in 1937. In 1950, it was adopted by the American Gynecological Society, by the American Association of Obstetricians, Gynecologists, and Abdominal Surgeons, by the Section of Obstetrics and Gynecology of the American Medical Association, and by the World Health Organization. The representatives of these organizations proposed a simplified definition and added a Stage 0 for carcinomas in situ.

Stage 0—*Carcinoma in situ, preinvasive carcinoma, intraepithelial carcinoma, and similar conditions*

All cases in which there is no evidence of infiltration should be placed in this category. Exact definition of histologic requirements has been deferred.

Stage I—*Carcinoma strictly confined to cervix*

The lesion is confined to the cervix if the ulceration or induration does not extend beyond the cervix and if the fornices appear free and the parametria are not indurated. This group may be subdivided by designating as Stage IA those lesions that are less than 2 cm in diameter and as Stage IB all other larger lesions still confined to the cervix.

Stage II—*Carcinoma extends beyond cervix but has not reached pelvic wall or involves vagina but not lower third*

The presence of a free space between the tumor and the pelvic wall on both sides satisfies the first requirement. Differences of opinion will take place in the estimation of what is the lower third of the vagina. It must not be forgotten that the anterior wall is much shorter than the posterior wall. This group may be subdivided into Stage IIA for cases of medial parametrial extension and for vaginal involvement and into Stage IIB for those with lateral parametrial involvement.

Stage III—*Carcinoma has extended on to pelvic wall or lower third of vagina*

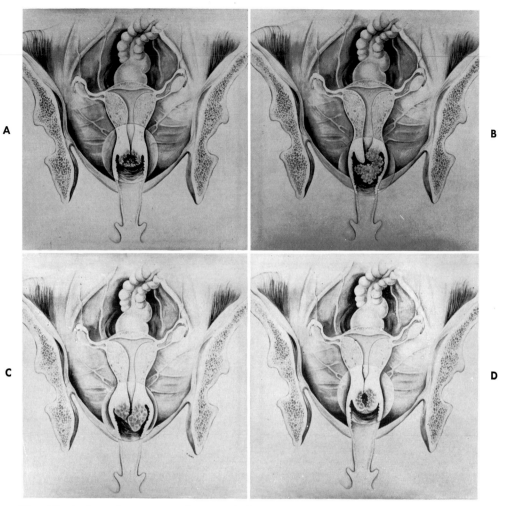

Fig. 602. **A,** Stage I carcinoma of cervix of ulcerating type. Tumor appears to be limited to cervix without invasion of fornices or parametria. **B,** Stage I carcinoma of cervix of exophytic type. Tumor is faintly pedunculated and fills upper third of vagina, but there is no invasion of fornices or parametria. **C,** Stage I carcinoma of cervix of nodular type. There is little ulceration and no invasion of fornices or parametria. **D,** Stage I carcinoma of endocervix. Tumor is not directly visible through speculum. There is no invasion of fornices, parametria, or uterine corpus.

On rectal palpation, no free space is found between the tumor and the pelvic wall. Invasion of the lower third of the vagina must be beyond doubt.

Stage IV—*Carcinoma involves mucosa of bladder or rectum or has extended beyond limits of true pelvis*

The bladder wall is involved long before the tumor breaks into the bladder lumen; indirect evidence of bladder wall involvement, such as *bullous edema,* should be accepted (Regato[168]; Heyman[88]). Involve-

ment of the rectal mucosa is also a relatively late occurrence as compared with involvement of the rectal wall, which may be ascertained by palpation.

Cherry et al.[31] compared the gross *operative* findings with *histopathologic* evidence in 199 patients with cancer of the cervix (Table 80). In most patients the disease was more advanced than expected, and in a few it was less advanced. Appraisal of lymph node involvement at operation proved very inaccurate. The Annual Re-

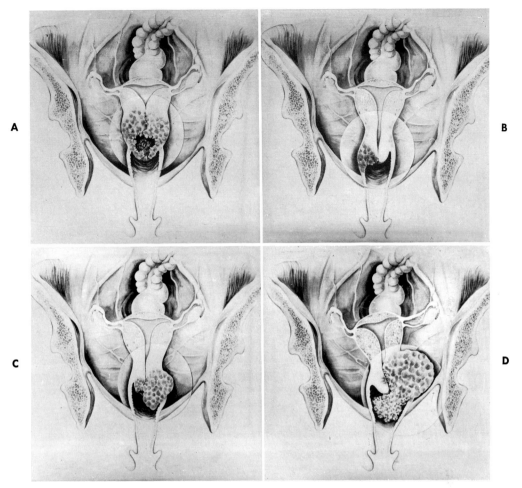

Fig. 603. **A,** Stage II carcinoma of endocervix with invasion of uterine corpus. **B,** Stage II carcinoma of cervix with early invasion of fornix. **C,** Stage II carcinoma of cervix. Nodular tumor with invasion of fornix and adjacent part of parametrium. **D,** Stage II carcinoma of cervix. Exophytic growth with invasion of fornix and almost entire left parametrium.

Table 80. Macroscopic assessment of node involvement*

	No.	% of all nodes
Total nodes studied	573	—
Palpable at operation and histologically involved with cancer	158	27
Palpable at operation and histologically not involved with cancer	113	20
Not palpable at operation and histologically involved with cancer	73	13
Not palpable at operation and histologically not involved with cancer	229	40

*From Cherry, C. P., et al.: Observations on lymph node involvement in carcinoma of the cervix, J. Obstet. Gynaec. Brit. Emp. 60:368-377, 1953.

ports of 124 institutions show a very slight increase in early cases treated in the past two decades. However, a breakdown of the figures reveal that for the decade of 1951 to 1960 the proportion of Stage I cases is much greater in thirty Canadian and American institutions than in ninety-six institutions in the twenty-four other reporting nations (Table 81). Perhaps this reflects a greater application of cytologic and screening technique.

The following general rules should be observed for stage grouping:

1 *When allocating a lesion to a stage, nothing but facts revealed by examination should be taken into account; if a patient is in bad general condition*

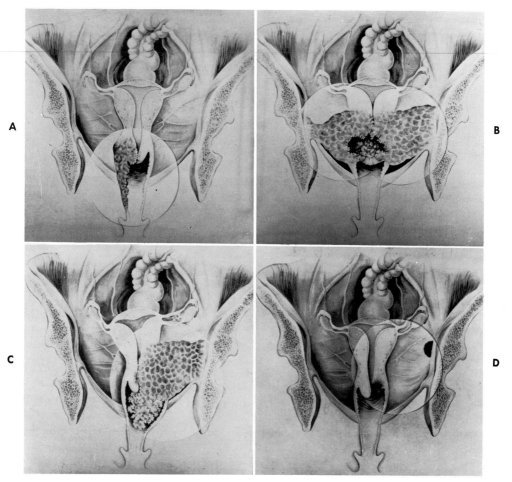

Fig. 604. **A,** Stage III carcinoma of cervix. Tumor has invaded lower third of vagina. **B,** Stage III carcinoma of cervix. Craterlike ulceration with invasion of both parametria in their entire length. Total invasion of one or both parametria relegates lesion to this stage. **C,** Stage III carcinoma of cervix. Exophytic tumor occupying upper half of vagina and extending to entire left parametrium. **D,** Stage III carcinoma of cervix. Small lesion that has already metastasized. Metastatic nodule can be felt against pelvic wall on rectal palpation.

because of hemorrhage, uremia, etc., her lesion is not necessarily a Stage IV.

2 *Allocation should be decided at an examination prior to treatment and should remain.* A change in staging is permissible only when a subsequent examination (cystoscopy, roentgenography), at the beginning of the treatment, reveals further extension.

3 *When it is doubtful to which stage a given lesion is to be allocated, the earlier stage should be chosen.* This rule provides the solution to reasonable doubts (or discrepancy between

equally qualified examiners) as to whether or not the pelvic or the lower third of the vagina has been reached.

4 *The presence of two or more conditions characterizing a stage does not affect the staging;* extension to both pelvic walls, or to the pelvic wall and lower third of the vagina, when present in the same patient, does not make the lesion more than a Stage III.

5 *Sarcomas, chorioepitheliomas, mixed tumors, etc. should be excluded from staging. Also, any carcinoma the cervical origin of which cannot be ascertained (vagina, endometrium) and all*

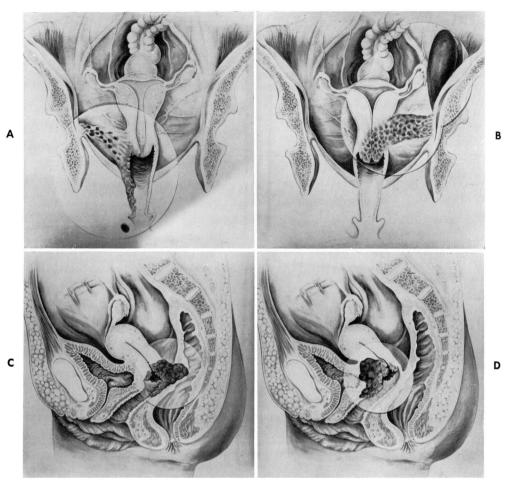

Fig. 605. **A,** Stage IV carcinoma of cervix. Tumor has extended to introitus, and there is metastatic nodule within labium majus. **B,** Stage IV carcinoma of cervix. Tumor has already metastasized to external iliac nodes, and there are large palpable masses above anatomic limits of pelvis. **C,** Stage IV carcinoma of cervix. Tumor has invaded posterior vaginal wall and rectovaginal septum. Bimanual vaginal and rectal palpation reveals evidence of induration within septum. **D,** Stage IV carcinoma of cervix. Tumor has invaded anterior fornix, vaginal wall, and wall of bladder.

postirradiation or postoperative cases should be excluded. This rule is applied when reporting the cases and permits the segregation of previously treated patients from those who are treated for the first time.

Cystoscopic examination

A routine cystoscopic examination of all patients with carcinoma of the cervix is indicated. This examination often reveals a deformity of the trigone area, small areas of ecchymosis and of cystitis may be observed, and there may be exaggeration of the rugae of the floor of the bladder and linear edema. But none of these findings is necessarily related to the extent of the tumor nor of significance in the staging. The cystoscopic examination may be extended to include a study of the ureteral meatus by means of an intravenously injected dye: the urine output may be diminished or abolished in case of ureteral compression. Aman-Jean[5] described a counterclockwise distortion of the bladder that results from the development of cervical tumors with consequent change in position of the ureteral meatuses.

Only the presence of *bullous edema* has been considered a significant cystoscopic

Table 81. Changing proportion of cases in different stages of carcinoma of cervix*

Stage	All institutions 1941-1945 24,032 cases	All institutions 1956-1960 65,051 cases	Twenty-four nations 1951-1960 110,365 cases	American and Canadian 1951-1960 15,590 cases
I	19%	26%	23%	35%
II	39%	38%	38%	36%
III	32%	30%	33%	23%
IV	9%	6%	5%	6%

*Compiled from data in Kottmeier, H.-L., editor: Annual report on the results of treatment in carcinoma of the uterus and vagina, vol. 14, Stockholm, 1967, P. A. Norstedt & Söner, and from data in previous annual reports.

finding. We believe that, with rare exception, it betrays the invasion of the bladder wall by the tumor and that it should be considered as a criterion for classification of the lesion as a Stage IV.

Roentgenologic examination

A roentgenogram of the pelvis is seldom of any value in carcinoma of the cervix. In advanced lesions it sometimes shows definite involvement of the pelvic bones by direct extension of the tumor; lesions observed in the pelvic bones in irradiated patients may have to be differentiated from avascular necroses (Rubin and Prabhasawat[181]).

Pyelograms are essential in the evaluation of cancer of the cervix in the pretreatment phase. In an unexpected proportion of patients the urograms will show some abnormality, usually of the ureters, but hydronephrosis and complete lack of kidney function may be found. Dearing[47] emphasized that an abnormal pretreatment pyelogram is a sign of grave significance, irrespective of the stage of the carcinoma of the cervix. Moss and Brand[139] emphasized that alterations in pretreatment pyelograms will be more common in the presence of more advanced disease but that changes can also occur in Stage I. Naturally, such alterations indicate much more advanced disease than is readily apparent on clinical examination (Parker and Friedman[155]). Abnormalities occur more frequently in undifferentiated tumors and often imply lymph node involvement. Brites Patricio and Baptista[22] performed 257 examinations of the kidney with hippuran[131] before or after radiotherapy for carcinoma of the cervix and concluded that these tests are useful in demonstrating parametrial invasion and in evaluating re-

sults of treatment. Follow-up pyelograms are of unquestionable value (Stander et al.[199]). Hittmair and Frick[90] demonstrated urographic abnormalities in the follow-up examination of twenty-six patients, with recurrent disease being the cause in eleven. *Retrograde pyelography* is indicated in all patients in whom the excretory pyelograms have shown a suspected abnormality. The procedure may not add any useful information or, on the contrary, may clearly show a point of ureteral obstruction or the presence of hydronephrosis.

Urovenogram has been advocated in order to obtain additional information (Kottmeier[106]). It may reveal compression of veins by involved lymph nodes. *Lymphangiography* has been used in an attempt to detect the presence of metastatic lymph nodes. Chavanne et al.[30] studied by lymphangiography seventy-five patients with Stage II carcinoma of the cervix. They subsequently removed the lymph nodes surgically and found nineteen patients to have metastases, in only six of whom involvement was suspected on the lymphangiography. The lymphographic study after surgery often reveals the inadequacy of the lymphadenectomy when postoperative roentgenograms are made (Vuksanovic et al.[211]).

Exfoliative cytology

The microscopic examination of vaginal smears is an essential procedure in the screening examination of women for cancer (p. 780). The procedure is highly accurate, more so in the presence of carcinoma in situ than in large ulcerated and infected invasive carcinoma; it yields few false positives. However, positive cytology in a patient without symptoms or findings is only grounds for further investigation by

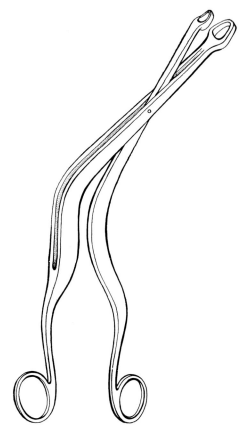

Fig. 606. Curved biopsy forceps with sharp cutting edges designed by Faure for purpose of removing specimens from nodular tumors of cervix.

biopsy or conization: *no definitive treatment should be instituted on the basis of positive cytology alone.*

Biopsy

A satisfactory biopsy is the most important step toward the diagnosis. The specimen should be taken from the border of the lesion as near as possible to normal tissue. A cutting forceps of the Faure type is preferable (Fig. 606). Large fragments removed by grasping forceps from the center of the lesion may prove to be composed mostly of necrotic tissue. Some infiltrating lesions of the endocervix cannot be biopsied with ease. In such instances, a dilatation and curettage are indicated. In patients without gross evidence of cancer or with only a cervical erosion, several specimens should be taken, preferably from the middle of the anterior and posterior

lips and near the commissures, as close as possible to the endocervix.

Patients with a positive cytologic examination should always be submitted to further tissue examination. A conization may be done, but adequate multiple biopsies are satisfactory for diagnosis in a high proportion of instances. Griffiths[76] studied the accuracy of cervical biopsies, using a sharp punch and endocervical curettements, in 159 cases of carcinoma in situ, with 97% positive results. He believes that the need for *diagnostic* conizations has been exaggerated, particularly when biopsies are accompanied by endocervical curettage (Kolstad[103]).

Differential diagnosis

Benign ulcerations of the cervix and *eversions of the endocervical mucosa* may be difficult to differentiate from early carcinoma. In many instances in which the inflammatory lesions fail to disappear under a short appropriate management, a biopsy is indicated to establish the diagnosis. Benign ulcerations due to trauma or other causes are easily recognizable when away from the cervical os, for they are not indurated. Breaking of *vaginal adhesions* may cause bleeding. They usually show corresponding areas with telangiectatic appearance. Inflammatory changes associated with *Trichomonas* infection may have to be differentiated from carcinoma in situ (Koss and Wolinska[104]).

Decidual reaction in the cervix during pregnancy may be confused with carcinoma. Decidual lesions may present multiple small yellow or reddish elevations of the cervical mucosa that are soft and friable and bleed easily on contact. Rarely, they may present as a fungating mass (Bausch et al.[11]), but the differential diagnosis on biopsy is not difficult.

Chancres of the cervix are rarely found. They are usually situated on the anterior lip and look like a clear-cut ulceration about 1 cm in diameter. The base is indurated, and there is little bleeding. Chancres may be found on a cervical erosion and circle around the os. Carefully taken specimens will reveal the *Treponema pallidum* in microscopic dark-field examination. Secondary syphilis is quite often accompanied by superficial wide ulcera-

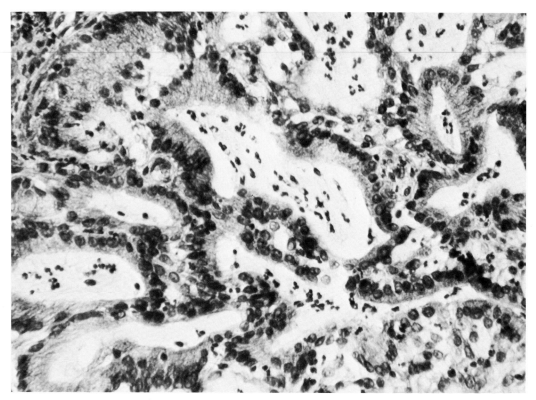

Fig. 607. Pronounced microglandular metaplasia related to progestogen effect. This change, although confusing, is benign and does not progress to cancer. (WU neg. 69-32.)

tions of the cervix that are covered by yellowish false membranes. In these cases, there are usually other manifestations of the disease, and the serologic tests show a positive reaction. *Leukoplakia* of the cervix is rare. In recent years, an increasing proportion of biopsies of the cervix has shown prominent *microglandular hyperplasia of the endocervix*. This change (Fig. 607) is associated with the use of cyclic artificial progestogens and can be easily mistaken for carcinoma (Kyriakos et al.[110]).

Tuberculous lesions of the cervix are mostly secondary. The diagnosis is facilitated by locating other indications of tuberculosis in the lungs or bladder. Whether ulcerative or proliferative, tuberculous lesions are accompanied by considerable secondary infection. Pyometra and endometritis may be present as well. Multiple lesions are easily recognized, but diagnosis of the proliferative type is possible only upon biopsy. Extensive involvement of the cervix by *bilharzial disease* may result in a clinical picture indistinguishable from

carcinoma; the correct diagnosis can only be made by biopsy (Skinner[188]).

Cervical polyps produce a scanty, spotty type of bleeding, are generally small, pedunculated, and nonulcerated, and protrude from the os (Plate 4). It may be accompanied by a more or less important degree of inflammation. In some instances, it may break down and become necrotic and thus be confused with carcinoma. Mezer[134] reported a study of 1639 cervical polyps in which five demonstrated carcinoma. The epithelium of a cervical polyp has no greater chance of developing a carcinoma than the epithelium of the cervix itself. As a rule, cervical polyps are easily removed.

Chronic cervicitis may offer great difficulty in differential diagnosis with an early carcinoma. In general, it occurs in a younger group than does carcinoma. The cervix is enlarged and indurated and presents a marked granulation around the os. Cervical erosions may be associated with some degree of pelvic inflammation. In re-

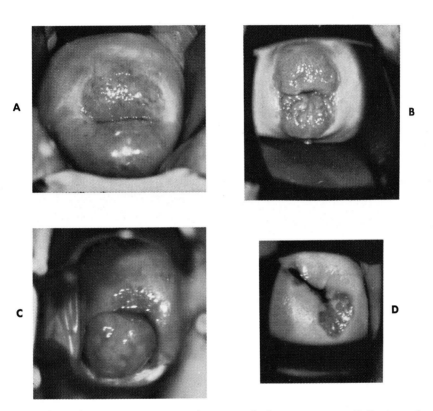

Plate 4. A, Cervical erosion. **B,** Eversion of cervix with chronic cervicitis. **C,** Benign polyp of cervix. **D,** Early carcinoma on lacerated cervix. (Courtesy Dr. B. Z. Cashman, Pittsburgh, Pa.)

moving a specimen for biopsy, the tissues are found fibrotic rather than friable. Negative biopsies should be complemented by dilatation and curettage to assure that a carcinoma is not present.

Treatment
Carcinoma in situ

In the context of carcinoma of the cervix, *prevention* means the discovery of carcinoma in situ by screening examinations, its adequate treatment, and its cure before it transgresses into an infiltrating, less curable lesion. In the presence of carcinoma in situ, the choice is among a therapeutic conization, a hysterectomy, and transvaginal roentgentherapy. When the diagnosis of carcinoma in situ is made during pregnancy, there should be no hurry—the patient should be permitted to deliver normally.

The *therapeutic conization* for carcinoma in situ can be adapted to the extent of the lesion in the ectocervix. When this is done, the recurrence rate after conization is not any higher than after hysterectomy. Christopherson and Parker[34] reported 124 cases of carcinoma in situ diagnosed by biopsy: 117 were confirmed by conization (fourteen microinvasive), three were negative, and four showed residual dysplasia. Conversely, in 117 cases of dysplasia diagnosed by biopsy, ninety-four were confirmed by conization and eighteen were diagnosed as carcinoma in situ (one microinvasive). Silbar and Woodruff[191] reported twenty-four instances in which biopsy, conization, and hysterectomy specimens were available: there were three instances in which invasive carcinoma was not suspected on biopsy but diagnosed on conization. Frozen section can be utilized with conizations with topographic plotting (Beyer[13]; Greenberg and Kaufman[73]). Step serial sectioning of conization specimens can be undertaken to eliminate the possibility of incomplete excision or the presence of early invasion. Lesser efforts frequently lead the pathologist to warn of probable incomplete removal and to an unnecessary hysterectomy. There are great differences of opinion in reference to what has come to be designated as *microinvasion*. Various observers have concluded that such evidence implies no greater gravity nor need for radicality than is usually the case in carcinoma in situ. All that seems necessary in such instances is the assurance, as in any other patient with carcinoma in situ treated conservatively, of periodic follow-up examinations and cytologic surveillance (Green[72]). Carcinoma in situ is multifocal, and adequacy of conization is best controlled by postconization cytology. Topographic plotting is not necessarily assurance that any carcinoma remains because of its multifocal nature (Krieger and McCormack[109]). However, Nichols et al.[144] believe that step serial sectioning of cervical cone biopsies is essential and accurate and that no cases of invasive carcinoma will be missed.

Hysterectomy is an effective treatment of carcinoma in situ. It can be done in women past the childbearing age or in those not desirous of having more children to remove the present carcinoma in situ and the possibility of further carcinomatous manifestations, but the procedure is not always necessary or advisable and certainly not without some risk. TeLinde et al.[204] reported on 211 patients treated with hysterectomy, 209 of whom were cured and two lost to follow-up. Others have had similar experiences (Pederson and Jeffries[157]). In a series of 561 patients followed for at least two years after hysterectomy, six developed subsequent carcinoma of the vaginal vault (Mussey and Soule[141]). There is an increased morbidity in postconization hysterectomy. Malinak et al.[126] believes that hysterectomy should be done immediately after frozen section examination of the conization specimen or after a delay of twenty-one days.

Transvaginal roentgentherapy is an effective treatment of carcinoma in situ in young women desirous to retain their menstrual function and fertility. Regato and Cox[171] reported on a series of twenty-seven patients followed for as long as eighteen years after roentgentherapy, with no instance of recurrence and no case of invasive transformation, and two of the patients subsequently became pregnant and delivered normal children. The procedure is, of course, applicable to other patients in whom, for any reason, a conization or hysterectomy is not advisable or possible.

Irrespective of treatment administered,

patients with carcinoma in situ should undergo periodic examinations, and vaginal smears should be examined at least once a year.

Invasive carcinoma
Surgery

The radical hysterectomy known as the Wertheim operation was used in the treatment of early carcinoma of the cervix over half a century ago, but it was almost generally abandoned due to its excessive operative mortality (Bonney[15]) and to the relative success of radiotherapy. Advances in the knowledge of anesthesia, prevention of shock, and infectious complications have reduced or almost entirely eliminated the operative mortality, and thus there has been renewed enthusiasm for the surgical treatment of early carcinoma of the cervix.

Advocates of surgery for early carcinoma of the cervix often base their position on

negative grounds such as many cases of carcinoma of the cervix are radioresistant. Baud[10] succeeded in the local sterilization of all but eight carcinomas in an *unselected* series of 105 cases of carcinoma of the cervix, Stage I, treated with radium. Such proportion of local recurrences does not necessarily imply radioresistance and could be explained by technical errors. The results of radiotherapy depend greatly on the skill with which it is applied. The statement has often been made that radiotherapy cannot destroy metastatic carcinoma in lymph nodes, but there is ample evidence that this statement is incorrect. Kottmeier[105] proved by preirradiation biopsy and long follow-up that patients with metastatic carcinoma of the cervix can be cured by radiotherapy. According to Navratil[142] the proportion of lymph node involvement is 11% in Stage I, 23% in Stage II, and 43% in Stage III. Rutledge and

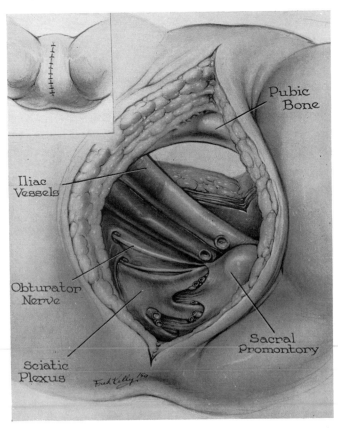

Fig. 608. Appearance of pelvis after evisceration for recurrent carcinoma of cervix. (From Bricker, E. M., and Modlin, J.: The role of pelvic evisceration in surgery, Surgery **30:**76-94, 1951.)

Fletcher[183] administered radiations to the entire pelvis in six weeks and submitted the patients to lymphadenectomy after a period of three months. Careful histologic study revealed sterilization of nodes, with the proportion of involved nodes found to be 50% lower than expected for the stage.

If surgery applied as a routine procedure is not sufficiently justified, there are definite cases of early carcinoma of the cervix in which the operation may be preferred to radiotherapy. Some endocervical carcinomas in conjunction with voluminous leiomyomas make radiotherapy difficult. Small carcinomas in very young women may be successfully treated by hysterectomy without removal of the ovaries, although in such cases transvaginal roentgentherapy alone may fill the same purposes. In the treatment of a large number of cases by radiotherapy, there is always a group that may not be controlled due to technical difficulties or errors and perhaps a small proportion of true "radioincurable" cases within the circumstances of the treatment given. Close follow-up and early surgical treatment of patients in whom radiotherapy fails may prove successful, although in many instances more than hysterectomy may be necessary.

Pelvic exenteration may be used in the treatment of advanced carcinoma of the cervix. It implies removal of the uterus, tubes, ovaries, rectum, and bladder, with the establishment of a colostomy and transplantation of the ureters. Bricker and Modlin[21] standardized a technique that includes removal of the hypogastric artery and the internal iliac vein, to facilitate removal of lymphatics, and the establishment of an artificial "ilial bladder" (Fig. 608). Pelvic exenteration should be reserved for, and the best results are obtained in, patients with recurrent carcinoma in the midpelvis (Ulfelder and Meigs[209]). It is also indicated in serious radionecrotic complications in the absence of cancer. Presence of para-aortic metastases contraindicates this operation. In a series of 218 exenterations reported by Bricker et al.,[20] there were twenty-five operative deaths but only five in the last seventy-five patients. This operation should be undertaken only by experienced surgical teams.

Surgery is the treatment of choice of sarcomas but rarely are they diagnosed in the operable stage.

Sarcoma botryoides grows by direct extension. Radiation therapy is usually ineffective. This tumor usually occurs in young children. At times, cure can be effected by pelvic exenteration. This tumor should be treated by surgery, which was used as initial therapy in five patients by Rutledge and Sullivan.[186]

Radiotherapy

Radiotherapy remains the outstanding treatment of cervical cancer. In the beginning, internal treatment by means of radium was given greater importance, but with the perfection of equipment and of techniques of irradiation, external pelvic irradiation has gained an important place, so that *if internal irradiation can be called the most important single factor in the treatment of early lesions, thorough external roentgentherapy is the most important single factor in the treatment of advanced disease* (Regato[167]).

External pelvic irradiation. We believe that *a thorough external irradiation of the pelvis is an important first step in the treatment of all cases.* The institution of external pelvic irradiation as a preliminary step has several definite advantages. Secondary infection and inflammation that accompany the tumor are greatly reduced. Any pain

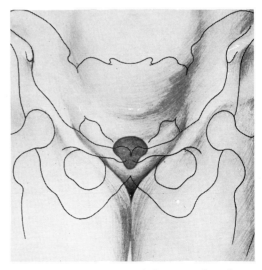

Fig. 609. Anterior approach for external irradiation of carcinoma of cervix. Note relatively low position of uterus.

that was present disappears, the patients become euphoric, and their general condition improves. Moreover, the physical dimensions of the tumor are reduced to boundaries within which their sterilization is possible by internal irradiation. It is true that as a consequence of the shrinkage of the tumor and vaginal fornices after external roentgentherapy, the intracavitary application of radium may be rendered more difficult, but this is overbalanced by the advantages previously mentioned.

External irradiation alone may reach the entire tumor area in sufficient quantities to sterilize the tumor without help of further internal irradiation. Baclesse[6] reported on a series of forty-five patients with Stage III and Stage IV carcinomas who received external pelvic roentgentherapy alone, with seven (15%) free of disease at the end of five years. Although these patients received a very thorough external irradiation, there obviously would have been a higher percentage of cures if the treatment had been completed by internal therapy. The series, however, proves that external irradiation is a powerful agent in the treatment of the two last stages of the disease.

The use of supervoltage roentgentherapy and cobalt[60] teletherapy has made possible a wide and effective administration of a sufficient amount of radiations throughout the potential area of involvement from the outside alone, but the *higher intensity* of the internal treatment, though limited in scope, remains a powerful weapon in circumscribed lesions.

In administering external roentgentherapy, the dimensions of the pelvis and the superficial projection of the uterus and parametria should be taken into consideration. With conventional roentgentherapy, most techniques of external irradiation utilize several fields of entry in order to minimize the skin reaction and to facilitate cross-firing of the tumor area. On the contrary, with supervoltage and cobalt[60] teletherapy, it has become more effective to utilize large fields, usually one anterior and one posterior. Because of the fact that some workers may start with the internal radium application, or simply to provide the possibility of an intense final application of radium, the midline is protected in some institutions during the external irradiation (Fletcher[56]). Thus, the core of the tumor, indeed the whole of the tumor, may receive very little irradiation during the course of external treatments. We prefer to start with the external treatment and to irradiate the entire tumor area. This procedure requires only a greater protraction of the final radiumtherapy and the diminishing somewhat of the radium dose to avoid excessive irradiation of the midline (Regato[169]).

The external irradiation must, of necessity, be fractionated over several weeks. This diminishes the systemic effects and, with conventional roentgentherapy, the intensity of the superficial reactions. Fractionation also diminishes the untoward effects on normal structures.

Intracavitary curietherapy. It is not advisable to allow a long period of time to elapse between the external treatments and their completion by intracavitary curietherapy. Although the tumor may have been reduced in size and generally affected by external irradiation, it has not, in all probability, received sufficient treatment to prevent a rapid recurrence. A period of ten days to two weeks may be considered a reasonable interval between treatments. Bosch and Marcial[16] believe that the time interval between external roentgentherapy and intracavitary radium should be two weeks. It permits recovery from radiation-induced normal tissue reactions. Longer intervals should be avoided in view of possible harmful influences on curability, particularly in Stage III and Stage IV.

There are numerous techniques of intracavitary curietherapy for the treatment of carcinoma of the cervix. They all have in common the use of an intrauterine applicator, flexible or rigid, and differ in the character of vaginal application, usually intended to be placed as far laterally on either side of the midline as possible. The differences in technique of application are beyond the scope of this discussion. We believe that protraction of the radium application to ten to twelve days permits a thorough irradiation and diminishes complications (Hunt[94]).

Interstitial curietherapy. Interstitial curietherapy consists of introducing needles containing radium or other radioactive sub-

stances into the tumor itself and the surrounding soft tissues of the pelvis. The
advantage of this procedure lies in the
fact that large doses may be administered
to the tumor area with great intensity, but
homogeneity of the irradiation so delivered
is lacking, and the treatment is sometimes
followed by radionecrotic accidents to the
surrounding structures.

The interstitial injection of *radioactive
colloidal gold* has been used in the treatment of carcinoma of the cervix. The results of this treatment have been comparable to those obtained by conventional
methods, but the complications have been
excessive—radionecrosis of the bowel,
bladder, and uréters, necessitating surgery.
It is technically very difficult to administer
a homogeneous dose by this means. The
possibilities of necrosis are all too great.

Transvaginal roentgentherapy. Transvaginal roentgentherapy can be utilized
alone for the irradiation of carcinomas in
situ or for very early infiltrating carcinomas
of the cervix. When used in conjunction
with external roentgentherapy, it should
not be considered as a mere substitute for
radiumtherapy (Fig. 610). However, the
use of transvaginal roentgentherapy, by
eliminating the unnecessary overirradiation
of the midline, permits a better utilization
of the external irradiation (Regato[169]). This
"integral" radiotherapy of carcinoma of the
cervix has proved capable of improving
the results in the treatment of advanced
cases while reducing the incidence of radionecrotic fistulas and other complications.

Transvaginal roentgentherapy, done
through lead specula to avoid irradiation
of the ovaries, is an excellent means of
irradiation for *carcinoma in situ* in young
women. This conservative procedure preserves menstrual function and the capability of subsequent fecundation and
delivery. Regato and Cox[171] have treated
young patients in this fashion who have
later become pregnant and delivered normal children without presenting subsequent manifestations of carcinoma.

Early complications of radiotherapy. Infectious complications have been responsible for a number of radiotherapeutic failures. These consist primarily of pelvic
cellulitis, peritonitis, pyometra, and urinary
infection. Particularly during curietherapy,

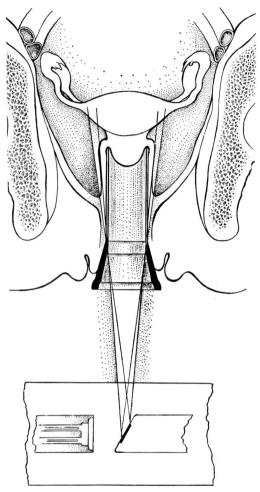

Fig. 610. Transvaginal roentgentherapy. Irradiation
through specially designed speculum (Regato)
which protects vulva while allowing dispersion of
beam through its walls.

infectious complications may force discontinuation of the treatment with resulting
failure (García and Schlosser[64]; Van Her-
ick[210]). Adequate use of antibiotics and
the institution of external irradiation as an
initial step have eliminated the majority
of these infectious complications and have
brought to better light the urinary complications that may hide behind them. It
appears evident that a number of patients
develop obstructions of the ureters due to
the presence of tumor in the parametria
and nodes that lie along their course.
Whereas such cases are advanced and
probably hopeless, a great deal of palliation and prolongation of life may be ob-

tained by ureteral catheterization and, in some instances, ureteral transplantation.

The administration of radiations through large fields at immoderately high daily doses results in anorexia, nausea, or vomiting, as well as malaise. Any degree of these symptoms is known as *radiation sickness*. This systemic effect of irradiations depends primarily on the proper balance of daily dose and size of fields to suit the necessities and tolerance of the individual patient. During the course of treatment, a more or less marked *diarrhea* usually appears. This symptom is quite variable in intensity, does not follow a recognizable chronology, and has no correlation with dosage. Administration of antidiarrheic medication is all that is required during the course of treatment. No correspondence should be established between this functional postirradiation reaction and permanent histopathologic effects that may be observed at autopsy or after surgery (Gricouroff and Potet[75]).

External irradiation with conventional roentgentherapy does result in *dry* or *moist epidermitis*. With supervoltage roentgentherapy and cobalt[60] teletherapy, the skin reaction does not reach the limits of dry or moist shedding of the epidermal layer, but after weeks of irradiation the devitalized dermis may become easily contaminated, particularly on the anterior field. Such contamination should be averted or properly medicated.

Following the application of radium, a mild degree of vaginal reaction always develops, appearing in the form of a diphtheroid membrane more or less limited to the upper third of the vagina. This mucosal reaction spontaneously subsides under proper antiseptic care but if neglected may develop into radionecrosis as in the skin. Fortunately, the vagina has a great ability to repair itself, and many localized radionecrotic accidents are passed unnoticed. Proper vaginal douches and antiseptic jellies are adequate preventive measures.

Following the application of radium, there may be a mild degree of *proctitis* caused by the reaction of the rectal mucosa (Dulac and Rousseau[50]). If the radium comes in contact with the rectum and the dose is large, a localized radionecrotic area may develop on the anterior rectal wall at the level of the cervix. A certain amount of rectal bleeding, accompanied by pain and tenesmus, may appear. These small areas of necrosis often heal spontaneously. Gricouroff and Potet[75] studied the rectum of sixteen patients who had had radiation therapy of cancer of the cervix and found superficial microulcerations of the mucosa, sclerohyalinosis of the submucosa, dilatation of the capillaries, and hyaline change in the muscularis. *Cystitis* is rarely observed.

A *rectovaginal* or a *vesicovaginal* fistula may appear in the course of treatments or immediately afterward but is not necessarily due to excessive irradiation. If tumor has invaded the rectovaginal septum or the bladder, the destruction of the tumor opens a passage that results in a urinary or fecal fistula. This is particularly evident in patients with advanced disease following a massive dose of radiations. The production of vesicovaginal or rectovaginal fistulas due to irradiation can be avoided by properly packing the radium applicators in the vagina.

Late complications of radiotherapy. External and intracavitary irradiations may result in an overirradiation of the vital organs of the pelvis. A small amount of rectal bleeding and sometimes a rectal hemorrhage, usually accompanied by "gas pains," may occur in patients who have been well for some time. The bleeding may be due to the *untoward effect of radiations on the large or small intestine* or both, but these symptoms are neither frequent nor necessarily fatal. Prompt administration of antibiotics, and, if necessary, blood transfusions may be sufficient to facilitate total and permanent recovery. Bowel obstruction occurs in a few patients, which may necessitate an enteroenterostomy or a colostomy.

In a study of 369 patients irradiated for carcinoma of the cervix, with reference to urologic complications, Cushing et al.[43] found no evidence of urologic complications before treatment in 286, of whom 248 remained free of such complications for as long as they lived. The literature reveals frequent references to postirradiation "injury" of the ureters. No such radiation effects have been experimentally reproduced within therapeutic limits of dose and frac-

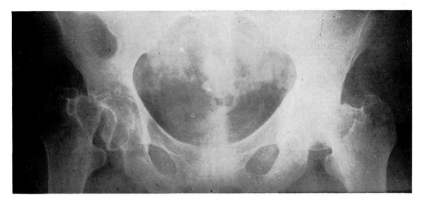

Fig. 611. Bilateral fractures of heads of femurs following irradiation through lateral pelvic fields for carcinoma of cervix. Patient remained cured of carcinoma.

tionation. Ureteral obstructions observed in patients treated for carcinoma of the cervix are often sequelae of preirradiation urinary complications or the result of compression by recurrent disease in the parametrium and nodes. Rarely, they may be due to postirradiation fibrosis in the parametrium compressing the ureter (Kottmeier[106]). When lateral fields of irradiation have been used or oversized fields of entry have been applied to a small pelvis, *avascular changes of the pelvic bones* and later spontaneous fractures may result, particularly at the head of the femur (Fig. 611). Avoidance of this portal of entry eliminates this complication.

An area of heavily irradiated skin may be the site of a *late radiodermitis* occurring several years after treatment. As a general rule, there is a history of trauma (or surgical incision) and subsequent secondary infection which, brought into a devitalized area of the skin, contributes as much to this accident as the radiations themselves. To avoid such late radionecrosis, the patient should be cautioned against allowing excessive dryness of the irradiated area of the skin.

Late *rectovaginal* or *vesicovaginal fistulas* may result years after the carcinoma has been controlled purely from the effects of irradiation of these structures. More frequently, however, these late complications accompany a recurrence, which causes secondary infection and consequent necrosis.

Causes of failure of radiotherapy. The most common cause of failure of radiotherapy of carcinoma of the cervix is insufficient irradiation at some point of the potential tumor area. Naturally, the proportion of failures increases with the extent of the tumor area, since the possibilities of technical error or of inability to deliver a sufficient dose throughout are lessened (Blomfield et al.[14]). The proportion of local recurrences following treatment of early cases is so small (Baud[10]; Baclesse and Fernandez-Colmeiro[7]; Cantril[25]) that it offers no comfort to those who would consider radioresistance as a factor in the choice of treatment. If some lesions are, in reality, biologically radioincurable, their number must be small. Compression or invasion of the ureters, resulting uremia, urinary dysfunction, and deterioration of the general condition are frequent causes of immediate failure.

Upper abdominal metastases outside of the field of irradiation may be present during the course of treatments and may result in generalization of the disease even when the tumor has been totally sterilized in the pelvis. With the improvement of radiotherapeutic techniques, this phenomenon is being observed more often. Finally, the untoward effect of radiations on the small or large bowel may result in a large area of necrosis that can cause death, but this is exceptional (Aldridge[3]). In general, most bowel complications properly handled medically or surgically are not fatal.

Estimation of radiosensitivity. Since the dawn of radiotherapy, attempts have been made to predict the relative radiosensitivity of tumors. In the case of carcinoma of the cervix, efforts have been made to choose the early lesions that should be treated by either surgery or radiotherapy. This approach assumes that the cases that are relatively unfavorable for the one are favorable for the other form of treatment. Although there are variations in radiosensitivity of carcinomas of the cervix, there are no radioresistant ones. The most radiosensitive carcinomas are precisely the most likely to recur and to metastasize. The more differentiated carcinomas are relatively less radiosensitive but more radiocurable. Repeated biopsies made during treatment may reveal variations in the effects of irradiation (Glücksmann and Way[68]), but these are not necessarily of prognostic value (Merrill[133]).

Follow-up exfoliative cytology. The pretension of guiding or deciding on the adequacy of treatment by means of cytologic examination has now been recognized as being unfounded (McLennan and McLennan[123]). Persistent "tumor" cells in the vaginal smears of irradiated patients have no prognostic value when found within the first four months of irradiation. An occasional patient may show abnormal cells for as long as twelve months after treatment and never show any evidence of recurrence (Marcial et al.[128]).

Combined surgery and radiotherapy

Surgeons and radiotherapists have considered the possibility of improving results by a combination of radiotherapy and surgery, in view of the fact that neither approach yields perfect results and that cases that are unfavorable to one form of treatment are also unyielding to the alternate approach. Rutledge et al.[184] randomized patients with Stage I, II, and III lesions in two groups, one group receiving radiation therapy alone and another receiving a radical hysterectomy and iliac lymphadenectomy following radiotherapy: the complications of surgery proved to be excessive and the results not improved (Table 82). Other such attempts have only shown evidence that radiotherapy sterilizes a good proportion of metastatic lymph nodes (Gray and Frick[71]; Decker et al.[48]; Morton et al.[138]; Gary et al.[65]). Although there is no evidence that adenocarcinomas of the cervix are less radiocurable than squamous cell carcinomas (Cuccia et al.[42]), Rutledge et al.[184] believe that the combined treat-

Table 82. Cancer of cervix—five-year survival by modified life table method*

Stage	Study group		Control group	
	No.	Survived	No.	Survived
I	30	86%	39	93%
IIA	39	77%	39	89%
IIB	25	54%	28	62%
IIIA	23	54%	28	33%
IIIB	25	54%	35	63%
	142		169	

*From Rutledge F. N., et al.: Pelvic lymphadenectomy as an adjunct to radiation therapy in treatment for cancer of the cervix, Amer. J. Roentgen. 93:607-614, 1965.

ment may be slightly more fruitful than radiotherapy alone.

Chemotherapy

Carcinoma of the cervix has shown response to the administration of *methotrexate*, and for this reason this medical approach has been advocated in areas of the world in which no radiotherapy is available. The response to methotrexate is ephemeral, however, even when administered intra-arterially (Bateman et al.[9]). Solidoro et al.[196] treated forty-two patients with *cyclophosphamide* and observed six "complete" but temporary remissions. Using the same drug, Smith et al.[192] treated 107 patients with recurrent disease. One-third of the patients showed subjective improvement, and one-fifth responded with some apparent increased survival.

Prognosis

In 1965, there were 8053 deaths from cancer of the cervix in the United States, a crude mortality rate of 7.4 for white and 14.0 for black women per 100,000 population. This represents a decrease from the observed rates of 9.8 and 21.9, respectively, in 1950. These declining figures have been confirmed in British Columbia (Boyes et al.[18]), Tennessee (Ruch et al.[182]), and California (Linden and Dunn[116]).

Carcinoma in situ, if treated adequately, is cured in 100% of cases, even when it shows extension to glands or microinvasion (Way[213]). The five-year survival for patients with microinvasive carcinoma has been found to be 95.8% (Ng and Reagan[143]).

Objective evidence of the value of screening through cytologic techniques is that recorded by Christopherson et al.[32]

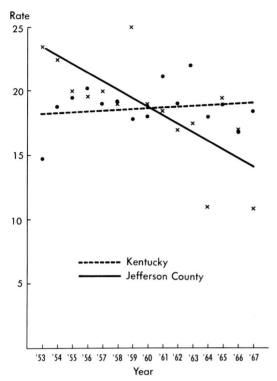

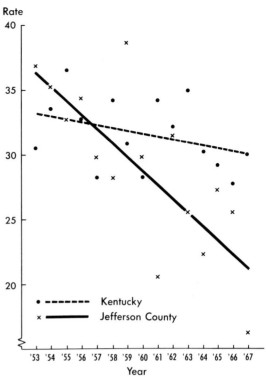

Fig. 612. Mortality rates in cancer of cervix, 1953-1967—Jefferson County versus remainder of Kentucky. (Courtesy Dr. W. M. Christopherson, Louisville, Ky.)

Fig. 613. Total uterine cancer mortality rates, 1953-1967—Jefferson County versus remainder of Kentucky. (Courtesy Dr. W. M. Christopherson, Louisville, Ky.)

Women in Jefferson County in Kentucky were thoroughly screened, but in the remainder of the state there was no attempt at mass screening. The decline of mortality rates for cancer of the cervix and total uterine cancer in a Kentucky community (Christopherson et al.[32]) is shown in Figs. 612 and 613. In California, the mortality rate for carcinoma of the cervix has steadily declined from 10.7 in 1950 to 5.5 in 1968; the reduction in death rate is still more remarkable in women 45 to 64 years of age (Breslow[18a]).

Carcinoma of the cervix treated adequately has the best prognosis of all major forms of cancer. Although an early diagnosis is desirable and offers a greater chance of cure, the curability of even advanced carcinomas of the cervix is remarkable.

Marcial[127a] reported a five-year survival of 59% in 261 patients with carcinoma of the cervix treated with cobalt[60] and radiotherapy at the Puerto Rico Nuclear Center at San Juan, Puerto Rico; the results ob-

tained in the different stages (Table 83) are remarkable when one considers the fact that the patients are, for the most part, indigents.

A five-year survival rate figure is a very satisfactory way to appraise results of treatment of carcinoma of the cervix since recurrences are not frequently seen after five years. But results vary considerably depending on whether there is selection of

Table 83. Results of radiotherapy for carcinoma of cervix (Radiotherapy and Cancer Division, Puerto Rico Nuclear Center)*

Stage	Patients	Well 5 yr†	%
I	41	35	87
II	118	79	66
III	81	37	45
IV	21	3	14
	261	154	59

*From Marcial, V.: Radiation therapy of carcinoma of the uterine cervix (presented at the Tenth International Cancer Congress, Houston, Texas, May, 1970).
†Six patients lost to follow-up.

the material reported. Also, the varying concepts on what constitutes early invasive carcinoma may influence the estimation of results. A series that contains a large proportion of patients with subclinical microscopically invasive carcinomas would naturally yield a high proportion of cures. In Latour's series,[113] the overall result in patients with Stage I lesions was 87.5% but only 73% if the preclinical cases were excluded.

The presence of ureteral abnormalities as shown by pyelography has an adverse effect on prognosis, particularly in patients with advanced disease (Table 84).

It has been suggested that carcinoma of the cervix has a less favorable prognosis in *younger women*, but Laborde[111] found no appreciable difference in the outcome of the different age groups in fifty-seven patients with Stage I carcinoma of the cervix. The *histologic grading* of epidermoid carcinomas of the cervix does not provide a basis for prognosis. It is possible that in a large group the most undifferentiated tumors may be found to have a poorer prognosis than other lesions in the same stage (Gilmour et al.[66]).

Adenocarcinomas have been regarded for a long time as having a less favorable prognosis than the more common epidermoid carcinomas. However, Baclesse and Fernandez-Colmeiro[7] reported on a series of forty patients with adenocarcinomas treated at the Radium Institute of Paris, twelve (30%) of whom remained well after five years. Then they compiled 420 cases of adenocarcinomas of the cervix from the world literature and found that 101 (24%) of the patients were reported well five

years after radiotherapy. Bergsjø[12] reported a five-year survival of 36% in a series of 113 patients treated for adenocarcinoma of the cervix; for the earlier stages, the survival was not so good as in squamous cell carcinomas. Cuccia et al.[42] and Ubiñas and Marcial[208a] reported that the results of radiotherapy were statistically similar in both forms. The response of clear cell mesonephric carcinomas to radiation therapy is at least as good as that of other adenocarcinomas (Fawcett et al.[53]; Hameed[80]).

The most important single factor influencing the prognosis of carcinoma of the cervix is the extent of the disease. The International Classification in four stages offers an excellent basis for prognosis.

Stage I. In their initial stage, carcinomas of the cervix are most curable, yet the best results of radiotherapy or surgery have never been above 90% five-year survival. Way[213] treated eighty-seven patients with Stage I carcinoma by hysterectomy and lymph node dissection, with fifty-one patients (86%) with no lymph node involvement surviving five years but only thirty-six (19%) with metastases surviving five years. In an attempt to improve his own results, Kottmeier[107] performed a radical hysterectomy four weeks after intracavitary radiumtherapy, with only five (17%) of twenty-nine patients with metastatic nodes living five years. It is obvious that in institutions in which surgery is done for the most favorable cases and radiotherapy for the remainder (Regato[170]), the results are not better than in those in which radiotherapy is administered to all (Table 86). Nevertheless, advocates of surgery persist (Lockwood and Stancke[118]).

Table 84. Pyelographic findings before irradiation and five-year results*

		Normal Findings			Hydronephrosis or nonfunctional kidney			
			Symptom free at 5 yr				Symptom free at 5 yr	
Stage	Patients examined	Cases	Cases	%	Cases	%	Cases	%
I	170	154	135	87.7	16	9.4	13	81.3
II A	373	330	231	70.0	43	11.5	27	62.8
II B	424	366	183	50.0	58	13.7	21	36.3
III	354	244	80	32.8	110	26.1	21	19.1
IV	81	40	2	5.0	41	59.1	6	12.2
I-IV	1402	1134	631	55.6%	268	19.1%	32.8%	88

*From Kottmeier, H.-L.: Surgical and radiation treatment of carcinoma of the uterine cervix, Acta Obstet. Gynec. Scand. 43(suppl. 2):1-47, 1964.

Stage II. The results of radiotherapy in moderately advanced carcinomas of the cervix are rather satisfying. In a series of 261 cases treated by radiotherapy alone at the M. D. Anderson Hospital in Houston from 1950 to 1954, 183 patients (70%) remained well after five years. Serious study of statistical data (Wheeler and Hertig[216]) has led to the conclusion that there is no evidence of any superiority of surgery over adequate radiotherapy. The results of institutions favoring surgery for some Stage

Table 85. Results of treatment of carcinoma of cervix in 124 institutions in twenty-six countries (1956-1960)*

Stage	Patients	Well 5 yr	%
I	17,016	12,881	75.7
II	24,553	13,329	54.3
III	19,892	6,261	31.5
IV	3,590	303	8.4
Total	65,051	32,774	50.4

*From Kottmeier, H.-L., editor: Annual report on the results of treatment in carcinoma of the uterus and vagina, vol. 14, Stockholm, 1967, P. A. Norstedt & Söner.

Table 86. Results of treatment of Stage I carcinoma of cervix (1956-1960)*

No. institutions	Treatment	Patients	Well 5 yr	%
Surgery in most favorable cases—93	Surgery	6,815	5,534	81
	Radiotherapy	6,446	4,540	70
	Total	13,261	10,074	75
Radiotherapy alone in all cases—26	Radiotherapy	3,430	2,578	75
All (119) institutions	Surgery or radiotherapy	16,691	12,652	75

*Compiled by Frank Wilson, M.D., from data in Kottmeier, H.-L., editor: Annual report on the results of treatment in carcinoma of the uterus and vagina, vol. 14, Stockholm, 1967, P. A. Norstedt & Söner.

Table 87. Results of treatment of stage II carcinoma of cervix (1956-1960)*

No. institutions	Treatment	Patients	Well 5 yr	%
Surgery in most favorable cases—76	Surgery	4,506	2,800	62
	Radiotherapy	9,564	4,645	48
	Total	14,070	7,445	52
Radiotherapy alone in all cases—43	Radiotherapy	10,152	5,728	56
All (119) institutions	Surgery or radiotherapy	24,222	13,173	54

*Compiled by Frank Wilson, M.D., from data in Kottmeier, H.-L., editor: Annual report on the results of treatment in carcinoma of the uterus and vagina, vol. 14, Stockholm, 1967, P. A. Norstedt & Söner.

Table 88. Results of radiotherapy in Stage III carcinoma of cervix (1956-1960)*

No. institutions	Treatment	Patients	Well 5 yr	%
Radiotherapy sometimes combined with surgery—46	Radiotherapy plus surgery	555	313	56
	Radiotherapy alone	6,039	1,705	28
	Total	6,594	2,018	30
Radiotherapy alone in all cases—73	Radiotherapy	12,938	4,195	32
All (119) institutions	Surgery and/or radiotherapy	19,532	6,213	31

*Compiled by Frank Wilson, M.D., from data in Kottmeier, H.-L., editor: Annual report on the results of treatment in carcinoma of the uterus and vagina, vol. 14, Stockholm, 1967, P. A. Norstedt & Söner.

Table 89. Results of treatment of Stage IV carcinoma of cervix (1956-1960)*

No. institutions	Treatment	Patients	Well 5 yr	%
Radiotherapy sometimes combined with surgery—30	Radiotherapy plus surgery	134	10	7.4
	Radiotherapy alone	789	64	8.1
	Total	923	74	8.0
Radiotherapy alone in all cases—89	Radiotherapy	2,634	228	8.6
All (119) institutions	Surgery and/or radiotherapy	3,557	302	8.4

*Compiled by Frank Wilson, M.D., from data in Kottmeier, H.-L., editor: Annual report on the results of treatment in carcinoma of the uterus and vagina, vol. 14, Stockholm, 1967, P. A. Norstedt & Söner.

Table 90. Cumulative survival rates following pelvic exenteration for postirradiational carcinoma of cervix (1950-1965)*

Interval after operation (yr)	Alive at beginning of interval	Died during interval	Lost or withdrawn during interval	Number exposed to risk of dying	Proportion dying	Proportion surviving	Cumulative % survival rates
0-1	207	45	5	204	0.221	0.779	78
1-2	153	35	10	148	0.236	0.764	60
2-3	109	15	5	106	0.142	0.858	51
3-4	88	12	7	84	0.143	0.857	44
4-5	68	7	3	66	0.106	0.894	39
5-6	59	2	6	56	0.036	0.964	38
6-7	51	1	10	46	0.022	0.978	37
7-8	40	1	8	36	0.028	0.972	36
8-9	31	0	2	30	0.0	1.000	36
9-10	29	0	6	26	0.0	1.000	36
10-11	21	2	6	20	0.100	0.900	32
11-12	15	0	3	13	0.0	1.000	32
12-13	12	0	4	10	0.0	1.000	32
13-14	8	0	5	5	0.0	1.000	32
14-15	3	0	2	2	0.0	1.000	32

Cutler, S. J., and Ederer, F.: Maximum utilization of the life table method in analyzing survival, J. Chronic Dis. 8:699-712, 1958.
*From Kiselow, M., et al.: Results of the radical surgical treatment of advanced pelvic cancer: a fifteen year study, Ann. Surg. 166:428-436, 1967.

II lesions are not so good as those of others administering radiotherapy to all (Table 87).

Stage III. It cannot be sufficiently emphasized *that a Stage III carcinoma of the cervix has a better prognosis than an operable carcinoma of the stomach* (Regato[164]). This fact ought to encourage and promote the attention given to this group of cases. What is usually called a "frozen pelvis" is often a curable Stage III carcinoma of the cervix and should never be considered as hopeless. The results obtained in this group, however, are invariably due to a thorough external irradiation. More than one in every three patients treated in special institutions may recover (Table 88).

Stage IV. A very restricted number of these carcinomas have been permanently sterilized even after tumor had perforated into the bladder or the rectum (Table 89). The results of external and internal treatment for the majority of these Stage IV cases yield only a worthwhile palliation.

• • •

Postoperative recurrences have challenged radiotherapists and unquestionable results have been shown. Friedman and Pearlman[62] treated thirty-eight consecutive patients with postoperative residual or recurrent carcinoma of the cervix, with 42% five-year survivals. Guttman[77] reported on seventy-five such cases, yielding a rather significant survival after radiotherapy. *Postirradiation recurrences* can, in turn, be rescued by surgery if the recurrences are limited (Kiselow et al.[101]) (Table 90). Gary et al.[65] reported on 299 patients with postirradiation recurrence who were operated upon, with only fourteen (4%) surviving. Tarlowska et al.[202] observed 1.5% recurrences after five years among 5671 patients treated at the Institute of Oncologie of Warsaw, or 3.3% of those observed to be well at five years. *Involvement of lymph nodes* hinders the possibilities of surgical success. Ingersoll and Ulfelder[95] reported on thirty-one patients with metastatic lymph nodes, only two of whom survived, whereas fifteen of thirty-nine with negative lymph nodes survived. Between 1950 and 1955, Bricker[19] reported seventy-five patients who underwent pelvic exenteration for persistent carcinoma of the cervix, with nineteen living and well five to ten years later.

In summary, it is clear that pessimism is not justified in the treatment of carcinoma of the cervix and that the time and expense involved in administering an adequate treatment to most of the patients will be amply rewarded by the satisfying results. A progressive improvement of results has been mainly due to the greater proportion of cases that are being diagnosed in earlier stages as well as to a better utilization of radiotherapeutic and surgical skills. Roman and Latour[175] showed an improvement of five-year results from 56% to 88% in the treatment of Stage I carcinoma, from 1943-1947 to 1953-1957, mostly due to earlier diagnosis.

The prognosis of *sarcomas* of the cervix is admittedly very poor (Ober and Edgcomb[150]). However, four patients with sarcoma botryoides were apparently cured by exenteration, and the fifth patient developed a recrudescence following exenteration that responded dramatically to vincristine (Rutledge and Sullivan[186]).

REFERENCES

1 Abou-Daoud, K. T.: Epidemiology of carcinoma of the cervix uteri in Lebanese Christians and Moslems, Cancer **20**:1706-1714, 1967.

2 Aitken-Swan, J., and Baird, D.: Cancer of the uterine cervix in Aberdeenshire; aetiological aspects, Brit. J. Cancer **20**:642-659, 1966.

3 Aldridge, A. H.: Intestinal injuries resulting from irradiation treatment of uterine carcinoma, Amer. J. Obstet. Gynec. **44**:833-857, 1942.

4 Allen, W. M., Sherman, A. I., and Camel, H. M.: Radiogold in the treatment of cancer of the cervix, Radiology **70**:523-527, 1958.

5 Aman-Jean, F.: La vessie au cours de l'évolution du cancer de l'utérus, Bull. Ass. Franc. Cancer **22**:556-590, 1933.

6 Baclesse, F.: Quelques considerations sur la roentgenthérapie employée seule dans le traitement des épithéliomas avancés du col de l'utérus et du vagin, Radiophys. Radiother. **3**:379-412, 1937.

7 Baclesse, F., and Fernandez-Colmeiro, J. M.: Quelques remarques sur le traitement radiothérapique des adénocarcinomes du col uterin, Bull. Ass. Franc. Cancer **30**:118-128, 1942.

8 Badib, A. O., Kurohara, S. S., Webster, J. H., and Pickren, J. W.: Metastasis to organs in carcinoma of the uterine cervix; influence of treatment on incidence and distribution, Cancer **21**:434-439, 1968.

9 Bateman, J. R., Hazen, J. G., Stolinsky, D. C., and Steinfeld, J. L.: Advanced carcinoma of the cervix treated by intra-arterial methotrexate, Amer. J. Obstet. Gynec. **96**:181-187, 1966.

10 Baud, J.: Carcinoma of the cervix (stage I) treated intracavitarily with radium alone. Five, ten and fifteen year results; recurrences after more than five years, J.A.M.A. **138**:1138-1142, 1948.

11 Bausch, R. G., Kaump, D. H., and Alles, R. W.: Observations on the decidual reaction of the cervix during pregnancy, Amer. J. Obstet. Gynec. **58**:777-783, 1949.

12 Bergsjø, P.: Adenocarcinoma cervicis uteri; a clinical study, Acta Obstet. Gynec. Scand. **42**(Fasc. 1):85-92, 1963.

13 Beyer, F. D., Jr.: Topographic study of in situ and microinvasive carcinoma of uterine cervix, Obstet. Gynec. **24**:116-121, 1964.

14 Blomfield, G. W., Cherry, C. P., and Glücksmann, A.: Biological factors influencing the radiotherapeutic results in carcinoma of the cervix, Brit. J. Radiol. **38**:241-254, 1965.

15 Bonney, F.: The results of 500 cases of Wertheim's operation for carcinoma of the cervix, J. Obstet. Gynaec. Brit. Emp. **48**:421-435, 1941.

16 Bosch, A., and Marcial, V. A.: Evaluation of the time interval between external irradiation and intracavitary curietherapy in carcinoma of the uterine cervix; influence on curability, Radiology **88**:563-567, 1967.

17 Boyes, D. A.: Personal communication, 1968.

18 Boyes, D. A., Fidler, H. K., and Lock, D. R.: Significance of in situ carcinoma of the uterine cervix, Brit. Med. J. **1**:203-210, 1962.

18a Breslow, L.: Cytology and the decline in uterine cervix mortality in California (presented at the Tenth International Cancer Congress, Houston, Texas, May, 1970).

19 Bricker, E. M.: Management of recurrent cancer of the cervix, Postgrad. Med. **35**:145-149, 1964.

20 Bricker, E. M., Butcher, H. R., Jr., Lawler,

W. H., Jr., and McAfee, C. A.: Surgical treatment of advanced and recurrent cancer of the pelvic viscera; an evaluation of ten years' experience, Ann. Surg. **152:**388-402, 1960.

21 Bricker, E. M., and Modlin, J.: The role of pelvic evisceration in surgery, Surgery **30:**76-94, 1951.

22 Brites Patricio M., and Baptista, A. M.: Renographic analyses in radiation therapy of carcinoma of the uterus, Acta Radiol. [Ther.] (Stockholm) **7:**97-107, 1968.

23 Brown, W. E., Meschan, I., Kerekes, E., and Sadler, J. M.: Effect of radiation on metastatic pelvic lymph node involvement in carcinoma of the cervix, Amer. J. Obstet. Gynec. **62:**871-889, 1951.

24 Bryans, F. E., Boyes, D. A., and Fidler, H. K.: The influence of a cytological screening program upon the incidence of invasive squamous cell carcinoma of the cervix in British Columbia, Amer. J. Obstet. Gynec. **88:**898-906, 1964.

25 Cantril, S. T.: Radiation therapy in the management of cancer of the uterine cervix, Springfield, Ill., 1950, Charles C Thomas, Publisher.

26 Carlson, V., Delclos, L., and Fletcher, G. H.: Distant metastases in squamous-cell carcinoma of the uterine cervix, Radiology **88:**961-966, 1967.

27 Carter, B., Cuyler, W. K., Kaufmann, L. A., Thomas, W. L., Creadick, R. N., Parker, R. T., Peete, C. H., Jr., and Cherny, W. B.: Clinical problems in Stage 0 (intraepithelial) cancer of the cervix, Amer. J. Obstet. Gynec. **71:**634-652, 1956.

28 Cartier, R.: Comparative colpophotographic and histopathological study of dystrophic and cancerous lesions of the cervix uteri, Gynec. Obstet. (Paris) **63:**451-476, 1964.

29 Caulk, R. M.: Review of ten years experience with transvaginal roentgen therapy, Radiology **52:**26-33, 1949.

30 Chavanne, G., Pellier, D., and Valette, M.: La lymphographie dans les stades I et II du cancer du col utérin; étude de 150 cas operés et verifiés histologiquement, J. Radiol. Electr. **48:**137-156, 1967.

31 Cherry, C. P., Glücksmann, A., Dearing, R., and Way, S.: Observations on lymph node involvement in carcinoma of the cervix, J. Obstet. Gynaec. Brit. Emp. **60:**368-377, 1953.

32 Christopherson, W. M., Mendez, W. M., Ahuja, E. M., Ludin, F. E., Jr., and Parker, J. E.: Cervix cancer control in Louisville, Kentucky, Cancer **26:**29-38, 1970.

33 Christopherson, W. M., and Parker, J. E.: A study of the relative frequency of carcinoma of the cervix in the Negro, Cancer **13:**711-713, 1960.

34 Christopherson, W. M., and Parker, J. E.: A critical study of cervical biopsies including serial sectioning, Cancer **14:**213-216, 1961.

35 Christopherson, W. M., and Parker, J. E.: Relation of cervical cancer to early marriage and childbearing, New Eng. J. Med. **273:**235-239, 1965.

36 Christopherson, W. M., and Parker, J. E.: Control of cervix cancer in women of low income in a community, Cancer **24:**64-69, 1969.

37 Clarke, R. L.: Carcinoma of the uterine cervix, Fifth Annual Clinical Conference on Cancer at the University of Texas, M. D. Anderson Hospital and Tumor Institute, Houston, Texas, 1960, Chicago, 1962, Year Book Publications.

38 Cole, S.: Pelvic cancer in Cincinnati; a 5-year study, Obstet. Gynec. **23:**274-278, 1964.

39 Constable, W. C., and Truskett, I. D.: Relationship of cytological screening facilities and cure rate in cancer of the cervix, Brit. J. Radiol. **40:**691-699, 1967.

40 Coppleson, M.: Colposcopy, cervical carcinoma in situ and the gynaecologist; based on experience with the method in 200 cases of carcinoma in situ, J. Obstet. Gynaec. Brit. Comm. **71:**854-870, 1964.

41 Cross, H. E., Kennel, E. E., and Lilienfeld, A. M.: Cancer of the cervix in an Amish population, Cancer **21:**102-108, 1968.

42 Cuccia, C. A., Bloedorn, F. G., and Onal, M.: Treatment of primary adenocarcinoma of the cervix, Amer. J. Roentgen. **49:**371-375, 1967.

43 Cushing, R. M., Tovell, H. M. M., and Liegner, L. M.: Major urologic complications following radium and x-ray therapy for carcinoma of the cervix, Amer. J. Obstet. Gynec. **101:**750-755, 1968.

44 Cutler, S. J.: Cancer illness among residents in Atlanta, Georgia, 1947, Cancer Morbidity Series no. 1, P.H.S. pub. 13, Washington, D. C., 1950, National Cancer Institute, United States Federal Security Agency, National Institutes of Health.

45 Davies, J. N. P., Knowelden, J., and Wilson, B. A.: Incidence rates of cancer in Kyadondo County, Uganda, 1954-1960, J. Nat. Cancer Inst. **35:**729-757, 1965.

46 Davis, H. J., and Jones, H. W., Jr.: Population screening for cancer of the cervix with irrigation smears, Amer. J. Obstet. Gynec. **96:**605-618, 1966.

47 Dearing, R.: A study of the renal tract in carcinoma of the cervix, J. Obstet. Gynaec. Brit. Emp. **60:**165-174, 1953.

48 Decker, D. G., Aaro, L. A., Hunt, A. B., Johnson, C. E., and Smith, R. A.: Sequential radiation and operation in carcinoma of the uterine cervix, Amer. J. Obstet. Gynec. **92:**35-42, 1965.

49 Díaz-Bazán, N.: Cancer del cuello uterino asociado con prolapso total en El Salvador, revision de la literatura y reporte complementario de 25 casos, Extrait Deuxième Congr. Int. Gynec. Obstet. Montréal (1958) **1:**1-24, 1958.

50 Dulac, G. L., and Rousseau, J.: Les conditions d'apparition et la prevention de la rectite post-radiothérapique au cours des traitements

pour cancer du col utérin, Arch. Mal. Appar. Dig. **52**:5-20, 1963.

51 Dunn, J. E., and Martin, P. L.: Morphogenesis of cervical cancer; findings from San Diego County Cytology Registry, Cancer **20**: 1899-1906, 1967.

52 Erickson, C. C., and others: Population screening for uterine cancer by vaginal cytology; preliminary summary of results of first examination of 108,000 women and second testing of 33,000 women, J.A.M.A. **162**:167-173, 1956.

53 Fawcett, K. J., Dockerty, M. B., and Hunt, A. B.: Mesonephric carcinomas and adenocarcinomas of the cervix in children, J. Pediat. **69**:104-110, 1966.

54 Feste, J. R., Kaufman, R. H., Skogland, H. L., and Topek, N. H.: Management of abnormal cytology late in pregnancy, Amer. J. Obstet. Gynec. **95**:763-768, 1968.

55 Fidler, H. K., Boyes, D. A., and Worth, A. J.: Cervical cancer detection in British Columbia, J. Obstet. Gyneac. Brit. Comm. **75**: 392-404, 1968.

56 Fletcher, G. H.: The planning of external irradiation in pelvic cancer, Amer. J. Roentgen. **64**:95-112, 1950.

57 Fletcher, G. H., Watanavit, T., and Rutledge, F. N.: Whole-pelvis irradiation with 4,000 rads in Stage and Stage II cancers of the uterine cervix, Radiology **86**:436-443, 1966.

58 Fontana-Donatelli, G., and Variati, G.: Amputation and conization of the cervix and their effects on the fertility of the woman; a clinical discussion, Ann. Ostet. Ginec. **88**: 622-630, 1966.

59 Foraker, A. G., and Denham, S. W.: Squamous-cell carcinoma of the uterine cervix; a histochemical review, Amer. J. Obstet. Gynec. **74**:13-24, 1957.

60 Friedell, G. H., and Graham, J. B.: Regional lymph node involvement in small carcinoma of the cervix, Surg. Gynec. Obstet. **108**:513-517, 1959.

61 Friedell, G. H., Hertig, A. T., and Younge, P. A.: Carcinoma in situ of the uterine cervix, Springfield, Ill., 1960, Charles C Thomas, Publisher (extensive bibliography).

62 Friedman, M., and Pearlman, A. W.: Carcinoma of the cervix; radiation salvage of surgical failures, Radiology **84**:801-811, 1965.

63 Gagnon, F.: Contribution to the study of the etiology and prevention of cancer of the cervix of the uterus, Amer. J. Obstet. Gynec. **60**:516-522, 1950.

64 Garcia, M., and Schlosser, J. V.: The treatment of carcinoma of the cervix at Charity Hospital, New Orleans Med. Surg. J. **98**:314-324, 1946.

65 Gary, R. K., Sala, J. M., and Spratt, J. S., Jr.: The detection and treatment of post-irradiationally recidivated cancers of the cervix uteri, Radiology **83**:208-218, 1964.

66 Gilmour, M., Glücksmann, A., and Spear, F. G.: The influence of tumour histology, duration of symptoms and age of patient on the radiocurability of cervix tumours, Brit. J. Radiol. **22**:90-95, 1949.

67 Glücksmann, A.: The influence of histological structure on the radio-sensitivity of tumours: symposium; the influence of systemic factors on the differentiation and radiocurability of cervical cancer, Brit. J. Radiol. **29**:483-487, 1956.

68 Glücksmann, A., and Way, S.: On the choice of treatment of individual carcinomas of the cervix based on the analysis of serial biopsies, J. Obstet. Gynaec. Brit. Emp. **55**:573-582, 1948.

69 Goldman, R. L., and Friedman, N. B.: Blue nevus of the uterine cervix, Cancer **20**:210-214, 1967.

70 Govan, A. D. T., Haines, R. M., Langley, F. A., Taylor, C. W., and Woodcock, A. S.: Changes in the epithelium of the cervix uteri; a study by the panel of pathologists engaged in the survey of carcinoma in situ carried out by the Royal College of Obstetricians and Gynaecologists, J. Obstet. Gynaec. Brit. Comm. **73**:883-896, 1966.

71 Gray, M. J., and Frick, H. C.: Pelvic lymph node dissection following radiotherapy for cancer of the cervix, Amer. J. Obstet. Gynec. **93**:110-114, 1965.

72 Green, G. H.: The significance of cervical carcinoma in situ, Amer. J. Obstet. Gynec. **94**:1009-1022, 1966.

73 Greenberg, S. D., and Kaufman, R. H.: Use of the cryostat in diagnosis with frozen sections of specimens from cervical conization, Amer. J. Clin. Path. **40**:500-507, 1963.

74 Gricouroff, G.: Répartition topographique et délai d'apparition des métastases extrapelviennes dans le cancer de l'utérus, Bull. Ass. Franc. Cancer **30**:90-117, 1942.

75 Gricouroff, G., and Potet, F.: Aspects histologiques des complications rectales de la radiothérapie du cancer du col de l'utérus, Arch. Mal. Appar. Dig. **52**:53-66, 1963.

76 Griffiths, A.: Punch biopsy of the cervix, Amer. J. Obstet. Gynec. **88**:695, 1964.

77 Guttman, R.: Significance of postoperative irradiation in carcinoma of the cervix; a ten-year study, Amer. J. Roentgen. **108**:102-108, 1970.

78 Habibi, A.: Cancer in Iran; a survey of the most common cases, J. Nat. Cancer Inst. **34**: 553-569, 1965.

79 Haenszel, W., and Hillhouse, M.: Uterine-cancer morbidity in New York City and its relation to the pattern of regional variation within the United States, J. Nat. Cancer Inst. **22**:1157-1181, 1959.

80 Hameed, K.: Clear cell carcinoma of the uterine cervix, Amer. J. Obstet. Gynec. **101**: 954-958, 1968.

81 Hammond, E. C., Burns, E. L., Seidman, H., and Percy, C.: Detection of uterine cancer, Cancer **22**:1096-1107, 1968.

82 Hamperl, H., and Kaufmann, C.: The cervix uteri at different ages, Obstet. Gynec. **14**: 621-631, 1959.

83 Hamperl, H., Kaufmann, C., and Ober, K. C.:

Histologische Untersuchungen an der Cervix schwangerer Frauen; die Erosion und das Carcinoma in situ, Arch. Gynaek. **184**:181-280, 1954.

84 Heckel, G. P.: Carcinoma of the cervix in the first year of life, Pediatrics **5**:924-929, 1950.

85 Henriksen, E.: The lymphatic spread of carcinoma of the cervix and of the body of the uterus, Amer. J. Obstet. Gynec. **58**:924-942, 1949.

86 Hertig, A. T., and Younge, P. A.: What is cancer in situ of the cervix? Is it the pre-invasive form of true carcinoma? Amer. J. Obstet. Gynec. **64**:807-815, 1952.

87 Hesselberg, E.: Cancer of the cervix associated with procidentia. S. Afr. Med. J. **37**:589-592, 1963.

88 Heyman, J.: Staging in carcinoma of the uterine cervix; a reply to Dr. del Regato, Amer. J. Roentgen. **70**:840-841, 1953.

89 Higginson, J., and Oettlé, A. G.: Cancer incidence in the Bantu and "Cape Colored" races of South Africa; report of a cancer survey in the Transvaal (1953-55), J. Nat. Cancer Inst. **24**:589-671, 1960.

90 Hittmair, A., and Frick, J.: Veränderungen an den oberen anleitenden Harnwegen bei der Strahlenbehandlung des Zervixkarzinom, Zbl. Gynaek. **89**:1466-1471, 1967.

91 Hochman, A., Ratzkowski, E., and Schreiber, H.: Incidence of carcinoma of cervix in Jewish women in Israel, Brit. J. Cancer **9**:358-364, 1955.

92 Howard, L., Jr., Erickson, C. C., and Stoddard, L. D.: A study of the incidence and histogenesis of endocervical metaplasia and intra-epithelial carcinoma; observations on 400 uteri removed for noncervical disease, Cancer **4**:1210-1223, 1951.

93 Hreshchyshyn, M. M., and Sheehan, F. R.: Collateral lymphatics in patients with gynecological cancer, Amer. J. Obstet. Gynec. **91**:118-121, 1965.

94 Hunt, H. B.: Response of carcinoma of the cervix uteri to fractionated radium and roentgen therapy given concurrently, Amer. J. Roentgen. **64**:446-464, 1950.

95 Ingersoll, F. M., and Ulfelder, H.: Pelvic exenteration for carcinoma of the cervix, New Eng. J. Med. **274**:648-651, 1966.

96 Javert, C. T.: Pathological classification for staging of squamous cancer of the cervix, Cancer **8**:225-294, 1955.

97 Jeffcoate, T. N. A.: Cervical cytology; its value and limitations, Brit. Med. J. **2**:1091-1094, 1966.

98 Jones, E. G., McDonald, I., and Breslow, L.: A study of epidemiologic factors in carcinoma of the uterine cervix, Amer. J. Obstet. Gynec. **76**:1-10, 1958.

99 Kaiser, R. F., Erickson, C. C., Everett, B. E., Jr., Gilliam, A. G., Graves, L. M., Walton, M., and Sprunt, D. H.: Initial effect of community-wide cytologic screening on clinical stage of cervical cancer detected in an entire community; results of Memphis-Shelby County, Tennessee, Study, J. Nat. Cancer Inst. **25**:863-881, 1960.

100 Kennaway, E. L.: The racial and social incidence of cancer of the uterus, Brit. J. Cancer **2**:177-212, 1948.

101 Kiselow, M., Butcher, H. R., Jr., and Bricker, E. M.: Results of the radical surgical treatment of advanced pelvic cancer: a fifteen year study, Ann. Surg. **166**:428-436, 1967.

102 Koch, F.: The population screening for cervical carcinoma in the Borough of Frederiksberg 1962-1963; application of the irrigation smear technique in a mass screening (thesis), Copenhagen, 1966, Ejnar Munksgaard.

103 Kolstad, P.: Carcinoma of the cervix, Stage O; diagnosis and treatment Amer. J. Obstet. Gynec. **96**:1098-1111, 1966.

104 Koss, L. G., and Wolinska, W. H.: Trichomonas vaginalis cervicitis and its relationship to cervical cancer, Cancer **12**:1171-1184, 1959.

105 Kottmeier, H.-L.: Current treatment of carcinoma of the cervix, Amer. J. Obstet. Gynec. **65**:243-251, 1958.

106 Kottmeier, H.-L.: Complications following radiation therapy in carcinoma of the cervix and their treatment, Amer. J. Obstet. Gynec. **88**:854-866, 1964.

107 Kottmeier, H.-L.: editor: Statements of results obtained in 1951 to 1960, inclusive (collated in 1966). Annual report on the results of treatment in carcinoma of the uterus and vagina, vol. 14, Stockholm, 1967, P. A. Norstedt & Söner.

108 Kottmeier, H.-L., and Moberger, G.: Experience with radioactive gold as an additional treatment in the radiotherapy of uterine cancer, Acta Obstet. Gynec. Scand. **34**:1-29, 1955.

109 Krieger, J. S., and McCormack, L. J.: Graded treatment for in situ carcinoma of the uterine cervix, Amer. J. Obstet. Gynec. **101**:171-183, 1968.

110 Kyriakos, M., Kempson, R. L., and Konikov, N. F.: A clinical and pathologic study of endocervical lesions associated with oral contraceptives, Cancer **21**:1345-1356, 1968.

111 Laborde, S.: Les résultats de la radiothérapie des cancers cervico-utérins du premier degré (statistique de l'Institut du Cancer), Bull. Ass. Franc. Cancer **30**:43-51, 1942.

112 Laborde, S., and Kritter, H.: Les metastases et les propagations neoplasiques au niveau du systeme osseux dans le cancer du col utérin, J. Radiol. Electr. **26**:1-3, 1945.

113 Latour, J. P. A.: Results in the management of preclinical carcinoma of the cervix, Amer. J. Obstet. Gynec. **81**:511-520, 1961.

114 Leveuf, J., and Godard, H.: Les lymphatiques de l'utérus, Rev. Chir. (Paris) **61**:219-248, 1923.

115 Levin, M. L., Kress, L. C., and Goldstein, H.: Syphilis and cancer, New York J. Med. **42**:1737-1745, 1942.

116 Linden, G., and Dunn, J. E., Jr.: Earlier diagnosis of cervical cancer; an analysis of

reports to the California Tumor Registry from 1942 to 1963, Calif. Med. **105**:331-336, 1966.

117 Lipin, T., and Davison, C.: Metastases of uterine carcinoma to the central nervous system; a clinicopathologic study, Arch. Neurol. Psychiat. **57**:186-198, 1947.

118 Lockwood, K., and Stancke, B.: Survival rates for uterine cancer of corpus and cervix treated in Denmark 1943-1952, Acta Radiol. [Ther.] (Stockholm) **6**:1-21, 1967.

119 Lombard, H. L., and Potter, E. A.: Epidemiological aspects of cancer of the cervix. II. Hereditary and environmental factors, Cancer **3**:960-968, 1950.

120 Lucas-Championnière, J.: Lymphatiques utérins et lymphangite utérine, Thesis, School of Medicine, University of Paris, 1870.

121 Lundin, F. E., Erickson, C. C., and Sprunt, D. H.: Socioeconomic distribution of cervical cancer, Public Health Monograph no. 73, Washington, D. C., 1964, U. S. Government Printing Office.

122 Macgregor, J. E.: Cervical carcinoma; the beginning of the end? Lancet **2**:1296-1299, 1967.

123 McLennan, M. T., and McLennan, C. E.: Cytologic radiation response in cervical cancer; a critical appraisal, including the effect of supervoltage radiation, Obstet. Gynec. **24**: 161-168, 1964.

124 Mackles, A., Wolfe, S. A., and Neigus, I.: Benign and malignant mesonephric lesions of the cervix, Cancer **11**:292-305, 1958.

125 Magner, J. W., and Bennett, M. J.: Cancer of the cervix uteri; incidence in Ireland, J. Irish Med. Ass. **57**:14-16, 1965.

126 Malinak, R. L., Jeffrey, R. A., Jr., and Dunn, W. J.: The conization-hysterectomy time interval; a clinical and pathological study, Obstet. Gynec. **23**:317-329, 1964.

127 Maliphant, R. G.: The incidence of cancer of the uterine cervix, Brit. Med. J. **1**:978-982, 1949.

127a Marcial, V.: Radiation therapy of carcinoma of the uterine cervix (presented at the Tenth International Cancer Congress, Houston, Texas, May, 1970).

128 Marcial, V. A., Blanco, M. S., and De León, E.: Persistent tumor cells in the vaginal smear during the first year after radiation therapy of carcinoma of the uterine cervix; prognostic significance, Amer. J. Roentgen. **102**:170-175, 1968.

129 Marshall, C. E.: A ten-year cervical-smear screening programme, Lancet **2**:1026-1029, 1968.

130 Masson, J. C.: Sarcoma of the uterus, Amer. J. Obstet. Gynec. **5**:345-357, 1923.

131 Meigs, J. V.: Radical hysterectomy with bilateral pelvic lymph node dissection; a report of 100 patients operated on five or more years ago, Amer. J. Obstet. Gynec. **62**:854-865, 1951.

132 Meigs, J. V.: The results of surgical treatment of cancer of the cervix uteri, Amer. J. Roentgen. **65**:698-708, 1951.

133 Merrill, J. A.: Radiosensitivity studies in treatment of cancer of the cervix, Cancer **19**:143-148, 1966.

134 Mezer, J.: Metaplasia and carcinoma in cervical polyps, Surg. Gynec Obstet. **75**:239-244, 1942.

135 Michaels, J. P.: Study of ureteral blood supply and its bearing on necrosis of the ureter following the Wertheim operation, Surg. Gynec. Obstet. **86**:36-44, 1948.

136 Mitani, Y., Yukinari, S., Jimi, S., and Iwasaki, H.: Carcinomatous infiltration into the uterine body in carcinoma of the uterine cervix, Amer. J. Obstet. Gynec. **89**:984-989, 1964.

137 Moghissi, K. S., and Mack, H. C.: Epidemiology of cervical cancer; study of a prison population, Amer. J. Obstet. Gynec. **100**: 607-614, 1968.

138 Morton, D. G., Lagasse, L. D., Moore, J. G., Jacobs, M., and Amromin, G. D.: Pelvic lymphnodectomy following radiation in cervical carcinoma, Amer. J. Obstet. Gynec. **88**: 932-943, 1964.

139 Moss, W. T., and Brand, W. N.: Therapeutic radiology, ed. 2, St. Louis, 1965, The C. V. Mosby Co.

140 Munnell, E. W., and Bonney, W. A.: Critical points of failure in the therapy of cancer of the cervix, Amer. J. Obstet. Gynec. **81**:521-534, 1961.

141 Mussey, E., and Soule, E. H.: Carcinoma in situ of the cervix, Amer. J. Obstet. Gynec. **77**:957-972, 1959.

142 Navratil, E.: In Meigs, J. V., editor: Surgical treatment of cancer of the cervix, vol. 6, New York, 1954, Grune & Stratton, Inc., pp. 218-247.

143 Ng, A. B. P., and Reagan, J. W.: Microinvasive carcinoma of the uterine cervix, Amer. J. Clin. Path. **52**:511-529, 1969.

144 Nichols, T. M., Boyes, D. A., and Fidler, H. K.: Advantages of routine step serial sectioning of cervical cone biopsies, Amer. J. Clin. Path. **49**:342-346, 1968.

145 Nieburgs, H. E., and Lund, E. R.: Detection of cancer of the cervix uteri, J.A.M.A. **142**: 221-225, 1950.

146 Nielson, I. C., Smith, R. R., McLaren, J. R., and Scarborough, J. E.: Carcinoma of the uterine cervix; a study of 864 patients, Cancer **20**:86-92, 1967.

147 Novak, E.: What constitutes an adequate cancer detection examination of the cervix? Amer. J. Obstet. Gynec. **58**:851-864, 1949.

148 Novak, E. R., and Galvin, G. A.: Mistakes in interpretations of intraepithelial carcinoma, Amer. J. Obstet. Gynec. **62**:1079-1085, 1951.

149 Nyberg, R., Törnberg, B., and Westin, B.: Colposcopy and Schiller's iodine test as an aid in the diagnosis of malignant and premalignant lesions of the cervix uteri, Acta Obstet. Gynec. Scand. **39**:540-556, 1960.

150 Ober, W. B., and Edgcomb, J. H.: Sarcoma botryoides in the female, Cancer **7**:75-91, 1954.

151 Ober, W. B., and Reiner, L.: Cancer of the cervix in Jewish women, New Eng. J. Med. **251**:555-559, 1954.

152 Östberg, H., and Darcis, L.: Study on sensitization response on 200 patients with carcinoma of the cervix treated at the Radiumhemmet by the current Stockholm technique, Acta Obstet. Gynec. Scand. 35:25-34, 1956.

153 Oettlé, A. G.: Cancer in Africa, especially in regions south of the Sahara, J. Nat. Cancer Inst. 33:383-439, 1964.

154 Papanicolaou, G. N.: A general survey of the vaginal smear and its use in research and diagnosis, Amer. J. Obstet Gynec. 51: 316-324, 1946.

155 Parker, R. G., and Friedman, R. F.: A critical evaluation of the roentgenologic examination of patients with carcinoma of the cervix, Amer. J. Roentgen. 96:100-107, 1966.

156 Pearson, B., and Garcia, M.: Intestinal obstruction as a phase of carcinoma of the cervix, Surgery 11:636-643, 1942.

157 Pederson, B. L., and Jeffries, F. W.: Cervical carcinoma in situ; a study of 144 patients, Obstet. Gynec. 26:725-730, 1965.

158 Peiser, E.: Anatomische und klinische Untersuchungen über den Lymphapparat der Uterus mit besonderer Beruchsichtigung der Totalexstirpation bei Carcinoma uteri, Z. Geburtsh. Gynaek. 39:259-325, 1898.

159 Perez-Mesa, C., and Spjut, H. J.: Persistent postirradiation carcinoma of cervix uteri, Arch. Path. (Chicago) 75:462-474, 1963.

159a Petersen, O.: Precancerous changes of cervical epithelium in relation to manifest cervical carcinoma; clinical and histological aspects, Acta Radiol. (Stockholm) (suppl. 127), pp. 1-168, 1955.

159b Petersen, O.: Spontaneous course of cervical precancerous conditions, Amer. J. Obstet. Gynec. 72:1063-1071, 1956.

160 Piquand, G.: Le sarcome de l'utérus, Rev. Gynec. Chir. Abd. 9:387-446, 1905.

161 Pitts, H. C., and Waterman, G. W.: Further report on the radium treatment of carcinoma of the cervix uteri, Amer. J. Roentgen. 43: 567-576, 1940.

162 Prates, M. D., and Torres, F. O.: A cancer survey in Lourenco Marques, Portuguese East Africa, J. Nat. Cancer Inst. 35:729-757, 1965.

163 Przybora, L. A., and Plutowa, A.: Histological topography of carcinoma in situ of the cervix uteri, Cancer 12:263-277, 1959.

164 del Regato, J. A.: The treatment of carcinoma of the cervix, Radiology 46:579-582, 1946.

165 del Regato, J. A.: Radioterapia de cancer del cuello uterino; Resultados de la roentgenoterapia transvaginal, Prensa Med. Argent. 36:2747-2755, 1949.

166 del Regato, J. A.: La roentgenthérapie transvaginale dans le traitement du cancer du col de l'utérus, Acta Un. Int. Cancr. 8:44-50, 1952.

167 del Regato, J. A.: The role of roentgen therapy in the treatment of cancer of the cervix uteri, Amer. J. Roentgen. 68:63-66, 1952.

168 del Regato, J. A.: The international classification of carcinoma of the uterine cervix, Amer. J. Roentgen. 69:652-653, 1953.

169 del Regato, J. A.: Integral roentgentherapy, Amer. J. Roentgen. 71:676-680, 1954.

170 del Regato, J. A.: Cancer of the cervix; radiation therapy, J.A.M.A. 193:15, 1965.

171 del Regato, J. A., and Cox, J. D.: Transvaginal roentgentherapy in the conservative management of carcinoma in situ of the uterine cervix, Radiology 84:1090-1095, 1965.

172 Regaud, C., Gricouroff, G., and Villela, E.: Sur l'histogenése et la classification des épithéliomas cervic-utérins: données nouvelles et rectifications, Bull. Ass. Franc. Cancer 22:668-677, 1933.

173 Roberts, T. W., and Linkins, T.: Differentiation between intramucosal and invasive carcinoma of the cervix smear; is it reliable? Acta Cytol. (Balt.) 8:280-283, 1964.

174 Røjel, J.: The interrelation between uterine cancer and syphilis, Acta Path. Microbiol. Scand. (suppl. 97), pp. 1-82, 1953.

175 Roman, T. N., and Latour, J. P. A.: The effect of early diagnosis on survival statistics in carcinoma of the uterine cervix, Amer. J. Obstet. Gynec. 97:739-749, 1967.

176 Rosh, R., and Strax, P.: Intravenous pyelography as an aid in classification of carcinoma of the cervix, Radiology 59:107-110, 1952.

177 Rotkin, I. D.: Further studies in cervical cancer inheritance, Cancer 19:1251-1268, 1966.

178 Rotkin, I. D.: Adolescent coitus and cervical cancer; associates of related events with increased risk, Cancer Res. 27:603-617, 1967.

179 Rotkin, I. D.: Epidemiology of cancer of the cervix. III. Sexual characteristics of a cervical cancer population, Amer. J. Public Health 57: 815-829, 1967.

180 Rouvière, H.: Anatomie des lymphatiques des l'homme, Paris, 1932, Masson et Cie.

181 Rubin, P., and Prabhasawat, D.: Characteristic bone lesions in postirradiated carcinoma of the cervix; metastases versus osteonecrosis, Radiology 76:703-717, 1961.

182 Ruch, R. M., Blake, C., Abou, A., Lado, M., and Ruch, W. A.: The changing incidence of cervical carcinoma, Amer. J. Obstet. Gynec. 89:727-731, 1964.

183 Rutledge, F. N., and Fletcher, G. H.: Transperitoneal pelvic lymphadenectomy following supervoltage irradiation for squamous-cell carcinoma of the cervix, Amer. J. Obstet. Gynec. 76:321-334, 1958.

184 Rutledge, F. N., Fletcher, G. H., and MacDonald, E. J.: Pelvic lymphadenectomy as an adjunct to radiation therapy in treatment for cancer of the cervix, Amer. J. Roentgen. 93: 607-614, 1965.

185 Rutledge, F. N., Gutierrez, A. G., and Fletcher, G. H.: Management of stage I and II adenocarcinomas of the uterine cervix on intact uterus, Amer. J. Roentgen. 102:161-164, 1968.

186 Rutledge, F., and Sullivan, M. P.: Sarcoma botryoides, Ann. N. Y. Acad. Sci. 142:694-708, 1967.

187 Sadugor, M. G., and Palmer, J. P.: Age, incidence, and distribution of 4,652 cases of

carcinoma of the cervix, Amer. J. Obstet. Gynec. **56**:680-686, 1948.

188 Skinner, M. E. G.: Personal communication, Bulawayo, Rhodesia, June, 1970.

189 Sukuraba, H.: Diagnosis of cervical cancer with special reference to the value of colposcopy, Hirosaki Med. J. **19**:374-387, 1967.

190 Schonberg, L. A., Carlin, F., Irwin, H. R., Juibel, F. J., and Maas, H. E.: Cancer of the cervix in a Mexican population, J.A.M.A. **191**:84-86, 1965.

191 Silbar, E. L., and Woodruff, J. D.: Evaluation of biopsy, cone and hysterectomy sequence in intraepithelial carcinoma of the cervix, Obstet. Gynec. **27**:89-97, 1966.

192 Smith, J. P., Rutledge, F., Burns, B. C., Jr., and Soffar, S.: Systemic chemotherapy for carcinoma of the cervix, Amer. J. Obstet. Gynec. **97**:800-807, 1967.

193 Smith, R. R., Ketchum, A. S., and Thomas, L. B.: Carcinoma of the uterine cervix, Cancer **16**:1105-1112, 1963.

194 Sneeden, V. D.: Mesonephric lesions of the cervix; a practical means of demonstration and a suggestion of incidence, Cancer **11**:334-336, 1958.

195 Sörensen, H. M., Petersen, O., Nielsen, J., Bang, F., and Koch, F.: The spontaneous course of praemalignant lesions on the vaginal portion of the uterus, Acta Obstet. Gynec. Scand. **43**(suppl. 7):103-104, 1964.

196 Solidoro, A. S., Esteves, L., Castellano, C., Valdivia, E., and Barriga, O.: Chemotherapy of advanced cancer of the cervix, Amer. J. Obstet. Gynec. **94**:208-213, 1966.

197 Speert, H.: Cervical cancer in young girls, Amer. J. Obstet. Gynec. **54**:982-986, 1947.

198 Spjut, J. H., Ruch, W. A., Jr., Martin, P. A., and Hobbs, J. E.: Exfoliative cytology during pregnancy for detection of carcinoma of the cervix, Obstet. Gynec. **15**:19-27, 1960.

199 Stander, R. W., Rhamy, R. K., Henderson, W. P., Lansford, K. G., and Pearcy, M.: The intravenous pyelogram and carcinoma of the cervix, Obstet. Gynec. **17**:26-29, 1961.

200 Stern, E., and Dixon, W. J.: Cancer of the cervix—a biometric approach to etiology, Cancer **14**:153-160, 1961.

201 Stocking, B. W.: Carcinoma of the cervix uteri in identical twins, Cancer **3**:969-971, 1950.

202 Tarlowska, L., Jentys, W., and Jablonska, M.: Récidives tardives du cancer du col utérin traité par irradiation, J. Radiol. Electr. **49**:807-812, 1968.

203 Taylor, R. S., Carroll, B. E., and Lloyd, J. W.: Mortality among women in 3 Catholic religious orders with special references to cancer, Cancer **12**:1207-1223, 1959.

204 TeLinde, R. W., Galvin, G. A., and Jones, H. W., Jr.: Therapy of carcinoma in situ, Amer. J. Obstet. Gynec. **74**:792-803, 1957.

205 Terris, M., and Oalmann, M. C.: Carcinoma of the cervix, J.A.M.A. **174**:1847-1851, 1960.

206 Terris, M., Wilson, F., Smith, H., Sprung, E., and Nelson, J. H., Jr.: Epidemiology of cancer of the cervix. V. The relationship of coitus to carcinoma of the cervix, Amer. J. Public Health **57**:840-847, 1967.

207 Testut, L.: Traité d'anatomic humaine, ed. 8, vol. 5, Paris, 1931, Gaston Doin.

208 Törnberg, B., Westin, B., and Norlander, A.: Fluorescence microscopy and acridin-orange staining in the cytological diagnosis of atypical epithelial changes in cervical epithelium, Acta Obstet. Gynec. Scand. **39**:517-527, 1960.

208a Ubiñas, J., and Marcial, V.: Adenocarcinoma of the cervix: a review of cases; Dr. I. Gonzalez-Martinez Oncologic Hospital, J. Amer. Med. Women Ass. **21**:571-574, 1966.

209 Ulfelder, H., and Meigs, J. V.: The surgery of advanced pelvic cancer in women, New Eng. J. Med. **246**:243-247, 1952.

210 Van Herik, M.: Fever as a complication of radiation therapy for carcinoma of the cervix, Amer. J. Roentgen. **43**:104-109, 1965.

211 Vuksanovic, M., Viamonte, M., and Martin, J. E.: The place of lymphangio-adenography in the diagnosis and during the treatment of malignant diseases, Amer. J. Roentgen. **96**:205-221, 1966.

212 Walter, L., Harrison, C. V., Glucksmann, A., and Cherry, C. P.: Assessment of response of cervical cancers to irradiation by routine histological methods, Brit. Med. J. **5399**:1673-1675, 1964.

213 Way, S.: Microinvasive carcinoma of the cervix, Acta Cytol. (Balt.) **8**:14-15, 1964.

214 Weiner, I., Burke, L., and Goldberger, M. A.: Carcinoma of the cervix in Jewish women, Amer. J. Obstet. Gynec. **61**:418-422, 1951.

215 Wertheim, E.: Zur Frage der Radicaloperation beim Uteruskrebs, Arch. Gynaek. **61**:627-668, 1900.

216 Wheeler, J. D., and Hertig, A. T.: The pathologic anatomy of carcinoma of the uterus. I. Squamous carcinoma of the cervix, Amer. J. Clin. Path. **25**:345-373, 1955.

217 Wieczorkiewicz, A., Hliniakowa, I., and Vorbrodtowa, J.: Complications following irradiation of patients with uterine cervix cancer; the influence of the general health condition before the treatment on the survival time, Pol. Med. J. **1**:368-376, 1962.

218 Wynder, E. L.: Environmental factors in cervical cancer, Brit. Med. J. **1**:743-747, 1955.

219 Younge, P. A., Hertig, A. T., and Armstrong, D.: A study of 135 cases of carcinoma in situ of the cervix at the Free Hospital for Women, Amer. J. Obstet. Gynec. **58**:867-895, 1949.

Cervical stump

The cervical stump is that portion of the cervix left after a supravaginal hysterectomy has been performed. The uterus is usually amputated at the isthmus, 1.5 cm to 2 cm above the free surface of the cervix. The cervical canal is obliterated to a maximum depth of 1.5 cm to 2 cm, but the lymphatic drainage of the remaining cervix is practically untouched.

Carcinoma may develop in the cervical stump twenty-five years or more after a subtotal hysterectomy. The actual incidence, however, is not known. Many of the cases reported in the literature as carcinoma of the cervical stump developed shortly after hysterectomy and were in all probability carcinomas of the cervix or the endocervix that were not suspected at the time of operation. The occurrence of true carcinoma of the cervical stump has decreased and is likely to continue decreasing since the practice of subtotal hysterectomies has declined.

If subtotal hysterectomies are performed in patients with vaginal bleeding without a previous dilatation and curettage for diagnostic purposes, a carcinoma of the endocervix may be severed, and the subsequent pathologic examination will reveal the error. In other patients, the entire tumor may be left behind and the diagnosis not established for some time. Some of these tumors, particularly the adenocarcinomas of the endocervix, may continue to develop so slowly that further treatment is not sought for two to three years. Such tumors do not constitute true carcinomas of the cervical stump. Carcinoma may, of course, develop on the remaining cervix at any time after the operation, but it is better for statistical purposes not to consider as carcinomas of the cervical stump those lesions presenting symptoms within three years. A uterine myoma present at the time of operation does not eliminate the possibility of a coexisting but overlooked carcinoma of the cervix.

Some authors report that, as a rule, the diagnosis of carcinoma of the cervical stump is made later than the diagnosis of carcinoma of the cervix in general. Cantril and Buschke,[3] however, found a large proportion of early cases and attributed this finding to the fact that patients presenting vaginal bleeding after a subtotal hysterectomy are more often alarmed than those with no previous operation. In a series of seventy-three cases of carcinoma of the cervical stump seen at the Radiumhemmet in Stockholm, Lachmann[5] found three-fourths in Stages I and II.

Treatment

It is in the practicability and the results of treatment that carcinoma of the cervical stump differs most from carcinoma of the cervix. An important step in the treatment of carcinomas of the cervix is intracavitary irradiation by the introduction of a tandem in the cervical canal. This procedure is practically impossible in patients with carcinoma of the cervical stump because of the shortness of the canal. The result is a diminution of the total dosage and a consequent greater possibility of local recurrence.

Transvaginal roentgentherapy as a complement to external irradiation is probably the best treatment for carcinomas of the cervical stump. Its use may become more widespread after its superiority is proved by statistics of results. $Cesium^{137}$ is used by Vaeth et al.[8] in the treatment of carcinoma of the cervical stump. They feel that this is preferable to low voltage roentgentherapy because of the better quality of its radiations and the improved depth dose.

Prognosis

The prognosis of carcinoma of the cervical stump seems to be the same, depending on extent of the lesion, as that of carcinoma of the cervix in general. Cantril[2] reported on a series of ten patients treated by roentgentherapy and radiumtherapy at the Tumor Institute of Seattle, with eight living after five years. Baud[1] reported fifty-one of 124 patients living and well (41%) five or more years after radiotherapy. Holmes[4] reported forty-one five-year survivals in 107 patients. The best results were obtained with intracavitary radiumtherapy and external radiotherapy. In a series of fifty-nine patients with infiltrating carcinoma treated by external and transvaginal roentgentherapy by Sala and Diaz de Leon,[7] the cumulative five-year survival was 38%. Similar good results have been obtained by others (Nielsen[6]).

REFERENCES

1 Baud, J.: Les resultats de la radiothérapie (curiethérapie et roentgenthérapie) de 124 cas d'épithéliomas sur col restant traités dans les services de la Fondation Curie, de 1919 à 1944 inclus, Bull. Ass. Franc. Cancer 39:100-104, 1952.
2 Cantril, S. T.: Radiation therapy in the manage-

ment of cancer of the uterine cervix, Springfield, Ill., 1950, Charles C Thomas, Publisher.

3 Cantril, S. T., and Buschke, F.: Carcinoma of the cervical stump, West. J. Surg. **50:**454-457, 1942.

4 Holmes, K. S.: Carcinoma of the cervical stump, Brit. J. Radiol. **34:**581-586, 1961.

5 Lachmann, A.: Cancer of the cervical stump, Acta Obstet. Gynec. Scand. **30:**169-185, 1950.

6 Nielsen, K.: Carcinoma of the cervix following supracervical hysterectomy, Acta Radiol. (Stockholm) **37:**335-340, 1952.

7 Sala, J. M., and Diaz, de Leon, A.: Treatment of carcinoma of the cervical stump, Radiology **81:**300-306, 1963.

8 Vaeth, J. M., Nussbaum, N., and Meurk, M. L.: Transvaginal cesium 137 therapy, Amer. J. Roentgen. **99:**376-378, 1967.

Cervix and pregnancy

Carcinoma of the cervix is an infrequent complication of pregnancy (Fig. 614). It is more often found when reproductivity is over, and pregnancy seldom occurs in a woman who already has carcinoma of the cervix. The occurrence of this association has been variously estimated as 1 in 1000 to 1 in 20,000 pregnancies. The average age of a pregnant patient with carcinoma of the cervix is about 31 years, or fifteen years younger than nonpregnant women with cervical cancer (Williams and Brack[30]). In a review of 4652 cases of carcinoma of the cervix at the Roswell Park Memorial Institute in a period of thirty years, 124 patients (2.6%) were pregnant or had been pregnant within the year preceeding admission (Sadugor et al.[25]).

During pregnancy, the cervix is subjected to an increased blood circulation with hypertrophy of the muscle and connective tissue. Moreover, the columnar epithelium of the endocervix is replaced by cuboidal cells, and there is marked subepithelial proliferation extending deep into the connective tissue. These histologic changes, no matter how impressive, do not necessarily lead to carcinoma, but carcinoma that develops on the cervix of a pregnant uterus is reputed to be able to develop much faster than in the absence of pregnancy. A few authors believe that carcinoma develops faster due to hormonal stimulation and have reported an arrest in the development of the tumor with the

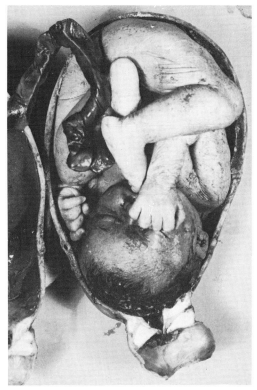

Fig. 614. Carcinoma of cervix and full-term pregnancy. (Courtesy Dr. W. N. Thornton, Charlottesville, Va.)

end of gestation, but this is not corroborated by the majority (Richman and Goodfriend[23]). The rapid development of carcinoma during pregnancy could be explained on the basis of increased blood supply and of added young connective tissue on which the tumor develops. This, however, is purely theoretic.

Routine cytologic examinations of pregnant women are advisable (Boutselis and Ullery[5]). Judicious biopsies may also be taken, with Lugol's solution used to pinpoint the areas to be biopsied. Colposcopy and colpophotography may be used.

When carcinoma of the cervix develops in the early stages of pregnancy or when pregnancy has occurred in spite of its presence, the chances of an early spontaneous abortion due to infection are great. Vaginal bleeding may persist and become alarming, but in the majority of instances it is rather mild. Lumbar pain spreading to the hip and thigh may be present after the tumor has invaded the parametrium.

Repeated or prolonged bleeding during gestation often leads to an early diagnosis of carcinoma of the cervix. In general, in order for impregnation to occur in the presence of a carcinoma of the cervix, the tumor must not be very advanced, and if impregnation has preceded the tumor, then it has not been present for long when it is discovered. The symptomatology is usually and unfortunately attributed to other more common complications of pregnancy. As a rule, bleeding is taken for a symptom of abortion, and the conservative management of threatened abortion is usually given. If inspection and palpation of the cervix reveal an area of ulceration and induration, the greatest care should be exercised to obtain a biopsy. In the early stages of pregnancy, a lacerated, everted cervix with an irregular easily bleeding center may be taken for a carcinoma. The decidual reaction of the endocervical epithelium could also be mistaken microscopically for early carcinomatous changes. Nonspecific proliferative lesions of the cervix can also be mistaken for carcinoma, but the biopsy will easily solve the problem of diagnosis. When the patient is first seen toward the end of pregnancy, a large, soft, exophytic carcinoma may be mistaken for a spongy placenta previa, an error possibly fatal to the patient. A small specimen may be removed from the cervix for biopsy without fear of complications (Hirst[13]). Various benign proliferative lesions may also be observed (Fluhmann[8]).

Hydatidiform moles and *choriocarcinoma* may occur during pregnancy. Choriocarcinoma is relatively rare in the United States, but its incidence is disproportionately high in the Philippines (Acosta-Sison[1]), Indonesia (Tjokronegoro[28]), and China (King[15]). In China, King[15] reported one hydatidiform mole in every 530 pregnancies and one choriocarcinoma in every 3708 pregnancies. Yuan-Ying et al.[31] believe that pregnancies in rapid succession and multiparity are causative factors. The hydatid mole is composed of cysts that are a product of cystic degeneration of the stroma of the villae. The cysts that are spontaneously eliminated have a characteristic appearance. Destructive hydatid moles (chorioadenoma destruens) may invade beyond the uterine wall and cause bleeding into the peritoneal cavity (Acosta-Sison[1]). Hysterotomy is indicated in such cases. Hydatidiform moles may give rise to choriocarcinomas. About half of all choriocarcinomas arise from moles, one-fourth after full-term pregnancies and one-fourth after abortions (Novak[19]). Thus, this tumor does not arise from the host but from the products of conception.

The differential diagnosis between mole and choriocarcinoma may not be difficult, but in a small proportion of cases a decision may require considerable judgment. In such instances, a conservative attitude is indicated. The diagnosis of choriocarcinoma may be difficult to establish due to spontaneous regression in the uterus and, at times, in its metastatic sites. In twenty-eight patients who came to autopsy, no lesion was found within the uterus in nine patients (Hou and Pang[14]). Thus, in the clinical investigation of suspected cases, a curettement may be negative because of complete regression or because the lesion is deep in the myometrium (Logan and Motyloff[16]). A rising titer of chorionic gonadotropin one month after evacuation of a hydatid mole is a significant finding. Equally, a return of positive reaction is also significant but may be due to the presence of luteal cysts or to a normal pregnancy. Repeated hormonal studies and histopathologic examinations may be necessary to establish the diagnosis (Hertig and Sheldon[11]). Reed et al.[22] reported one such case with resection of the pulmonary metastases. Yuan-Ying et al.[31] reported spontaneous regression and disappearance of pulmonary metastases in patients with malignant moles but not in those with choriocarcinomas. Radiotherapy has caused the disappearance of pulmonary metastases.

Effective drugs have transformed the outlook for patients with gestational choriocarcinoma (Fig. 615). Ross et al.[24] reported that remission occurred in about 75% of patients treated at the National Institute of Health following treatment with methotrexate and actinomycin D. They emphasize the importance of early diagnosis with prompt institution of therapy, for there is a direct correlation between delay in treatment and survival. It is important to monitor the effects of treatment with

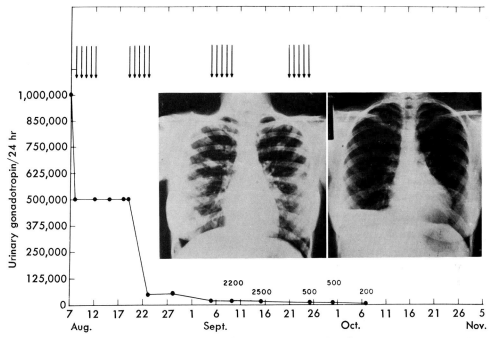

Fig. 615. Graphic representation of gonadotropin excretion and pulmonary metastases in 18-year-old patient with choriocarcinoma treated with methotrexate. Patient remained without evidence of disease for somewhat over three years. (From Hertz, R., et al.: Chemotherapy of choriocarcinoma and related trophoblastic tumors in women, J.A.M.A. **168**:845-854, 1958; follow-up information from Dr. R. Hertz in March, 1961.)

effective and sequential quantitative determination of chorionic gonadotropin production (Hammond et al.[10]). Surgery is not indicated in chorioadenoma destruens or choriocarcinoma unless there is rupture of the uterus or death is threatened because of hemorrhage. Notably, methotrexate is not effective in choriocarcinoma of the male.

Treatment

When the tumor is not discovered and delivery *per vias naturales* is allowed to occur, deep lacerations and fatal hemorrhage may follow. However, uncomplicated delivery has occurred in the presence of small carcinomas. In some instances, patients have died undelivered because of obstruction by the tumor.

If *carcinoma in situ* is diagnosed during the first trimester of pregnancy, conization may cause abortion in about 40% of cases. It is preferable to wait until the pregnancy has reached the thirty-eighth or thirty-ninth week, when conization can be done with little risk. A histologic diagnosis of

carcinoma in situ during pregnancy need not cause precipitous action, for treatment may await delivery without detriment (Feste et al.[7]). There is no evidence that delivery through a cervix with carcinoma in situ is deleterious (Mikuta et al.[17]). The one excuse to do a conization during pregnancy is the possibility or the suspicion of infiltrating carcinoma (Moore et al.[18]). Fontana-Donatelli and Variati[9] reported on conization or cervical amputation in seventy-four patients with eighteen subsequent pregnancies. If the specimen shows infiltrating carcinoma, the course of treatment should be as presented below (Bosch and Marcial[4]; Prem et al.[21]).

Treatment of carcinoma of the cervix during gestation may imply dramatic decisions. Two important factors are involved: the life of the infant and the risk incurred by the usually young mother. In addition, the stage of advancement of the tumor and the stage of development of the pregnancy must both be considered.

First half of gestation. It is generally accepted that during the first four or five months of pregnancy, the fetus should be sacrificed in the interest of the mother. When this decision is reached, treatment should be started by external pelvic roentgentherapy (Fig. 616), just as for carcinoma of the cervix in the nonpregnant uterus. After a period of four to six weeks, abortion occurs in the majority of patients. After the abortion, treatment should be continued in the usual manner. In the early lesions that are commonly associated with early pregnancies, a total hysterectomy may be equally successful. It has the advantage of being expeditive.

The application of small amounts of radium may not cause an abortion but does not have sufficient effect on the tumor to cure it. The only alternative left under these circumstances is absolute abstention of therapy in order to allow development of the fetus and delivery by cesarean section. This procedure, which is directed to protect the life of the infant at the risk of the mother, often results in the loss of both.

Second half of gestation. During the last half of pregnancy, it is generally accepted that an effort can be made to preserve the life of the infant without endangering the

life of the mother or without considerably reducing her chances of being cured.

The procedure generally consists of a preliminary intravaginal application of radium. At this stage, the possible damage to the child is considerably less than in the early stages because the relative distance of the fetus from the cervix is much greater (Fig. 617). If the diagnosis of carcinoma is made during the fifth or sixth month of gestation, it may be best to wait a month or six weeks before the radium is applied. Following the application of radium, a cesarean section should be done as soon as the infant is viable. After cesarean section, treatment should be continued by intra-uterine curietherapy. Another procedure to be used in the presence of early lesions consists of applying radium while awaiting the viability of the infant and then performing a cesarean section followed by hysterectomy (Porro section). Berkeley[3] reported a case so treated. The infant was born with bald patches on her head which later were covered by hair,

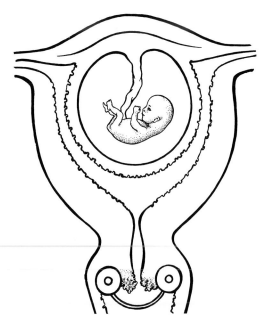

Fig. 616. Intravaginal curietherapy for carcinoma of cervix in early pregnancy. Small fetus is inevitably close to cervix so that most of it is heavily and dangerously irradiated.

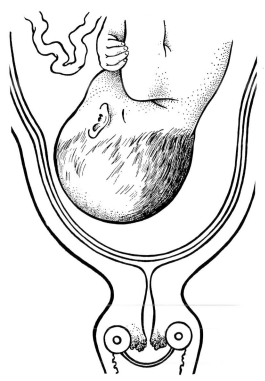

Fig. 617. Intravaginal application of radium in late pregnancy. Only presenting part of fetus is irradiated, and permanent damage is not necessarily implied by therapy.

and she grew to be an outstanding athlete. If the tumor is advanced, the intravaginal application of radium without previous external pelvic roentgentherapy is of little value. Consequently, it may be preferable to do a cesarean operation first (as soon as the infant is viable) and then proceed with the regular course of treatment. Hysterectomies are accompanied by a greater operative mortality when done on these patients.

Term of gestation. Many carcinomas of the cervix are diagnosed at the time pregnancy has reached its full development. If the carcinoma is a very early one, delivery may be chanced per vias naturales with the use of forceps as a protective measure against possible lacerations. If, however, the lesion does not warrant this risk, a cesarean section should be done and the carcinoma treated later by the regular radiotherapeutic methods.

During labor. Carcinoma of the cervix discovered during the first stage of labor affords little opportunity for deliberation. If the tumor does not appear to allow complete dilatation of the cervix and a cesarean section is still possible, it should be performed immediately. A Porro section is preferable (Danforth[6]). If the cervix is already considerably dilated, the use of forceps is indicated to avoid lacerations as much as possible, but the consequences are usually grave. If the patient survives delivery, external roentgentherapy should be administered at the earliest possible time and later complemented by internal treatments.

During puerperium. Carcinoma of the cervix diagnosed following delivery requires no special technique of treatment and should be managed like all other carcinomas of the cervix.

Prognosis

In 1907, Sarwey[26] reported a mortality of 53% in pregnant patients with carcinoma of the cervix who were allowed to develop to term and be delivered per vias naturales, 8% of whom died undelivered. Today, the prognosis for the mother is much better than it used to be because the mortality rate has been reduced and the radiotherapeutic results improved.

The prognosis for the fetus improves with the duration of pregnancy at the time of treatment. In the early stages, the fetus must be lost, but the outlook is better as the fetus reaches viability and there is the possibility of a successful cesarean section. If the tumor is advanced when the cesarean section is done, the infant mortality is, however, high. Conversely, the prognosis for the mother is best in the early stages of pregnancy and decreases toward term. Obviously, the prognosis of these patients also depends on the stage of development of the tumor, which, in the majority of cases, falls within the definition of a Stage I or Stage II. Truelsen[29] reported that nine of sixteen patients treated in the first three months of pregnancy were well. Patients treated in this period yielded the best results. Further, he reported that the condition was controlled in four of sixteen patients treated in the fourth to sixth month and in only one of seven patients treated later than the seventh month of pregnancy.

Large statistics of five-year results are not available, for the reports of these cases are usually concerned with the technique of management rather than with the long-term results. Of twenty-four patients with invasive carcinoma of the cervix during pregnancy, eighteen were living and well more than five years (Williams and Brack[30]). Treatment of forty-eight patients reported by Sadugor et al.[25] yielded eighteen (37%) five-year survivals. The main obstacle is the delay in diagnosis and in the institution of early treatment (Baud[2]).

REFERENCES

1 Acosta-Sison, H.: Changing attitudes in the management of hydatiform mole; a report on 196 patients admitted to the Philippine General Hospital from April 10, 1959, to March 27, 1963, Amer. J. Obstet. Gynec. **88**:634-636, 1964.

2 Baud, J., and Blanchet, F.: Évolution clinique de 44 cas d'épithéliomas du col utérin au cours de la gestation, traités, par radiothérapie à la Fondation Curie de 1929 à 1950, Bull. Ass. Franc. Cancer **39**:48-62, 1952.

3 Berkeley, C.: Carcinoma of the cervix uteri in pregnancy and labor. III. Wertheim's operation at term, following the classical caesarean section preceded by radium treatment during pregnancy, J. Obstet. Gynaec. Brit. Emp. **41**:402-404, 1934.

4 Bosch, A., and Marcial, V. A.: Carcinoma of

the uterine cervix associated with pregnancy, Amer. J. Roentgen. 96:92-99, 1966.

5 Boutselis, J. G., and Ullery, J. C.: Intraepithelial carcinoma of the cervix in pregnancy, Amer. J. Obstet. Gynec. 90:593-609, 1964.

6 Danforth, W. C.: Carcinoma of the cervix during pregnancy, Amer. J. Obstet. Gynec. 34: 365-379, 1937.

7 Feste, J. R., Kaufman, R. H., Skogland, H. L., and Topek, N. H.: Management of abnormal cytology late in pregnancy, Amer. J. Obstet. Gynec. 95:763-768, 1968.

8 Fluhmann, C. F.: A clinical and histopathologic study of lesions of the cervix uteri during pregnancy, Amer. J. Obstet. Gynec. 55: 133-147, 1948.

9 Fontana-Donatelli, G., and Variati, G.: Amputation and conization of the cervix and their effects on the fertility of the woman; a clinical discussion, Ann. Ostet. Ginec. 88: 622-630, 1966.

10 Hammond, C. B., Hertz, R., Ross, G. T., Lipsett, M. B., and O'Dell, W. D.: Diagnostic problems of choriocarcinoma and related trophoblastic neoplasms, Obstet. Gynec. 29:224-229, 1967.

11 Hertig, A. T., and Sheldon, W. H.: Hydatidiform mole; a pathologico-clinical correlation of 200 cases, Amer. J. Obstet. Gynec. 53:1-36, 1947.

12 Hesselberg, E.: Cancer of the cervix associated with procidentia, S. Afr. Med. J. 37:589-592, 1963.

13 Hirst, J. C.: Carcinoma of the uterine cervix complicating pregnancy, J.A.M.A. 142:230-234, 1950.

14 Hou, P. C., and Pang, S. C.: Chorionepithelioma; an analytical study of 28 necropsied cases, with special reference to the possibility of spontaneous retrogression, J. Path. Bact. 72: 95-104, 1956.

15 King, G.: Hydatidiform mole and chorionepithelioma; the problem of the borderline cases, Proc. Roy. Soc. Med. 49:381-390, 1956.

16 Logan, B. J., and Motyloff, L.: Hydatidiform mole, Amer. J. Obstet. Gynec. 75:1134-1148, 1958.

17 Mikuta, J. J., Enterline, H. T., and Braun, T. E., Jr.: Carcinoma in situ of the cervix associated with pregnancy, J.A.M.A. 204:763-766, 1968.

18 Moore, J. G., Wells, R. G., and Morton, D. G.: Management of superficial cervical cancer in pregnancy, Obstet. Gynec. 27:307-318, 1966.

19 Novak, E.: Hydatidiform mole and chorioepithelioma, J.A.M.A. 78:1771-1779, 1922.

20 Park, W. W., and Lees, J. C.: Choriocarcinoma, Arch. Path. (Chicago) 49:73-104, 205-241, 1950.

21 Prem, K. A., Makowski, E. L., and McKelvey, J. L.: Carcinoma of the cervix associated with pregnancy, Amer. J. Obstet. Gynec. 95:99-108, 1966.

22 Reed, S., Coe, J. I., and Bergquist, J.: Invasive hydatidiform mole metastatic to the lungs; report of a case, Obstet. Gynec. 13: 749-753, 1959.

23 Richman, S., and Goodfriend, M. J.: Cancer of the cervix uteri associated with pregnancy, Amer. J. Roentgen. 48:677-684, 1942.

24 Ross, G. T., Goldstein, D. P., Hertz, R., Lipsett, M. B., and Odell, W. D.: Sequential use of methotrexate and actinomycin D in the treatment of metastatic choriocarcinoma and related trophoblastic diseases in women, Amer. J. Obstet. Gynec. 93:223-229, 1965.

25 Sadugor, M. G., Palmer, J. P., and Reinhard, M. C.: Carcinoma of the cervix concomitant with pregnancy, Amer. J. Obstet. Gynec. 57: 933-938, 1949.

26 Sarwey, O.: In Handbuch der Gynäkologie (revised by Anton et al.: edited by J. Veit), Wiesbaden, 1907, J. F. Bergmann.

27 Thornton, W. N., Jr., Nokes, J. M., Wilson, L. A., and Brown, D. J., Jr.: Epidermoid carcinoma of the cervix complicating pregnancy, Amer. J. Obstet. Gynec. 64:573-580, 1952.

28 Tjokronegoro, S.: Choriocarcinoma in Indonesia (unpublished data).

29 Truelsen, F.: Radiation treatment of carcinoma in the cervix coincident with pregnancy; presented to Seventh International Congress of Radiology, Copenhagen, July, 1953 (unpublished).

30 Williams, T. B., and Brack, C. B.: Carcinoma of the cervix in pregnancy, Cancer 17:1486-1491, 1964.

31 Yuan-Ying, L., Li-Wu, T., and Chen-Wei, H.: Uterine chorionic neoplasm; a study of 22 cases, Chin. Med. J. (Peking) 77:30-42, 1958.

Vagina

Anatomy

The vagina, a muscular, membranous, very elastic tube, extends from the vulva to the uterus and lies immediately posterior to the bladder and the urethra and anterior to the rectum. Its internal surface presents numerous transverse folds. Its upper extremity reflects upon itself to become continuous with the uterine cervix, forming a circular cuff that is arbitrarily divided into four arcs, the anterior, the posterior, and the lateral fornices. The vagina is in contact with the peritoneum only at the level of the posterior fornix, where it is in relation with the cul-de-sac of Douglas. Its lower or outer extremity is its narrowest part and is surrounded by the constrictor muscles.

The vaginal wall is 3 mm or 4 mm thick and is formed by three layers of tissue: an outer fibrous layer, a middle muscular layer, and an inner mucosa. The mucosa is a stratified squamous epithelium on an irregularly wavy basement membrane. Normally, the mucosa has no horny layer and no glands, but these may occasionally be found in the fornices.

Lymphatics. The lymphatics of the vaginal wall may be divided into two main groups, one accompanying the uterine artery and the other following the course of the vaginal artery (Rouvière[22]). Those that follow the *uterine artery* drain the superior part of the vagina and empty into one of the nodes of the external iliac chain. Those that follow the *vaginal artery* drain, for the most part, the lower half of the vagina and empty into one of the hypogastric lymph nodes. In addition, the lymphatics of the vagina anastomose with those of the cervix and of the vulva. Rarely, some of them may also penetrate into the rectal wall and terminate in perirectal lymph nodes.

Epidemiology

Cancer of the vagina is rare, being considerably less frequent than cancer of the cervix or even cancer of the vulva. Higginson[9] reported a high incidence of vaginal carcinoma among the Bantus in South Africa. It is rare among blacks and Jews in the United States (Marcus[14]). No causal factor has been incriminated for its development. It is usually found in women between 45 and 65 years of age. Sarcomas of the vaginal wall are relatively more frequent in young girls under 6 years of age. Other forms of sarcoma are rarely observed in women. Primary malignant melanomas of the vagina are rare (Norris and Taylor[19]).

Pathology

Gross pathology

Carcinoma of the vagina most often develops on the upper third of the posterior wall but is also found on the lateral and anterior walls. This tumor may easily invade the rectovaginal septum and the paracystium, yet actual involvement of the

bladder or rectal walls has not frequently been reported. It may also secondarily invade the cervix and the vulva.

Vaginal sarcomas occurring in young girls are of the botryoid (grapelike) type and arise most often on the anterior wall. The sarcoma occurring in adults may arise from any part of the wall and is most often of parietal rather than mucous origin. These tumors rapidly spread to the paracystium and paraproctium, producing constriction of the bladder and the rectum.

Microscopic pathology

The overwhelming majority of tumors of the vagina are undifferentiated epidermoid carcinomas. Carcinomas in situ may be an extension of such lesions originating in the cervix (Copenhaver et al.[4]) or may arise independently from the vaginal mucosa (Ferguson and Maclure[7]). Adenocarcinomas of mesonephric origin may arise in the vagina (Truskett and Constable[26]). Vawter[29] reported two cases of embryonal carcinoma, but adenocarcinomas of the vaginal wall are, as a rule, metastatic from primary lesions elsewhere. The botryoid sarcoma demonstrates a variable microscopic pattern and is often myxomatous with striated tumor cells. Leiomyosarcomas are often rather undifferentiated (Malkasian et al.[13]). Malignant melanomas seem to arise from melanoblasts in the vaginal wall (Nigogosyan et al.[18]), and their pattern is similar to that of malignant melanomas elsewhere.

Metastatic spread

Carcinomas of the vagina metastasize to the lymph nodes of the external iliac and hypogastric chains, with inguinal node involvement observed only when the vulva has been invaded. Distant visceral metastases are rare except with sarcomas in the adult.

Clinical evolution

The clinical onset of *carcinoma* of the vagina is often manifested by vaginal bleeding (Livingstone[12]) of variable intensity. The second most frequent complaint is vaginal discharge. Pain appears only when the tumor has spread to the subperitoneal areolar tissue of the parametrium and the paracystium. Extension to the cervix and parametria is more frequently observed than extension to the urethra and vulva. Inguinal, pelvic, and abdominal lymph node metastases are commonly observed, but distant blood-borne metastases are exceptional.

A bloody vaginal discharge may be the first symptom of a *sarcoma* of the vagina. In the young girl, tumor may be seen protruding through the vulva. There is immediate local pain followed later by dysuria and constipation due to constriction of the bladder and rectum. Hematuria and edema of the lower extremities may be observed. Distant metastases are rare with sarcoma in the child but are not uncommon with that in the adult. Deterioration of the general condition with anemia and uremia rapidly develops.

Diagnosis

Gray and Christopherson[7a] described the appearance of vaginal carcinoma in situ as a "blush with pink granulations" or as a white plaque.

It should be kept in mind that a primary carcinoma of the vagina occurs less frequently than direct involvement or metastases from primary lesions in other organs. Because of the frequent involvement of the vaginal wall by carcinomas of the cervix, a diagnosis of primary carcinoma of the vagina should not be made unless the cervix is found intact. When an exploration of the cervix is not possible through the vagina, a diagnosis of carcinoma of the vagina should be made only when, on rectal palpation, the region of the cervix appears normal and the parametria are not involved (Radiological Subcommission, Committee on Hygiene of the League of Nations). These strict rules are justified because of the rarity of carcinoma of the vagina. Carcinomas of the endometrium may also directly involve or metastasize to the vagina (Price et al.[21]). Because some of these metastatic tumors are undifferentiated and do not show distinct adenoid arrangements, an erroneous diagnosis of primary carcinoma of the vagina is often made, particularly when the cervix is not affected. Vaginal metastases are common in uterine chorioepitheliomas, but the differential diagnosis can be based on a recent pregnancy or on the recent elimination of typical hydatid cysts. Malignant tumors of the ovary and carcinomas of the gastrointestinal tract may produce abdominal implants that gravitate to the cul-de-sac of Douglas, where the tumor easily invades the posterior wall of the vagina and simulates a primary tumor of the wall. A dilatation of the cervix and curettage of the endometrium should always be done when the carcinoma is not frankly epidermoid. Very rarely, an unsuspected carcinoma of the bladder invades the vagina, and in such advanced lesions there may be a difficulty in establishing the true point of origin. Primary lymphosarcomas and reticulum cell sarcomas have been observed in the vagina (Weseley and Berrigan[31]). This diagnosis may have to be differentiated from secondary lymphosarcomatous or leukemic manifestations. A glomus tumor causing dyspareunia has been reported (Banner and Winkelmann[1]).

Sarcoma in the child is easily recognized. Sarcoma in the adult may present itself as a submucous nonulcerated mass of the vaginal wall or as an already ulcerated necrotic tumor. The diagnosis is made on biopsy. Norris and Taylor[20] reported twenty-four vaginal polyps, benign in nature, which in many instances were incorrectly diagnosed as sarcoma botryoides. Malignant melanomas grow rapidly and may be recognized by their dark blue or black appearance (Collantes et al.[3]).

Most of the benign lesions of the vaginal wall are pedunculated and nonulcerated and consequently easily diagnosed. Condyloma acuminata usually spread into the vagina from the vulva. Benign ulcerations are superficial and often tender. Tuberculosis and syphilitic ulcerations are rare. Teratomas (dermoid cysts) occur usually in the rectovaginal septum and may be confused in the adult with sarcomas. However, the latter develop faster and are often accompanied by pain. Primary sarcomas of the vesicovaginal septum are rare.

Treatment
Surgery

A surgical excision is well indicated for the treatment of carcinomas in situ or small superficial carcinomas, particularly of the lower third of the vagina. Herbst et al.[8] reported on the surgical treatment of carcinoma of the vagina in which results were favorable. In the treatment of post-irradiation recurrences of sarcomas (Ulfelder and Quan[28]) and melanomas (Desai and Cavanagh[5]), a surgical approach is often the only justifiable course, but then the surgical procedure is often radical and mutilating. Unfortunately, when such radical procedures are justified, the tumor is seldom curable. Pelvic exenterations carry with them considerable operable mortality and morbidity. Cosmetic reconstructions of the vagina usually fail.

Radiotherapy

Irradiation of carcinomas of the vagina by means of intracavitary radioactive sources has motivated the design of a variety of vaginal applicators. Among the most widely utilized is the Bloedorn applicator (Rutledge[24]). Intracavitary irradiation may be complemented by interstitial implantation of radioactive sources in the substance of the tumor (Chau[2]; Way[30]). Transvaginal roentgentherapy may be useful for the irradiation of lesions of the upper third of the vagina. Although atresia of the vagina is often the price of postirradiation healing, radiotherapy may preserve a vaginal canal.

For the treatment of most carcinomas of the vagina, a thorough external irradiation, by means of cobalt[60] or supervoltage roentgentherapy, is a more logical and satisfactory approach. External pelvic irradiation may utilize a complementary perineal portal of entry, thus favoring a more homogeneous irradiation of the vaginal lesion and extravaginal infiltration and metastatic implants. Homogeneity of irradiation allows for a higher minimum dose and eventual success.

Prognosis

The prognosis of vaginal carcinomas is much better now than has been reported in the past. In a group of 135 patients treated by Murphy,[16] thirty-five were living without cancer after five years. There was correlation between the stage of disease and the number of patients cured, but, as he emphasized, even extensive cancer of the vagina may be cured.

Unfortunately, many of the articles reporting end results of primary carcinoma

Table 91. Treatment results in invasive carcinoma*

Years observed		Patients
Less than three years		15
Minimum three years		55
Not treated	5	
Dead not of carcinoma	7	}35
Dead of carcinoma or lost	23	
Alive	20	(36%)
Minimum five years		43
Not treated	5	
Dead not of carcinoma	4	}28
Dead of carcinoma or lost	19	
Alive	15	(35%)

*From Rutledge, F.: Cancer of the vagina, Amer. J. Obstet. Gynec. 97:635-655, 1967.

of the vagina do not give any information concerning the extent of the tumor or exactly how it was treated. The five-year survival rates, overall are about the same. In thirty-nine patients reported by Roy,[23] the five-year survival rate after radiotherapy was 30%. Jentys and Rustowski[10] reported an overall cure rate of 38% in ninety patients with vaginal cancer. Wolff and Douyon[32] reported a 21% five-year recovery, and Kratochwil[11] reported 28%. Rutledge[24] gave the details of treatment in all of his patients, and the overall results in those with invasive carcinoma followed for a minimum of five years was 35% (Table 91).

The prognosis of sarcomas is invariably poor. The patient with botryoid sarcoma reported by Ulfelder and Quan[28] remained well over five years after surgical excision.

REFERENCES

1 Banner, E. A., and Winkelmann, R. K.: Glomus tumor of the vagina, Obstet. Gynec. 9:326-328, 1957.
2 Chau, P. M.: Radiotherapeutic management of malignant tumors of the vagina, Amer. J. Roentgen. 89:502-523, 1963.
3 Collantes, T. M., Pratt, J. H., and Dockerty, M. B.: Primary malignant melanoma of the vagina, Obstet. Gynec. 29:508-514, 1967.
4 Copenhaver, E. H., Salsman, F. A., and Wright, K. A.: Carcinoma in situ of the vagina, Amer. J. Obstet. Gynec. 89:962-969, 1964.
5 Desai, S., and Cavanagh, D.: Malignant melanoma of the vagina, Cancer 19:632-636, 1966.
6 Dunn, L. J., and Napier, J. G.: Primary carcinoma of the vagina, Amer. J. Obstet. Gynec. 96:1112-1116, 1966.
7 Ferguson, J. H., and Maclure, J. G.: Intraepithelial carcinoma, dysplasia, and exfoliation

of cancer cells in the vaginal mucosa, Amer. J. Obstet. Gynec. **87**:326-336, 1963.

7a Gray, L. A., and Christopherson, W. M.: Insitu and early invasive carcinoma of the vagina, Obstet. Gynec. **34**:226-230, 1969.

8 Herbst, A. L., Green, T. H., Jr., and Ulfelder, H.: Primary carcinoma of the vagina, Amer. J. Obstet. Gynec. **106**:210-218, 1970.

9 Higginson, J.: Malignant neoplastic disease in the South African Bantu, Cancer **4**:1224-1231, 1951.

10 Jentys, W., and Rustowski, J.: Wyniki leczenia pierwotnego raka pochwy w Instytucie Onkologii w Warszawie, Nowotwory **14**:401-404, 1964.

11 Kratochwil, A.: Therapeutische Ergebnisse beim primären Karzinom der Vagina, Krebsarzt **20**: 94-98, 1965.

12 Livingstone, R. G.: Primary carcinoma of the vagina, Springfield, Ill., 1950, Charles C Thomas, Publisher.

13 Malkasian, G. D., Jr., Welch, J. S., and Soule, E. H.: Primary leiomyosarcoma of the vagina, Amer. J. Obstet. Gynec. **86**:730-736, 1963.

14 Marcus, S. L.: Primary carcinoma of the vagina, Obstet. Gynec. **15**:673-689, 1960.

15 Merrill, J. A., and Bender, W. T.: Primary carcinoma of the vagina, Obstet. Gynec. **11**:3-11, 1958.

16 Murphy, W. T.: Primary vaginal cancer; irradiation management and end-results, Radiology **68**:157-168, 1957.

17 Murphy, W. T., and Bozzini, M. A.: End results in the irradiation of primary carcinoma of the vagina, Radiology **80**:566-567, 1963.

18 Nigogosyan, G., de la Pava, S., and Pickren, J. W.: Melanoblasts in vaginal mucosa; origin for primary malignant melanoma, Cancer **17**: 912-913, 1964.

19 Norris, H. J., and Taylor, H. B.: Melanomas of the vagina, Amer. J. Clin. Path. **46**:420-426, 1966.

20 Norris, H. J., and Taylor, H. B.: Polyps of the vagina, Cancer **19**:227-232, 1966.

21 Price, J. J., Hahn, G. A., and Rominger, C. J.: Vaginal involvement in endometrial carcinoma, Amer. J. Obstet. Gynec. **91**:1060-1065, 1965.

22 Rouvière, H.: Anatomie des lymphatiques de l'homme, Paris, 1922, Masson et Cie.

23 Roy, D. K.: Primary carcinoma of the vagina, J. Obstet. Gynaec. India **13**:504-510, 1963.

24 Rutledge, F.: Cancer of the vagina, Amer. J. Obstet. Gynec. **97**:635-655, 1967.

25 Taylor, R. W.: Pessaries and carcinoma of the vagina, Lancet **1**:831, 1964.

26 Truskett, I. D., and Constable, W. C.: Clear cell adenocarcinoma of the cervix and vaginal vault of mesonephric origin, Cancer **21**:249-254, 1968.

27 Ulfelder, H.: Personal communication, 1952.

28 Ulfelder, H., and Quan, S. H.: Sarcoma botryoides vaginae, complete excision of the tumor in an infant by the combined abdominal and perineal approach, Surg. Clin. N. Amer. **27**:1240-1245, 1947.

29 Vawter, G. F.: Carcinoma of the vagina in infancy, Cancer **18**:1479-1484, 1965.

30 Way, S.: Primary carcinoma of the vagina, J. Obstet. Gynaec. Brit. Emp. **55**:739-755, 1948.

31 Weseley, A. C., and Berrigan, M. V.: Reticulum-cell sarcoma of the vagina; report of a case, Obstet. Gynec. **11**:192-195, 1958.

32 Wolff, J.-P., and Douyon, E.: Primary cancer of the vagina, Gynec. Obstet. (Paris) **63**:565-584, 1964.

Vulva

Anatomy

The vulva is formed by the labia majora, labia minora, vestibule, clitoris, and greater vestibular glands. The labia majora are paired folds of skin that lie medial to the thighs. Anteriorly, they merge and become continuous with the mons pubis, whereas posteriorly they narrow and end 3 cm in front of the anus. The labia minora are smaller folds situated medially to the labia majora. They join anteriorly to form the anterior commissure, beneath the symphysis pubis, and to surround the erectile clitoris (Fig. 618). The vestibule is the triangular space between the labia minora and the clitoris and urethral meatus. It contains Skene's glands which end in a small orifice near the meatus. The labia majora are lined by slightly pigmented skin with glands and hair follicles. The labia minora and vestibule are covered by thin moist epithelium without sweat glands or follicles. The Bartholin glands are situated in the posterolateral quadrant of the vaginal orifice.

Lymphatics. The lymphatics of the vulva arise from a very fine and diffuse network that covers the entire surface except the lateral surface of the labia majora. They gather in the direction of the mons veneris and then turn laterally toward the superficial inguinal nodes. The lymphatics of the clitoris and vestibule ascend along the midline to a presymphyseal plexus, per-

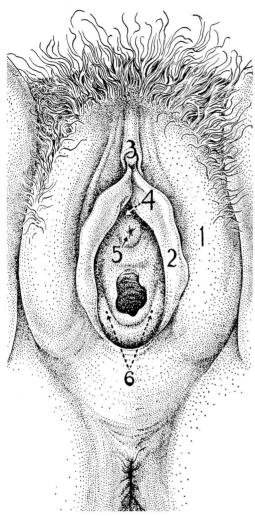

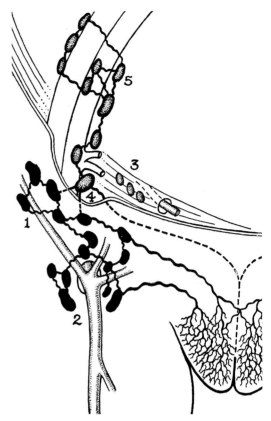

Fig. 619. Lymphatics of vulva leading to superficial inguinal nodes, **1**; superficial femoral nodes, **2**; deep inguinal nodes through main clearing station, **3**; node of Cloquet, **4**; external iliac nodes, **5**.

Fig. 618. Vulva showing labium majus, **1**; labium minus, **2**; clitoris, **3**; vestibule, **4**; urethra, **5**; orifice of Bartholin glands, **6**.

forate the fascia, and end in the deep inguinal and retrofemoral nodes. Another group follows the round ligament and empties into the lateral retrofemoral node and may communicate with the hypogastric nodes through the network of the lymphatics of the urethra. The lymphatics of the Bartholin glands end in the inguinal nodes (Rouvière[43]). Parry-Jones[40] found no evidence of lateral drainage of vulvar lymphatics. Way[51] divides the lymph nodes draining the vulva into four groups (Fig. 619):

1 The *superficial inguinal nodes* lie along the inguinal ligament and slight-ly below it and are arranged in a *lateral* elongated group and a *medial* cluster just below the superficial inguinal ring.

2 The *deep inguinal nodes* lie in the inguinal canal along the course of the round ligament and are inconstant.

3 The *superficial femoral nodes* are grouped around the great saphenous vein just before it passes through the fossa ovalis to join the femoral vein and are arranged in a *medial* group near the entry of the superficial veins into the saphenous vein and a *lateral* group on the lateral side of the vein. Some of their efferent lymphatics follow the femoral vessels to deep femoral nodes.

4 The *deep femoral nodes* are often represented by mere fusiform enlargements of the vessels. The upper node

of this group, called the *node of Clo-quet*, lies at the upper end of the inguinal canal under the inguinal ligament and receives the lymphatics from the clitoris and superficial inguinal nodes, thus draining a great part of the lymph from the vulva.

Epidemiology

The age-sex adjusted incidence of cancer of the vulva is relatively low, of the order of 1.4 to 1.8 per 100,000 population in the United States. The incidence is negligible in patients under 50 years of age and then rises sharply in the later decades of life, showing no decline. In a series of 238 cases reported by Green et al.,[20] 70% occurred in patients 60 years of age or older. In El Salvador, 19% of patients observed by Díaz-Bazán[16] were under 40 years of age. In Lunin's series[30] of fifty patients admitted to the Charity Hospital of New Orleans, thirty-one were black. It seems that carcinoma of the vulva appears, as an average, at an earlier age in black women.

Taussig[47] found that vestibular carcinomas predominated among black women, with syphilis or granulomatous venereal diseases frequently the precursors in his patients (Collins et al.[14]; Birch[7]). In a series of thirteen cases of vulvar carcinoma following granulomatous lesions reported by Saltzstein et al.,[44] twelve had a history of syphilis and twelve were in black patients. In the African with carcinoma of the vulva, there is a high associated occurrence of syphilis (Lithgow and Farrell[29]). Concomitant diabetes (Saltzstein et al.[44]), hypertension, and obesity (Green et al.[20]) have been noted.

A high proportion of patients with carcinoma of the vulva give a history of dryness and shrinkage of the vulva. These changes are initiated by the menopause and probably obey to endocrine causes. Carcinomas arising on this basis are often multicentric. Lichen sclerosus et atrophicus (kraurosis vulvae) is not a precancerous condition (Clark[13]). Leukoplakia has been often presented as a precancerous condition frequently leading to the development of carcinoma: leukoplakia is a clinical appearance that may be produced by benign dyskeratosis, early superficial carcinomatous changes, or frank carcinoma.

Pathology
Gross pathology

The greater majority of carcinomas of the vulva develop on the labia (Figs. 620 and 621). Taussig[47] divided 155 cases of carcinoma of the vulva into groups according to point of origin (Table 92).

Carcinomas of the vulva tend to spread submucosally. The large superficial masses later become ulcerated and secondarily infected. Vestibular lesions are usually excavating with hard nodular borders. When the ulcerations become deep and necrotic, the underlying blood vessels may be eroded, and hemorrhage may result. Leukoplakia is associated with carcinomas of the vulva in a large proportion of the cases.

Microscopic pathology

Carcinomas of the vulva are squamous in nature with the exception of Bartholin gland carcinomas and some of those developing in the vestibule that may be adenocarcinomas. Most of the carcinomas arising from the labia are rather well differentiated, but those that arise from the clitoris and vestibular region usually are not.

Bowen's disease may also be present, showing hyperplasia, disorderly pattern of the architecture, numerous mitotic figures, and foam cells (Jeffcoate et al.[26]). The basement membrane, however, remains intact in Bowen's disease, the carcinoma remaining strictly intraepidermal. Barclay et al.[4] reported twenty-one cases of intraepithelial cancer of the vulva. This situation may not remain as such, and the carcinoma may transgress through the basement membrane. In the twenty-four patients reported by Abell and Gosling,[2] ten showed infiltrative growth. Furthermore, 37.5% of this group showed other malignant neoplasms,

Table 92. Point of origin of carcinoma of vulva*

Origin	Cases
Epidermal	104
Vestibular	11
Periurethral	12
Bartholin gland	9
Glans clitoris	2
Unclassified (advanced cases)	17

*From Taussig. F. J.: Cancer of the vulva, Amer. J. Obstet. Gynec. **40:**764-779, 1940.

particularly squamous cell carcinoma of the uterus, cervix, and upper vagina. Helwig and Graham[22] reported forty cases of Paget's disease of the anogenital area, fifteen occurring on the vulva. The histochemical differentiation of anogenital Paget's disease from malignant melanoma, Bowen's disease, and erythroplasia of Queyrat is firmly based on a positive aldehyde-fuchsin reaction in the Paget cells and a negative reaction in the other three lesions. Intradermal migration of the tumor cells occurs in Paget's disease (Adamsons and Reisfield[3]).

Melanocarcinomas of the vulva are relatively infrequent. They may arise from a preexisting nevus. Only one-half of nevi of the vulva are junctional in type. Benign tumors arising from the blood vessels, muscles, and connective tissue are rare. The so-called hidradenoma that arises from the sweat glands is often confused with carcinoma grossly. It is well circumscribed but has a tendency to ulcerate. Microscopically, hidradenomas show the evidence of their sweat gland origin with papillary-like projections and never extend beyond the basement membrane (Rothman and Gray[42]; Novak and Stevenson[37]). They are never malignant. The adenoid cystic form of carcinoma can arise from the vestibular glands of the vulva (Abell[1]). We have found this tumor to be highly malignant and difficult to cure.

True basal cell carcinomas of the vulva are rare (Wilson[54]). Metastatic lesions from other genital carcinomas, particularly chorioepitheliomas and carcinomas of the endometrium, have been encountered but are uncommon. Carcinoma of the cervix and rectum may directly invade the vulva, but ovarian neoplasms rarely involve it.

Metastatic spread

Over half of all patients seen with carcinoma of the vulva present metastases in the inguinal lymph nodes (Díaz-Bazán[16]). Metastases are often bilateral, and the deep inguinal nodes are not uncommonly involved. Metastases to the abdominal

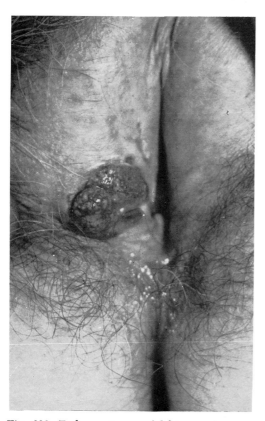

Fig. 620. Early carcinoma of labium majus near fourchette. Note atrophy of labia and narrowing of introitus.

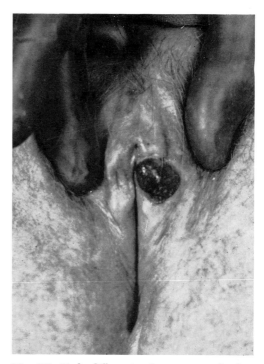

Fig. 621. Early differentiated carcinoma of vulva. Note general atrophy of labia.

lymph nodes, as well as blood-borne metastases to the liver and lungs, may occur.

Clinical evolution

Most cases of carcinoma of the vulva are preceded or accompanied by *pruritus*. This symptom, however, is often due to the development of kraurosis rather than to the carcinoma itself. The pruritus is most marked at night and seems to center about the clitoris and the anal folds. Scratching makes further excoriation which, in turn, aggravates the pruritus and leads to insomnia. These symptoms may have been present for several years before the appearance of carcinoma. In addition, the kraurosis may result in shrinkage of the vaginal orifice and in marked *dyspareunia*. In some instances, there is an intermittent bleeding that may become hemorrhagic. In addition, the hair may become brittle, and the skin is abnormally dry and parchment-thin. Shrinkage with flattening and atrophy of the clitoris and narrowing of the vaginal orifice may have occurred, as well as a red mottling in the region of the labia minora on either side of the introitus.

In general, carcinomas of the vulva are papillary outgrowths that may become very extensive. Some cases, however, have a tendency to ulcerate and diffusely infiltrate and may present a large crater instead of an exophytic mass. A constant complication of carcinomas of the vulva is the presence of secondary infection that may be more or less marked, depending on the case. In uncontrolled cases, the patients rapidly become cachectic and may die as a consequence of complications rather than because of generalization of the disease. Diffuse cellulitis and phlebitis are not uncommon complications.

Tumors of the Bartholin gland may be adenocarcinoma or epidermoid carcinoma. They usually present as an indurated swelling within the labium majoris near the fourchette, the skin not usually being involved. Their evolution may be slow. Basal cell carcinomas of the vulva may present as ulcerated lesions or simply as erythematous lesions without ulceration (Siegler and Greene[45]). Lesions of the vulva identified as extramammary Paget's disease are usually confined to the skin and are reddened, eczematoid, ulcerated, and sharply

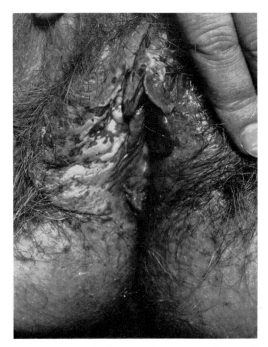

Fig. 622. Paget's disease of vulva in 67-year-old woman. Note mottled eczematoid appearance covered by numerous white macerated patches. (From Rosser, E. ap I., and Hamlin, I. M. E.: Paget's disease of the vulva, J. Obstet. Gynaec. Brit. Emp. **64:**127-130, 1957.)

delineated (Casper[12]). This lesion represents invasion of the overlying epidermis from an underlying carcinoma arising from apocrine glands (Huber et al.[23]; Rosser and Hamlin[41] (Fig. 622). *Malignant melanoma* of the vulva may arise from a pre-existing junctional-type nevus. It has the clinical characteristics of a malignant melanoma of the skin. On the vulva, it is often seen late as an ulcerating, deeply pigmented tumor. The clinical evolution is invariably rapid (Wilson[55]), but some rare cases metastasize late (Symmonds et al.[46]). *Reticulum cell sarcoma* of the vulva has been reported (Buckingham and McClure[10]).

Involvement of the inguinal nodes occurs rather early in the development of the disease. However, these nodes may also be enlarged because of secondary infection. The larger and more undifferentiated the lesion is, the higher the frequency of involved lymph nodes. Ulceration is also associated with a high frequency of lymph node involvement. In a series reported by Green et al.,[20] one-third of the carcinomas measuring 1 cm in diameter had metastases. Way[53] reported thirty-six patients with enlarged lymph nodes and no metastases and thirty-three patients with metastases in nonpalpable lymph nodes. Since metastases are greatly dependent on size and location, the following staging proposed by McKelvey and Adcock[33] may have its usefulness:

Stage I

Carcinomas less than 10 cm² and not involving the urethra, vagina or anus

Stage II

Carcinomas more than 10 cm² but not involving the urethra, vagina, or anus

Stage III

Carcinomas of any size involving the urethra, vagina, or anus

Stage IV

Carcinomas with clinically ostensible intra-abdominal or distant metastases

Diagnosis

Lichen sclerosus et atrophicus can be recognized by the characteristic acellular band of homogenized tissue beneath the thinned-out epidermis (Fig. 623). The pattern is similar to that of Peyronie's disease. The clinical term *leukoplakia* has no histopathologic significance—only a biopsy will reveal whether the "white patch" is due to a benign or actually to a malignant lesion. Large whitish areas may cover the labia and extend to the perianal region. These areas are usually pearly gray and sharply demarcated. This appearance is often described as "precancerous." It is more correct, however, to state that it may be associated with cancer of the vulva. Woodruff and Baens[56] studied eighty cases of "leukoplakia," with limited or radical excision in sixty and biopsy only in twenty. Of forty-four patients traced, three subsequently had carcinoma of the vulva. Toluidine blue stain is useful for detecting areas of malignant transformation in the vulvar epithelium.

The history and physical findings in carcinomas of the vulva make the clinical diagnosis rather simple. However, a few other conditions might offer a problem of

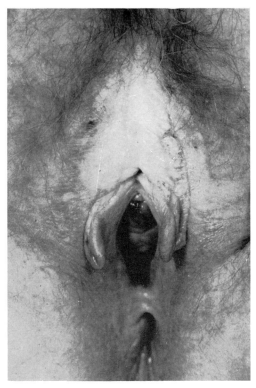

Fig. 623. Lichen sclerosus atrophicus of vestibular region of vulva with atrophy of clitoris and marked narrowing of vaginal orifice.

differential diagnosis. Benign lesions such as *condyloma* usually occur in young women (Fig. 624). These are soft, nonulcerated, papillary outgrowths that become pedunculated and are usually associated with other venereal diseases. They do not become malignant. *Lymphogranuloma venereum* is often also associated with rectal lesions and may be ruled out because of a positive Frei test. However, it should not be forgotten that this, as any other venereal disease, is compatible with a concomitant carcinoma of the vulva. Other benign tumors, such as hemangiomas, leiomyomas, lipomas, and fibromas, are very rare in the vulva. They are easily differentiated because of the absence of ulceration or infiltration and because of the slow rate of their growth. The *hidradenoma* of sweat gland origin is a well-circumscribed lesion usually of long duration. When it becomes ulcerated, it may be confused with carcinoma, but the biopsy will be conclusive.

Granular cell myoblastoma, a rare lesion

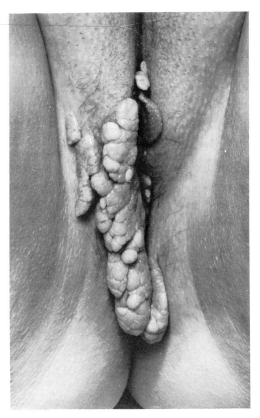

Fig. 624. Condyloma of vulva. (Courtesy Maud E. Jacobs, London, England.)

in the vulva, may be mistaken microscopically for carcinoma because of overlying pseudoepitheliomatous proliferation. *Ectopic breast tissue* (twenty-one instances recorded by Fouchee and Pruitt[18]) and *endometriosis* may lead to confusion when found in the vulva.

Primary carcinomas of the female urethra are rare. They usually manifest themselves by dysuria, urethrorrhagia, or the presence of a tumor at the urethral meatus. The urethral tumor may enlarge the urethral canal and transform it into a hard tube (Brack and Farber[8]) but also may present as a nodule or a red, easily bleeding mass at the urethral meatus (Walker and Huffman[50]). It may be adenocarcinoma or epidermoid carcinoma and does not metastasize frequently (Desaive and Ramioul[15]). Treatment of carcinomas of the urethra is successfully carried out by means of radium (Fricke and McMillan[19]) or roentgentherapy (Buschke and Cantril[11]) with excellent results. Involvement of the prox-

imal urethra is said to carry a bad prognosis (Antoniades[3a]). Confusion with urethral caruncle may be avoided by biopsying all of these lesions. The so-called *urethral caruncle* is the most common lesion of the urethra, but rarely it may represent a malignant tumor (Marshall et al.[34]).

Treatment
Surgery

In the presence of a variety of vulvar lesions which may be encountered, an adequate biopsy is a necessary first step that may lead to a proper therapeutic decision. Areas of "leukoplakia" may prove to be due to simple hyperkeratosis or may show widespread atypical proliferation or carcinoma in situ. Paget's disease or lichen sclerosus et atrophicus may also be present. In all of these instances, a wide local excision is justified and easily practicable (Janovski and Ames[24]; Jeffcoate[25]). Some malignant melanomas of the vulva may arise from preexisting junctional nevi. Therefore, as a preventive measure, such nevi should be removed.

In recognized carcinomas, as well as in Bowen's disease and melanomas of the vulva, a *radical vulvectomy* is the treatment of choice. This implies ample removal of all vulvar skin, including perianal skin (Brunchswig and Brockunier[9]). The resulting defect may heal with surprising rapidity. McGregor[31] advised the use of split-skin grafts to cover the raw surface. Lesser procedures, in consideration of advanced age, etc., usually lead to recurrences and to the enforced need for a delayed radical procedure with lessened chances of success.

A *bilateral inguinal dissection* carried out in continuity with the vulvectomy is now the accepted procedure (Green et al.[21]) in view of the multicentricity of many carcinomas, the inadequacy of clinical judgment as to the presence or absence of metastases (Way[53]), and the frequency and bilaterality of metastatic involvement (Table 93). The mortality and morbidity of the single-stage operation is relatively low. The inguinal dissection is usually augmented by an extraperitoneal *iliac lymphadenectomy*. This is particularly justified in carcinomas of or invading the clitoris, in which there may be deep metastases with-

Table 93. Relative accuracy of clinical estimate of lymph node involvement*

	No palpable nodes	*Palpable nodes*
Total	82	65
Histologically positive	35	45
Histologically negative	38	16
Not recorded	9	4
Relative accuracy	52% (38/73)	37% (23/61)

*Data from Green, T. H., Jr., et al.: Epidermoid carcinoma; an analysis of 238 cases, Amer. J. Obstet. Gynec. 75:834-847, 1958.

out superficial node involvement. Some surgeons limit the extent of the dissection if the superficial inguinal nodes are not involved (Way[52]; Ulfelder[49]), but others advocate the larger operation in any event (Merrill and Ross[35]).

Rutledge et al.[43a] feel that total vulvectomy and lymphadenectomy should be the standard treatment for carcinoma of the vulva. They also believe that iliac lymphadenectomy does not need to be done routinely, for if the inguinal lymph nodes are not involved, the nodes of the pelvic wall are practically never involved.

Radiotherapy

Most vulvar tumors are radiosensitive but their irradiation is not, for the most part, justified on several counts: fractionated irradiation may prove more onerous to the usually elderly patients than a surgical procedure; short intensive treatments of this moist area usually result in unwarranted reactions and great possibility of extensive superficial necroses (Baud[6]; Ellis[17]); and there is no important functional or esthetic disadvantage to the surgical removal. It is possible that a case might be made for the preoperative irradiation of metastatic areas by means of cobalt[60] or supervoltage roentgentherapy (Mousseau and Barbin[36]). A careful and extensive irradiation of inoperable cases may prove fruitful (Lisse[28]).

Prognosis

In 1965, there was a total of 531 deaths in the United States due to cancer of the vulva, or a crude death rate of 0.5 per 100,000 population. Carcinoma of the vulva

has a relatively favorable prognosis, second only to carcinoma of the endometrium among tumors of the female genital tract. McKelvey and Adcock[33] reported on 124 consecutive patients with cancer of the vulva, not previously treated, seen at the University of Minnesota Hospital from 1938 to 1960: eight had melanomas (only one patient survived five years), one an adenocarcinoma, one a basal cell carcinoma, one a fibrosarcoma, and one Paget's disease; 113 of these patients had a radical vulvectomy and bilateral inguinal and femoral lymphadenectomy, three had pelvic exenterations, six others had various limited or conservative procedures, and two were not treated by virtue of pathology, age, etc. A total of sixty-five patients (56%) were well and free of tumor five or more years after treatment. There were six operative deaths, ten deaths from intercurrent disease, and thirty-four deaths from cancer. Of 106 patients with carcinoma of the vulva who received the standard vulvectomy and bilateral dissection, thirty were found to have lymph node metastases. There were two operative deaths, three deaths from intercurrent disease, and sixteen deaths from cancer, and nine (30%) patients were well five years or more. Bruchschwig and Brockunier[9] operated on 115 patients with an aim to cure, twenty-four of whom had some form of pelvic exenteration. Of thirty-four patients who had inguinal metastases, only twelve survived.

Green et al.[21] reported excellent results for surgery of cancer of the vulva. With adequate surgical treatment twenty-five of twenty-nine patients with negative lymph nodes were alive and well more than five years, and seventeen of thirty-six patients with positive lymph nodes were alive and well more than five years. With the one-stage radical vulvectomy with bilateral superficial groin and deep pelvic node dissection, the results as reported by Ulfelder[49] are excellent, and there has also been little morbidity (Table 94). Way[53] reported sixty-nine patients with carcinoma of the vulva treated by surgery, with forty-two (61%) surviving five years, twenty-eight (41%) surviving ten years, and twenty (30%) surviving fifteen years.

Carcinomas of the vestibular area of the

Table 94. Results of one-stage radical vulvectomy with bilateral groin dissection on thirty-six patients with epidermoid carcinoma of vulva*

	Patients	Dead of cancer	Dead of intercurrent disease	Alive and well 5 yr or more	%
Negative nodes	16	1[1]	1[2]	14[3]	88
Positive nodes	20	7[4]	5[5]	8[6]	40
Total	36	8[7]	6	22	60

*Massachusetts General Hospital and Pondville Hospital, 1949-1956; Courtesy Dr. Howard Ulfelder, Boston, Mass., April, 1961.
[1]Local recurrence at seven years.
[2]At one and one-half years.
[3]Four for ten years.
[4]Four "deliberate" palliative operation; three attempts at cure.
[5]Two at two years, two at three years, and one at four years—none with recurrence.
[6]Three for ten years.
[7]One operative death.

vulva have a poorer prognosis than those arising from the labia. The dimensions of the primary lesion and the duration of its presence also have a bearing on the prognosis. The larger the tumor and the longer it has been present, the greater the possibilities of intra-abdominal metastasis. The outlook for the cure of malignant melanoma of the vulva is poor (Pack and Oropeza[38]).

REFERENCES

1 Abell, M. R.: Adenocystic (pseudoadenomatous) basal cell carcinoma of vestibular glands of vulva, Amer. J. Obstet. Gynec. **86**:470-482, 1963.

2 Abell, M. R., and Gosling, J. R. G.: Intraepithelial and infiltrative carcinoma of vulva; Bowen's type, Cancer **14**:318-329, 1961.

3 Adamsons, K., Jr., and Reisfield, D.: Observations on intradermal migration of Paget cells, Amer. J. Obstet. Gynec. **90**:1274-1280, 1964.

3a Antoniades, J.: Radiation therapy in carcinoma of the female urethra, Cancer **24**:70-76, 1969.

4 Barclay, D. L., Collins, C. G., and Hansen, L. H.: Problem patients with vulvar malignancy, Clin. Obstet. Gynec. **10**:641-654, 1967.

5 Barclay, D. L., Collins, C. G., and Macey, H. B., Jr.: Cancer of the Bartholin gland, Obstet. Gynec. **24**:329-336, 1964.

6 Baud, D. J.: Le traitement des épithéliomas de la vulve. Resultats obtenus dans 63 cas traités de 1920 á 1943 inclus par radiothérapie dans les services de la Fondation Curie, Bull. Ass. Franc. Cancer **36**:104-116, 1949.

7 Birch, H. W.: Premalignant lesions of the vulva, South. Med. J. **58**:1487-1492, 1955.

8 Brack, G. B., and Farber, G. J.: Carcinoma of the female urethra, J. Urol. **64**:710-715, 1950.

9 Brunschwig, A., and Brockunier, A., Jr.: Surgical treatment of squamous-cell carcinoma of the vulva, Obstet. Gynec. **29**:362-368, 1967.

10 Buckingham, J. C., and McClure, J. H.: Reticulum cell sarcoma of the vulva; report of a case, Obstet. Gynec. **6**:138-143, 1955.

11 Buschke, F., and Cantril, S. T.: Roentgen therapy of carcinoma of female urethra and vulva, Radiology **51**:155-165, 1948.

12 Casper, W. A.: Paget's disease of the vulva, Arch. Derm. Syph. (Chicago) **57**:668-678, 1948.

13 Clark, W. H., Jr.: A histological study of kraurosis vulvae, lichen sclerosus et atrophicus and leukoplakia of the vulva—a preliminary report; a fresh review of a stubborn problem, Bull. Tulane Med. Fac. **16**:123-128, 1957.

14 Collins, C. G., Collins, J. H., Nelson, E. W., Smith, R. C., and MacCallum, E. A.: Malignant tumors involving the vulva, Amer. J. Obstet. Gynec. **62**:1198-1208, 1951.

15 Desaive, P., and Ramioul, H.: Le cancer de l'urétre feminin (étude de 21 cas), Soc. Belg. Urol., no. 2, December, 1948.

16 Díaz-Bazán, N.: Cancer de la Vulva en El Salvador, Arch. Col. Med. El Salvador **9**:42-74, 1956.

17 Ellis, F.: Carcinoma of vulva: cancer of the vulva treated by radiation, an analysis of 127 cases; symposium, Brit. J. Radiol. **22**:513-520, 1949.

18 Foushee, J. H. S., and Pruitt, A. B., Jr.: Vulvar fibroadenoma from aberrant breast tissue, Obstet. Gynec. **29**:819-823, 1967.

19 Fricke, R. E., and McMillan, J. T.: Radium therapy in carcinoma of the female urethra, Radiology **52**:533-540, 1949.

20 Green, T. H., Jr., Ulfelder, H., and Meigs, J. V.: Epidermoid carcinoma; an analysis of 238 cases. Part I. Etiology and diagnosis, Amer. J. Obstet. Gynec. **75**:834-847, 1958.

21 Green, T. H., Jr., Ulfelder, H., and Meigs, J. V.: Epidermoid carcinoma; an analysis of 238 cases. Part II. Therapy and end results, Amer. J. Obstet. Gynec. **75**:848-864, 1958.

22 Helwig, E. B., and Graham, J. H.: Anogenital (extramammary) Paget's disease, Cancer **16**:387-403, 1963.

23 Huber, C. P., Gardiner, S. H., and Michael,

A.: Paget's disease of the vulva, Amer. J. Obstet. Gynec. 62:778-792, 1951.

24 Janovski, N. A., and Ames, S.: Lichen sclerosus et atrophicus of the vulva; a poorly understood disease entity, Obstet. Gynec. 22:697-708, 1963.

25 Jeffcoate, T. N. A.: Chronic vulval dystrophies, Amer. J. Obstet. Gynec. 95:61-74, 1966.

26 Jeffcoate, T. N. A., Davie, T. B., and Harrison, C. V.: Intra-epidermal carcinoma (Bowen's disease) of the vulva, J. Obstet. Gynaec. Brit. Emp. 51:377-385, 1944.

27 Lacour, J., and Cohen, J.: Cancer of the vulva; prognostic and therapeutic remarks with reference to 163 cases, Gynec. Obstet. (Paris) 63:69-83, 1964.

28 Lisse, K.: Ergebnisse der chirurgischen Behandlung und der Betatrontherapie des Vulvakarzinom, Zbl. Gynaek. 86:681-687, 1964.

29 Lithgow, D. M., and Farrell, A. G. W.: Vulval malignancy at Edendale Hospital from June, 1954 to July, 1963, S. Afr. Med. J. 38:186-191, 1964.

30 Lunin, A. B.: Carcinoma of the vulva, Amer. J. Obstet. Gynec. 57:742-747, 1949.

31 McGregor, I. A.: Skin grafting after radical vulvectomy, J. Obstet. Gynaec. Brit. Comm. 73:599-604, 1966.

32 McKelvey, J. L.: The treatment of carcinoma of the vulva, Amer. J. Obstet. Gynec. 54:626-633, 1947.

33 McKelvey, J. L., and Adcock, L. L.: Cancer of the vulva, Obstet. Gynec. 26:455-466, 1965.

34 Marshall, F. C., Uson, A. C., and Melicow, M. M.: Neoplasms and caruncles of the female urethra, Surg. Gynec. Obstet. 110:723-733, 1960.

35 Merrill, J. A., and Ross, N. L.: Cancer of the vulva, Cancer 14:13-20, 1961.

36 Mousseau, M., and Barbin, J.-Y.: Cancer de la vulve, Gaz. Med. France 2:2239-2248, 1966.

37 Novak, E., and Stevenson, R. R.: Sweat gland tumors of the vulva, benign (hidra-adenoma) and malignant (adenocarcinoma), Amer. J. Obstet. Gynec. 50:641-659, 1945.

38 Pack, G. T., and Oropeza, R.: A comparative study of melanomas and epidermoid carcinomas of the vulva, Rev. Surg. (Phila.) 24:305-324, 1967.

39 Palmer, J. P., Saducor, M. G., and Reinhard, M. C.: Carcinoma of the vulva, Surg. Gynec. Obstet. 88:435-440, 1949.

40 Parry-Jones, E. H. M.: Lymphatics of the vulva, J. Obstet. Gynaec. Brit. Comm. 70:751-765, 1963.

41 Rosser, E. ap I., and Hamlin, I. M. E.: Paget's disease of the vulva, J. Obstet. Gynaec. Brit. Emp. 64:127-130, 1957.

42 Rothman, D., and Gray, S. H.: Hidradenoma of the vulva, Amer. J. Obstet. Gynec. 38:509-514, 1939.

43 Rouvière, H.: Anatomie des lymphatiques de l'homme, Paris, 1932, Masson et Cie.

43a Rutledge, F., Smith, J. P., and Franklin, E. W.: Carcinoma of the vulva, Amer. J. Obstet. Gynec. 106:1117-1130, 1970.

44 Saltzstein, S. L., Woodruff, J. D., and Novak, E. R.: Postgranulomatous carcinoma of the vulva, Obstet. Gynec. 7:80-90, 1956.

45 Siegler, A. M., and Greene, H. J.: Basal-cell carcinoma of the vulva, Amer. J. Obstet. Gynec. 62:1219-1224, 1951.

46 Symmonds, R. E., Pratt, J. H., and Dockerty, M. B.: Melanoma of the vulva, Obstet. Gynec. 15:543-553, 1960.

47 Taussig, F. J.: Cancer of the vulva, Amer. J. Obstet. Gynec. 40:764-779, 1940.

48 Taussig, F. J.: Prevention of cancer of the vulva, Cancer Res. 1:901-904, 1941.

49 Ulfelder, H.: Radical vulvectomy with bilateral, inguinal, femoral and iliac node resection, Amer. J. Obstet. Gynec. 78:1074-1082, 1959.

50 Walker, L. M., and Huffman, J. W.: Adenocarcinoma of the female urethra; a review, Quart. Bull. Northwestern Univ. Med. Sch. 21:115-126, 1947.

51 Way, S.: The anatomy of the lymphatic drainage of the vulva and its influence on the radical operation for carcinoma, Ann. Roy. Coll. Surg. Eng. 3:187-209, 1948.

52 Way, S.: Carcinoma of the vulva, Amer. J. Obstet. Gynec. 79:692-697, 1960.

53 Way, S.: The late results of extended radical vulvectomy for carcinoma of the vulva, J. Obstet. Gynaec. Brit. Comm. 73:594-598, 1966.

54 Wilson, J. M.: Basal cell carcinoma of the vulva, Arch. Surg. (Chicago) 43:101-112, 1941.

55 Wilson, K. M.: Melanoma of the vulva with report of two cases, J. Mt. Sinai Hosp. 14:688-694, 1947.

56 Woodruff, J. D., and Baens, J. S.: Interpretations of atrophic and hypertrophic alterations in the vulvar epithelium, Amer. J. Obstet. Gynec. 86:713-723, 1963.

Chapter 15

Cancer of the mammary gland

Anatomy

The mammary glands lie directly over the pectoralis major muscles from the second to the sixth rib anteriorly and from the sternum to the anterior axillary line. Each gland is made up of twelve to twenty glandular lobes with a ramified duct. The ducts are irregular and tortuous and travel in the direction of the nipple dilating to form the ampullae and dividing into minute ducts that finally end in small openings in the nipple. The ducts and acini have two fibrous coverings: an inner periductal or periacinar layer and an outer layer, the perilobular connective tissue. The cells of the acini are cuboidal in shape, whereas those of the lactiferous ducts are columnar. The gland is encased in a layer of fat which allows its movement over the pectoral muscle (Fig. 625). Each gland appears as a hemisphere in the middle of which there is a salient papilla, the nipple, and a circular area of pigmented skin, the areola. Anteriorly, its convex surface is irregular due to the presence of salient fibrous crests. These crests form the deep attachment of fibrous septa (Cooper's ligaments), which run between the superficial and deep fascia. The superficial fascia is attached to the skin.

In men, the mammary glands remain in a functionless infantile state, neither useful nor esthetic. The gland is reduced in size with a nipple and areola of corresponding dimensions. Microscopically, there is a rudimentary gland containing short, narrow ducts but no well-developed acini.

Supernumerary breasts, with or without corresponding nipples, are observed in men and women. Most frequently, supernumerary glands are found below and medial to the normal breast, overlying the pectoralis major muscle at the anterior axillary line, or in the hollow of the axilla.

Lymphatics. The *lymphatics of the skin of the breast* form a dense network under the areola. This network is continuous with the lymphatics of the skin of the surrounding regions, forming an uninterrupted network over the entire surface of the chest, neck, and abdomen. Thus, the lymphatics of the skin of one breast communicate with the lymphatics of the skin of the opposite breast. In addition, some lymphatic trunks originating in the skin may cross the mid-

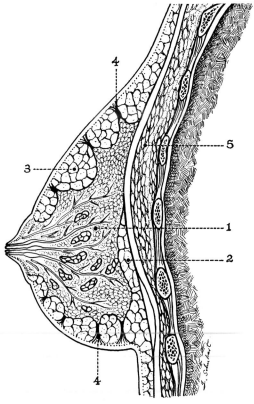

Fig. 625. Section of normal breast showing, 1, mammary gland; 2, retromammary fat; 3, superficial fat; 4, fibrous septa called Cooper's ligaments; 5, fat.

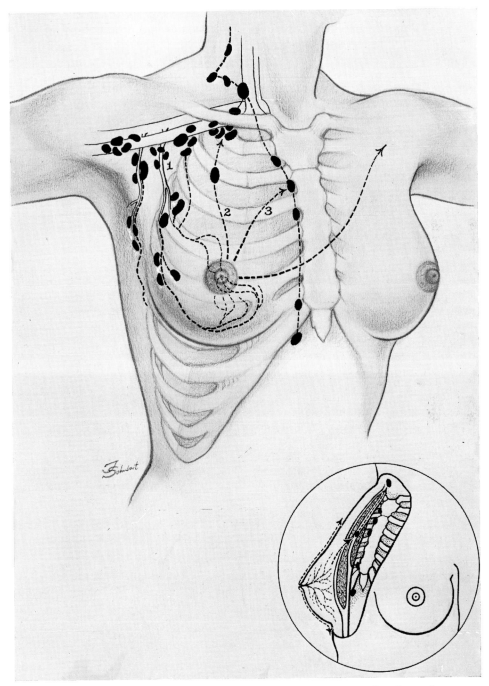

Fig. 626. Lymphatics of breast leading to axillary nodes which are distributed over large area from lateral aspects of breast proper to axillary vessels, 1; interpectoral chain leading to interpectoral node (Rotter's node: circle detail) and to high nodes in axilla, 2; internal mammary chain leading frequently to node in second interspace and to supraclavicular and cervical nodes, 3. Lymphatics of breast may empty into opposite axillary nodes.

line and drain into the axillary nodes of the opposite side (Oelsner[271]).

The *lymphatics of the mammary gland* rise from the interlobular or perilobular spaces. Some follow the ducts and end in the subareolar network of lymphatics of the skin, but the majority originate in the base of the breast and travel toward the axillary lymph nodes. Others end in the internal mammary chain, and still others end on the transverse cervical chain of lymph nodes (Rouvière[301]). The lymphatics of glandular origin may follow these pathways:

1   The *axillary* or *principal pathway* is formed by several trunks coming from the upper and lower half of the gland, passing through the fascia, and ending in the lateral mammary chain of nodes situated between the second and third intercostal spaces. Some of these lymphatics, however, do not stop in these nodes but follow directly to the group of nodes of the axillary vein or to a central group of nodes in the axilla (Fig. 626).

2   The *transpectoral pathway* is formed by the lymphatics that pass through the pectoralis major muscle with the branches of the lateral thoracic artery and end in the supraclavicular lymph nodes. Some of these may follow the inferior borders of the pectoralis major muscle and ascend directly to the infraclavicular lymph nodes behind the pectoralis minor muscle or between the two pectoral muscles. In this last instance, they may be interrupted by a few interpectoral lymph nodes.

3   The *internal mammary pathway* runs toward the midline, passes through the pectoralis major and the intercostal muscles, usually close to the sternum, and ends in the nodes of the internal mammary chain. The latter chain lies deep to the plane of the costal cartilages, winding around the internal mammary blood vessels. Lymph nodes are usually present opposite the first, second, third, and sixth intercostal spaces. In addition to these nodes, there are frequently (in this network) many smaller ones composed of only a few follicles (Stibbe[329]). The internal mammary chain usually communicates with a single lymph node situated just above the medial end of the clavicle and closely related to the great veins. An important lymph node terminus is at the confluence of the internal jugular and supraclavicular veins. If tumor involves the sentinel node at the confluence, retrograde spread takes place to involve the supraclavicular nodes (McDonald et al.[230]).

The lymphatics originating in the mammary gland also follow an anterolateral pathway (Rouvière[301]) and end in the lymph nodes of the opposite axilla. Grant et al.[121] emphasized the surgical significance of the subareolar plexus, for the interlobular and interductal lymphatics drain to this plexus. This plexus communicates between the parenchymal, cutaneous, and fascial groups of lymphatics.

Epidemiology

Carcinoma of the breast is the most common form of cancer occurring in white women over 40 years of age in the United States. In the 1947 cancer survey in the United States, the sex-age adjusted incidence rate was 53.9 for nonwhites and 72.6 for whites per 100,000 females. The rate for women 35 to 39 years of age in the state of New York is 42.3 and rises grad-

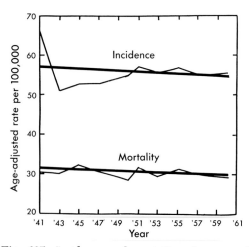

Fig. 627. Incidence and mortality of cancer of breast, New York exclusive of New York City, 1941-1960. (From Shimkin, M. B.: End results in cancer of the breast, Cancer **20**:1039-1043, 1967; partly based on data from Shimkin, M. B.: Cancer of the breast; some old facts and new prospectives, J.A.M.A. **183**:358-361, 1963.)

ually to 365.5 in women 80 to 84 years old; this incidence rate has remained rather constant for the past thirty years (Fig. 627). This form of cancer very rarely occurs in children. McDivitt and Stewart[226] reported seven cases in children 3 to 15 years of age. It is rarely found in women under the age of 25 years. The proportion of women with cancer of the breast in each age group shows a progressive rise with each age group and then a decline after 60 years of age (Fig. 628), but the same number of cases plotted against the total population in each age group shows a continued increase up to the age group 80 to 89 years (Berkson et al.[28]).

The relative occurrence of mammary cancer is greater among single, divorced, and widowed than among married women. It has been suggested that the occurrence of cancer of the breast is inversely proportional to fertility (Smithers et al.[319]; Stocks[330]). In the Netherlands, there has been a decrease in fertility and a definite increase in the incidence of cancer of the breast, but, some populations have shown a simultaneous increase in fertility and in cancer of the breast (MacMahon[233]). "Age at first pregnancy is a significant factor in breast cancer risk. *Women who have their first child prior to the age of 20 have only about one-third of the breast cancer risk of women whose first birth is delayed until 35 years or older.*"* The relative levels of the individual estrogen fractions produced in the first decade after puberty are possibly important determinants in a women's lifetime breast cancer risk (Cole and Mac-Mahon[66]). The hypothesis is advanced by Lemon[213] that estriol plays a significant anticarcinogenic role in the human female, accounting in part for the reduced expectancy of mammary cancer in women with multiple pregnancies in their early child-bearing years. A woman who has suffered from carcinoma of the breast has a greater than average chance of developing carcinoma of the remaining breast (Robbins and Berg[299]).

Versluys[356] believes that a comparison of incidence rates between countries or re-

*From MacMahon, B., et al.: Age at first birth and breast cancer risk, Bull. W.H.O (in press).

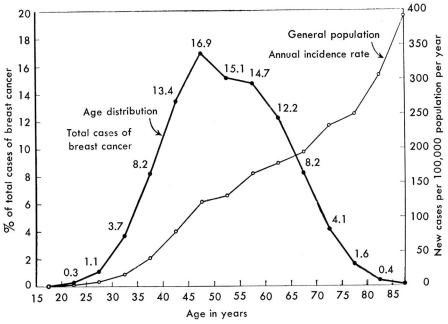

Fig. 628. Age distribution of total cases of cancer of breast (scale on left) and annual incidence rate for general population (scale on right). Annual incidence rate rises correspondingly with age. (From Berkson, J., et al.: Mortality and survival in surgically treated cancer of the breast: a statistical summary of some experience of the Mayo Clinic, Proc. Staff Meet. Mayo Clin. **32:**645-674, 1957.)

gions is acceptable only if observed in single women, for otherwise it must take into consideration the differences in fertility. The lesser incidence in the fertile has been attributed to the suppression during pregnancy of the mammary cellular changes during each menstrual cycle (Macklin[243]) or to the protection afforded by repeated periods of lactation. A history of abnormal lactation is often given by mothers with cancer of the breast (Regato[296]). A comparison has shown a greater proportion of women with premenstrual engorgement and a shorter duration of breast feeding of their babies among women with cancer of the breast than among others (Schwartz et al.[308]). A low incidence of cancer of the breast among Japanese women has been attributed to the habit of prolonged lactation of their children, but this has been shown to be incorrect. The incidence among immigrant Japanese in the United States and among Japanese-Americans shows no apparent tendency to rise to the host country levels. The different lactating habits among American women, as well as the prolonged use of estrogens, have no demonstrable effects on incidence rates (Shimkin[312]). In Egypt, the incidence of cancer of the breast is several times greater than that of cancer of the cervix, although women lactate their babies for two or more years. In India, the reported frequency of cancer of the breast is three times greater among Parsi women, who usually marry early, than among Hindus and Moslems (Paymaster[286]). Cancer of the breast is found more frequently in women of higher than average economic position (Kennaway[189]; Clemmesen and Nielsen[64]), a fact attributed to lesser fertility or greater longevity of this group. An apparent relative decrease along the age occurrence curves is observed between 48 and 52 years of age (Clemmesen and Nielsen[64]). Wagoner et al.[361] and de Waard et al.[360] emphasize the bimodal distribution of mammary cancer patients (Fig. 629). They believe that the type associated with hypertension is probably influenced by heredity.

Bucalossi and Veronessi[45] studied the families of eighty-one patients with cancer of the breast whose mothers also had mammary cancer and found, among their sisters,

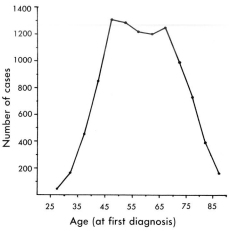

Fig. 629. Age distribution of 10,047 women with mammary carcinoma registered by the Central Cancer Registry, Amsterdam, during 1954-1960. Number of cases registered annually has increased from 891 cases in 1954 to 1811 in 1960. It is estimated that about 70% of cases diagnosed in the Netherlands during 1960 have been registered. (From de Waard, F., et al.: The bimodal age distribution of patients with mammary carcinoma, Cancer 17:141-151, 1964; data courtesy Dr. L. Meinsma, Amsterdam, The Netherlands.)

an occurrence fifteen times greater than in the general population. A similar finding has been reported by others, particularly in the unmarried female relatives of mammary cancer patients. The tumors seem to occur at an earlier age among the descendants (Papadrianos et al.[276]). Wood and Darling[378] reported a family in which several members developed bilateral carcinoma of the breast, one of them an 18-year-old girl and three in the same generation. We have observed the family of a woman who had cancer of the breast at the age of 47 years. Three of her daughters* presented cancer of the breast when 40, 43, and 47 years of age and another daughter† had cancer of the ovary when 49 years of age. A fifth daughter,‡ now 62 years of age, is apparently in good health, but one of her own daughters§ has already developed carcinoma of the ovary at the age of 41. There were also four sons who are now 53, 57, 60, and 70 years of age and in good health (in 1970). None of

*PCH 53-194, PCH 53-367, and PCH 53-839.
†PCH 53-1027.
‡PCH 54-889.
§PCH 70-657.

these patients was obese or hypertensive, and all had children. These family occurrences cannot be attributed to bias selection, to lesser fertility of the families, or to environment, for the excess is larger than accountable by these factors.

MacMahon and Feinleib[236] reported the relative rarity of carcinoma of the breast among women who had undergone an oophorectomy. As a result of the experimental demonstration of the carcinogenic effect of estrogens in lower animals, a great deal has been said on the subject of the possible injudicious clinical use of estrogens and their potential for carcinogenesis in women. There are few cases in the medical literature that would support such a thesis (Auchincloss and Haagenson[17]; Parsons and McCall[279]). It is perhaps prudent to avoid the use of estrogens in women with a family history of cancer of the breast. Goldenberg et al.[119] reported prominent epithelial proliferation in fibroadenomas of patients taking oral contraceptives, but Fechner[100a] could not support this. It remains to be seen whether the wide use of oral contraceptives will alter the incidence of mammary carcinoma.

Chalstrey and Benjamin[58] reported a high frequency of carcinoma of the breast among women treated for carcinoma of the thyroid gland. Mackenzie[231] reported fifty cases of carcinoma of the breast in women who had previously been treated for tuberculosis and he speculated on the possible role of repeated fluoroscopies as a cause of cancer of the breast. Berg et al.[26] found seven carcinomas of the breast among 396 patients with malignant tumors of the salivary glands. A greater than expected occurrence of carcinoma of the breast and of the endometrium in the same patient has been noted (MacMahon and Austin[234]).

There is about one case of cancer of the male breast for every 100 in women. The age distribution is almost identical except for a larger relative proportion among elderly males. Cancer of the male breast may be associated with gynecomastia (Liechty et al.[219]), and there may be frequently a history of benign breast disease, orchitis, or orchiectomy (Lilienfeld[221]). Symmers[332] reported two cases of carcinoma of the breast in men who had submitted to castration and penectomy and who sought to change their secondary sex characteristics by prolonged use of hormones.

Sarcomas make up between 0.5% and 3% of all malignant tumors of the breast. They occur at any age but predominantly in the fifth decade of life.

The relationship of *chronic cystic disease* and cancer of the breast continues to be debated. In the first place, there is no generally accepted histopathologic criteria of chronic cystic disease. Second, there is discrepancy (Frantz et al.[110]) between the clinical occurrence of cystic disease (18%) and the microscopic evidence (52%). Third, the reported proportion of specimens showing both conditions concomitantly varies with the authors (Semb[311]). However, it is certain that the frequency of microscopically observed cystic disease is greater in the cancerous than in the noncancerous breast. Both conditions are rare in Japanese women (Strode[331]). Fourth, histologic evidence that a malignant lesion arises from a benign one is lacking. Bonser et al.[39] believe that there is a relationship between cystic disease, epithelial proliferation, and carcinoma. Foote and Stewart[107] have seen carcinoma arising in duct papillomatosis, in single and in multiple cysts, in blunt duct adenosis, and in apocrine epithelium. McDivitt et al.[228] have reported twenty-six cases of carcinoma of the breast arising from *fibroadenomas*. In summary, there is no doubt that carcinoma is accompanied by proliferative lesions of the breast in greater proportion than normally expected and that infrequently the benign lesions seem to be the point of departure of carcinoma (Davis et al.[81]).

Pathology
Gross and microscopic pathology

It is of utmost importance that the surgical specimen of a radical mastectomy be so sectioned and so studied that, when the examination is completed, the extent of the tumor, the character of its local invasion, and the distribution of its metastases (and thereby its prognosis) are known. The specimen should be oriented, the tumor located, and the condition of the nipple noted, as well as the presence or absence of ulceration and edema of the skin overlying the tumor. Dissection should start with the nipple, using care to ascertain whether or not the main ducts are dilated and whether or not tumor is arising from or involving that area. The primary tumor should be measured in three dimensions and its relation to skin, nipple, pectoral fascia, and quadrants of the breast given. Step sections should be made of the tumor, including the overlying skin, and the individual characteristics should be observed. Other sections should be made of the transition points between apparently uninvolved breast tissue and the diseased area. If the tumor arises in proximity to the nipple or has extended to involve the pectoral fascia, appropriate sections of these areas should be selected. Multiple sections should be taken from the other three quadrants of the breast where the parenchyma is most prominent.

At the time of operation, the high point of the axilla should be tagged. Later, at gross examination, this will facilitate division of the axilla into high, mid, and low portions. Lymph nodes obtained from these areas should be kept separately so that the extent of axillary involvement can be ascertained microscopically. Rotter's nodes located between the pectoral muscles should always be looked for, since they may be the only ones involved (Kay[186]). In our experience, nodes are most easily found by palpating small amounts of axillary fat against a strong light. By this means, nodes only 5 mm in diameter may be seen as fairly distinct gray nodules well delineated against the translucent background.

All nodes must be sectioned. If examination of the axilla is rushed, only a small fraction of the existing nodes will be found. We have seen numerous instances in which only one of twenty-five or thirty nodes was involved by carcinoma, but these cases were and should be classified as having axillary involvement. An average of between twenty and thirty nodes should be found in every axillary specimen. As many as eighty nodes have been studied in one case. *Incomplete examination of the axillary area after radical mastectomy is probably one of the main reasons why statistics on this subject vary so greatly.* Although this search for nodes is time consuming, the information so obtained is valuable enough to warrant it.

The gross appearance of the nodes varies with the presence or absence of tumor and of inflammation. If the nodes are negative with no inflammation, they are often small, soft, and consequently difficult to find. On section, they are homogeneous and gray in color and infrequently give cause for error. When the primary tumor is ulcerated and inflamed, then the axillary nodes are enlarged and hard, even though they may not contain carcinoma. Sharply delineated grayish yellow areas within nodes almost certainly represent metastatic carcinoma.

In the past, certain proliferative lesions of chronic cystic disease, such as sclerosing adenosis and intraductal papilloma, were erroneously diagnosed as carcinoma. In consequence, clinicians have questioned the reliability of the pathologist's diagnosis of early carcinomas in the absence of metastases. The study made by Linden et al.[222] showed a high degree of accuracy in the diagnosis of practicing pathologists. With a series of consecutive breast lesions, we have been able to verify the fact that the accuracy of diagnoses varies with the pathologists and their background of experience. Pathologists with incomplete training or not particularly interested in surgical pathology show a low degree of accuracy, whereas those skilled in surgical pathology were in about 98% agreement.

There are some special problems to be faced in the histopathologic examination of surgical specimens of breast tumors. A crucial one is the appreciation of *effects of irradiation.* A heavy irradiation followed shortly by surgical excision may not permit appreciation of the full effects of radiations or of the eventual destruction of the tumor. The viability of irradiated tumor cells cannot be predicted histologically. Depending on the radiosensitivity, thoroughness of the irradiation, and interval allowed before excision, the changes observed may vary considerably. Bone metastases that are clinically and radiographically benefited by radiotherapy may be found to contain residual tumor, but much of such palliative treatment is not aimed at sterilization of the tumor. We have been convinced that adequate irradiation is capable of sterilizing primary and metastatic carcinoma of the breast in proved cases. Pathologists have also been concerned with the response of carcinoma of the breast to *hormone therapy*. The hormone dependence of mammary carcinomas is not identified with any histopathologic type. Emerson et al.[98] found that tumors with low or median degree of malignancy have a greater chance of response than highly malignant tumors. The study of the noncancerous tissue of the breast is not helpful in determining response. In patients who do respond to hormone therapy, there are objective histologic changes that are rather similar to the effects of irradiation: dissolution and death of cells, fibrosis, and often an increase of elastic tissue. In order to learn something of the possible relationship of cancer of the breast to the endocrine glands, Sommers[322] examined 207 women who died of mammary cancer and 248 others for control. He found a disproportionately greater number of cases of hyperplasia of the ovarian stroma, adrenal cortex, endometrium, pituitary amphophils and basophils, and uninvolved breast epithelium among the women who died of cancer of the breast.

A high percentage of carcinomas of the breast arise from duct epithelium. In many cases the tumor is advanced, and consequently the exact histogenesis is obscured. The form that a carcinoma takes depends largely on whether the tumor arises from duct or terminal duct epithelium, whether it is confined to the ducts by dense connective tissue, whether it produces large amounts of mucin, or whether it has some specific pattern. The tumor may remain localized in the ducts for months or even years, depending on the ability of the connective and elastic tissue to prevent spread into the breast parenchyma. In patients in the older age groups, in whom atrophy of the breast parenchyma has taken place, the tumor arises from duct epithelium. In those in the younger age groups, in whom acinar tissue is prominent and in whom the tumor is more frequently undifferentiated, the neoplasm can arise from acinar epithelium or terminal duct epithelium and spread quickly over a wide area. The tumor also grows rapidly during pregnancy and lactation because of increased vascularization and perhaps also because of other unknown factors, possibly hormonal in nature. Simultaneous involvement of both breasts with apparent multiple foci of origin can occur in pregnancy, as shown by Siegmund.[315]

It is important to divide breast carcinomas into different types. If these types can be identified, then some statement can be made of the probable extent of the lymph node metastases and thereby prognosis and treatment. We have somewhat modified Törnberg's classification of mammary carcinoma as follows:

Type I—Nonmetastasizing (not invasive)

1 Intraductal (comedo) carcinoma without stromal invasion

When this type of neoplasm affects the epithelium of the nipple, the signs of Paget's disease of the breast may exist. It would also include papillary cancer and lobular carcinoma without evidence of invasion.

Type II—Rarely metastasizing (always invasive)

1 Pure extracellular mucinous or colloid carcinomas

These are recognized easily. They are seen to be circumscribed, are homogenously gelatinous, are soft, and have a gray to reddish brown color. The mucin is always extracellular.

2 Medullary carcinomas with lymphocytic infiltration

These have sharply delimited margins, are uniformly soft, have a light gray color, and may contain small focal necroses. Lymphocytic infiltration is prominent. Medullary carcinomas may be mistaken grossly for fibroadenoma.

3 Well-differentiated adenocarcinomas (Fig. 630)

Microscopically, these tumors have discretely circumscribed borders and are highly and uniformly cellularly differentiated. They would include papillary carcinomas extending outside of the ducts.

Type III—Moderately metastasizing (always invasive)

1 Adenocarcinoma

2 Intraductal carcinoma with stromal invasion

Actually, all carcinomas not definitely

classified as Type I, II, or IV constitute Type III.

Type IV—Highly metastasizing (always invasive)

1 Undifferentiated carcinoma

The undifferentiated carcinomas having cells without ductal or tubular arrangement and without cellular inflammatory response about them *and all types of tumors indisputably invading blood vessels.*

The differentiation of mammary cancer into these types can be made solely from properly prepared and selected "permanent" tissue sections of the primary tumor. In fact, the differentiation of the first two types (I and II) from the last two (III and IV) can be effected with a high degree of certainty by visual examination and from *frozen sections.*

This typing of breast cancer is based on grading. Grading of breast cancer has been done by Haagensen,[139] Bloom,[35] Gricouroff,[124] and Törnberg.[343] There have been a number of papers on the importance of a pushing border as compared to an infiltrating border in the cancer (Lane et al.[207]), and Berg[25] emphasized the degenerative changes in the neoplasm at the point of contact between the infiltrating cancer and normal tissue. He also emphasized that a plasma cellular reaction is a favorable sign. In the grading of carcinomas that are not of a specific type (medullary cancer, Paget's disease, etc.), the most important factors are the ability of the tumor to form a well-defined glandular structure (Fig. 630) and the tendency of the cancer to diffuse unrestrained growth. Törnberg[343] also listed the delimitation of the cancer, degree of peripheral infiltration (mainly lymphocytes and plasma cells), degree of cellular and nuclear polymorphism, and frequency of mitoses. Grading is done on the basis of the changes in the border. Only three grades are used, and in Törnberg's grading, Grade I comprised approximately 10%; Grade II, 50%; and Grade III, 40% (Hultborn and Törnberg[174]).

In the common type of carcinoma of the breast, the findings on section may be somewhat variable. If the tumor is soft and cellular with little stroma, then areas of re-

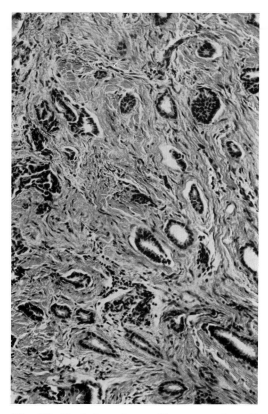

Fig. 630. Grade I carcinoma. Note extremely well-differentiated glands in tumor with pushing borders. (×140; WU neg. 59-7302A.)

cent and old hemorrhage may be present. Much more frequently, however, the tumor is hard with poorly defined, chalky yellow areas seen against the dense background of almost cartilaginous stroma. In fact, if the tumor has been present for many years, areas of calcification may be present. Not infrequently, there are areas of chronic cystic disease either intimately associated with, or distinct from, the tumor. Such changes are more common in the young patients. The reported proportion of associated chronic cystic disease and carcinoma varies with the liberality of the pathologist in his diagnosis of such lesions. If lesions due to degenerative phenomena and also obvious lesions that have not been shown to bear any relation to cancer, such as fat necrosis, fibrosis, or periductal mastitis, are omitted, then the frequency of association drops sharply. Foote and Stewart[107] studied 300 cases of mammary carcinoma and found 59% associated with at least one of five proliferative changes (cysts, duct papillomatosis, blunt duct adenosis, sclerosing adenosis, apocrine epithelium), 35% with two or more, and 17% with three or more of these changes.

Within the breast, the carcinoma spreads with a variable rate of growth. With increase in size, ramifying fingers of tumor extend out into the breast parenchyma. The main tumor mass may enlarge to involve the skin, which becomes thin and taut and finally ulcerates. The tumor may also extend downward to the pectoral fascia which, for a time, restrains its extension. After growth through the pectoral fascia, the tumor becomes fixed, and further extension may involve the pectoral muscles. In advanced disease, when the tumor approximates the axilla, it may directly invade it, and the tumor and axillary masses become continuous and fixed.

The microscopic appearance of carcinoma of the breast of the most common type can vary considerably. In many instances, the duct origin can be traced. The cellular nature of the tumor often varies in different areas. In the large tumors, zones of necrosis and hemorrhage are common. The amount of connective tissue stroma present is extremely variable, and on the age of this connective tissue will depend its relative cellularity. Of considerable importance is how the tumor appears under low power. It is important to note whether the lesion has a circumscribed or an infiltrating border. The well-differentiated lesions have a fairly orderly pattern with a tendency toward adenoid formation. The undifferentiated carcinomas have an extremely disorderly pattern, marked variation in cell size and shape, and innumerable mitotic figures, many of which are abnormal.

In *Paget's disease,* there is a weeping eczematoid lesion involving the nipple, areola, and occasionally a large area of contiguous skin. On section, definite carcinoma is found directly beneath the nipple. The disease is often poorly circumscribed but very hard because of increased connective tissue. The tumor has chalky yellow streaks and is usually confined to the ducts.

The microscopic examination always shows the presence of intraductal carcinoma. Muir[258] reported that intraductal carcinoma was present in the nipple alone in all of his thirty-nine patients and in the breast and nipple in thirty-four and was accompanied by infiltrating carcinoma of the breast in thirty. Cells present in the ducts are also present in the overlying epidermis (Fig. 631). These cells are malignant, arise from duct epithelium, and directly invade the nipple. This invasion of the contiguous epithelium is what gives the clinical appearance of Paget's disease (Fig. 641). Spread to the overlying skin probably occurs because of the migration of these cells. If enough sections are made, communication between duct carcinoma and tumor cells growing in the overlying epithelium can always be demonstrated. Carcinoma arises within the ducts and invades the nipple rather than the reverse. In several of our cases, a specific stain showed epithelial mucin in the tumor cells within the ducts and in the tumor cells within the overlying epidermis (Neubecker and Bradshaw[261]). This supports the concept of the origin of this tumor from the underlying duct epithelium and is further evidence against the theory that Paget's disease may arise independently from the overlying epidermis.

Intraductal (comedo) carcinoma is often large, rarely ulcerates through the skin, and is accompanied by evidence of infection. On cut section, the tumor shows well-delineated plugs of carcinoma within dilated ducts (Fig. 632). However, these plugs may spread diffusely and give an impression of irregular nodularity in the breast. On compressing the breast, wormlike masses of tumor can be extruded from the involved ducts. In a few isolated areas, invasion of the surrounding breast tissue may have occurred. The intraductal carcinoma usually shows well-differentiated tumor cells confined to the ducts. Focal calcification and dilatation of the ducts is common; these changes can be seen by mammography (Wolfe[376]). It is not infrequent for these ducts to be greatly distended by the tumor, and it is common to see considerable thickening of their walls (Fig. 633). This thickening is due to connective tissue production, and elastic tissue stains often show very large amounts of it. This particular quality of the intraductal

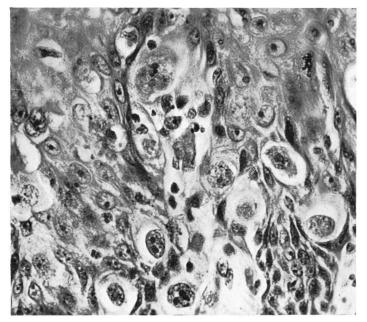

Fig. 631. Large so-called Paget cells with clear cytoplasm in overlying epithelium. (High-power enlargement.)

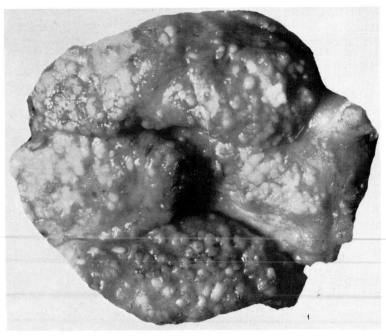

Fig. 632. Intraductal (comedo) carcinoma of breast. Note nodular, comedo-like rings of carcinoma within ducts.

carcinoma is unexplained, but the tendency of the connective and elastic tissues to wall in the tumor no doubt explains its gross and microscopic appearance. Breakthrough occurs in some of these tumors, and a typical infiltrating carcinoma of duct-epithelial origin is observed.

Papillary carcinomas do not arise from preexisting intraductal papillomas and usually present well-delineated cystic masses. Such areas may be multiple within the breast. On section, areas of hemorrhage are often present. The tumors may transgress the wall of the cyst and may grow over a wide area within the breast parenchyma. Multiple foci of origin may be present. These tumors are malignant from the start rather than arising from a preexisting intraductal papilloma. The papillary carcinoma is made up of papillary projections with layering of the epithelium, associated hemorrhage, increased vascularity, and growth of the tumor through the surrounding, often thick, connective tissue walls.

Lobular carcinomas are infrequent, often forming a diffuse mass within the breast. Lobular carcinoma in situ is concentrated in the upper quadrants beneath the areolar periphery (Lambird and Shelley[206]). At times, it is difficult to see any abnormality except what appears to be very large lobules. There are no chalky streaks present. After infiltration develops, it assumes the characteristics of any mammary carcinoma (Foote and Stewart[106]). The lobular carcinoma follows a distinct pattern. In a lobule or in a group of lobules, there may be increased numbers of cells with a disorderly pattern and usually with a few mitoses. Occasionally, there are small zones of necrosis and, as the process continues, more and more lobules become involved until microscopically there is invasion of the parenchyma (Fig. 634). It apparently has multiple foci of origin. Lobular carcinoma in situ has a cumulative risk of invasion which reaches 35% after twenty years (McDivitt et al.[225]).

The *mucinous carcinoma* is usually quite

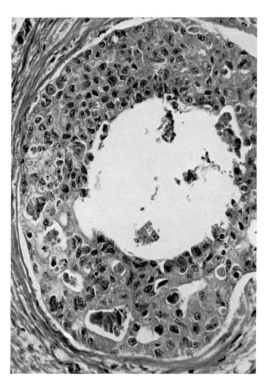

Fig. 633. Intraductal (comedo) carcinoma of breast showing variations in size and shape of cells with thick-walled duct and central necrosis.

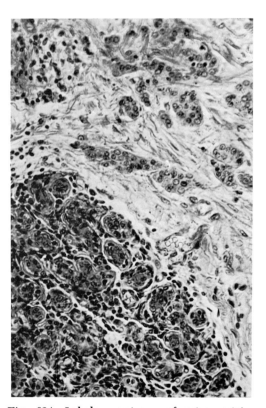

Fig. 634. Lobular carcinoma of acinar origin. Note tumor growing around prominent lobule.

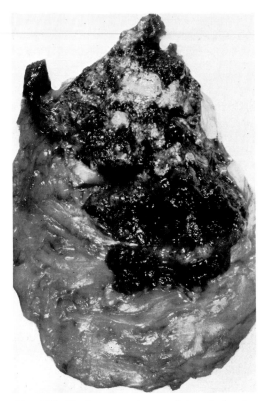

Fig. 635. Mucinous carcinoma of breast showing gelatinous-like quality and sharply delimited margins.

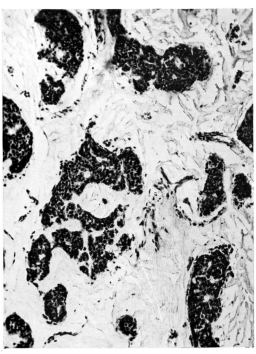

Fig. 636. Mucinous carcinoma of breast. "Nests of tumor cells floating in a sea of mucus." Individual cells are well differentiated.

large when first seen. On palpation, it feels somewhat cystic. On section, it frequently appears circumscribed and encapsulated. The mucin may dominate the gross appearance, and it may have a currant jelly, gelatinous, glistening, glary appearance (Fig. 635). This may be patchy in distribution or may cover the whole surface. The tumor varies in color from purple to reddish brown to gray. The amount of mucin present in different stages of the carcinoma is variable. Not too infrequently, only small nests of cells are present in large masses of acellular mucin (Fig. 636). The mucin is a product of the cell rather than of the stroma, for it is present in the metastases to lymph nodes. Electron microscopy demonstrates that the mucin is produced by the cells of the tumor (Tellem et al.[338]). Mucin may distend the cells so that they have a signet-ring appearance similar to that seen in some carcinomas of

the stomach. When this appearance is present, growth is very rapid. This rare type usually shows well-preserved, mucin-secreting cells (Saphir[303a]). The incidence of lymph node metastases is low, somewhat comparable to medullary carcinoma (Norris and Taylor[266]).

Moore and Foote[254] described a variant of mammary carcinoma which they designate as *medullary carcinoma*. This tumor often suggests a fibroadenoma on clinical examination and grossly may be so diagnosed because of its apparent encapsulation. Close inspection of its cut surface usually shows small areas of necrosis. These tumors may be small but can measure up to 8 cm or more. Microscopically, they are made up of anastomosing nests of tumor cells with large nuclei, delicate cytoplasm, and numerous mitotic figures (Fig. 637). A lymphoid infiltrate is common. It has sharp borders.

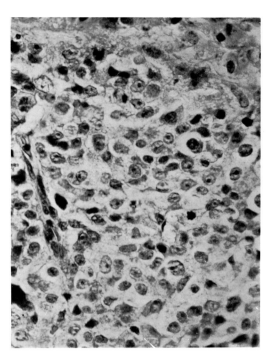

Fig. 637. Medullary carcinoma of breast of circumscribed type. Only one of thirteen nodes was found invaded. (High power.)

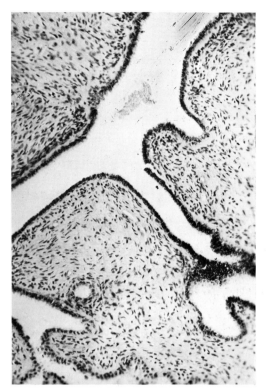

Fig. 638. Giant cystosarcoma phyllodes (benign pattern). (From Cooper, W. G., Jr., and Ackerman, L. V.: Cystosarcoma phylloides, with a consideration of its more malignant variant, Surg. Gynec. Obstet. **77:**279-283, 1943; by permission of Surgery, Gynecology & Obstetrics.)

The acute or *inflammatory carcinoma* invariably shows a diffuse edema of the overlying skin much larger than the localized tumor. Ulceration is practically never present. Frequently the tumor is fairly diffuse within the breast parenchyma. The axillary nodes are invariably involved. This type of carcinoma is usually extremely undifferentiated, often associated with inflammatory cells. Most important, however, there is usually widespread involvement of the subdermal lymphatics together with hyperemia of the subpapillary plexus. These changes account for the edema and erythema of the overlying skin.

Epidermoid carcinoma is rare and is usually far advanced when first seen. When it does occur it is frequently found in a black patient. On section, the tumor usually gives evidence of origin from duct epithelium. An epidermoid carcinoma arising from duct epithelium is a pathologic curiosity. We have seen only two cases in 413 consecutive breast carcinomas. The gradual metaplasia of this epithelium to well-differentiated squamous epithelium can usually be traced. The tumor has the histologic appearance of a squamous carcinoma, forms epithelial pearls and intercellular bridges, and has the characteristics of epidermoid carcinomas elsewhere.

Adenoid cystic cancer of the breast is an extremely rare lesion, and we have not seen it metastasize. If recognized at frozen section, probably it could be treated by adequate local excision. At a seminar at which approximately one thousand pathologists were present, about twenty-five instances of this type of tumor had been seen, and in no instance was there regional lymph node involvement. Metastases have been reported (Wilson and Spell[374]; Cavanzo and Taylor[57a]).

Sarcomas of the breast are of two main

varieties, the most common arising in the form of a pericanalicular or intracanalicular adenofibroma and the other arising from the interlobar and interlobular fibrous tissue. The first variant, designated as *cystosarcoma phyllodes,* usually becomes very large. On section, it may present a frond-like appearance with numerous clefts, cyst-like spaces, zones of hemorrhage, and mucinous degeneration (Fig. 638). The cystosarcoma phyllodes usually remains well localized but, after many months of growth, can eventually rupture through the skin and, on rare occasion, may invade the underlying muscle. The epithelial elements play only a passive role. In the malignant variant, the stroma shows all the changes of a sarcoma. The earliest change is in the subepithelial stromal tissue.

The *fibrosarcomas* are usually well circumscribed, firm, and grayish white and

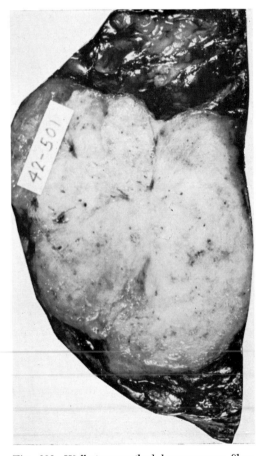

Fig. 639. Well-circumscribed homogeneous fibrosarcoma of breast.

often reveal zones of necrosis and hemorrhage (Fig. 639). These sarcomas do not, as a rule, cause nipple retraction or skin involvement. The fibrosarcoma has a much greater tendency toward local invasive growth. The typical fibrosarcoma arising from connective tissue shows cells varying from well differentiated to extremely undifferentiated, and tumor giant cells are often present. These sarcomas may show cartilage or bone and for that reason are called chondrosarcomas or osteosarcomas, but there is no justification for such a nomenclature. The connective tissue is the primary source of the tumor.

Sarcomas arising from other components of breast tissue are pathologic curiosities. Liposarcoma (Stewart[327]), lymphosarcoma (Harrington and Miller[158]), myosarcoma, and angiosarcoma are rarely encountered (Hill and Stout[168]). Lymphangiosarcoma can occur as a complication of prolonged postmastectomy lymphedema (Stewart and Treves[328]). The time interval from edema to the development of the sarcoma is variable. It is manifested early by the presence of small, elevated, pink subcutaneous nodules. Microscopically, these nodules may be difficult to diagnose as lymphangiosarcoma (McSwain and Stephenson[237]). Lymphosarcomas may occur within the breast as a part of the generalized process, or they may be localized within the breast parenchyma. Melanocarcinomas in the breast are undoubtedly not primary but occur either as metastases or as an extension from a melanocarcinoma arising in the overlying epithelium. Hodgkin's disease of the breast has been reported.

Metastatic spread

Involvement of the axilla by carcinoma of the breast develops in three stages: first, tumor reaches the axillary lymph nodes by emboli and gradually fills up a node or nodes; second, it breaks through the capsule of these involved nodes and begins growing in the loose fat of the axilla; and finally, tumor in the axilla becomes so advanced that fixation occurs (Fig. 640). With growth out into the loose fat, the tumor then has an opportunity to involve contiguous veins. At times, the metastases to the axilla are restricted to a single large node that may even reach a diameter of

5 cm. In relatively few instances, the axillary node groups will be bypassed, and the first nodes involved will be those of the infraclavicular or supraclavicular areas. It is also not too rare for the nodes of the anterior mediastinum or even the opposite axilla to be involved. These metastatic lesions occur particularly from tumors located in the inner quadrants of the breast and from those with axillary metastases. Vogt-Hoerner and Contesso[358] found metastases in the Rotter group of interpectoral nodes in 12% of 530 specimens of radical mastectomy. These nodes are seldom found invaded in the absence of axillary or internal mammary metastases.

After regional lymph node involvement, the lungs and pleura are commonly implicated. Tumor spreads directly to the pleura through the lymphatics that travel by the internal mammary chain. With pleural involvement, the lymphatics are widely invaded, and this process takes on all the characteristics of lymphangitic metastases. The liver and bones may also become involved. The dorsal spine may even be involved without lung metastases because of spread through the vertebral vein plexus. Metastases to the sternum may take place by direct venous extension or

through the internal mammary lymphatics. These metastases within the vertebrae, pelvis, and skull (sites of predilection) are almost invariably osteolytic in type. Involvement of other organs such as the suprarenal glands, ovaries, and spleen is not unusual. Gurling et al.[130] reported a surprisingly high proportion (eleven of forty-four) of pituitary metastases in patients subject to hypophysectomy for advanced carcinoma of the breast. The anterior lobe was more often involved than the posterior lobe, and the metastases had not been betrayed by any symptoms, except very rarely. Lumb and Mackenzie[223] reported ninety-two cases of adrenal metastases (39%) in 235 adrenalectomy specimens and fifty-six metastases to the ovary (29%) in 190 oophorectomy specimens.

Cystosarcomas of the breast only rarely metastasize to the axillary lymph nodes (Cooper and Ackerman[68]). Postoperative recurrences of cystosarcoma phyllodes may involve the chest wall and spread to the pleura and lung. *Liposarcomas* of the breast may metastasize to regional lymph nodes (Stewart[327]). *Fibrosarcomas*, however, metastasize, much more commonly, particularly to lungs, liver, and brain.

Clinical evolution

There are few early symptoms of carcinoma of the breast. The most important single presenting sign is a lump, usually painless. Infrequently, the first symptom is a large mass in the axilla or a sensation of heaviness in the breast, or there may be pain due to metastases to the vertebrae (Table 95).

The rate of growth of breast tumors is extremely variable. As the tumor increases, local pain, edema of the skin, and satellite skin nodules may appear, though at very variable intervals. Ulceration, secondary infection, and hemorrhage may also result. When axillary metastases are present and the nodes have become fixed, edema of the arm may occur. Pain in the thoracic cage, dorsolumbar spine, or hips is usually due to bone metastases in those areas and usually precedes the radiographic demonstration of such lesions. Cough, pleurisy, and dyspnea may be symptoms of hydrothorax due to pulmonary and mediastinal

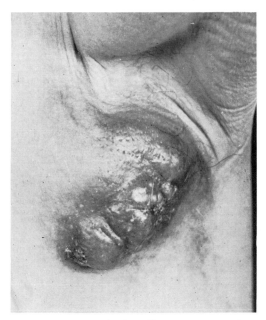

Fig. 640. Large fixed axillary metastases from carcinoma of breast.

metastases. Weight loss and secondary anemia usually follow generalization of disease. Cardiorespiratory failure is the most common cause of death from carcinoma of the breast, but in a few cases death is the result of cachexia caused by the widespread dissemination of the disease with metastases to viscera. Infrequently, neurologic signs may develop before death, suggesting brain metastases.

The evolution of some of the specific types of carcinoma of the breast varies. *Paget's disease* of the nipple makes up only slightly more than 2% of all breast carcinomas. It occurs most frequently in women of middle age. The duration of the symptoms averages about three years. The clinical history is usually that of a slowly spreading, rosy red, dry rash with fine white scales *appearing first on the nipple* and later spreading to the areola and adjacent skin (Fig. 641). As the disease progresses, the nipple retracts to the level of the areola. Often no definite mass is felt but, if present, will be directly beneath the nipple. Sometimes the lesion is bilateral. Axillary nodes are involved in about 50% of the patients but are often clinically intangible.

Intraductal (comedo) carcinoma is relatively infrequent, making up only about 4% of all carcinomas of the breast. The

patients give a long history of a slowly growing tumor often accompanied by discharge from the nipple. The tumor feels fairly firm and often grows just beneath the thinned-out overlying skin. Dimpling of the skin or retraction of the nipple is rare, however. After the growth reaches a large size, it may ulcerate through the skin, and infection with bleeding from the tumor may take place. With ulceration, the nodes may increase in size because of infection. In spite of the large size of the tumor and the long duration, axillary node involvement is infrequent.

Papillary carcinomas are fairly distinct clinically and occur predominantly in women 40 to 60 years of age. These tumors tend to grow to a large size, are centrally located, often involve skin, and may be cystic but rarely become fixed to the deeper structures. Despite their large size, the incidence of axillary metastases is surprisingly low.

Lobular carcinomas of the breast occurs in patients in the younger age groups. The tumors do not form a definite mass, for the carcinoma is confined to a lobule early in its evolution. There may be multiple foci of origin. However, late in the disease, invasion of the breast parenchyma occurs, and the usual clinical picture of carcinoma of the breast appears.

Medullary carcinoma occurs in the younger age group. Thirty-one of the fifty-two patients reported by Moore and Foote[254] were under 50 years of age. The

Table 95. Relative frequency of common clinical symptoms and signs in 100 consecutive patients with cancer of mammary gland

Symptom	Order of appearance of symptom			Total frequency
	First	Second	Third	
Lump	78	9	1	88
Local pain	12	28	8	48
Enlargement of lump		16	4	20
Lump in axilla	4	3	1	8
Soreness of nipple	6	2		8
Discharge from nipple	4	2	2	8
Retraction of nipple	1	5	2	8
Ulceration		5		5
Enlargement of breast	1	3		4
Attachment to skin		2		2
Weight loss			3	3
Hemorrhage			1	1

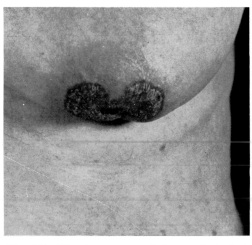

Fig. 641. Weeping eczematoid lesion of nipple in Paget's disease.

tumors may reach a large size, frequently appear encapsulated, and are not unlike a fibroadenoma (Fig. 644).

Inflammatory carcinoma of the breast is a relatively rare form of mammary cancer. According to Taylor and Meltzer,[334] it has two forms, primary and secondary. In the primary form, the changes occur where a lump has been present for some time. The secondary type occurs following radical

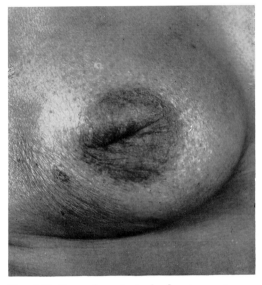

Fig. 642. Retraction of nipple due to carcinoma.

mastectomy. It has a rapid evolution with increase in the size of the breast. The axillary nodes quickly enlarge, and the skin of the breast becomes edematous and warm. Fever invariably accompanies the tumor.

Mucinous carcinoma usually occurs in women over 60 years of age and makes up only about 2% of all carcinomas of the breast. The tumors grow very slowly. In a series of seventy-five patients reported by Lange,[208] an average of thirty-four months elapsed before fixation of the skin occurred, and ulceration appeared after fifty-eight months. The tumor is smaller than might be expected from the long period of growth. It is found most commonly in the center of the breast or in the upper outer quadrant directly beneath the skin. The overlying fat is atrophied, the nipple protruding and enlarged.

Adenoid cystic carcinoma is a rare neoplasm of the breast similar in microscopic pattern to the same tumor in the salivary gland and often appears in the region of the nipple and areola. For all practical purposes, it does not involve the axillary lymph nodes and can, therefore, be treated conservatively (Friedman and Oberman[112a]).

Carcinoma of the male breast occurs, on the whole, in a slightly older group of pa-

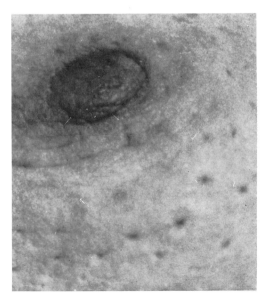

Fig. 643. Retraction of nipple and periareolar edema with pigskin appearance in carcinoma of breast.

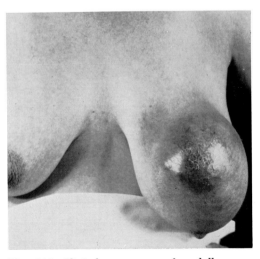

Fig. 644. Clinical appearance of medullary carcinoma of breast. In spite of appearance, prognosis is relatively good. (From Moore, O. S., Jr., and Foote, F. W., Jr.: The relatively favorable prognosis of medullary carcinoma of the breast, Cancer **2:**635-642, 1949.)

tients, but it does not differ in its evolution except in minor details (Wainright[362]). Cuenca and Becker[74] reported one case and found five additional reported ones of coincidence of cancer of the breast in men with a Klinefelter's syndrome. The tumors have a slower evolution than carcinoma of the female breast, but they are not usually seen until late. By that time, the tumor has usually extended to the underlying pectoral fascia and muscle because of the relatively

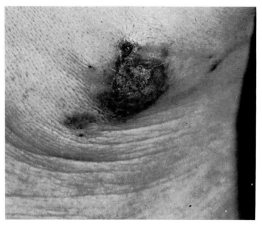

Fig. 645. Advanced ulcerating fixed carcinoma of male breast with satellite skin nodules.

small amount of breast parenchyma (Greening and Aichroth[122]). For this same reason, satellite skin nodules and metastases to the axilla are invariably present (Fig. 645). Their terminal course is similar to that of carcinoma of the female breast.

The presence of *regional and distant metastases* is always a strong possibility in the majority of patients of carcinoma of the breast, even under unimpressive circumstances of short history and small growths. Frequently, axillary and internal mammary nodes are found invaded. A systematic biopsy of the twelfth rib in sixty-three patients by Guillaud-Bourgeois et al.[128] revealed evidence of involvement in 38%. Bone metastases are frequently observed also in the dorsal vertebrae. Snell and Beals[320] found metastases to the femur in half of the patients with osseous manifestations. Postoperative supraclavicular metastases may be the first manifestation of surgical failure and usually imply widely disseminated decrease (Jackson[179]). Simon et al.[316] reported fifty-five cases of intracranial metastases, twenty-six of which appeared unique.

The clinical history of a patient with *cystosarcoma* is that of a small, painless nodule in the breast which, after many

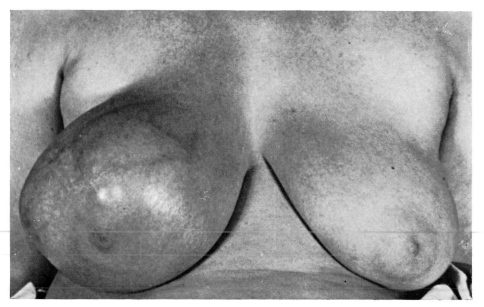

Fig. 646. Typical teardrop cystosarcoma phyllodes of breast. Note effacement of nipple without retraction. (From Cooper, W. G., Jr., and Ackerman, L. V.: Cystosarcoma phylloides, with a consideration of its more malignant variant, Surg. Gynec. Obstet. **77:**279-283, 1943; by permission of Surgery, Gynecology & Obstetrics.)

years of quiescence, suddenly begins to grow. This tumor gradually forms a large mass within the breast, causes very few symptoms except heaviness, and usually remains localized (Fig. 646). McDivitt et al.[229] reported on seventy-three cases, fifty-nine of which were benign and only fourteen malignant. Oberman[270] and Norris and Taylor[269] have reported large collections of cases. Ulceration through the skin may eventually take place, with resultant hemorrhage and infection. This may cause systemic symptoms with weight loss, anorexia, and anemia. Death comes from local recurrence, ulceration, and hemorrhage and in about 15% is caused by distant metastases (Treves and Sunderland[346]). The *fibrosarcoma* has a more rapid evolution without any previous history of an existing lump. It usually develops distant metastases, particularly to the lung, liver, and brain and, at times, may be widely disseminated. Local recurrence is common.

Diagnosis

Self-examination

Successful treatment of carcinoma of the breast depends, to a considerable extent, on early diagnosis (Bloom[36]), yet in spite of public education and a greater desire on the part of modern women to seek medical advice, a large proportion of carcinomas diagnosed today have already progressed beyond the site of origin in the mammary gland. Periodic examinations of symptomless women are desirable, but they cannot be done frequently enough nor is the number that would or could seek these examinations large enough to be of real consequence. Self-examination of the breasts, if done systematically and intelligently, could aid many patients to an earlier discovery of a tumor, to earlier treatment, and to consequent improved prognosis. In 1927, Auchincloss[14] suggested teaching women a simple technique for frequent periodic self-palpation of the breasts. He felt certain of the great importance of this step and expressed his conviction that "it is highly probable that they can and would discover breast lumps . . . far sooner than they would be felt by a doctor in a routine examination. . . . There is a way and, with our present knowledge, but one way to reduce the frightful mortality of breast cancer. Every girl of twenty or thereabouts should be taught to intentionally feel her breast tissue for a lump, every few weeks, all her life."*

Self-examination is best carried out once a month, in the middle of the menstrual cycle, when mammary engorgement is minimal (Haagensen[137]). The subject should be in supine position with a hard pillow under the shoulder and the arm raised above the head. This position favors the spread of the breast over the chest wall and facilitates its palpation with the fingers of the opposite hand placed flat against the breast. An excellent motion picture film has been produced by the American Cancer Society and the National Cancer Institute to promote the self-examination of breasts among women of all ages.

Laboratory discriminants

Testing patients with early carcinomas of the breast, Hayward[161] found that half of them excreted subnormal amounts of urinary metabolites of androgen and cortisol. This finding suggested that patients about to develop cancer, or with early subclinical carcinomas of the breast, may be discovered by this excretory deficiency. In a painstaking and praiseworthy test on 4800 women between 35 and 55 years of age, Bulbrook and Hayward[49] confirmed such predictability or early detection. Lemon et al.[214] noted a reduced estriol excretion in patients with mammary cancer and reasoned also that this metabolic deficit could be recognized early by quantitative analysis of labeled precursors in "cancer-predisposed" individuals. Smith and Smith[318a] believe that extensive studies in urinary estrogen profiles in relation to breast cancer risk as proposed by Cole and MacMahon[66] are worth doing. They believe that interpretation of the results should take into consideration the role of the pituitary gland.

Clinical examination

In the clinical examination of a patient with suspected carcinoma of the breast, certain clinical information is absolutely

---

*From Auchincloss, H., Jr.: Surgery of the breast. In Nelson's loose-leaf living surgery, vol. 4, New York, 1927, Thomas Nelson & Sons, pp. 1-99.

necessary. A first step in the clinical examination is a careful *inspection* of both breasts, which should include notations of size, form, and symmetry. In addition, inspection may reveal pigmentation, scaling, or eczematoid lesions of the nipple and dilated veins or edema of the skin. The presence or absence of edema or ulceration should be recorded. The inspection will be most helpful in revealing *retraction phenomena,* which are extremely important in the diagnosis of early cancer. These phenomena are due to a tension on the fibrous septa ("Cooper's ligament") that are superficially attached to the skin. When the pectoral fascia is stretched, the fibrous septa are pulled in, with resulting dimpling of the skin. Retraction of the nipple may also result. In some instances of early carcinoma of the breast, the retraction phenomenon is observable only when the patient is invited to contract the pectoral muscles (by placing her arms akimbo and exercising pressure on the hips). Raising the arms above the head or leaning forward may facilitate the search for areas of retraction. In some instances, gentle compression of the breast by the examiner may also bring out a retraction sign (Fig. 647). Retraction phenomena are obvious in most patients with advanced cancer (Fig. 648).

The next step in the examination is a methodical and thorough but *gentle palpation* of both breasts. Rough handling or repeated examinations in inexperienced hands are to be condemned because dissemination of the tumor is possible with manipulation. A satisfactory palpation of the breasts is seldom possible with the patient in an erect position. Best results may be obtained with the patient in supine position and the shoulder raised so as to permit the breast to flatten evenly over the chest wall. It is advantageous to palpate the medial half of the breast when the patient's arm is raised above the head (Fig. 649). When a tumor is found, palpation should establish whether there is fixation to underlying structures or skin and whether the nipple's excursion is the same as on the normal side. The dimensions of the tumor should be recorded. Its consistency, shape, and character of outline and increased temperature of the skin should also be noted.

A lump is the first symptom in over 80% of all patients with cancer of the breast. Consequently, the finding of any lump in the breast is a highly significant sign and warrants a thorough investigation. In more than half of the patients with breast cancer, the lump is entirely painless. The tumor

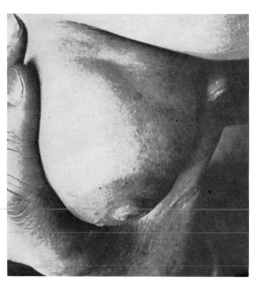

Fig. 647. Slight retraction of skin elicited by gentle compression of breast. (From Haagensen, C. D.: Carcinoma of the breast, New York, 1950, American Cancer Society, Inc.)

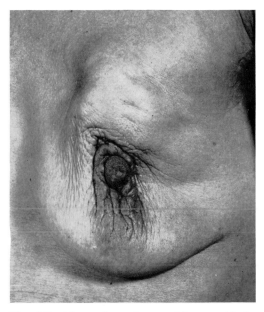

Fig. 648. Advanced carcinoma of breast with infiltration of skin and retraction of nipple.

is usually hard with an irregular outline, but it may be astonishingly soft and have a perfectly smooth contour. Palpation of mucinous carcinoma may suggest a cystic lesion sometimes not unlike an area of subcutaneous emphysema, "a delicate swish or crush of a jellylike structure under ten-

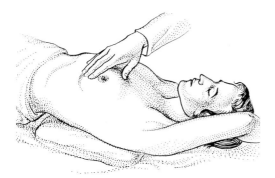

Fig. 649. With patient lying on back with hard pillow under shoulder and arm raised, examiner may easily palpate breast against relaxed chest wall and discover early lesions. (Courtesy Cancer Seminar.)

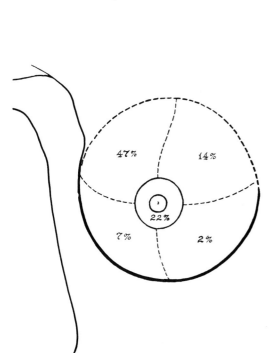

Fig. 650. Distribution of carcinomas in different areas of breast.

sion" (Halsted[149]). The clinical evaluation of a mass found in the breast is fraught with difficulty, and the most experienced examiner can diagnose accurately only some 70% of carcinomas at clinical examination. Even well-trained hospital interns and residents are seldom able to diagnose more than one-half of them. Carcinomas of the breast are most frequently located in the upper outer quadrant but may be found in any of the other quadrants (Fig. 650), in the inframammary region, or in the axillary extension of the breast. Rarely, carcinomas arise in an axillary supernumerary breast (de Cholnoky[61]), in which instances the tumor is usually taken for an axillary adenopathy from an undiscovered primary lesion.

Palpation of the breast should be complemented by a careful *palpation of the axillae and the supraclavicular regions.* Palpation of the axilla is best done with the patient erect and at a higher level than the examiner. The patient's forearm should be held by the examiner to allow relaxation of the muscles (Fig. 651), and the cupped fingers of the examiner should be rolled in all directions against the deep axillary tissues. The evaluation of axillary lymph nodes is most difficult. It is remarkable how incorrect clinical impressions can be. An analysis of the results in a series of cases examined at the Ellis Fischel State Cancer Hospital (Ackerman[1]) is shown in

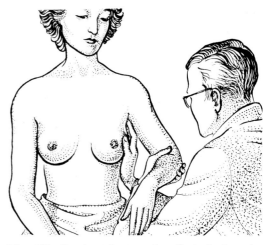

Fig. 651. Gentle palpation of axilla is facilitated when examiner is slightly lower than patient. (Courtesy Cancer Seminar.)

Table 96. Evaluation of axillary metastases—clinical impression versus microscopic findings*

Clinical findings	Cases	Examiner correct
Clinically and microscopically negative	84	54% of cases
Clinically negative and microscopically positive	71	
Clinically and microscopically positive	124	85% of cases
Clinically positive and microscopically negative	22	

*From Ackerman, L. V.: Clinical and pathological correlation of carcinoma of the breast, Amer. Pract. Digest Treat. 1:124-131, 1950.

Table 96. Certain general conclusions can be drawn from the figures. The most common error is the clinical inability to detect nodes already invaded by cancer, the examiner being correct in only 54% of the instances when he believed there was no axillary adenopathy. When metastases were diagnosed, the examiner was more often found right. Minute metastases may be too deeply situated to be reached by palpation, or their consistency may not be greater than that of axillary fat. Consequently, they were often missed. Large inflammatory nodes may, of course, mislead the examiner in the other extreme. Particular care should be taken to examine the opposite axilla. Palpation of the supraclavicular regions is best done with the examiner standing behind the seated patient (Fig. 652), for nodes may often be hidden behind the clavicular insertion of the sternocleidomastoid muscle. Palpation should be extended to the jugular and spinal chain of nodes of the cervical region.

Transillumination of the breast may give additional information for the differential diagnosis of breast lesions. This should be done in a totally dark room with an intense light so that good visualization of any mass within the breast is possible. It is of particular value for the recognition of cysts and hematomas and for the localization of duct papillomas. Cysts containing clear fluid are translucent, but if the fluid is milky or bloody, then they may be opaque. Hematomas do not transilluminate. Transillumination is of no value in differentiating between a benign solid tumor and a malignant tumor.

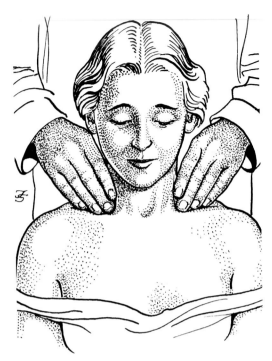

Fig. 652. Palpation of supraclavicular areas is best carried out when examiner stands behind seated patient. (Courtesy Cancer Seminar.)

Clinical staging of breast cancer has been done by many individuals. In order for such staging to have practical value, it must not be so complicated that there will be tremendous variability in staging of a given case. The best clinical staging is one that would be reproducible by skilled clinical examiners. We believe the following clinical staging as devised by Haagensen et al.* is workable from the standpoint of the clinician.

Stage I

No skin edema, ulceration, or solid fixation of tumor to chest wall. Axillary nodes not clinically involved.

Stage II

No skin edema, ulceration, or solid fixation of tumor to chest wall. Clinically involved axillary nodes, but less than 2.5 cm in transverse diameter and not fixed to overlying skin or deeper structures of axilla.

*From Haagensen, C. D. et al.: Treatment of early mammary carcinoma; a cooperative international study, Ann. Surg. **157**:157-179, 1963.

Stage III

Any *one* of five grave signs of comparatively advanced carcinoma:

1 Edema of skin of limited extent (involving less than one-third of the skin over the breast)
2 Skin ulceration
3 Solid fixation of tumor to chest wall
4 Massive involvement of axillary lymph nodes (measuring 2.5 cm or more in transverse diameter)
5 Fixation of the axillary nodes to overlying skin or deeper structures of axilla

Stage IV

All other patients with more advanced breast carcinoma, including:

1 A combination of any *two or more* of the five grave signs listed in Stage C
2 Extensive edema of skin (involving more than one-third of the skin over the breast)
3 Satellite skin nodules
4 The inflammatory type of carcinoma
5 Supraclavicular metastases (clinically apparent)
6 Parasternal metastases (clinically apparent)
7 Edema of the arm
8 Distant metastases

"It should be noted that no distinction as to the size of the primary tumor and its position in the breast has been made in the classification. Pathologic type or grade is likewise ignored. These and other features of breast carcinoma are, of course, of prognostic significance, but to subdivide cases on these grounds makes our classification too complex."[*]

The clinical examination of a male patient with carcinoma of the breast does not differ from that of carcinoma of the female breast. The tumor, however, is more frequently seen within the region of the nipple, often has a longer history, and frequently shows ulceration. This occurred in 38% of the 418 patients reported by Wainright.[362] The presence of a breast mass and a nipple discharge in a male is almost certain evidence that the lesion is cancer (Treves and Holleb[345]). It is the most frequent neoplasm affecting the male breast.

Biopsy

Franzén and Zajicek[111] performed 3119 *aspiration biopsies* on lesions of the breast without significant complications. In 867 cases, a diagnosis of carcinoma was made and confirmed histologically, whereas in ninety-four cases of cancer, a false negative diagnosis was rendered. A *needle biopsy* may be successful, particularly in

[*]From Haagensen, C. D. et al.: Treatment of early mammary carcinoma; a cooperative international study, Ann. Surg. **157**:157-179, 1963.

Table 97. Clinicopathologic correlations in carcinoma of breast

Clinical findings	Pathologic findings
Lump: small, painless, hard	Smaller the cancer, less chance of axillary metastasis; hardness directly related to amount of connective tissue or inflammation present
Attachment to skin	Tumor growing just beneath skin
Discharge from nipple	If bloody, cancer has grown into a major duct, is Paget's disease or intraductal cancer
Prominent veins in region of tumor	Tumor blocking venous return
Edema, orange-skin appearance to skin	Tumor growing in subdermal and dermal lymphatics
Fixation to chest wall	Invasion of pectoral fascia and rarely of muscle
Satellite nodules	Extensive dermal and subdermal lymphatic involvement
Hard supraclavicular node	Usually metastasis; rule out benign lesions by biopsy
Contralateral axillary lymph nodes	Usually metastasis; rule out benign lesions by aspiration or formal biopsy
Fixed masses in axilla	Tumor growing in nodes, breaking through capsule, and growing in loose fat
Edema of arm	Tumor blocking lymphatics and venous return
Horner's syndrome (miosis, enophthalmos, and narrowing of palpebral fissure)	Metastatic tumor pressing on or invading cervical sympathetic chain
Diffuse chest pain, dyspnea	Tumor involving pleura and probably lung
Girdle chest pains (lumbar or sciatic pains)	Questionable metastasis to vertebrae or sacroiliac region
Marked, extreme weight loss	May mean distant metastasis, possible to liver

large tumors (Salzstein[303]). When the neo-plasm is small, it is preferable to submit the patient to a surgical exploration with an understanding that it may lead to a radical mastectomy. On surgical exposure of the lesion, an experienced surgeon can recognize at least three-fourths of all malignant tumors. In practically all cases, frozen section should be done for microscopic diagnosis. If the mass is 2 cm or less in diameter, it is preferable to excise it in toto. If the lesion is larger, a careful *incisional biopsy* should be taken and frozen section made. In most instances, the pathologist will be able to diagnose the malignant tumors, and the surgeon may proceed with a radical mastectomy. In 1006 consecutive lesions of the breast, frozen section diagnosis was correct in 97%; in the other 3% it was necessary to await the paraffin sections (Desai[87]). However, in a few instances, there may be difficulty in establishing a definite diagnosis on frozen section, and then it is preferable to adopt a conservative attitude. If the lesion proves to be malignant, no harm is done by waiting twenty-four hours for the thorough study of multiple sections processed in the usual manner. An effort should be made to obtain histopathologic confirmation of metastatic lesions to be treated by roentgentherapy. This is usually possible by means of needle biopsy. In all patients who are operated upon, a histopathologic diagnosis is assured. In inoperable cases, a histopathologic diagnosis should be secured for the sake of the record. Incisional biopsies may be obtained in skin nodules and ulcerations and needle biopsies in obvious inoperable tumors; cytologic diagnosis may be possible in centrifugated pleural fluid. Scalene node biopsy is a valid approach in advanced cases to establish the diagnosis and decide on inoperability (Paparoannou and Urban[278]).

Cytologic study of breast secretions has been done in an effort to diagnose benign and malignant tumors in this manner. The cases presenting a nipple discharge are few, and considerable experience is necessary for this interpretation. Consequently, this study is of little practical value. In some rare cases with nipple discharge and no palpable tumor, or Paget's disease with intraductal carcinoma, the finding of can-

cer cells in the secretion may reemphasize the necessity of a surgical exploration of the area immediately beneath the nipple (Masukawa et al.[248]).

Roentgenologic examination

The radiographic examination of the breast called *mammography* is now extensively used in the United States and France for the early detection of mammary carcinoma, often before it can be

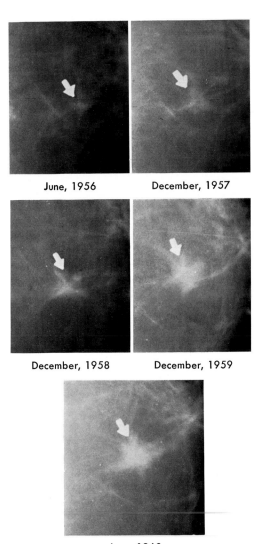

June, 1956   December, 1957

December, 1958   December, 1959

June, 1960

Fig. 653. Serial roentgenograms of patient with nonpalpable carcinoma of breast first seen by roentgenologist in December, 1958, and finally operated upon in June, 1960. At no time was this lesion felt clinically. (Courtesy Dr. J. Gershon-Cohen, Philadelphia, Pa.)

palpated by the clinician (Egan[96]; Gros[127]). Mammography requires exacting technique, special material and equipment, and skillful interpretation. Leborgne,[210] in his comprehensive monograph, set forth very early the necessary requirements. Gershon-Cohen et al.[114, 116] reemphasized the radiographic signs of malignant tumors of the breast: opacity with spiculated margins, circumscribed densities with irregular margins, and punctate calcifications along the duct lines (Fig. 653). Calcifications may be found in benign lesions (Black and Young[29]), but the pattern differs. Radiographic examinations of specimens of benign and malignant disease of the breast demonstrate calcification in about 25% of the benign lesions and over 60% of the malignant lesions (Koehl et al.[201]). Artifacts (Selby[310]) and fat necrosis may be the cause of misinterpretation (Minagi and Youker[250]). The procedure is highly accurate in slow-growing carcinomas but may easily miss the fast-growing tumors. In young women, the abundant parenchyma and corresponding lack of contrasts render the diagnosis of cancer difficult. The most successful diagnoses are made in women over 55 years of age and in those with fatty breasts.

Mammography is too elaborate and expensive to be used as a routine screening procedure (Saxen and Hakama[306]) (Fig. 654), but it is certainly well indicated in any patient with a palpable mass or nodules in the breast and in the follow-up of the opposite breast after radical mastectomy (Chavanne et al.[59]; Missakian et al.[251]).

In a study of 1543 patients reported by Barker et al.,[20] biopsy was recorded in seventy-nine patients, and twenty-nine carcinomas were found. Although twenty-one of the tumors were probably capable of being diagnosed without mammography, eight were nonpalpable prior to radiographic localization. In 2000 patients with carcinoma of the breast examined at the Radium Institute of Paris, nineteen were found to have a contralateral tumor as revealed by mammography. Gershon-Cohen et al.[116] examined 1120 women over 35 years of age at intervals of six months and found carcinoma of the breast in thirty-three. The average diameter of the tumors found was 1.1 cm, and lymph node metastases were present in only 30% of them. Snyder[321] reported detection of lobular carcinoma in situ by mammography in thirty-

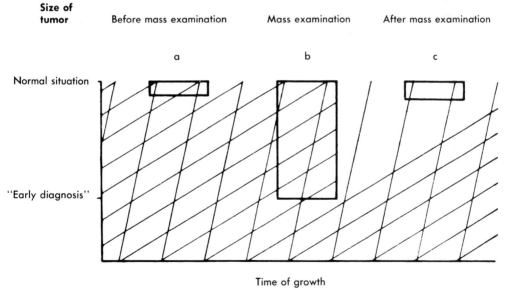

Fig. 654. Diagram forcibly illustrating that with screening of breast cancer, slow-growing tumors will be identified and fast-moving tumors, as shown by vertical lines, will be missed. Cost of finding single case in asymptomatic women with palpable breast mass is prohibitive. (From Saxén, E., and Hakama, M.: Cancer incidence in Finland with a note on difficulties in comparing epidemiological data, Cancro **19**:88-96, 1966; WU neg. 68-10861.)

five breasts of twenty-seven patients. The calcification in this lesion is usually spherical and often in normal tissue near the lobular carcinoma (Hutter et al.[177]). In 1000 mammographic examinations in 634 patients reported by Egan,[97] two malignant lesions were missed out of 240 that were present, and nineteen carcinomas were found in breasts that had been considered clinically negative. Wolfe[375] found 11% false positive results on mammography and twenty carcinomas found at surgery that cound not be seen in mammography. Leborgne et al.[211] have made an interesting soft tissue radiographic study of axillary lymph nodes. The practice of mammography has brought renewed need for cooperation between the radiologist, pathologist, and surgeon (Siegelman et al.[314]; Patton et al.[285]; Berger et al.[27]). By screening women without detectable masses, carcinomas can be found by mammography (Figs. 655 and 656). The optimal interval between mammographic examinations remains to be established (Stevens and Weigen[326]). Gershon-Cohen et al.[115] measured the doubling time of breast cancer by mammography and found a variation of twenty-three to 209 days. This finding could influence the optimum interval between mammographic examinations.

Xerography, a procedure based on selenium-coated plates, has certain advantages over mammography. Xerograms are easier to interpret, breast structures are recorded with clarity on one image, less irradiation is required, and the procedure is quick (Wolfe[377]).

Thermography, a procedure based on the measure of small differences in temperature, is another exploitable method in the early detection of cancer of the breast. It is more expeditious and economical than mammography, the false negative rate is similar but the proportion of false positives is greater, and there is often no spatial relationship between the location of the thermographic lesion and the lesion (Wallace and Dodd[363]). The value of mass screening through mammography is debatable (Hitchcock et al.[169]). Strax et al.[330a] have been carrying on a large mass screening program, and the long-term results of this should be helpful in making a decision.

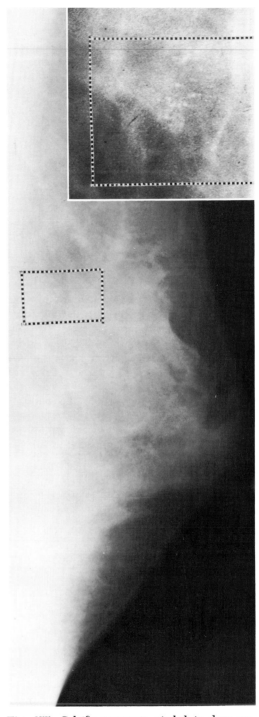

Fig. 655. Calcific aggregate circled in deep upper outer quadrant of left breast indicates locale of 3 mm to 4 mm clinically undetectable carcinoma. **Inset,** Enlargement of calcific aggregate ×4. Actual tumor mass not discernible. (From Stevens, G. M., and Weigen, J. F.: Mammography survey for breast cancer detection; a 2-year study of 1,223 clinically negative asymptomatic women over 40, Cancer **19:**51-59, 1966.)

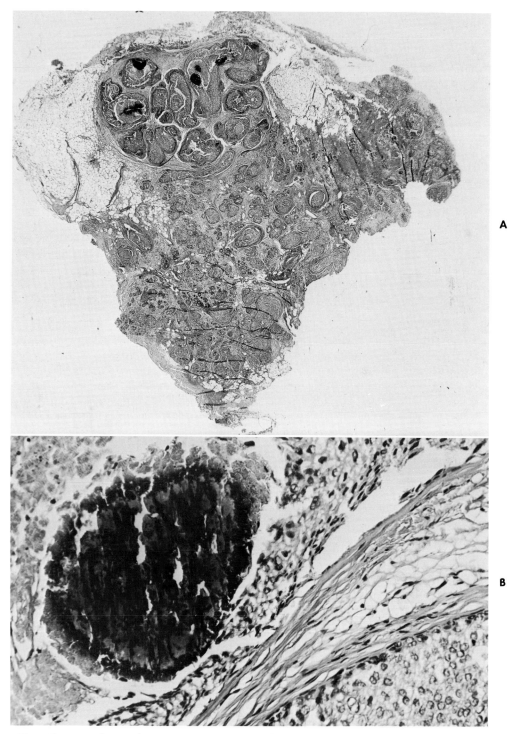

Fig. 656. Same lesion shown in Fig. 655. **A,** Predominantly intraductal carcinoma of breast. It is fairly well circumscribed. Calcification can be seen. **B,** Tumor is better observed under high power. Focal area of calcification is observed. Calcification seen is also observed in mammogram. (From Stevens, G. M., and Weigen, J. F.: Mammography survey for breast cancer detection; a 2-year study of 1,223 clinically negative asymptomatic women over 40, Cancer **19:**51-59, 1966; **A,** ×15; WU neg. 65-3704; **B,** ×275, WU neg. 65-3707.)

A routine roentgenogram of the chest is advisable in all patients with breast cancer on first examination and, of course, periodically following treatment. Pulmonary metastases from carcinoma are frequently of the nodular variety, presenting as rounded shadows of moderate density that may be found anywhere throughout both lung fields long before any symptom betrays their presence. Small lesions superimposed on the rib shadows may pass unnoticed, but larger ones are obvious and, if they grow near the surface of the lung, may be overshadowed by associated pleural effusion. Less often, pulmonary invasion presents the pattern of *lymphangitic metastases* (Schattenberg and Ryan[307]), which is more commonly observed in carcinoma of the stomach. The roentgenographic appearance of lymphangitic metastases is that of a stringlike design radiating from the hilus of either lung toward the periphery and branching to become a fine webbing of delicate striations. This reticular appearance is punctuated by denser miliary nodules apparently corresponding to the points of intersection. The pattern is more marked in the middle and lower lobes, and concomitantly enlarged hilar lymph nodes may be observed (Mueller and Sniffin[257]). This radiographic appearance is often so uniform that it may be misinterpreted as pulmonary fibrosis or may be confused with sarcoidosis or pneumoconiosis.

The roentgenologic appearance of bone metastases from carcinoma of the breast is rather constant (Bouchard[41]). The majority of the bone lesions are of the osteolytic type, a few are osteolytic and osteoblastic, and very few are purely osteoblastic. The latter are found in the slowly growing tumors. Pain usually calls attention to the presence of bone metastases, but several weeks may elapse between the onset of pain and the radiographic verification of a metastatic lesion. The most common sites of bone metastases from carcinoma of the breast are, in order of decreasing frequency, the spine, pelvis, ribs, skull, humerus, and scapula. In only very few cases are metastases found below the elbow or knee, and then only after the lower half of the humerus or femur has been invaded (Carnett and Howell[57]). The typical lesion is a rounded, localized area

of destruction of the medulla of the bone. Medullary lesions growing near the cortex produce a rounded, sharply circumscribed destruction of the inner table, giving a punched-out appearance. In some bones, a generalized demineralization occurs with no apparent limits. The thinned dense cortex contrasts with the rest of the bone where normal trabeculation has disappeared. The cortex is then expanded (ribs and skull), and the bone fractures (humerus and femur) or collapses (vertebrae). This diffuse decalcification is often confused with demineralization of disuse that may or may not be associated with osteoarthritis. Conversely, radiation-induced avascular bone necrosis may be taken for metastases (Ratzkowski et al.[292]). If a patient has symptoms suggesting involvement of bone, such as in the vertebral area, appropriate roentgenograms should be taken. In addition, routine preoperative roentgenograms of the chest should always be requested; routine so-called skeletal series, in the absence of symptoms, are seldom useful and often onerous. Axial skeletal *scintigraphy* with fluorine[18] is very helpful in detecting metastatic osseous lesions not seen in conventional radiography (Galasko et al.[112c]). Twelve of fifty patients with inoperable carcinoma of the breast (24%) showed a positive scan, and there were no false positive results (Galasko[112b]).

Differential diagnosis

Fibroadenomas are common lesions of the breast. That some relationship exists between these tumors and hyperestrogenism is supported by the fact that they can be produced with estrogens in animals. Fibroadenomas occur at a much earlier age than does cancer, being most common in patients between 20 and 35 years of age (peak age incidence, from 21 to 25 years). The lesions are usually painless but may be tender, the nipple itself is usually normal, there is no discharge, and there are no skin changes unless the tumor has reached a large size. They are freely movable and firm, with smoothly lobulated boundaries, in contrast to the indefinite outlines of carcinoma. Unlike carcinoma, they move independently of breast tissue. In young girls, extreme enlargement of the

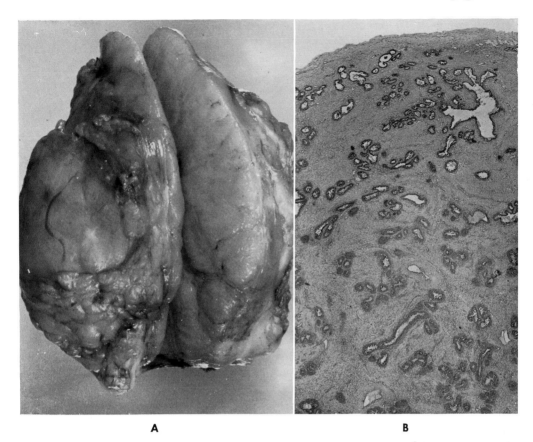

A   **B**

Fig. 657. A, Large breast tumor in 14-year-old black girl, probably best designated as virginal hypertrophy. Tumor measured 10 cm × 15 cm. **B,** Note proliferating ducts and stroma. (From Wulsin, J. H.: Large breast tumors in adolescent females, Ann. Surg. **152:**151-159, 1960.)

breast *(virginal hypertrophy)* has been reported (Fig. 657). Rapid growth of one breast can occur, and the lesion is mistaken for a malignant tumor (Wulsin[379]). These tumors often grow rapidly at the time of pregnancy or lactation. Multiple tumors occur in about 15% of the patients. Additional fibroadenomas frequently appear in the breast that has contained the disease but may occur in either breast. On gross examination, fibroadenomas exhibit a well-defined capsule with a slightly nodular surface. The cut section shows them to be lobulated, yellowish gray, and homogeneous in character. There are none of the chalky streaks so characteristic of carcinoma. At times, fibroadenomas are associated with cystic disease of the breast. Microscopically, they are classified as pericanalicular or intracanalicular. Because of the rapid growth of connective tissue in the latter variety, there are intracanalicular invaginations. Conservative surgical treatment is curative. In some instances, it is clinically impossible to be certain that the lesion is a fibroadenoma, and it is always simpler to excise it locally. At the time of operation, its characteristic appearance is easily recognized. If there is any doubt as to the gross diagnosis, frozen section can determine its character in almost 100% of the cases.

Adenomas of the nipple are an example of a highly proliferative lesion that ulcerates the nipple and is often confused clinically with Paget's disease (Fig. 659). There is a prominent overgrowth of ductal, papillary, and epithelial structures. There is no necrosis, and there is a double layer of the ducts (Taylor and Robertson[336]).

Sclerosing adenosis infrequently forms a palpable tumor. This benign breast lesion

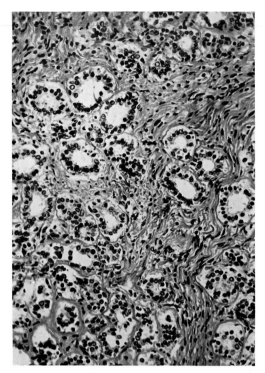

Fig. 658. So-called fetal type of fibroadenoma. (Low power.)

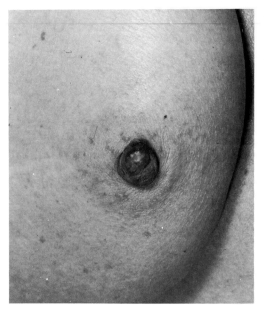

Fig. 659. Adenoma (papilloma) of nipple. Note resemblance to Paget's disease. (From Haagensen, C. D.: Diseases of the breast, ed. 2, Philadelphia, W. B. Saunders Co.; in press, 1970.)

is often mistaken for carcinoma. At the Memorial Hospital for Cancer and Allied Diseases in New York, only about one example of this process is seen in every seventy-five benign breast lesions (Urban and Adair[353]), the disease usually occurring in patients between 20 and 30 years of age. Consistency of the lesion is less rubbery than a fibroadenoma and less firm than carcinoma of the breast. The process is usually discrete but not definitely encapsulated and is grayish white or pinkish yellow. On gross examination, the most characteristic finding is the definite lobulation. If lobulation and circumscription are not clear or if, in addition, the lesion is somewhat firm with chalky streaks, it may be impossible to tell it from carcinoma. The changes are particularly difficult to interpret when the process has been present for a long period of time and there has been great overproduction of fibrous connective tissue. This causes distortion of the lobules, giving a false impression of invasion. Because of the activity of this process, an occasional mitotic figure may also be observed. Frequently, there is ex-

cessive multiplication of ductlike structures. In the series reported by Urban and Adair,[353] the average age of twenty-two patients with well-defined nodules was 31 years. If the clinical impression of carcinoma is carried to a surgical exploration with frozen section, there is danger that the microscopic examination will add further confusion. On section, sclerosing adenosis shows indefinite encapsulation and a grayish white or pinkish yellow surface, but the chalky streaks so commonly observed in carcinoma are usually absent.

Chronic cystic disease is often confused with carcinoma of the breast (cystic mastitis is a misnomer, for there is no inflammation). It usually occurs in parous women with small breasts. It is present most commonly in the upper outer quadrant but may occur in other parts and eventually involve the entire breast. It is often painful, particularly in the premenstrual period, and accompanying menstrual disturbances are common. Nipple discharge, usually serous, occurs in approximately 15% of the cases, but there are no changes in the nipple itself. The lesion is diffuse without sharp demarcation and without fixation to the overlying skin. Multiple cysts are firm,

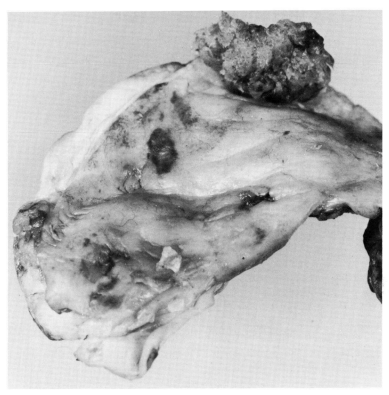

Fig. 660. Intraductal papilloma in 55-year-old woman. (WU neg. 68-10805.)

round, and fluctuant and may transilluminate if they contain clear fluid. A large cyst in an area of chronic cystic disease feels like a tumor, but it is usually smoother and well delimited. The axillary lymph nodes are usually not enlarged.

Chronic cystic disease infrequently shows large bluish cysts (blue dome cysts of Bloodgood). More often, the cysts are multiple and small, with intervening increased yellowish gray parenchyma, containing serous or viscid liquid. The yellowish gray tissue cuts smoothly and does not show the chalky streaks of carcinoma. Many changes can be observed in the ducts, acini, and connective tissue stroma, some of which may be due to advancing age and nonspecific inflammatory processes. The proliferative changes are most important and include apocrine epithelium, blunt duct adenosis, papillomatosis, and sclerosing adenosis. There is proliferation of the acini, and the connective tissue may increase and distort the architectural pattern so that a false impression of proliferation and invasion is given. However, mitoses are absent, and the nuclei are very regular in appearance. This process is due to an excessive multiplication of both extralobular and intralobular portions of the mammary parenchyma (Foote and Stewart[107]).

The treatment of chronic cystic disease requires considerable judgment. Patients should be followed and examined at properly timed intervals. If a dominant lump develops, it should be removed and examined microscopically. Simple mastectomy has been recommended for this lesion, but we feel that it is not indicated for several reasons. Chronic cystic disease is invariably a bilateral process (Reclus[295]); if the development of cancer is feared, both breasts would have to be excised. Also, in doing the usual simple mastectomy, all the breast tissue is not removed (Hicken[167]). A cyst of the breast can be treated by aspiration with certain precautions. In a series reported by Goode et al.,[120] 267 breast aspirations were done on 202 women considered to have a cyst in the breast. There were fifty-seven dry taps, and forty of these were due to benign lesions. After the tapping, many lesions will completely disappear because there is *no lining* to the cyst wall. If blood or no fluid is obtained, this would indicate surgical exploration.

Intraductal papillomas occur in women between the ages of 20 and 65 years. About 75% are located centrally and about 25% peripherally (Fig. 660). The papilloma is often soft and located in the central portion of the breast beneath the nipple, which is usually normal. The mass is movable unless infection has caused fixation and retraction of the nipple. The axillary lymph nodes may be enlarged if infection is present. A sporadic discharge occurs in half of the patients, and this is more frequently bloody, or greenish, than serous. Pain occurs when hemorrhage takes place into a dilated obstructed duct; the tumor may enlarge but, if discharge follows, may diminish and no longer be felt, with reduction or complete relief of pain. If a patient has only a small palpable mass and bleeding from the nipple, the chances are

over 95% that this bleeding represents an intraductal papilloma. If no mass at all is felt, careful repeated examination of the patient may eventually demonstrate the area of papilloma. Paget's disease of the nipple and intraductal carcinoma may cause bleeding from the nipple. A carcinoma of the breast may erode into a main duct and cause bleeding, or an intraductal papilloma may be associated with a mammary cancer. However, 100 consecutive cases of carcinoma of the breast will yield only about 1.5% with bleeding from the nipple. Nipple discharge can occur in chronic cystic disease and in patients who have been receiving hormone therapy. Women taking tranquilizer drugs may also have nipple discharge. When the discharge or bleeding is bilateral and a careful palpation fails to detect a tumor, the chances are great that the symptom is due to a benign lesion. If there is a unilateral bloody discharge and a large, firm mass, carcinoma may be present. Fitts et al.[102] reported on twenty-four patients with cancer of the

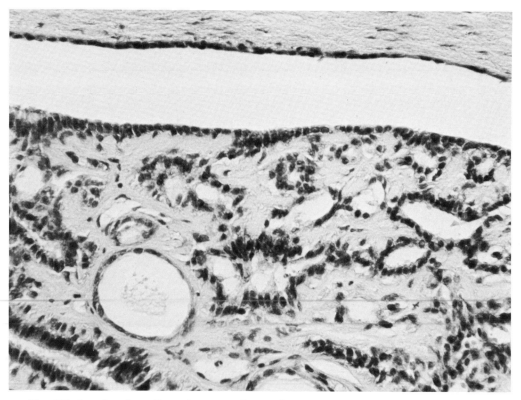

Fig. 661. Intraductal papilloma. Note complexity of pattern. However, glands are well differentiated with double layer. (×300; WU neg. 68-11134.)

breast in whom there was a nipple discharge; twenty-two of them had a palpable mass, and two others had Paget's disease.

Intraductal papillomas are usually small, measuring up to 4 mm and extending along the ducts for 1 cm or 2 cm. Infrequently, they are seen protruding from a cyst and measuring up to 10 cm in diameter. They are almost always single. When infection develops, even with frozen section, the lesion may be mistaken for cancer because of the diffuse epithelial growth (Fig. 661). If the sections are cut tangentially, remnants of acini or ducts may be seen beyond the apparent wall of the cyst, suggesting invasion. If, at operation, the lesion is grossly an intraductal papilloma, it should be removed by wedge excision. Because of its localization to a single quadrant and because it does not undergo transition to cancer, there is no justification for simple or radical mastectomy (Forrest[109]). Haagensen et al.[147] treated seventy-six patients with intraductal papilloma by wedge resection. There were five recurrences and some instances of new papillomas, but carcinoma did not develop in any patient (Table 98). In Hendrick's series[164] of 208 patients observed from 1933 to 1951, none of the papillomas became malignant. Papillomas should not be confused with the diffuse microscopic intraductal papillomatous changes often associated with other proliferative phenomena of chronic cystic disease. Multiple papillary tumors within the breast usually represent papillary carcinoma. McDivitt et al.[224] believe that a papillary carcinoma is malignant from its inception and does not arise from preexisting intraductal papilloma. The differential diagnosis between this lesion and papillary carcinoma has been well defined by Kraus and Neubecker.[203]

Fat necrosis is relatively infrequent in the breast. It arises following trauma, and its clinical characteristics mimic with great exactitude those of carcinoma. Occasionally, fat necrosis occurs on the scar of a mastectomy, and it is prone to occur in large, fatty, pendulous breasts. It may be attached to the skin, feel superficial, have indefinite margins, and be almost stony hard and is usually accompanied by severe pain. On gross examination, these lesions resemble carcinoma except for their somewhat greasy surface. Frozen section will reveal their true nature. Microscopically, these cases always show duct stasis with periductal inflammation. If trauma occurred to a breast showing these pathologic alterations, the development of fat necrosis would seem logical (Stewart[327]). Simple excision is sufficient treatment. Extensive fat necrosis with the formation of sinuses may, in rare instances, necessitate simple mastectomy (Slaughter and Peterson[318]). *Mammary duct ectasia* is a lesion of the aging breast that may be impossible to differentiate grossly from carcinoma because of signs of redness and retraction of the skin (Haagensen[138]). It may arise following trauma, and in almost half of all cases the clinical appearance is that of a carcinoma of the breast (Adair[6]).

Plasma cell mastitis is a rare benign condition of the breast frequently diagnosed as cancer (Cheatle and Cutler[60]). It almost invariably occurs in married women. The average age of 100 patients reported by Adair[5] was 36 years. The first symptom is usually pain, accompanied by localized redness and sometimes nipple discharge. Retraction of the nipple, edema, skin adherence, and enlarged axillary lymph nodes may be present. Because of these findings, a clinical diagnosis of cancer may be made, followed by radical mastectomy. Grossly, the changes may involve large areas of

Table 98. Follow-up of seventy-six patients with intraductal papilloma treated by local excision (Presbyterian Hospital, New York, 1916-1941)*

Site in breast	Total treated by local excision	Recurrence of papilloma		Developed carcinoma	% follow-up
		Under 5 yr	*After 5 yr*		
Central	56	2	0	0	94.6
Peripheral	20	0	1	0	95.0
All sites	76	2	1	0	94.7

*From Haagensen, C. D., et al.: The papillary neoplasms of the breast. I. Benign intraductal papilloma, Ann. Surg. 133: 18-36, 1951.

breast parenchyma. Microscopically, subacute inflammation of the duct system is
found and sheets of plasma cells are extremely abundant. Bacteria are infrequently present. Deep incisional biopsies may
be necessary to differentiate from carcinoma. We have observed a case in which
biopsies showed a picture of plasma cell
mastitis masking an underlying carcinoma.
In mammary duct ectasia, fat necrosis, and
plasma cell mastitis, duct stasis is present.
These three processes are all related, and
trauma associated with duct stasis may initiate fat necrosis and plasma cell mastitis.
All three may be mistaken for cancer.

Fibrosis of the breast may form a definitive, firm mass within the breast, usually
without dimpling of the overlying skin. It
measures between 3 cm and 5 cm, is usually unilateral, and clinically is often
thought to be cancer. Microscopically, it is
not associated with epithelial hyperplasia
or cyst formation but consists of diffuse
hyalinized stroma and fibrosis. Haagensen[139]
described this lesion, and Vassar and Culling[355] reported twenty cases.

*Circumscribed chronic suppurative mas-
titis*, a rare condition in our experience,
can exactly simulate cancer clinically and
grossly. It can follow lactation (Tuttle and
Kean[347]). Patients with this lesion may
have a hard, circumscribed, encapsulated
mass, adherent to the skin, with edema, and
grossly it may cut with resistance and suggest cancer. It contains a central abscess.

Tuberculosis of the breast is rare in the
United States. It occurs at an earlier age
than cancer, usually between 20 and 40
years, and is probably a secondary manifestation of pulmonary tuberculosis. As a
rule, the infection is hematogenous in origin, but occasionally it represents a direct
extension from a tuberculous empyema.
The lesion is nearly always unilateral, presenting multiple irregular, slowly growing
nodules. Some of these coalesce and rupture with persistent sinus formation. In
rare cases, the tumor may be very hard
because of the overproduction of connective tissue, may have indefinite margins,
and may be attached to the skin. It is impossible to differentiate these cases from
cancer on physical examination. Biopsy
alone gives the diagnosis, although the history does give important clues as to the
nature of the lesion. Tuberculosis of the
breast associated with carcinoma has been
observed (Raven[293]).

Inflammatory lesions of the skin of the
nipple or areola may be confused with
Paget's disease, but the former appear in
young women, and they usually respond
to anti-inflammatory treatment.

Erysipelas of the skin of the breast,
which often occurs during pregnancy and
lactation, may suggest inflammatory carcinoma, but the leukocytosis, fever, and systemic reaction that often accompany erysipelas frequently facilitate the differential
diagnosis.

Treatment

The treatment of cancer of the breast
has motivated innumerable modalities of
approach and has stimulated perennial
controversies. Unlike patients with other
forms of cancer, the patient with mammary
carcinoma seems to have benefitted little
by earlier diagnosis and by the advances
of surgery and radiotherapy of the past
decades. The advent of hormone therapy
and chemotherapy has contributed, only
relatively, to the management of the incurable patient. The mortality rates have
remained unchanged for several decades.

In any group of patients who are first
seen with cancer of the breast, a shockingly high proportion already has distant
metastases (Habif[148]) (Fig. 662). In a
good number of such patients, the presence
of distant metastases is obvious or definitely
predictable on the basis of local or regional
findings which have been recognized as
signs of "inoperability" or, rather, of incurability. Among those judged operable,
an additional rather large proportion of
patients also has distant metastases, but
only time will reveal these metastases at
variable intervals following operation; in
this sizable group, any and all forms of
treatment will fail. The remainder is composed of patients with tumors of different
character, behavior, and extent on which
details the chance of cure does depend: a
few may present tumors which by chance
or, more often, by rule remain confined
to the breast; they are curable by radical
or simple mastectomy, and any surgical
adjuvant is superfluous. An additional
group of patients may have carcinomas

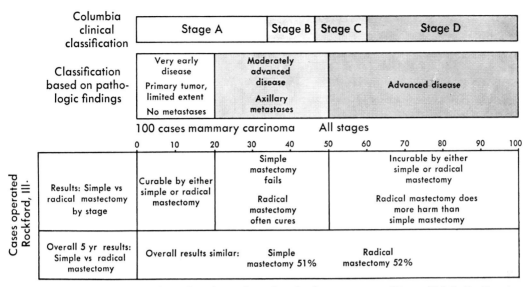

Columbia clinical classification	Stage A			Stage B	Stage C	Stage D	

Fig. 662. Comparison of results of simple and radical mastectomy. (From Habif, D. V.: Selection of treatment for primary breast cancer, Postgrad. Med. **35**:300-306, 1964.)

limited to the breast and low axillary nodes; they are also curable by radical or modified mastectomy, and it is questionable that any additional treatment is needed. Those with carcinomas that have metastasized to the high nodes in the axilla or to the supraclavicular and/or to the internal mammary chain of nodes constitute a group not curable by radical mastectomy alone. Extensions of the radical mastectomy and considerations of surgical adjuvants are concerned only with this group; *their true proportion within the overall group of operable cases may be rather small* (Regato[296b]).

Hormone therapy and chemotherapy are not, at present, expected to contribute to the curability of any of these groups. In some instances, they do, as does palliative radiotherapy, improve the lot and prolong the life of some incurable patients with primary lesions and those with postoperative recurrences and metastases.

Surgery

Various surgical procedures were utilized for the extirpation of malignant tumors of the breast until Halstead and Meyer independently evolved the technique of *radical mastectomy* and placed emphasis on the following classical requisites:

1 Wide excision of the skin
2 Extirpation of both pectoral muscles
3 Thorough axillary dissection
4 Removal of all tissues in one block

The extent of the skin removed and the utilization of vast skin grafts have been thought to be inversely related to the proportion of local recurrences. We know now, however, that local recurrences are more related to the original extent of the tumor (Auchincloss[15]; Oliver and Sugarbaker[273]) and probably also to the extent of internal mammary node involvement. Another point of surgical technique, frequently emphasized as required, is the thinness of the skin flaps left after mastectomy. There is no evidence that this fact alone improves the results (Crile[70]).

A retrospective study of results of radical mastectomy has led to the establishing of criteria of operability, mostly based on the probability of failure due to distant metastases (Haagensen and Stout[146]). Absolute contraindications are as follows:

1 Presence of distant metastases
2 Proved supraclavicular metastases
3 Edema of the arm
4 Extensive edema of the skin of the breast
5 Intercostal or parasternal nodules
6 Satellite tumor nodules
7 Inflammatory type of carcinoma

These contraindications are valid insofar as the likelihood of failure, but it is doubtful that a radical mastectomy may harm any of these patients. In some instances, it is best to operate and give the patient the benefit of doubt. Distant metastases should be above doubt to rule out an operation; supraclavicular metastases should be proved by biopsy. Carcinoma of the breast developing during pregnancy or lactation, once considered by Haagensen and Stout as inoperable, is no longer so considered for, with limited extent and a favorable histologic type, cure is possible. It is questionable whether the patient may gain anything by interruption of pregnancy (Haagensen[140]). Haagensen and Obeid[142] devised a so-called *triple biopsy* as a preliminary procedure before radical mastec-

Table 99. Apex of axilla and internal mammary biopsies (Presbyterian and Francis Delafield Hospitals, New York, Jan., 1955— July, 1957)*

Group	Classification of cases	Cases
1	Neither internal mammary nor apex of axilla nodes involved	65
2	Both internal mammary and apex of axilla nodes involved	13
3	Internal mammary nodes involved Apex of axilla nodes uninvolved	10
3	Internal mammary nodes uninvolved Apex of axilla nodes involved	12
	Total cases with triple biopsy	100
	Total internal mammary nodes involved	23†
	Total apex of axilla nodes involved	25

*From Haagensen, C. D., and Obeid, S. J.: Biopsy of the apex of the axilla in carcinoma of the breast, Ann. Surg. 149:149-161, 1959.
†This does not represent the true frequency of internal mammary metastases found in the studies, because the patients who had internal mammary biopsy only are not included here. The true frequency of internal mammary metastasis is at least 30%.

tomy. It consists of biopsy of the breast tumor, the first three intercostal spaces, and the apex of the axilla. If the apex of the axilla or the internal mammary nodes are involved, they do not proceed with the operation. We have no evidence that this superselection through a rather prolonged preliminary procedure is, in fact, beneficial.

Handley[152] explored the internal mammary nodes during mastectomy, merely as a reconnaissance for prognostic purposes, and tabulated his findings in 300 cases according to location of the primary tumor (Table 100). As a consequence of the acquisition of this knowledge, and the understanding of one more cause of failure of radical mastectomies, *superradical* procedures have been devised and advocated. Wangensteen et al.[366] practiced an *en bloc* dissection of the breast, axillary, internal mammary, supraclavicular, and mediastinal nodes. There was high mortality and morbidity and the end results were poor. The procedure was abandoned. Urban[348-350] modified this approach with removal of half of the sternum and applied the procedure to patients with central and inner quadrant tumors; he had little operative mortality and morbidity.

A *simple mastectomy*, as applied to the treatment of these tumors, implies the resection of the breast without removal of pectoral muscles or axillary contents. Recently, various types of *modified simple mastectomy* have been advocated. In Patey's operation,[284] the breast is removed with the pectoralis minor, Rotter's interpectoral nodes, and the axillary nodes. Auchincloss' procedure[16] implies also the removal of Rotter's and axillary nodes but not of the pectoralis minor. It is a more difficult operation than the radical mas-

Table 100. Invasion of internal mammary chain; biopsy results (300 cases)*

	Inner hemisphere primary tumor (and central area)	Outer hemisphere primary tumor	Total
All nodes free	49	52	101
Axilla only invaded	37	65	102
Internal mammary only invaded	16 ⎫ 43%	3 ⎫ 21%	19 ⎫ 32%
Both internal mammary and axilla invaded	50 ⎭	28 ⎭	78 ⎭
Total	152	148	300

*From Handley, R. S.: Prognosis according to involvement of internal mammary lymph nodes, Acta Un. Int. Cancr. 15:1030-1031, 1959.

tectomy. This operation offers unquestionable advantages, from a functional point of view, over the radical procedure: the arm remains strong, there is no postoperative edema, and dissimulation of the defect is easier. Lymphographic studies have been adduced to show that it is possible to remove, by these means, all involved nodes (Ackland[4]; Kendall et al.[188]) (Fig. 663). However, the lymphographic evaluation is not always accurate. Auchincloss[16] reasons that whenever the apical axillary nodes are involved, the radical mastectomy does not contribute to survival and, on the contrary, the modified simple mastectomy is sufficient to extirpate low axillary nodes. Kouchoukos et al.[202] reviewed 482 specimens of radical mastectomy in an effort to relate the extent of lymph node involvement to the character of the primary tumor. In spite of an appreciable margin of error, they showed that a simple mastectomy could have been decided upon in a number of cases of predictable lack of lymph node involvement, which forms about one-fifth of all cases.

Cystosarcoma phyllodes, both the benign and malignant varieties, should be treated surgically. The clinical suspicion of this entity may be confirmed by frozen section. The essential is to adequately remove the neoplasm. If the tumor extends near the fascia, it may be necessary to excise the muscle. Involvement of axillary lymph nodes is rare, but if the tumor is extensive or involves the muscle, additional dissection of the low axilla should be carried out. Díaz-Bazán and Astacio[90] prefer a systematic radical mastectomy. Local recurrences from the benign variety can occur depending on the adequacy of excision. The malignant variety may recur for the same reason and extend to the chest wall, pleura, and lung. Norris and Taylor[267] indicated that patients with cystosarcoma have a good prognosis if the tumor is small (less than 4 cm in diameter) and has a low mitotic rate and a pushing border. *Sarcomas* of the breast should be treated surgically following the same principles (Steingaszner et al.[324]; Norris and Taylor[268]).

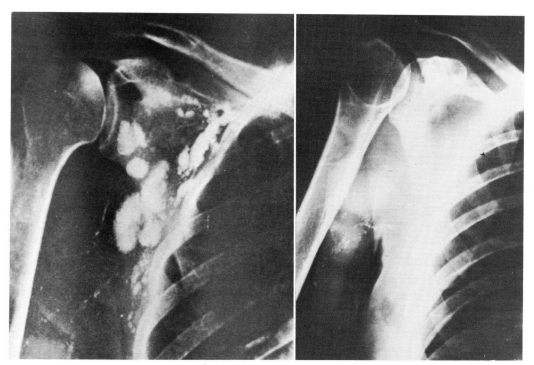

Fig. 663. A, Preoperative axillary lymphography. **B,** Same patient after Patey's dissection. Note adequacy of lymph node dissection. (Courtesy Dr. Thomas H. Ackland, Melbourne, Australia; **A,** WU neg. 69-2732; **B,** WU neg. 69-2731.)

Radiotherapy

It is possible to sterilize carcinomas of the breast by means of radiations, but the systematic application of this form of treatment as an alternative to surgery is not justified in operable lesions. The usefulness of radiotherapy as an adjunct to surgery in the treatment of operable carcinomas of the breast is of questionable value. Radiotherapy plays a very important role in the treatment of inoperable patients, who constitute a large proportion of the cases diagnosed today (Fig. 664). In addition, irradiation of postoperative local recurrences is of great value. Finally, radiotherapy is extremely valuable in the management of bone metastases. In bone metastases a relatively small amount of radiations may relieve pain or even promote bone healing. Radiographic evidence of bone reconstruction is not so constant as relief of pain.

At the present time, the following combinations of surgery and radiotherapy are being advocated:

1 Radical mastectomy plus postoperative radiotherapy
2 Preoperative radiotherapy plus radical mastectomy
3 Simple mastectomy plus postoperative radiotherapy
4 Wedge resection plus postoperative radiotherapy

Despite the careful selection of cases and high surgical skill, about a third of the patients with carcinoma of the breast and axillary metastases who fail to be cured present regional recurrences. Bruce et al.[44a] analyzed the pattern of recurrent disease in 423 potentially curable patients who had simple mastectomy followed by radiotherapy. They pointed out that distant metastasis is the most important feature of therapeutic failure and that often local recrudescence of the disease appears at the same time. Because of this, the support of radiations has been sought as a *postoperative* measure following radical mastectomy. The purpose is to destroy any tumor cells that might be left and thus avoid these recurrences. Pusey and Caldwell[291] applied this principle of "prophylactic" roentgentherapy following radical mastectomy in the very early days after the discovery of the roentgen rays. This conduct has been ardently defended, and it has been the subject of lively controversy for decades. Convincing arguments in favor of systematic postoperative irradiation have been based on a greater percentage of five-year survivals and a relative prolongation of life (Harrington[155]). Actually, the life expec-

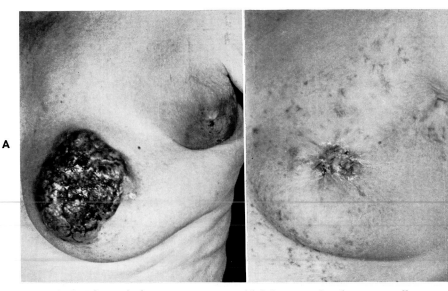

Fig. 664. A, Advanced ulcerative carcinoma of left breast with voluminous axillary metastases. **B,** Same lesion showing healing and clinical disappearance of axillary adenopathy following intensive radiotherapy. Patient later developed supraclavicular and distant metastases.

tancy of failures and the percentage of five-year survivals depend greatly on the widely different concepts of operability and operative skills. Radiotherapy, on the other hand, cannot be expected to have any influence upon the failures that are due to distant metastases.

On a purely radiophysiologic basis and in spite of statistics, doubt may be expressed as to the value of systematic postoperative irradiation. There is no proof that disseminated tumor cells, no matter how few in number, are more radiosensitive or radiocurable than the tumors from which they originate. Serious studies and reports of series of cases have remained unconvincing (Harrington[155]; Gricouroff et al.[125]). Paterson and Russell[283] reported on a random experiment based on 1461 patients with carcinoma of the breast treated at the Christy Hospital of Manchester from 1949 to 1955. These patients were or were not given routine postoperative irradiation, depending only on whether the day of their birth was an even or uneven number. The irradiated patients were divided into two groups. In the first group, the radiations were directed to the operative area only. In the second group, only the supraclavic-

ular and parasternal regions were irradiated. Doses employed were moderate, and treatments were administered with conventional roentgentherapy. The authors of this interesting experiment reported no statistically significant difference in five-year survivals of these patients (Fig. 665), *but there were statistically significant and interesting differences in the proportion of recurrences*, the site of which corresponded well with the technique of irradiation employed (Cole[65]). The randomized study stands to be repeated with supervoltage roentgentherapy or cobalt[60] and a larger dose at the level of the potential metastatic nodes of the apex of the axilla, supraclavicular region, and internal mammary chain. As indicated previously, the potential beneficiaries constitute a small group among the operable patients and consequently only a large material and a long follow-up of cases may give the answer. Whereas the ultimate aim is to improve the overall results, an early sign of the radiotherapeutic effectiveness may be obtained by demonstation of a lesser proportion of regional recurrences. Many of the patients so benefited may die anyway because of the presence of distant metastases,

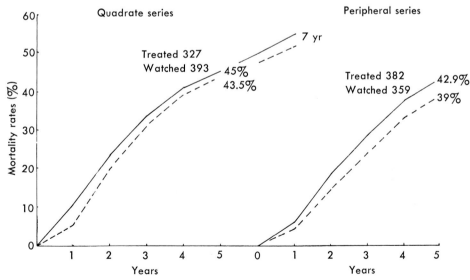

Fig. 665. Mortality in two series of patients with cancer of breast treated by radical mastectomy and randomized between postoperative roentgentherapy (two different techniques) and no irradiation. Note similarity in overall mortality rates in treated (solid lines) and untreated (broken lines) groups. (From Paterson, R., and Russell, M. H.: Clinical trials in malignant disease. Part III—Breast cancer: evaluation of post-operative radiotherapy, J. Fac. Radiol. **10:**175-180, 1959.)

but no one can gainsay the possibility that in a few cases this additional benefit over surgery may result in cure (Regato[296a]).

Even those who would not practice routine postoperative irradiation may find some compelling circumstances. Upon dissection of the axilla, the surgeon may realize that the tumor has been cut through or that it extended beyond the limits of resectability or, following operation, thorough pathologic study of the surgical specimen reveals this same ominous finding. In such cases, a thorough postoperative irradiation of the axilla is indicated as an additional recourse. But then the radiations must be administered in sufficient dosage if a permanent effect upon the remaining tumor is to be expected. The results of the procedure are questionable, but the unfavorable prognosis of such cases justifies it. Recurrences in the axilla following radical mastectomy are infrequent. On the other hand, about half of all patients with axillary metastases also present internal mammary involvement. On the basis of these facts, a rational approach is the irradiation of the apex of the axilla, the supraclavicular region, and the internal mammary nodes following radical mastectomy.

As a *preoperative* measure, radiotherapy has been advocated and studied (Baclesse[18]; Delarue et al.[84]; Fletcher et al.[105]) but has never gained any great number of advocates. In the treatment of operable lesions, few have been willing to delay the operative intervention. Preoperative irradiation has been evaluated on the basis of its ability to destroy completely the present tumor. In reality, the irradiation might be useful even if it failed to do so, but, moreover, the histologic verification of complete destruction depends on the intensity of the irradiation and the time interval before surgical removal. Guttmann[133] employed supervoltage radiations in a group of patients who were considered operable but rejected after biopsy of the apex of the axilla and internal mammary chain (Haagensen and Obeid[142]); the five-year results are notable. Bouchard[42] irradiated advanced inoperable carcinomas of the breast, with complete clinical regression in sixty-one of 109 patients treated and complete regression of palpable lymphadenopathy in half of the cases. In isolated instances, we have verified the ability of radiations to sterilize proved carcinomas and their lymph node metastases. A more important question yet would be to test the usefulness of systematic preoperative irradiation in a random series of operable patients. The borderline inoperable lesions offer an extremely fruitful opportunity to employ this approach without fear of harm. Supervoltage equipment and cobalt[60] permit the administration of large amounts of radiations to the mammary area and the axillary draining area.

Radical radiotherapy has been applied successfully to the treatment of inoperable lesions (Delclos and Johnson[85]; Edelman et al.[93]; Montague[252]). An extensive irradiation of the breast, axilla, and supraclavicular region is required, an irradiation capable of administering at any point of the tumor a minimum dose of several thousand rads in a few weeks (Sarrazin and Lalanne[305]). A fractionated irradiation diminishes the possible untoward effects on the lung. The results of these painstaking efforts are not often rewarding. Baclesse[19] reported that 133 patients (31%) appeared well at the end of five years in a series of 431 cases in all stages treated by radiotherapy only. Gummel and Widow[129] found no relationship between the effects of radiations, as judged histologically, and the prognosis of the case.

A combination of *simple mastectomy and wide roentgentherapy* has been courageously advocated by McWhirter[238] *in lieu of* radical mastectomy for operable tumors. He based this innovation on the idea that when the axilla is not invaded, an axillary dissection is not necessary, whereas when the axilla is invaded, "the radical mastectomy often fails." This statement can be widely disproved. Deaths during the first two years following diagnosis or treatment are predominantly due to far-advanced or highly malignant tumors. Johnson[182] shows that when these first two years are excluded, there is little difference in survival rates between McWhirter's series of radical mastectomy and the experimental series with simple mastectomy plus roentgentherapy. Johnson[182] concludes that the apparent difference is due only to the varying proportions of highly malignant tumors in the series. In order to accept the practice of

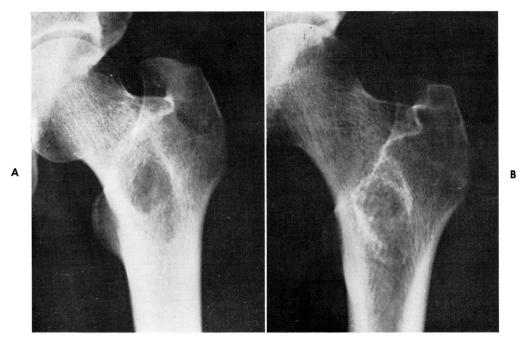

Fig. 666. A, Metastatic carcinoma of head of femur producing osteolytic transparency. **B,** Same lesion eighteen months after roentgentherapy showing reformation of bone.

this procedure, one would have to agree that a radical mastectomy may actually be harmful and that radiotherapy may control a greater proportion of axillary metastases than is the case with radical surgery and without greater morbidity or mortality.

Radiotherapy finds its most useful indication in the treatment of *bone metastases* from carcinomas of the breast. Early roentgentherapy to metastatic lesions of the vertebrae rapidly eliminates pain and avoids collapse of the vertebrae and subsequent paraplegia. Elsewhere, radiotherapy to a metastatic lesion of the bone may circumvent a fracture or help to recalcify one that has already occurred (Fig. 666). The recalcification of these lesions occurs with a variable intensity in different individuals. Radiotherapy has an unquestionable anodyne effect in the treatment of osseous metastases which, in itself, is sufficient reason for its indication. Local recurrences on the chest wall may be controlled successfully by irradiation and assure the patient of a long survival. The irradiation of limited areas may be sufficient, but in some instances it is best to include a large area of the chest wall. In order to do this without excessive exposure of the lung, several techniques have been proposed.

Endocrine therapy

In the palliative management of incurable mammary cancer, one may have recourse to fruitful alterations of the hormonal environment. These purposes may be approached by *hormone therapy* (i.e., the administration of androgens, estrogens, progestogens, and corticosteroids) or by surgery (i.e., *endocrine organ ablations*, such as oophorectomy, orchiectomy, adrenalectomy, and hypophysectomy) (Figs. 667 and 668). The choice of procedure to follow may be perplexing, and any hint of tumor hormone dependence, or lack of it, may save the patient unnecessary difficulties. Bulbrook et al.[47, 50] found that patients with cancer of the breast who show a subnormal urinary excretion of androgen and corticosteroid metabolites have a greater recurrence rate after mastectomy than patients with normal excretions; in a clinical trial, they confirmed the predictability of response to endocrine ablations. Crowley et al.[73] studied the excretion patterns of urinary metabolites of estradiol-

4-C[14] and noted a lower amount among women with cancer than in those with cystic disease, but the differences found between those who responded to estrogen therapy and those who did not were insufficient for discrimination. Miller et al.[249] described a method that would permit prediction of response. Atkins et al.[12] have used discriminant function for the prediction of response to adrenalectomy or hypophysectomy. The combination of various clinical factors with discriminant function helps to identify a group of patients who are not responsive to endocrine ablation. Unfortunately, many of the urinary excretion tests are not easily done in any laboratory. One fact is clear: if the patient responds favorably to the first endocrine therapy, other measures are likely to meet a similar favorable response (Kennedy and Fortuny[196]). The scheme devised by Kennedy[194] (Figs. 669 and 670) is a practical approach to the problem. In any event, the decisions to be made on behalf of the patient may be onerous rather than helpful. These decisions should be pondered seriously by those with an understanding of neoplasia and of the significance of the various manifestations.

Hormone therapy of advanced cancer of the breast may prove very fruitful: A carefully controlled cooperative study was carried out for twelve years under the Therapeutic Trials Committee of the American Medical Association[340]: *androgens* produced objective regressions in 20% of the premenopausal and 21% of the postmenopausal patients, and *estrogens* produced 36% regressions in the postmenopausal patients. Estrogens were relatively more effective in the soft tissue lesions, whereas androgens were more effective on skeletal metastases. The results of studies of the Cooperative Breast Cancer Group[339] carried out from 1956 to 1963 revealed 112 responses out of 521 patients treated with testosterone. Androgens have undesirable side effects which often cause rejection of its use by the patients. Kennedy[194] advises the use of estrogens as the initial approach for postmenopausal women. A patient who fails to improve with androgens may do so with estrogens. The reverse is less often true. If a remission occurs with one hormone, the even-

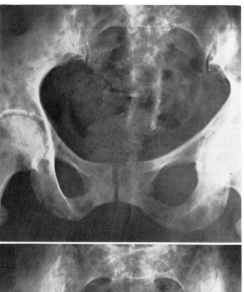

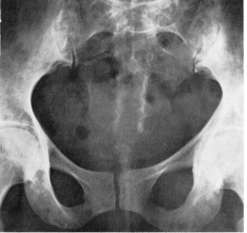

Fig. 667. **A,** Extensive osteolytic metastases from rapidly growing carcinoma of breast in young woman who was confined to bed. **B,** Noticeable regression of bone lesions after irradiation of ovaries. Patient regained weight, large breast lesion almost disappeared, and she resumed work for year before death.

tual reactivation of the disease may respond to the other one. Administration of both hormones may yield some good results (Kennedy and Brown[195]). *Corticosteroids* are suppressors of adrenal function which, when effective, give remarkable objective and subjective regressions and considerable prolongation of life, particularly in patients who have previously responded favorably to estrogens, androgens, or ovarian ablation. The corticosteroids seem to be of particular value in the rapid relief of serious symptoms such as effusions, edema, jaundice, hypercalcemia, and pain.

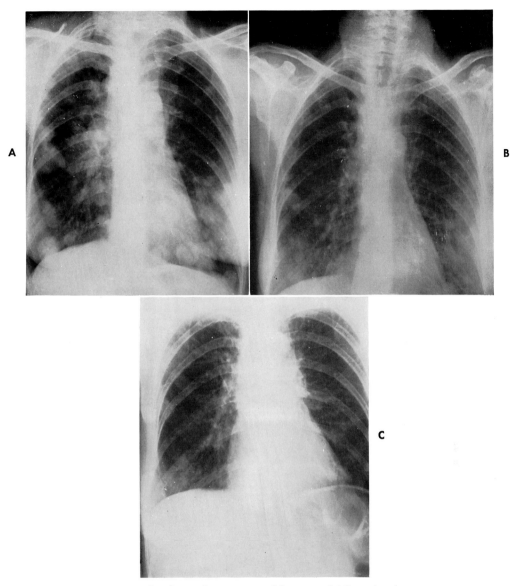

Fig. 668. A, Patient with advanced carcinoma of breast and bilateral pulmonary metastases. B, Same patient five weeks after short period on estrogen therapy. C, Same patient six months later, still on estrogen therapy. (PCH 60-245.)

The use of *progestogens* has not been, as yet, sufficiently warranted to be used as an alternative to other hormones.

Endocrine organ ablations can also be used in the management of cancer of the breast. However, greater information and observation are needed to decide on their indications. *Oophorectomy* has been advised as a routine procedure following or concomitantly with a radical mastectomy in young women. Such routine ablation imposes an unnecessary artificial menopause in women who may be cured. It also eliminates any discrimination as to the hormone dependence of the tumor which could be utilized later if the tumor is not controlled by surgery. Lewison[217] favors routine oophorectomy for women with cancer of the breast with axillary metastases who are under 40 years of age and also for those over 40 years with a high estrogenic index in the vaginal cyto-

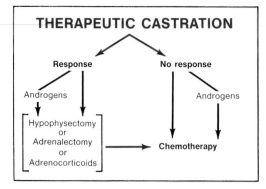

Fig. 669. Pattern of sequential hormone therapy for advanced breast cancer in premenopausal women. (From Kennedy, B. J.: Endocrine therapy of breast cancer, J.A.M.A. **200:**971-972, 1967.)

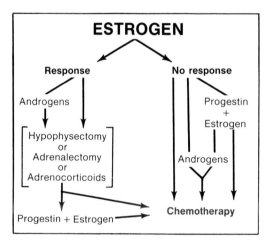

Fig. 670. Pattern of sequential hormone therapy for advanced breast cancer in postmenopausal women. (From Kennedy, B. J.: Endocrine therapy of breast cancer, J.A.M.A. **200:**971-972, 1967.)

gram. Kennedy[191] has thoroughly demonstrated that there is no advantage to the routine ovarian ablation. We are also of this opinion.

Oophorectomy or *radiotherapeutic suppression of ovarian function* is the first indication in the management of young women with disseminated disease. Ovarian ablation is of no value in women who have undergone complete involution of ovarian function following cessation of menstruation. There continues to be some ovarian function for several years after the menopause. Barlow et al.[21a] find that postmenopausal ovaries make no contribution to estrogen production. Estrogen activity in early postmenopausal women may be

Table 101. Comparative survival after adrenalectomy—objective responders versus nonresponders*

Type of response	Survival (yr)				
	1	2	3	4	5
Responders (110 cases)	89	41	29	20	15
%	80.9	37.2	26.3	18.1	13.6
Nonresponders (170 cases)	51	14	5	2	0
%	30	8.2	2.9	1.2	0

Of 306 cases, seventeen postoperative deaths, two male cases, and seven cases in which response classification was impossible were excluded from this table.

*From Yonemoto, R. H., et al.: Long-term survival after adrenalectomy for advanced cancer of the breast, Cancer **20:**254-259, 1967.

determined by vaginal smears or urine bioassay, but hormone excretion studies of the urine are difficult and costly (Rubin[302]). Irradiation of the ovary results in the arrest of ovulation. The eventual hormonal change results from the radiophysiologic involution of the organ following cessation of menstruation. Large doses of radiations cannot affect the internal secretion of the irradiated ovary; only time achieves it. Thus, the oophorectomy is a faster way of achieving the aim. Irradiation is less immediate (Debois[82]) but not less effective.

Bilateral adrenalectomy may be effective particularly in patients who have shown favorable responses to orchiectomy (McLaughlin et al.[232]), oophorectomy, or hormone therapy (Harris and Spratt[160]). A greater proportion of premenopausal women who have reacted favorably to castration will respond to adrenalectomy also, whereas a small proportion of the nonresponders will be favorably affected by it (Yonemoto et al.[380]) (Table 101). This has brought into consideration whether adrenalectomy should not be done first in certain patients, such as in those with inflammatory carcinomas (Johnson[182]), rather than as a secondary procedure, but this is disputed by others (Atkins et al.[13]). Adrenalectomy is now safely carried out with the aid of cortisone acetate. The longer the time interval between the radical mastectomy and adrenalectomy, the longer the survival (Mye and Neal[260]). In cancer of the male breast with metastases, *bilateral orchiectomy* yields excellent palliation in a high proportion of cases (Houttuin et al.[171]). Adrenalectomy may also result in remission in metastatic carcinoma of the male breast (McLaughlin et al.[232]).

Hypophysectomy is a useful palliative operation. A joint committee of the American College of Physicians and of the American College of Surgeons evaluated the results in 358 patients who survived hypophysectomy: 112 (31%) showed definite improvement, with the best results being obtained in women in the first decade after cessation of periods (Jessiman et al.[181]). The greater morbidity and mortality of the operation may be minimized in skilled hands, but many patients would not be eligible for the operation. Atkins et al.[10, 11] and Hayward and Bulbrook[162, 163] have used a positive discriminate function to predict the response to adrenalectomy or hypophysectomy over a ten-year period. They have found it useful when combined with other factors such as the cancer-free period and menopausal status in the selection of patients. For instance, patients without a previous mastectomy do not respond so well to adrenalectomy as they do to hypophysectomy. Significant atrophy of the adrenal glands may be observed after hypophysectomy (Jantet et al.[180]). Implementation of radioactive yttrium through a transethmoidal approach may destroy the pituitary gland and yield favorable results (Greening and Thompson[123]; Critchley[72]).

Chemotherapy

Antineoplastic drugs have been disappointingly ineffective in cancer of the breast. In a cooperative clinical trial at thirty institutions, Thio-TEPA was administered as a surgical adjuvant to patients undergoing radical mastectomy, and the results were compared with those following the administration of 5-fluorouracil and of a placebo. There was no difference in the rate of recurrences and metastases and in survival between those who received Thio-TEPA or a placebo (Noer[265]). The toxicity of 5-fluorouracil made its use unwarranted (Fisher et al.[101]). Ansfield[8] found both drugs ineffective. Melphalan and methotrexate (Vogler et al.[357]) have been tried and produced short-term regressions.

Prognosis

In 1965 there were in the United States 27,048 deaths from cancer of the breast or a crude rate of 14.0 per 100,000 population. The rate was 28.4 for white and 18.3 for nonwhite females. The mortality rates for 1955, 1960, and 1965 are essentially the same as they have been for thirty-five years. The highest age-adjusted mortality rate, about 50% higher than the United States white female rate, is reported from LaPlata, Argentina. The lowest mortality rates are found in the Union of Socialist Soviet Republics and a few countries of Eastern Asia, Africa, and the Caribbean. The Japanese rate is about one-sixth that of the United States.

An estimation of the average duration of life of untreated patients with cancer of the breast would require the observation of a large number of *consecutive* patients, without selection for age, race, economic status, etc. who would not be given any form of treatment. Such series of patients is not likely to be produced. Instead, we have observations of patients who refused or were not eligible for treatment and series of "consecutive" numbers of such cases. Such series naturally contain an abnormal number of elderly or indigent patients with slow-growing tumors that cause no alarm or symptoms for a long time. Daland's analysis[77] of 100 untreated patients is a classic series to which reference often is made—22% of the patients survived five years and 5% were living at the end of ten years (Fig. 671). Bloom et al.[38] reviewed the records of 250 patients (seen from 1805 to 1933) who were given no treatment for cancer of the breast and found that 18% survived five years, 3.6% survived ten years, and 0.8% were living at the end of fifteen years. Comparison with a more recent series of treated patients showed definite improvement in the survival of that group (Table 102).

The age of the patient does not have in itself any prognostic value. The prognosis of women under 30 years of age with cancer of the breast is similar to that of older women with tumors of comparable extent (Moore and Lewis[255]). However, Papadrianos et al.[275] have shown that women over 65 years of age, as a group, do better. Escher and Kaufman[99] reported a poorer

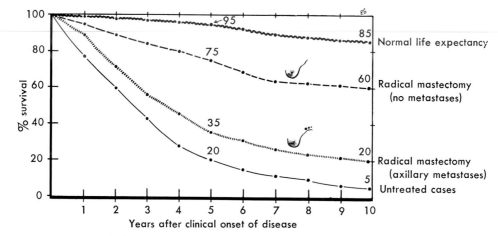

Fig. 671. Survival of patients with cancer of breast after radical mastectomy compared with untreated patients (Daland[77]) and with normal life expectancy of women at 47 years of age.

Table 102. Survival from onset of symptoms in treated and untreated patients with cancer of breast*

	Survival		
	5 yr	10 yr	15 yr
Untreated patients 1805-1933	46/250 (18%)	9/250 (3.6%)	2/250 (0.8%)
Treated patients 1936-1949	683/1246 (55%)	244/714 (34%)	68/303 (22%)

*From Bloom, H. J. G., et al.: Natural history of untreated breast cancer (1805-1933), Brit. Med. J. 2:213-221, 1962; reprinted by permission of authors and editor.

prognosis for patients within five years after cessation of periods as compared with those in subsequent years or before the menopause. Patients who had an artificial premature menopause have an unfavorable prognosis when they subsequently develop carcinoma of the breast (Dargent[79]; Ackerman[1]).

The prognosis of patients with carcinoma of the breast diagnosed during *pregnancy* or *lactation* is poor. Harrington[157] found that the prognosis of those diagnosed during pregnancy was relatively better. Of twelve patients with carcinomas confined to the breast, White and White[370] reported six survivors, but only two of twenty-five with axillary metastases survived. Rissanen[297] reported thirty-three patients with mammary carcinoma during pregnancy or lactation: three-fourths had axillary metastases and 43% of them survived five years. Peters[289] studied 126 patients with mammary cancer associated with pregnancy. She found that patients who became pregnant subsequent to treated mammary cancer did best, whereas those in whom cancer became clinically apparent during the lactation period did worst. She found no evidence that interruption of pregnancy coexisting with mammary cancer was of value. In her series, there was no evidence that immediate *prophylactic castration* in patients of the premenopausal age group was of value. It appeared best to delay definitive treatment until the postpartum period.

Clinical classifications of cancer of the breast have been often discarded as inadequate in relating prognosis due to the variations in clinical behavior and response to treatment which may be observed. The clinical classification proposed by Haagensen et al.[141] (p. 852) has the merits of its application to the material of seven institutions with apparently consistent results.

Patients who have had a *radical mastectomy* should be followed indefinitely because local recurrence or distant metastases may appear many years (up to forty-five) after operation. However, the most important reason for continuing follow-up in these patients is that they have a three to four times greater chance of developing a second carcinoma in the opposite breast than a woman of the same age has of developing her first cancer. Urban[352] biopsied

Table 103. Five-year and ten-year results of radical mastectomy*

	5 yr results 1935-1950		10 yr results 1935-1945	
	No.	%	No.	%
Number of radical mastectomies	356		216	
Operative deaths	0		0	
Lost track of before end of period	0		0	
Died of unknown cause before end of period	3	0.8	2	0.9
Died of intercurrent disease before end of period	13	3.7	9	4.2
Died of breast carcinoma before end of period	103	28.9	98	45.4
Alive at end of period (relative survival rates)	237	66.6	107	49.5
Alive without recurrence at end of period (relative clinical cure rates)	202	56.7	95	44.0

*From Haagensen, C. D.: Diseases of the breast, Philadelphia, 1956, W. B. Saunders Co., and personal communication.

the opposite breast of 159 patients with mammary carcinoma, in ninety-nine instances because of minimal clinical or mammographic suspicion: twelve cases of infiltrating carcinoma and twelve of noninfiltrating carcinoma were diagnosed. In 1199 patients who had a radical mastectomy and 573 of whom were living after five years, Kilgore et al.[199] reported thirty-one (2.6%) carcinomas of the opposite breast eighteen months to eighteen years later. Patients who originally had a limited lesion, a greater proportion of whom lived longer, were more often subject to a second lesion.

Haagensen's personal series[139] of operable carcinomas of the breast demonstrates the best results that can be obtained with a selected series (Table 103). A single surgeon reported on the results of 930 radical mastectomies, done between 1920 and 1955 and without operative mortality after 1944, with an absolute five-year survival of 50% and ten-year survival of 34% (Buchanan[46]). Early lesions confined to the breast yield an even better result (Shimkin[312]). In eight cases of carcinoma detected through mammography, Stevens and Weigen[326] found none with axillary metastases. However, it must be stressed that only a rare fast-growing tumor will be detected by this method. In thirty-four patients whose carcinoma was found early during a cancer screening examination, twenty-six had no evidence of lymph node involvement and twenty-five survived five years, and six of eight who had lymph node metastases also survived (Gilbertson[118]).

Cáceres[54] reported the results of "extended" radical mastectomy on 616 patients: 386 (62%) survived five years; 183 (47%) patients of 387 at risk survived ten years. Of a total of 115 patients with proved metastases to the internal mammary nodes, thirty-six (31%) survived five years, and of seventy-six at risk, twelve (16%) survived ten years. In the few patients with internal mammary but no axillary involvement, eight of sixteen survived five years and five of seven survived ten years.

The larger the tumor, the worse the prognosis (Fig. 672). The presence or absence of lymph node involvement is, of course, important. The degree of the involvement is also of some relative importance. The prognosis of patients with only one lymph node involved, in the low or mid axilla, is almost the same as for those patients without lymphatic metastases (Kouchoukos et al.[202]). Fitts et al.[103] reported on eleven patients with mammary carcinomas in whom the only manifestation was an enlarged axillary node. Such patients have a good prognosis because often only that node is involved. When more than three axillary nodes are involved, the survival drops precipitously (Harvey and Auchincloss[160a]). Extension of tumor outside the nodes is also unfavorable. Hultborn and Törnberg[174] reported a 52% five-year survival when perinodular involvement was not present and only 19% when perinodular involvement was present. Absence of axillary involvement does not exclude the possibility of internal mammary metastases and consequent poor prognosis. Handley[152, 153] reported forty-one five-year survivals (84%) in a series of forty-nine patients in whom no axillary or internal mammary involvement was found. In contrast, only two in a series of forty-one patients with both axillary and internal mammary involvement were living (Table 104).

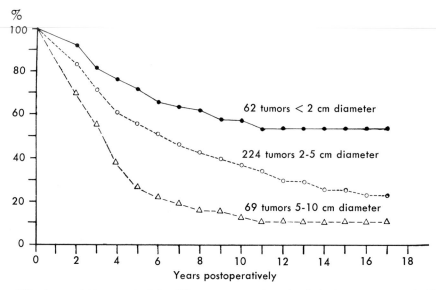

Fig. 672. Accumulative survival in different tumor sizes (pathologic measurement). Note prominent difference in prognosis according to size. (Group of cases from Ellis Fischel State Cancer Hospital, Columbia, Mo., studied by Dr. H. R. Butcher, Jr., and Dr. Bo Törnberg in 1960; WU neg. 60-3975.)

Table 104. Invasion of internal mammary chain—five-year results (200 cases with 100% follow-up)*†

	Total	Alive and well	Alive with recurrence	Dead
No nodes involved	68	53 (78%)	3	12
Axilla only invaded	66	36	8	22
Internal mammary nodes only invaded	12	6	1	5
Both axillary and internal mammary nodes invaded	54	7 (13%)	8	39

*From Handley, R.: Observations and reflections on breast cancer, J. Roy. Coll. Surg. Edinb. 6:1-12, 1960.
†Patients were treated by modified radical mastectomy, leaving the pectoralis major muscle. Internal mammary nodes were removed by dissection. Note poor prognosis when internal mammary nodes were involved.

The prognosis of any given series of cases reported depends, above all, on the proportion of low metastasizing tumors included in the group. These are the medullary, papillary, intraductal, and well-differentiated carcinomas plus the lobular carcinomas in situ and those with excess mucin production. *In any large series of patients, this group constitutes about 15% of the whole. Medullary carcinomas* may metastasize in 25% of cases, usually to only one lymph node. *Papillary carcinomas*, even when invasive, have a low rate of metastases. *Intraductal carcinomas* that are confined to the ducts and *lobular carcinomas* that are confined to lobules do not metastasize at all. *Well-differentiated adenocarcinomas* have only a 10% chance of metastases. All of these carcinomas may

be cured by modified simple mastectomy (Kouchoukos et al.[202]).

Bilateral or *simultaneous carcinomas* of the breast have a prognosis that is also dependent on the presence or absence of axillary lymph node metastases. If the carcinoma is both bilateral and simultaneous, the prognosis is much worse (Farrow[100]). A patient with a carcinoma in the medial half of the breast without axillary lymph node metastases has a poorer prognosis than one with a similar tumor located elsewhere in the breast.

There is no proof that postoperative radiotherapy is of value in the treatment of carcinoma of the breast; neither is there proof that it is not. An additional self-evident statement is that postoperative irradiation is unnecessary in the treatment of carcinomas limited to the breast or to the breast and low axilla (when that is actually the case). It should also be self-evident that postoperative radiotherapy (administered before the facts are known) could not possibly help the rather large proportion of operable patients who already have distant metastases when operated upon. An appraisal of any benefits derived from postoperative radiotherapy would concern those few patients with high axillary or supraclavicular or internal mammary involvement *who do not already have distant metastases.* Although their proportion may be indeed small, no one can deny the possibility that they may benefit importantly. Differences that affect such small groups are clouded when considering the results of *all* patients treated (Regato[296b]). Unwarranted conclusions on the basis of limited or inappropriate material (Getzen et al.[117]; Hutchinson[176]) continue to cloud the issues. Cooperative clinical trials could reveal the differences, but they are not above suspicion of bias and not infrequently attempt to give old prejudices a new dignity (Regato[296a]). Statisticians often simplify their task by comparing survival in the entire sample, ignoring the undeterminable number of the few that may benefit. Clinician's preconceived ideas of what is right bring false scruples and false moral connotations into clinical research which devalue the significance of the findings. Statisticians as well as clinicians may overlook the protean ingredient—the unrandomizable diversity of biologic behaviors exhibited by mammary tumors.

The observation has been variously made that groups of patients receiving postoperative radiotherapy may show a lesser rate of regional recurrences but may more often die from distant metastases than those not so treated (Forrest et al.[108]; Norris and Taylor[266]; Fisher et al.[101a]). In everyday practice it is the patients with more rapidly growing, more malignant, and more extensive tumors who are likely to be referred for postoperative radiotherapy: often they are subsequently found to harbor disseminated disease. The group they are compared with contains all of the tumors which are small or remain confined to the breast and low axilla. Even in randomized clinical trials, surgeons have been

found avoiding the irradiation of their more favorable cases. The differences should be analyzed in the light of this bias and of the arguments in the preceding paragraph. Instead, the retrospective explanation is quickly advanced that the differences are due to untoward effects on the "barrier of immunity" of lymph nodes and to "systemic effects" of radiations that would facilitate generalization of the tumor. There is no valid support, experimental or clinical, for these assumptions. Bond,[38a] in another retrospective study, has noted no such difference when the axillary nodes were involved; however, he has observed an increase in the occurrence of metastatic disease in patients with clinically negative nodes who received "prophylactic" irradiation following surgery, with a 7% to 9% fall in survival rate. Enticing though the sophisticated ideas of "host immunity" may be, we suggest that the partisans of this explanation attempt to test it on the basis of a prospective scientific design rather than be satisfied with retrospective study.

Using a rather limited simple mastectomy and postoperative roentgentherapy as a systematic form of treatment on a large series of unselected cases, McWhirter[240] obtained an impressive rate of five-year and ten-year survivals at the Royal Infirmary of Edinburgh (Table 105). Kaae[183] reported 219 patients treated by simple mastectomy plus radiotherapy and compared them with 206 patients treated by radical mastectomy plus dissection of supraclavicular and internal mammary nodes: the ten-year survival rates, local and regional recurrence rates, and distant metastases rates were identical in both series. Brinkley and Haybittle[43] compared two series of patients with carcinomas confined to the breast and axilla; ninety-one patients were treated by radical mastectomy plus radiotherapy and 113 patients were treated by simple mastectomy followed by postoperative radiotherapy; no statistically significant difference in results was observed. The difficulty with such comparison is that in the first group radiotherapy is intended as a postoperative surgical *adjuvant,* whereas in the second radiotherapy was done *in lieu of* axillary dissection: regional recurrences may or

Table 105. Results of simple mastectomy plus radiotherapy*

Stage of disease	1941-1947 5-year crude survival rate			1941-1942 10-yr crude survival rate		
	Total	*Alive*	*% alive*	*Total*	*Alive*	*% alive*
Operable	1063	612	58	254	99	39
Locally advanced	546	162	30	157	23	15
Distant metastases present	273	12	4	69	0	0
Total	1882	786	42	480	122	25

*From McWhirter, R.: Simple mastectomy and radiotherapy in the treatment of breast cancer, Brit. J. Radiol. 28: 128-139, 1955.

Table 106. Comparison of results of simple mastectomy plus radiotherapy (Edinburgh[240]) and of radical mastectomy plus radiotherapy (Saskatchewan[367])

Factors	Edinburgh	Saskatchewan
Period under review	1941-1947	1944-1952
Selection of patients	None	None
Percentage "seen" of all cases occurring in a circumscribed geographic region	Nearly all	Nearly all
Percentage of patients appearing originally with distant metastases	15%	13%
Percentage of patients, pathologically unproved, who survived five years	0.4%	1%
Intercurrent deaths under five years	Counted as "deaths from cancer"	Counted as "deaths from cancer"
Untraced patients	None	6 (all counted as "dead from cancer")
Total number of primary cases seen	1882	1055
Gross five-year survival rate	42%	52%

may not be an early index of usefulness of radiotherapy in the first group, whereas only a long follow-up may decide the validity of the substitution in the second (Regato[296b]).

Watson,[367] a radiotherapist, insists on the advantage of radical mastectomy combined with postoperative radiotherapy over the McWhirter technique, as demonstrated on a large series in Saskatchewan, Canada (Table 106). In a series of 592 patients with carcinoma of the breast and verified axillary involvement treated by radical mastectomy plus postoperative radiotherapy (Watson[368]), 303 (51%) survived five years.

Delarue et al.[84] reported on the results of *preoperative irradiation* followed by radical mastectomy at the Ontario Cancer Institute and the Toronto General Hospital with significant improvement in survival noted particularly in patients with the "locally advanced" tumors: of 370 patients so treated, sixty-nine (18.6%) survived ten years. Kaae[183] compared a group of 308 patients treated by preoperative irradia-tion and radical mastectomy with another group of 180 patients treated by "extended" radical mastectomy without benefit of irradiation. The irradiated patients showed fewer local recurrences. As one would expect, the proportion of patients in both series who developed distant metastases was about the same.

Guttman[133, 134] reported on a series of 148 cases found inoperable by Haagensen's triple biopsy technique and treated with supervoltage roentgentherapy, with eighty-nine patients (60%) surviving five years. After more than fifteen years of this approach, Haagensen et al.[140a] have decided to follow Handley's example: to proceed with a radical mastectomy in spite of internal mammary involvement and to administer postoperative radiotherapy to this area. This is a belated acceptance of our long-held point of view that a radical mastectomy may prove often useless but not necessarily harmful. The fact is that the extensive irradiation of the entire breast, axilla, and supraclavicular and internal

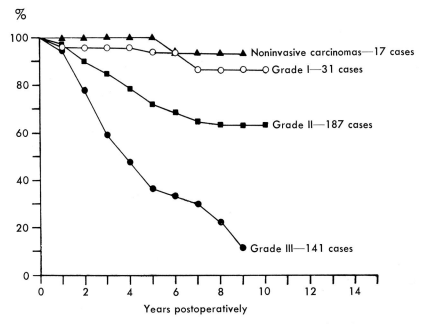

Fig. 673. Survival rates after radical mastectomy for different grades of mammary cancer (accumulative; Barnes Hospital, St. Louis, Mo.).

mammary regions, to a meaningful dose, is not in itself innocuous. Radical irradiation of advanced cancer of the breast may prove worthwhile: Fletcher and Montague[104] reported ninety-nine patients (20%) living and well in a series of irradiated patients.

After operation, the prognosis may be related to the gross findings and to histopathology. The actual dimensions of the tumor, as measured on the specimen, correlates well with the proportion of lymph node metastases found. The histologic grading of the tumor may prove fruitful when used in the light of the size of the primary lesion and the extent of the regional involvement. Lane et al.[207] felt that the histologic character of the periphery of the tumor is of prognostic importance. In forty-six patients with well-delineated carcinomas, the five-year survival was 80%, whereas in 158 with lesions with irregular borders, the five-year survival was 38%. Hultburn and Törnberg[174] emphasized the importance of grading in prognosis and reported five-year survivals of 98% for Grade I, 78% for Grade II, and 37% for Grade III (Fig. 673). Extensive edema, satellite nodules, and metastases to the supraclavicular region or the opposite axilla imply no hope of cure.

Clinical fixation to the pectoral fascia may not be due to tumor extension.

Microscopic examination of the specimen helps determine the prognosis by establishing the number and position of the involved axillary nodes. Black et al.[31] proposed that sinus histiocytoses found in radical mastectomy specimens in the axillary lymph nodes represent host resistance. Patients with inflammatory carcinoma do poorly. The lesion recurs rapidly after mastectomy and usually develops brain and liver metastases. There is no correlation of this tumor with endocrine therapy and chemotherapy response. Local control of inflammatory carcinoma and prolonged survival may be obtained by irradiation (Wang and Griscom[364]).

If the microscopic examination demonstrates invasion of the muscle, the outlook is extremely poor. Blood vessel invasion by tumor, as shown in the surgical specimen, significantly reduces the ten-year survival when in the presence of lymph node metastases (Kister et al.[200]). Certain well-defined, circumscribed types of carcinoma (intraductal, papillary cystadenocarcinoma, gelatinous carcinoma) have a better prognosis than the rest because their evolution is longer and they metastasize late. The

Table 107. Carcinoma of breast—occurrence of regional recurrences within ten years*

Columbia clinical classification	Method of treatment	Parasternal recurrence % 10 yr	Chest wall recurrence % 10 yr	Axillary recurrence % 10 yr	Recurrence % 10 yr
Stage A	Total mastectomy + axillary dissection + irradiation Williams and Stone	0	12	10	22
	Conservative radical mastectomy Handley and Thackray	5	12	2	16
	McWhirter method Kaae and Johansen	1	10	8	19
	Extended radical mastectomy Dahl-Iversen and Tobiassen	2	10	8	20
	Radical mastectomy Haagensen and Cooley	4	3	0	7
Stage B	Total mastectomy + axillary dissection + irradiation Williams and Stone	0	12	14	26
	Conservative radical mastectomy Handley and Thackray	6	22	0	26
	McWhirter method Kaae and Johansen	0	11	18	29
	Extended radical mastectomy Dahl-Iversen and Tobiassen	0	16	16	32
	Radical mastectomy Haagensen and Cooley	5	13	1	18

*From Haagensen, C. D., et al.: Treatment of early mammary carcinoma; a cooperative international study, Ann. Surg. **170:**875-899, 1969.

same is true of the medullary type of carcinoma (Moore and Foote[254]). In the presence of a palpable tumor in Paget's disease, the prognosis is poor (Rissanen and Holsti[298]).

Gricouroff[124] proposed a microscopic classification of carcinomas of the breast in four grades based on (1) anaplasia of the cells, (2) absence of glandlike formation, and (3) infiltration of adjacent structures. This classification takes no notice of the number of mitoses, composition of the stroma, or invasion of blood and lymphatic vessels. An assessment of results in comparison with the histologic grade in 281 cases showed that the five-year survival rates were 75%, 50%, 33%, and 14% for Grades I, II, III, and IV, respectively, permitting histopathologic discrimination between cases of similar gross extension. Later, Bloom[35] proposed a classification that would take into consideration both the clinical stage and the histologic grading.

Recurrences after radical mastectomy appear most frequently on the chest wall, whereas after lesser mastectomies, they occur most frequently in the axilla (Table 107). A group of twenty-nine patients treated by radical mastectomy following simple mastectomy for carcinoma of the breast was reported by Donegan.[92] The five-year and ten-year survival rates were 54% and 37%, respectively. The prognosis of patients with recurrences or metastases, following initial treatment, implies consideration of the apparently cancer-free interval, the menstrual status, the site of recurrence or metastases, the hormonal response, etc. The longer the cancer-free period, the longer the expected life span reflecting the rate of growth of the tumor. However, Papaioannou et al.[277] did not find significant differences in the survival of two groups of patients with recurrent or metastatic carcinomas occurring within the second year or after five years. Patients with a local recurrence have a relatively better prognosis, whereas those with visceral metastases have a very bad outlook. Patients with a radiographic demonstration of bone metastases have a 35% chance of survival for one year and a 10% chance for a two-year survival (Ariel and Lehman[9]). An important prognostic factor for these patients is their potential response to endocrine therapy. Kaufman et al.[185] found that radiation therapy helps the prognosis of recurrences in patients who show no favorable response to hormone therapy.

Den Besten and Ziffren[86] demonstrated no statistical difference in the five-year survival in patients undergoing simple mastectomy and those undergoing radical mastectomy irrespective of the presence or absence of clinically detectable nodes. Copher et al.[69] compared the results of treatment of 210 patients at Barnes Hospital in St. Louis during 1912 to 1933 with those of 739 patients treated at the Ellis Fischel Cancer Hospital during 1940 to 1955: the latter group showed a better survival apparently due to a greater proportion of earlier lesions in the series.

Carcinomas of the male breast have a much worse prognosis than those of the female breast. This is almost entirely related to the fact that when first seen they invariably present axillary lymph node metastases. Norris and Taylor[269] reported 113 cases of carcinoma of the male breast, seventy-five of which proved inoperable. Of the twenty-nine patients without axillary metastases, only 14% died, whereas of forty-six with lymph node involvement, 80% died. Early involvement of the dermal lymphatics seems to be responsible for the darker outlook of mammary cancer in males.

It is very difficult to draw conclusions on the results of treatments by comparisons of any two series of cases, for they are seldom comparable (Smithers et al.[319]). Often, two periods of work at the same institution show a favorable result for the more recent one which may be simply explained by earlier diagnosis (Collins and Adams[67]). Patients treated at an earlier stage of the disease, even when unsuccessfully, may yield a longer survival *after treatment.*

In evaluating the results of treatment, it may be appropriate to use *the point* of biologic truncation of the probit line (Bliss and Stevens[32])—i.e., the point in the follow-up where the annual death rate of a group of treated patients become equal to that of the general population of the same age. Thus, simple mastectomy may be reckoned the therapeutic equal of radical mastectomy in the following categories: those without axillary metastases whether they subsequently die of cancer or not and those with axillary metastases who die before the point of truncation of the probit line. Similarly, radical mastectomy must be reckoned superior to simple mastectomy in those patients with axillary metastases who lived beyond the point of truncation. Applying these principles and using a large group of patients with cancer of the breast, Butcher[51] found that the proportion of patients that may survive as well by a simple as by a radical mastectomy is rather high (75%). He also found in the remaining group a proportion of patients (36%) treated by radical mastectomy and who were alive beyond the point of truncation.

In carcinoma of the breast, the five-year survivals after surgery are considerably influenced by the extent of the tumor operated upon. Obviously, if cases are taken that are not truly operable, then five-year results will be extremely poor. Usually such statistics are made on the basis of those with axillary node metastases and those without. The number of cases falling in the first group depends on the thoroughness of the pathologic examination of the axilla. A lymphoid infiltrate in association with a cancer such as the medullary type implies host resistance, and this host resistance Hamlin[150] believes is the highest in the presence of germinal centers. Opler[274a] has described the changes in the lymph nodes as immune reactive lymphadenopathy in association with hyperplastic histiocytes as evidence of increased host immunity. Black and Asire[30] and Cutler et al.[74a] have also insisted on these findings, but Berg[24] and Di Re and Lane[91] have been unable to confirm them. The presence of bilateral "palpable" adenopathy in a series of 100 patients with mammary carcinoma was judged to be associated with "favorable" prognosis by Cutler et al.,[76] who theorized that "the bilateral palpable nodes may be a manifestation of host defensive response." Crile[71] reported the results of mastectomy in patients without clinical evidence of axillary metastases and found them to be 13% higher when the nodes were left in place than when they were removed. He suggested that this was due to the fact that uninvolved lymph nodes contribute to the "host's immunological resistance." Bloom[37] found round cell infiltration in only 5% to 10% of cases of medullary carcinoma, of known favorable prognosis, and concluded that his finding throws doubt on the significance of histologic criteria of "host resistance." Webster and Sabbadini[369] showed that the presence of circulating tumor cells in the peripheral blood does not affect the prognosis. It must be understood that what is identified as "tumor cells" are often monocytes, megakaryocytes, etc. In evaluating the end results of carcinoma of the breast, patients who have been lost to follow-up or who have died with intercurrent disease without evidence of cancer should not be excluded.

In seventy-seven cases of cystosarcoma phyllodes reported by Treves and Sunderland,[346] the forty-one patients with benign tumors did well. The eighteen with borderline lesions also did well, but four developed local recurrence. Of the eighteen patients with obviously malignant lesions, eight died with metastases. The prognosis for patients with lymphangiosarcoma is extremely poor. In thirty-seven cases collected by McSwain and Stephenson,[237] two patients were successfully treated, one by irradiation and one by surgery.

REFERENCES

1 Ackerman, L. V.: Clinical and pathological correlation of carcinoma of the breast; preliminary report of the pathologic study of 318 radical mastectomy specimens, Amer. Pract. Digest Treat. 1:124-131, 1950.

2 Ackerman, L. V.: Carcinoma of the breast; pathologic changes correlated with diagnosis, treatment and prognosis, J. Indiana Med. Ass. 45:891-899, 1952.

3 Ackermann, W.: Vertebral trephine biopsy, Ann. Surg. 143:373-385, 1956.

4 Ackland, T. H.: Dilemma and decision; problems of breast cancer, Med. J. Aust. 1:945-955, 1967.

5 Adair, F. E.: Plasma cell mastitis—a lesion simulating mammary carcinoma, Arch. Surg. (Chicago) 26:735-749, 1933.

6 Adair, F. E.: Fat necrosis of the female breast; report of 110 cases, Amer. J. Surg. 74:117-128, 1947.

7 Anonymous: Adrenalectomy and hypophysectomy in disseminated mammary carcinoma; a preliminary statement by the Joint Committee on Endocrine Ablative Procedures in Disseminated Mammary Carcinoma, J.A.M.A. 175:787-790, 1961.

8 Ansfield, F. J.: Chemotherapy in primary therapy of cancer of the breast, Cancer 20: 1054-1055, 1967.

9 Ariel, I. M., and Lehman, W. B.: Prognosis in patients with metastases to bone from primary breast cancer, Bull. Hosp. Joint Dis. 26:40-46, 1965.

10 Atkins, H., Bulbrook, R. D., Falconer, M. A., Hayward, J. L., MacLean, K. S., and Schurr, P. H.: Urinary steroid estimations in the prediction of response to adrenalectomy or hypophysectomy, Lancet 2:1133-1136, 1964.

11 Atkins, H., Bulbrook, R. D., Falconer, M. A., Hayward, J. L., MacLean, K. S., and Schurr, P. H.: Ten years' experience of steroid assays in the management of breast cancer; a review, Lancet 2:1255-1260, 1968.

12 Atkins, H., Bulbrook, R. D., Falconer, M. A., Hayward, J. L., MacLean, K. C., and Schurr, P. H.: Urinary steroids in the prediction of response to adrenalectomy or hypophysectomy; a second clinical trial, Lancet 2:1263-1264, 1968.

13 Atkins, H., Falconer, M. A., Hayward, J. L., MacLean, K. S., and Schurr, P. H.: The timing of adrenalectomy and of hypophysectomy in the treatment of advanced breast cancer, Lancet 1:827-830, 1966.

14 Auchincloss, H., Jr.: Surgery of the breast. In Nelson's loose-leaf living surgery, vol. 4, New York, 1927, Thomas Nelson & Sons, pp. 1-99.

15 Auchincloss, H., Jr.: The nature of local recurrence following radical mastectomy, Cancer 11:611-619, 1958.

16 Auchincloss, H.: Significance of location and number of axillary metastases in carcinoma of the breast, Ann. Surg. 158:37-46, 1963.

17 Auchincloss, H., and Haagensen, C. D.: Cancer of the breast possibly induced by estrogenic substance, J.A.M.A. 114:1517-1523, 1940.

18 Baclesse, F.: Roentgenthérapie préopératoire à dose élevée suivie de chirurgie large dans les cancers du sein, recul de dix ans, J. Radiol. Electr. 36:680-690, 1955.

19 Baclesse, F.: Five-year results in 431 breast cancers treated solely by roentgen rays, Ann. Surg. 161:103-104, 1965.

20 Barker, W. F., Sperling, L., Dawdy, A. H., Zeldis, L. J., and Longmire, W. P., Jr.: Management of nonpalpable breast carcinoma discovered by mammography, Ann. Surg. 170: 385-393, 1969.

21 Barlow, J. J., Emerson, K., Jr., and Saxena, B. N.: Estradiol production after ovariectomy

for carcinoma of the breast; relevance to the treatment of menopausal women, New Eng. J. Med. **280**:633-637, 1969.

22 Baron, D. N., Gurling, K. J., and Smith, E. J. Radley: The effect of hypophysectomy in advanced carcinoma of the breast, Brit. J. Surg. **65**:593-606, 1958.

23 Batley, F., and Holloway, A. F.: The moving-strip technique in the roentgen treatment of carcinoma of the breast, Amer. J. Roentgen. **83**:533-537, 1960.

24 Berg, J. W.: Sinus histiocytosis; a fallacious measure of host resistance to cancer, Cancer **9**:935-939, 1956.

25 Berg, J. W.: Inflammation and prognosis in breast cancer; a search for host resistance, Cancer **12**:714-720, 1959.

26 Berg, J. W., Hutter, R. V. P., and Foote, F. W.: The unique association between salivary gland cancer and breast cancer, J.A.M.A. **204**:771-774, 1968.

27 Berger, S. M., Curcio, B. M., Gershon-Cohen, J., and Isard, H. F.: Mammographic localization of unsuspected breast cancer, Amer. J. Roentgen. **96**:1046-1052, 1966.

28 Berkson, J., Harrington, S. W., Clagett, O. T., Kirklin, J. W., Dockerty, M. B., and McDonald, J. R.: Mortality and survival in surgically treated cancer of the breast: a statistical summary of some experience of the Mayo Clinic. I. Relation of survival to various biometric factors. II. Comparison of radical mastectomy (Mayo Clinic) with simple mastectomy and radiotherapy (McWhirter), Proc. Staff Meet. Mayo Clin. **32**:645-674, 1957.

29 Black, J. W., and Young, B.: A radiological and pathological study of the incidence of calcification in diseases of the breast and neoplasms of other tissues, Brit. J. Radiol. **38**:596-598, 1965.

30 Black, M. M., and Asire, A. J.: Palpable axillary lymph nodes in cancer of the breast; structural and biologic considerations, Cancer **23**:251-259, 1969.

31 Black, M. M., Kerpe, S., and Speer, F. D.: Lymph node structure in patients with cancer of the breast, Amer. J. Path. **29**:505-521, 1953.

32 Bliss, C. I., and Stevens, W. L.: The calculation of the time-mortality curve, Ann. Appl. Biol. **24**:815-852, 1937.

33 Block, G. E., Lampe, I., Vial, A., and Coller, F.: Therapeutic castration for advanced mammary cancer, Surgery **47**:877-884, 1960.

34 Block, G. E., Vial, A. B., McCarthy, J. D., Porter, C. W., and Coller, F. A.: Adrenalectomy in advanced mammary cancer, Surg. Gynec. Obstet. **108**:651-668, 1959.

35 Bloom, H. J. G.: Prognosis in carcinoma of the breast, Brit. J. Cancer **4**:259-288, 1950.

36 Bloom, H. J. G.: The influence of delay on the natural history and prognosis of breast cancer, Brit. J. Cancer **19**:228-262, 1965.

37 Bloom, H. J. G.: Host resistance and survival in medullary carcinoma of the breast, Brit. J. Med. (to be published).

38 Bloom, H. J. G., Richardson, W. W., and Harries, E. J.: Natural history of untreated breast cancer (1805-1933), Brit. J. Med. **2**:213-221, 1962.

38a Bond, W. H.: The prognostic implication of treatment, Proc. Roy. Soc. Med. **63**:111-113, 1970.

39 Bonser, G. M., Dossett, J. A., and Jull, J. W.: Human and experimental breast cancer, London, 1961, Sir Isaac Pitman & Sons, Ltd.

40 Borden, A. G. B., and Gershon-Cohen, J.: Mammography of lobular carcinoma, Radiology **81**:17-23, 1963.

41 Bouchard, J.: Skeletal metastases in cancer of the breast, study of the character, incidence and response to roentgen therapy, Amer. J. Roentgen. **54**:156-171, 1945.

42 Bouchard, J.: Advanced cancer of the breast treated primarily with irradiation, Radiology **84**:823-842, 1965.

43 Brinkley, D., and Haybittle, J. L.: Treatment of stage-II carcinoma of the female breast, Lancet **2**:291-295, 1966.

44 Brinkley, D. M., and Pillers, E. K.: Treatment of advanced carcinoma of the breast by bilateral oophorectomy and prednisone, Lancet **1**:123-126, 1960.

44a Bruce, J., Carter, D. C., and Fraser, J.: Patterns of recurrent disease in breast cancer, Lancet **1**:433-435, 1970.

45 Bucalossi, P., and Veronesi, U.: Some observations on cancer of the breast in mothers and daughters, Brit. J. Cancer **11**:337-347, 1957.

46 Buchanan, E. B.: Cancer of the breast, Amer. J. Surg. **122**:879-887, 1966.

47 Bulbrook, R. D., Greenwood, R. C., and Hayward, J. L.: Selection of breast-cancer patients for adrenalectomy or hypophysectomy by determination of urinary 17-hydroxycorticosteroids and aetiocholanolone, Lancet **1**:1154-1157, 1960.

48 Bulbrook, R. D., and Hayward, J. L.: The possibility of predicting the response of patients with early breast cancer to subsequent endocrine ablation, Cancer Res. **25**:1135-1139, 1965.

49 Bulbrook, R. D., and Hayward, J. L.: Abnormal urinary steroid excretion and subsequent breast cancer; a prospective study in the Island of Guernsey, Lancet **1**:519-525, 1967.

50 Bulbrook, R. D., Hayward, J. L., and Thomas, B. S.: The relation between the urinary 17-hydroxycorticosteroids and 11-deoxy-17-oxosteroids and the fate of patients after mastectomy, Lancet **1**:945-947, 1964.

51 Butcher, H. R., Jr.: Effectiveness of radical mastectomy for mammary cancer; an analysis of mortalities by the methods of probits, Ann. Surg. **154**:383-392, 1961.

52 Butcher, H. R., Jr., Seaman, W. B., Eckert, C., and Saltzstein, S.: An assessment of radical mastectomy and postoperative irradiation therapy in the treatment of mammary cancer, Cancer **17**:480-485, 1964.

53 Cáceres, E.: Incidence of metastasis in the

internal mammary chain in operable cancer of the breast, Surg. Gynec. Obstet. 108:715-720, 1959.

54 Cáceres, E. E.: Indications and limitations of radical mastectomy combined with internal mammary node dissection (presented at the Tenth International Cancer Congress, Houston, Texas, May, 1970).

55 Cade, S.: Treatment and results in cancer of the breast, Amer. J. Roentgen. 62:326-327, 1949.

56 Cantril, S. T.: The care of the patient with advanced cancer of the breast, Radiology 66:46-54, 1956.

57 Carnett, J. B., and Howell, J. C.: Bone metastases in cancer of the breast, Ann. Surg. 91:811-832, 1930.

57a Cavanzo, F. J., and Taylor, H. B.: Adenoid cystic carcinoma of the breast; an analysis of 21 cases, Cancer 24:740-745, 1969.

58 Chalstrey, L. J., and Benjamin, B.: High incidence of breast cancer in thyroid cancer patients, Brit. J. Cancer 20:670-675, 1966.

59 Chavanne, G., Galle, R., and Gatto, I.: Le cancer mammaire "bilatéral d'emblée." Découverte de la deuzième localisation par la mammographie bilatérale systématique, J. Radiol. Electr. 45:447-450, 1964.

60 Cheatle, G. L., and Cutler, M.: Tumours of the breast, London, 1931, Edward Arnold (Publishers), Ltd.

61 de Cholnoky, T.: Mammary cancer in youth, Surg. Gynec. Obstet. 77:55-60, 1943.

62 Chu, F. C. H., Scheer, A. C., and Gaspar-Landero, J.: Electron-beam therapy in the management of carcinoma of the breast, Radiology 75:559-567, 1960.

63 Chu, F. C. H., Sved, D. W., Escher, G. C., Nickson, J. J., and Phillips, R.: Management of advanced breast carcinoma with special reference to combined radiation and hormone therapy, Amer. J. Roentgen. 77:438-447, 1957.

64 Clemmesen, J., and Nielsen, A.: The social distribution of cancer in Copenhagen, 1943 to 1947, Brit. J. Cancer 5:159-171, 1951.

65 Cole, M. P.: The place of radiotherapy in the management of early breast cancer; a report of two clinical trials, Brit. J. Surg. 51:216-220, 1964.

66 Cole, P., and MacMahon, B.: Oestrogen fractions during early reproductive life in the aetiology of breast cancer, Lancet 1:604-606, 1969.

67 Collins, V. P., and Adams, R. M.: The paradox of breast cancer, Amer. J. Roentgen. 99:965-972, 1967.

68 Cooper, W. G., Jr., and Ackerman, L. V.: Cystosarcoma phylloides, with a consideration of its more malignant variant, Surg. Gynec. Obstet. 77:279-283, 1943.

69 Copher, G. H., Chenard, J., and Butcher, H. R., Jr.: Factors influencing mortality from mammary cancer, Arch. Surg. (Chicago) 85:73-81, 1962.

70 Crile, G.: Rationale for cutting thick skin flaps and not grafting skin in operations for cancer of the breast, Cancer 18:795-799, 1965.

71 Crile, G.: Results of simple mastectomy without irradiation in the treatment of operative stage I cancer of the breast, Ann. Surg. 168:330-336, 1968.

72 Critchley, E. M. R.: Hypophysectomy for metastatic carcinoma of the breast; some electroencephalographic and clinical observations, Brit. J. Cancer 18:634-647, 1964.

73 Crowley, L. G., Demetriou, J. A., Kotin, P., Donovan, A. J., and Kushinsky, S.: Excretion patterns of urinary metabolites of estradiol-4-C^{14} in postmenopausal women with benign and malignant disease of the breast, Cancer Res. 25:371-376, 1965.

74 Cuenca, C. R., and Becker, K. L.: Klinefelter's syndrome and cancer of the breast, Arch. Intern. Med. (Chicago) 121:159-162, 1968.

74a Cutler, S. J., Black, M. M., Mork, T., Harvei, S., and Freeman, C.: Further observations on prognostic factors in cancer of the female breast, Cancer 24:653-667, 1969.

75 Cutler, S. J., and Myers, M. H.: Clinical classification of extent of disease in cancer of the breast, J. Nat. Cancer Inst. 39:193-207, 1967.

76 Cutler, S. J., Zippin, C., and Asire, A. J.: The prognostic significance of palpable lymph nodes in cancer of the breast, Cancer 23:243-250, 1969.

77 Daland, E. M.: Untreated cancer of the breast, Surg. Gynec. Obstet. 44:264-268, 1927.

78 Dao, T. L. Y.: Cancer of the male breast treated by adrenalectomy, Surg. Clin. N. Amer. 35:1663-1667, 1955.

79 Dargent, M.: Carcinoma of the breast in castrated women, Brit. Med. J. 2:54-56, 1949.

80 Davies, F. L., and Buston, P. H.: Pituitary destruction by injection of radioactive substance and section of the pituitary stalk for advanced cancer, Brit. J. Cancer 11:8-17, 1957.

81 Davis, H. H., Simons, M., and Davis, J. B.: Cystic disease of the breast; relationship to carcinoma, Cancer 17:957-978, 1964.

82 Debois, J. M.: Les techniques d'irradiation de l'ovaire dans le traitement du cancer du sein, Proceedings of the Eleventh International Congress of Radiology, Rome, September, 1965, Excerpta Medica International Congress Series No. 105, pp. 953-966, 1967.

83 Dedrick, M. M., Taft, P. D., Lojananond, P., and Hall, T. C.: Effect of therapy upon vaginal smears in breast cancer patients, Surg. Gynec. Obstet. 118:1019-1023, 1964.

84 Delarue, N. C., Ash, C. L., Peters, V., and Fielden, R.: Preoperative irradiation in management of locally advanced breast cancer, Arch. Surg. (Chicago) 91:136-154, 1965.

85 Delclos, L., and Johnson, G. C.: Palliative irradiation in breast cancer; the place of radiotherapy in the palliation of local recurrences and distant metastases, Radiology 83:272-276, 1964.

86 Den Besten, L., and Ziffren, S. E.: Simple and radical mastectomy, Arch. Surg. (Chicago) 90:755-759, 1965.

87 Desai, S. B.: Uses and limitations of frozen section in diagnosis of lesions of the breast, Brit. J. Surg. 53:1038-1042, 1966.

88 Devitt, J. E.: The significance of regional lymph node metastases in breast carcinoma, Canad. Med. Ass. J. 93:289-293, 1965.

89 Devitt, J. E., and Catton, G. E.: Successful estrogen therapy for post-adrenalectomy relapses of breast cancer, Canad. Med. Ass. J. 94:929-932, 1966.

90 Díaz-Bazán, N., and Astacio, J. N.: Cistosarcoma filodio de la mama. Análisis clínicopatológico; tratamiento con cirugía radical, Arch. Col. Med. El Salvador 20:39-60, 1967.

91 Di Re, J. J., and Lane, N.: The relation of sinus histiocytosis in axillary lymph nodes to surgical curability of carcinoma of the breast, Amer. J. Clin. Path. 40:508-515, 1963.

92 Donegan, W. L.: An evaluation of radical mastectomy following simple mastectomy for carcinoma of the breast, Missouri Med. 61:1014-1018, 1964.

93 Edelman, A. H., Holtz, S., and Powers, W. E.: Rapid radiotherapy for inoperable carcinoma of the breast; benefits and complications, Amer. J. Roentgen. 93:585-599, 1965.

94 Edelstyn, G. A., Gleadhill, C. A., and Lyons, A. R.: Attempted total hypophysectomy in advanced breast cancer; report on a new method of using both surgery and radiation, Brit. J. Surg. 51:32-35, 1964.

95 Editorial: Mammography—a radiological challenge, Brit. J. Radiol. 40:721-723, 1967.

96 Egan, R. L.: Experience with mammography in a tumor institution, Radiology 75:894-900, 1960.

97 Egan, R. L.: Mammography, Amer. J. Surg. 106:421-429, 1963.

98 Emerson, W. J., Kennedy, B. J., and Taft, E. B.: Correlation of histological alterations in breast cancer with hormone therapy, Cancer 13:1047-1052, 1960.

99 Escher, G. C., and Kaufman, R. J.: Advanced breast carcinoma; factors influencing survival, Acta Un. Int. Cancr. 19:1039-1043, 1963.

100 Farrow, J. H.: Bilateral mammary cancer, Cancer 9:1182-1188, 1956.

100a Fechner, R. E.: Fibroadenomas in patients receiving oral contraceptives; a clinical and pathologic study, Amer. J. Clin. Path. 53:857-864, 1970.

101 Fisher, B., Ravdin, R. G., Ausman, R. K., Slack, N. H., Moore, G. E., and Noer, R. J.: Surgical adjuvant chemotherapy in cancer of the breast; results of a decade of cooperative investigation, Ann. Surg. 168:337-356, 1968.

101a Fisher, B., Slack, N. H., and Ravdin, R. G.: The worth of post-operative irradiation for breast cancer; results of the National Surgical Adjuvant Breast Project (presented at the Annual Meeting of the American Surgical Association, April, 1970).

102 Fitts, W. T., Maxwell, J. T., and Horn, R. C.: The significance of nipple discharge, Ann. Surg. 134:29-39, 1951.

103 Fitts, W. T., Jr., Steiner, G. C., and Enterline, H. T.: Prognosis of occult carcinoma of the breast, Amer. J. Surg. 106:460-463, 1963.

104 Fletcher, G. H., and Montague, E. D.: Radical irradiation of advanced breast cancer, Amer. J. Roentgen. 93:573-584, 1965.

105 Fletcher, G. H., Montague, E. D., and White, E. C.: Evaluation of irradiation of the peripheral lymphatics in conjunction with radical mastectomy for cancer of the breast, Cancer 21:791-797, 1968.

106 Foote, F. W., and Stewart, F. W.: Lobular carcinoma in situ, Amer. J. Path. 17:491-496, 1941.

107 Foote, F. W., and Stewart, F. W.: Comparative studies of cancerous versus noncancerous breasts, Ann. Surg. 121:6-79, 1945.

108 Forrest, A. P. M., Gleave, E. N., Roberts, M. M., Henk, J. M., and Gravelle, I. H.: Management of early carcinoma of the breast; a controlled trial of conservative treatment for early breast cancer, Proc. Roy. Soc. Med. 63:107-110, 1970.

109 Forrest, H.: Intraduct papilloma of the breast, Brit. J. Surg. 53:1028-1032, 1966.

110 Frantz, V. K., Pickren, J. W., Melcher, G. W., and Auchincloss, H., Jr.: Incidence of chronic cystic disease in so-called "normal breast," Cancer 4:762-783, 1951.

111 Franzén, S., and Zajicek, J.: Aspiration biopsy in diagnosis of palpable lesions of the breast, Acta Radiol. [Ther.] (Stockholm) 7:241-262, 1968.

112 Friedman, A. K., Askovitz, S. I., Berger, S. M., Dodd, G. D., Fisher, M. S., Lapayowker, M. S., Moore, J. P., Parlee, D. E., Stein, G. N., and Pendergrass, E. P.: A co-operative evaluation of mammography in seven teaching hospitals, Radiology 86:886-891, 1966.

112a Friedman, B. A., and Oberman, H. A.: Adenoid cystic carcinoma of the breast, Amer. J. Clin. Path. 54:1-14, 1970.

112b Galasko, C. S. B.: The detection of skeletal metastases from mammary cancer by gamma camera scintigraphy, Brit. J. Surg. 56:757-764, 1969.

112c Galasko, C. S. B., Westerman, B., Li, J., Sellwood, R. A., and Burn, J. I.: Use of the gamma camera for early detection of osseous metastases from mammary cancer, Brit. J. Surg. 55:613-615, 1968.

113 Gershon-Cohen, J., and Berger, S. M.: Mastography, Radiol. Clin. N. Amer. 1:115-143, 1963.

114 Gershon-Cohen, J., Berger, S. M., and Hermel, M. B.: Roentgenography and the management of breast cancer, Amer. J. Roentgen. 89:51-57, 1963.

115 Gershon-Cohen, J., Berger, S. M., and Klickstein, H. S.: Roentgenography of breast cancer moderating concept of biologic "predeterminism," Cancer 16:961-964, 1963.

116 Gershon-Cohen, J., Ingleby, H., Berger, S. M., Forman, M., and Curcio, B. M.: Mam-

mographic screening for breast cancer, Radiology **88**:663-667, 1967.

117 Getzen, L. G., Lobpreis, E. L., and Holloway, C. K.: The treatment of primary breast cancer, Arch. Surg. (Chicago) **98**:131-137, 1969.

118 Gilbertsen, V. A.: Improving breast cancer prognosis, Geriatrics **21**:128-132, 1966.

119 Goldenberg, V. E., Wiegenstein, L., and Mottet, N. K.: Florid breast fibroadenomas in patients taking hormonal oral contraceptives, Amer. J. Clin. Path. **49**:52-59, 1968.

120 Goode, J. V., McNeill, J. P., and Gordon, C. E.: Routine aspiration of discrete breast cysts; report of two hundred sixty-seven breast aspirations, Arch. Surg. (Chicago) **70**: 686-690, 1955.

121 Grant, R. N., Tabah, E. J., and Adair, F. I.: The surgical significance of the subareolar lymph plexus in cancer of the breast, Surgery **33**:71-78, 1953.

122 Greening, W. P., and Aichroth, P. M.: Cancer of the male breast, Brit. J. Cancer **19**: 92-100, 1965.

123 Greening, W. P., and Thompson, S. G.: Interstitial irradiation of the pituitary gland for advanced carcinoma of the breast using the transethmoidal approach, Brit. J. Cancer **20**: 703-709, 1966.

124 Gricouroff, G.: Du pronostic histologique dans le cancer du sein, Bull. Ass. Franc. Cancer **35**:275-290, 1948.

125 Gricouroff, G., Ennuyer, A., and Fautrel, M.: Quelle est l'efficacité de la radiothérapie postoperatoire dans le cancer mammaire traité par amputation large avec curage axillaire? Bull. Ass. Franc. Cancer **46**:701-721, 1959.

126 Gricouroff, G., Fautrel, M., Faverge, J. M., and Zrzur, J.: Precisions statistiques sur le rôle de l'histologie dans le pronostic postoperatoire du cancer du sein, Presse Med. **57**:118-120, 1949.

127 Gros, C.: Les maladies du sein, Paris, 1963, Masson et Cie.

128 Guillaurd-Bourgeois, M., Tuaillon, P., Dargent,, M., and Mayer, M.: Étude systématique de la 12ᵉ côte chez des malades atteintes d'une tumeur du sein en phase advancée. I. Données anatomo-pathologiques, Bull. Cancer (Paris) **51**:235-242, 1964.

129 Gummel, H., and Widow, W.: Preoperative irradiation of breast cancer, Zbl. Chir. **89**: 1473-1480, 1964.

130 Gurling, K. J., Scott, G. B. D., and Baron, D. N.: Metastases in pituitary tissue removed at hypophysectomy in women with mammary carcinoma, Brit. J. Cancer **11**:519-522, 1957.

131 Guttmann, R. J.: Survival and results after 2-million volt irradiation in the treatment of primary operable carcinoma of the breast with proved positive internal mammary and/or highest axillar nodes, Cancer **15**:383-386, 1962.

132 Guttmann, R.: Radiotherapy in the treatment of primary operable carcinoma of the breast

with proved lymph node metastases, Amer. J. Roentgen. **89**:58-63, 1963.

133 Guttmann, R. J.: Role of supervoltage irradiation of regional lymph node bearing areas in breast cancer, Amer. J. Roentgen. **96**:560-564, 1966.

134 Guttmann, R.: Radiotherapy in locally advanced cancer of the breast, Cancer **20**:1046-1050, 1967.

135 Haagensen, C. D.: Carcinoma of the breast, J.A.M.A. **138**:195-205, 279-292, 1948.

136 Haagensen, C. D.: The treatment and results in cancer of the breast at the Presbyterian Hospital, New York, Amer. J. Roentgen. **62**:328-334, 1949.

137 Haagensen, C. D.: Carcinoma of the breast (fifth of a series on the early recognition of cancer), New York, 1950, American Cancer Society, Inc.

138 Haagensen, C. D.: Mammary-duct ectasis, Cancer **4**:749-761, 1951.

139 Haagensen, C. D.: Diseases of the breast, Philadelphia, 1956, W. B. Saunders Co.

140 Haagensen, C. D.: Cancer of the breast in pregnancy and during lactation, Amer. J. Obstet. Gynec. **98**:141-149, 1967.

140a Haagensen, C. D., Bronslay, S. B., Guttmann, R. J., Habif, D. V., Kister, S. J., Markowitz, A. M., Sanger, G., Tretter, P., Wiedel, P. D., and Cooley, E.: Metastasis of carcinoma of the breast to the periphery of the regional lymph node filter, Ann. Surg. **169**:174-190, 1969.

141 Haagensen, C. D., Cooley, E., Kennedy, C. S., Miller, E., Handley, R. S., Thackray, A. C., Butcher, H. R., Jr., Dahl-Iversen, E., Tobiassen, T., Williams, I. C., Curwen, M. P., Kaae, S., and Johansen, H.: Treatment of early mammary carcinoma; a cooperative international study, Ann. Surg. **157**:157-179, 1963.

142 Haagensen, C. D., and Obeid, S. J.: Biopsy of the apex of the axilla in carcinoma of the breast, Ann. Surg. **149**:149-161, 1959.

143 Haagensen, C. D., and Stout, A. P.: Carcinoma of the breast, Ann. Surg. **116**:801-815, 1942.

144 Haagensen, C. D., and Stout, A. P.: Carcinoma of the breast, Ann. Surg. **118**:1-32, 1943.

145 Haagensen, C. D., and Stout, A. P.: Granular cell myoblastoma of the mammary gland, Ann. Surg. **124**:218-227, 1946.

146 Haagensen, C. D., and Stout, A. P.: Carcinoma of the breast. III. Results of treatment 1935-1942, Ann. Surg. **134**:151-172, 1951.

147 Haagensen, C. D., Stout, A. P., and Phillips, J. S.: The papillary neoplasms of the breast, I. Benign intraductal papilloma, Ann. Surg. **133**:18-36, 1951.

148 Habif, D. V.: Selection of treatment for primary breast cancer, Postgrad. Med. **35**: 300-306, 1964.

149 Halsted, W. S.: A diagnostic sign of gelatinous carcinoma of the breast, J.A.M.A. **64**: 1653, 1915.

150 Hamlin, I. M. E.: Possible host resistance in

carcinoma of the breast; a histological study, Brit. J. Cancer 22:383-401, 1968.

151 Hamperl, H., Huhn, F. O., Kaufmann, C., and Ober, K.-G.: Histologische Untersuchungen präoperative bestrahlter Mammakarzinome, Deutsch. Med. Wschr. 88:616-620, 1963.

152 Handley, R. S.: Prognosis according to involvement of internal mammary lymph nodes, Acta Un. Int. Cancr. 15:1030-1031, 1959.

153 Handley, R. S.: The early spread of breast carcinoma and its bearing on operative treatment, Brit. J. Surg. 51:206-208, 1964.

154 Handley, R. S., and Thackray, A. C.: Internal mammary lymph chain in carcinoma of the breast, Lancet 2:276-278, 1949.

155 Harrington, S. W.: Survival rates of radical mastectomy for unilateral and bilateral carcinoma of the breast, Surgery 19:154-166, 1946.

156 Harrington, S. W.: Results of surgical treatment of unilateral carcinoma of breast in women, J.A.M.A. 148:1007-1011, 1952.

157 Harrington, S. W.: In the discussion of White, T. T., and White, W. C.: Breast cancer and pregnancy; report of 49 cases followed 5 years, Ann. Surg. 144:384-393, 1956.

158 Harrington, S. W., and Miller, J. M.: Lymphosarcoma of the mammary glands, Amer. J. Surg. 48:346-352, 1940.

159 Harris, D. L., Greening, W. P., and Aichroth, P. M.: Infra-red in the diagnosis of a lump in the breast, Brit. J. Cancer 20:710-721, 1966.

160 Harris, H. S., and Spratt, J. S.: Bilateral adrenalectomy in metastatic mammary cancer; an analysis of sixty-four cases, Cancer 23:145-151, 1969.

160a Harvey, H. D., and Auchincloss, H.: Metastases to lymph nodes from carcinomas that were arrested, Cancer 21:684-691, 1968.

161 Hayward, J. L.: Steroid excretion in the early breast cancer, Brit. J. Surg. 51:224-227, 1964.

162 Hayward, J. L., and Bulbrook, R. D.: The value of urinary steroid estimations in the prediction of response to adrenalectomy or hyphophysectomy, Cancer Res. 25:1129-1134, 1965.

163 Hayward, J. L., and Bulbrook, R. D., editors: Clinical evaluation in breast cancer, proceedings of the first Imperial cancer research fund symposium held in London, Oct. 21-23, 1965, New York, 1966, Academic Press, Inc.

164 Hendrick, J. W.: Intraductal papilloma of the breast, Surg. Gynec. Obstet. 105:215-223, 1957.

165 Hendrick, J. W.: Results of treatment of cystic disease of the breast, Surgery 44:457-482, 1958.

166 Hessler, C., and Gershon-Cohen, J.: Mastography—evaluation in 215 proven lesions, Acta Radiol. [Diag.] (Stockholm) 3:249-256, 1965.

167 Hicken, N. F.: Mastectomy; a clinical pathologic study demonstrating why most mastectomies result in incomplete removal of the mammary gland, Arch. Surg. (Chicago) 40:6-14, 1940.

168 Hill, R. P., and Stout, A. P.: Sarcoma of the breast, Arch. Surg. (Chicago) 44:723-759, 1942.

169 Hitchcock, C. R., Hickok, D. F., Soucheray, J., Moulton, T., and Baker, R. C.: Thermography in mass screening for occult breast cancer, J.A.M.A. 204:419-422, 1968.

170 Hochman, A., and Robinson, E.: Eighty-two cases of mammary cancer treated exclusively with roentgen therapy, Cancer 13:670-673, 1960.

171 Houttuin, E., Van Prohaska, J., and Taxman, P.: Response of male mammary carcinoma metastases to bilateral adrenalectomy, Surg. Gynec. Obstet. 125:279-283, 1967.

172 Huggins, C. B.: Adrenalectomy as palliative treatment, J.A.M.A. 200:973, 1967.

173 Hultborn, K. A., Larsson, L. G., and Ragnhult, I.: The lymph drainage from the breast to the axillary and parasternal lymph nodes, studied with the aid of colloidal Au^{198}, Acta Radiol. (Stockholm) 43:52-64, 1955.

174 Hultborn, K. A., and Törnberg, B.: Mammary carcinoma; the biologic character of mammary carcinoma studied in 517 cases by a new form of malignancy grading, Acta Radiol. (Stockholm) (suppl. 196), pp. 1-143, 1960.

175 Huseby, R. A.: The endocrinologic treatment of advanced breast cancer, Ann. Surg. 26:87-94, 1960.

176 Hutchison, G. B.: Treatment of breast cancer, J.A.M.A. 208:855, 1969.

177 Hutter, R. V. P., Snyder, R. E., Lucas, J. C., Foote, F. W., and Farrow, J. H.: Clinical and pathologic correlation with mammographic findings in lobular carcinoma in situ, Cancer 23:829-839, 1969.

178 Ingleby, H., Moore, L., and Gershon-Cohen, J.: A roentgenographic study of the growth rate of 6 "early" cancers of the breast, Cancer 11:726-730, 1958.

179 Jackson, S. M.: Carcinoma of the breast—the significance of supraclavicular lymph node metastases, Clin. Radiol. 17:107-114, 1966.

180 Jantet, G., Crocker, D. W., Shiraki, M., and Moore, F. D.: Adrenal suppression in disseminated carcinoma of the breast. I. The effect on adrenal morphology of hypophysectomy and corticosteroid treatment, New Eng. J. Med. 269:1-7, 1963.

181 Jessiman, A. G., Matson, D. D., and Moore, F. D.: Hypophysectomy in the treatment of breast cancer, New Eng. J. Med. 261:1199-1207, 1959.

182 Johnson, R. E.: Breast cancer, measurements of treatment, Cancer 5:267-270, 1952.

183 Kaae, S.: Role of radiation therapy in the treatment of breast carcinoma (presented at the Tenth International Cancer Congress, Houston, Texas, May, 1970).

184 Kaae, S., and Johansen, H.: In Progress in clinical cancer (edited by I. Ariel), New York, 1965, Grune & Stratton, Inc.

185 Kaufman, R. J., Chu, F. C. H., and Escher, G. C.: The effect of radiation therapy on the survival time of women with recurrent mam-

mary carcinoma, Amer. J. Roentgen. **93**:600-606, 1965.

186 Kay, S.: Evaluation of Rotter's lymph nodes in radical mastectomy specimens as a guide to prognosis, Cancer **18**:1441-1444, 1965.

187 Keller, A. Z.: Demographic, clinical and survivorship characteristics of males with primary cancer of the breast, Amer. J. Epidem. **85**:183-199, 1967.

188 Kendall, B. E., Arthur, J. F., and Patey, D. H.: Lymphangiography in carcinoma of the breast, Cancer **16**:1233-1242, 1963.

189 Kennaway, E. L.: The data relating to cancer in the publications of the General Register Office, Brit. J. Cancer **4**:158-172, 1950.

190 Kennedy, B. J.: The control of advanced breast cancer, Amer. J. Surg. **106**:413-419, 1963.

191 Kennedy, B. J.: The role of castration in breast cancer, Arch. Surg. (Chicago) **88**: 743-746, 1964.

192 Kennedy, B. J.: Hormone therapy for advanced breast cancer, Cancer **18**:1551-1557, 1965.

193 Kennedy, B. J.: Systemic effects of androgenic and estrogenic hormones in advanced breast cancer, J. Amer. Geriat. Soc. **13**:230-235, 1965.

194 Kennedy, B. J.: Endocrine therapy of breast cancer, J.A.M.A. **200**:971-972, 1967.

195 Kennedy, B. J., and Brown, J. H.: Combined estrogenic and androgenic hormone therapy in advanced breast cancer, Cancer **18**:431-435, 1965.

196 Kennedy, B. J., and Fortuny, I. E.: Therapeutic castration in the treatment of advanced breast cancer, Cancer **17**:1197-1202, 1964.

197 Kennedy, B. J., French, L. A., and Peyton, W. T.: Hypophysectomy in advanced breast cancer, New Eng. J. Med. **255**:1165-1172, 1956.

198 Kennedy, B. J., Mielke, P. W., and Fortuny, I. E.: Therapeutic castration versus prophylactic castration in breast cancer, Surg. Gynec. Obstet. **118**:524-540, 1964.

199 Kilgore, A. R., Bell, H. G., and Ahlquist, R. E., Jr.: Cancer in the second breast, Amer. J. Surg. **92**:156-161, 1956.

200 Kister, S. J., Sommers, S. C., Haagensen, C. D., and Cooley, E.: Reevaluation of blood-vessel invasion as a prognostic factor in carcinoma of the breast, Cancer **19**:1213-1216, 1966.

201 Koehl, R. H., Snyder, R. E., Hutter, R. V. P., and Foote, F. W., Jr.: The incidence and significance of calcifications within operative breast specimens, Amer. J. Clin. Path. **53**: 3-14, 1970.

202 Kouchoukos, N. T., Ackerman, L. V., and Butcher, H. R., Jr.: Prediction of axillary nodal mestastases from the morphology of primary mammary carcinomas, Cancer **20**: 948-960, 1967.

203 Kraus, F. T., and Neubecker, R. D.: The differential diagnosis of papillary tumors of the breast, Cancer **15**:444-455, 1962.

204 Lalanne, C. M., Juret, P., Hourtoule, F., and Sarrazin, D.: La castration dans le cancer du sein: chirurgie ou radiations, Acta Radiol. [Ther.] (Stockholm) **6**:323-334, 1967.

205 Lamarque, P., Pourquier, H., and Leenhardt, P.: Analyse des possibilities techniques dans la télécobalthérapie des tumeurs du sein, J. Radiol. Electr. **40**:15-23, 1959.

206 Lambird, P. A., and Shelley, W. M.: The spatial distribution of lobular in situ mammary carcinoma, J.A.M.A. **210**:689-693, 1969.

207 Lane, N., Goksen, H., Salerno, R. A., and Haagensen, C. D.: Clinico-pathologic analysis of the surgical curability of breast cancers, Ann. Surg. **153**:483-498, 1961.

208 Lange, F.: Der Gallertkrebs der Brustdrüse, Beitr. Klin. Chir. **16**:1-60, 1896.

209 Leborgne, R.: Intraductal biopsy of certain pathologic processes of the breast, Surgery **19**:47-54, 1946.

210 Leborgne, R.: The breast in roentgen diagnosis, Montevideo, 1953, Impresora Uruguaya.

211 Leborgne, R., Leborgne, F., and Leborgne, J. H.: Soft-tissue radiography of axillary nodes with fatty infiltration, Radiology **84**: 513-515, 1965.

212 Lemon, H. M.: Medical treatment of cancer of the breast and prostate, Disease-a-Month (Chicago), May, 1959.

213 Lemon, H. M.: Abnormal estrogen metabolism and tissue estrogen receptor proteins in breast cancer, Cancer **25**:423-435, 1970.

214 Lemon, H. M., Wotiz, H. H., Parsons, L., and Mozden, P. J.: Reduced estriol excretion in patients with breast cancer prior to endocrine therapy, J.A.M.A. **196**:1128-1136, 1966.

215 Lewis, D., and Rienhoff, W. F., Jr.: A study of the results of operations for cure of cancer of the breast performed at Johns Hopkins Hospital from 1889 to 1931, Ann. Surg. **95**: 336-400, 1932.

216 Lewison, E. F.: An appraisal of long-term results in surgical treatment of breast cancer, J.A.M.A. **186**:975-978, 1963.

217 Lewison, E. F.: Castration in the treatment of advanced breast cancer, Cancer **18**:1558-1562, 1965.

218 Lewison, E. F., and Smith, R. T.: Results of breast cancer treatment at Johns Hopkins Hospital, 1946-1950, Surgery **53**:644-656, 1963.

219 Liechty, R. D., Davis, J., and Gleysteen, J.: Cancer of the male breast, Cancer **20**:1617-1624, 1967.

220 Lilienfeld, A. M.: The relationship of cancer of the female breast to artificial menopause and marital status, Cancer **9**:927-934, 1956.

221 Lilienfeld, A. M.: The epidemiology of breast cancer, Cancer Res. **23**:1503-1513, 1963.

222 Linden, G., Cline, J. W., Wood, D. A., Guiss, L. W., and Breslow, L.: Validity of pathological diagnosis of breast cancer, J.A.M.A. **173**:143-147, 1960.

223 Lumb, G., and Mackenzie, D. H.: The incidence of metastasis in adrenal glands and ovaries removed for carcinoma of the breast, Cancer **12**:521-526, 1959.

224 McDivitt, R. W., Holleb, A. I., and Foote, F. W., Jr.: Prior breast disease in patients treated for papillary carcinoma, Arch. Path. (Chicago) **85**:117-124, 1968.

225 McDivitt, R. W., Hutter, R. V. P., Foote, F. W., Jr., and Stewart, F. W.: In situ lobular carcinoma, J.A.M.A. **201**:82-86, 1967.

226 McDivitt, R. W., and Stewart, F. W.: Breast carcinoma in children, J.A.M.A. **195**:388-390, 1966.

227 McDivitt, R. W., Stewart, F. W., and Berg, J. W.: Tumors of the breast. In Atlas of tumor pathology, second series 2, Fasc. 2, Washington, D. C., 1967, Armed Forces Institute of Pathology.

228 McDivitt, R. W., Stewart, F. W., and Farrow, J. H.: Breast carcinoma arising in solitary fibroadenomas, Surg. Gynec. Obstet. **125**:572-576, 1967.

229 McDivitt, R. W., Urban, J. A., and Farrow, J. H.: Cystosarcoma phyllodes, Johns Hopkins Med. J. **120**:33-45, 1967.

230 McDonald, J. J., Haagensen, C. D., and Stout, A. P.: Metastasis from mammary carcinoma to the supraclavicular and internal mammary lymph nodes, Surgery **34**:521-542, 1953.

231 Mackenzie, I.: Breast cancer following multiple fluoroscopies, Brit. J. Cancer **19**:1-8, 1965.

232 McLaughlin, J. S., Hull, H. C., Oda, F., and Buxton, R. W.: Metastatic carcinoma of the male breast; remission of adrenalectomy, Ann. Surg. **162**:9-14, 1965.

233 MacMahon, B.: Cohort fertility and increasing breast cancer incidence, Cancer **11**:250-254, 1958.

234 MacMahon, B., and Austin, J. H.: Association of carcinomas of the breast and corpus uteri, Cancer **23**:275-280, 1969.

235 MacMahon, B., Cole, P., Lin, T. M., Lowe, C. R., Mirra, A. P., Ravnihar, B., Salber, E. J., Balaoras, V. G., and Yuasa, S.: Age at first birth and breast cancer risk, Bull. W.H.O. (in press).

236 MacMahon, B., and Feinleib, M.: Breast cancer in relation to nursing and menopausal history, J. Nat. Cancer Inst. **24**:733-753, 1960.

237 McSwain, B., and Stephenson, S.: Lymphangiosarcoma of the edematous extremity, Ann. Surg. **151**:649-656, 1960.

238 McWhirter, R.: The value of simple mastectomy and radiotherapy in the treatment of cancer of the breast, Brit. J. Radiol. **21**:599-610, 1948.

239 McWhirter, R.: Cancer of the breast, Amer. J. Roentgen. **62**:335-340, 1949.

240 McWhirter, R.: Simple mastectomy and radiotherapy in the treatment of breast cancer, Brit. J. Radiol. **28**:128-139, 1955.

241 Macklin, M. T.: The genetic basis of human mammary cancer, Proc. Nat. Cancer Conf. **2**:1074-1084, 1952.

242 Macklin, M. T.: Comparison of the number of breast-cancer deaths observed in relatives of breast-cancer patients and the number

243 Macklin, M. T.: Relative status of parity and genetic background in producing human breast cancer, J. Nat. Cancer Inst. **23**:1179-1188, 1959.

244 Maisin, J.: Le traitement du cancerdu sein par curietherapie et roentgenographie, Acta Radiol. (Stockholm) **28**:593-610, 1947.

245 Mannheimer, I. H.: Hypercalcemia of breast cancer; management with corticosteroids, Cancer **18**:679-691, 1965.

246 Marmorston, J., Crowley, L. G., Myers, S. M., Stern, E., and Hopkins, C. E.: Urinary excretion of neutral 17-ketosteroids and pregnanediol by patients with breast cancer and benign breast disease, Amer. J. Obstet. Gynec. **92**:447-459, 1965.

247 Marmorston, J., Crowley, L. G., Myers, S. M., Stern, E., and Hopkins, C. E.: Urinary excretion of estrone, estradiol and estriol by patients with breast cancer and benign breast disease, Amer. J. Obstet. Gynec. **92**:460-467, 1965.

248 Masukawa, T., Lewison, E. F., and Frost, J. K.: The cytologic examination of breast secretions, Acta Cytol. (Balt.) **10**:261-265, 1966.

249 Miller, H., Durant, J. A., Jacobs, A. G., and Allison, J. F.: Alternative discriminating function for determining hormone dependency of breast cancer, Brit. Med. J. **1**:147-149, 1967.

250 Minagi, H., and Youker, J. E.: Roentgen appearance of fat necrosis in the breast, Radiology **90**:62-65, 1968.

251 Missakian, M. M., Witten, D. M., and Harrison, E. G., Jr.: Mammography after mastectomy, J.A.M.A. **191**:1045-1048, 1965.

252 Montague, E. D.: Physical and clinical parameters in the management of advanced breast cancer with radiation therapy alone, Amer. J. Roentgen. **99**:995-1001, 1967.

253 Moore, F. D., Woodrow, S. I., Aliapoulios, M. A., and Wilson, R. E.: Carcinoma of the breast, New Eng. J. Med. **277**:293-295, 1967.

254 Moore, O. S., Jr., and Foote, F. W., Jr.: The relatively favorable prognosis of medullary carcinoma of the breast, Cancer **2**:635-642, 1949.

255 Moore, S. W., and Lewis, R. J.: Carcinoma of the breast in women 30 years of age and under, Surg. Gynec. Obstet. **119**:1253-1255, 1964.

256 Moseley, R. D., Jr., Ironside, W. M. S., Harper, P. V., and McCrea, A.: Transsphenoidal destruction of the hypophysis with radioactive yttrium, Amer. J. Roentgen. **82**:604-611, 1959.

257 Mueller, H. P., and Sniffen, R. C.: Roentgenologic appearance and pathology of intrapulmonary lymphatic spread of metastatic cancer, Amer. J. Roentgen. **53**:109-123, 1945.

258 Muir, R.: Pathogenesis of Paget's disease of the nipple and associated lesions, Brit. J. Surg. **22**:728-737, 1935.

259 Muir, R.: Further observations on Paget's

disease of the nipple, J. Path. Bact. **49**:299-312, 1939.

260 Mye, G. L., Jr., and Neal, W., Jr.: Bilateral adrenalectomy for advanced mammary cancer, Amer. Surg. **31**:621-624, 1965.

261 Neubecker, R. E., and Bradshaw, R. P.: Mucin, melanin and glycogen in Paget's disease of the breast, Amer. J. Clin. Path. **36**:40-53, 1961.

262 Newell, F. W., and Ironside, W. M. S.: Ocular complications of transsphenoidal yttrium-90 hypophysectomy, Amer. J. Ophthal. **49**:476-483, 1960.

263 Newman, W.: In situ lobular carcinoma of the breast, Ann. Surg. **157**:591-599, 1963.

264 Newman, W.: Lobular carcinoma of the female breast, Ann. Surg. **164**:305-314, 1966.

265 Noer, R. J.: Breast adjuvant chemotherapy: effectiveness of Thio-TEPA (Triethylene-thiophosphoramide) as adjuvant to radical mastectomy for breast cancer, Ann. Surg. **154**:629-647, 1961.

266 Norris, H. J., and Taylor, H. B.: Prognosis of mucinous (gelatinous) carcinoma of the breast, Cancer **18**:879-885, 1965.

267 Norris, H. J., and Taylor, H. B.: Relationship of histologic features to behavior of cystosarcoma phyllodes—an analysis of 94 cases, Cancer **20**:2090-2099, 1967.

268 Norris, H. J., and Taylor, H. B.: Sarcomas and related mesenchymal tumors of the breast, Cancer **22**:22-28, 1968.

269 Norris, H. J., and Taylor, H. B.: Carcinoma of the male breast, Cancer **23**:1428-1435, 1969.

270 Oberman, H. A.: Cystosarcoma phyllodes of the breast, Cancer **18**:697-710, 1965.

271 Oelsner, L.: Anatomische Untersuchungen uber die Lymphwege der Brust mit Bezug auf die Ausbritung des Mammacarcinoms. (Inaugural dissertation, Breslau, 1901), Arch. Klin. Chir. **64**:134-158, 1901.

272 Olivecrona, H., and Luft, R.: Experiences with hypophysectomy in cancer of the breast, Ann. Roy. Coll. Surg. Eng. **20**:267-279, 1957.

273 Oliver, D. R., and Sugarbaker, E. D.: The significance of skin recurrences following radical mastectomy, Surg. Gynec. Obstet. **85**:360-367, 1947.

274 O'Mara, R. E., Ruzicka, F. F., Jr., Osborn, A., and Connell, J., Jr.: Xeromammography and film mammography, Radiology **88**:1121-1126, 1967.

274a Opler, S. R.: Immunological significance of histologic alterations of the lymph nodes associated with long-term survival in human beings with breast cancer (presented at the Tenth International Cancer Congress, Houston, Texas, May, 1970) (to be published).

275 Papadrianos, E., Cooley, E., and Haagenson, C. D.: Mammary carcinoma in old age, Ann. Surg. **161**:189-194, 1965.

276 Papadrianos, E., Haagenson, C. D., and Cooley, E.: Cancer of the breast as a familial disease, Ann. Surg. **165**:10-19, 1967.

277 Papaioannou, A. N., Tanz, F. J., and Volk, H.: Fate of patients with recurrent carcinoma of the breast; recurrence five or more years after initial treatment, Cancer **20**:371-376, 1967.

278 Papaioannou, A. N., and Urban, J. A.: Scalene node biopsy in locally advanced primary breast cancer of questionable operability, Cancer **17**:1006-1011, 1964.

279 Parsons, W. H., and McCall, E. F.: The role of estrogenic substances in the production of malignant mammary lesions, Surgery **9**:780-786, 1941.

280 Paterson, R.: The treatment of malignant disease by radium and x-rays, London, 1948, Edward Arnold (Publishers), Ltd.

281 Paterson, R.: Clinical trials in malignant disease; principles of random selection, J. Fac. Radiol. **9**:80-83, 1958.

282 Paterson, R., and Russell, M. H.: Clinical trials in malignant disease. Part II—Breast cancer: value of irradiation of the ovaries, J. Fac. Radiol. **10**:130-133, 1959.

283 Paterson, R., and Russell, M. H.: Clinical trials in malignant disease. Part III—Breast cancer: evaluation of post-operative radiotherapy, J. Fac. Radiol. **10**:175-180, 1960.

284 Patey, D. H.: A review of 146 cases of carcinoma of the breast operated on between 1930 and 1943, Brit. J. Cancer **21**:260-269, 1967.

285 Patton, R. B., Poznanski, A. K., and Zylak, C. J.: Pathologic examination of specimens containing nonpalpable breast cancers discovered by radiography, Amer. J. Clin. Path. **46**:330-334, 1966.

286 Paymaster, J. C.: Cancer of the breast in Indian women, Surgery **40**:372-377, 1956.

287 Pearson, O. H., and Ray, B. S.: Hypophysectomy in the treatment of metastatic mammary cancer, Amer. J. Surg. **99**:544-552, 1960.

288 Persson, B. H., and Risholm, L.: Treatment of metastasizing cancer of the breast with oophorectomy and cortisone, Acta Chir. Scand. **118**:217-224, 1959/1960.

289 Peters, M. V.: Carcinoma of the breast associated with pregnancy, Radiology **78**:58-67, 1962.

290 Phillips, A. J.: A comparison of treated and untreated cases of cancer of the breast, Brit. J. Cancer **13**:20-25, 1959.

291 Pusey, W. A., and Caldwell, E. W.: The practical application of roentgen rays in therapeutics and diagnosis, Philadelphia, 1903, W. B. Saunders Co.

292 Ratzkowski, E., Frankel, M., and Hochman, A.: Bone metastases, osteoporosis and radiation necrosis in breast cancer, Clin. Radiol. **18**:146-153, 1967.

293 Raven, R. W.: Tuberculosis of the breast, Brit. Med. J. **2**:734-736, 1949.

294 Ray, B. S.: Hypophysectomy as palliative treatment, J.A.M.A. **200**:974-975, 1967.

295 Reclus, P.: La maladie kystique des mamelles, Bull. Mem. Soc. Anat. Paris **58**:428-433, 1833.

296 del Regato, J. A.: El cancer del seno en relación con la vida sexual de la mujer en

Cuba. Influencia de la raza, edad, estado civil, esterilidad y lactancia. Conclusiones sobre 150 casos de cánceres de la mama, Vida Nueva **27**:413-418, 1931.

296a del Regato, J. A.: Letter to Dr. Bernard Fisher, April, 1970.

296b del Regato, J. A.: Radiotherapy as a post-operative surgical adjuvant in the treatment of carcinoma of the breast, Radiology (to be published).

297 Rissanen, P. M.: Carcinoma of the breast during pregnancy and lactation, Brit. J. Cancer **22**:663-668, 1968.

298 Rissanen, P. M., and Holsti, P.: Paget's disease of the breast; the influence of the presence or absence of an underlying palpable tumor on the prognosis and on the choice of treatment, Oncology **23**:209-216, 1969.

299 Robbins, G. F., and Berg, J. W.: Bilateral primary breast cancer, Cancer **17**:1501-1527, 1964.

300 Roper, C. L., Camp, F. A., and Kempson, R. L.: Atrial myxoma associated with fibroadenomas of the breast, Missouri Med. **62**: 113-116, 1965.

301 Rouvière H.: Anatomy of the human lymphatic system, Ann Arbor, Mich., 1938, Edwards Brothers, Inc.

302 Rubin, P.: Comment: the basis for selection of hormonal addition or subtraction, J.A.M.A. **200**:977-978, 1967.

303 Saltzstein, S. L.: Histologic diagnosis of breast carcinoma with the Silverman needle biopsy, Surgery **48**:366-374, 1960.

303a Saphir, O.: Mucinous carcinoma of the breast, Surg. Gynec. Obstet. **72**:908-914, 1941.

304 Saphir, O., and Parker, M. L.: Intracystic papilloma of the breast, Amer. J. Path. **16**: 189-210, 1940.

305 Sarrazin, D., and Lalanne, C. M.: La télécobalthérapie à doses élevées des cancers mammaires; évolution locale et séquelles, Ann. Radiol. (Paris) **9**:377-389, 1966.

306 Saxén, E., and Hakama, M.: Cancer incidence in Finland with a note on difficulties in comparing epidemiological data, Cancro **19**:88-96, 1966.

307 Schattenberg, H. J., and Ryan, J. F.: Lymphangitic carcinomatosis of lung; case report with autopsy findings, Ann. Intern. Med. **14**: 1710-1721, 1941.

308 Schwartz, D., Denoix, P. F., and Rouquette, C.: Enquete sur l'etiologie des cancer genitaux de la femme; cancer du sein, Bull. Ass. Franc. Cancer **45**:476-493, 1958.

309 Sears, M. E., Haut, A., and Eckles, N.: Melphalan (NSC-8806) in advanced breast cancer, Cancer Chemother. Rep. **50**:271-279, 1966.

310 Selby, H. M.: Mammographic pseudocalcifications, Cancer **17**:187-188, 1967.

311 Semb, C.: Fibro-adenomatosis cystica mammae, Acta Path. Microbiol. Scand. **5**(suppl.): 62-70, 1928.

312 Shimkin, M. B.: End results in cancer of the breast, Cancer **20**:1039-1043, 1967.

313 Shimkin, M. B., Lucia, E. L., E. L., Stone, R. S., and Bell, H. G.: Cancer of the breast; analysis of frequency, distribution and mortality at the University of California Hospital, 1918 to 1947 inclusive, Surg. Gynec. Obstet. **94**:645-661, 1952.

314 Siegelman, S. S., Rubinstein, B. M., and Schwartz, A.: Elusive carcinoma of the breast, Amer. J. Surg. **113**:401-403, 1967.

315 Siegmund, H.: Extragenitale Krebse in der Schwangerschaft. Ein Beitrag zur Frage der diffusen Krebsbildung in Brustdruse und Magen, Klin. Wschr. **27**:681-684, 1949.

316 Simon, J., Fischgold, H., and Bernard-Weil, E.: Les métastases encéphaliques du cancer du sein, Ann. Radiol. (Paris) **11**:651-661, 1968.

317 Sirtori, C., and Veronesi, U.: Gynecomastia; a review of 218 cases, Cancer **10**:645-654, 1957.

318 Slaughter, D. P., and Peterson, L. W.: Indications for simple mastectomy, Surg. Gynec. Obstet. **85**:456-466, 1947.

318a Smith, O. W., and Smith, G. V.: Urinary oestrogen profiles and aetiology of breast cancer, Lancet **1**:1152-1155, 1970.

319 Smithers, D. W., Rigby-Jones, P., Galton, D. A. G., and Payne, P. M.: Cancer of the breast; a review, Brit. J. Radiol. (suppl. 4), pp. i-xiii; 1-90, 1952.

320 Snell, W., and Beals, R. K.: Femoral metastases and fractures from breast cancer, Surg. Gynec. Obstet. **119**:22-24, 1964.

321 Snyder, R. E.: Mammography and lobular carcinoma in situ, Surg. Gynec. Obstet. **122**: 255-260, 1966.

322 Sommers, S. C.: Endocrine abnormalities in women with breast cancer, Lab. Invest. **4**: 160-174, 1955.

323 Spratt, J. S.: Locally recurrent cancer after radical mastectomy, Cancer **20**:1051-1053, 1967.

324 Steingaszner, L. C., Enzinger, F. M., and Taylor, H. B.: Hemangiosarcoma of the breast, Cancer **18**:352-361, 1965.

325 Sternby, N. H., Gynning, I., and Hogeman, K. E.: Postmastectomy angiosarcoma, Acta Chir. Scand. **121**:420-432, 1961.

326 Stevens, G. M., and Weigen, J. F.: Mammography survey for breast cancer detection; a 2-year study of 1,223 clinically negative asymptomatic women over 40, Cancer **19**: 51-59, 1966.

327 Stewart, F. W.: Tumors of the breast; Subcommittee of Oncology of the Committee of Pathology of the National Research Council, Sect. IX, Fasc. 34, Washington, D. C., 1950, Armed Forces Institute of Pathology.

328 Stewart, F. W., and Treves, N.: Lymphangiosarcoma in postmastectomy lymphedema, Cancer **1**:64-81, 1948.

329 Stibbe, E. P.: The internal mammary lymphatic glands, J. Anat. **52**:257-264, 1918.

330 Stocks, P.: Studies of cancer death rates at different ages in England and Wales in 1921 to 1950; uterus, breast and lung, Brit. J. Cancer **7**:283-302, 1953.

330a Strax, P., Venet, L., Shapiro, S., Gross, F., and Venet, W.: Breast cancer found on repetitive examination and mass screening, Arch. Environ. Health (Chicago) **20**:758-763, 1970.

331 Strode, J. E.: Tumors of the breast occurring in Hawaii, Ann. Surg. **144**:872-879, 1956.

332 Symmers, W. St. C.: Carcinoma of breast in trans-sexual individuals after surgical and hormonal interference with the primary and secondary sex characteristics, Brit. Med. J. **2**:83-85, 1968.

333 Taylor, G. W.: Carcinoma of the breast in young women, New Eng. J. Med. **215**:1276-1278, 1936.

334 Taylor, G. W., and Meltzer, A.: "Inflammatory carcinoma" of the breast, Amer. J. Cancer **33**:33-49, 1938.

335 Taylor, H. B., and Norris, H. J.: Well-differentiated carcinoma of the breast, Cancer **25**:687-692, 1970.

335a Taylor, H. B., and Norris, H. J.: Carcinoma of the breast in women less than 30 years old, Cancer (in press).

336 Taylor, H. B., and Robertson, A. G.: Adenomas of the nipple, Cancer **18**:995-1002, 1965.

337 Taylor, S. G., III, Eckles, N., Slaughter, D. P., and McDonald, J. H.: Effect of surgical Addison's disease on advanced carcinoma of the breast and prostate, Cancer **6**:997-1009, 1953.

338 Tellem, M., Nedwich, A., Amenta, P. S., and Imbriglia, J. E.: Mucin-producing carcinoma of the breast, Cancer **19**:573-584, 1966.

339 Testosterone propionate therapy in breast cancer, J.A.M.A. **188**:1069-1072, 1964.

340 Therapeutic Trials Committee, American Medical Association: Androgens and estrogens in the treatment of disseminated mammary carcinoma, J.A.M.A. **172**:1271-1283, 1960.

341 Tice, G. M.: Cancer of the breast; radiation therapy of carcinoma of the breast supplementing surgery, J. Kansas Med. Soc. **61**:122-127, 1960.

342 Tobias, C. A., Lawrence, J. H., Born, J. L., McCombs, R. K., Roberts, J. E., Anger, H. O., Low-Beer, B. V. A., and Huggins, C. B.: Pituitary irradiation with high-energy proton beams; a preliminary report, Cancer Res. **18**: 121-132, 1958.

343 Törnberg, B.: See Hultborn and Törnberg.[174]

344 Tough, I. C. K.: The significance of recurrence in breast cancer, Brit. J. Surg. **53**:897-900, 1966.

345 Treves, N., and Holleb, A. I.: Cancer of the male breast, Cancer **8**:1239-1250, 1955.

346 Treves, N., and Sunderland, D. A.: Cystosarcoma phyllodes of the breast; a malignant and a benign tumor, Cancer **4**:1286-1332, 1951.

347 Tuttle, H. K., and Kean, B. H.: Circumscribed chronic suppurative mastitis simulating cancer, Surg. Gynec. Obstet. **84**:933-938, 1947.

348 Urban, J. A.: Radical mastectomy with en bloc in continuity resection of the internal

mammary lymph node chain, Surg. Clin. N. Amer. **36**:1065-1082, 1956.

349 Urban, J. A.: Radical mastectomy with en bloc in continuity resection of the internal mammary lymph node chain, Amer. J. Roentgen. **77**:431-437, 1957.

350 Urban, J. A.: Clinical experience and results of excision of the internal mammary lymph node chain in primary operable breast cancer, Cancer **12**:14-22, 1959.

351 Urban, J. A.: Excision of the major duct system of the breast, Cancer **16**:516-520, 1963.

352 Urban, J. A.: Bilaterality of cancer of the breast; biopsy of the opposite breast, Cancer **20**:1867-1870, 1967.

353 Urban, J. A., and Adair, F.: Sclerosing adenosis, Cancer **2**:625-634, 1949.

354 Urban, J. A., and Baker, H. W.: Radical mastectomy in continuity with en bloc resection of the internal mammary lymph-node chain, Cancer **5**:992-1008, 1952.

355 Vassar, P. S., and Culling, C. F. A.: Fibrosis of the breast, Arch. Path. (Chicago) **67**:128-133, 1959.

356 Versluys, J. J.: Marriage fertility and cancer mortality of the specifically female organs; mammary carcinoma, Brit. J. Cancer **9**:239-245, 1955.

357 Vogler, W. R., Furtado, V. P., and Huguley, C. M.: Methotrexate for advanced cancer of the breast, Cancer **21**:26-30, 1968.

358 Vogt-Hoerner, G., and Contesso, G.: Localisation anatomique du premier ganglion axillaire métastatique de cancer du sein (A propos de 73 observations n'ayant qu'un seul ganglion axillaire envahi), J. Chir. (Paris) **86**:37-42, 1963.

359 Vogt-Hoerner, G., and Contesso, G.: Ganglions interpectoraux et cancers du sein, Int. J. Cancer **3**:35-38, 1968.

360 de Waard, F., Baanders-Van Halewijn, E. A., and Huizinga, J.: The bimodal age distribution of patients with mammary carcinoma; evidence for the existence of 2 types of human breast cancer, Cancer **17**:141-151, 1964.

361 Wagoner, J. K., Chiazze, L., and Lloyd, J. W.: Cancer of the breast at menopausal ages, Cancer **20**:354-362, 1967.

362 Wainwright, J. M.: Carcinoma of the male breast, Arch. Surg. (Chicago) **14**:836-958, 1927.

363 Wallace, J. D., and Dodd, G. D.: Thermography in the diagnosis of breast cancer, Radiology **91**:679-685, 1968.

364 Wang, C. C., and Griscom, N. T.: Inflammatory carcinoma of the breast; results following orthovoltage and supervoltage radiation therapy, Clin. Radiol. **15**:168-174, 1964.

365 Wangensteen, O. H.: In discussion of Bell, H.: Cancer of the breast, Ann. Surg. **130**: 310-317, 1949.

366 Wangensteen, O. H., Lewis, F. J., and Arheiger, S. W.: The extended or superficial mastectomy for carcinoma of the breast, Surg. Clin. N. Amer. **36**:1051-1063, 1956.

367 Watson, T. A.: Treatment of breast cancer;

comparison of results of simple mastectomy and radiotherapy with results of radical mastectomy and radiotherapy, Lancet 1:1191-1194, 1959.

368 Watson, T. W.: Cancer of the breast (the Janeway lecture—1965), Amer. J. Roentgen. 96:547-559, 1966.

369 Webster, D. R., and Sabbadini, E.: The prognostic significance of circulating tumour cells, Canad. Med. Ass. J. 96:129-131, 1967.

370 White, T. T., and White, W. C.: Breast cancer and pregnancy; report of 49 cases followed 5 years, Ann. Surg. 144:384-393, 1956.

371 Whitney, D. G., Smith, R. F., and Szilagyi, D. E.: Meaning of five-year cure in cancer of the breast, Arch. Surg. (Chicago) 88:637-644, 1964.

372 Wilkinson, L., and Green, W. O., Jr.: Infarction of breast lesions during pregnancy and lactation, Cancer 17:1567-1572, 1964.

373 Williams, I. G., and Cunningham, G. J.: Histological changes in irradiated carcinoma of the breast, Brit. J. Radiol. 24:123-133, 1951.

374 Wilson, W. B., and Spell, J. P.: Adenoid cystic carcinoma of breast; a case with recurrence and regional metastasis, Ann. Surg. 166:861-864, 1967.

375 Wolfe, J. N.: Mammography; errors in diagnosis, Radiology 87:214-219, 1966.

376 Wolfe, J. N.: Mammography; ducts as a sole indicator of breast carcinoma, Radiology 89:206-210, 1967.

377 Wolfe, J. N.: Xerography of the breast, Cancer 23:791-796, 1969.

378 Wood, D. A., and Darling, H. H.: Cancer family manifesting multiple occurrences of bilateral carcinoma of the breast, Cancer Res. 3:509-514, 1943.

379 Wulsin, J. H.: Large breast tumors in adolescent females, Ann. Surg. 152:151-159, 1960.

380 Yonemoto, R. H., Byron, R. L., Jr., and Keating, J. L.: Long-term survival after adrenalectomy for advanced cancer of the breast, Cancer 20:254-259, 1967.

Chapter 16

Malignant tumors of bone

Anatomy

A knowledge of the fundamental development and histology of bone is necessary for an understanding of bone neoplasms. The long bones, which are most often the sites of primary tumors, are made up of two types of bone: compact and spongy. The compact bone is a continuous sheath of bone in which no space can be observed except microscopically, whereas the spongy bone is made up of a latticelike network of bone. The bone is covered by periosteum that cannot be stripped away because of its strong attachment by Sharpey's fibers.

The shaft of the bone is the diaphysis, its extremity is the epiphysis, and the portion of the shaft near the epiphyseal line is the metaphysis (Fig. 674). The epiphysis is made up of cartilage, but it becomes calcified at varying ages in the different bones. The degree of calcification depends on other factors. After calcification, the epiphyseal line is no longer a barrier to the spread of tumor, and therefore the age of the calcification is important.

The blood supply of the bones is of particular interest from the standpoint of metastases. The arteries enter the flat bones in various areas, and the veins leave these bones by separate canals. In the long bones, branches from the articular arteries enter the foramina at the extremities. Through the fibrous attachments of Sharpey's fibers, blood vessels extend into the compact bone, creating a rich network that unites to form the haversian canals which, in turn, communicate directly with Volkmann's canals, penetrating through the periosteum. The walls of the medullary cavity and the medulla are supplied by nutrient arteries. The nutrient arteries enter the medullary cavity through a special canal and divide into proximal and distal branches that anastomose with the articular arteries. The large veins of the medulla leave the bone through the same foramina that the nutrient artery enters.

Lymphatics. The lymphatics of the bones of the upper and lower extremities leave by the nutrient foramina, traverse the periosteum, and empty into the nearest deep collecting trunk. The lymphatics of the periosteum of the tibia terminate, for the most part, in the popliteal nodes, but some empty into superficial inguinal lymph nodes.

Epidemiology

Giant cell tumors are rarely found in patients under 20 or over 55 years of age. Such tumors reported outside of this age group should be viewed with suspicion. Giant cell tumors are more common in female than in male individuals and may be associated with Paget's disease (Hutter et al.[85]).

Ewing's sarcoma makes up between 7% and 15% of all malignant bone tumors. About 60% of the cases are in male individuals. This tumor is infrequently reported in patients past 30 years of age, the majority of patients being 4 to 25 years old. Two instances of Ewing's sarcoma in siblings have been reported (Hutter et al.[86]).

Osteosarcomas make up about 30% of all malignant bone tumors. A traumatic etiology of bone sarcoma remains unproved (Stewart[205]). Major trauma (fracture, surgery, particularly amputation, and exodontia) does not cause osteogenic sarcoma. It is difficult to understand, therefore, how the relatively insignificant trauma often cited could possibly cause this neoplasm. Sarcomas of bone have been produced experimentally by means of *roentgen rays* and *radium*. Lacassagne[112] produced fibrosarcoma of the tibia in a rabbit thirty-six months after administration of radiations to an abscess near the bone. Osteosarcomas can be induced into miniature swine by

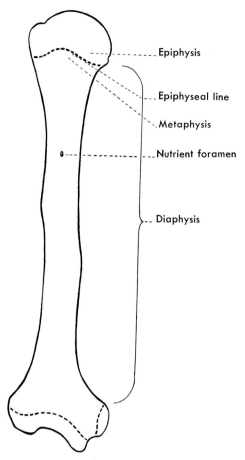

Epiphysis

Epiphyseal line

Metaphysis

Nutrient foramen

Diaphysis

Fig. 674. Sketch of humerus identifying different anatomic landmarks in long bone.

strontium[90] (Howard et al.[82]). Hatcher[72] collected twenty-seven cases of bone sarcoma that developed in apparent connection with the local administration of large amounts of radiations. Usually the interval between irradiation and the development of the tumor is rather long (Cruz et al.[32]). Fortunately, the complication is rare (Cahan et al.[18]). Nine of the seventeen post-irradiation sarcomas of bone reported from the Mayo Clinic seemingly arose following irradiation of supposedly benign giant cell tumors (Sabanas et al.[181]). Martland and Humphries[143] reported a series of eighteen patients who died from *radium* poisoning, five of whom had developed osteosarcoma. The victims were young women employed in the painting of clock dials with luminous paint made of zinc sulfide and 1 part in 40,000 of radium, mesothorium, and radiothorium. It was the custom of the work-

ers to moisten the bristles of the brush between their lips, and this resulted in the ingestion of a certain amount of radioactive material. Oral administration of minute amounts of radium for questionable therapeutic purposes has resulted in the development of osteosarcomas in the past (Looney et al.[133]; Hems[76]).

There is no doubt that Paget's disease has a definite relationship with osteosarcoma of the adult, considerably more frequently in men than in women. In a group of 1753 patients with Paget's disease, osteosarcoma was present in sixteen at the time of reporting. Undetected or subclinical Paget's disease is often found at autopsy. These facts make any percentage evaluation of the association with osteosarcomas rather difficult. Although osteosarcomas predominate, chondrosarcomas, fibrosarcomas, and giant cell tumors have been found in association with Paget's disease (Summey and Pressly[208]; Goldenberg[65]; Snapper[200, 201]). The extreme stromal activity that accompanies Paget's disease may serve as a focus for malignant transformation. When osteosarcoma develops on Paget's disease, it occurs in the areas in which Paget's disease is most advanced and has been present for years (Coley and Sharp[30]). Osteosarcomas of the skull almost always occur in male individuals suffering from Paget's disease. Paget's disease is very rare in Scandinavia, Greece, and Japan. In these countries, osteosarcoma is mainly a disease of adolescents (Price[175]). Schwartz and Alpert[191] collected twenty-eight cases of osteosarcoma apparently secondary to fibrous dysplasia, often of the polyostotic type. Fraumeni[56] found that youngsters under 18 years of age with osteosarcomas were significantly taller than those in a control group with nonosseous malignant tumors.

Chondrosarcomas are considered separately from osteosarcomas because their clinical behavior, pathology, treatment, and prognosis are distinctive. Henderson and Dahlin[77] reported 181 cases in males and 107 in females. Chondrosarcomas are one-half as common as osteosarcomas and twice as common as Ewing's sarcomas. Schajowicz and Bessone[187] reported chondrosarcomas occurring in three brothers. A fairly good proportion of cases of mul-

tiple cartilaginous exostoses (chondrodysplasia) may develop chondrosarcoma arising from the cartilaginous cap (Jaffe[92]).
Chondrodysplasia is inherited in two-thirds
of the cases (Solomon[202]) and is equally
distributed between the sexes. McKenna
et al.[140] reported twelve cases of secondary
chondrosarcoma, all of which arose on
hereditary multiple exostoses. It is frequently stated that chondrosarcomas may
also arise from enchondromas, but this almost never occurs in cartilaginous tumors
of the small bones (Lansche and Spjut[114]).
Infrequently, chondrosarcomas arise from
the cartilaginous cap of exostoses but most
arise primarily. Of 288 cases reported by
Henderson and Dahlin,[77] twenty-five developed in exostoses, fifteen of these in
multiple exostoses of the hereditary type.
In the series reported by McKenna et al.,[140]
there were 139 primary chondrosarcomas
and twelve arising from hereditary multiple
exostoses. Infrequently, chondrosarcomas
arise in Ollier's disease or are found in
association with Paget's disease.

Multiple myeloma occurs predominantly
in men. In a series studied by us, there
were sixty men and thirty women. The
youngest patient was 25 years old, and
most cases occurred in patients 50 to 70
years of age. These tumors have rarely
been reported in children or adolescents
(Slavens[198]). Talerman[209a] reported a high
occurrence of myeloma among Jamaican
blacks; no such higher occurrence has been
reported among African or American
blacks.

Reticulum cell sarcoma also predominates in male patients in a ratio of 2:1.
More than half of the cases are found in
patients 10 to 30 years of age (Coley et
al.[28]). *Fibrosarcoma* of bone is most common in the second to fourth decade of life.

Pathology
Gross and microscopic pathology

A classification of bone tumors modified
from Lichtenstein's classification is presented in Table 108.

Giant cell tumors arise in the epiphyseal
end of the long bones. These tumors are
globular in shape, have a well-defined capsule, and contain numerous well-vascularized loculations. The large tumors thin out
the cortex and infrequently fracture. In the

Table 108. Classification of primary benign
and malignant neoplasms of bone*

Tissue of origin	Benign neoplasm	Malignant counterpart
Fat	Lipoma	Liposarcoma
Blood vessels	Hemangioma	Angiosarcoma
Lymph vessels	Lymphangioma	—
Nerve sheath	Neurilemoma	—
Fibrous tissue	Desmoplastic fibroma	Fibrosarcoma
Uncertain	Giant cell tumor	Giant cell tumor
Cartilage	Chondro-blastoma	—
	Chondro-myxoid fibroma	—
	Enchondroma	Chondrosarcoma (1) Primary (2) Secondary
	Osteochon-droma	—
Bone	Osteoid osteoma	Osteosarcoma (1) Juxtacortical (2) Arising in Paget's disease (3) Arising in irradiated bone
	Giant osteoid osteoma (osteoblastoma)	—
Bone marrow elements	—	Plasma cell myeloma
	—	Reticulum cell sarcoma
	—	Ewing's sarcoma
Tumors of uncertain histologic origin (?epithelial)	—	Adamantinoma

*Modified from Lichtenstein, L.: Classification of primary
tumors of bone, Cancer 4:335-341, 1951.

medullary cavity, they usually have a sharp
dividing line. Only rarely will periosteal
reaction occur. They may invade the metaphysis but only rarely affect the joint. An
area of sclerosed bone usually develops
beneath the articular cartilage. Windeyer
and Woodyatt[227] reported a giant cell tumor that extended from the proximal end
of the femur across the joint space by way
of the ligamentum teres, to involve the
bones of the pelvis. Microscopic examination reveals the tumor to be made up of
two elements: stroma and giant cells. The

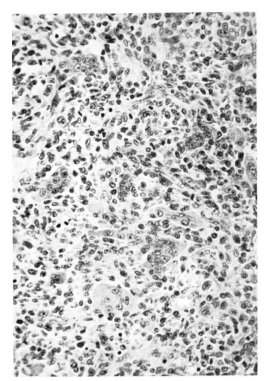

Fig. 675. Giant cell tumor showing numerous giant cells with multiple, regular, identical nuclei. Stroma reveals increased cellularity, but individual cells are uniform. (Moderate enlargement.)

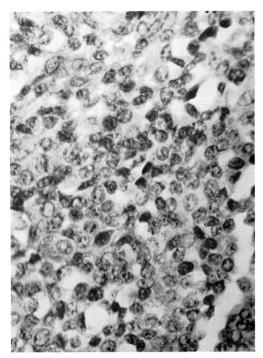

Fig. 676. Ewing's sarcoma with uniform cells, fine nucleoli, and inconspicuous cytoplasm. (High-power enlargement.)

giant cells are presumably products of fusion of nuclei from the stromal cells. Many of these giant cells contain twenty to thirty-five nuclei identical in appearance (Fig. 675). The predominance of giant cells has given them unprecedented importance, but the stroma is of much greater importance and should be examined carefully from the standpoint of cellularity, mitotic activity, and variation. Thorough sectioning of these tumors should be done, for the variations in appearance may be great. Jaffe et al.[97] outlined criteria for the grading of giant cell tumors. We do not believe grading has practical value (Schajowicz[186]). By electron microscopy, the giant cells are shown to be osteoclasts.

Ewing's sarcoma has an obscure histogenesis. Some authorities believe that it is probably derived from the young reticular cells (Lichtenstein and Jaffe[128]). In the long bones, the tumor takes origin in the shaft *and never primarily involves the epiphysis.* In the early stages, there is con-

densation of the shaft of the bone, and the widened cortex is made up of subperiosteal and endosteal formation of new bone. This new bone is a reaction to the tumor rather than a specific product of it. With further growth, the tumor spreads to involve a greater portion of the shaft and finally extends through the periosteum into the soft tissue. This involvement of the shaft is characteristic, and widespread involvement is the rule. With separation of the periosteum, spicules of new bone from the subperiosteal layer are laid down at right angles to the shaft. These changes occur because Volkmann's canals unite the periosteal blood supply with the haversian vessels. There may be necrosis, cyst formation, and increase of connective tissue with focal spontaneous regression of the tumor. On microscopic examination, Ewing's sarcoma is made up of broad sheaths of tumor with polyhedral-shaped cells with very scanty or pale cytoplasm. The individual cells are monotonously similar, with small nuclei and fine nucleoli (Fig. 676). There is no intercellular substance, and *the tumor never produces osteoid.* The histochemical demonstration of glycogen in Ewing's sarcoma and its absence in reticulum cell sarcoma proved to be an important method of differentiation in the hands of Schajowicz.[185] The haversian canals are frequently infiltrated.

The gross appearance of an *osteosarcoma* is exceedingly variable and depends upon bone production, vascularity, extent, and duration of the lesion. Osteosarcomas are sometimes divided into sclerosing and osteolytic varieties, but all gradations of each occur, and one blends into the other. The cut section of a predominantly sclerosing osteosarcoma shows a fan-shaped tumor usually involving the end of a long bone. The tumor is made up of dense connective and osteoid tissue. It will usually have extended through the periosteum to involve the surrounding soft tissue and muscle, and it may have extended down the marrow cavity without, however, having involved the joint cavity. The predominantly osteolytic tumor may be cut with ease and may present large areas of hemorrhage and necrosis. Fragmentation of the periosteum and invasion of the soft tissues are early phenomena in this type of tumor. Osteosarcomas usually do not invade the epiphysis until after ossification of the epiphyseal line has occurred, and they may involve the joint secondarily after fracture or perforation of the periosteum in the metaphyseal region. In many instances, there may be laying down of bone at right angles to the shaft because of extension of the tumor beneath the periosteum. The periosteum confines the tumor and gives it a spindle shape that is altered if the neoplasm grows through it. The microscopic appearance of osteosarcoma is extremely variable and differs from area to area (Fig. 677). If large or multiple sections are taken, the variation is more apparent. There is, therefore, little justification for

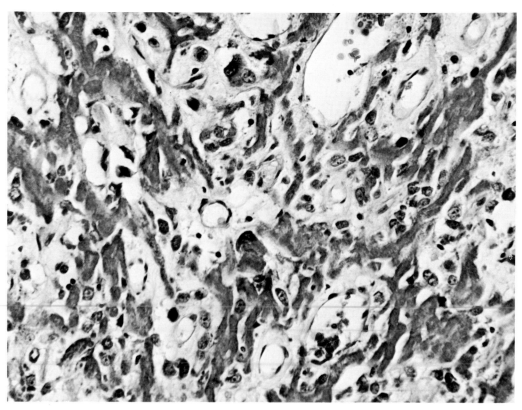

Fig. 677. Extremely well-differentiated osteosarcoma with pattern of atypical osteoid. Stroma is not particularly alarming. (×350; WU neg. 67-9896.)

any complicated classification for, fundamentally speaking, the osteosarcoma arises from bone-forming mesenchyme which can give rise to spindlelike cells, mucoid material, cartilage, and bone. In the typical osteosarcoma, osteoid tissue is usually seen evolving directly from a sarcomatous stroma. *This does not occur in the chondrosarcoma.* The presence of giant cells and well-differentiated fibrous areas may be confusing.

Chondrosarcomas must be separated from osteosarcomas. They are made up of cartilage and are not associated with osteoid. Grossly, they may become large and sometimes cystic. Characteristically, they may grow into the large veins. Tumor thrombi may extend over long distances, as far as the lungs (Warren[223]). The evaluation of whether a cartilaginous tumor is benign or malignant is very difficult. Often, the decision considers clinical and radiographic, as well as gross and microscopic, evidence. The presence of mucoid changes points strongly to malignancy. Jaffe[92] indicated that the diagnosis of chondrosarcoma can be made in the presence of plump, atypical, or double nuclei (Fig. 678). However, some of the benign cartilaginous tumors of the small bones and the tumors of Ollier's disease may show disturbing cellularity. By contrast, the voluminous tumors arising in the pelvis may be formed by well-differentiated cartilage of benign appearance but of frequent malignant evolution. Distinct microscopic types of chondrosarcoma designated as mesenchymal, and often found in flat bones, have been reported by Dahlin and Coventry[35] and Dowling.[43] Furthermore, in synovial chrondromatosis it is common for the nuclei to appear extremely bizarre (Murphy et al.[154]), but this lesion is practically never malignant (Goldman and Lichtenstein[66]).

The *myeloma* tends to produce extensive areas of patchy destruction. The involved bone may have a preserved paper-thin cortex. The areas of destruction are more often patchy than diffuse, and zones of hemorrhage, infarction, and necrosis are not unusual. The tumor is usually grayish red in color. At times, this tumor may be first seen as an apparently single focus within a flat bone or in the pelvis, vertebra, or femur. The widespread replacement often seen in the end stages may be due to multiple foci of origin. There may be wide variations in the degree of destruction. In some instances, the bones architecturally appear normal. Microscopically,

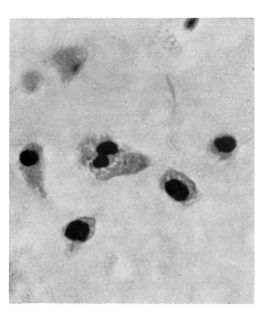

Fig. 678. Chondosarcoma showing multinucleated cells and plump nuclei. (Moderate enlargement.)

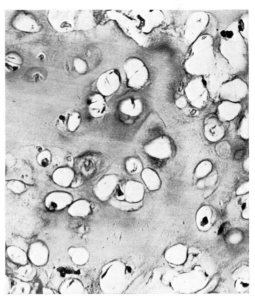

Fig. 679. Chondroma with no multinucleated forms and very regular pattern. Note contrast with photomicrograph shown in Fig. 678. (Moderate enlargement.)

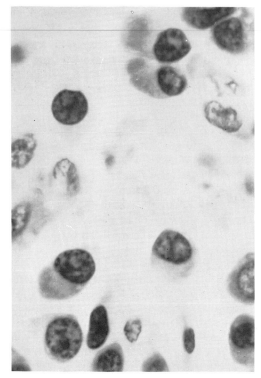

Fig. 680. Well-differentiated plasma cell myeloma. Nuclei are eccentric with cartwheel arrangement of chromatin. (High-power enlargement.)

the bone shows replacement by tumor cells. In the vertebrae, this often results in complete replacement. Plasma cells have eccentric nuclei with a cartwheel arrangement of the chromatin (Fig. 680). Frequently, they are multinucleated, and their cytoplasm is pink with a perinuclear halo. They may be large or small and are rarely highly undifferentiated. Electron microscopically, they present a typical pattern. Primary *reticulum cell sarcoma* of bone was first described by Oberling[159] and later by Jackson and Parker,[89] who reported twenty-five cases. The medullary cavity is often extensively invaded by pinkish gray tissue which, in advanced stages, is accompanied by areas of bone destruction. Areas of necrosis are frequent (Parker and Jackson[169]). The tumor cells are larger than the cells in Ewing's sarcoma, and they have eosinophilic cytoplasm and rather prominent nucleoli. They also show an abundant reticulin network. Phagocytosis may be present.

Fibrosarcoma is a rare primary bone tumor. It may arise in preexisting benign fibrous dysplasia (Perkinson and Higinbotham[171]; Eyre-Brook and Price[51]). The tumors vary in their microscopic pattern from exceedingly well differentiated to poorly differentiated (Cunningham and Arlen[34]). True *liposarcoma* of bone is extremely rare. Dawson's[38] case is unequivocal. The histogenesis of *adamantinomas* of bone is in doubt (Changus et al.[20]). They arise in the shaft of long bones, usually the tibia, do not involve the epiphysis, and extend through the cortex to invade the soft tissues. Microscopically, they have a variable pattern. Rosai[178] reported an adamantinoma that appeared to have an epithelial pattern (Fig. 681). Electron microscopically, it was shown to be epithelial in origin with tonofibrils and desmosomes (Fig. 682). *Hemangioendotheliomas* of bone may be observed. Malignant bone tumors may have more than one distinct component and be designated as *malignant mesenchymomas* (Schajowicz et al.[188]). Hutter et al.[84] reported twenty-five tumors designated as "primitive multipotential primary sarcoma of bone," and Evans and Sanerkin[48] have reported a leiomyosarcoma.

Metastatic spread

Malignant giant cell tumors metastasize primarily to the lungs. Morphologically, "benign" varieties of giant cell tumors have been reported to have metastasized (Jaffe et al.[97]; Murphy and Ackerman[155]; Jewell and Bush[101]).

Ewing's sarcomas metastasize early and widely, and the distribution of metastases is characteristic. The lungs, lymph nodes, and bones of the skull, in that order, are most frequently involved. Widespread bone metastases may occur in the skull, spine, scapula, and clavicle. This ability to metastasize to other bones is unique, and it is still a questionable point whether the bone lesions represent metastases from the primary lesion or multiple foci of origin. *Osteosarcoma* and *chondrosarcoma* only rarely metastasize to regional lymph nodes. Osteosarcoma primarily spreads by blood vessels most often to the lungs.

Multiple myeloma is invariably discovered only after it has spread to many

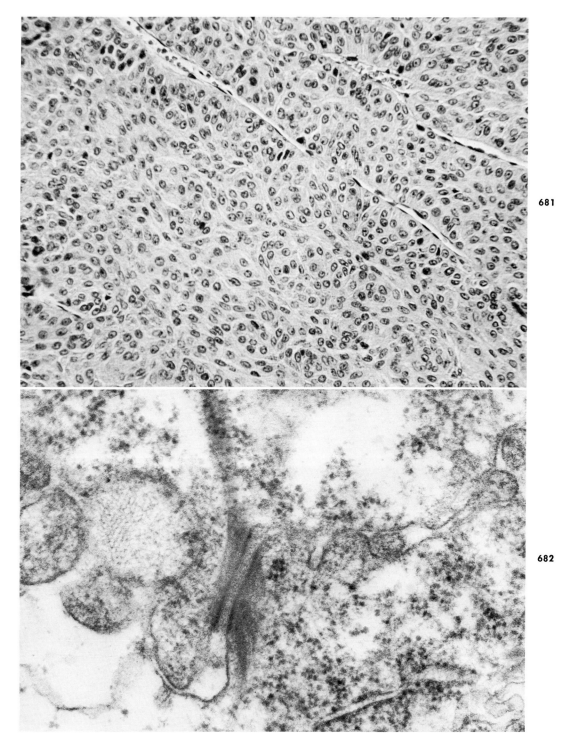

681

682

Fig. 681. Adamantinoma. Area showing definite squamoid appearance. Note bland appearance of nuclei and absence of mitoses. (From Rosai, J.: Adamantinoma of the tibia; electron microscopic evidence of its epithelial origin, Amer. J. Clin. Path. **51**:786-792, 1969; © 1969, The Williams & Wilkins Co., Baltimore, Md., U.S.A.; WU neg. 68-7293.)

Fig. 682. Adamantinoma. Typical desmosome is seen connecting two tumor cells. Note two opposing dense plates, tonofibrils converging upon them, and thin parallel lines present in intercellular space. (From Rosai, J.: Adamantinoma of the tibia; electron microscopic evidence of its epithelial origin, Amer. J. Clin. Path. **51**:786-792, 1969; © 1969, The Williams & Wilkins Co., Baltimore, Md., U.S.A.)

bones. Most frequently affected are the vertebrae, bones of the pelvis, skull, ribs, clavicle, and sternum. Infrequently, lymph nodes, spleen, liver, and other organs can be implicated. Pulmonary involvement is rare.

Reticulum cell sarcomas metastasize predominantly to other bones (ribs, vertebrae, and pelvic bones), lymph nodes, and lungs.

Clinical evolution

Giant cell tumors begin insidiously. Their first symptoms usually suggest a mild arthritis or neuritis, and later definite local pain may appear that produces increased disability. They develop frequently in the distal end of the femur and radius and the proximal end of the tibia but are also found in numerous other bones: proximal end of the femur, proximal end of the humerus, proximal end of the radius, distal end of the ulna, proximal end of the fibula, small bones of the hands and feet, patella, sacrum (Johnson et al.[103]), and ilium. The very large giant cell tumors occurring in the lower end of the femur or tibia may cause complete disability. Fractures may occur in the weight-bearing bones (10% to 15%). These tumors alone infrequently cause death. Death may occur when an inadequately treated malignant giant cell tumor disseminates. Lichtenstein[121] believes that cases of giant cell tumor reported arising from the shaft of long bones, the maxillae (Dechaume[39]), ribs, and flat bones of the skull, pelvis, or vertebrae are more likely to be aneurysmal bone cysts. He does not believe that genuine giant cell tumors develop in patients under 20 years of age.

The first symptom of *Ewing's sarcoma* is often pain, which almost invariably appears at some time during the course of the disease. Tumor without pain is unusual. The pain is deceptive and intermittent. As the disease progresses, the attacks of pain become more frequent and intense. It is usually more severe at night and is accompanied by a temperature ranging from 99° to 103° F. This elevation is somewhat proportional to the duration of the tumor and its size. Frequent primary manifestations are seen in the long bones of the lower extremities, femur, tibia, and

fibula, but also in the pelvic bones (Uehlinger et al.[215]), ribs (Coley et al.[27]), ulna, clavicle, metacarpal bones, radius, mandible, metatarsal bones, and skull. Spontaneous fractures in cases of Ewing's sarcoma have a tendency to heal spontaneously (Unander-Scharin[216]). The authenticity of Ewing's sarcoma is disputed by Willis,[226] who believes that cases reported as such are reticulum cell sarcomas or metastatic lesions from neuroblastomas and other tumors. We certainly agree that in some instances metastatic tumors arising from the adrenal gland, lung, or other organs, as well as reticulum cell sarcoma, can be mistaken for Ewing's tumor.

The onset of *osteosarcoma* often resembles rheumatism, a sprain, or arthritis. The pain is minimal in most instances and precedes the appearance of tumor by days, weeks, or months. It is undoubtedly due to the tension placed on the periosteum by underlying tumor and may abruptly be alleviated if rupture of the periosteum occurs. In the lower extremities, it may be relieved by drawing up the legs and thus relaxing the muscles overlying the taut periostetum. As the tumor increases in size, the pain becomes severe and worse at night, which contributes in some degree to the progressive weight loss.

Osteosarcomas occur twice as frequently in men as in women (Ross[179]). They most commonly begin in the metaphysis of long bones. About half of all cases are found in the femur, and four of five arise in the distal end. In the shoulder girdle, the scapula is the seat of predilection. Other frequent sites are the tibia, humerus, pelvic bones, fibula, bones of hand and foot, ribs, jaws, and vertebrae. The distal end of the humerus and fibula and the phalanges and toes are rarely the site of osteosarcoma (Kolodny[109]).

Osteosarcomas have a variable speed of growth, the osteolytic varieties developing much more rapidly than the sclerosing types. The osteolytic type causes elevated temperature with increase in pulse rate. If the tumor is not treated, dissemination of the disease to the lungs occurs, followed by further dissemination, extreme weight loss, and death. Cases of multiple simultaneous manifestations of bone sarcoma have been reported often arising on the basis of Paget's disease (Ackerman[1]; Derman et al.[41]).

Chondrosarcomas arise most frequently from the ends of long bones and from pre-existing chondrodysplasia. In Henderson and Dahlin's series,[77] there were eighty cases in the innominate bones, fifty in the ribs, forty-eight in the femur, twenty-five in the humerus, twenty-one in the spine, eighteen in the scapula, and fifteen in the tibia or fibula. They rarely arise in the small bones of the hand and foot but exceptionally may be found in the calcaneous (Barnes and Catto[10]). When found in the long bones, cartilaginous tumors are often malignant, as they are in the ribs and sternum (O'Neal and Ackerman[161]). Multiple areas of simultaneous malignant transformation may occur. Evidence suggestive of malignant changes in the cartilaginous tumors includes the presence of large peripheral tumors (greater than 8 cm in diameter with a thick cartilaginous cap) and the presence of acceleration of growth of an osteochondroma after the age of 20 years. We view with suspicion enchondromatous lesions other than those of the bones of hands and feet.

The first symptoms of a *myeloma* are intermittent, usually in the form of local pain, suggesting neuralgia and arthritis. This pain often becomes worse with exercise. As the disease progresses and disseminates, there may be episodes of extreme pain followed by collapse. The tumors frequently occur in the ribs, vertebrae, pelvis, and flat bones of the skull. Fracture is common in this type of bone tumor and occurred in approximately 20% of the patients with multiple myeloma. Paraplegia may be the first sign of disease because of collapsed vertebrae. Fractures often occur in nonweight-bearing bones, appearing most frequently in the ribs, usually between the fifth and twelfth. A multiple myeloma may begin as an extramedullary tumor, to be followed later by multiple bone lesions. Extensive soft tissue involvement may be observed (Edwards and Zawadzki[45]). In still other instances, the tumor begins as an apparent single focus within a bone. Treatment of one of these areas may relieve the symptoms, but years later there may be widespread dissemination. In the late stages of multiple mye-

loma, there is excessive pain due to multiple fractures and is also extreme weight loss and anemia. Thoracic deformities, kyphosis, and shortening of stature due to the involvement of the vertebrae may also develop. Renal failure due to tubular changes specific to multiple myeloma can occur (Snapper[200, 201]). Pulmonary complications are common and usually secondary to multiple rib fractures and a flail chest. Cases of multiple myeloma associated with polycythemia vera have been reported.

Reticulum cell sarcoma of bone usually begins with pain localized to the site of the disease. As the process continues, the pain becomes more and more prominent, and weight loss ensues. Local swelling is often a first symptom or is rapidly added to the clinical picture. Local heat and fever are not infrequently observed. Patients with reticulum cell sarcoma are often in excellent general condition, even with widespread involvement, and may live much longer than one would expect from the extent of bone involvement. This tumor occurs in patients of all ages and frequently in the long or flat bones but particularly in the femur, clavicle, tibia, and humerus. In the long bones, it frequently starts in the metaphysis and extends to involve a large area of the diaphysis.

Four of five of the *fibrosarcomas* of bone arise in the femur or proximal end of the tibia (Gilmer and McEwen[64]), but this tumor has also been reported arising in the radius, ulna, and pelvic bones. One case of fibrosarcoma was reported arising at the site of infarct in the femoral shaft of a caisson worker (Dorfman et al.[42]) (Fig. 683). *Liposarcomas* of bone are very rare. *Adamantinomas* of bone typically arise in the tibia but also in the ulna, fibula, and radius (Moon[148]). *Hemangioendotheliomas* have been reported in long and flat bones and presenting apparent multiple foci of origin (Otis et al.[166]).

Diagnosis

The diagnosis of bone tumors requires the combined efforts of an experienced clinician, roentgenologist, and pathologist. If the clinical history and examination are deficient, if roentgenograms are of inferior quality or badly interpreted, if biopsies are poorly prepared and the histologic opinion

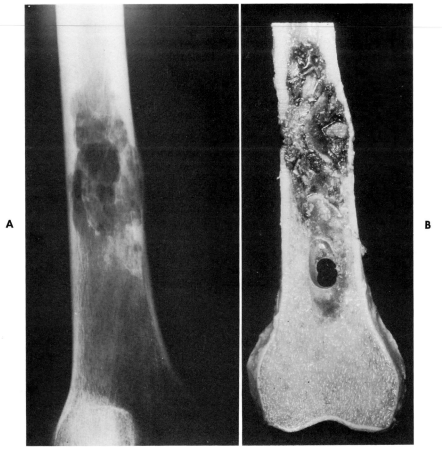

Fig. 683. **A,** Area of destruction in region of bone infarction in femur. **B,** Tumor occupying medullary cavity and eroding cortex. Old infarct occupies center of tumor. (From Dorfman, H. D., et al.: Fibrosarcoma complicating bone infarction in a caisson worker, J. Bone Joint Surg. **48-A:**528-532, 1966.)

is not expert, then an accurate diagnosis is seldom made. The clinical history must be taken carefully from the viewpoint of exact time of onset, presence or absence of pain and fever, and rate of growth of the tumor. The clinical examination should estimate the exact limits of the tumor and its relationship to the bone, joint, and skin. The presence or absence of increased vascularity and the relationship of the tumor to the surrounding muscles should be ascertained. Roentgenograms must be taken carefully. Several views may be necessary. The pathologist should report only on well-selected and well-prepared biopsies. When all this information is put together, an accurate diagnosis can usually be made. Efforts to make a diagnosis on just clinical,

roentgenographic, or pathologic grounds alone often result in errors.

Once the presence of a bone tumor is established, there are further identifying factors that are not, however, absolute. The *age* of the patient may help in diagnosis. Giant cell tumors are most frequently observed in patients 20 to 35 years old. Ewing's sarcomas are very infrequent after the age of 30 years. On the other hand, myelomas practically never develop before 40 years. The majority of osteosarcomas appear between the ages of 10 and 30 years. Like multiple myelomas, they can occur in aged patients, in which case they are often associated with Paget's disease. The *sex* of the patient may have a slight bearing on the diagnosis. The giant cell

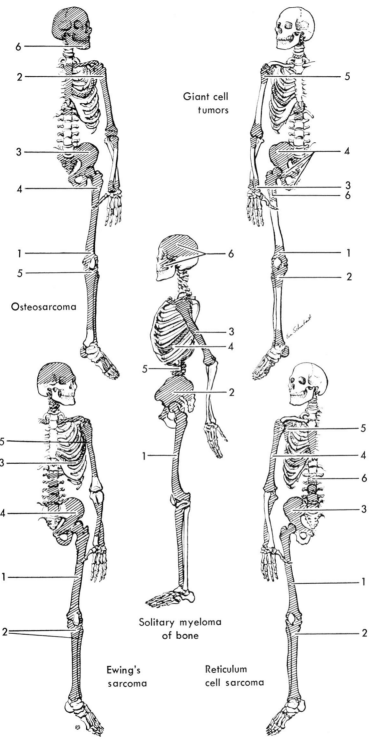

Fig. 684. Most frequent site of origin of five most common bone tumors (figure for osteosarcoma includes chondrosarcomas), with six most frequent sites of origin indicated. (Based on data from Coley and others.)

tumor is more often found in female than in male patients. Ewing's sarcoma, osteosarcoma, and multiple myeloma predominate in male patients. A knowledge of the usual *distribution* of bone tumors in the skeletal system is of relative value (Fig. 684). The *location* of a tumor in a long bone is also of differential value in that giant cell tumors of the long bones occur in the epiphysis, Ewing's sarcoma in the shaft, osteosarcomas in the metaphysis, and multiple myelomas in the shaft.

The *giant cell tumor* may present areas of tenderness at local examination but usually no increased temperature of the skin and no dilated veins. It may have a bulky, spherical shape, and eggshell crackling may be present on palpation. In the very vascular type, a bruit may be heard. A *Ewing's sarcoma* of the long bones often forms a fusiform mass over the involved shaft. The temperature of the overlying skin is increased, and small superficial blood vessels are often prominent. The skin moves freely over the surface of the tumor, but on pressure exquisite pain is elicited. Evidence of fracture is infrequent. In the rapidly growing *osteosarcoma*, the tumor mass often is relatively small, the temperature of the overlying skin (bluish red) is elevated, and pain may be very marked with movement. Any factor that produces tension on the periosteum results in increased pain. With the osteolytic variety, vascularization is rich, and pulsation of the tumor mass can often be felt. Dilated superficial veins may be present. The larger tumors stretch the skin taut but do not ulcerate it. A *reticulum cell sarcoma* is suggested when the tumor is of slow growth and the patient is young and in relatively good condition in spite of advanced local disease. Usually, however, the diagnosis is not made until biopsy is done.

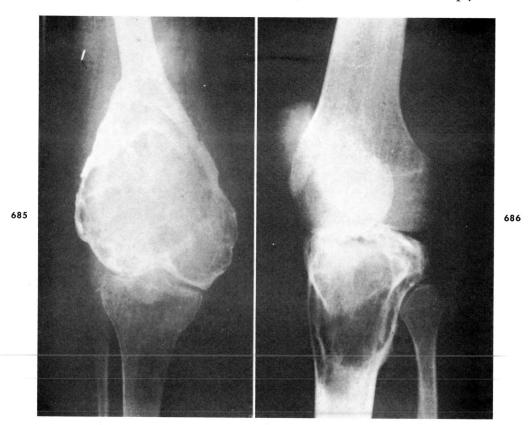

685

686

Fig. 685. Giant cell tumor of lower end of femur showing characteristic loculated appearance and no evidence of periosteal reaction.

Fig. 686. Giant cell tumor in epiphyseal region of upper end of tibia with sharply delineated osteolytic appearance and without periosteal reaction.

Roentgenologic examination

The radiologic examination of bone lesions offers valuable data. In some instances, the findings may be sufficient to make a diagnosis of probability. In general, however, too much emphasis has been put on the possibilities of this examination (Brailsford[15]). It must be taken into consideration that bone lesions have to destroy a good portion of the bone before their presence is roentgenologically appreciable (Ardran[5]), that it is impossible to make a diagnosis of multiple myeloma, for instance, in the absence of any roentgenologic evidence of bone destruction (Heiser and Schwartzman[75]), and that very often the changes found associated with the same variety of tumor are not constant nor characteristic (McSwain et al.[142]).

Roentgenographic examination of *giant cell tumors* reveals a well-delineated cystic lesion with abrupt transition from normal bone. The area of rarefaction is usually eccentrically situated at the end of a long bone, but exceptions to this rule are frequent (Gee and Pugh[62]). As the tumor grows in the long bones, the involved area becomes club-shaped. There is usually no periosteal thickening (Fig. 685). A fine irregular network of trabeculation may traverse the tumor, but only osteolysis is apparent in some instances (Fig. 686). Baclesse[6] emphasizes that in the growth of the tumor there is a peripheral advance of osteolysis followed by a period of recalcification. These phenomena may take place three or four times in eight to twelve years, producing an effect described as "accordion-like." The osteolytic phase may give an erroneous impression of malignant change. Changes in the bony architecture following curettage and roentgentherapy may be confusing, so that a knowledge of these changes is of value in describing follow-up roentgenograms. If fracture occurs in a weight-bearing bone, the fragments are telescoped.

In *Ewing's sarcoma*, the earliest alterations are seen in the marrow cavity, with differences in density due to breakdown of architectural framework. Slight roughening of the periosteum may be observed,

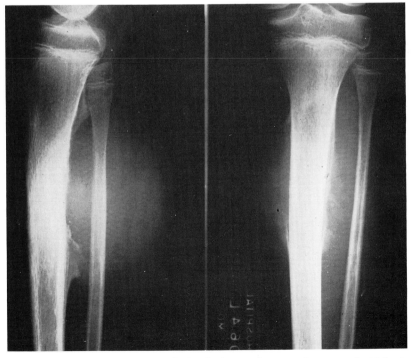

Fig. 687. Ewing's sarcoma arising in shaft of tibia without involvement of epiphysis. Note increased density in medullary portion of bone with subperiosteal new bone formation and soft tissue mass.

and this may lead to the erroneous diagnosis of osteomyelitis. As the process continues, the tumor extends parallel to the long axis of the bone and involves more and more of the shaft (Fig. 687). Because these changes are so evenly distributed, the pathologic findings often show more involvement than the roentgenologic examination reveals. There may also be an accentuation of changes in the cortical bone and periosteum without much change in the shaft. These changes are due to permeation of tumor cells through the haversian canals (Swenson[209]). An apparently normal marrow shadow does not rule out the possibility of a central origin. When the tumor has become extensive, endosteal defects occur, and marrow abnormalities become apparent. Some evidence of the central origin of a Ewing's sarcoma is found when the metaphysis of a long bone is affected and the involvement of the cancellous bone in the subepiphyseal zone occurs simultaneously with involvement of the thin cortex and subperiosteal space in this region. In twenty-six patients with Ewing's sarcoma reported on by Swenson,[209] bone destruction was revealed in twenty-four, increased density within the bone in five, increased width in eight, subperiosteal new bone in eleven, a layering effect in four, and a prominent soft tissue mass in seven. Varying amounts of periosteal thickening may be present and sometimes accompanied by a laminar deposit and subperiosteal new bone of so-called onionskin appearance. This onionskin feature, often considered as diagnostic, is inconstant. As the tumor grows, the medullary cavity reveals extreme osteoporosis, and the cortex shows prominent evidence of bone destruction. The periosteum becomes separated, and new bone is laid down at right angles to the shaft. At times, a Ewing's sarcoma may simulate a soft tissue sarcoma because of apparent absence of bone changes (Falk and Alpert[52]). In 111 patients with Ewing's tumor, Sherman and Soong[193] emphasized

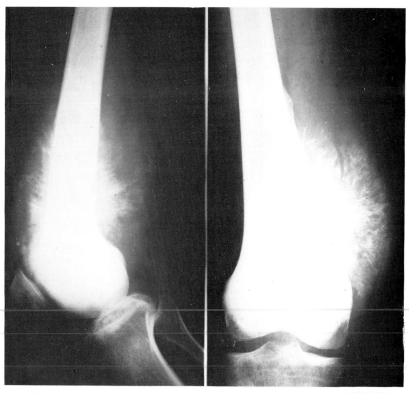

Fig. 688. Sclerosing osteosarcoma arising in lower end of femur in 17-year-old girl. Tumor is fan-shaped with radiating spicules of new bone. Periosteal reaction has extended up along shaft, and already ossified epiphyseal line has been invaded.

that only one of four presented a classic radiographic appearance. This lesion is particularly difficult to diagnose in the flat bones and in the metaphyseal areas.

In *osteosarcoma*, the variable changes are a reflection of the summation of changes rather than an indication of specific tumor type. The sclerosing type of osteosarcoma is much more common than the osteolytic, and the tumor may be either peripheral or central (Fig. 688). A type of sclerosing osteogenic sarcomatosis affecting numerous bones has been described as a radiologic entity (Moseley and Bass[150]). Unilateral forms affecting successive bones of one extremity may be incorrectly described as cases of *melorheostosis*; histologically, they appear as highly differentiated, low-grade osteosarcomas (Smithers and Gowing[199]). The peripheral type is classic,

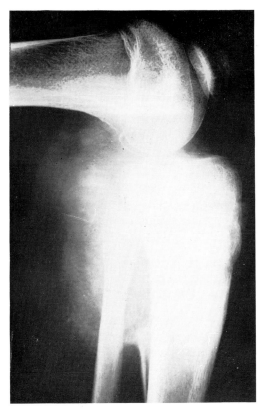

Fig. 689. Osteolytic, rapidly growing osteosarcoma of upper end of tibia in 15-year-old girl. Tumor arose in metaphysis and shows no invasion of still cartilaginous epiphyseal line. There are fragmentation of periosteum and formation of large soft tissue mass. Codman's reactive triangle is clearly defined.

with Codman's reactive triangle (elevation of periosteum), dense obliteration of cortical striae, secondary destruction of the medulla, and mottled areas (Fig. 689). The osteolytic variety shows irregular expansile destruction of the cortex, varied periosteal reaction, early perforation, and a bulky mass (Macdonald and Budd[136]). As the tumor increases beneath the periosteum, needlelike new bone may be observed growing at right angles to the shaft. The radiographic characteristics of advanced *parosteal osteosarcomas* are considered to be diagnostic. These unusual tumors arise and proliferate densely. The main features are the lobular encircling and juxtacortical character of the growth, its failure to destroy the cortex or to cause periosteal elevation, and the heterogeneity of the ossification (Fig. 690). The presence of new bone parallel to the long axis is thought by some to be diagnostic of osteosarcoma. These changes represent fairly advanced disease. New bone can be deposited in any process, neoplastic or inflammatory, which causes elevation of the periosteum (Fig. 703). The epiphysis of the long bones is rarely invaded by osteosarcoma unless the epiphyseal cartilage has become ossified (Figs. 688 and 689). In advanced stages, the osteosarcoma may take on a reputed characteristic sunray appearance, a configuration modeled by the periosteum. After the tumor breaks through the periosteum, the pattern is altered again as the tumor speedily grows in the surrounding structures. There is a variable degree of osteolytic change within the involved bone combined with a variable amount of osteoblastic changes. In the advanced stages, fractures may infrequently be seen in the weight-bearing bones, particularly in the osteolytic varieties. Metastatic osteosarcoma in the lungs is often preceded by roentgenologic evidence of pleural effusion due to pleural involvement. Later, the lungs may be packed with innumerable spherical homogeneous nodules.

Two-thirds of osteosarcomas can be diagnosed roentgenographically without too much difficulty. However, the remaining third may present the appearance considered characteristic of other bone tumors (Lindbom et al.[132]) (Fig. 691). Lagergren et al.[113] demonstrated with combined mi-

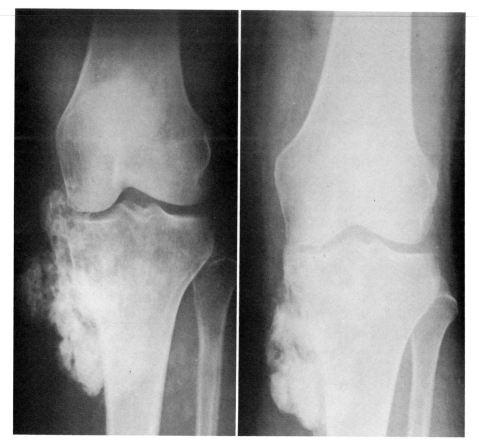

Fig. 690. Typical juxtacortical osteosarcoma. Lesion has usual configuration and forms well-delimited tumor in close apposition to cortical surface. (WU neg. 57-5271.)

croangiography and histologic techniques that all osteosarcomas are more vascular than the surrounding tissues and that angiography can show how far the neoplasm extends into the medullary cavity.

The *chondrosarcomas* can arise de novo or from a preexisting enchondroma (central type) or from a cartilaginous exostosis (peripheral type) (Fig. 692). The central chondrosarcomas arise from the femur and humerus or in the region of the metaphysis and show blotchy or scattered small areas of calcification (Pendergrass et al.[170]). In the long bones, they produce an expansile swelling of the shaft that results first in thickening of the cortex. The tumor may become very large, and often there are cystic spaces within it. Blotchy areas are particularly characteristic (Fig. 693, *B*). An enchondroma of a long bone demonstrates a granular or flocculent de-

posit in the medulla, in or adjacent to the metaphysis, surrounded by normal cancellous bone (Lawrence and Franklin[116]). In peripheral chondrosarcomas, there are often other lesions indicative of chondrodysplasia. In general, benign or malignant cartilaginous tumors can be easily recognized radiographically. In some instances, the differentiation between these may be easier radiographically than histopathologically (Middlemiss[145]).

Fibrosarcoma roentgenologically presents as an osteolytic lesion, well delimited, totally enclosed by reactive subperiosteal bone (Fig. 694), and confined within the bone. It is often taken for a cyst or a giant cell tumor (Eyre-Brook and Price[51]).

A *myeloma* usually presents many areas of punched-out bone destruction with little periosteal reaction and thinning of the cortex of bone (Fig. 695). The lesions are

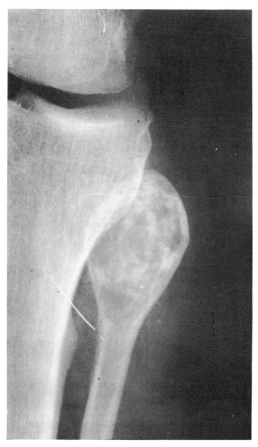

Fig. 691. Cystic lesion of fibula thought radiographically to be giant cell tumor but proved to be osteosarcoma on biopsy. (Courtesy Dr. Ake Lindbom, Stockholm, Sweden.)

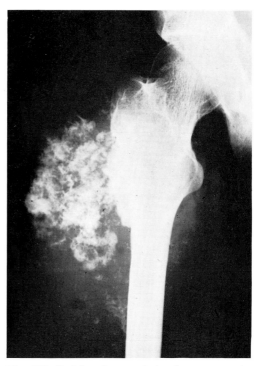

Fig. 692. Peripheral type of chondrosarcoma arising from cartilaginous cap of preexisting cartilaginous exostosis in 21-year-old girl.

most prominent in the pelvis, skull, ribs, vertebrae, sternum, and clavicle. If multiple myeloma is suspected, roentgenograms of all these regions should be taken. In certain rare instances, involvement of these bones may be diffuse, suggesting osteoporosis. Rib fractures are commonly seen. The solitary myeloma may be perplexing because, at times, it presents a cystic trabeculated appearance resembling a giant cell tumor (Gootnick[68]). It can also show bone formation (Lewin and Stein[119]). The humerus, mandible, femur, bones of the pelvis, and cervical and thoracic vertebrae are frequent sites of so-called single myeloma (Raven and Willis[177]). Most, if not all, of the so-called solitary myelomas eventually become widely disseminated. The time interval between the first clinical manifestation and dissemination may be

from five to ten years. Moseley[149] stresses the frequency of involvement of the outer end of the acromion even when the remaining portions of the clavicle and scapula are uninvolved. Bone sclerosis is very rarely encountered, mostly in the form of thickening on the borders of an osteolytic lesion (Evison and Evans[49]).

The roentgenographic appearance of primary *reticulum cell sarcoma* of bone is variable (Sherman and Snyder[192]). Usually an osteolytic process is observed in the metaphysis of long bones, extending to the diaphysis. In early cases, only mottled areas of medullary destruction may be observed. Later, widening of the shaft and fragmentation of the cortex may be observed. Patchy new bone formation may be present in early lesions, giving the tumor a mottled appearance (Medill[144]). Periosteal thickening is seen both early and late in the disease. Invasion of the surrounding soft structures is not unusual (Jackson and Parker[89]).

Arteriography has proved valuable in the diagnosis of bone tumors. At times, it can resolve the difference between benign

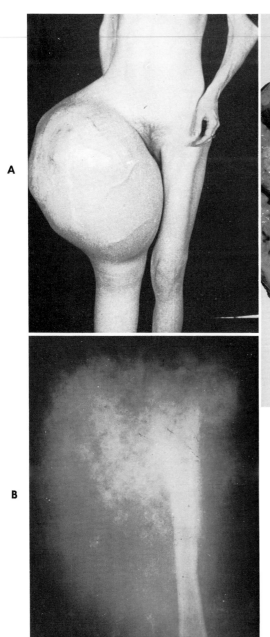

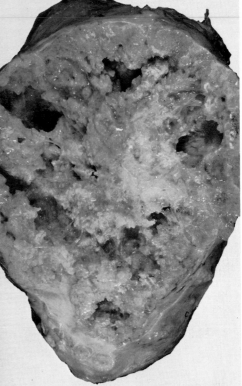

Fig. 693. **A,** Huge chondrosarcoma of head of femur in young woman. Patient remains well over fifteen years after hemipelvectomy. **B,** Note blotchy appearance of lesion. **C,** Surgical specimen revealing cartilaginous framework with numerous cystic spaces. (**A** and **B,** From Sugarbaker, E. D., and Ackerman, L. V.: Disarticulation of the innominate bone for malignant tumors of the pelvic parietes and upper thigh, Surg. Gynec. Obstet. 81:36-52, 1945; by permission of Surgery, Gynecology & Obstetrics.)

and malignant neoplasms, although one must remember that a normal arteriogram does not exclude the possibility of a malignant lesion (Strickland[206]). It is also helpful in determining the extent of the lesion (Fig. 696).

Scintiscanning. Scintiscanning with strontium[85] may be helpful in the diagnosis of bone lesions. The radioactive strontium concentrates in areas of elevated bone production: Paget's disease, fractures, osteomyelitis, and bone metastases. It is helpful in delineating the extent of bone involvement (Fig. 697). It is unquestionably capable of detecting metastases before they are seen by conventional radiographic techniques (Sklaroff and Charkes[196]). It is an excellent ancillary diagnostic procedure (DeNardo and Volpe[40]).

Laboratory examinations

In *myeloma*, there are often abnormal proteins in the plasma and/or urine that may be identified by paper electrophoresis

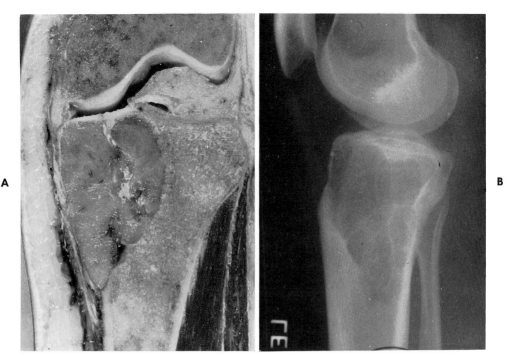

Fig. 694. A, Hemisection of fibrosarcoma of proximal end of left tibia in 27-year-old woman. There was previous history of trauma with subsequent swelling of knee. Lesion demonstrates characteristic discrete delineation of tumor with scalloped margins. Cortex had been destroyed. Lesion still appears confined by periosteum. B, Scalloped margins and destruction of cortical and cancellous bone are evident. Lesion has multicystic appearance upon roentgenographic examination. (A, WU neg. 57-789; B, WU neg. 57-893.)

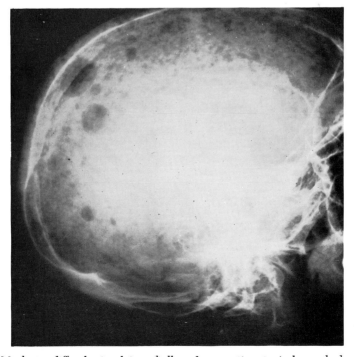

Fig. 695. Myeloma diffusely involving skull and presenting typical punched-out areas of osteolytic destruction.

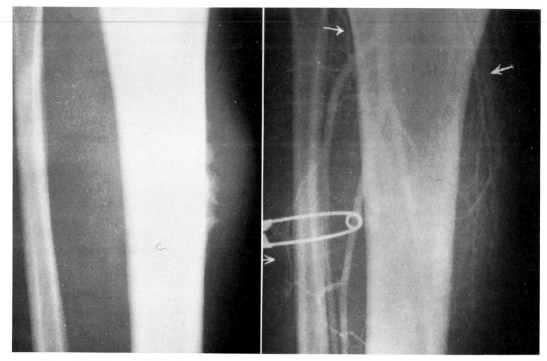

Fig. 696. Lesion in boy about 15 years of age, seen following injury and thought to be reactive. Arteriogram shows many arteriovenous shunts with irregular networks of vessels. There are also superficial arteriovenous communications present in soft tissues lateral to fibula. Lesion was therefore called osteosarcoma, which it proved to be on biopsy. (From Margulis, A. R., and Murphy, T. O.: Arteriography in neoplasms of extremities, Amer. J. Roentgen. **80:**330-339, 1958.)

(Osserman and Takatsuki[165]). However, it is possible to have a focal myelomatous lesion without any laboratory manifestations. With advanced involvement of bone, there may be hypercalcemia. If there is bone production, the alkaline phosphatase level may be elevated, but this is a nonspecific finding. *Giant cell tumors* contain the enzyme acid phosphatase (Gomori[67]). In a patient with giant cell tumor, an elevation of the serum acid phosphatase level was found (Lasser and Tetewsky[115]). In *osteosarcoma*, the bone production results in an elevated alkaline phosphatase level, and the return to normal after surgical removal is a relatively favorable sign. In *Ewing's sarcoma*, the leukocyte count may be elevated to 10,000 to 15,000. The sedimentation rate is also constantly elevated and may be the first sign of recurrence.

Histochemical tests may be helpful in diagnosis. Osteosarcoma and some of the associated fibroblasts may produce considerable alkaline phosphatase. However, neither benign nor malignant cartilage tumors produce alkaline phosphatase; the same is true of fibrosarcoma. The giant cells of giant cell tumors are rich in acid phosphatase, but the stroma is inert (Jeffree and Price[99]).

Biopsy

Biopsy of bone lesions is an essential and most important step in the clarification of diagnostic problems presented by these lesions. Biopsy should be done in the overwhelming majority of cases and before definitive therapy is executed. In some instances, as in osteoid osteoma, no further treatment may be indicated. In others, biopsy may reveal the malignant or benign nature of the lesion and indicate the radical or conservative character of the treatment of choice in the particular case. We would advise against biopsy in the obviously cartilaginous tumors in and around

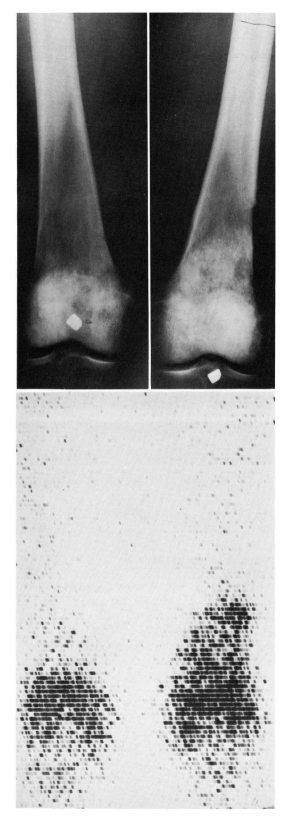

the pelvis. The incision into the tumor may imply contamination of the operative field and, conceivably, increase the magnitude of the operative procedure. But it is proper to remember that implantation of tumor in the soft tissues can result from biopsy (Dahlin and Coventry[35]; Thompson and Steggall[212]). There is no objective evidence that biopsy may increase the possibilities of metastases.

Needle biopsy may be utilized in the soft tissue extensions of bone tumors. Fragments of bone may also be obtained with special drills (Schajowicz and Derqui[189]). Needle biopsy is particularly helpful in lesions of the vertebrae.

Frozen section of the soft tissue extension is possible and, at times, fruitful. This is particularly true in osteosarcomas. If a definite diagnosis is possible, it gives strength and direction to definitive therapy. The differential diagnosis of Ewing's tumor and eosinophilic granuloma absolves the patient from unnecessary radical treatment in the latter case.

Biopsy should not be done by inexperienced surgeons not capable of coping with all of the therapeutic issues that may result. Preferably, also, biopsy should not be done unless the patient and his relatives are ready to follow, without dangerous waste of time, whatever decision is to be taken. Rather than allow delay in the administration of definitive treatment, the patient should be advised to seek biopsy and treatment at an institution of his trust.

Differential diagnosis

Most of the confusion that has existed regarding the giant cell tumor has been due to the fact that there are numerous other lesions that crudely caricature it. It is imperative that the giant cell tumor be identified and isolated from this group, for its pathologic behavior and clinical evolution are distinctive.

The *metaphyseal fibrous defect* (nonosteogenic fibroma) occurs almost invariably

Fig. 697. Bilateral involvement of distal ends of both femurs by reticulum cell sarcoma in 42-year-old man. Radioactive strontium scintigram shows extent of involvement. (WU negs. 68-6576 and 68-6577.)

Table 109. Differential character of four most common malignant bone tumors

	Giant cell tumor	*Ewing's sarcoma*	*Osteosarcoma*	*Multiple myeloma*
Sex	Females predominate	Males predominate	Males predominate	Males predominate
Age (highest incidence)	20 to 35 yr	4 to 20 yr	10 to 30 yr	Usually over 40 yr
Location in bone	Epiphysis and metaphysis	Shaft	Metaphysis	Shaft
Most common sites	Lower end of femur, upper end of tibia, lower end of radius	Femur, tibia, humerus, mandible	Lower end of femur, upper end of tibia, upper end of humerus	Bones of pelvis and femur
Metastases	Infrequent	Lymph nodes, lung, skull, ribs, vertebrae	Lungs; practically never in lymph nodes	Skull, ribs, vertebrae; practically never in lungs
Most important differential diagnoses	Metaphyseal fibrous defect	Osteomyelitis; metastatic neuroblastoma	Other primary malignant bone tumors	Metastatic carcinoma

in children and, for this reason, should seldom be confused with giant cell tumors. It has a distinctive radiologic appearance, and it is the pathologic diagnosis that is often in error due to the ubiquitous giant cell in its microscopic pattern (Fig. 698). *Hemangiomas* occur most frequently in the spine and skull. In flat bones they may show a sunburst appearance, and in the rib and clavicle they can resemble a malignant bone tumor (Sherman and Wilner[195]). We have also seen such changes in the fibula.

Aneurysmal bone cysts have also been recognized as distinctive from giant cell tumors (Lichtenstein[126]). These cystic lesions occur more commonly in the second and third decades of life but have been seen in infants and aged patients (Sherman and Soong[194]). They may occur in any bone. In the long bones, the lesion is usually eccentric and expands into the soft tissues from either end of the shaft. When it occurs in a vertebra, it may be thought to be a giant cell tumor radiographically, and large lesions may be considered malignant (Fig. 699). The pathologist may make a diagnosis of giant cell tumor if he fails to recognize the islands of hemorrhage, the thin trabeculae frequently containing new bone formation, and the arrangement of the giant cells toward the hemorrhagic cavities (Ackerman and Spjut[3]). It must be remembered that the gross and microscopic pattern of aneurysmal bone cyst may complicate the pattern of osteosarcoma, chondrosarcoma,

Table 110. Differential characteristics of bone cysts and giant cell tumors

	Solitary bone cyst	*Giant cell tumor*
Age of greatest frequency	5 to 15 yr (under 20 yr)	20 to 35 yr (over 20 yr)
Sex	M > F	F > M
Site of origin	Metaphyseal	Epiphyseal
Bones of election	Humerus (upper end) Femur (upper end)	Femur (lower end) Tibia (upper end) Radius (lower end)
Clinical course	Fracture (common) with spontaneous healing	Fracture (uncommon) with no spontaneous healing

chondromyxoid fibroma, and giant cell tumor. We have seen one case of chondroblastoma and five of osteosarcoma of the telangiectatic type in which the dominant pattern was that of an aneurysmal bone cyst. Treatment of aneurysmal bone cyst has, for the most part, been surgical, sometimes radical (Phelan[172]). Radiotherapy has been proved to be consistently successful (Nobler et al.[157]).

Another lesion frequently misinterpreted as a giant cell tumor is the *bone cyst*. Bone cysts occur predominantly in patients under 20 years of age and are found more frequently in male than in female patients. About 75% of all bone cysts are found in the humerus and the femur (Garceau and Gregory[59]). They are located in the meta-

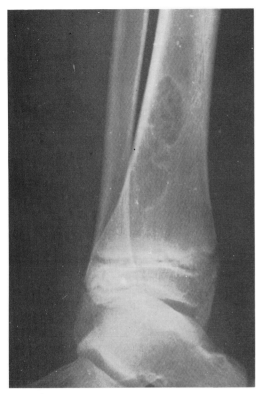

Fig. 698. Typical metaphyseal fibrous defect. Note eccentric location in metaphysis of distal portion of tibia, sharply defined periphery, and orientation in longitudinal axis.

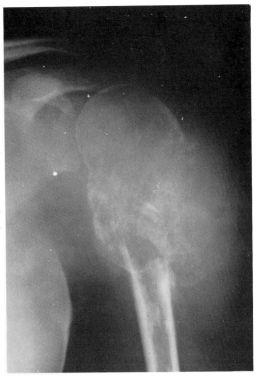

Fig. 699. Aneurysmal bone cyst of proximal end of humerus in 15-year-old girl with extension into soft tissue. Diagnosis was difficult both radiographically and pathologically but was eventually established as aneurysmal bone cyst. (WU neg. 59-7985.)

physeal area, usually close to the epiphyseal plate (Table 110). *Osteitis fibrosa cystica* shows multiple lesions that occasionally may be confused with giant cell tumors, particularly when a roentgenogram is made of a single bone with a cystic lesion. These cystic lesions, like the single bone cysts, do not involve the epiphysis and are associated with striking changes in blood chemistry. They are the result of functioning parathyroid adenomas (Albright et al.[4]). In patients with bone involvement, the alkaline phosphatase level is invariably elevated. Benign *chondroblastomas*, once designated as epiphyseal chondromatous giant cell tumors (Codman[21]), are a rare form of tumor usually found in male patients under 20 years of age. They may be mistaken for giant cell tumors on microscopic examination (Jaffee and Lichtenstein[93]), but small areas of calcification and focal necrosis are always present. This lesion is usually treated by curettement and replacement by bone chips. However, it may locally recur in the soft tissues (Coleman[24]). We have seen three instances of distant metastases. Chondromyxoidfibroma usually occurs in young adults, often in a long bone (Feldman et al.[54]). It can extend into the soft tissues and can recur after inadequate treatment (Benedetti et al.[11]).

Fibrous dysplasia of bone may be diagnosed as a giant cell tumor, mostly because of the presence of giant cells. *Osteoid osteoma* is a distinctive benign bone lesion often confused with chronic bone abscess and other tumors. It occurs in long bones and is accompanied by overgrowth of bone. It is often painful. It is also common in the spine; a painful scoliosis in an adolescent should suggest the possibility of a vertebral osteoid osteoma (MacLellan and Wilson[135]). The diagnosis should be highly suspected in adequate radiographs (Fowles[55]). The lesion is highly vascular and has a bewildering microscopic pattern with new bone formation. This pattern is exactly mimicked by another lesion called *osteoblastoma* (Lichtenstein and Sawyer[131]) or *giant osteoid osteoma* (Dahlin and Johnson[37]). The variations in symptoms and location in other bones such as vertebrae and the lack of pain are responsible for the variations (Byers[16]). This tumor may be misdiagnosed as osteosarcoma.

Osteomyelitis is most often confused with Ewing's sarcoma and reticulum cell sarcoma due to the presence of pain and constitutional reactions. The Garré type of sclerosing osteomyelitis mimics the tumor in some respects, but it is sudden in onset and rapidly becomes chronic, whereas Ewing's sarcoma has a mild onset and usually becomes acute. In acute osteomyelitis, the temperature and the leukocyte count are elevated, and a primary focus of infection is present. In chronic osteomyelitis, an involucrum, never seen in Ewing's sarcoma, is often present. Metastatic *neuroblastoma of the suprarenal gland* may be impossible to differentiate from Ewing's sarcoma (Barden[9]). In some instances, only an autopsy may reveal the presence of a suprarenal primary tumor (Willis[226]). Biopsy of metastatic lesions may not reveal the rosettes of neuroblastoma, but intravenous pyelograms may reveal displacement of the kidney on the affected side. Furthermore, tissue culture may show the formation of neurites. Glycogen stains are positive in Ewing's tumor and are negative in metastatic neuroblastoma (Schajowicz[185]).

Bone tuberculosis may be considered in the differential diagnosis of bone tumors, but usually roentgenograms of the chest reveal evidence of healed pulmonary tuberculosis. Aspiration of any fluid with guinea pig inoculation is also diagnostic. In tuberculosis, the upper portions of the bone show destruction of the epiphysis, involvement of the joint cavity, and calcification of the soft parts. Infection plus tuberculosis is harder to diagnose because the excessive new bone production simulates the sclerosing type of osteosarcoma. The

differential diagnosis between osteolytic osteosarcoma and a single *bone cyst* may be very difficult. Patients are usually under 20 years of age, both lesions may develop in the metaphysis of long bones, and complicating fractures may occur also in both. Osteosarcoma is often asymmetrical and does not expand the cortex, whereas bone cysts are symmetrical and expand the cortex of the bone (Luck[134]). Periosteal reaction or constitutional repercussions are not present in bone cysts. The sclerosing form of *syphilis of bones* may resemble osteosarcoma in the roentgenogram (Figs. 700 and 701), but syphilitic changes are often symmetrical, are not confined to a single bone, and respond to antisyphilitic therapy (Westermark and Hellerstrom[225]).

Myositis ossificans is a poorly defined entity that has frequently been confused with osteosarcoma. This error in diagnosis has usually been made by the pathologist. These lesions may or may not be associated with the periosteum, and there may be no history of trauma. The lesion most frequently occurs in the flexor muscles of the upper arm and the quadriceps femoris as well as the adductor muscles of the thigh (Fig. 702). Early in its evolution, the

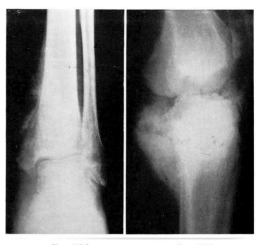

Fig. 700 Fig. 701

Fig. 700. Bone formation at right angles to shaft in syphilis of lower end of tibia. These changes resolved followed antisyphilitic therapy.

Fig. 701. Syphilitic lesion of upper end of tibia with bone destruction and bone production. This tumor was first erroneously considered as osteosarcoma. (Courtesy Dr. Murray Stone, Springfield, Mo.)

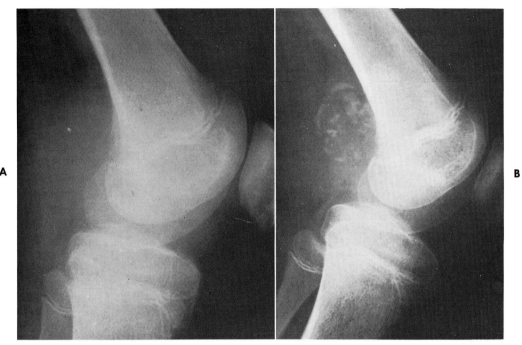

Fig. 702. **A,** Soft tissue mass in region of knee joint in 11-year-old girl. Lesion was biopsied and diagnosed as possible osteosarcoma. **B,** Fourteen days later, showing obvious bone formation within soft tissue mass. There was peripheral maturation, and lesion was then diagnosed as myositis ossificans. (AFIP acc. no. 918115; **A,** WU neg. 59-4048; **B,** WU neg. 59-4047.)

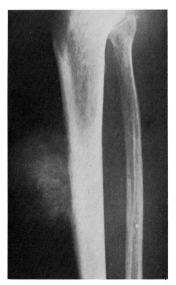

Fig. 703. Bone-producing lesion in tibia suggesting osteosarcoma but actually due to metastatic adenocarcinoma. Primary lesion was located in sigmoid.

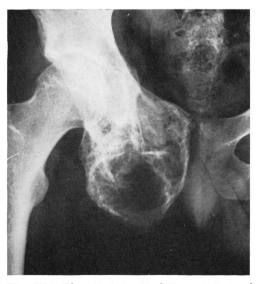

Fig. 704. Characteristic osteolytic metastasis of innominate bone. Primary tumor was adenocarcinoma of kidney.

central portion of this process is impossible to differentiate from sarcoma. With the passage of time, there is progressive maturation toward the periphery. Therefore, biopsy taken from the periphery in a well-established lesion will show well-oriented bone. This finding is in contrast to parosteal sarcoma in which there is no orientation. This confusion with parosteal sarcoma has led to the impression in the past that myositis ossificans may become malignant. We have not seen such a transition. *Metastatic carcinoma* developing in long bones, particularly when slow in growth and hence osteoblastic, may closely mimic an osteogenic tumor (Figs. 703 and 704). It must be remembered that metastatic carcinoma is the most common malignant tumor involving bone.

The *enchondroma* must be differentiated from the chondrosarcoma, but it is a benign cartilaginous growth appearing mainly in the phalanges of the metacarpal bones, femur, and humerus. In the small bones, it produces an area of rarefaction with thinning and bulging of the cortex. In the long bones, it appears in the region of the metaphysis and probably arises from islands of cartilage cells derived from the epiphyseal cartilage. In twenty-eight cases reported by Jaffe and Lichtenstein,[96] thirteen occurred in a finger phalanx, five in the metacarpal bone, five in the humerus, three in the femur, one in a toe phalanx, and one in a metatarsal bone. The enchondromas arising in teminal phalanges practically never become chondrosarcomas. By contrast, enchondroma located in long bones should always be suspected of being chondrosarcoma until proved otherwise. *Epiphyseal chondroblastomas* are most often confused with giant cell tumors and are invariably benign (Valls et al.[220]; Lichtenstein and Kaplan[130]).

Eosinophilic granuloma, Hand-Schüller-Christian disease, and *Letterer-Siwe disease* are clinical entities originating in the reticuloendothelial system (Hansen[70]; Lichtenstein[124]). Eosinophilic granuloma is usually first identified in roentgenograms and may mimic other benign and malignant bone lesions (Ochsner[160]). More than half of the cases are seen in children under 10 years of age (Lieberman et al.[131a]). It usually produces local pain and disa-

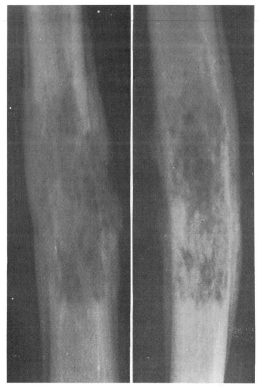

Fig. 705. Eosinophilic granuloma of right humerus with extensive cortical destruction and periosteal reaction simulating Ewing's sarcoma or osteosarcoma in 9-year-old boy. Lesion was biopsied and irradiated. (From McGavran, M. H., and Spady, H. A.: Eosinophilic granuloma of bone, J. Bone Joint Surg. **42-A:**979-992, 1960; WU neg. 51-5164.)

bility. It is frequently found in the bones of the skull and spine but may occur in the long bones (Fig. 705). Letterer-Siwe disease is an expression of the disseminated form of the process occurring in infants (Wallace[222]). Because of their localized character and, at times, prominent periosteal proliferation, the single lesions in the long bones of a child are often mistaken for Ewing's tumor or osteosarcoma (Jaffe[92]; Hansen[70]; McGavran and Spady[137]). The disseminated form of reticuloendotheliosis may be mistaken for myeloma radiographically. Clinically, the differentiation, because of age and other factors, should not be difficult. In young adults, single destructive osteolytic lesions of eosinophilic granuloma, particularly in the skull, have been diagnosed radiographically as metastatic carcinoma. Biopsy is definitive.

Clinically, multiple myeloma can be confused with *Paget's disease* because of the thoracic deformities. However, in patients with Paget's disease the alkaline phosphatase level is elevated, and in those with multiple myeloma it is normal. Paget's disease is characterized by other phenomena such as bowing of the legs and increased size of the skull. In attempting to differentiate *metastatic carcinoma* from myeloma of the vertebrae, Jacobson et al.[90] found that the pedicle of the vertebrae is involved more frequently in metastatic carcinoma than in myeloma.

Treatment

Surgery

Surgical resection of *giant cell tumors* may be done when the resection does not imply impairment of function (involvement of ulna, ribs, metatarsal bones, patella, and fibula). Complete surgical excision is preferred by many surgeons (Mnaymneh et al.[147]). Of forty-seven patients reported by Dahlin et al.[36] treated by less than excision or amputation, tumor recurred in twenty (43%). Also, a radical surgical resection of giant cell tumors may be indicated when biopsy shows evidence of malignancy or when radiotherapy has previously failed. If resection implies impairment of function, curettage with replacement by bone chips is recommended. Curettage alone is often followed by recrudescence, and this occurred in 85% of the patients treated by this method in the large series reported by Goldenberg et al.[65a] They also cited several instances of cure following resection of pulmonary metastases. Cases of "malignant transformation" following surgical treatment have been not infrequently noted (Verbiest[221]). Joynt and Ortved[106] reported the accidental operative transplantation of a giant cell tumor of the tibia to the soft tissues.

The overall cure rate of *Ewing's sarcoma* used to be dismal. At the present time, there is uniform agreement that radiation therapy, often supported by chemotherapy, gives by far the best results, and there is no indication for surgery (Boyer et al.[13]).

The only successful treatment of *osteo-*

sarcomas and *chondrosarcomas* is adequate surgical resection (Henderson and Dahlin[77]; McKenna et al.[140]). An amputation above the proximal joint of the affected bone is accepted generally as the procedure of choice. This treatment applies in all instances except when the tumor is located in the distal end of the femur. In this instance, an amputation at the level of the femoral neck is usually done. The formidable operative procedure of hemipelvectomy (hind quarter amputation) is not indicated for malignant bone tumors such as plasma cell myeloma, Ewing's tumor, or undifferentiated osteosarcoma. It finds its best indication in chondrosarcoma, and most of the reported cures are in this category (Sugarbaker and Ackerman[207]; Coley et al.[29]). The results are best in patients with bulky chondrosarcomas arising in the upper end of the femur, not suitable for disarticulation (Lewis and Bickel[120]). With careful selection of patients, particularly from the standpoint of operative risk and type of tumor, there is now little or no operative mortality (Taylor and Rogers[210]), and satisfactory prosthesis allows walking without a cane (Higinbotham and Coley[79]). Interscapulothoracic amputations may also be justified for tumors occurring in the shoulder girdle (Pack et al.[167]; Levinthal and Grossman[118]).

The treatment of *parosteal osteosarcoma* is often difficult. Local resection is possible and successful when the diagnosis is established early in the evolution of the case, but this tumor tends to surround the bone, rendering local resection difficult or impossible (Scaglietti and Calandriello[183]). Local resections will undoubtedly be extended as substitute prostheses are improved (Kraft and Levinthal[110]). Local resection of *adamantinoma* of the tibia is not frequently curative. Local resections of *chondrosarcomas* are possible at times, particularly when the tumor is situated peripherally. When the radiographic diagnosis is that of a cartilaginous tumor, resection should be done without resorting to biopsy, for the danger of soft tissue implantation is real (Fig. 706). Cartilaginous tumors of the ribs should also be resected without previous biopsy.

Medullary fibrosarcomas are best treated

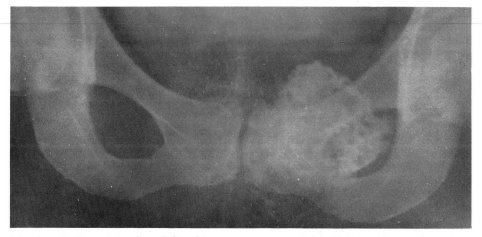

Fig. 706. Lesion arising from left pubic ramus near symphysis. Patient, 31-year-old woman, had had progresssive urinary frequency for eight weeks. Pelvic examination disclosed hard mass. Roentgenograms were interpreted as chondrosarcoma. Without biopsy, bloc excision was done. (WU neg. 54-3577.)

by appropriate amputation (Cunningham and Arlen[34]). Local excision is justified in *periosteal fibrosarcomas*. But the number of malignant tumors that may be treated by local resection is unfortunately small. On the other hand, such a decision should not be taken because of age or emotional reasons but on the basis of sound histopathologic judgment (Coley and Higinbotham[26]).

Liposarcomas and *angiosarcomas* of the bone should be treated by radical surgery.

Radiotherapy

Radiotherapy of *giant cell tumors* should always be given preference in the treatment whenever the surgical excision would imply impairment or dysfunction (Berman[12]). That radiotherapy is the treatment of choice of these tumors is well substantiated by serious work that has been sporadically published (Baclesse[6]; Jansson[98]; Windeyer and Woodyall[227]; Ellis[47]; Bradshaw[14]). The histopathologic identity of many of these cases is disputed (Lichtenstein[121]), but authenticated cases have been definitely and permanently sterilized by roentgentherapy (Gershon-Cohen[63]). The response of giant cell tumors to irradiation is usually slow, and the daily and total doses administered need not be very large. If radiotherapy fails, surgical treatment is always possible. Total doses need to be relatively large to assure frequent control, although good results have been obtained with small doses (Papillon et al.[168]; Friedman and Pearlman[57]).

Radiotherapy is the treatment of choice for *Ewing's sarcoma*, for it is an extremely radiosensitive tumor capable of being cured locally. Cobalt[60] and supervoltage roentgentherapy have made it possible to irradiate large areas of adjacent soft tissue, as well as the entire long bones, to a sufficiently high dosage of radiations, thus improving results and discouraging unwarranted surgery (Boyer et al.[13]). Local radiotherapy has been combined with total body irradiation (Millburn et al.[146]). Combinations of radiotherapy and chemotherapy are presently advocated (Hustu et al.[83]; Johnson and Humphreys[104]). Subjective improvement follows the first treatments, and, in addition, roentgentherapy may avoid compression of the spine and the development of paraplegia when the tumor develops in vertebrae. The tumor regresses rapidly and becomes densely calcified. Failure of treatment is most often due to the appearance of other bone lesions or pulmonary metastases. Radiotherapy is the treatment of choice of *reticulum cell sarcoma* (Fig. 708). Ivins and Dahlin[88] found no basis to recommend surgery. Irradiation is followed by scar formation (Sherman and Snyder[192]).

Myelomas are radiosensitive and locally radiocurable. Conservative treatment of

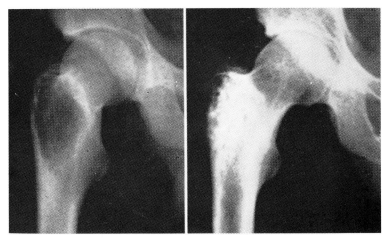

Fig. 707. Giant cell tumor before and ten years after radiotherapy. (From Leucutia, T., et al.: Late results in benign giant-cell tumor of bone obtained by radiation therapy, Radiology 37:1-17, 1941.)

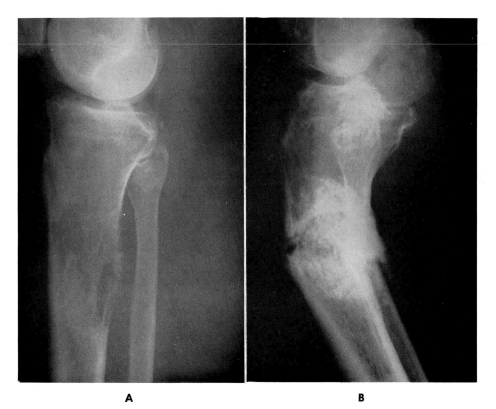

A   B

Fig. 708. A, Reticulum cell sarcoma of tibia of 70-year-old man. Patient had suffered pain for two weeks prior to hospital admission. Pathologic fracture is evident. B, Five years after roentgentherapy. Patient now has useful limb. (A, WU neg. 57-6921; B, WU neg. 57-6922.)

multiple new lesions increases life expectancy. In the single-focus myeloma, radiotherapy may control the disease for long time periods. In order to attain total local sterilization, treatment should be continued even after the clinical disappearance of the tumor, for most failures may be laid to an insufficient total dose.

Osteosarcomas have long been considered to be radioresistant, but the frequent failure of surgical treatment has motivated trials of radiotherapy which have revealed unquestionable radiosensitivity. These effects have been utilized by some authors to delay radical surgery and thus avoid unnecessary mutilation when metastases reveal themselves in the interim (Cade[17]). Massive preoperative irradiation has also given some promise (Lee and Mackenzie[117]). Six survivals of over five years, in histologically verified cases treated by roentgentherapy, have been put on record (Baclesse[6]). Supervoltage roentgentherapy has given encouraging long remissions (Cade[17]). This has given basis to its advocates as a curative procedure (Tudway[213]).

Chemotherapy

L-phenylalanine mustard (sarcolysin, melphalan) has resulted in long-standing regressions of *myeloma* (Hoogstraten et al.[81]). Striking regressions have also been obtained with cyclophosphamides (Skoog and Adams[197]). Skeletal fluorosis has been induced in patients with myeloma for palliation (Cohen[22]). Cyclophosphamides and vincristine have been used as adjuvants to radiotherapy in the treatment of Ewing's sarcoma (Johnson et al.[105]; Jenkin[100]; Hustu et al.[83]).

Prognosis

Prognosis of *giant cell tumor* is usually good. However, curettage does not appear to be an ideal treatment. Further, if the patients are followed long enough, the recurrence rate is high. In Johnson and Dahlin's series,[102] it reached over 50%. It is also not realized that about one in ten of these tumors is malignant or may become malignant and cause death. These lesions can be cured by well-planned irradiation (Windeyer and Woodyatt[227]; Ellis[47]; Berman[12]) or surgery (Johnson and Dahlin[102]).

In the past, the curability of *Ewing's sarcoma* has been disappointing. In recent years, the use of supervoltage roentgentherapy and its combination with chemotherapy have yielded encouraging results. Phillips and Higinbotham[173] treated thirty-nine patients, thirteen of whom survived five or more years. Eleven of twenty-four patients with Ewing's sarcoma of the long bones did well as compared with only two of fifteen others with tumors of the bones of the trunk. Pulmonary metastases may be successfully irradiated (Heald et al.[74]; Phillips and Higinbotham[173]).

The prognosis of *reticulum cell sarcomas* is, on the contrary, relatively good. Coley et al.[28] reported ten five-year survivals (48%) in a series of twenty patients treated. In a group of thirty-nine patients with reticulum cell sarcoma reported by Ivins and Dahlin,[87] ten of twenty-nine followed for five years or more survived. Most had been treated by radiotherapy. Jackson and Parker[89] reported six patients with reticulum cell sarcoma of bone treated by amputation followed by postoperative irradiation. One died at the end of two years, and five were living between six and sixteen years. Sarrazin et al.[182] reported fifty-five cases of reticulosarcoma treated by radiotherapy at the Institut Gustave-Roussy with a five-year survival rate of 18%.

The prognosis of *osteosarcoma* is related to many factors, and only when the majority of these are known can a prediction of the end results be made. The case with a long clinical history and a well-localized large tumor has a much better prognosis than the case with a very short history and a rapidly growing tumor. The osteolytic osteosarcoma grows so fast and metastasizes so early that it has no time to attain any considerable size. Patients under 20 or over 50 years of age do much more poorly than those between the ages of 20 and 40 years. McKenna et al.[138] found that the prognosis in 130 children under 16 years of age was similar to that of adults (18.5% survival at five years). Those over 50 years have a poor prognosis probably because of the relatively high incidence of associated Paget's disease. In fact, if osteosarcoma is superimposed upon Paget's disease, then the prognosis is poor—less than 2% five-year survival (McKenna et al.[139]). Coley and Sharp[30] reported fifty-nine patients with bone sarcoma who presented no evidence of recurrence or metastases for five or more years. Most of these patients were treated by radical surgical procedures, but a few received conservative forms of surgery.

The type of operation may influence the prognosis. Conservative surgery performed for a rapidly growing tumor offers practically no hope of cure. If the tumor is not resected above the involved joint, then tumor may be left to grow within the remaining segment of bone marrow (Fig. 709). The location of the tumor is also impor-

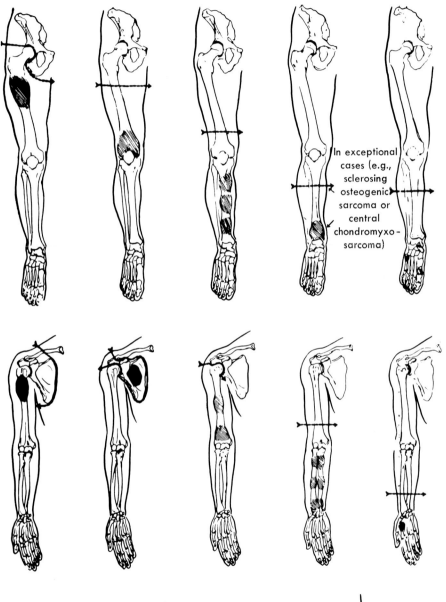

In exceptional cases (e.g., sclerosing osteogenic sarcoma or central chondromyxo-sarcoma)

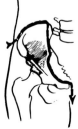

Fig. 709. Indications for amputation or disarticulation according to place and nature of osteosarcoma. (From Coley, B. L., and Higinbotham, N. L.: Tumors of bone. In Advances in surgery, vol. 1, New York/London, 1949, Interscience Publishers, Inc.)

tant, for if it develops in an area in which it cannot be surgically removed (skull, vertebra, and some pelvic bones), the condition is hopeless. Generally speaking, the nearer the tumor is to the trunk, the worse the prognosis. Osteosarcomas of the scapula, clavicle, and middle and upper thirds of the femur have a poor prognosis. Conversely, patients with osteosarcomas arising from the small bones of the feet or forearm have a better than 50% five-year survival after surgical treatment.

The pathology of a bone tumor is significant in regard to prognosis. The well-differentiated osteosarcomas, particularly those made up predominantly of adult fibrous tissue and cartilage, do better than the undifferentiated rapidly growing osteolytic type of tumor. Price[176] has correlated the degree of mitotic activity with survival.

Dahlin and Coventry[35] reviewed a series of 600 cases of *osteosarcoma* (exclusive of tumors of the jaw and parosteal osteosarcomas): of 408 patients, eighty-three (20.3%) survived more than five years. Usually, patients with Paget's disease have a hopeless prognosis, but three of twenty patients with Paget's disease and osteosarcoma in Dahlin and Coventry's series[35] were long-term survivors. Of the sixteen patients who had osteosarcoma arising in previously irradiated bones, none survived more than three years. The prognosis is not apparently affected by site of origin except perhaps in the mandible, where an earlier diagnosis may favor it (Garrington et al.[61]). The prognosis in men with lesions adjacent to an open epiphysis seems to be worse than in women (Nosanchuk et al.[158]). Patients with predominantly chondroblastic or fibroblastic sarcomas did better than those with osteoblastic sarcomas. The five-year survival rate of ninety-six patients with osteosarcoma treated at the Radiumhemmet was 18.5% (Lindbom et al.[132]).

Chondrosarcomas have a much better prognosis than osteosarcomas, particularly when they arise from osteochondromas (O'Neal and Ackerman[162]). The prognosis of chondrosarcoma is directly related to the primary therapy. If adequate surgery is done, a ten-year survival of 69% can be anticipated (Henderson and Dahlin[77]); inadequate surgery resulted in a ten-year survival of only 19%.

The five-year survival rate of *fibrosarcomas* is about 25% (McLeod et al.[141]). The well-differentiated tumors have the best prognosis (Cunningham and Arlen[34]). In Gilmer and McEwen's[64] series, no patient with undifferentiated fibrosarcoma survived. The well-differentiated *periosteal fibrosarcoma* has a good prognosis (Lichtenstein[127]). The parosteal *(juxtacortical) sarcoma* has the best prognosis of all. Approximately 80% of patients with juxtacortical osteosarcoma survive five years (Van der Heul and Von Ronnen[219]).

Plasma cell myeloma has an extremely poor prognosis. Of sixty patients with multiple bone involvement, thirty-one (52%) died within three months of the diagnosis, and only three lived more than two years. Patients with single-focus myelomas live longer, but eventually almost all die of disseminated disease (Carson et al.[19]).

Osgood[163] calculated the survival time from the onset of symptoms of 600 cases of plasmocytic myeloma gathered from the literature (Fig. 710). For instance, he compared the results of treatment with urethan,

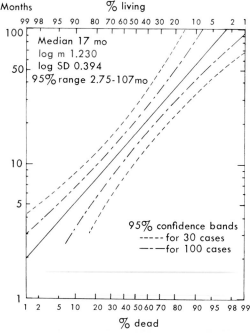

Fig. 710. Plasmocytic myeloma. Survival time from onset of symptoms based on 600 cases from literature. (From Osgood, E. E.: The survival time of patients with plasmocytic myeloma, Cancer Chemother. Rep. 9:1-10, 1960.)

11-oxycorticoids, and P^{32} and found they did not differ significantly from the median, suggesting but not proving that none of the therapeutic methods now in use is different from any other in survival time. We know, however, that therapy may relieve pain, lead to recalcification of osteolytic lesions, and increase the number of months of useful life. Osteosarcomas of the jaw seem to have a favorable prognosis (Kragh et al.[111]).

REFERENCES

1 Ackerman, A. J.: Multiple osteogenic sarcoma; report of two cases, Amer. J. Roentgen. **60**:623-632, 1948.

2 Ackerman, L. V.: Extra-osseous localized non-neoplastic bone and cartilage formation (so-called myositis ossificans); clinical and pathological confusion with malignant neoplasms, J. Bone Joint Surg. **40-A**:279-298, 1958.

3 Ackerman, L. V., and Spjut, H. J.: Tumors of bone and cartilage. In Atlas of tumor pathology, Sect. II, Fasc. 4, Washington, D. C., 1962, Armed Forces Institute of Pathology.

4 Albright, F., Aub, J. C., and Bauer, W.: Hyperparathyroidism; common and polymorphic condition as illustrated by seventeen proved cases from one clinic, J.A.M.A. **102**:1276-1287, 1934.

5 Ardran, G. M.: Bone destruction not demonstrable by radiography, Brit. J. Radiol. **24**:107-109, 1951.

6 Baclesse, F.: Quelques remarques sur les tumeurs à myéloplaxes et leur traitement radiothérapique considéré à longue échéance, J. Radiol. Electr. **26**:41-46, 1944-45.

7 Baird, R. J., and Krause, V. W.: Ewing's tumour; a review of 33 cases, Canad. J. Surg. **6**:136-140, 1963.

8 Baker, P. L., Dockerty, M. B., and Coventry, M. B.: Adamantinoma (so-called) of the long bones; review of the literature and a report of three new cases, J. Bone Joint Surg. **36-A**:704-720, 1954.

9 Barden, R. P.: The similarity of clinical and roentgen findings in children with Ewing's sarcoma (endothelial myeloma) and sympathetic neuroblastoma, Amer. J. Roentgen. **50**:575-581, 1943.

10 Barnes, R., and Catto, M.: Chondrosarcoma of bone, J. Bone Joint Surg. **48-B**:729-764, 1966.

11 Benedetti, G. B., Canepa, G., and Garcia, M.: Il fibroma condromixoide dell'osso. Revisione critica delle letterature de indagini istologiche ed istochimiche su 8 casi, Arch. Putti **17**:44-72, 1962.

12 Berman, H. L.: The treatment of benign giant-cell tumors of the vertebrae by irradiation, Radiology **83**:202-207, 1964.

13 Boyer, C. W., Jr., Bricker, T. J., Jr., and Perry, R. H.: Ewing's sarcoma; case against surgery, Cancer **20**:1602-1606, 1967.

14 Bradshaw, J. D.: The value of x-ray therapy in the management of osteoclastoma, Clin. Radiol. **15**:70-74, 1964.

15 Brailsford, J. F.: The serious limitations and erroneous indications of biopsy in the diagnosis of tumours of bone, Proc. Roy. Soc. Med. **41**:225-236, 1948.

16 Byers, P. D.: Solitary benign osteoblastic lesions of bone—osteoid osteoma and benign osteoblastoma, Cancer **22**:43-57, 1968.

17 Cade, S.: Osteogenic sarcoma, J. Roy Coll. Surg. Edinb. **1**:79-111, 1955.

18 Cahan, W. C., Woodard, H. Q., Higinbotham, N. L., Stewart, F. W., and Coley, B. L.: Sarcoma arising in irradiated bone; report of eleven cases, Cancer **1**:3-29, 1948.

19 Carson, C. P., Ackerman, L. V., and Maltby, J. D.: Plasma cell myeloma; a clinical pathologic and roentgenologic review of 90 cases, Amer. J. Clin. Path. **25**:849-888, 1955 (extensive bibliography).

20 Changus, G. W., Speed, J. S., and Stewart, F. W.: Malignant angioblastoma of bone, Cancer **10**:540-559, 1957.

21 Codman, E. A.: Epiphyseal chondromatous giant cell tumors of the upper end of the humerus, Surg. Gynec. Obstet. **52**:543-548, 1931.

22 Cohen, P.: Fluoride and calcium therapy for myeloma bone lesions, J.A.M.A. **198**:583-586, 1966.

23 Cohen, D. M., Dahlin, D. C., and MacCarty, S. C.: Apparently solitary tumors of the vertebral column, Mayo Clin. Proc. **39**:509-528, 1964.

24 Coleman, S. S.: Benign chondroblastoma with recurrent soft-tissue and intra-articular lesions, J. Bone Joint Surg. **48-A**:1554-1560, 1966.

25 Coley, B. L.: Atypical forms of bone sarcoma, Bull. Hosp. Joint Dis. **12**:148-173, 1951.

26 Coley, B. L., and Higinbotham, N. L.: Conservative surgery in tumors of bone with special reference to segmental resection, Ann. Surg. **127**:231-242, 1948.

27 Coley, B. L., Higinbotham, N. L., and Bowden, L.: Endothelioma of bone (Ewing's sarcoma), Ann. Surg. **128**:533-560, 1948.

28 Coley, B. L., Higinbotham, N. L., and Groesbeck, H. P.: Primary reticulum-cell sarcoma of bone; summary of 37 cases, Radiology **55**:641-658, 1959.

29 Coley, B. L., Higinbotham, N. L., and Romeiu, C.: Hemipelvectomy for tumors of bone; report of fourteen cases, Amer. J. Surg. **82**:27-43, 1951.

30 Coley, B. L., and Sharp, G. S.: Paget's disease; a predisposing factor to osteogenic sarcoma, Arch. Surg. (Chicago) **23**:918-936, 1931.

31 Collins, D. H.: Paget's disease of bone, Lancet **2**:51-57, 1956.

32 Cruz, M., Coley, B. L., and Stewart, F. W.: Postradiation bone sarcoma, Cancer **10**:72-88, 1957.

33 Cunningham, J. B., and Ackerman, L. V.: Metaphyseal fibrous defects, J. Bone Joint Surg. **38-A**:797-808, 1956.

34 Cunningham, M. P., and Arlen, M.: Medullary fibrosarcoma of bone, Cancer **21**:31-37, 1968.

35 Dahlin, D. C., and Coventry, M. B.: Osteogenic sarcoma; a study of six hundred cases, J. Bone Joint Surg. **49-A**:101-110, 1967.

36 Dahlin, D. C., Cupps, R. E., and Johnson, E. W., Jr.: Giant-cell tumor; a study of 195 cases, Cancer **25**:1061-1070, 1970.

37 Dahlin, D. C., and Johnson, E. W., Jr.: Giant osteoid osteoma, J. Bone Joint Surg. **36-A**: 559-572, 1954.

38 Dawson, E. K.: Liposarcoma of bone, J. Path. Bact. **70**:513-520, 1955.

39 Dechaume, M.: Les tumeurs à myéloplaxes des maxillaires; considérations pathogéniques et thérapetiques, Rev. Stomat. (Paris) **50**: 670-693, 1949.

40 DeNardo, G. L., and Volpe, J. A.: Detection of bone lesions with the strontium-85 scintiscan, J. Nucl. Med. **7**:219-236, 1966.

41 Derman, H., Pizzolato, P., and Ziskind, J.: Multicentric osteogenic sarcoma in Paget's disease with cerebral extensions, Amer. J. Roentgen. **65**:221-226, 1951.

42 Dorfman, H. D., Norman, A., and Wolff, H.: Fibrosarcoma complicating bone infarction in a caisson worker; a case report, J. Bone Joint Surg. **48-A**:528-532, 1966.

43 Dowling, E. A.: Mesenchymal chondrosarcoma, J. Bone Joint Surg. **46-A**:747-754, 1964.

44 Dunlap, C. E., Aub, J. C., Evans, R. D., and Harris, R. S.: Transplantable osteogenic sarcoma induced in rats by feeding radium, Amer. J. Path. **20**:1-21, 1944.

45 Edwards, G. A., and Zawadzki, Z. A.: Extraosseous lesions in plasma cell myeloma; a report of six cases, Amer. J. Med. **43**:194-205, 1967.

46 Ehrenfried, A.: Multiple cartilaginous exotoses-hereditary deforming chondrodysplasia, J.A.M.A. **64**:1642-1646, 1915.

47 Ellis, F.: Treatment of osteoclastoma by radiation, J. Bone Joint Surg. **31-B**:268-280, 1949.

48 Evans, D. M. D., and Sanerkin, N. G.: Primary leiomyosarcoma of bone, J. Path. Bact. **90**:348-350, 1965.

49 Evison, G., and Evans, K. T.: Bone sclerosis in multiple myeloma, Brit. J. Radiol. **40**:81-89, 1967.

50 Ewing, J.: Diffuse endothelioma of bone, Proc. N. Y. Path. Soc. **21**:17-24, 1921.

51 Eyre-Brook, A. L., and Price, C. H.: Fibrosarcoma of bone; review of fifty consecutive cases from the Bristol Bone Tumour Registry, J. Bone Joint Surg. **51**:20-37, 1969.

52 Falk, S., and Alpert, M.: The clinical and roentgen aspects of Ewing's sarcoma, Amer. J. Med. Sci. **250**:492-508, 1965.

53 Falk, S., and Alpert, M.: Five-year survival of patients with Ewing's sarcoma, Surg. Gynec. Obstet. **124**:319-324, 1967.

54 Feldman, F., Hecht, H. L., and Johnson, A. D.: Chondromyxoid fibroma of bone, Radiology **94**:249-260, 1970.

55 Fowles, S. J.: Osteoid osteoma, Brit. J. Radiol. **37**:245-252, 1964.

56 Fraumeni, J. F., Jr.: Stature and malignant tumors of bone in childhood and adolescence, Cancer **20**:967-973, 1967.

57 Friedman, M., and Pearlman, A. W.: Benign giant-cell tumor of bone; radiation dosage for each type, Radiology **91**:1151-1158, 1968.

58 Fruhling, L., and Chadli, A.: Le sarcome plasmocytaire extrasquellettique, Ann. Anat. Path. (Paris) **8**:317-376, 1963.

59 Garceau, G. J., and Gregory, C. F.: Solitary unicameral bone cyst, J. Bone Joint Surg. **36-A**:267-280, 1954.

60 Garré, C.: Ueber besondere Formen and Folgezustande der akuten infektiösen Osteomyelitis, Beitr. Klin. Chir. **10**:241-298, 1893.

61 Garrington, G. E., Scofield, H. H., Cornyn, J., and Hooker, S. P.: Osteosarcoma of the jaws; analysis of 56 cases, Cancer **20**:377-391, 1967.

62 Gee, V. R., and Pugh, D. G.: Giant-cell tumor of bone, Radiology **70**:33-45, 1958.

63 Gershon-Cohen, J.: Giant-cell tumors; radiation therapy and late results, Radiology **41**: 261-267, 1943.

64 Gilmer, W. S., Jr., and McEwen, G. D.: Central (medullary) fibrosarcoma of bone, J. Bone Joint Surg. **40-A**:121-141, 1958.

65 Goldenberg, R. R.: The skeleton in Paget's disease, Bull. Hosp. Joint Dis. **12**:229-255, 1951.

65a Goldenberg, R. R., Campbell, C. J., and Bonfiglio, M.: Giant-cell tumor of bone, J. Bone Joint Surg. **52-A**:619-664, 1970.

66 Goldman, R. L., and Lichtenstein, L.: Synovial condrosarcoma, Cancer **12**:1233-1240, 1964.

67 Gomori, G. H.: Distribution of acid phosphatase in tissues under normal and under pathologic conditions, Arch. Path. (Chicago) **32**:189-199, 1941.

68 Gootnick, L. T.: Solitary myeloma; review of sixty-one cases, Radiology **45**:385-391, 1945.

69 Green, W. T., and Farber, S.: "Eosinophilic or solitary granuloma" of bone, J. Bone Joint Surg. **24**:499-526, 1942.

70 Hansen, P. B.: The relationship of Hand-Schuller-Christian's disease; Letterer-Siwe's disease and eosinophilic granulomas of bone, Acta Radiol. (Stockholm) **32**:89-112, 1949.

71 Hartman, W. H., and Stewart, F. W.: Hemangioendothelioma of bone; unusual tumor characterized by indolent course, Cancer **15**: 846-854, 1962.

72 Hatcher, C. H.: The development of sarcoma in bone subjected to roentgen or radium irradiation, J. Bone Joint Surg. **27**:179-195, 1945 (extensive bibliography).

73 Hatcher, C. H.: Pathogenesis of localized fibrous lesions in the metaphyses of long bone, Ann. Surg. **122**:1016-1030, 1945.

74 Heald, J. H., Soto-Hall, R., and Hill, H. A.: Ewing's sarcoma, Amer. J. Roentgen. **91**:1167-1171, 1964.

75 Heiser, S., and Schwartzman, J. J.: Variations in the roentgen appearance of the

skeletal system in myeloma, Radiology **58**: 178-191, 1952.

76 Hems, G.: The risk of bone cancer in man from internally deposited radium, Brit. J. Radiol. 40:506-511, 1967.

77 Henderson, E. D., and Dahlin, D. C.: Chondrosarcoma of bone—a study of two hundred and eighty-eight cases, J. Bone Joint Surg. **45-A**:1450-1458, 1963.

78 Heremans, E. P., and Waldenström, J.: Cytology and electrophoretic pattern in myeloma, Acta Med. Scand. **170**:575-589, 1961.

79 Higinbotham, N. L., and Coley, B. L.: Hemipelvectomy; experience in a series of thirtynine cases, Cancer 9:1233-1238, 1956.

80 Hochheim, W.: Malignant evolution of osteochondromatosis type Ollier, Acta Chir. Orthop. Traum. Cech. 33:161-163, 1966.

81 Hoogstraten, B., Sheehe, P. R., Cuttner, J., Cooper, T., Kyle, R. A., Oberfield, R. A., Townsend, S. R., Harley, J. B., Hayes, D. M., Costa, G., and Holland, J. F.: Melphalan in multiple myeloma, Blood 30:74-83, 1967.

82 Howard, E. B., Clarke, W. J., Karagianes, M. T., and Palmer, R. F.: Strontium-90-induced bone tumors in miniature swine, Radiat. Res. 39:594-607, 1969.

83 Hustu, H. O., Holton, C., James, D., Jr., and Pinkel, D.: Treatment of Ewing's sarcoma with concurrent radiotherapy and chemotherapy, J. Pediat. 73:249-251, 1968.

84 Hutter, R. V. P., Foote, F. W., Francis, K. C., and Sherman, R. S.: Primitive multi-potential primary sarcoma of bone, Cancer 19:1-25, 1966.

85 Hutter, R. V. P., Foote, F. W., Jr., Frazell, E. L., and Francis, K. C.: Giant cell tumors complicating Paget's disease of bone, Cancer 16:1044-1056, 1963.

86 Hutter, R. V. P., Francis, K. C., and Foote, F. W.: Ewing's sarcoma in siblings; report of the second known occurrence, Amer. J. Surg. 107:598-603, 1964.

87 Ivins, J. C., and Dahlin, D. C.: Reticulum-cell sarcoma of bone, J. Bone Joint Surg. **35-A**:835-842, 1953.

88 Ivins, J. C., and Dahlin, D. C.: Malignant lymphoma (reticulum cell sarcoma) of bone, Mayo Clin. Proc. 38:375-396, 1963.

89 Jackson, H., Jr., and Parker, F., Jr.: Reticulum cell sarcoma, New York, 1944, Oxford University Press, chap. I-A, pp. 68-94.

90 Jacobson, H. G., Poppel, M. H., Shapiro, J. H., and Grossberger, S.: The vertebral pedicle sign; a roentgen finding to differentiate metastatic carcinoma from multiple myeloma, Amer. J. Roentgen. 80:817-821, 1958.

91 Jaffe, H. L.: Osteoid-osteoma of bone, Radiology **45**:319-334, 1945.

92 Jaffe, H. L.: Tumors and tumorous conditions of the bones and joints, Philadelphia, 1958, Lea & Febiger (excellent reference book).

93 Jaffe, H. L., and Lichtenstein, L.: Benign chondroblastoma of bone, Amer. J. Path. **18**: 969-991, 1942.

94 Jaffe, H. L., and Lichtenstein, L.: Solitary unicameral bone cyst; with emphasis on the roentgen picture, pathologic appearance and pathogenesis, Arch. Surg. (Chicago) 44:1004-1025, 1942.

95 Jaffe, H. L., and Lichtenstein, L.: Non-osteogenic fibroma of bone, Amer. J. Path. 18:205-221, 1942.

96 Jaffe, H. L., and Lichtenstein, L.: Solitary benign enchondroma of bone, Arch. Surg. (Chicago) 46:480-493, 1943.

97 Jaffe, H. L., Lichtenstein, L., and Portis, R. B.: Giant cell tumor of bone, Arch. Path. (Chicago) 30:993-1031, 1940.

98 Jansson, G.: Roentgen treatment and the course of cure of giant cell tumor in the osseous system, Acta Radiol. (Stockholm) 25: 569-579, 1944.

99 Jeffree, G. M., and Price, C. H.: Bone tumours and their enzymes; a study of phosphatases, non-specific esterases and beta-glucuronidase of osteogenic and cartilaginous tumours, fibroblastic and giant-cell lesions, J. Bone Joint Surg. **47-B**:120-136, 1965.

100 Jenkin, R. D. T.: Ewing's sarcoma; a study of treatment methods, Clin. Radiol. 17:97-106, 1966.

101 Jewell, J. H., and Bush, L. F.: "Benign" giant-cell tumor of bone with a solitary pulmonary metastasis; a case report, J. Bone Joint Surg. **46-A**:848-852, 1964.

102 Johnson, E. W., Jr., and Dahlin, D. C.: Treatment of giant-cell tumor of bone, J. Bone Joint Surg. **41-A**:895-904, 1959.

103 Johnson, E. W., Gee, V. R., and Dahlin, D. C.: Giant-cell tumors of the sacrum, Amer. J. Orthop. 4:302-305, 1962.

104 Johnson, R., and Humphreys, S. R.: Past failures and future possibilities in Ewing's sarcoma; experimental and preliminary clinical results, Cancer 23:161-166, 1969.

105 Johnson, R. E., Senyszyn, J. J., Rabson, A. S., and Peterson, K. A.: Treatment of Ewing's sarcoma with local irradiation and systemic chemotherapy; a progress report, Radiology **95**:195-197, 1970.

106 Joynt, G. H. C., and Ortved, W. E.: The accidental operative transplantation of benign giant cell tumor, Ann. Surg. 127:1232-1239, 1948.

107 Keith, A.: Studies on the anatomical changes which accompany certain growth disorders of the human body. I. The nature of the structural alterations in the disorder known as multiple exostoses, J. Anat. 54:101-115, 1919.

108 Kempson, R. L.: Ossifying fibroma of the long bones; A light and electron microscopic study, Arch. Path. (Chicago) 82:218-233, 1966.

109 Kolodny, A.: Bone sarcoma; primary malignant tumors of bone and giant cell sarcoma, Surg. Gynec. Obstet. 44:1-214, 1927.

110 Kraft, G. L., and Levinthal, D. H.: Acrylic prosthesis replacing lower end of the femur for benign giant cell tumor, J. Bone Joint Surg. **36-A**:368-374, 1954.

111 Kragh, L. V., Dahlin, D. C., and Erich, J. B.:

Osteogenic sarcoma of the jaws and facial bones, Amer. J. Surg. 96:496-505, 1958.

112 Lacassagne, A.: Conditions dans lesquelles ont été obtenus, chez le lapin, des cancers par action des rayons X sur des foyers inflammatoires, C. R. Soc. Biol. (Paris) 112:562-564, 1933.

113 Lagergren, C., Lindbom, A., and Soderberg, G.: The blood vessels of osteogenic sarcomas, Acta Radiol. (Stockholm) 55:161-176, 1961.

114 Lansche, W. E., and Spjut, H. J.: Chondrosarcoma of the small bones of the hand, J. Bone Joint Surg. 40-A:1139-1145, 1958.

115 Lasser, E. C., and Tetewsky, H.: Metastasizing giant cell tumor; report of an unusual case with indolent bone and pulmonary metastases, Amer. J. Roentgen. 78:804-811, 1957.

116 Lawrence, W., and Franklin, E. L.: Calcifying enchondroma of long bones, J. Bone Joint Surg. 35-B:224-228, 1953.

117 Lee, E. S., and MacKenzie, D. H.: Osteosarcoma; a study of the value of preoperative megavoltage radiotherapy, Brit. J. Surg. 51:252-274, 1964.

118 Levinthal, D. H., and Grossman, A.: Interscapulothoracic amputation for malignant tumors of the shoulder region, Surg. Gynec. Obstet. 69:234-239, 1939.

119 Lewin, H., and Stein, J. M.: Solitary plasma cell myeloma with new bone formation, Amer. J. Roentgen. 79:630-637, 1958.

120 Lewis, R. C., Jr., and Bickel, W. H.: Hemipelvectomy for malignant disease, J.A.M.A. 165:8-12, 1957.

121 Lichtenstein, L.: Giant-cell tumor of bone; current status of problems in diagnosis and treatment, J. Bone Joint Surg. 33-A:143-150, 1951.

122 Lichtenstein, L.: Classification of primary tumors of bone, Cancer 4:335-341, 1951.

123 Lichtenstein, L.: Aneurysmal bone cyst; further observations, Cancer 6:1228-1237, 1953.

124 Lichtenstein, L.: Histocytosis X, integration of eosinophilic granuloma of bone, "Letterer-Siwe disease," and "Schüller-Christian disease" as related manifestations of a single nosologic entity, Arch. Path. (Chicago) 56:84-102, 1953.

125 Lichtenstein, L.: Benign osteoblastoma; a category of osteoid- and bone-forming tumors other than classical osteoid osteoma, which may be mistaken for giant-cell tumor or osteogenic sarcoma, Cancer 9:1044-1052, 1956.

126 Lichentstein, L.: Aneurysmal bone cyst; observations on fifty cases, J. Bone Joint Surg. 39-A:873-882, 1957.

127 Lichtenstein, L.: Bone tumors, ed. 3, St. Louis, 1965, The C. V. Mosby Co.

128 Lichtenstein, L., and Jaffe, H. L.: Ewing's sarcoma, Amer. J. Path. 23:43-78, 1947.

129 Lichtenstein, L., and Jaffe, H. L.: Multiple myeloma; a survey based on thirty-five cases, eighteen of which came at autopsy, Arch. Path. (Chicago) 44:207-246, 1947.

130 Lichtenstein, L.. and Kaplan, L.: Benign chondroblastoma of bone; unusual localization in femoral capital epiphysis, Cancer 2:793-798, 1949.

131 Lichtenstein, L., and Sawyer, W. R.: Benign osteoblastoma, J. Bone Joint Surg. 46-A:755-765, 1964.

131a Lieberman, P. H., Jones, C. R., Dargeon, H. W. K., and Begg, C. F.: A reappraisal of eosinophilic granuloma of bone, Hand-Schüller-Christian syndrome and Letterer-Siwe syndrome, Medicine (Balt.) 48:375-400, 1969.

132 Lindbom, A., Soderberg, G., and Spjut, H. J.: Osteosarcoma; a review of 96 cases, Acta Radiol. (Stockholm) 56:1-19, 1961.

133 Looney, W. B., Hasterlik, R. J., Brues, A. M., and Skirmont, E.: A clinical investigation of the chronic effects of radium salts administered therapeutically (1915-1930), Amer. J. Roentgen. 73:1006-1037, 1955.

134 Luck, J. V.: Bone and joint diseases, Springfield, Ill., 1950, Charles C Thomas, Publisher.

135 MacLellan, D. I., and Wilson, F. C., Jr.: Osteoid osteoma of the spine, J. Bone Joint Surg. 49-A:111-121, 1967.

136 Macdonald, I., and Budd, J. W.: Osteogenic sarcoma. II. Roentgenographic interpretation of growth patterns in bone sarcoma, Surg. Gynec. Obstet. 82:81-86, 1948.

137 McGavran, M. H., and Spady, H. A.: Eosinophilic granuloma of bone, J. Bone Joint Surg. 42-A:979-992, 1960.

138 McKenna, R. J., Schwinn, C. P., and Higinbotham, N. L.: Osteogenic sarcoma in children, Calif. Med. 103:165-170, 1965.

139 McKenna, R. J., Schwinn, C. P., Soong, K. Y., and Higinbotham, N. L.: Osteogenic sarcoma arising in Paget's disease, Cancer 17:42-66, 1964.

140 McKenna, R. J., Schwinn, C. P., Soong, K. Y., and Higinbotham, N. L.: Sarcomata of the osteogenic series (osteosarcoma, fibrosarcoma, chondrosarcoma, parosteal osteogenic sarcoma, and sarcomata arising in abnormal bone); an analysis of 552 cases, J. Bone Joint Surg. 48-A:1-26, 1966.

141 McLeod, J. J., Dahlin, D. C., and Ivins, J. C.: Fibrosarcoma of bone, Amer. J. Surg. 94:431-437, 1957.

142 McSwain, B., Byrd, B. F., Jr., and Inman, W. O., Jr.: Ewing's tumor, Surg. Gynec. Obstet, 89:209-221, 1949.

143 Martland, H. S., and Humphries, R. E.: Osteogenic sarcoma in dial painters using luminous paint, Arch. Path. (Chicago) 7:406-417, 1929.

144 Medill, E. V.: Primary reticulum-cell sarcoma of bone, J. Fac. Radiol. 8:102-117, 1956.

145 Middlemiss, J. H.: Cartilage tumours, Brit. J. Radiol. 37:277-286, 1964.

146 Millburn, L. F., O'Grady, L., and Hendrickson, F. R.: Radical radiation therapy and total body irradiation in the treatment of Ewing's sarcoma, Cancer 22:919-925, 1968.

147 Mnaymneh, W. A., Dudley, H. R., and Mnaymneh, L. G.: Giant-cell tumor of bone; an analysis and follow-up study of the forty-

one cases observed at the Massachusetts General Hospital between 1925 and 1960, J. Bone Joint Surg. **46-A:**63-75, 1964.

148 Moon, N. F.: Adamantinoma of the appendicular skeleton; a statistical review of reported cases and inclusion of 10 new cases, Clin. Orthop. **43:**189-213, 1965.

149 Moseley, J. E.: Patterns of bone change in multiple myeloma, J. Mt. Sinai Hosp. **28:**511-536, 1961.

150 Moseley, J. E., and Bass, M. H.: Sclerosing osteogenic sarcomatosis, Radiology **66:**41-45, 1956.

151 Moseley, J. E., and Starobin, S. G.: Cystic angiomatosis of bone; manifestation of hamartomatous disease entity, Amer. J. Roentgen. **91:**1114-1120, 1964.

152 Mukerjea, S. K.: Traumatic aneurysm of the popliteal artery due to osteochondroma, Brit. J. Surg. **54:**810-811, 1967.

153 Murphy, F. D., Jr., and Blount, W. P.: Cartilaginous exostoses following irradiation, J. Bone Joint Surg. **44-A:**662-668, 1962.

154 Murphy, F. P., Dahlin, D. C., and Sullivan, C. R.: Articular synovial chondromatosis, J. Bone Joint Surg. **44-A:**77-86, 1962.

155 Murphy, W. R., and Ackerman, L. V.: Benign and malignant giant-cell tumors of bone; a clinical-pathological evaluation of thirty-one cases, Cancer **9:**317-339, 1956.

156 Nielsen, A. R., and Poulsen, H.: Multiple diffuse fibrosarcomata of the bones, Acta Path. Microbiol. Scand. **55:**265-272, 1962.

157 Nobler, M. P., Higinbotham, N. L., and Phillips, R. F.: The cure of aneurysmal bone cyst; irradiation superior to surgery in an analysis of 33 cases, Radiology **90:**1185-1192, 1968.

158 Nosanchuk, J. S., Weatherbee, L., and Brody, G. L.: Osteogenic sarcoma; prognosis related to epiphyseal closure, J.A.M.A. **208:**2439-2441, 1969.

159 Oberling, C.: Les réticulosarcomes et les réticulo-endothéliosarcomes de la moelle osseuse (sarcomes d'Ewing), Bull. Ass. Franc. Cancer **17:**259-296, 1928.

160 Ochsner, S. F.: Eosinophilic granuloma of bone; experience with 20 cases, Amer. J. Roentgen. **97:**719-726, 1966.

161 O'Neal, L. W., and Ackerman, L. V.: Cartilaginous tumors of ribs and sternum, J. Thorac. Surg. **21:**71-108, 1951.

162 O'Neal, L. W., and Ackerman, L. V.: Chondrosarcoma of bone, Cancer **5:**551-577, 1952.

163 Osgood, E. E.: The survival time of patients with plasmocytic myeloma, Cancer Chemother. Rep. **9:**1-10, 1960.

164 Osserman, E. F.: Multiple myeloma; current clinical and chemical concepts, Amer. J. Med. **23:**283-309, 1957 (extensive bibliography).

165 Osserman, E. F., and Takatsuki, K.: Plasma cell myeloma: gamma globulin synthesis and structure; a review of biochemical and clinical data, with the description of a newly-recognized and related syndrome, "H-gamma-2-chain (Franklin's) disease," Medicine (Balt.) **42:**357-384, 1963.

166 Otis, J., Hutter, R. V. P., Foote, F. W., Marcove, R. C., and Stewart, F. W.: Hemangioendothelioma of bone, Surg. Gynec. Obstet. **127:**295-305, 1968.

167 Pack, G. T., McNeer, G., and Coley, B. L.: Interscapulothoracic amputation for malignant tumors of the upper extremity; a report of thirty-one consecutive cases, Surg. Gynec. Obstet. **74:**161-175, 1942.

168 Papillon, J., Montbarbon, J.-F., and Chollat, L.: La roentgenthérapie des tumeurs à myéloplaxes, J. Radiol. Electr. **4:**288-299, 1958.

169 Parker, F., Jr., and Jackson, H., Jr.: Primary reticulum cell sarcoma of bone, Surg. Gynec. Obstet. **68:**45-53, 1939.

170 Pendergrass, E. P., Lafferty, J. O., and Horn, R. C.: Osteogenic sarcoma and chondrosarcoma; with special reference to the roentgen diagnosis, Amer. J. Roentgen. **54:**234-256, 1946.

171 Perkinson, N. G., and Higinbotham, N. L.: Osteogenic sarcoma arising in polyostotic fibrous dysplasia; report of a case, Cancer **8:**396-402, 1955.

172 Phelan, J. T.: Aneurysmal bone cyst, Surg. Gynec. Obstet. **119:**979-983, 1964.

173 Phillips, R. F., and Higinbotham, N. L.: The curability of Ewing's endothelioma of bone in children, J. Pediat. **70:**391-397, 1967.

174 Potozky, H., and Freid, J. R.: Ewing's tumor simulating sarcoma of soft-tissue origin, Amer. J. Cancer **36:**1-11, 1939.

175 Price, C. H. G.: Osteogenic sarcoma; an analysis of the age and sex incidence, Brit. J. Cancer **9:**558-574, 1955.

176 Price, C. H. G.: The prognosis of osteosarcoma, Brit. J. Radiol. **39:**181-188, 1966.

177 Raven, R. W., and Willis, R. A.: Solitary plasmocytoma of the spine, J. Bone Joint Surg. **31-B:**369-375, 1949.

178 Rosai, J.: Adamantinoma of the tibia; electron microscopic evidence of its epithelial origin, Amer. J. Clin. Path. **51:**786-792, 1969.

179 Ross, F. G. M.: Osteogenic sarcoma, Brit. J. Radiol. **37:**259-276, 1964.

180 Rundles, R. W., Dillon, M. L., and Dillon, E. S.: Multiple myeloma. III. Effect of urethane therapy on plasma cell growth, abnormal serum protein components and Bence Jones proteinuria, J. Clin. Invest. **29:**1243-1260, 1950.

181 Sabanas, A. O., Dahlin, D. C., Childs, D. S., Jr., and Ivins, J. C.: Postradiation sarcoma of bone, Cancer **9:**528-542, 1956.

182 Sarrazin, D., Schweisguth, O., and Hourtelle, F.-G.: Radiotherapy of reticulosarcoma of bone; technique and results, Ann. Radiol. **10:**401-418, 1967.

183 Scaglietti, O., and Calandriello, B.: Ossifying parosteal sarcoma; parosteal osteoma or juxtacortical osteogenic sarcoma, J. Bone Joint Surg. **44-A:**635-647, 1962.

184 Schajowicz, F.: Aspiration biopsy in bone lesions, J. Bone Joint Surg. **37-A:**465-471, 1955.

185 Schajowicz, F.: Ewing's sarcoma and reticulum cell sarcoma of bone; with special refer-

ence to the histochemical demonstration of glycogen as an aid to differential diagnosis, J. Bone Joint Surg. **41-A**:349-356, 1959.

186 Schajowicz, F.: Giant-cell tumors of bone (osteoclastoma), J. Bone Joint Surg. **43-A**: 1-29, 1961.

187 Schajowicz, F., and Bessone, J. E.: Chondrosarcoma in three brothers, J. Bone Joint Surg. **49-A**:129-141, 1967.

188 Schajowicz, F., Cuevillas, A. R., and Silberman, F. S.: Primary malignant mesenchymoma of bone; a new tumor entity, Cancer **19**:1423-1428, 1966.

189 Schajowicz, F., and Derqui, J. C.: Puncture biopsy in lesions of the locomotor system, Cancer **21**:531-548, 1968.

190 Schlumberger, H. G.: Fibrous dysplasia of single bones (monostotic fibrous dysplasia), Milit. Surg. **99**:504-527, 1946.

191 Schwartz, D. T., and Alpert, M.: The malignant transformation of fibrous dysplasia, Amer. J. Med. Sci. **247**:1-20, 1964 (extensive bibliography).

192 Sherman, R. S., and Snyder, R. E.: The roentgen appearance of primary reticulum cell sarcoma of bone, Amer. J. Roentgen. **58**:291-306, 1947.

193 Sherman, R. S., and Soong, K. Y.: Ewing's sarcoma; its roentgen classification and diagnosis, Radiology **66**:529-539, 1956.

194 Sherman, R. S., and Soong, K. Y.: Aneurysmal bone cyst; its roentgen diagnosis, Radiology **68**:54-64, 1957.

195 Sherman, R. S., and Wilner, D.: The roentgen diagnosis of hemangioma of bone, Amer. J. Roentgen. **86**:1146-1159, 1961.

196 Sklaroff, D. M., and Charkes, N. D.: The value of strontium 85 bone scanning in radiation therapy, Amer. J. Roentgen. **99**:415-421, 1967.

197 Skoog, W. A., and Adams, W. S.: Clinical and metabolic investigations of eight cases of multiple myeloma during prolonged cyclophosphamide administration, Amer. J. Med. **41**:76-95, 1966.

198 Slavens, J. J.: Multiple myeloma in a child, Amer. J. Dis. Child. **47**:821-836, 1934.

199 Smithers, D. W., and Gowing, N. F. C.: Melorheostosis, Cancer Seminar **2**:166-168, 1959.

200 Snapper, I.: Medical clinics on bone diseases, New York, 1943, Interscience Publishers, Inc.

201 Snapper, I.: Medical clinics on bone diseases, ed. 2, New York, 1949, Interscience Publishers, Inc.

202 Solomon, I.: Hereditary multiple exostosis, J. Bone Joint Surg. **45-B**:292-304, 1963.

203 Spjut, H. J., and Lindbom, A.: Skeletal angiomatosis; report of two cases, Acta Path. Microbiol. Scand. **55**:49-58, 1962.

204 Stevens, G. M., Pugh, D. G., and Dahlin, D. C.: Roentgenographic recognition and differentiation of parosteal osteogenic sarcoma, Amer. J. Roentgen. **78**:1-12, 1957.

205 Stewart, F. W.: Occupational and post-traumatic cancer, Bull. N. Y. Acad. Med. **23**:145-162, 1947.

206 Strickland, B.: The value of arteriography in the diagnosis of bone tumors, Brit. J. Radiol. **32**:705-713, 1959.

207 Sugarbaker, E. D., and Ackerman, L. V.: Disarticulation of the innominate bone for malignant tumors of the pelvic parietes and upper thigh, Surg. Gynec. Obstet. **81**:36-52, 1945.

208 Summey, T. J., and Pressly, C. L.: Sarcoma complicating Paget's disease of bone, Ann. Surg. **123**:135-153, 1946.

209 Swenson, P. C.: The roentgenological aspects of Ewing's tumor of bone marrow. Amer. J. Roentgen. **50**:343-353, 1943.

209a Talerman, A.: Clinico-pathological study of multiple myeloma in Jamaica, Brit. J. Cancer **23**:285-293, 1969.

210 Taylor, G. W., and Rogers, W. P., Jr.: Hindquarter amputation; experience with eighteen cases, New Eng. J. Med. **249**:963-969, 1953.

211 Teitelbaum, S. L.: Tumors of the chest wall, Surg. Gynec. Obstet. **129**:1059-1073, 1969.

212 Thompson, V. P., and Steggall, C. T.: Chondrosarcoma of the proximal portion of the femur treated by resection and bone replacement, J. Bone Joint Surg. **38-A**:357-367, 1956.

213 Tudway, R. C.: The place of external irradiation in the treatment of osteogenic sarcoma, J. Bone Joint Surg. **35-B**:9-21, 1953.

214 Tudway, R. C.: Giant cell tumour of bone, Brit. J. Radiol. **32**:315-321, 1959.

215 Uehlinger, E., Botsztejn, C., and Schinz, H. R.: Ewingsarkom und Knochenretikulosarkom; Klinik, Diagnose und Differential-diagnose, Oncologia (Basel) **1**:193-245, 1948.

216 Unander-Scharin, L.: On the tendency of Ewing's sarcoma to heal spontaneously, and on the alterations due to irradiation, Acta Orthop. Scand. **18**:436-476, 1949.

217 Upshaw, J. E., McDonald, J. R., and Ghormley, R. K.: Extension of primary neoplasms of bone to bone marrow, Surg. Gynec. Obstet. **89**:704-714, 1949.

218 Van Horn, P. E., Johnson, E. W., and Dahlin, D. C.: Fibrous dysplasia of the femur with sarcomatous change, Amer. J. Orthop. **5**:165-167, 1963.

219 van der Heul, R. O., and von Ronnen, J. R.: Juxtacortical osteosarcoma, J. Bone Joint Surg. **49-A**:415-439, 1967.

220 Valls, J., Ottolenghi, C. E., and Schajowicz, F.: Epiphyseal chondroblastoma of bone, J. Bone Joint Surg. **33-A**:997-1009, 1951.

221 Verbiest, H.: Giant-cell tumours and aneurysmal bone cysts of the spine with special reference to the problems related to the removal of a vertebral body, J. Bone Joint Surg. **47-B**:699-713, 1965.

222 Wallace, W. S.: Reticulo-endotheliosis: Hand-Schüller-Christian disease and the rarer manifestations, Amer. J. Roentgen. **62**:189-207, 1949.

223 Warren, S.: Chondrosarcoma with intravascular growth and tumor emboli to lungs, Amer. J. Path. **7**:161-168, 1931.

224 Welsh, R. A., and Meyer, A. T.: A histo-

Bone **935**

genetic study of chondroblastoma, Cancer 17:
578-589, 1964.
225 Westermark, N., and Hellerstrom, S.: Zwei
Fälle von Osteitis luetica osteogenes Sarkom
vortäuschend, Acta Radiol. (Stockholm) 18:
422-427, 1937.

226 Willis, R. A.: Pathology of tumours, ed. 4,
London, 1967, Butterworth & Co. (Publishers) Ltd.
227 Windeyer, B. W., and Woodyatt, P. B.:
Osteoclastoma; a study of thirty-eight cases,
J. Bone Joint Surg. 31-B:252-267, 1949.

Chapter 17

Sarcomas of the soft tissues

Epidemiology

Soft tissue sarcomas are a small and exclusive group of tumors of mesodermal origin (smooth muscle, striated muscle, fat, connective tissue, cartilage, and blood vessels). They appear at any site the parent tissue is present. Their rate of growth is unpredictable. Not included in this chapter are the lymphosarcomas and the sarcomas of special organs (e.g., leiomyosarcoma of the uterus). Kaposi's sarcomas are described in the chapter on the skin (p. 135). Malignant tumors of nerve sheath origin are discussed in the chapter on the mediastinum (p. 396).

In the retroperitoneal space, liposarcomas are the most frequent primary lesion (Farbman[34]), followed by the leiomyosarcomas (Ackerman[3]). Fibrosarcomas are the most frequently found tumors in the extremities. Rhabdomyosarcomas are predominant among neoplasms found in the orbit (Kassel et al.[50]) and the gluteal and interscapular regions. Synovial sarcomas are the most frequent tumors occurring around the ankles and knees.

Data on sex incidence, mean age, common locations, origins, and gross and microscopic characteristics of the five most common types of soft tissue sarcomas are presented in Table 111.

Fibrosarcomas occur at all ages and seem to present no sex predilection (Stout[105]). *Liposarcomas* are found predominantly between 40 and 60 years of age in both male and females (Reszel et al.[88]). *Rhabdomyosarcomas* are found at all ages but most commonly in the second and third decades of life (Cade[13]). However, those occurring in the orbit are primarily found in young children (Dito and Batsakis[27]), and there seems to be a different average age for the various types (Patton and Horn[78]). *Synovial sarcomas* occur predominantly in young adults. *Alveolar soft parts sarcomas* occur in men at an average age of 30

and in women at an average age of 20 years (Lieberman et al.[59]).

Trauma has never been proved to be a causative factor of soft tissue sarcomas. Fibrosarcoma has been reported within a sinus tract of chronic osteomyelitis (Morris and Lucas[69]). Irradiation for benign conditions such as tuberculosis of the skin and thyroid disease may give rise to fibromatosis or to fibrosarcoma after long time periods (Marques et al.[67]; Pettit et al.[82]; Gentele[39]). Frequently, the irradiation is poorly conceived or intensive. Lymphangiosarcomas may develop as a rare complication of prolonged, massive postmastectomy lymphedema (Stewart and Treves[96]). This type of sarcoma can also develop in a chronically edematous extremity (Herrmann and Gruhn[44]).

Pathology
Gross and microscopic pathology

The pathology of the soft tissue sarcomas may be varied because of their mesodermal origin. However, differentiation of the specific types can usually be made because of the location of the tumor and its pathologic characteristics. Exact histogenesis may be determined with special stains and, in a few instances, by tissue culture (Murray and Stout[72]; Murray et al.[73]) and electron microscopy. All of these tumors are capable of producing reticulin.

Soft tissue tumors may have a characteristic reticulin pattern. Intermingling of different types of sarcomas may, though rarely, occur in the same neoplasm. Such tumors have been designated as malignant mesenchymomas (Stout[104]).

Fibrosarcomas may arise in the extremities, trunk, head, and neck. They arise from subcutaneous fibrous tissue, from deep connective tissue around tendon sheaths, or from other areas in which connective tissue is found. Grossly, they are firm and homogeneous (Fig. 711), forming round

Table 111. Summarized characteristics of most common varieties of soft tissue sarcomas

	Fibrosarcoma	*Liposarcoma*	*Rhabdomysarcoma*	*Synovial sarcoma*	*Angiosarcoma (hemangioendothelioma)*
Sex	No definite preponderance	No definite preponderance	Slight male preponderance	Men 3:2	Data insufficient
Mean age	50 yr	All ages	All ages	32 (Haagensen)	Data insufficient
Common locations	Extremities and trunk	Gluteal region, thighs, and popliteal and retroperitoneal regions	Popliteal, inguinal, gluteal and interscapular regions	About tendon sheaths and immediate vicinity of knee and ankle joints	Subcutaneous tissue and muscle
Parent tissue of origin	Connective tissue or nerve sheath	Adipose tissue	Striated muscle	Synovium	Blood vessels
Gross characteristics	Firm or soft; pseudoencapsulated; grayish white	May be very large; resembles brain tissue; often pseudoencapsulated	Rather soft; pseudoencapsulated; often hemorrhagic	Pseudocircumscribed; grayish pink; hemorrhagic, fibrous, and calcified at times	Very vascular; bleed within themselves or externally
Microscopic characteristics	Connective tissue cells of varying ages; phosphotungstic acid–hematoxylin stain demonstrates fibroglia and fibrils	Nucleus often compressed to crescentic shape by fat; cytoplasmic fat prominent with fat stains; sudan IV and scharlach R helpful in diagnosis	Cross striations infrequent: best seen with phosphotungstic acid–hematoxylin stain; giant cells common; vacuolation of nuclei; transition from normal muscles at times seen	Two types of tissue forms present, one resembling synovial structures and other suggesting fibrosarcoma; silver stains helpful in diagnosis	Silver stain demonstrates usually layering of endothelial tumor cells and anastomosing vascular channels

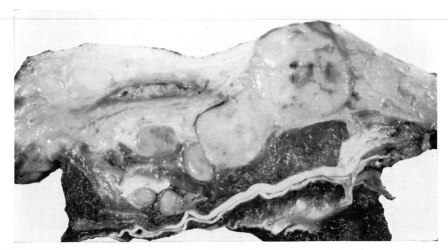

Fig. 711. Fibrosarcoma of thigh recurring after inadequate surgery. Note deep extension.

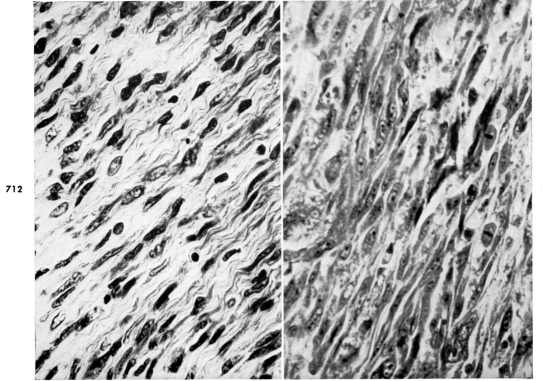

712

713

Fig. 712. Well-differentiated fibrosarcoma showing characteristic spindle-shaped cells. (Moderate enlargement.)

Fig. 713. Moderately differentiated fibrosarcoma. Note numerous mitotic figures.

or spindle-shaped masses that may appear encapsulated. On section, they are pale grayish white. Poorly differentiated tumors frequently show hemorrhages and necrosis. The majority of fibrosarcomas are well differentiated, and the remainder show considerable variation in pattern with many mitotic figures (Figs. 712 and 713). Giant cells are not frequently seen. These tumors form collagen and reticulin fibers. In the

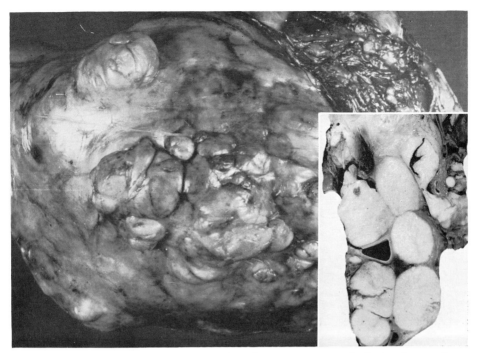

Fig. 714. Liposarcoma showing typical surface that caricatures cerebral convolutions. **Inset,** cross section of involved retroperitoneal lymph nodes. Note close resemblance to brain tissue.

well-differentiated fibrosarcomas, the reticulin wraps itself around the cells (Stout[105]). In florid Recklinghausen's disease, malignant change can occur. The resulting malignant tumors often produce a fusiform enlargement in a nerve and are best designated as malignant schwannomas (neurofibrosarcomas). Close association of a tumor with a nerve does not suffice to establish its nerve origin. Neurogenous tumors can be identified in tissue culture (Murray[71]).

Liposarcomas are malignant from their inception and frequently grow to a large size. Grossly, their surface may show convolutions that crudely caricature cerebral cortex (Fig. 714). On section, the tumor is usually yellowish white and often has a slimy appearance. Satellite nodules may be observed around the main mass. Occasionally, liposarcomas have multiple foci of origin (Ackerman[2]). The infrequent form

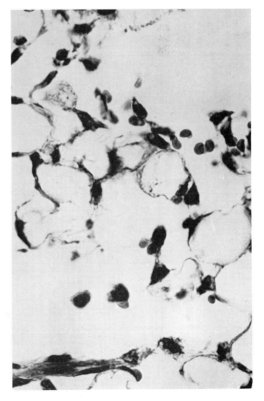

Fig. 715. Liposarcoma with cytoplasmic vacuolation and compression of nuclei to crescentic ring. (High-power enlargement.)

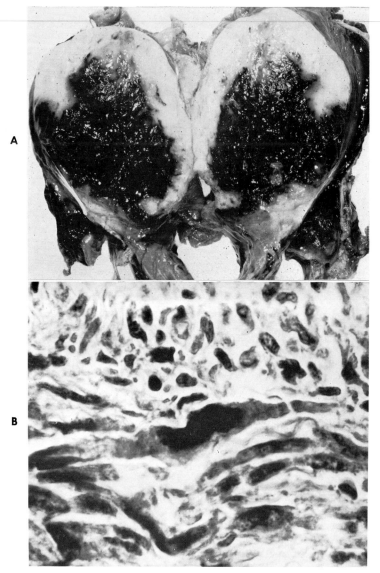

Fig. 716. A, Rhabdomyosarcoma of psoas muscle showing areas of hemorrhage. **B,** Note central giant cell with fingerlike cytoplasmic process.

of exceedingly well-differentiated liposarcoma grossly resembles a lipoma. Intramuscular lipomas can occur (Greenberg et al.[40]). We have seen one of the soft tissue of the arm that was inadequately excised and regrew after a twenty-year interval.

Microscopically, liposarcoma may have an extremely variable pattern. In a few instances, it may be well differentiated (Enzinger and Winslow[33a]). This type and the myxoid variant tend to remain localized. Liposarcomas with signet-ring cells showing cytoplasmic fat are easily recognized (Fig. 715). There are also highly undifferentiated small cell types and those with bizarre giant cells.

Rhabdomyosarcomas are infrequent malignant soft tissue sarcomas, are deep seated, and may take the shape of the muscle from which they arise (Fig. 716, A). They often become large and may ulcerate through the skin to form a fungating hemorrhagic mass (Fig. 717). Microscopic ex-

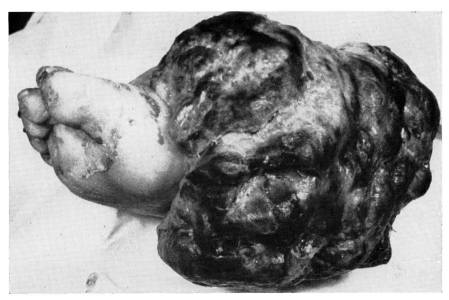

Fig. 717. Large fungating rhabdomyosarcoma of foot.

amination reveals tumor growing in close proximity to, or in intimate relation with, striated muscle. Tennis racket–shaped cells in particular may present cross striations or longitudinal myofibrils, and giant cells with peripherally arranged vacuolation resemble spiders or spider webs (Stout[102]) (Fig. 716, *B*). The cytoplasm is invariably strongly acidophilic. The alveolar form may be mistaken microscopically for reticulum cell sarcoma (Riopelle and Theriault[90]).

Granular cell myoblastoma is a rare lesion, probably a neoplasm. Grossly, on cut section, it mimics a malignant tumor, for it is poorly defined and firm with grayish white streaks. Frequently, there are bizarre epithelial alterations overlying the lesion that may be mistaken for carcinoma. Thus far, we have seen these changes in granular cell myoblastoma of the tongue, skin, larynx, vulva, and anus. We believe that these lesions are, with rare exception, benign (Mackenzie[64]). Microscopically, individual cells have prominent granular cytoplasm, and frequently there is an intimate association with nerve filaments suggesting a neurogenic origin. Histogenesis of this tumor is unknown (Pearse[79]; Stout[110]).

Synovial sarcomas arise in close proximity to tendons, tendon sheaths, and the exterior walls of the bursal pouches and joint capsules (Wright[118]) but only rarely involve the joint synovia. This is an important point in the differential diagnosis because synovial hyperplasia, hemangiomas, and other lesions show involvement of the synovia. Grossly, the synovial sarcoma is fairly firm, appears encapsulated, and is grayish pink. On section, it remains grayish pink but may show areas of hemorrhage and calcification. It is often firmly fixed to a neighboring structure (joint, bursa, or tendon sheath). Microscopically, there must be two elements present: an intimate intermingling web of adenomatous structures and a sarcomatous-like stroma (Fig. 718). These adenomatous areas may look very much like synovial membrane. The cells secrete a sticky mucoid substance, hyaluronic acid, which is usually found in joints. A single section may contain only one of these elements so that multiple sections should be studied in order to differentiate synovial sarcomas from adenocarcinomas or fibrosarcomas.

Angiosarcoma (hemangioendothelioma) is a malignant tumor of blood vessel origin which, although rare, may arise wherever there are blood vessels. A malignant blood vessel tumor does not arise from a hemangioma. The apparent encapsulation of the tumor is a false one. The cut section is hemorrhagic in appearance. The

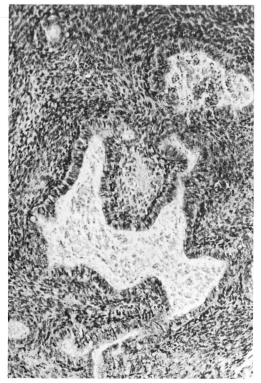

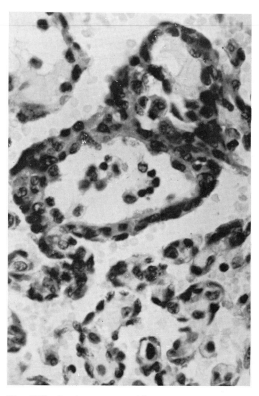

Fig. 718. Synovial sarcoma with mingling of pseudoglandular elements and sarcomatous stroma. (High-power enlargement.)

Fig. 719. Angiosarcoma with anastomosing vascular channels and layering of cells. (High-power enlargement.)

microscopic findings are characteristic. Silver stains clarify the picture by demonstrating a layering of the endothelial cells and the invariable presence of anastomosing vascular channels (Fig. 719). *Hemangiopericytoma* (a vascular tumor usually of low malignancy) has been described by Stout[107] and O'Brien and Brasfield.[74]

Alveolar soft part sarcoma is a rare tumor of the soft tissue. Grossly, it forms a soft, yellowish gray well-delimited mass. Microscopically, it shows nests of cells with granular cytoplasm surrounded by delicate connective tissue septa, giving it an organoid pattern. Its histogenesis is unknown (Fisher[36]).

Rarely, *osteosarcoma* and *chondrosarcoma* arise from soft tissues (Fine and Stout[35]). They behave as malignant tumors. *Leiomyosarcomas* are rare. Grossly, particularly in the retroperitoneal area, they show cystic degeneration (Lumb[61]). Microscopically, differential fiber stains may be necessary to reveal myofibrils.

Lymphomas and *plasma cell tumors* have been rarely reported as arising in soft tissues. Many of these lesions are not true neoplasms (Lattes and Pochter[55]). Detailed review of the pathologic characteristics of this entire group of neoplasms is available (Enzinger et al.[32a]; Stout and Lattes[112]). Elastofibroma is a rare lesion, probably not a true neoplasm, that occurs most frequently in the subscapular area (Jarvi et al.[48]). Myxosarcoma probably does not exist as an entity, but intramuscular myxomas which are benign are most common in the vastus lateralis muscle (Enzinger[31a]).

Metastatic spread

Regional lymph node metastases in *fibrosarcomas* occur rather frequently. However, distant metastases are infrequent in dermatofibrosarcoma protuberans (McPeak et al.[65]). The *synovial sarcoma* also metastasizes to regional nodes. In 104 collected cases, the inguinal nodes were involved in seven and the axillary nodes in four (Haagensen and Stout[42]). *Rhabdomyosarcomas* and *liposarcomas* also involve regional lymph nodes, but not nearly so frequently, and the extraosseous *osteosarcomas* practically never have node metastases. *Leiomyosarcomas* often recur locally and may have distant metastases. All of these sarcomas tend to metastasize distantly, particularly to the lungs, and not infrequently to other organs such as liver and bone. Occasionally, the metastases are widely disseminated to many organs.

Clinical evolution

Soft tissue sarcomas are discovered either by accident or because of symptoms due to their encroachment upon vital organs or nerves. Those arising in the soft tissues of the leg, thigh, or upper extremity may reach a fairly large size before pain or disability occurs. In the retroperitoneal area and particularly around the kidney, the sarcomas may become huge before they provoke symptoms by infringing upon the function of the neighboring organs (kidneys, ureters, bladder, or intestinal tract). If treatment is not instituted, they may rupture through the skin to ulcerate and become infected. Hemorrhages from their surface with resultant secondary anemia and infection may cause general symptoms with fever and weight loss. Local pain is invariably present with advanced disease. With distant metastases, a rather profound weight loss may quickly ensue.

Fibrosarcomas occur predominantly in the trunk and lower extremities but are occasionally found in the upper extremity, head, or neck (Stout[105]). In the skin, they may present as a single nodule (Darier[23]) or take the multinodular character of *dermatofibroma protuberans* of Hoffmann (Fig. 720). *Liposarcomas* may arise in any area in which there is fat—gluteal regions, popliteal spaces, thighs, retroperitoneal space, upper extremity, and neck in that approximate order of frequency (Stout[101]). *Rhabdomyosarcomas* develop in the lower and upper extremities, head, and trunk (Cappell[15]). The botryoid variety predominates in the urogenital tracts of children, and the embryonal variety develops in the extremities and orbit (Kassel et al.[50]) and middle ear (Davison[24]) of children. Rhab-

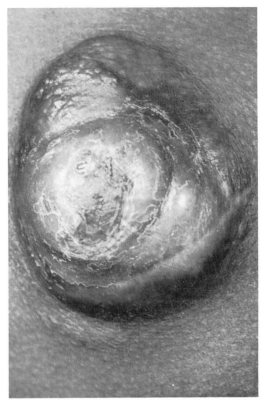

Fig. 720. Dermatofibrosarcoma protuberans occurring on buttock of black patient. (WU neg. neg. 57-5168.)

domyosarcomas may infiltrate the skin surface, become reddened, ulcerate, and bleed (Fig. 721). *Granular cell myoblastomas* occur most frequently in the tongue (Crane and Tremblay[18]) but also in the skin, vulva, breast, larynx, esophagus, bronchus, rectum, bladder, etc.

Synovial sarcomas arise predominantly in the lower extremities, mostly in the knee and ankle joint (Haagensen and Stout[42]) but may also present at the hand, wrist, and elbow (Cadman et al.[14]). *Angiosarcomas* are frequently found in muscles and subcutaneous tissues but also occur in the breast, liver, pleura, and other structures. Their origin from postsurgical (Stewart and Treves[96]) or chronic lymphedema (Eby et al.[28]; Danese et al.[22]) has been noted. *Alveolar soft parts sarcomas* are most frequently found in the extremities. *Leiomyosarcomas* may arise in the retroperitoneal space and, very rarely, in the extremities (Stout[110]). Leiomyosarcomas in children

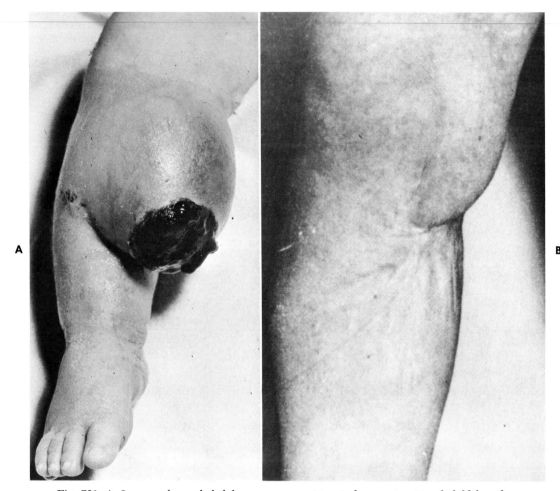

Fig. 721. A, Large embryonal rhabdomyosarcoma arising in lower extremity of child less than 1 month of age (tumor was present at birth). Treatment was local excision. **B,** Eight years after operation. (**A,** From Pack, G. T., and Eberhart, W. F.: Rhabdomyosarcoma of skeletal muscle, Surgery **32**:1023-1064, 1952; **B,** from Lawrence, W., Jr., et al.: Embryonal rhabdomyosarcoma; a clinicopathological study, Cancer **17**:361-376, 1964.)

do not differ in evolution from those in adults (Botting et al.[12]). Enzinger[31] reported a rare but definite sarcoma arising from tendons and aponeuroses, which he designated as a clear cell type.

Diagnosis

The diagnosis of soft tissue sarcomas may be difficult in the early stages of evolution because often they may appear encapsulated on palpation, and the diagnosis of sarcoma is not considered. At the time of examination, an attempt should be made to determine whether the tumor is attached to the overlying skin, muscle, or underlying bone, for this may determine operability. The retroperitoneal sarcoma is often very large at the time of the first examination and palpates as a rather large, indefinite mass of variable consistency. Rhabdomyosarcomas may appear mobile when the involved muscle is at rest but become fixed on contraction. The liposarcoma is often deep, bulky, and nodular. Nerve sheath tumors may have fusiform configuration, movable from side to side, but not on the long axis of the extremity. Angiosarcomas occur predominantly in the lower extremities, as do many other soft tissue sarcomas.

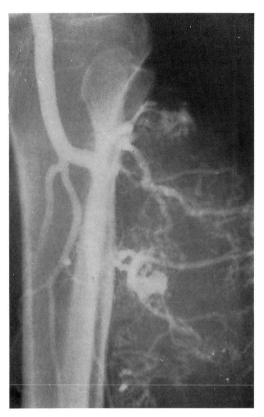

Fig. 722. Arteriogram of large sarcoma (hemangiopericytoma) of leg in 67-year-old man. Extent of tumor and its vascular pattern demonstrated that amputation was necessary. (Courtesy Dr. A. R. Margulis, San Francisco, Calif.)

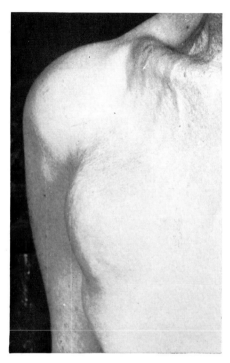

Fig. 723. Liposarcoma arising in region of anterior axillary border—soft, fairly well circumscribed, and impossible to differentiate clinically from lipoma. Patient remains well five years after radical excision.

Roentgenologic examination

Roentgenologic examination frequently shows the extent of the tumor, often seen as a somewhat circumscribed shadow with slightly increased density over the surrounding soft tissue. This examination is of greatest help in determining whether there is bone destruction or thinning of the cortex of the underlying bone due to pressure atrophy by the tumor. The presence of periosteal thickening, together with an irregularity of contour, might suggest that the tumor is attached to the bone. Careful soft tissue roentgenographic studies are helpful in synovial tumors, showing at times the presence of calcification, but usually the mass is a homogeneous water density mass often closely associated with a joint, particularly the knee joint (Sherman and Chu[94]). However, in the series reported by Cadman et al.,[14] calcification

was demonstrated in one-third. In the diagnosis of retroperitoneal sarcomas, intravenous pyelography (anterior and lateral views) is the most useful diagnostic procedure (DeWeerd and Dockerty[26]). Liposarcomas of the retroperitoneal space and other areas may be revealed by areas of radiolucency (Schick and Rogers[93]). Hemangiopericytoma may cause pressure erosion on bones (Mujahed et al.[70]).

Arteriography has been increasingly used in the study of these tumors. The procedure can be done expeditiously without morbidity (Margulis and Murphy[66]). In malignant tumors, the vascularity is greatly increased, the vessels are large and run at different angles, and arteriovenous shunts are present. Hemangiopericytoma has particularly prominent vascularization (Pinet et al.[84]). The more malignant the tumor, the greater may be the vascularization

(Lagergren et al.[54]). Thus, arteriography may be sufficiently conclusive to determine the extent of an excision (Rosenberg[91]) (Fig. 722).

Differential diagnosis

Soft tissue sarcomas may be confused with *benign tumors* such as lipomas, neurofibromas, hemangiomas, and leiomyomas (Fig. 723). These benign tumors usually have a long clinical evolution with very slow increase in size. They are freely movable and not firmly attached to underlying structures. The sarcoma, on the other hand, ordinarily grows fairly rapidly and becomes fixed to the underlying tissue. A *sebaceous cyst* can become fastened to the overlying skin. In rare instances, *Ewing's sarcoma* may have inconspicuous symptoms referable to bone and may masquerade as a soft tissue sarcoma. Myxopapillary ependymomas can be present in the soft tissue over the sacrococcygeal region and can be mistaken for a chondroma or a sweat gland tumor (Anderson[7]). *Aneurysms* of large blood vessels can also be confused with a sarcoma, but the roentgenographic examination may help in differentiation. *Subcutaneous abscesses* are usually painful and are associated with fever and other signs of infection. Liposarcomas of the popliteal space are often incorrectly diagnosed as *Baker's cysts*.

Fibrosarcomas of soft tissues must be differentiated from the numerous highly proliferative fibrous tissue lesions with which they are confused. During the past few years, numerous lesions have been separated from true sarcomas. The synovial aponeurotic fibroma is the cartilage analogue of fibromatosis and may be confused with sarcoma (Lichtenstein and Goldman[58]). A much more common lesion, however, is *nodular fasciitis* (Konwaler et al.[52]). Price et al.[85] described sixty-five cases, forty-five of which were in men. The lesions were most common on the upper extremities and trunk and usually occurred in a subcutaneous location (thirteen were in the deep fascia). In our experience, these lesions often have a rather rapid growth with poorly defined margins and are usually incorrectly diagnosed as fibrosarcoma or liposarcoma. They do not, as a rule, reach a large size. In children, Stout[109] described

proliferations of the fibrous tissue forming indistinct masses and designated them *juvenile fibromatosis*. *Desmoids* are found on the abdominal wall of women during pregnancy but may occur in other locations (Pearman and Mayo[80]) and may be found in children. The region of the shoulder is a frequent location. Desmoids grossly infiltrate the muscle and may have poorly defined margins but, although poorly encapsulated, they are not called malignant (Figs. 724 and 725) and never metastasize (Hunt et al.[46]). As many as half of them recur after excision (Enzinger and Shiraki[33]).

Myositis ossificans is a poor name for a group of lesions appearing in the soft tissue that may or may not be associated with periosteum. It is a poor designation established by custom. There is no inflammation and often no bone and, in some instances, muscle is not included in the pathologic process. The localized lesion, classic "myositis ossificans," occurs particularly in young and vigorous male adults. "Strauss' statistics dealing with 127 cases of traumatic myositis ossificans show the following anatomic distribution: sixty-four of these occurred in the flexor muscles of the upper arm, the brachialis anticus being the one most frequently affected; forty-three occurred in the quadriceps femoris; thirteen in the adductor muscles of the thigh; two in the gluteal muscles; one in the muscles of the ball of the thumb; and one in the temporal muscle."[*]

We have seen myositis ossificans in atypical locations such as the buttock; frequently, an incorrect diagnosis of sarcoma is first made and amputation recommended (Ackerman[4]). The diagnosis of these lesions is difficult for many reasons. In only about half the patients is there a history of trauma. The lesion may first present as a rather large soft tissue tumor. The pathologist may call it sarcoma because of the excessive cellularity and great variation in cell size and shape. A correct diagnosis can be made by paying strict attention microscopically to evidence of maturation. This maturation progresses from the center to the periphery (Fig.

---

[*]From Lewis, D.: Myositis ossificans, J.A.M.A. 80:1281-1287, 1923.

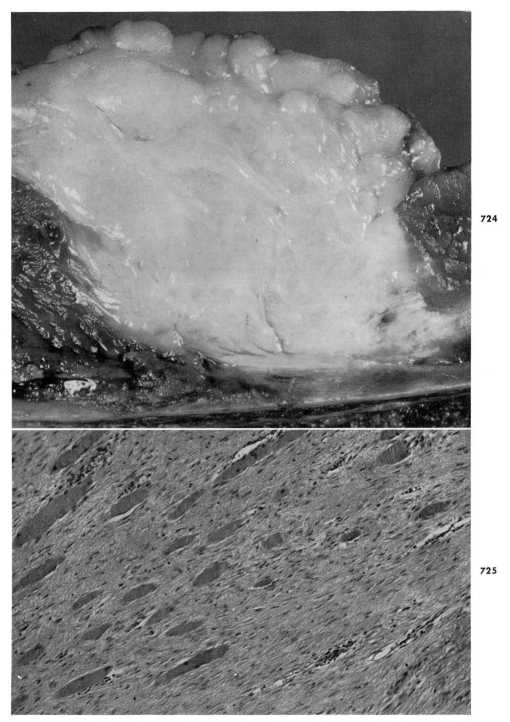

Fig. 724. Large desmoid tumor of arm with poorly defined margins that became firmly attached to periosteum of humerus, necessitating partial resection of this bone. (WU neg. 58-5952.)

Fig. 725. Desmoid tumor with well-differentiated fibrous tissue infiltrating muscle bundles. Note lack of delimitation. (Low power; WU neg. 59-3743.)

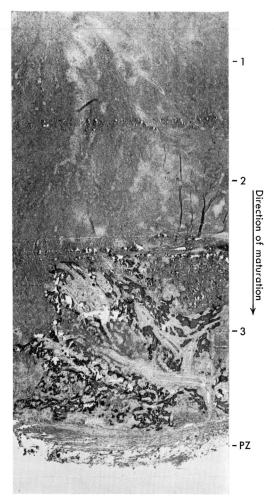

Direction of maturation

- 1

- 2

- 3

- PZ

Fig. 726. Myositis ossificans. Encapsulation and different pattern of zones from innermost cellular zone to outermost (peripheral) zone showing well-delimited bone. (Low power; WU neg. 57-1317.)

726). The central portion suggests undifferentiated sarcoma, the midportion demonstrates osteoid that has some degree of orientation, and the periphery shows well-oriented bone. With the passage of time, progressive maturation of the bone is seen and can be demonstrated roentgenologically. In the rare extraosteosarcoma of soft tissue, there is no evidence of zone phenomena or maturation, and sections from these tumors show a similar pattern throughout (Fine and Stout[35]). *Proliferative myositis* may form a poorly defined mass with extremely bizarre microscopic pattern. This pattern is probably related

to trauma to the muscle. There is sarcolemmal proliferation, attempts at muscle regeneration, and extremely disorderly appearance (Enzinger and Dulcey[32]).

Giant cell tumors of the tendon sheaths may be confused with fibrosarcomas when they become large or are extremely cellular (Galloway et al.[38]; Jaffe et al.[47]; Stewart[97]). They infrequently recur locally and invade bone (Fletcher and Horn[37]) but do not metastasize. D'Agostino et al.[20] reported twenty-one patients with Recklinghausen's disease in whom sarcomas developed. These sarcomas usually develop in the soft tissue of the extremities, posterior mediastinum, or retroperitoneal area. These tumors usually recur locally a number of times before distant metastases appear. Therefore, if the lesion is in the extremity, a local recrudescence often may be treated with hope of cure.

Metastatic carcinomas growing in the soft tissues, particularly in the thigh, may simulate a soft tissue sarcoma. When the primary lesion has remained asymptomatic, the diagnosis may be difficult. Carcinomas of the kidney are most prone to produce such a clinical picture. Patients with metastatic carcinoma usually present a rapidly deteriorating general condition that is unusual in those with the well-localized soft tissue sarcoma.

Treatment
Surgery

The treatment of choice of soft tissue sarcomas is adequate surgical excision. In any clinically suspicious lesion, an incisional biopsy should be done before definitive treatment is decided upon. Rarely, a diagnosis can be made on a needle biopsy. Whenever a definitive diagnosis can be reached on frozen section, this is, of course, proper basis for a decision. Often, permanent sections are required (Lieberman and Ackerman[60]). But it is wrong to proceed to a biopsy without discussing the possible issues with the patient and his relatives, for if amputation were a necessary definitive treatment, there should be no delay between diagnosis and any necessary surgery. Likewise, whenever the surgeon enucleates what turns out to be pseudoencapsulated sarcoma, delay and incurability may ensue (Ariel and Pack[8]).

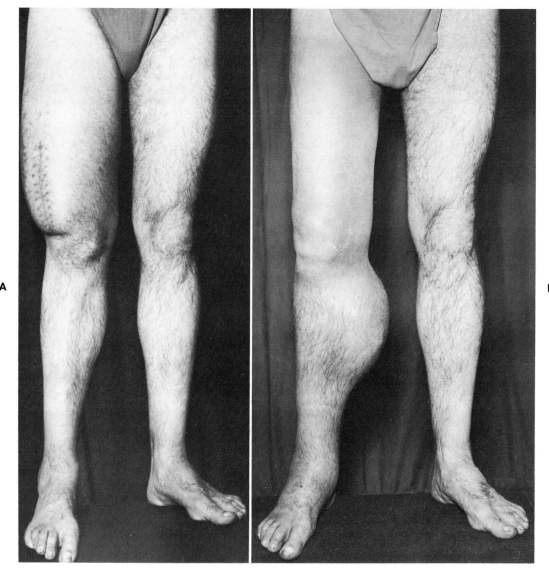

Fig. 727. **A,** Synovial sarcoma appearing in typical location in 33-year-old man. **B,** Local recrudescence after inadequate surgical incision. (From Cade, Sir Stanford: Synovial sarcoma, J. Roy. Coll. Surg. Edinb. **8:**1-51, 1962.)

In certain locations, such as the inner aspects of the thigh, if primary inadequate enucleation is done, then further treatment may necessitate amputation or even hemi-pelvectomy (Fig. 727). In the well-differentiated tumors without extension to deeper structures and with a favorable location, local excision can be done without amputation. If the tumor is large and adherent to skeletal structures or located in unfavorable places, such as deep in the thigh, primary amputation may have to be done (Pack and Ariel[76]). The largest proportion of these tumors develop in the extremities (Clark et al.[17]). Thus, their surgical treatment often involves consideration of pathology, anatomy, and function. We do not adhere to the point of view that site rather than histopathology should be the determining factor of the type of surgery to be used in all cases (Fig. 728).

Fibrosarcoma, rhabdomyosarcoma, liposarcoma, and particularly synovial sarcoma may metastasize to the regional lymph

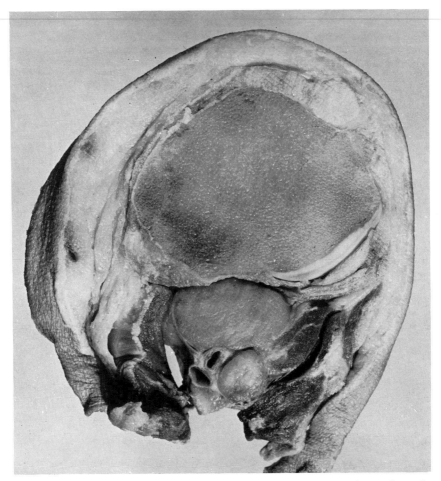

Fig. 728. Pseudoencapsulated fibrosarcoma of popliteal space. Note close relationship to bone and vessels. It would have been impossible to locally excise this neoplasm. (WU neg. 53-5763.)

nodes. The occurrence of such metastases, however, is low, and radical regional lymph node dissection is indicated only in the presence of clinically enlarged nodes. Metastasis should be properly proved by incisional or needle aspiration before doing such dissection.

Radiotherapy

For a long time, the false concept of *"radioresistance"* of soft tissue sarcomas has been widely accepted. This view was based upon the fact that the majority of these tumors regress slowly after irradiation (Regato[87]) and that seldom are they sufficiently irradiated to test their curability by this means (Windeyer et al.[119]). Evidence has accumulated slowly from various sources that many of these tumors are radiosensitive and that some are definitely radiocurable. Radiotherapy should not be considered as an alternative to surgery. In some special circumstances of location and character of tumor, it may be the treatment of choice. In others, radiotherapy has been established as an important surgical adjunct. In some cases of postsurgical recurrence, radiotherapy may be the only recourse. Patients with inoperable *fibrosarcomas* have been cured by radiotherapy and others have been afforded considerable palliation. Windeyer et al.[119] consider preoperative radiotherapy preferable to postoperative.

The radiosensitivity and radiocurability of *liposarcomas* have long been recognized. Thorough postoperative irradiation of the tumor area is now widely recommended as a procedure of choice if the excision has been inadequate (Pack and Ariel[76]). Edland[30] reported his observations on fifteen cases of liposarcoma treated by radiotherapy, noting that few liposarcomas are totally radioresistant. He advocates routine postoperative irradiation in all cases of liposarcoma.

Most *rhabdomyosarcomas* are radioresponsive (Edland[29]; Perry and Chu[81]). Radiotherapy is most effective in the embryonal type of rhabdomyosarcoma (Albores-Saavedra et al.[6]). Some cases of long-standing control have been reported (Horn and Enterline[45]). Cassady et al.[16] conclude that adequately planned radiotherapy is the treatment of choice of rhabdomyosarcomas of the orbit.

The radiosensitivity of *synovial sarcomas* has been long disputed (Haagensen and Stout[42]; Pack and Ariel[75]), probably due to differences in histopathologic concepts. Preoperative and postoperative irradiation have come to be considered of value (Cade[13]; Berman[10]; Raben et al.[86]), and occasional cases of cure by means of radiations alone have been obtained (Pack and Ariel[75]).

We have observed a case of *hemangiosarcoma* of the breast that was completely destroyed locally by irradiation. *Leiomyosarcomas* may be radiosensitive in their primary or metastatic manifestations (Gunn and Kramer[41]). Despite the foregoing considerations, in the present state of our experience seldom is it justified to offer radiotherapy as an alternative to surgery. Frequently, however, adjuvant radiotherapy may be indicated.

Palliative treatment

Attempts at palliation by means of perfusion of antineoplastic drugs (Krementz and Shaver[53]) or combination of chemotherapy and radiotherapy (Molander[68]) may prove demanding but, at times, rewarding.

Prognosis

The prognosis of soft tissue sarcomas depends on various factors—type of sarcoma, degree of differentiation or undifferentiation of the tumor, location of the neoplasm, age of the patient, and adequacy of the treatment. A favorable combination of these circumstances may result in the cure of a patient, whereas a single unfavorable factor in another may decide his fate. Sarcomas located in the retroperitoneal space or mediastinum can rarely be adequately excised. Amputation or disarticulation of an extremity succeeds in the cure of rather malignant sarcomas provided surgery is done before metastases have occurred, whereas "enucleation" or attempts at conservative excision may fail to control a rather differentiated or localized neoplasm.

Fibrosarcomas that are found at birth or in young children have a very good prognosis (Stout[111]; Balsaver et al.[9]). There is very good correlation between the relative differentiation of fibrosarcomas and their prognoses. van der Werf-Messing and van Unnik[116] have shown that this differentiation can be assessed through the mitotic index. *Liposarcomas* that develop superficially have the best prognosis (Phelan and Perez-Mesa[83]), whereas those that arise in the retroperitoneal space are seldom cured (DeWeerd and Dockerty[26]). The degree of differentiation of liposarcomas correlates very well with their prognosis. Enzinger and Winslow[33] reported a series of patients with liposarcomas with a five-year survival rate of 85% for patients with well-differentiated tumors, 77% for those with the myxoid type, 21% for those with the pleomorphic type, and 18% for those with the round-cell type. Well-differentiated liposarcomas in children have an excellent prognosis (Kauffman and Stout[49]).

Most patients with rhabdomyosarcomas do poorly no matter what the location or the treatment. Under exceptionally favorable circumstances, however, a few are cured. Lawrence et al.[56] reported seven of forty-four patients with embryonal rhabdomyosarcoma living five years following treatment. The prognosis of *synovial sarcomas* is usually somber. Haagensen and Stout[42] collected 104 cases in which, for the most part, treatment had been conservative and found that only three patients survived more than five years. At times, adequate local excision of synovial sarcomas in children results in cure. Crocker and Stout[19] reported nine cases of five-year survival in children. Cadman et al.[14] reported 107 patients with synovial sarcoma, twenty-seven (25%) of whom survived five years. Twelve patients lived for more than ten years, three of whom died of tumor—one after eleven years and two after fourteen years.

The prognosis of *hemangiosarcomas* is invariably poor. *Leiomyosarcomas*, depending on location, may be amenable to cure. Malignant schwannomas do surprisingly well with adequate surgery (White[117]).

REFERENCES

1 Abrikossoff, A. I.: Weitere Untersuchungen über Myoblastenmyome, Virchow Arch. Path. Anat. **280**:723-740, 1931.

2 Ackerman, L. V.: Multiple primary liposarcomas, Amer. J. Path. **20**:789-798, 1944.

3 Ackerman, L. V.: Tumors of the peritoneum, mesentery, and retroperitoneum. In Atlas of tumor pathology, Sect. VI, Fascs. 23 and 24, Washington, D. C., 1953, Armed Forces Institute of Pathology.

4 Ackerman, L. V.: Extra-osseous localized non-neoplastic bone and cartilage formation (so-called myositis ossificans), J. Bone Joint Surg. **40-A**:279-298, 1958.

5 Aird, I., Weinbren, K., and Walter, L.: Angiosarcoma in a limb—the seat of spontaneous lymphoedema, Brit. J. Cancer **10**:424-430, 1956.

6 Albores-Saavedra, J., Martin, R. G., and Smith, J. L., Jr.: Rhabdomyosarcoma; a study of 35 cases, Ann. Surg. **157**:186-197, 1963.

7 Anderson, M. S.: Myxopapillary ependymomas presenting in the soft tissue over the sacrococcygeal region, Cancer **19**:585-590, 1966.

8 Ariel, I. M., and Pack, G. T.: Synovial sarcoma; review of 25 cases, New Eng. J. Med. **268**:1272-1275, 1963.

9 Balsaver, A. M., Butler, J. J., and Martin, R. G.: Congenital fibrosarcoma, Cancer **20**:1607-1616, 1967.

10 Berman, H. L.: The role of raliation therapy in the management of synovial sarcoma, Radiology **81**:997-1002, 1963.

11 Black, W. C., McGavran, M. H., and Graham, P.: Nodular subepidermal fibrosis; a clinical pathologic study emphasizing the frequency of clinical misdiagnoses, Arch. Surg. (Chicago) **98**:296-300, 1969.

12 Botting, A. J., Soule, E. H., and Brown, A. L., Jr.: Smooth muscle tumors in children, Cancer **18**:711-720, 1965.

13 Cade, S.: Synovial sarcoma, J. Roy. Coll. Surg. Edinb. **8**:1-51, 1962.

14 Cadman, N. L., Soule, E. H., and Kelley, P. J.: Synovial sarcoma: an analysis of 134 tumors, Cancer **18**:613-627, 1965.

15 Cappell, D. F.: Tumours of striated muscle, Ann. Roy. Coll. Surg. Eng. **2**:80-82, 1948.

16 Cassady, J. R., Sagerman, R. H., Tretter, P., and Ellsworth, R. M.: Radiation therapy for

rhabdomyosarcoma, Radiology **91**:116-120, 1968.

17 Clark, R. L., Martin, R. G., White, E. C., and Old, J. W.: Clinical aspects of soft-tissue tumors, Arch. Surg. (Chicago) **74**:859-870, 1957.

18 Crane, A. R., and Tremblay, R. G.: Myoblastoma, Amer. J. Path. **21**:357-375, 1945.

19 Crocker, D. W., and Stout, A. P.: Synovial sarcoma in children, Cancer **12**:1123-1133, 1959.

20 D'Agostino, A. N., Soule, E. H., and Miller, R. H.: Sarcomas of the peripheral nerves and somatic soft tissues associated with multiple neurofibromas (von Recklinghausen's disease), Cancer **16**:1015-1027, 1963.

21 Dahn, I., Johnson, N., and Lundh, G.: Desmoid tumors; a series of 33 cases, Acta Chir. Scand. **126**:305-314, 1963.

22 Danese, C. A., Grishman, E., Oh, C., and Dreiling, D. A.: Malignant vascular tumors of the lymphedematous extremity, Ann. Surg. **166**:245-253, 1967.

23 Darier, J.: Dermatofibromes progressifs et recidvants ou fibrosarcomes de la peau, Ann. Derm. Syph. (Paris) **5**:545-562, 1924.

24 Davison, R. C.: Rhabdomyosarcoma of the middle ear, Laryngoscope **76**:1889-1920, 1966.

25 DeForest, E. H.: Synovioma; with special reference to the clinical and roentgenologic aspects, Amer. J. Roentgen. **65**:769-777, 1951.

26 DeWeerd, J. H., and Dockerty, M. B.: Lipomatous retroperitoneal tumors, Amer. J. Surg. **84**:397-407, 1952.

27 Dito, W. R., and Batsakis, J. G.: Rhabdomyosarcoma of the head and neck; an appraisal of the biologic behavior in 170 cases, Arch. Surg. (Chicago) **84**:582-588, 1962.

28 Eby, C. S., Brennan, M. J., and Fine, G.: Lymphangiosarcoma; a lethal complication of chronic lymphedema—report of two cases and review of the literature, Arch. Surg. (Chicago) **94**:223-230, 1967.

29 Edland, R. W.: Embryonal rhabdomyosarcoma, Amer. J. Roentgen. **93**:671-685, 1965.

30 Edland, R. W.: Liposarcoma; a retrospective study of fifteen cases, a review of the literature and a discussion of radiosensitivity, Amer. J. Roentgen. **103**:778-791, 1968.

31 Enzinger, F. M.: Clear-cell sarcoma of tendons and aponeuroses; an analysis of 21 cases, Cancer **18**:1163-1174, 1965.

31a Enzinger, F. M.: Intramuscular myxoma, Amer. J. Clin. Path. **43**:104-113, 1965.

32 Enzinger, F. M., and Dulcey, F.: Proliferative myositis; a report of 33 cases, Cancer **20**:2213-2223, 1967.

32a Enzinger, F. M., Lattes, R., and Torloni, H.: International Classification of Tumours, No. 3: Histological typing of soft tissue tumours, Geneva, 1969, World Health Organization.

33 Enzinger, F. M., and Shiraki, M.: Musculo-aponeurotic fibromatosis of the shoulder girdle (extra-abdominal desmoid), Cancer **20**:1131-1140, 1967.

33a Enzinger, F. M., and Winslow, D. J.: Liposarcoma; a study of 103 cases, Virchow Arch. Path. Anat. **335**:367-388, 1962.

34 Farbman, A. A.: Retroperitoneal fatty tumors; a report of case and collective review of literature from 1937 to 1947, Arch. Surg. (Chicago) **60**:343-362, 1950.

35 Fine, G., and Stout, A. P.: Osteogenic sarcoma of the extraskeletal soft tissues, Cancer **9**:1027-1043, 1956.

36 Fisher, E. R.: Histochemical observations on alveolar soft-part sarcoma with reference to histogenesis, Amer. J. Path. **32**:721-737, 1956.

37 Fletcher, A. G., Jr., and Horn, R. C., Jr.: Giant cell tumors of tendon sheath origin; a consideration of bone involvement and report of two cases with extensive bone destruction, Ann. Surg. **133**:374-385, 1951.

38 Galloway, J. D. B., Broder, A. C., and Ghormley, R.: Xanthoma of tendon sheaths and synovial membrane; clinical and pathologic study, Arch. Surg. (Chicago) **40**:485-538, 1940.

39 Gentele, H.: Malignant, fibroblastic tumors of the skin; clinical and pathological-anatomical studies of 129 cases of malignant, fibroblastic tumors from the cutaneous and subcutaneous layers observed at Radiumhemmet during the period 1927-1947, Acta Dermatovener. (Stockholm) **31**(suppl. 27):1-180, 1951 (extensive bibliography).

40 Greenberg, S. D., Isensee, C., Gonzalez-Angulo, A., and Wallace, S. A.: Infiltrating lipomas of the thigh, Amer. J. Clin. Path. **39**:66-72, 1963.

41 Gunn, W. G., and Kramer, S.: The value of radiation therapy in leiomyosarcoma of the uterus, Radiology **81**:854-860, 1963.

42 Haagensen, C. D., and Stout, A. P.: Synovial sarcoma, Ann. Surg. **120**:826-842, 1944.

43 Herrmann, J.: Sarcomatous transformation in multiple neurofibromatosis (von Recklinghausen's disease); report of four cases, Ann. Surg. **131**:206-217, 1950.

44 Herrmann, J. B., and Gruhn, J. G.: Lymphangiosarcoma secondary to chronic lymphedema, Surg. Gynec. Obstet. **105**:665-674, 1957.

45 Horn, R. C., and Enterline, H. T.: Rhabdomyosarcoma; a clinicopathological study and classification of 39 cases, Cancer **2**:181-199, 1958.

46 Hunt, R. T., Morgan, H. C., and Ackerman, L. V.: Principles in the management of extra-abdominal desmoids, Cancer **13**:825-836, 1960.

47 Jaffe, H. L., Lichtenstein, L., and Sutro, C. J.: Pigmented villo-nodular synovitis, bursitis, and tenosynovitis, Arch. Path. (Chicago) **31**:731-765, 1941.

48 Jarvi, O. H., Saxen, A. E., Hopsu-Havu, V. K., Wartiovaara, J. J., and Caissalo, V. T.: Elastofibroma—a degenerative pseudotumor, Cancer **23**:42-63, 1969.

49 Kauffman, S. L., and Stout, A. P.: Lipoblastic tumors of children, Cancer **12**:912-925, 1959.

50 Kassel, S. H., Copenhaver, R., and Areán, V. M.: Orbital rhabdomyosarcoma, Amer. J. Ophthal. **60**:811-818, 1965.

51 Kleinstiver, B. J., and Rodriguez, H. A.: Nodular fasciitis; a study of forty-five cases and review of the literature, J. Bone Joint Surg. **50-A**:1204-1212, 1968.

52 Konwaler, B. E., Keasbey, L. E., and Kaplan, L.: Subcutaneous pseudocarcinomatous fibromatosis (fasciitis), Amer. J. Clin. Path. **25**:241-252, 1955.

53 Krementz, E. T., and Shaver, J. O.: Behavior and treatment of soft tissue sarcomas, Ann. Surg. **157**:770-784, 1963.

54 Lagergren, C., Lindbom, A., and Söderberg, G.: Vascularization of fibromatous and fibrosarcomatous tumors, Acta Radiol. (Stockholm) **53**:1-16, 1960.

55 Lattes, R., and Pochter, M. R.: Benign lymphoid masses of probable hamartomatous nature; analysis of 12 cases, Cancer **15**:197-214, 1962.

56 Lawrence, W., Jr., Jegge, G., and Foote, F. W.: Embryonal rhabdomyosarcoma; a clinicopathological study, Cancer **17**:361-376, 1964.

57 Lewis, D.: Myositis ossificans, J.A.M.A. **80**:1281-1287, 1923.

58 Lichtenstein, L., and Goldman, R. L.: The cartilage analogue of fibromatosis; a reinterpretation of the condition called "juvenile aponeurotic fibroma," Cancer **17**:810-816, 1964.

59 Lieberman, P. H., Foote, F. W., Stewart, F. W., and Berg, J. W.: Alveolar soft-part sarcoma, J.A.M.A. **198**:1047-1051, 1966.

60 Lieberman, Z., and Ackerman, L. V.: Principles in management of soft tissue sarcomas, Surgery **35**:350-365, 1954.

61 Lumb, G.: Smooth-muscle tumours of the gastro-intestinal tract and retroperitoneal tissues presenting as large cystic masses, J. Path. Bact. **63**:139-147, 1951.

62 McCarthy, W. D., and Pack, G. T.: Malignant blood vessel tumors; a report of 56 cases of angiosarcoma and Kaposi's sarcoma, Surg. Gynec. Obstet. **91**:465-482, 1950.

63 Mackenzie, D. H.: Synovial sarcoma, Cancer **19**:169-180, 1966.

64 Mackenzie, D. H.: Malignant granular cell myoblastoma, J. Clin. Path. **20**:739-742, 1967.

65 McPeak, C. J., Cruz, T., and Nicastri, A. D.: Dermatofibrosarcoma protuberans; an analysis of 86 cases-five with metastasis, Ann. Surg. **166**:803-816, 1967.

66 Margulis, A. R., and Murphy, T. O.: Arteriography in neoplasms of extremities, Amer. J. Roentgen. **80**:330-339, 1958.

67 Marques, P., Planel, H., and Hemous, G.: Sarcome fibroblastique de le langue aprés curiethérapie pour épithélioma spinocellulaire, Bull. Ass. Franc. Cancer **39**:214-216, 1952.

68 Molander, D. W.: Palliative treatment of metastatic tumors of the soft somatic tissues with irradiation and chemotherapy, Amer. J. Roentgen. **96**:150-157, 1966.

69 Morris, J. M., and Lucas, D. B.: Fibrosarcoma within a sinus tract of chronic draining

osteomyelitis; a case report and review of literature, J. Bone Joint Surg. **46-A**:853-857, 1964.

70 Mujahed, Z., Vasilas, A., and Evans, J. A.: Hemangiopericytoma; a report of four cases with a review of the literature, Amer. J. Roentgen. **82**:658-666, 1959.

71 Murray, M. R.: Cultural characteristics of three granular-cell myoblastomas, Cancer **4**:857-865, 1951.

72 Murray, M. R., and Stout, A. P.: Characteristics of liposarcoma grown in vitro, Amer. J. Path. **19**:751-763, 1943.

73 Murray, M. R., Stout, A. P., and Pogogeff, I. A.: Synovial sarcoma and normal synovial tissue cultivated in vitro, Ann. Surg. **120**:843-851, 1944.

74 O'Brien, P., and Brasfield, R. D.: Hemangiopericytoma, Cancer **18**:249-252, 1965.

75 Pack, G. T., and Ariel, I. M.: Synovial sarcoma (malignant synovioma), Surgery **28**:1047-1084, 1950.

76 Pack, G. T., and Ariel, I. M.: Tumors of the soft tissues, New York, 1958, Hoeber Medical Division, Harper & Row, Publishers.

77 Pack, G. T., and Eberhart, W. F.: Rhabdomyosarcoma of skeletal muscle, Surgery **32**:1023-1064, 1952.

78 Patton, R. B., and Horn, R. C., Jr.: Rhabdomyosarcoma; clinical and pathological features and comparison with human fetal and embryonal skeletal muscle, Surgery **52**:572-584, 1962.

79 Pearse, A. G. E.: The histogenesis of granular cell myoblastoma (? granular cell perineural fibroblastoma), J. Path. Bact. **62**:351-362, 1950.

80 Pearman, R. O., and Mayo, C. W.: Desmoid tumors, Ann. Surg. **115**:114-125, 1942.

81 Perry, H., and Chu, F. C. H.: Radiation therapy in the palliative management of soft tissue sarcomas, Cancer **15**:179-183, 1962.

82 Pettit, V. D., Chamness, J. T., and Ackerman, L. V.: Fibromatosis and fibrosarcoma following irradiation therapy, Cancer **7**:149-158, 1959.

83 Phelan, J. T., and Perez-Mesa, C.: Liposarcoma of the superficial soft tissues, Surg. Gynec. Obstet. **115**:609-614, 1962.

84 Pinet, F., Schlienger, R., Schemla, R., and Gravier, J.: Arteriography of soft tissue tumors, J. Radiol. Electr. **44**:590-593, 1963.

85 Price, E. B., Silliphant, W. M., and Shuman, R.: Nodular fasciitis, Amer. J. Clin. Path. **35**:122-136, 1961.

86 Raben, M., Calabrese, A., Higinbotham, N. L., and Phillips, R.: Malignant synovioma, Amer. J. Roentgen. **93**:145-153, 1965.

87 del Regato, J. A.: Radiotherapy of soft-tissue sarcomas, J.A.M.A. **185**:216-218, 1963.

88 Reszel, P. A., Soule, E. H., and Coventry, M. B.: Liposarcoma of the extremities and limb girdles, J. Bone Joint Surg. **48-A**:229-244, 1966.

89 Richardson, W. R., and Dewar, J. P.: Problems in managing fibrous tissue tumors in infants and children, Surgery **56**:426-435, 1964.

90 Riopelle, J. L., and Theriault, J. P.: Sur une forme meconnue de sarcome des parties molles; le rhabdomyosarcoma alveolaire, Ann. Anat. Path. (Paris) **1**:88-111, 1956.

91 Rosenberg, J. C.: The value of arteriography in the treatment of soft tissue tumors of the extremities, J. Int. Coll. Surg. **41**:405-414, 1964.

92 Ross, R. C., Miller, T. R., and Foote, F. W., Jr.: Malignant granular-cell myoblastoma, Cancer **5**:112-121, 1952.

93 Schick, A., and Rogers, L. S.: Liposarcoma; case reports and discussion of its pathology, diagnosis and treatment, Amer. J. Roentgen. **80**:799-806, 1958.

94 Sherman, R. S., and Chu, F. C. H.: A roentgenographic study of synovioma, Amer. J. Roentgen. **67**:80-89, 1952.

95 Stein, A. H., Jr.: The alveolar soft-part sarcoma, J. Bone Joint Surg. **38-A**:1126-1130, 1956.

96 Stewart, F. W., and Treves, N.: Lymphangiosarcoma in postmastectomy lymphedema, Cancer **1**:64-81, 1948.

97 Stewart, M. J.: Benign giant-cell synovioma and its relation to "xanthoma," J. Bone Joint Surg. **30-B**:522-527, 1948.

98 Stout, A. P.: The malignant tumors of the peripheral nerves, Amer. J. Cancer **25**:1-36, 1935.

99 Stout, A. P.: Solitary cutaneous and subcutaneous leiomyoma, Amer. J. Cancer **29**:435-469, 1937.

100 Stout, A. P.: Hemangio-endothelioma; a tumor of blood vessels featuring vascular endothelial cells, Ann. Surg. **118**:445-464, 1943.

101 Stout, A. P.: Liposarcoma—the malignant tumor of lipoblasts, Ann. Surg. **119**:86-107, 1944.

102 Stout, A. P.: Rhabdomyosarcoma of the skeletal muscles, Ann. Surg. **123**:447-472, 1946.

103 Stout, A. P.: Sarcomas of the soft parts, J. Missouri Med. Ass. **44**:329, 1947.

104 Stout, A. P.: Mesenchymoma, the mixed tumor of mesenchymal derivatives, Ann. Surg. **127**:278-290, 1948.

105 Stout, A. P.: Fibrosarcoma; the malignant tumor of fibroblasts, Cancer **1**:30-63, 1948.

106 Stout, A. P.: Myxoma, the tumor of primitive mesenchyme, Ann. Surg. **127**:706-719, 1948.

107 Stout, A. P.: Hemangiopericytoma; a study of twenty-five new cases, Cancer **2**:1027-1054, 1949.

108 Stout, A. P.: Tumors of the peripheral nervous system. In Atlas of tumor pathology, Sect. II, Fasc. 6, Washington, D. C., 1949, Armed Forces Institute of Pathology.

109 Stout, A. P.: Juvenile fibromatoses, Cancer **7**:953-978, 1954.

110 Stout, A. P.: Tumors of the soft tissues. In Atlas of tumor pathology, Sect. II, Fasc. 5, Washington, D. C., 1968, Armed Forces Institute of Pathology.

111 Stout, A. P.: Fibrosarcoma in infants and children, Cancer **15**:1028-1040, 1962.

112 Stout, A. P., and Lattes, R.: Tumors of the soft tissues. In Atlas of tumor pathology, Sect. II, Washington, D. C., 1967, Armed Forces Institute of Pathology.

113 Stout, A. P., and Murray, M. R.: Hemangiopericytoma, Ann. Surg. **116**:26-33, 1942.

114 Stout, A. P., and Verner, E. W.: Chondrosarcoma of the extraskeletal soft tissues, Cancer **6**:581-590, 1953.

115 Sugarbaker, E. D., and Ackerman, L. V.: Disarticulation of the innominate bone for malignant tumors of the pelvic parietes and upper thigh, Surg. Gynec. Obstet. **81**:36-52, 1945.

116 van der Werf-Messing, B., and van Unnik, J. A. M.: Fibrosarcoma of the soft tissue; a clinicopathologic study, Cancer **18**:1113-1123, 1965.

117 White, H. R., Jr.: Survival in malignant schwannoma; an 18 year study with some unusual metastatic patterns, Cancer 1970 (in press).

118 Wright, C. J. E.: Malignant synovioma, J. Path. Bact. **64**:585-603, 1952.

119 Windeyer, B., Dische, S., and Mansfield, C. M.: The place of radiotherapy in the management of fibrosarcoma of the soft tissues, Clin. Radiol. **17**:32-40, 1966.

Chapter 18

Cancer of the eye

Anatomy

A sketch of the eye, with the different structures labeled, is presented in Fig. 729. A more detailed anatomic description is not necessary for our purposes.

Lymphatics. True lymphatics have not been demonstrated in the cornea, sclera, uveal tract, lens, retina, or orbit. The lymphatics of the eyelids are drained by two groups of vessels: a medial group, which follows the course of the facial vein to the submaxillary lymph nodes, and a lateral group, which ends in the deep parotid lymph node. The lymphatics of the conjunctiva form two systems: a superficial network in the conjunctiva proper and a deep network in the fibrous layer. Both of these systems drain toward the lateral and medial canthi. The vessels in the region of the lateral canthus then drain into the preauricular lymph nodes, whereas those of the medial canthus drain into the submaxillary nodes. The lymphatics of the lacrimal gland join the conjunctival lymphatic system and pass to the preauricular nodes.

Epidemiology

Malignant melanomas are the most common intraocular malignant tumors of the eye, although they make up a relatively small proportion of all malignant melanomas. They present a peak incidence between 50 and 60 years of age. The tumors are almost always primary, single, and uniocular with no preference for male or female and are extremely rare in blacks (Templeton[87]). Melanomas arise from the pigmented or potentially pigment-producing cells of the uveal tract, with the choroid being the most common site. Virtually all malignant melanomas of the uveal tract appear to develop from preexisting nevi (Yanoff and Zimmerman[100]). Eyes with excessive congenital pigmentation (melanosis oculi) are particularly prone to develop malignant melanoma (Makley and King[60]). Familial occurrence of intraocular melanoma is rare. But if it does occur, the lesion follows an autosomal dominant mode of inheritance (Lynch et al.[59]). Malignant melanoma of the conjunctiva arises from three different sources: preexisting nevi, areas of acquired melanosis, or de novo.

Retinoblastomas are the most common intraocular neoplasms of children. Nearly all cases are diagnosed before the age of 4 years (Merriam[62]). Jensen[51] studied sixty-nine patients with retinoblastoma seen in Denmark over a sixteen-year period. There was one case for every 18,000 births. The frequency of the tumor has shown a steady increase from 1 in 34,000 births in 1931 to 1 in 14,000 in 1961 (François and Matton-Van Leuven[38]). Factors to be reckoned with in this increase are a greater number of cured adult survivors producing affected offspring and improved investigation and diagnosis. The tumors are bilateral in about 30% of cases (Weller[92]). The tumor is believed to be congenital and derived from the incompletely differentiated retinal cells. Although most cases arise sporadically, the influence of heredity has been well shown in many. It appears that the tumor may arise as an expression of a spontaneous gene mutation, which then may be transmitted to the offspring as a dominant trait with about 80% penetrance. The tumor is not uncommon in African children (Kodilinye[53]). In a study of 550 patients with retinoblastoma, Hemmes et al.[42] reported that: (1) with the first case in a family, the chance of a brother or sister being afflicted was 1 in 100; (2) in families otherwise free of retinoblastoma, fifty-eight patients with unilateral tumor had healthy children and ten others had a total of twenty-six healthy children and sixteen with retinoblastoma; (3) of the patients with a bilateral process, two had children

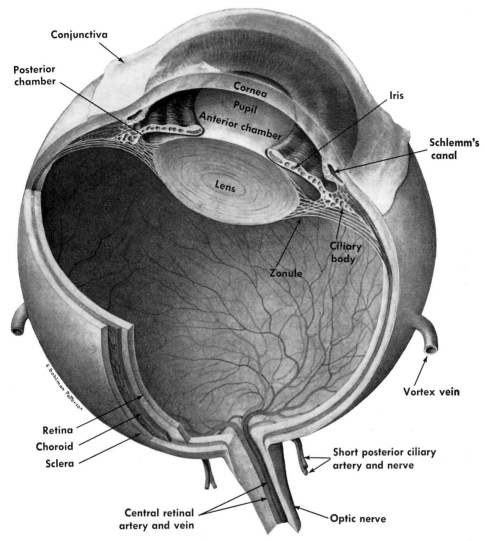

Conjunctiva

Posterior chamber

Cornea
Pupil
Anterior chamber

Iris

Schlemm's canal

Lens

Ciliary body

Zonule

E. Bohlman Patterson

Vortex vein

Retina
Choroid
Sclera

Short posterior ciliary artery and nerve

Central retinal artery and vein

Optic nerve

Fig. 729. Human eye. (From Newell, F. W.: Ophthalmology, ed. 2, St. Louis, 1969, The C. V. Mosby Co.)

without tumor and five had twelve children with tumor and six without it.

Epidermoid carcinomas of the conjunctiva are rare. These tumors may arise from a variety of dyskeratotic, acanthotic lesions of the conjunctival epithelium. In the Bantu, these tumors are frequent and often arise in association with a pterygium (Kaufmann[52a]).

Pathology

Gross and microscopic pathology

Malignant melanomas arise most frequently in the choroid and ciliary body and less frequently in the iris and conjunctiva. Brihaye-Van Geer-Truyden[18] concluded that all uveal melanomas are of neuroectodermal origin. Uveal melanomas arise from preexisting nevi in almost 100% of instances. In seventy-three of 100 consecutive melanomas of the choroid and ciliary body, evidence of such origin was found (Yanoff and Zimmerman[99]). The melanomas in the choroid increase in size and grow into the vitreous cavity, causing detachment and degeneration of the overlying retina, and present as the characteristic mound-shaped or mushroom-shaped

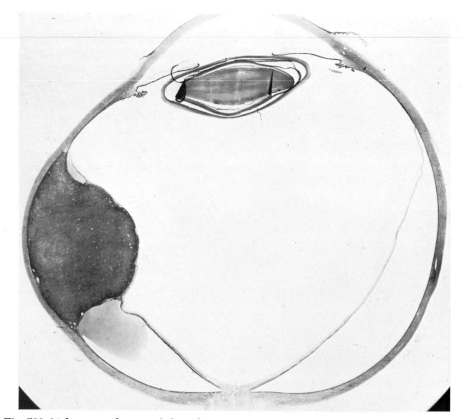

Fig. 730. Malignant melanoma of choroid.

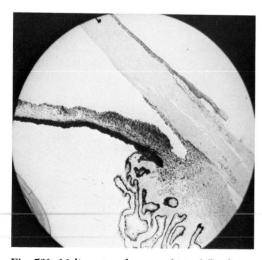

Fig. 731. Malignant melanoma of iris diffusely involving stroma. (From Zimmerman, L. E.: Clinical pathology of iris tumors, Amer. J. Clin. Path. 39:214-228, 1963; © 1963, The Williams & Wilkins Co., Baltimore, Md., U.S.A.; AFIP neg. 56-17963.)

tumor (Fig. 730). Further growth may lead to extraocular extension, closure of the angle with secondary glaucoma, and/or necrosis with inflammation. Tumors of the iris may be diffuse throughout the iris stroma or may extend into the anterior chamber and/or angle structures (Zimmerman[103]) (Fig. 731).

Uveal melanomas show three main cell types that have prognostic significance. The spindle A cells are slender spindle-shaped cells with small fusiform nuclei and chromatin often arranged in a linear fashion along the central axis of the nucleus (Fig. 732). Spindle B cells are larger and more pleomorphic and possess large ovoid nuclei with prominent nucleoli (Fig. 733). Under low magnification, they often present a fascicular pattern (Fig. 734). Epithelioid cells are still larger and more irregular. They have abundant cytoplasm, the nuclei are large, and the nucleoli are prominent (Fig. 735). There is often a mixture of

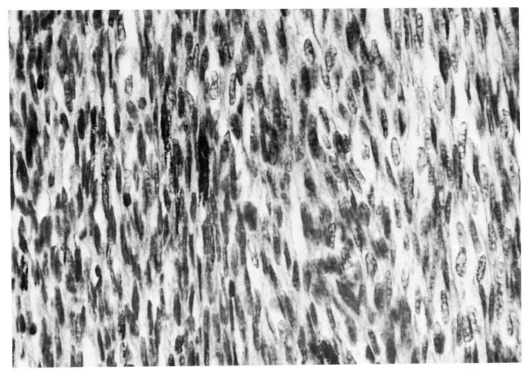

Fig. 732. Spindle A cells with small fusiform nuclei and chromatin arranged in linear fashion along central axis of nucleus. (×600; WU neg. 70-183.)

these cell types. In fact, the so-called mixed cell tumor (i.e., containing spindle B and epithelioid cells) is the most common type. Pigment content varies considerably. Melanomas of the iris are almost always of the spindle A or B variety.

Malignant melanomas of the conjunctiva are usually of the epithelioid type, although a mixture of epithelioid and spindle cell types may also be seen. The degree of pigmentation varies. Those arising from benign nevi may show areas of the pre-existing lesion (Fig. 736). The association of malignant melanoma of the conjunctiva with acquired melanosis is an interesting one. There are actually four classifications here which are based on the histopathologic appearance of the lesion: benign acquired melanosis with (1) minimal junctional activity and (2) marked junctional activity and cancerous acquired melanosis with (1) minimal invasion and (2) marked invasion (Zimmerman[107]).

Retinoblastomas may be flat and diffuse or elevated. They may protrude into the vitreous (endophytic type) or between the retina and the pigment epithelium (exophytic type). Since the tumors tend to outgrow their blood supply, necrosis is often extensive. Many minute foci of calcification are often present in these areas of necrosis (Fig. 737). The tumors are composed of dense masses of small round cells with scanty cytoplasm and hyperchromatic nuclei. Often the cells are arranged in the form of rosettes (Fig. 738). At times, they are undifferentiated and it is difficult to make a specific diagnosis (Fig. 739). The tumors tend to invade the choroid and/or the optic nerve with subsequent involvement of the meninges. If allowed to grow unhampered, the tumor extends outside the globe, fills the orbit, and invades the facial bones and base of the skull. It may invade the subdural space but more commonly may spread along the subarachnoid space. The spinal cord may be involved.

Epidermoid carcinomas arise from the conjunctival epithelium and form a solid grayish white tumor (Fig. 740). There is considerable tendency for these tumors to become papillomatous and spread along

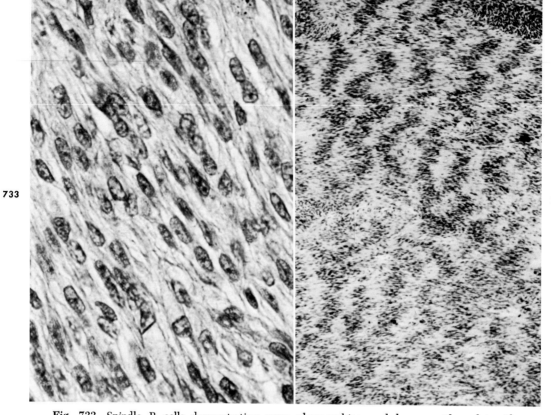

Fig. 733. Spindle B cells demonstrating some pleomorphism and large ovoid nuclei with prominent nucleoli. (×720; WU neg. 69-7514.)

Fig. 734. Spindle B cells with fascicular pattern. (WU neg. 69-3061.)

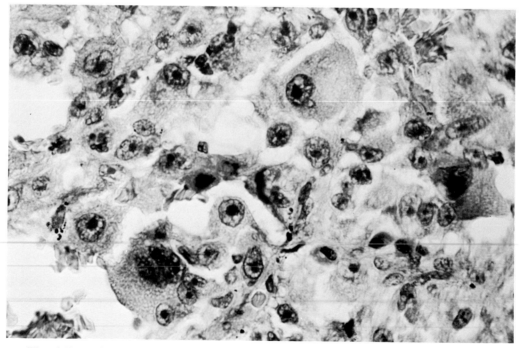

Fig. 735. Epithelioid cells with abundant cytoplasm, large nuclei, and extremely prominent nucleoli. (× 600; WU neg. 69-7517.)

the epithelial surface of the cornea. Many are classified as carcinoma in situ and invariably are well differentiated, and the diagnosis between a benign and malignant lesion is often difficult. Invasion of the globe itself is rare.

Metastatic spread

A *malignant melanoma* of the eye may have a very characteristic evolution in that a long time interval may elapse between

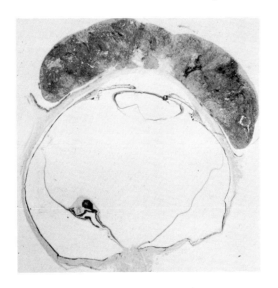

Fig. 736. Extensive flat malignant melanoma of conjunctiva. (Courtesy Registry of Ophthalmic Pathology, Armed Forces Institute of Pathology; WU neg. 69-2212.)

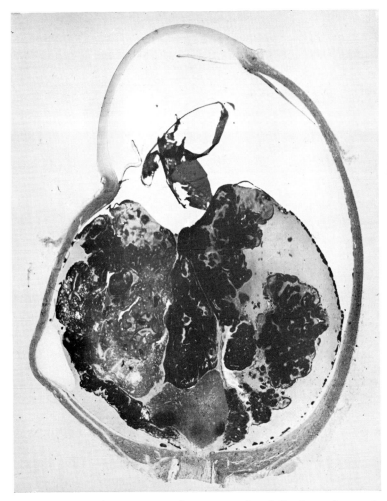

Fig. 737. Retinoblastoma showing areas of necrosis with calcification and extension to optic nerve.

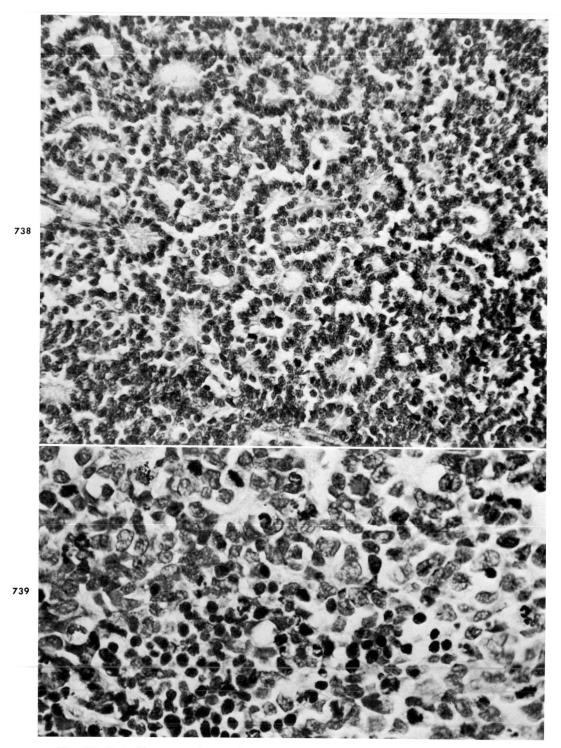

Fig. 738. Retinoblastoma with typical rosettes. (×350; WU neg. 69-7513.)

Fig. 739. Undifferentiated retinoblastoma showing several mitotic figures. (×600; WU neg. 69-7519.)

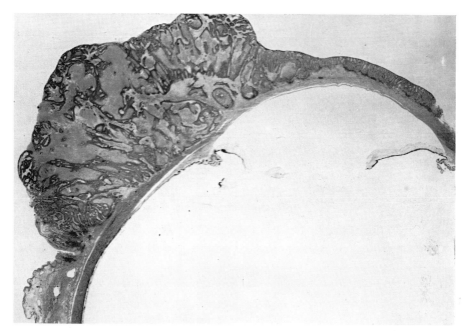

Fig. 740. Papillary squamous cell carcinoma of conjunctiva with involvement of cornea. (From Ash, J. E., and Wilder, H. C.: Epithelial tumors of the limbus, Amer. J. Ophthal. **25:**926-932, 1942.)

enucleation and the appearance of distant metastases. It is not too rare for twenty or more years to elapse before the tumor again becomes apparent invariably in the liver, and fairly often in the brain. Widespread dissemination may take place. Melanomas arising in the conjunctiva may involve the cervical lymph nodes.

Retinoblastomas may metastasize in terminal stages. Of seventeen autopsy cases reported by Merriam,[62] nine had distant metastases in bones, lymph nodes, and liver. Retinoblastomas may spread through the lymphatics, the blood, or the cerebrospinal fluid.

Epidermoid carcinomas remain localized for long periods of time and only rarely metastasize to preauricular lymph nodes.

Clinical evolution

Malignant melanoma arising in the choroid may produce a retinal detachment with consequent visual impairment. If the tumor is in or close to the macula, visual disturbance may develop quite early, even when the tumor is only minimally elevated. This visual impairment is usually the first symptom. Another presenting symptom may be pain from a secondary glaucoma caused by a forward displacement of the iris root against the outflow channels. Necrosis of the tumor may produce a marked inflammation and a clinical picture of uveitis. The tumor may break through the sclera and present under the conjunctiva (Fig. 741) or may present as an orbital tumor (Fig. 742). Tumors of the iris are often noticed by the patient before symptoms develop (Fig. 743). Progressive growth, however, may lead to secondary glaucoma.

Malignant melanoma of the conjunctiva is rare. It arises from three different sources: preexisting nevi, areas of acquired melanosis, or de novo. Those arising from nevi are usually at the limbus, where benign nevi are common (Figs. 744). These melanomas grow in an exophytic fashion and range in color from pink or tan to black. Melanomas arising from acquired melanosis are often in multiple sites (Fig. 745).

Retinoblastoma characteristically presents as a leukocoria (white pupillary reflex) (Fig. 746). The usual age of the patient is 2 years, and progressive blindness can be noticed only by indirect signs such as a strabismus or anisocoria. As the tumor

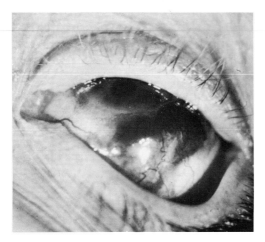

Fig. 741. Malignant melanoma of choroid breaking through sclera and presenting under conjunctiva. (Courtesy Registry of Ophthalmic Pathology, Armed Forces Institute of Pathology; WU neg. 69-2213.)

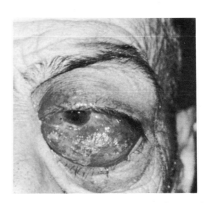

Fig. 742. Malignant melanoma involving choroid presenting as orbital mass. (WU neg. 69-7634.)

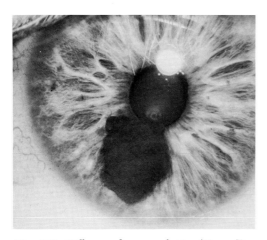

Fig. 743. Diffuse melanoma of iris. (From Zimmerman, L. E.: Clinical pathology of iris tumors, Amer. J. Clin. Path. **39:**214-228, 1963; © 1963, The Williams & Wilkins Co., Baltimore, Md., U.S.A.; AFIP neg. 58-900.)

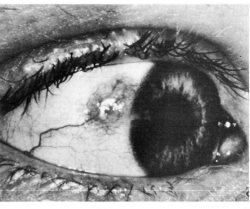

Fig. 744. Pigmented lesion at limbus which proved to be benign nevus. (Courtesy Registry of Ophthalmic Pathology, Armed Forces Institute of Pathology; WU neg. 69-2209.)

replaces the eye, it erupts from the orbit to form a fungating, ulcerated, infected mass and is extremely painful. Once the cells of this highly malignant tumor have escaped from the eye, death is almost certain. In approximately one-third of the patients, the opposite eye may also be affected. In 759 cases reported by Merriam,[62] 210 (27%) were bilateral. Ultimately, without institution of treatment, vision is lost in both eyes. Metastasis to the lung, brain, and other organs takes place, and the child usually dies blind and in considerable pain.

Epidermoid carcinoma of the conjunctiva usually starts at the limbus and grows as an exophytic gray-white tumor along the surface of the cornea and/or into the conjunctival fornices. Eventually, it may invade the globe and orbit and may even metastasize via lymphatics or blood (Fig. 747).

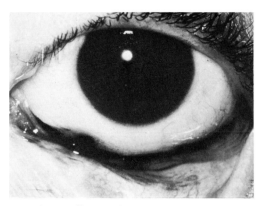

Fig. 745. Diffuse malignant melanoma of conjunctiva in lower cul-de-sac. (From Zimmerman, L. E.: Discussion of Pigmented tumors of the conjunctiva; courtesy Registry of Ophthalmic Pathology, Armed Forces Institute of Pathology. In Boniuk, M., editor: Ocular and adnexal tumors, St. Louis, 1964, The C. V. Mosby Co.; WU neg. 69-2211.)

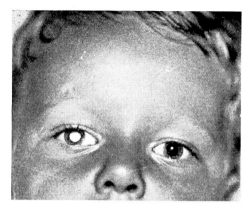

Fig. 746. Prominent white reflex present in dilated pupil of right eye due to retinoblastoma. (From Martin, H., and Reese, A. B.: Treatment of retinoblastoma [retinal glioma] surgically and by radiation, Arch. Ophthal. [Chicago] 27:40-72, 1942.)

Diagnosis

The diagnosis of intraocular tumors may be difficult, and examination under anesthesia is definitely indicated in children. The diagnosis of a malignant melanoma of the posterior uveal tract depends chiefly on the ophthalmoscopic appearance, and examination should be done with both the direct and the indirect ophthalmoscope. This will usually reveal a retinal detachment overlying a slate gray choroidal mass elevated toward the vitreous cavity. If the tumor is peripheral, scleral transillumination should be done and the light will characteristically be blocked by the solid tumor. Sometimes, the tumor grows swiftly, causing a massive retinal detachment with rapid progression of blindness. Peripheral lesions may be unnoticed by the patient for some time. Tumors of the ciliary body may present as changes in the refractive error (Foos et al.[36]). The diagnosis may be obscured by the presence of secondary glaucoma, uveitis, a massively detached retina, or vitreous hemorrhage. At times, a patient who has undergone enucleation of an eye consults a physician many years later for an abdominal complaint and presents an enlarged nodular liver. In such cases, a melanoma should be suspected. By contrast, the malignant melanoma of the iris has an extremely slow growth rate and

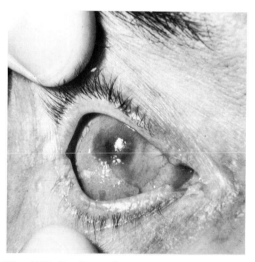

Fig. 747. Epidermoid carcinoma of conjunctiva growing along surface of cornea. (WU neg. 67-4283.)

practically never metastasizes. The diagnosis can be made by localized surgical excision. Patients with a blind eye with opaque media should be suspected of having malignant melanoma of the choroid or ciliary body, since it has been shown that blind painful eyes will often contain an occult malignant melanoma (Makley and Teed[61]).

The early diagnosis of *retinoblastomas* depends on the parents of the child recognizing a squint or noticing a light reflex (Fig. 746). The usual age of the patients is 2 years, and progressive blindness can be noticed only by indirect signs, such as esotropia or inequality in size of the pupils. Examination should be done under general anesthesia, for small tumors situated near the equator are easily missed. Frequent examination of the apparently unaffected eye should be done especially in familial cases, in which the incidence of bilaterality is about 75%. On ophthalmoscopic examination, the retinoblastoma presents as a rather characteristic creamy "cauliflower" tumor behind the usually clear lens. Henderson Brown[43] reported the urinary excretion of vanilmandelic acid (VMA) and homovanillic acid (HVA) in children with retinoblastoma. Patients with well-differentiated tumors with true rosettes excreted more vanilmandelic and homovanillic acid than those with less differentiated tumors. It appears obvious that this evidence of excretion can be useful in evaluating adequacy of treatment and evidence of recrudescence.

The *epidermoid carcinomas* of the eye usually arise in the region of the limbus and spread to the cornea and bulbar conjunctiva. They have a grayish white color. Epidermoid carcinomas may also arise in the palpebral conjunctiva.

Roentgenologic examination

In general, the radiographic examination is not of great value in tumors of the eye. But in three-fourths of the cases of retinoblastoma, carefully taken roentgenograms may show mottled, irregular calcification within the eye (Pfeiffer[70]). Enlargement of the optic canal has been noted particularly in gliomas of the chiasma or optic nerve. Various procedures such as tomography and arteriography may be fruitfully employed in the investigation of lesions of the eye and surrounding structures (Bertelsen[14]).

Differential diagnosis

There are numerous conditions that may mimic intraocular malignant melanoma of the eye and lead to enucleation (François[37]). These include *retinal detachment* secondary to holes or tears in the retina, localized granulomas of the choroid, localized hemorrhage beneath the retina or between the pigment epithelium and the retina, cysts of the retina, ciliary body or iris, serous detachment of the iris, staphylomas, focal areas of proliferation of the retinal pigment epithelium, and benign tumors such as nevi and hemangiomas.

Metastatic carcinoma is rare but is still the second most common intraocular tumor in adults. It usually involves the choroid and only rarely the anterior segment. Although the lesions are usually more diffuse and flat than malignant melanomas, they still may mimic melanomas enough to cause a problem in differential diagnosis. The site of the primary lesion is usually the breast or bronchus.

It is sometimes difficult to differentiate a *serous retinal detachment* from a retinal detachment secondary to a choroidal tumor. In a study of 204 enucleated eyes, following unsuccessful operations for reattachment of the retina, sixty were found to contain tumors, of which fifty-six were melanomas (Boniuk and Zimmerman[17]). In nine cases, the eye had been suspected of containing tumor; histopathologic studies demonstrated that the lesions represented scar tissue, proliferative pigmented epithelium, hemorrhage, and other benign lesions. In another study in which enucleation was done with a diagnosis of malignant melanoma of the iris or choroid, there were numerous errors. Of sixty-nine patients in whom a diagnosis of malignant melanoma of the iris was made, no tumor was found in 35%, and in the 529 eyes removed with a diagnosis of malignant melanoma of the choroid, pathologic examination showed that melanoma was not present in 19% (Ferry[32, 33]).

Fluorescein angiography of the ocular fundus has aided in differentiating tumors from other lesions (Norton et al.[66]). Radioactive phosphorus uptake may also be of help in determining the nature of lesions of the posterior pole (Thomas et al.[88]).

Retinoblastomas have a characteristic age incidence and symptomatology, yet errors in diagnosis lead to unwarranted enucleation in a substantial percentage of patients. Any disease process (congenital malformations, developmental disorders, inflammatory processes, trauma) that leads to a retinal detachment or a retrolental mass in a child under 6 years of age must be suspected of being a possible retinoblastoma.

In a study of 1000 enucleations performed on children under 15 years of age, eighty-four eyes were removed because of non-neoplastic lesions that simulated retinoblastoma (Kogan and Boniuk[54]). Lesions in this category include *retrolental fibroplasia,* in which there is virtually always a history of prematurity and oxygen administration. Persistent hyperplastic primary vitreous produces a leukokoria, but the involved eye is almost always microphthalmic, whereas the eye with retinoblastoma is of normal size. Nematode infestation produces an inflammatory retinal detachment. Massive *retinal gliosis* is a relatively uncommon condition in which a large elevated scar develops near the disk and posterior pole following hemorrhage (e.g., in newborn infants) or inflammation. *Coats's disease* is an exudative retinopathy associated with retinal detachment and foci of telangiectatic retinal vessels. Rare tumors of the eye of infants, called *diktyomas* and resembling histologically the embryonic retina, are often confused with retinoblastomas (Andersen[4]).

Benign papillomas of the conjunctiva may be mistaken for carcinomas. *Leukoplakia* or *hyperkeratosis* of the limbus may grow and appear grossly as a carcinoma. A biopsy or excision biopsy will clarify diagnosis. *Lymphomas* of the conjunctiva are usually benign, grow slowly, and occur in elderly patients. Some true lymphomas may be present, and it may be difficult to evaluate whether they are benign or malignant. Follow-up of four patients by Mortada[63] revealed that most orbital, eyelid, lacrimal gland, and conjunctiva masses made up of mature lymphocytes represent lymphocytic hyperplasia rather than malignant lymphoma. *Plasmacytomas* are often found in young women, represent granulomatous lesions rather than true neoplasms (Andersen[3]), and often are associated with trachoma.

The most common presenting sign of *orbital disease* is exophthalmos. Most of the lesions that produce exophthalmos are not malignant (Table 112). In fact, the most common cause is "endocrine ophthalmopathy," in which there is some dysfunction of the pituitary-thyroid axis. Other benign conditions causing exophthalmos include inflammatory masses ("pseudotu-

Table 112. Clinical series of 230 consecutive cases of unilateral expanding lesions of orbit*

Diagnosis	Orbital surgery	Total
Endocrine ophthalmopathy	9	37
Hemangiomas	18	28
Malignant lymphomas	18	22
Chronic granulomas (pseudotumors)	13	18
Lacrimal gland epithelial tumors	17	17
Meningiomas	2	11
Lymphangiomas	10	10
Gliomas of optic nerve	6	8
Metastatic malignant tumors	4	8
Peripheral nerve tumors	7	7
Dermoid cysts	4	7
Mucocele or sinusitis	3	6
Rhabdomyosarcomas	5	5
Vascular aneurysm or fistula	–	5
Angiosarcomas	5	5
Osteomas	1	2
Histiocytomas	2	2
Sarcoids	2	2
Other lesions (one each)—fibrous dysplasia, encephalocele liposarcoma, tuberculoma, myxoma, and dacryoadenitis	3	6
Exophthalmos of unknown cause	4	23
Totals	133	230

*From Moss, H. M.: Expanding lesions of the orbit; a clinical study of 230 consecutive cases, Amer. J. Ophthal. 54:761-770, 1962.

mor") (Fig. 748), hemangiomas, lymphangiomas, benign cysts, mucoceles, neurofibromas, neurilemomas, and arteriovenous malformations. Rarer conditions include Hans-Schüller-Christian disease, Letterer-Siwe disease, and eosinophilic granuloma. The orbital bones may also be affected by osteomas or fibrous dysplasia. Juvenile xanthogranuloma, a benign disease of the skin of children, has also been reported to occur in the orbit (Sanders[79]).

Malignant tumors of the orbit may be metastatic, usually from primary lesions in the breast or lung.

Rhabdomyosarcomas of the orbit are rare, but they are the most common primary malignant tumor of the orbit in children (Jones et al.[52]). They are found slightly more frequently in males, and the are range is between 3½ months and 40 years. The tumor apparently originates in embryonic mesenchymal tissue, which is either prospective muscle or undifferentiated mesenchyme capable of heteroplastic muscle differentiation.

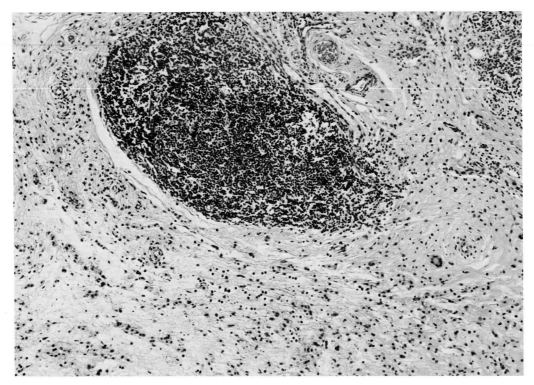

Fig. 748. Inflammatory "pseudotumor" of orbit showing lymphocytes, epithelioid cells, plasma cells, giant cells, and fibrosis. (×90; from Ackerman, L. V.: Surgical pathology, ed. 4, St. Louis, 1968, The C. V. Mosby Co.; WU neg. 67-4223.)

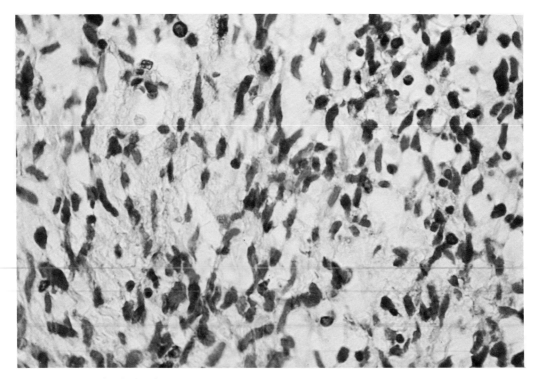

Fig. 749. Orbital rhabdomyosarcoma showing cells arranged in syncytium. (×600; WU neg. 69-7520.)

Porterfield and Zimmerman[71] have divided orbital rhabdomyosarcomas into three histologic types: embryonal, alveolar, and differentiated. The embryonal type is the commonest and is characterized by poorly differentiated mesenchymal cells arranged in a syncytium (Fig. 749). The cells are round, oval, elongated, or stellate with nuclei that are rich in chromatin. Cross-striations may be found in those cells which have a long ribbon of eosinophilic cytoplasm. The alveolar type is the next commonest, and the cells are separated into alveolar spaces by septae, with the cytoplasmic processes of the cells merging into these septae. Tadpole-shaped and multinucleated tumor giant cells are often seen, but cross-striations are rarely found. In the differentiated type, virtually every cell has a ribbon of eosinophilic cytoplasm, and cross-striations are easily detected.

Virtually all the patients present with painless unilateral exophthalmos, often striking in its rapid progression. The tumor may occur anywhere in the orbit, but a discrete mass can be palpated in only about one-third of the patients (Fig. 750). The presenting sign is sometimes an orbital cellulitis probably secondary to necrosis of the tumor. Roentgenograms are usually of no help unless the tumor has grown to cause bony erosion or optic foramen enlargement. Differential diagnosis includes hemangioma, leukemia, and neuro-blastoma. Exenteration has been shown to be effective in the control of a good proportion of these cases (Jones et al.[52]). There is also evidence that radiotherapy alone is curative in many cases (Fig. 751) (Regato[76a]; Sagerman et al.[78]). This is especially important since it preserves the eye and avoids the disfiguring procedure of exenteration in a child. There appears to be no definite correlation between histologic cell type and prognosis.

Other sarcomas, (fibrosarcomas, liposarcomas, chondrosarcomas, osteosarcomas, and osteoclastomas) are even rarer than rhabdomyosarcoma. They have all been reported occurring primarily in the orbit (Hogan and Zimmerman[44]; Yanoff and Scheie[98]; Eifrig and Foos[30]). These tumors can arise at any age, and they present as a unilateral exophthalmos. Treatment consists of exenteration sometimes combined with radiotherapy.

A *malignant lymphoma* or a *leukemic infiltrate* usually presents as a somewhat

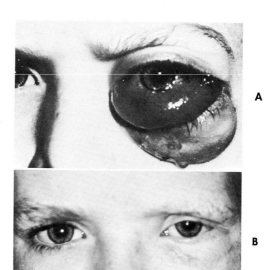

Fig. 751. A, Young patient with inoperable rhabdomyosarcoma of orbit and marked chemosis. B, Marked regression of tumor following cobalt[60] teletherapy irradiation. (Courtesy Dr. P. P. Ellis, University of Colorado Medical Center, Denver, Colo., and Dr. R. Perez-Tamayo, Loyola University Hospital, Hines, Ill.; from del Regato, J. A.: Radiotherapy of soft-tissue sarcomas, J.A.M.A. **185**:216-218, 1963.)

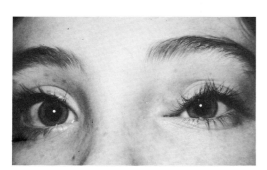

Fig. 750. Rhabdomyosarcoma presenting as palpable mass in upper medial quadrant of left orbit with only minimal downward and lateral displacement of eye. (From Smith, M. E.: The differential diagnosis of unilateral exophthalmos. In Gay, A. J., and Burde, R. M., editors: Clinical concepts in neuroophthalmology, International Opthalmology Clinics, vol. 7, no. 4, Boston, 1967, Little, Brown and Co., pp. 911-933; WU neg. 67-3507.)

soft mass in the eyelid or orbit or as a salmon-colored nodule beneath the conjunctiva. It can occur at any age, but the peak incidences are seen in childhood and in the sixth and seventh decades of life.

The pathologic evaluation of lymphomatous lesions is often exceedingly difficult. If the lesion shows mature cells with an admixture of other inflammatory cells, such as plasma cells, histiocytes, and epithelioid cells, then the lesion should be classified as a benign reactive lymphocytic hyperplasia or "pseudolymphoma." Furthermore, most lymphocytic infiltrations in the lacrimal gland are benign (Zimmerman[104]).

Epithelial tumors of the lacrimal gland comprise half of the tumor masses occupying the lacrimal fossa. The other half includes lymphomas, chronic inflammatory lesions, benign adenomas, and dermoid cysts. Of the epithelial tumors, 60% are benign mixed cell, 25% are adenoid cystic carcinomas, 8% are malignant mixed tumors, and 7% are other carcinomas. Their cytologic characteristics resemble the same tumors of the salivary gland (Zimmerman et al.[110]). Epithelial tumors of the lacrimal gland usually present as a painless mass in the upper outer quadrant of the orbit. The globe may be displaced downward and medially; the exophthalmos is usually minimal. Bone invasion is frequent with malignant tumors. Surgical resection is the treatment of choice. The prognosis is good for patients with benign mixed tumor, but recurrences may appear years later. In malignant tumors, exenteration of the orbit is recommended after diagnosis is established by biopsy. The prognosis is extremely poor in these cases.

Optic nerve gliomas occur in the first decade of life and usually present as a slowly progressing, painless, unilateral exophthalmos associated with optic nerve atrophy and roentgenographic evidence of an enlarged optic foramen. This tumor may be a feature of Recklinghausen's disease.

Certain clues aid in the differential diagnosis of orbital tumors (Smith[81]). For example, the direction of the proptosed eye may be important. A mucocele in the upper medial quadrant of the orbit displaces the eye downward and laterally (Fig. 752), while a lacrimal gland tumor displaces the eye downward and medially (Fig. 753).

Tumors usually located in the apex of the orbit, such as gliomas and hemangiomas, displace the eye directly forward. Those arising behind the eye may produce such secondary changes as retinal striae, papilledema, or optic atrophy. An enlarged optic foramen as seen in the roentgenograms is almost pathognomonic of optic nerve glioma. Hyperostosis of the bone is present in 85% of the patients with meningiomas.

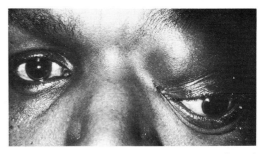

Fig. 752. Mucocele producing downward and lateral displacement of left eye. (WU neg. 69-7637.)

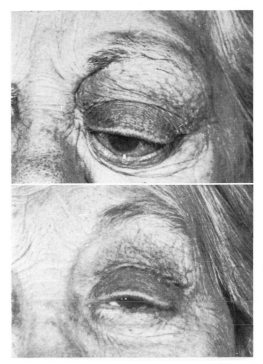

Fig. 753. A, Mixed tumor arising from lacrimal gland producing exophthalmos and displacement of eye downward and medially. **B,** Following surgical excision. Patient remained well for seven years and died of carcinoma of bladder.

Congenital benign lesions such as hemangiomas may show enlargement of the bony orbit on the involved side. Special tests that sometimes aid the clinician include angiography, venography, pneumography, and ultrasonography (Krayenbuhl[55]; Weidner and Hanofee[91]; Wheeler and Baker[93]; Hanafee et al.[41]; Lombardi and Passerini[58]; Bertelsen[15]; Coscas and Butex[24]; Baum[12]; Baum and Greenwood[13]). Through orbital angiography, Vladyka et al.[90] showed that, unlike benign orbital tumors, malignant tumors presented abnormal vascularization in addition to pressure symptoms. Carotid angiography facilitates the localization of angiomas and the definition of vascular lesions (Isfort and Küper[48]). Ossoinig and Seher[67] have used ultrasonography to evaluate size, shape, and location of orbital tumors. Bertelson[15] described the various radiographic examinations utilized in the diagnosis of orbital tumefactions (Fig. 754).

Although a presumptive diagnosis can often be made on an orbital tumor, it is often necessary to obtain tissue for biopsy. Treatment is then dependent upon the re-

sults of the biopsy. Certain benign lesions such as hemangiomas and lymphangiomas will often spontaneously subside. Inflammatory lesions should not be excised but should be treated with proper medication. Other benign lesions may be removed surgically without disturbing the eye. Malignant tumors such as primary sarcomas may necessitate exenteration, sometimes combined with radiotherapy. Lymphomas usually respond to radiotherapy alone or to systemic chemotherapy.

Treatment

Malignant melanoma of the posterior uvea should be treated by enucleation. Very small, minimally elevated choroidal tumors should be followed by repeated observations (including serial photographs) until there is an indication of growth and functional change (visual field studies). The value of diathermy, photocoagulation, cobalt[60] applicators, radon seeds, chemotherapy, and cryotherapy remains to be established.

Exenteration of the orbit is indicated in cases of obvious extension of the tumor out of the eye into the surrounding orbital tissues. If evidence of extraocular extension is so minimal that it is discovered only at the time of enucleation or later upon histopathologic examination, then the question of whether exenteration should be done remains controversial (Starr and Zimmerman[85]).

Iridectomy has become widely accepted as the treatment of choice for resectable iris tumor. However, if this tumor produces glaucoma or extends out of the eye, then local excision is no longer feasible and enucleation is indicated. Recently, segmental resection of localized tumors involving the ciliary body has met with encouraging success (Stallard[84]; Winter[95, 96]; Ashton and Wybar[8]).

The small isolated melanoma arising from a nevus or apparently de novo can be treated by simple excision (Jay[49]). Lederman[57] also claims good results with irradiation. Melanomas arising from acquired melanosis may require multiple repeated excisions. Lederman[57] reported good results from radiotherapy in limbal and conjunctival melanoma. Jay[49] reported forty-eight malignant melanomas of the limbus treated

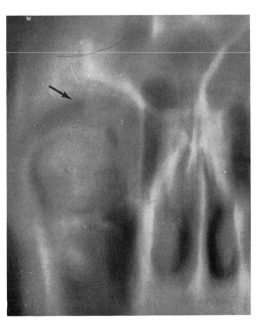

Fig. 754. Orbital pneumotomography demonstrating tumor lying above orbit. Arrow indicates neoplasm which was mixed tumor of lacrimal gland origin. (From Bertelsen, T. I.: The use of radiographic contrast media in diagnosing orbital tumors, Acta Ophthal. [Kobenhavn] 34:355-366, 1956.)

by a variety of means: local excision, enucleation, exenteration, and radiotherapy; he believes that enucleation is seldom justified and that local excision is usually the treatment of choice.

By the time most *retinoblastomas* are diagnosed, the tumor has filled much of the vitreous cavity and the eye is blind. This fact has justified the common attitude of enucleating the eye both for diagnosis and for treatment. In general, only an enucleation is necessary, but as much of the optic nerve as possible should also be excised. Careful histologic examination may reveal need for postoperative irradiation. In patients with bilateral retinoblastoma, the second, or less affected, eye is usually treated by radiotherapy, for it can cure the patient and preserve the vision. This formula has been allowed to become established so that one eye is always sacrificed even when it has salvageable vision. The fact is that a clinical diagnosis of retinoblastoma is seldom in error and that it takes the loss of an eye to disprove it. It is

justified in many instances to proceed with irradiation of one or both eyes on a clinical diagnosis in order to preserve vision.

The components of the eye have a great deal of resistance to irradiation (Skeggs and Williams[80]) with the exception of the lens, which may be affected by radiations and develop various degrees of cataract depending on the total dose, fractionation, daily intensity, and personal susceptibility. The use of cobalt[60] and supervoltage roentgentherapy through small fields has permitted successful irradiation without loss of vision in an increasing proportion of patients (Williams[94]; Bagshaw and Kaplan[10]; Paterson and Charteris[68]).

Triethylenemelamine (TEM) has been associated with radiotherapy for the treatment of retinoblastomas (Reese and Ellsworth[75]), but no evidence has been produced that it is, in itself, of additional value. Skeggs and Williams[80] have used cyclophosphamide as a radiotherapeutic adjuvant. Krementz et al.[56] have utilized the intra-arterial infusion of triethylene-

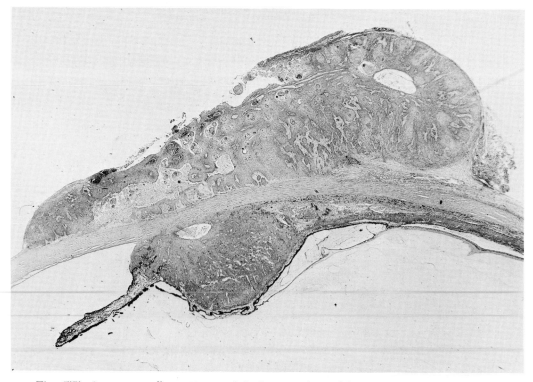

Fig. 755. Squamous cell carcinoma of limbus invading globe, necessitating enucleation. (Courtesy Registry of Ophthalmic Pathology, Armed Forces Institute of Pathology; WU neg. 67-4232.)

melamine combined with radiotherapy. This approach favors a greater utilization of the employed drug (Hyman et al.[46]). In postirradiation recurrences, photocoagulation and cryotherapy may be useful (Ellsworth[31]; Nadel and Lincoff[65]).

Small *epidermoid carcinomas* of the conjunctiva may be treated by excision, but in those which invade the globe, enucleation is necessary (Fig. 755). Radiotherapy can successfully eradicate these lesions and should be instituted in preference to an enucleation in spite of the possibility that cataract may develop. Fractionation of treatment will result in a longer interval before the cataract develops; radiation cataracts are surgically correctable.

Prognosis

The prognosis of intraocular *malignant melanomas* depends on many variables. It was shown by Callender[21] many years ago that uveal melanomas could be classified cytologically in such a way that their prognosis could be estimated. This classification has stood the test of time (Paul et al.[69]). There is a much higher five-year survival rate in patients with the pure spindle cell type of tumor than in those with a tumor with a predominance of epithelioid cells. More than half the patients with predominantly epithelioid cell malignant melanomas succumb within five years after enucleation. Other significant factors influencing prognosis are size of the tumor, extraocular extension, and vascular invasion. Of less prognostic significance are the degree of pigmentation and the reticulum content (Flocks et al.[34]). The more diffuse malignant melanomas of the choroid also have a poorer prognosis (Font et al.[35]). If a malignant melanoma of the choroid involves the posterior ciliary vessels or extends to the optic nerve or sclera at the level of the vortex vein, the prognosis is usually poor (Sorato[83]).

Tumors of the iris have a much more favorable prognosis than those of the posterior uvea and, in fact, practically never metastasize. Ashton and Wybar[8] reported on the follow-up of 105 patients with malignant melanoma of the iris. There were no deaths from the tumor, and no metastases even in the presence of extraocular extension. Malignant melanoma of the conjunctiva is often cured with simple excision. Lederman's results[57] of treatment of epibulbar malignant melanoma by irradiation are excellent (Table 113). He also treated the group designated as cancerous melanosis and precancerous melanosis with excellent results. In twenty-one leiomyomas of the iris which were locally invasive at times, all patients were cured by surgery. Jay[49] reported a series of forty-eight patients with malignant melanomas of the limbus. Of twenty-five patients treated by local excision alone, fourteen had been followed for more than five years and one had died of distant metastases. In fourteen of the patients in this series, the tumor apparently arose in a congenital nevus. Seven of the fourteen patients were followed for over five years, and one died.

The most important factor influencing the prognosis of *retinoblastoma* is the extent of its spread when treated. The prognosis has improved recently mainly because of earlier detection and diagnosis as well as improved methods of therapy. If the tumor is unilateral and confined to the retina and vitreous, the cure rate obtained by enucleation approaches 85%. Brown[19] indicated that if there was involvement of the entire choroidal thickness, there was a 60% mortality. When there was scleral involvement, the mortality was 75%. If there is true epibulbar involvement, there is even a higher mortality. Optic nerve involvement is highly unfavorable. A less important factor is cell differentiation, for the prognosis in tumors with a large number of rosettes or pseudorosettes is slightly better

Table 113. Cancerous melanosis—results of treatment by radiotherapy, 1941-1961*

Number treated		26
Alive and well (2 patients after removal of eye)	22	
1—over 12 yr		
10—5 yr and over		
5—3 yr and over		
6—2 yr and less		
Dead		4
All died of disease		
1 after 7 yr		
3 at 2 yr and less		

*From Lederman, M.: Discussion of Pigmented tumors of the conjunctiva. In Boniuk, M., editor: Ocular and adnexal tumors, St. Louis, 1964, The C. V. Mosby Co.

than that in the more anaplastic types with necrosis and calcification. In Brown's series,[19] all of the fatalities in the patients with unilateral involvement occurred within two years of enucleation, whereas in those with bilateral involvement, only 76% of the fatalities occurred in the first three years. In patients with bilateral tumors, prognosis depends upon the size, location, and number of lesions in the second eye. Reese and Ellsworth[74] have classified these into five groups from "very favorable" to "very unfavorable." In the former group, radiotherapy alone usually results in an 85% cure rate with preservation of vision. In the "very unfavorable" group, survival beyond five years, in spite of irradiation, chemotherapy, photocoagulation, and cryotherapy, is no more than 23%. Paterson and Charteris[68] treated nineteen patients with bilateral retinoblastoma with radiotherapy, thirteen of whom survived; five of these had vision of 6/12, and three had vision of less than this. Skeggs and Williams[80] treated forty children with external cobalt combined with cyclophosphamide. These patients all had bilateral disease; thirty-five had had one eye removed. Follow-up on thirty patients revealed that twenty-one had some degree of vision and no sign of tumor activity; in twelve of the patients, the condition had been controlled between eighteen months and three years.

The prognosis for life in epibulbar *epidermoid carcinomas* is good. Most of the lesions are noninvasive and may often be classified merely as "dyskeratotic" tumors (Irvine[47]). They virtually never metastasize. In a series of forty-eight patients with carcinomas reported by Ash,[5] local excision completely eradicated the tumor in twenty-three. In two additional patients, control was obtained by further excision, in twenty-three others, an enucleation was done. Only one of the forty-eight patients was presumed to have died as a consequence of cancer. Among a group of nine patients with small carcinomas of the bulbar conjunctiva treated with contact radiotherapy by Baclesse et al.,[9] there were nine recoveries followed five years or more. The results, in a series of eight patients with more extensive lesions were not nearly so good, with only three recoveries.

REFERENCES

1 Ackerman, L. V.: Surgical pathology, ed. 4, St. Louis, 1968, The C. V. Mosby Co.
2 Allen, J. C., and Jaeschke, W. H.: Recurrence of malignant melanoma in an orbit after 28 years, Arch. Ophthal. (Chicago) 76:79-81, 1966.
3 Andersen, P. E.: Extramedullary plasmocytomas, Acta Radiol. (Stockholm) 32:365-374, 1949.
4 Andersen, S. R.: Medullo-epitheliomas. Diktyoma and malignant epithelioma of the ciliary body; a general review and a new case of diktyoma, Acta Ophthal. (Kobenhavn) 26: 313-330, 1948.
5 Ash, J. E.: Epibulbar tumor, Amer. J. Ophthal. 33:1203-1219, 1950.
6 Ashton, N.: Primary tumors of the iris, Brit. J. Ophthal. 48:650-668, 1964.
7 Ashton, N., and Morgan, G.: Embryonal sarcoma and embryonal rhabdomyosarcoma of the orbit, J. Clin. Path. 18:699-714, 1965.
8 Ashton, N., and Wybar, K.: Primary tumours of the iris, Ophthalmologica (Basel) 151: 97-113, 1966.
9 Baclesse, F., Dollfus, M.-A., and Haye, C.: Les épithéliomas de la conjonctive bulbaire. Traitement par les radiations. Resultats eloignés, Bull. Soc. Franc. Ophthal. 17:147-154, 1958.
10 Bagshaw, M. A., and Kaplan, H. S.: Supervoltage linear accelerator radiation therapy. VIII. Retinoblastoma, Radiology 86:242-246, 1966.
11 Bagshaw, M., and Kaplan, H. S.: Retinoblastoma; megavoltage therapy and unilateral disease, Trans. Amer. Acad. Ophthal. Otolaryng. 70:944-950, 1966.
12 Baum, G.: A reappraisal of orbital ultrasonography, Trans. Amer. Acad. Ophthal. Otolaryng. 69:943, 1965.
13 Baum, G., and Greenwood, I.: Orbital lesion localization by three-dimensional ultrasonography, New York J. Med. 61:4149, 1961.
14 Bertelsen, T. I.: The use of radiographic contrast media in diagnosing orbital tumors, Acta Ophthal. (Kobenhavn) 34:355-366, 1956.
15 Bertelsen, T. I.: A new and improved technique in orbital pneumography, Acta Ophthal. (Kobenhavn) 38:57, 1960.
16 Boniuk, M., editor: Ocular and adnexal tumors: new and controversial aspects (symposium sponsored by Department of Ophthalmology, Baylor University College of Medicine), St. Louis, 1964, The C. V. Mosby Co.
17 Boniuk, M., and Zimmerman, L. E.: Pathological anatomy of complications. In Schepens, C. L., and Regan, C. D. J.: Controversial aspects of the management of retinal detachment, Boston, 1965, Little Brown and Co., chap. 13.
18 Brihaye-Van Geer-Truyden, M.: Melanotic tumours of the uvea and their origin, Docum. Ophthal. 17:163-248, 1963.
19 Brown, D. H.: The clinicopathology of retino-

blastoma, Amer. J. Ophthal. **61**:508-514, 1966.

20 Burns, R. P., Fraunfelder, F. T., and Klass, A. M.: A laboratory evaluation of enucleation in treatment of intraocular malignant melanoma, Arch. Ophthal. (Chicago) **67**:490-500, 1962.

21 Callender, G. R.: Malignant melanotic tumors of the eye; a study of histologic types in 111 cases, Trans. Amer. Acad. Ophthal. Otolaryng. **36**:131-142, 1931.

22 Callender, G. R., Wilder, H., and Ash, J. E.: Five hundred melanomas of the choroid and ciliary body followed five years or longer, Amer. J. Ophthal. **25**:962-967, 1942.

23 Cancer Registration in Norway: Norwegian Cancer Society, Oslo, 1961.

24 Coscas, G., and Butex, J.: Orbit tomography with injection of oil and water soluble iodized contrast substances, Arch. Ophthal. (Chicago) **24**:235, 1964.

25 Craig, W. McK., and Gogela, L. J.: Intraorbital meningiomas; a clinico-pathologic study, Amer. J. Ophthal. **32**:1663-1680, 1949.

26 Duke, J. R., and Dunn, S. N.: Primary tumours of the iris, Arch. Ophthal. (Chicago) **59**:204-214, 1958.

27 Duke, J. R., and Walsh, F. B.: Metastatic carcinoma to the retina, Amer. J. Ophthal. **47**:44-48, 1959.

28 Dunphy, E. B.: The story of retinoblastoma, Trans. Amer. Acad. Ophthal. Otolaryng. **68**:249-264, 1964.

29 Dunphy, E. B., Forrest, A. W., Leopold, I. H., Reese, A. B., and Zimmerman, L. E.: The diagnosis and management of intraocular melanomas (a symposium), Trans. Amer. Acad. Ophthal. Otolaryng. **62**:517-555, 1958.

30 Eifrig, D., and Foos, R.: Fibrosarcoma of the orbit, Amer. J. Ophthal. **67**:244-248, 1969.

31 Ellsworth, R. M.: Treatment of retinoblastoma, Amer. J. Ophthal. **66**:49-51, 1968.

32 Ferry, A. P.: Lesions mistaken for malignant melanoma of the posterior uvea; a clinicopathologic analysis of 100 cases with ophthalmoscopically visible lesions, Arch. Ophthal. (Chicago) **72**:463-469, 1964.

33 Ferry, A. P.: Lesions mistaken for malignant melanoma or iris, Arch. Ophthal. (Chicago) **74**:9-18, 1965.

34 Flocks, M., Gerend, J. H., and Zimmerman, L. E.: The size and shape of malignant melanomas of the choroid and ciliary body in relation to prognosis and histologic characteristics; a statistical study of 210 tumors, Trans. Amer. Acad. Ophthal. Otolaryng. **59**:740-758, 1955.

35 Font, R. L., Spaulding, A. G., and Zimmerman, L. E.: Diffuse malignant melanoma of the uveal tract, Trans. Amer. Acad. Ophthal. Otolaryng. **68**:877-894, 1968.

36 Foos, R. Y., Hull, S. N., and Straatsma, B. R.: Early diagnosis of ciliary body melanomas, Arch. Ophthal. (Chicago) **81**:336, 1969.

37 François, J.: The diagnosis of malignant melanoma of the choroid, Ophthalmologica (Basel) **151**:114-134, 1966.

38 François, J., and Matton-Van Leuven, M. T.: Recent data on the heredity of retinoblastoma. In Boniuk, M., editor: Ocular and adnexal tumors: new and controversial aspects (symposium sponsored by Department of Ophthalmology, Baylor University College of Medicine), St. Louis, 1964, The C. V. Mosby Co.

39 Halama, J.: Die Strahlenbehandlung des Retinoblastoms, Strahlentherapie **128**:87-92, 1965.

40 Hale, P. N., Allen, R. A., and Straatsma, B. R.: Benign melanomas (nevi) of the choroid and ciliary body, Arch. Ophthal. (Kobenhavn) **74**:532-538, 1965.

41 Hanafee, W., Shin, P., and Dayton, G.: Orbital venography, Amer. J. Roentgen. **104**:29, 1968.

42 Hemmes, G. D., Nijland, R., and Schappert-Kimmijser, J.: De kans op ontwikkeling van retinoblastoma bij kinderen uit gezinnen waarin deze ziekte is voorgekomen, Nederl. T. Geneesk. **108**:1906-1908, 1964.

43 Henderson Brown, D.: The urinary excretion of vanilmandelic acid (VMA) and homovanillic acid (HVA) in children and retinoblastoma, Amer. J. Ophthal. **62**:239-243, 1966.

44 Hogan, M. J., and Zimmerman, L. E.: Ophthalmic pathology: an atlas and textbook, ed. 2, Philadelphia, 1962, W. B. Saunders Co.

45 Howard, G. M., and Ellsworth, R. M.: Differential diagnosis of retinoblastoma; a statistical survey of 500 children, Amer. J. Ophthal. **60**:610-612, 1965.

46 Hyman, G. A., Feind, C. R., Spalter, H. F., and Finkel, M. P.: Chemotherapy of retinoblastoma; intracarotid arterial infusion and isolation head and neck perfusion—tracer studies, Cancer **17**:992-996, 1964.

47 Irvine, A. R.: Dyskeratotic epibulbar tumors, Trans. Amer. Ophthal. Soc. **61**:243-273, 1963.

48 Isfort, A., and Küper, J.: Zur Diagnose und Therapie der Orbitaangiome, Arch. Psychiat. Nervenkr. **204**:317-327, 1963.

49 Jay, B.: Current developments in ophthalmology; a follow-up of limbal melanomata, Proc. Roy. Soc. Med. **57**:497-500, 1964.

50 Jay, B.: Naevi and melanomata of the conjunctiva, Brit. J. Ophthal. **49**:169-204, 1965.

51 Jensen, O. A.: Retinoblastoma in Denmark, 1943-1958; a clinical histopathological, and prognostic study, Acta Ophthal. (Kobenhavn) **43**:821-840, 1965.

52 Jones, I. S., Reese, A. B., and Kraut, J.: Orbital rhabdomyosarcoma, Amer. J. Ophthal. **61**:721-736, 1966.

52a Kaufmann, J. C. E.: Racial differences and similarities in tumors of the eye: evaluation of 2,000 cases from the National Ocular Tumor Registry of South Africa (presented at the Tenth International Cancer Congress, Houston, Texas, May, 1970).

53 Kodilinye, H. D.: Retinoblastoma in Nigeria; problems of treatment, Amer. J. Ophthal. **63**:469-481, 1967.

54 Kogan, L., and Boniuk, M.: Causes for enucleation in childhood with special reference to pseudogliomas and unsuspected retinoblastomas. In Zimmerman, L. E.: Tumors of the eye and adnexa, International Ophthalmology Clinics, vol. 2, no. 2, Boston, 1962, Little, Brown and Co.

55 Krayenbuhl, H.: Value of orbital angiography for diagnosis of unilateral exophthalmos, J. Neurosurg. 19:289, 1962.

56 Krementz, E. T., Schlosser, J. V., Rumage, J. P., and Herring, L.: Retinoblastoma; behavior and treatment with fractional irradiation and intra-arterial triethylenemelamine, Ann. N. Y. Acad. Sci. 114:963-975, 1964.

57 Lederman, M.: Discussion of Pigmented tumors of the conjunctiva. In Boniuk, M., editor: Ocular and adnexal tumors: new and controversial aspects (symposium sponsored by Department of Ophthalmology, Baylor University College of Medicine), St. Louis, 1964, The C. V. Mosby Co., pp. 24-48.

58 Lombardi, G., and Passerini, A.: Venography of the orbit, technique and anatomy, Brit. J. Radiol. 41:282, 1968.

59 Lynch, H. T., Anderson, D. E., and Krush, A. J.: Heredity and intraocular malignant melanoma; study of two families and review of forty-five cases, Cancer 21:119-125, 1968.

60 Makley, T. A., and King, C. M.: Malignant melanoma in melanosis oculi, Trans. Amer. Acad. Ophthal. Otolaryng. 71:638-641, 1967.

61 Makley, T. A., and Teed, R. W.: Unsuspected intraocular malignant melanomas, Arch. Ophthal. (Chicago) 60:475-478, 1958.

62 Merriam, G. R., Jr.: Retinoblastoma; analysis of seventeen autopsies, Arch. Ophthal. (Chicago) 44:71-108, 1950.

63 Mortada, A.: Reactive lymphocytic hyperplasia of orbit, lids, conjunctiva and lacrimal gland, Amer. J. Ophthal. 56:649-652, 1963.

64 Moss, H. M.: Expanding lesions of the orbit; a clinical study of 230 consecutive cases, Amer. J. Ophthal. 54:761-770, 1962.

65 Nadel, A., and Lincoff, H.: Cryosurgical treatment of eye tumors, Geriatrics 23:89-97, 1968.

66 Norton, E. W. D., Smith, J. L., and Justice, J., Jr.: Fluorescein fundus photography; an aid in the differential diagnosis of posterior ocular lesion, Trans. Amer. Acad. Ophthal. Otolaryng. 68:755-765, 1964.

67 Ossoinig, K., and Seher, K.: Ergebnisse der Ultraschalldiagnostik orbitaler Tumoren, Klin. Mbl. Augenheilk. 151:519-524, 1967.

68 Paterson, M. W., and Charteris, A. A.: Retinoblastoma; report on 19 patients treated with radiotherapy, Brit. J. Ophthal. 49:347-358, 1965.

69 Paul, E. V., Parnell, B. L., and Fraker, M.: Prognosis of malignant melanomas of the choroid and ciliary body. In Zimmerman, L. E.: Tumors of the eye and adnexa, International Ophthalmology Clinics, vol. 2, no. 2, Boston, 1962, Little, Brown and Co., pp. 387-402.

70 Pfeiffer, R. L.: Roentgenographic diagnosis of retinoblastoma, Arch. Ophthal. (Chicago) 15:811-821, 1936.

71 Porterfield, J. G., and Zimmerman, L. E.: Rhabdomyosarcoma of the orbit; a clinicopathologic study of 55 cases, Virchow Arch. Path. Anat. 335:329-344, 1962.

72 Reese, A. B.: Tumors of the eye, ed. 2, New York, 1963, Harper & Row, Publishers.

73 Reese, A. B.: Precancerous and cancerous melanosis, Amer. J. Ophthal. 61:1272-1277, 1966.

74 Reese, A. B., and Ellsworth, R. M.: The evaluation and current concept of retinoblastoma therapy, Trans. Amer. Acad. Ophthal. Otolaryng. 172:164, 1963.

75 Reese, A. B., and Ellsworth, R. M.: Management of retinoblastoma, Ann. N. Y. Acad. Sci. 114:958-962, 1964.

76 Reese, A. B., and Howard, G. M.: Flat uveal melanomas, Amer. J. Ophthal. 64:1021-1028, 1967.

76a del Regato, J. A.: Radiotherapy of soft-tissue sarcomas, J.A.M.A. 185:216-218, 1963.

77 Rouvière, H.: Anatomie des lymphatiques de l'homme, Paris, 1932, Masson et Cie.

78 Sagerman, R., Cassady, J. R., and Tretter, P.: Radiation therapy for rhabdomyosarcoma of the orbit, Trans. Amer. Acad. Ophthal. Otolaryng. 72:849, 1968.

79 Sanders, T. E.: Infantile xanthogranuloma of the orbit, Amer. J. Ophthal. 61:1299-1306, 1966.

80 Skeggs, D. B. L., and Williams, I. G.: The treatment of advanced retinoblastoma by means of external irradiation combined with chemotherapy, Clin. Radiol. 17:169-172, 1966.

81 Smith, M. E.: The differential diagnosis of unilateral exophthalmos. In Gay, A. J., and Burde, R. M., editors: Clinical concepts in neuroophthalmology, International Ophthalmology Clinics, vol. 7, no. 4, Boston, 1967, Little, Brown and Co., pp. 911-933.

82 Soloway, H. B.: Radiation-induced neoplasms following curative therapy for retinoblastoma, Cancer 19:1984-1988, 1966.

83 Sorato, M.: Prognosis of malignant melanomas of the choroid, Ann. Oculist. (Paris) 197:44-51, 1964.

84 Stallard, H. B.: The treatment of retinoblastoma, Ophthalmologica (Basel) 151:214-230, 1966.

85 Starr, H. J., and Zimmerman, L. E.: Extrascleral extension and orbital recurrence of malignant melanomas of the choroid and ciliary body. In Zimmerman, L. E.: Tumors of the eye and adnexa, International Ophthalmology Clinics, vol. 2, no. 2, Boston, 1962, Little, Brown and Co., pp. 369-385.

86 Tapley, N.: The treatment of bilateral retinoblastoma with radiation and chemotherapy. In Boniuk, M., editor: Ocular and adnexal tumors: new and controversial aspects (symposium sponsored by Department of Ophthalmology, Baylor University College of Medicine), St. Louis, 1964, The C. V. Mosby Co.

87 Templeton, A. C.: Tumors of the eye and

adnexa in Africans of Uganda, Cancer **20:** 1689-1698, 1967.

88 Thomas, C. L., Storaasli, J. P., and Friedell, H. L.: Radioactive phosphorus in the detection of intraocular neoplasms, Amer. J. Roentgen. **95:**935-941, 1965.

89 Vision and Its Disorders: National Institute of Neurological Diseases and Blindness Monograph no. 4, P.H.S. pub. no. 1688, Washington, D. C., 1967, United States Government Printing Office.

90 Vladyka, V., Fusek, I., and Bret, J.: Orbital angiography, Sborn. Lek. **65:**225-229, 1963.

91 Weidner, W., and Hanafee, W.: Special neuroradiological techniques for the ophthalmologist, Arch. Ophthal. (Chicago) **71:**793, 1964.

92 Weller, C. V.: The inheritance of retinoblastoma and its relationship to practical eugenics, Cancer Res. **1:**517-535, 1941.

93 Wheeler, E. C., and Baker, H. L.: The ophthalmic arterial complex in angiographic diagnosis, Radiology **83:**26, 1964.

94 Williams, I. G.: 'Let there be light.' The treatment of advanced retinoblastoma by external irradiation, Proc. Roy. Soc. Med. **60:** 189-196, 1967.

95 Winter, F. C.: Surgical excision of tumours of the ciliary body and iris, Arch. Ophthal. (Chicago) **70:**19-29, 1963.

96 Winter, F. C.: Iridocyclectomy for malignant melanomas of the iris and ciliary body. In Boniuk, M., editor: Ocular and adnexal tumors: new and controversial aspects (symposium sponsored by Department of Ophthalmology, Baylor University College of Medicine), St. Louis, 1964, The C. V. Mosby Co., pp. 341-352.

97 Wybar, K.: The management of primary iris tumours, An. Inst. Barraquer **7:**579-594, 1967.

98 Yanoff, M., and Scheie, H.: Fibrosarcoma of orbit, Cancer **19:**1711, 1966.

99 Yanoff, M., and Zimmerman, L. E.: Histogenesis of malignant melanomas of the uvea. I. Nevi of choroid and ciliary body, Arch. Ophthal. (Chicago) **76:**784-796, 1966.

100 Yanoff, M., and Zimmerman, L. E.: Histogenesis of malignant melanomas of the uvea. II. The relationship of uveal nevi to malignant melanoma, Cancer **20:**493-507, 1967.

101 Yanoff, M., and Zimmerman, L. E.: Histogenesis of malignant melanomas of the uvea. III. The relationship of congenital ocular melanocytosis and neurofibromatosis to uveal melanomas, Arch. Ophthal. (Chicago) **77:** 331-336, 1967.

102 Zimmerman, L. E.: Tumors of the eye and adnexa, International Ophthalmology Clinics, vol. 2, no. 2, Boston, 1962, Little, Brown and Co.

103 Zimmerman, L. E.: Clinical pathology of iris tumors, Amer. J. Clin. Path. **39:**214-228, 1963.

104 Zimmerman, L. E.: Lymphoid tumors. In Boniuk, M., editor: Ocular and adnexal tumors: new and controversial aspects (symposium sponsored by Department of Ophthalmology, Baylor University College of Medicine), St. Louis, 1964, The C. V. Mosby Co., pp. 429-446.

105 Zimmerman, L. E.: Melanocytes, melanocytic nevi and melanocytomas, Invest. Ophthal. **4:** 11-41, 1965.

106 Zimmerman, L. E.: Ocular lesions of xanthogranuloma, Amer. J. Ophthal. **60:**1011-1035, 1965.

107 Zimmerman, L. E.: Criteria for management of melanosis (correspondence), Arch. Ophthal. (Chicago) **76:**307-308, 1966.

108 Zimmerman, L. E.: Changing concepts concerning the malignancy of ocular tumors, Arch. Ophthal. (Chicago) **78:**166-173, 1967.

109 Zimmerman, L. E., and DeBuen, S.: Tumors of the eye in South America, Highlights Ophthal. **7:**no. 3, 1964 (editorial).

110 Zimmerman, L. E., Sanders, T. E., and Ackerman, L. V.: Tumors of the lacrimal gland. In Zimmerman, L. E.: Tumors of the eye and adnexa, International Ophthalmology Clinics, vol. 2, no. 2, Boston, 1962, Little Brown and Co., p. 337.

Chapter 19

Hodgkin's disease

Epidemiology

"Hodgkin's disease is a disease of unproven aetiology, varied histological appearances and protean clinical manifestations."*

In the 1947 cancer survey in the United States, the incidence of Hodgkin's disease was 3.3 for males and 2.3 for females per 100,000 population. The male incidence in the state of Connecticut rose from 2.4 in 1945-1949 to 3.6 in 1960-1962. In the state of New York, the incidence rose from 2.2 and 1.4 in 1941-1943 to 3.2 and 2.1 in 1958-1960 in males and females, respectively. The disease is more common in Denmark and the Netherlands than in the United States. It is rare in Japan (MacMahon[95]). It is reputedly frequent in children in Peru (Solidoro et al.[134]) and in Lebanon (Azzam[9]).

The predominance in men is most marked in adults 35 to 55 years of age and in children. Of 713 cases reported by Diamond,[28] 362 were found in patients 20 to 39 years old (Fig. 756). Between the ages of 5 and 15 years, there is a fairly uniform age incidence (Jenkin et al.[73]). The diagnosis of Hodgkin's disease in infants under 2 years of age should be strongly doubted. The occurrence of this disease is only slightly higher in whites than in blacks (Marcus[97]). In a study of 440 patients, fifteen instances of other familial manifestations were found (De Vore and Doan[27]), but the evidence does not support any more than possible familial susceptibility (Schier et al.[125]) or the possible role of environment (Razis et al.[144]). Aisenberg[2] presented evidence of an immunologic defect in patients with early Hodgkin's disease. Hoffbrand,[60] however, found no convincing evidence of autoimmune disease in thirty-nine patients with

Hodgkin's disease. Bowdler and Glick[20] reported a patient with assumed autoimmune hemolytic anemia who developed Hodgkin's disease. Pirofsky[111] reported thirteen other instances.

Kassel[82] and Aisenberg,[2, 3] as well as others, have reviewed reports on the etiology of Hodgkin's disease. There is no proof of a viral etiology. There is a questionable increased frequency of the disease among close relatives. Saltzstein and Ackerman[123] have reported the association of anticonvulsant drugs with atypical lymphoid hyperplasias. Hyman and Sommers[67] have also reported the occurrence of Hodgkin's disease in patients receiving anticonvulsant drugs. Other aspects and etiologic theories have been summarized by Ultmann.[142]

Pathology
Gross pathology

Practically every organ of the body has been cited as the apparent primary site of Hodgkin's disease. The overwhelming majority of cases seem to originate within the lymph nodes. These nodes show strikingly significant alterations. On section, their architecture is usually obliterated, and they have a homogeneous grayish yellow appearance that may or may not show zones

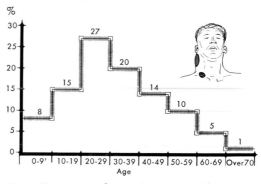

Fig. 756. Age incidence of patients of both sexes with Hodgkin's disease.

---

*From Jelliffe, A. M., and Thomson, A. D.: The prognosis in Hodgkin's disease, Brit. J. Cancer 9: 21-36, 1955.

of necrosis. These diseased lymph nodes may grow to involve adjacent structures. The cervical nodes may obstruct veins or invade the muscle. Those of the mediastinum and hilar region are frequently the point of departure for secondary involvement of the trachea, bronchi, pleura, or lungs. The retroperitoneal nodes may involve nerves and the vertebral bodies and, at times, may displace or occlude the ureters. The iliac nodes may obstruct venous return. Other lymph nodes lying in contiguity to viscera may invade them. Periportal lymph nodes rarely obstruct the biliary tract.

Lung involvement is frequently observed at autopsy. It may occur because of direct invasion of lung tissue from hilar lymph nodes and may result in intrabronchial and peribronchial spread. The lymphogranulomatous tissue may involve the interalveolar walls and spread luxuriantly within the lung parenchyma. At times, lobar infiltration with variable bronchomediastinal involvement, together with confluent lobular foci and associated involvement of lymph nodes, is present. Miliary dissemination and cavitation (Perttala and Svinhufvud[107]) can occur.

At postmortem examination, bone involvement is also found in a large number of cases, the incidence reported depending on the thoroughness of the examination and the number of sections taken. Ueh-

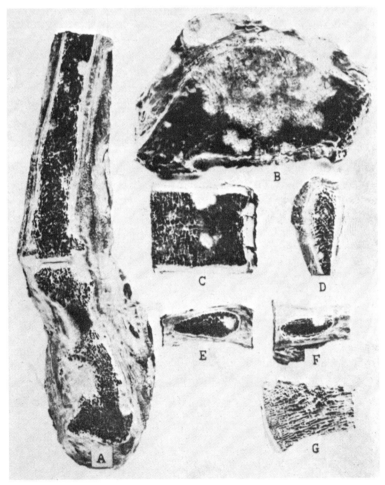

Fig. 757. Sections of different bones showing medullary and cortical involvement by Hodgkin's disease in single postmortem examination. **A,** Manubrium. **B,** Lumbar vertebra. **C,** Dorsal vertebra. **D,** Iliac crest. **E** and **F,** Ribs. **G,** Normal metatarsal bone. (From Steiner, P. E.: Hodgkin's disease, Arch. Path. [Chicago] 36:627-637, 1943.)

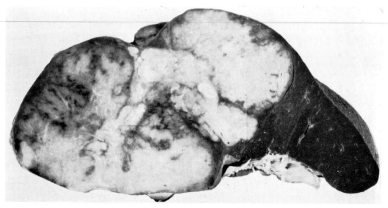

Fig. 758. Massive involvement of spleen by Hodgkin's disease.

linger[141] emphasized that the involvement of bone is often a secondary phenomenon due to direct invasion from diseased lymph nodes (Papillon et al.[105]). Involvement, therefore, of the vertebrae, ribs, and sternum is common (Fig. 757). Bone involvement may also take place through the bloodstream and result in pathologic alterations within the marrow cavity wherever red marrow is present—e.g., the vertebrae, sternum, femoral head, and, rarely, the ribs, pelvis, and skull. Steiner[136] felt that the distribution of bone lesions corresponded to the distribution of the reticuloendothelial system. Bone changes are predominantly osteolytic in the vertebrae and in the skull (Dresser and Spencer[30]). Osteoblastic changes, however, may be present, although their gross appearance does not permit differentiation from malignant tumors, either primary or metastatic.

Involvement of the spinal cord may occur. Weil[147] observed a high incidence of secondary invasion of the spinal canal by epidural lymphogranulomatous masses. In some patients in whom paraplegia had been treated by radiotherapy, postmortem examination revealed only scar tissue.

The spleen is found involved at autopsy in about 75% of the cases (Fig. 758). It is not usually greatly enlarged but presents involvement in the form of nodular masses. According to Klemperer,[85] the macroscopic and microscopic appearances of the spleen may often prove or disprove the diagnosis of Hodgkin's disease. Liver involvement occurs in about 50% of the patients without producing marked enlargement of the

organ (average weight, 2,000 gm). Primary involvement of the gastrointestinal tract is extremely rare.

Microscopic pathology

Hodgkin's disease, no matter where it may be present, has a sameness to its pathologic pattern. It may vary, however, within wide limits, depending upon cellularity, fibrosis, necrosis, and previous radiation therapy. The only cell that must be present in order to make a diagnosis of Hodgkin's disease in a lymph node is the *Sternberg-Reed* cell (Fig. 759). This cell may vary between 12μ and 40μ and may have an irregular shape, and its nucleus may be lobulated or multilobed. The chromatin of the nucleus appears in dense aggregates, and large nucleoli are the rule. The cytoplasm varies from eosinophilic to basophilic, and reticulin stains often reveal reticulin within it. It probably has its origin from sinus endothelium and reticulum cells. It is often confused with other multinucleated cells and is particularly difficult to differentiate from the megakaryocyte, whose nuclei are always single and whose nucleoli are fine and delicate (Jackson and Parker[68]). However, this problem practically never arises except in patients with extreme extramedullary hematopoiesis in whom a lymph node biopsy has been done. Megakaryocytes contain an intracytoplasmic substance that gives a strongly positive reaction when stained by the periodic acid–Schiff method, but this positive reaction does not occur in the Sternberg-Reed cell (Fisher and Hazard[39]).

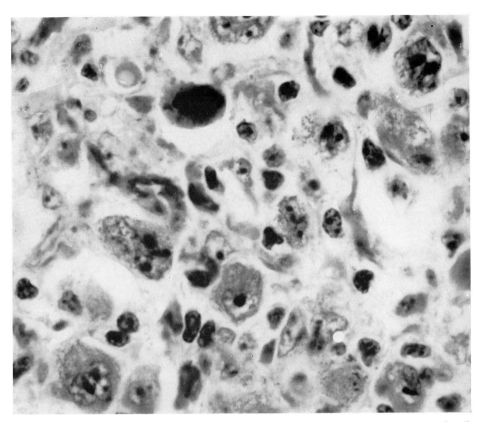

Fig. 759. Typical case of Hodgkin's disease with Sternberg-Reed cells. Sternberg-Reed cells have polylobated nuclei with prominent nucleoli. (High-power enlargement.)

The presence of other changes may be helpful in diagnosis, but they are not specific. Fibrosis and eosinophilia are not constant, for the eosinophilia may appear and disappear during the disease and will not parallel the peripheral blood count. Necrosis is also variable. At times, there may be innumerable plasma cells, and near areas of necrosis, polymorphonuclear leukocytes and reticular cells are abundant. Radiotherapy alters the histologic picture, at times causing complete sterilization. When nodes are not sterilized by the radiotherapy, Sternberg-Reed cells may be left surrounded by dense connective tissue (Brunschwig and Kandel[21]). Local recurrences usually take origin from nests of granulomatous islands (Gilbert[44]).

The microscopic diagnosis of Hodgkin's disease may be difficult, and there are many conditions under which there may be excessive reticuloendothelial proliferation within a lymph node. This may occur in patients with rheumatoid arthritis (Motulsky et al.[100]), and confusing changes can occur in lymph nodes draining an area of chronic inflammation of the skin (Laipply[87]). Lymph nodes and skin lesions related to insect bites are often difficult to interpret (Allen[7]), as are enlarged lymph nodes following vaccination. However, unless unequivocal Sternberg-Reed cells can be seen, a microscopic diagnosis of Hodgkin's disease should not be made. Even Sternberg-Reed cells can be mimicked rather successfully in a few conditions other than Hodgkin's disease, such as infectious mononucleosis, plasma cell myeloma, carcinoma of the breast, and malignant melanoma (Strum et al.[136a]). The term "atypical Hodgkin's" should never be used, for it may obscure the correct diagnosis and result in insufficient therapy.

Focal involvement of lymph nodes can occur (Strum et al.[136b]). Attempts have been made to divide Hodgkin's disease into various categories according to the microscopic characteristics.

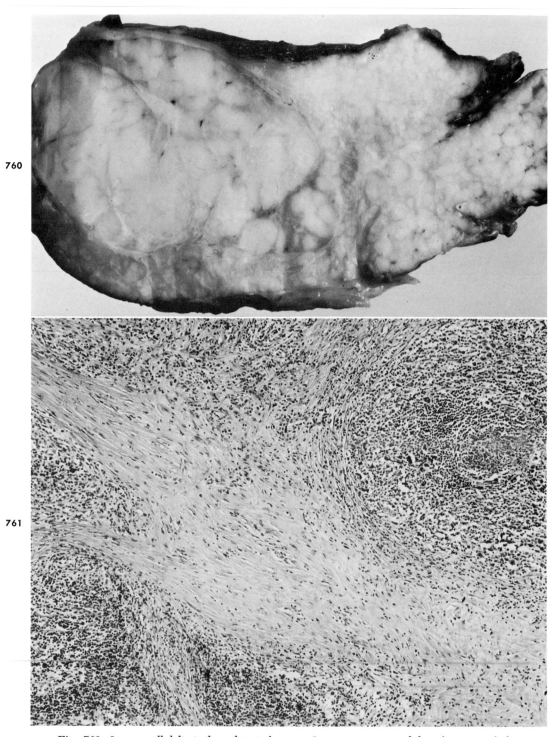

Fig. 760. Large well-delimited mediastinal mass. On cut section, nodular character of this distinctive type of Hodgkin's disease is clearly depicted. (WU neg. 68-3232.)

Fig. 761. Nodular sclerosing Hodgkin's disease demonstrating broad bands of relatively acellular fibrous tissue separating proliferating nodules. (Low power; WU neg. 68-2935.)

In the past, Hodgkin's disease was classified as paragranuloma, granuloma, and sarcoma. This classification was of little value in prognosis. The few cases in the paragranuloma group had an excellent prognosis (Bonenfant[17]; Dawson and Harrison[26]), and the even fewer cases in the sarcoma group had an extremely poor outlook. This left most of the cases in the granuloma group, and this group has now been shown to be of heterogeneous character. Lukes and Butler[93] have been very helpful in more accurately classifying Hodgkin's disease. They point out that a lymphocytic and histiocytic predominance is a favorable pattern. They have also well defined the nodular sclerosing type which has an excellent outlook (Figs. 760 and

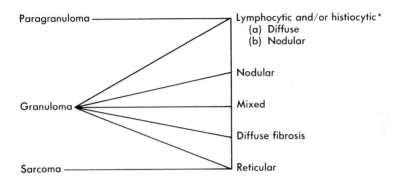

*L and H types may have predominance of either lymphocytes or histiocytes.

Fig. 762. Comparison of histologic classifications of Hodgkin's disease—left, Jackson and Parker[68]; right, Lukes[92] and Lukes et al.[94]. (From Lukes, R. J., and Butler, J. J.: The pathology and nomenclature of Hodgkin's disease, Cancer Res. **26**:1063-1081, 1966.)

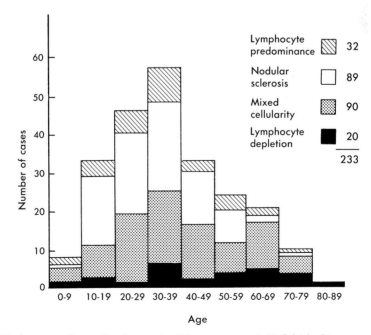

Fig. 763. Rather typical age distribution in different types of Hodgkin's disease emphasizing that favorable pathologic type makes up almost 50% of total. (Courtesy Dr. R. Dorfman, St. Louis, Mo.)

761). If diffuse fibrosis or a reticular pattern exists, the outlook for the patient worsens (Fig. 762). The age distribution in the different types of Hodgkin's disease emphasizes that the favorable types make up about 50% of the total group (Fig. 763). The presence of a favorable histologic type often correlates well with a favorable stage; e.g., young females often have mediastinal involvement of the nodular sclerosing type with an extremely favorable prognosis (Hanson[57]; Lukes[92]; Di Pietro and Pizzetti[29]). The classification we are using is as follows:

1 Hodgkin's disease with lymphocyte predominance
2 Hodgkin's disease with nodular sclerosis
3 Hodgkin's disease with mixed cellularity
4 Hodgkin's disease with lymphocyte depletion

Clinical evolution

The most frequent first symptom of Hodgkin's disease is a painless enlargement of a peripheral lymph node. In a few cases, a rapidly progressive anemia may be the first indication of the disease. In more than one-third of the patients, the first adenopathy is noted in the left cervical region, often in the left supraclavicular region (Table 114). With the development of routine roentgenographic chest surveys, the proportion of cases apparently starting with a symptomless mediastinal adenopathy has relatively increased. The cervical, axillary, inguinal, and retroperitoneal lymph nodes are most commonly affected

Table 114. Lymph node involvement in Hodgkin's disease*

First enlarged lymph node	Cases	%
Left cervical region	99	37.5
Right cervical region	55	20.8
Both sides of neck	19	6.8
Mediastinum	18	6.7
Right axilla	17	6.5
Left axilla	14	—
Left inguinal region	10	—
Right inguinal region	9	—
Total	241	

*Slightly modified from Slaughter, D. P., and Craver, L. F.: Hodgkin's disease, Amer. J. Roentgen. **47:**596-606, 1942.

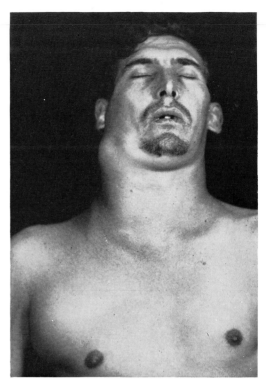

Fig. 764. Typical cervical and right axillary adenopathy in Hodgkin's disease. Note characteristic involvement of nodes of anterior cervical chain. (Courtesy Dr. N. Puente Duany, Roanoke, Va.)

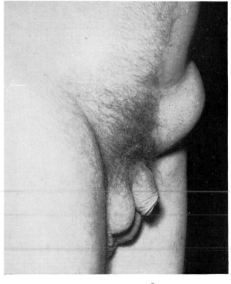

Fig. 765. Left inguinal adenopathy was first clinical manifestation of Hodgkin's disease in this patient.

(Figs. 764 and 765). The epitrochlear, submaxillary, antebrachial, and popliteal lymph nodes are only rarely involved. Interpectoral lymphadenopathy, presenting in the form of a diffuse infraclavicular swelling, is sometimes observed (Goldman[54]) and is rather characteristic of Hodgkin's disease. The nodes may grow slowly and progressively or may suddenly increase during attacks of fever. In many cases, the enlargement of various lymph node groups may be the only clinical manifestation for years. The nodes may regress spontaneously temporarily and cause clinical doubt as to the diagnosis (Johnson[74]).

Growth of lymph nodes in various locations may cause variegated symptoms. A lumbar ache usually is due to the enlargement of retroperitoneal nodes. Edema and pain of the lower extremity may be due to enlargement of pelvic and inguinal nodes. Dyspnea may be produced by mediastinal adenopathy, mostly because of compression, but sometimes also because of involvement of lung parenchyma. Enlargement of the spleen is noted at some time during the course of disease in most patients, causing pain or dull ache in the left hypochondrium. Enlargement of the liver is not clinically evident except in patients in the terminal stage of disease. Involvement of the esophagus (Ennuyer et al.[34]), stomach, and small intestine is very rare in our experience. Pruritus and excoriation due to scratching may be present in a majority of patients at some time during the course but are rarely an early symptom before the appearance of adenopathy. Goldman[52] reported a high percentage of cutaneous manifestations ranging from simple pruritus to exfoliative dermatitis and multiple nodules. Secondary skeletal involvement of vertebrae, sternum, or ribs from contiguous lymph nodes may cause pain as well as collapse of bone structure and fracture. The presence of herpes zoster usually indicates impending involvement of the epidural space. Bichel[13] reported herpes zoster in eleven of 240 patients with Hodgkin's disease. Invasion of the epidural space through the vertebral foramina may give symptoms of compression of the spinal cord (Smith and Stenstrom[131]). Cerebral involvement is rarely observed.

There are three different clinical forms of Hodgkin's disease:

1 A *chronic form*, which includes one-fourth of the cases, with very slow development in which the peripheral or purely lymphatic manifestations predominate

2 An *intermediate form*, which includes about half of all cases, with faster development and early visceral manifestations

3 An *acute form*, which includes fewer than one-fourth of all cases, with early anemia and rapid weight loss

These clinical forms roughly correspond to the three groups described long ago by Gilbert.[45]

Since Hodgkin's disease predominates in young individuals, it is not surprising that a number of cases may be complicated by pregnancy. Better treatment with longer survival will naturally increase the number of patients with this complication (Gilbert[47]). In general, pregnancy does not influence the course of Hodgkin's disease except when it occurs during one of the acute flare-ups. The disease does not affect gestation unfavorably. Myles[102] reviewed the world's literature and reported 166 patients who had had 218 pregnancies. There was no increase of abortions or premature births in this group. Difficulties may arise from inability to administer radiotherapy to the abdomen or pelvis during the term of pregnancy.

Lassitude, weight loss, anemia, and fever occur usually after the disease has become disseminated. The Pel-Ebstein type of fever (a relatively rare finding) is characterized by elevation of temperature followed by remissions that shorten progressively until the fever becomes continuous (Fig. 766). Anemia occurs particularly with invasion of the bone marrow. Weight loss is observed with every new manifestation. It becomes marked in patients in the terminal stage of disease. In patients with the acute form, lymph node involvement may be minimal, but the bone marrow and viscera may be extensively infiltrated at autopsy.

Hoster[63] first noted the occurrence of pain in patients with Hodgkin's disease immediately after they had ingested alcoholic beverages. Pain occurs in the diseased

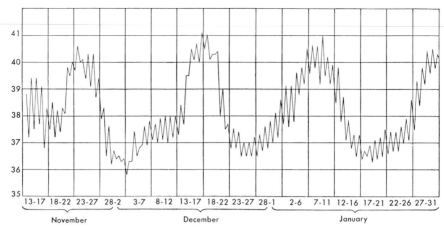

Fig. 766. Reproduction of original temperature chart of patient with Hodgkin's disease reported by Ebstein in 1887. Note that time period between paroxysms of fever progressively shortens.

areas and disappears after adequate treatment, but it may return with recrudescences of the disease. James[70] found frequent leukocytosis and spontaneous pain in these patients, as well as fewer reticulum cell mitoses, more eosinophils, and more fibrosis in the specimens. He suggested that they constituted a separate entity.

Diagnosis

In examining a patient with Hodgkin's disease, the general condition should be carefully noted and all lymph node areas meticulously explored. It is important to note the patient's weight as well as all symptoms that at first may appear irrelevant. The examination should include careful palpation of the spleen and liver areas.

The enlarged lymph nodes in Hodgkin's disease are generally smooth and present moderate induration. They are usually painless, and although they distend the skin, they rarely invade it. The nodes are usually surrounded by periadenitis and have a tendency to become matted but always conserve some of their own outline, giving the tumor mass a characteristic polylobated appearance.

In general, the findings are concentrated in one region (neck, mediastinum, or abdomen), and there is seldom discrete or generalized adenopathy characteristic of other lymphatic disturbances. Popliteal and epitrochlear lymph nodes are rarely involved in Hodgkin's disease.

Roentgenologic examination

Roentgenograms of the chest should be taken in every patient suspected of having Hodgkin's disease because of the frequent involvement of the mediastinum and lung parenchyma. Positive findings will often be revealed in spite of the absence of clinical symptoms. Wolpaw et al.[148] found intrathoracic involvement in thirty-five of fifty-five patients. It is imperative that oblique and lateral roentgenograms be taken in addition to the conventional ones so that the extent of the involvement may be accurately determined. The involvement of the mediastinal nodes may be discrete or massive (Fig. 767), but the disease is usually first confined to these nodes, from which it may spread to the lung. This type of involvement is sometimes observed along the course of the bronchi and interlobar or interlobular septa. Less frequently, a third type of involvement may exactly mimic a primary neoplasm of the lung with replacement of an entire lobe and, under the influence of bronchial block or infection, it may even cavitate. Rarely, the roentgenograms will show diffuse, scattered nodules throughout the lung parenchyma (Fig. 768). Not too rarely will the pleura be involved and signs of pleural effusion be present. The great variability of the pulmonary manifestations (Scheinmel et al.[124]), including rare cavitation, would cloud the diagnosis if other manifestations did not permit an easy histopathologic confirmation. Apparent primary manifestations

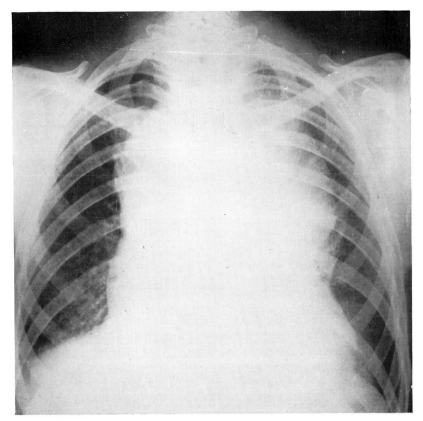

Fig. 767. Massive mediastinal involvement in Hodgkin's disease.

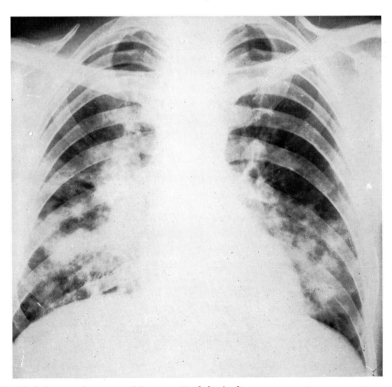

Fig. 768. Nodular involvement of lung in Hodgkin's disease suggesting metastatic carcinoma.

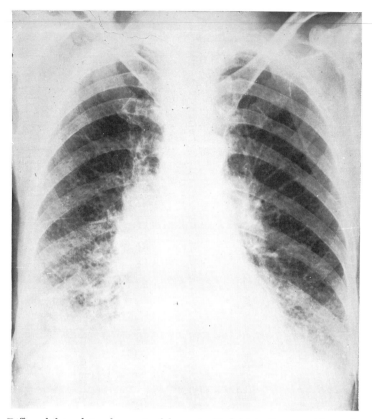

Fig. 769. Diffuse bilateral involvement of lungs in Hodgkin's disease with peribronchial distribution together with mediastinal involvement.

of Hodgkin's disease in the lung (Yardumian and Myers[151]) may offer considerable difficulty in diagnosis (Fig. 769). Grossman et al.[56] reported the radiographic changes observed in a series of forty-five cases of Hodgkin's disease in children 4 to 15 years of age: six of these patients presented pulmonary involvement when first seen and five presented it one to five years later.

Roentgenologic evidence of bone involvement may be found in a surprisingly high number of cases. Vieta et al.[144] demonstrated lesions of the bone in 14.8% of 257 patients on roentgenographic examination. Grossman et al.[56] reported eleven cases of bone involvement in a series of forty-five children with Hodgkin's disease. The higher percentage of bone involvement reported from autopsies indicates that many bone lesions escape detection by roentgenographic examination. Also, symptoms may precede positive roent-

genologic evidence of involvement for a long period of time, particularly in the blood-borne medullary lesions. When the involvement occurs from contiguous lymph nodes, destruction of the cortex will be easily demonstrated. Bone lesions are usually of a mixed osteoblastic and osteolytic type. Romeo and Leonardi[118] emphasized that apparent primary bone lesions may be mistaken for eosinophilic granuloma. Lesions of the skull are invariably osteolytic (Dresser and Spencer[30]). The changes in the extremities tend to be more variable, occurring usually at the ends of long bones, most frequently in the femur. The distribution of bone lesions in a study reported by Dresser and Spencer[30] is shown in Table 115. The presence of retroperitoneal manifestations of Hodgkin's disease may be detected roentgenologically because of displacement of the kidney or pressure defects on the stomach and duodenum (Richman[117]).

Table 115. Distribution of bone lesions in Hodgkin's disease in order of frequency*

Bone involved	Cases		% of total
Vertebrae		29	24.1
Cervical	3		
Dorsal	8		
Lumbar	18		
Pelvis		23	19.1
Femur		19	15.8
Skull		11	9.1
Ribs		11	9.1
Sternum		9	7.5
Clavicle		4	3.3
Tibia		4	3.3
Humerus		4	3.3
Scapula		3	2.5
Os calcis		1	0.8
Radius		1	0.8
Maxilla		1	0.8
Total		120	

*Data from Dresser, R., and Spencer, J.: Hodgkin's disease and allied conditions of bone, Amer. J. Roentgen. **36**:809-815, 1936.

Table 116. Lymphography in Hodgkin's disease—initial study lymphograms*

No. studied	Staging	Abnormal	Normal	Suspicious	Percentage staging advanced due to abnormal lymphography
33	IA	9	17	1	36%
	IB	3	3	0	
57	IIA	14	10	7	51%
	IIB	15	8	3	
9	III and IV	5	4	0	Staging not advanced
99		46	42	11	

*From Davidson, J. W.: Lymphography in malignant disease, Canad. Med. Ass. J. **97**:1282-1289, 1967.

Lymphangiography

In the assessment of the extent of Hodgkin's disease, at the time of initial examination, the ordinary clinical and radiographic examinations are insufficient. Lymphangiography has become an essential part of the examination (Table 116) (Fig. 770). It may be useful in any case but may be particularly fruitful in those patients in whom the disease is apparently of limited extent and who have few symptoms (Lee et al.[88]; Bismuth et al.[15]; Davidson[25]). The contrast material injected in the lower extremity enters the thoracic duct below the second lumbar segment and thus may fail to demonstrate the involvement of nodes above this level: *inferior venacavagrams* may reveal the involvement of high para-aortic node involvement and enhances the effectiveness of lymphangiography (Lee et al.[88]). Since the opaque material may remain in the nodes for weeks or months, repeated radiographic examinations during the course of radiotherapy may show the effect of treatments (Wallace et al.[146]; Marchal et al.[96]) (Fig. 771).

Laboratory examination

The hematologic findings in Hodgkin's disease are not diagnostic. Eosinophilia is found in approximately 20% of all patients, but it is exceedingly variable. It changes during the evolution of the disease

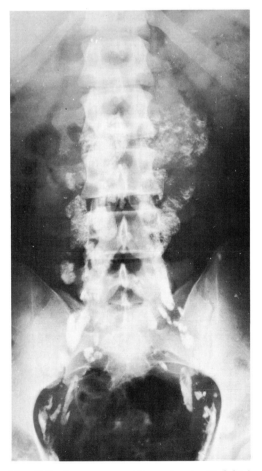

Fig. 770. Large para-aortic nodes in Hodgkin's disease. (From Davidson, J. W.: Lymphography in malignant disease, Canad. Med. Ass. J. **97**: 1282-1289, 1967.)

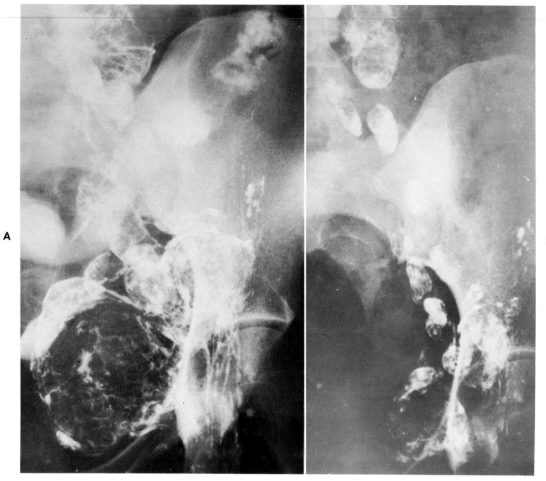

Fig. 771. **A,** Large iliac nodes in Hodgkin's disease. **B,** Same nodes three weeks after irradiation showing marked shrinkage. (From Davidson, J. W.: Lymphography in malignant disease, Canad. Med. Ass. J. **97:**1282-1289, 1967.)

and may or may not coincide with pruritus. The eosinophilia rarely rises to a high figure, averaging from 4% to 6%. The number of platelets and monocytes is increased in the earlier stages of the disease. Thrombocytopenia, as well as anemia, may be observed in early disease of the acute variety. In patients who have been extensively irradiated, hypochromic anemia may result.

Elevation of the serum *alkaline phosphatase* level is highly suggestive of bone involvement. Woodard[149] demonstrated a high incidence of elevated alkaline phosphatase among patients with bone involvement and reported little relationship between the degree of elevation and the type (osteolytic, osteoblastic) of lesion. She concluded that whenever the alkaline phosphatase level is elevated, it probably indicates bone pathology even in the absence of roentgenologic evidence. Cases of hypercalcemia have been reported (Kabakow et al.[78]).

In patients with alcohol-induced pain, an intravenous injection of ethyl alcohol may be used as a means of detecting recurrences in the absence of clinical findings (Godden et al.[51]). Unfortunately, this test is not specific, for the phenomenon is also present, though rarely, in cases of metastatic carcinoma.

Biopsy

A definite diagnosis of Hodgkin's disease can be obtained only by biopsy, and no case, no matter how clear the clinical diagnosis may be, should be treated without benefit of it. The node selected for pathologic examination should be carefully chosen. Because of the tendency of inguinal lymph nodes to be associated with inflammation, it is preferable to choose some other node area. Moreover, very small, easily accessible lymph nodes often overlying the main tumor mass may also reveal only evidence of inflammation. Moderately enlarged nodes that can be completely excised should therefore be selected. On the other hand, incision of a bulky mass for purposes of biopsy should be avoided. Any material obtained should be quickly put in a good fixative. Proper staining allows a careful study of histologic detail. Needle biopsy of Hodgkin's disease lesions is seldom conclusive.

Bone marrow biopsy is not diagnostic in Hodgkin's disease, but secondary findings may be of interest. In general, myeloid and megakaryocytic hyperplasia may be found. Eosinophilia of the bone marrow may be found without any correlation in the peripheral blood picture.

If Sternberg-Reed cells are observed in the bone marrow, they have to be distinguished from megakaryocytes (Yang and Palmer[150]).

Staging

The classification of malignant tumors in several degrees of development, offering some basis for the prognosis of a given case, is a desirable routine. Even when the prognosis of the lesion does not necessarily follow the staging progression, the staging of lesions establishes a possibility of comparison of material and sets a basis for understanding of treatment plans. In recent years, a clinical staging of Hodgkin's disease has been adopted and rather generally practiced:

Stage I

Tumor limited to one or two contiguous anatomic regions above or below the diaphragm

Stage II

Tumor in two separate regions or two noncontiguous regions on the same side of the diaphragm

Stage III

Tumor on both sides of the diaphragm but not outside of lymph nodes or spleen

Stage IV

Tumor involvement of skin, bones, pleura, and viscera, in addition to lymph nodes, or positive bone marrow biopsy

Evidently this segregation requires not only a careful clinical exploration, but also radiographic, lymphographic, and bone marrow studies. Rare cases of visceral manifestations in the absence of lymph node involvement are not eligible for this staging. Systemic symptoms, often an important qualification, are not susceptible to appraisal from one stage to the other, yet must be noted. It has been suggested that lesions in each stage be designated as A or B depending on the absence or presence of systemic symptoms. Liver and spleen scanning may be of value in the clarification of the extent of some cases (Smithers[133]). Advanced cases may not require lymphangiography.

A *clinical* staging fulfills a useful function as a simplified description of the physical findings; hopefully, it may also serve as a basis for prognosis, but its value should rest on a simple clinical basis. Almost without exception, attempts are made to seek a *histologic* accuracy that was not originally intended, nor can it be uniformly applied. Surgical procedures intended primarily to enhance the accuracy of the staging (Enright et al.[34a]) would appear unwarranted.

Differential diagnosis

It is possible to establish a diagnosis of Hodgkin's disease with considerable certainty on clinical examination. Several considerations will help this clinical diagnosis. In the first place, the lymphadenopathy in Hodgkin's disease, no matter how voluminous, is usually polylobated. The nodes are not stony hard as in *metastatic carcinoma*. The mass is usually found on the anterior lower part of the neck (Fig. 764), unlike metastatic carcinoma, which occupies the upper portion of the neck, and unlike lymphosarcoma, which is often found in the upper posterior cervical lymph nodes. In an early case, good general condition of the patient is always in favor of the diag-

Table 117. Clinical differences between lymphosarcoma and Hodgkin's disease

	Lymphosarcoma	*Hodgkin's disease*
Age	Common at extremes of life	Peak between 18 and 38 yr; rare at puberty
General condition of patient (early stages)	Often affected	Usually excellent
Pruritus	Usually not present	May precede and fairly frequently accompanies
Fever	Very rarely observed in early cases	May be found in early cases
Presence of lesion in upper air passages or gastrointestinal tract	Strong suggestion of primary lymphosarcoma of these structures	Rarely involves these structures secondarily
Lymph node involvement	Often symmetrical	Often unilateral
Cervical lymph nodes	Often bilateral, upper cervical, spinal, and jugular chains	Often unilateral, lower cervical and jugular chains
Physical character	Often voluminous, ovoid mass	Often polylobated
Sternal lymph nodes (Goldman and Victor[53])	Practically never involved	When involved, probably Hodgkin's disease
Epitrochlear lymph nodes	May be involved	Practically never involved
Basal metabolic rate (afebrile cases)	May be elevated	Invariably normal
Response to radiations	Great radiosensitivity; immediate response	Marked radiosensitivity; delayed response

nosis of Hodgkin's disease and a generalized adenopathy is against it.

Lymphocytic leukemia can be differentiated from Hodgkin's disease in that it usually presents generalized lymphadenopathy, and the nodes are usually small and have no tendency to be matted together. The basal metabolic rate will be elevated, the spleen will be found enlarged, and a bone marrow biopsy will frequently show leukemic infiltration.

A lymphosarcomatous mass with no demonstrable primary lesion offers the greatest difficulty in differentiation. In *lymphosarcoma*, however, the matted nodes become entirely united, and there is no polylobated appearance. The general condition of the patient is usually affected, and when the disease has spread widely, symmetrical lymph node areas are often involved. These differential points are summarized in Table 117.

The clinical evolution of *giant follicle lymphoma* is rather characteristic because of its slow evolution. This entity can be designated as nodular lymphoma. When first seen, the patients usually have generalized lymphadenopathy, often have lost weight, and fairly often show moderate enlargement of the spleen. The blood count is normal, and bone marrow biopsy is not remarkable. In contrast to patients with other lymphosarcomas, rarely is there involvement of the gastrointestinal or upper respiratory tract; often there is involvement of areas in which lymphoid tissue is not prominent. Tumor nodules can arise in the lacrimal gland, retro-orbital tissue, breast, loose connective tissue of the pelvis, subcutaneous fat, scalp, and bone marrow. Chylous ascites and hydrothorax are fairly frequent. Involvement of the lungs is practically never primary, in contrast to Hodgkin's disease. However, the symptoms and signs of secondary involvement of retroperitoneal lymph nodes and lungs are directly comparable with those observed in Hodgkin's disease. Giant follicle lymphoma responds rather dramatically to small doses of radiations. In sixty-three patients reported by Gall et al.,[42] the total duration of the disease was six years. Seventeen were alive, with an average duration of six years and eight months. The patients who died had lived five years and two months. These figures are in contrast with those of the other types of lymphosarcoma, in which long-time survival is possible in only 2% to 3% of the patients (Klemperer[85]). Patients with giant follicle lymphoma eventually die of their disease. In a high percentage of instances, the disease undergoes transition to lymphocytic leukemia, lymphosarcoma, or reticulum cell sarcoma (Rappaport et al.[113]).

When the lymphadenopathy is fluctuant, particularly in the cervical region, and discharging sinuses occur, *tuberculosis* may be coexistent with Hodgkin's disease. Tuberculosis of the cervical lymph nodes tends to localize to a single large node. If a superficial adenopathy is absent, it may be very difficult to determine whether the patient is suffering from Hodgkin's disease. When lung lesions are present, they may masquerade as a miliary tuberculosis or even primary bronchiogenic tumors (Moolten[99]). The enlargement of lymph nodes in the submaxillary or submental regions is seldom due to Hodgkin's disease but is more often related to tumors or infections of the oral cavity. There are other diseases of the lymph nodes which, at times, may also be hard to differentiate from Hodgkin's disease. Hyperplastic tuberculous lymphadenitis may be confused with Hodgkin's disease. Clinically, *Boeck's sarcoid* may simulate Hodgkin's disease, particularly when it involves mediastinal lymph nodes. If skin manifestations, uveitis, bone changes, or peripheral lymphadenopathy occur with it, then clinical or pathologic recognition is relatively simple. Oppenheim and Pollack[104] reported forty-two patients with Boeck's sarcoid, thirty-four of whom had mediastinal manifestations. The majority of patients were 20 to 35 years of age, and twelve were black. The roentgenologic appearance of pulmonary sarcoidosis may be easily confused with the lung infiltrations of Hodgkin's disease. In sarcoidosis, however, there is usually bilateral *symmetrical* hilar adenopathy and right paratracheal lymph node enlargement (Garland[43]) (Fig. 772). *Infectious mononucleosis* can be ruled out by its clinical course, the differential white blood cell count, and the heterophile antibody reaction. The interpretation of a lymph node in infectious mononucleosis is difficult.

In the absence of other manifestations, a bone lesion of Hodgkin's disease may suggest osteomyelitis, metastatic carcinoma, or primary osteogenic sarcoma. Bone lesions may also simulate multiple myeloma, Ewing's sarcoma, or bone cyst. Gastrointestinal lesions, when they are present, do

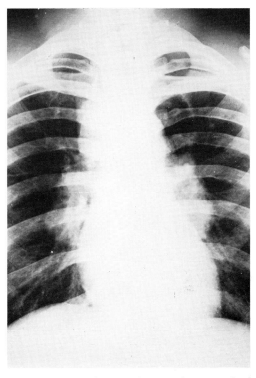

Fig. 772. Sarcoidosis with typical paratracheal adenopathy.

not present any characteristic roentgenologic picture and cannot be differentiated from ulcerative colitis, enteritis, or obstructions of the bowel (Sherman[127]). They are usually associated with peripheral enlargement of lymph nodes and other symptoms of Hodgkin's disease. When disease is confined to the abdominal cavity, the differential diagnosis may be particularly perplexing. Occasionally, because of its bizarre manifestations and absence of peripheral lymphadenopathy, Hodgkin's disease may be impossible to diagnose except at biopsy, laparotomy, or postmortem examination.

Treatment
Surgery

There is no indication for surgery as definitive treatment for Hodgkin's disease. Invariably, articles written quote a few examples of excellent results, but in practically all instances, surgery has been combined with radiation therapy (Lacher[86]; Slaughter and Craver[128]; Molander and Pack[98]). In the presence of gastric hemorrhage, intestinal obstruction, and secondary hypersplenism, surgery may have temporary palliative benefit. It has been shown that surgery cannot include as large a potentially involved area as irradiation, and no one now doubts the ability of radiation therapy to locally control the disease. In the few patients we have seen in whom surgery was done by an enthusiastic surgeon, local recurrence followed promptly. In patients with a single asymptomatic mediastinal mass, exploration may be necessary to make a diagnosis. This mass is often caused by Hodgkin's disease and is easily removed by the thoracic surgeon. Removal is uniformly followed by radiation therapy. Whether such a removal has benefit is doubtful.

Radiotherapy

The unquestionable treatment of choice of Hodgkin's disease is radiotherapy. The disease is invariably radiosensitive and locally radiocurable. Adequacy of radiotherapy requires serious considerations of approach and dosimetry without which the patient's outlook may be greatly compromised.

An important consideration is that of *dosage*, for, although clinical regression may be observed at times with the administration of a relatively small dose (Fayos et al.[38]), local sterilization requires, in general, a much larger one (Fig. 773). However, the necessary dose of radiations is not so large as in the treatment of car-

cinomas. A second important consideration is the *fractionation* of the dose in time. Since patients with Hodgkin's disease are frequently young and may be expected to survive for many years, irradiation should be conducted over a reasonably long period of time to minimize the untoward effects of radiations over the irradiated normal structures. The tumor does not require great intensity in the daily treatments. It is only important to accumulate a moderate total amount of radiations which may be increased with the total time in which it is administered. It is reasonable to administer a moderate dose of radiations at the level of the suspected tumor involvement in a period of no less than four to five weeks. Larger doses are often not necessary. But irradiation of the strictly clinical or radiographically ostensible involvement is not sufficient.

"The ideas behind modern treatment for this disease go back to the early 1920's and to the pioneer work of René Gilbert, of Geneva, who was the father of radiotherapy for Hodgkin's disease."[*] The principle advanced by Gilbert,[44] and now generally accepted, of "*prophylactic irradiation*" of potential areas of adjacent regional involvement has unquestionably resulted in better survival and even the hope of complete cure of some cases (Easson[31]) (Fig. 774).

We have practiced and advocated these principles of relatively high dosage, reasonable fractionation, and extended ("prophylactic") irradiation for over thirty years, following the example of Gilbert.[45] Even when the disease appears strictly localized to an area such as the supraclavicular or axillary region, the minimum irradiation should include the entire side of the neck, the homolateral axilla, and the upper mediastinum. When the mediastinum is ostensibly involved, both supraclavicular and axillary regions, as well as the para-aortic nodes, should be irradiated. With the help of lymphangiography and the discovery of abdominal involvement in an apparently localized case, the areas to be irradiated may be rather extensive and require, in our view, treatments fraction-

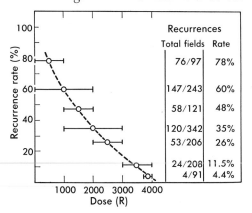

Fig. 773. Composite data on recurrence rate in radiation-treated fields as function of dose without reference to time of delivery. (From Kaplan, H. S.: Evidence for tumoricidal dose level in the radiotherapy of Hodgkin's disease, Cancer Res. **26:**1221-1224, 1966; WU neg. 68-4682.)

---

[*]From Smithers, D. W.: Factors influencing survival in patients with Hodgkin's disease, Clin. Radiol. **20:**124-132, 1969.

ated over several months. The principle of prophylactic or extended irradiation has been confused with an unwarranted and assumed need for *intensive* and *simultaneous* irradiation of a number of given areas. The simultaneous irradiation of both sides of the neck, supraclavicular and axillary regions, and mediastinum through a single anteroposterior field, dubbed "the mantle," is an artifact of mistaken pragmatism that has nothing to do with the principle of extended irradiation. In fact, the irradiation of such a field even in moderate doses is fraught with definite hazards in the irradiation of normal structures such as the lung, spinal cord, heart, and pericardium; the approach limits the irradiation to an anteroposterior and/or posteroanterior field. In addition, the use of this single field implies a greater than desirable daily intensity of irradiations. Better results are obtained by the irradiation of carefully planned regional fields which reduce the areas of untoward irradiation and fractionate the treatment over a desirable longer time (Regato[115]).

Johnson[75] has been impressed with the relative frequency of noncontiguous recurrences. He advocates irradiation of all lymph node areas in succession, rather than simultaneously, as we have ourselves advocated. He allows for periods of rest in between series of treatments for recovery of the irradiated bone marrow.

Although good results have long been obtained with conventional roentgentherapy when the foregoing principles were applied, cobalt[60] teletherapy and supervoltage roentgentherapy have made the irradiation of patients with Hodgkin's disease more tolerable and more efficient. It must be said also that these new sources have brought to the treatment a greater morbidity (Vogel et al.[145]) and even some mortality due to excessive reliance on their virtues (Kaplan and Rosenberg[80]).

A point seldom made in the considerations of radiotherapy of Hodgkin's disease is that of informing the patient of the hopefulness of his condition provided only that he submits to regular and frequent follow-up examinations for the rest of his life. Most patients, frequently young, are willing to submit to treatment but thereafter wish to forget their condition and its serious implications. They must be convinced that their best interest lies in not forgetting about it and that prompt diagnosis and adequate treatment of any new manifestation is the only basis for long survival.

Favorable results have been obtained even in apparently hopeless cases. Intrathoracic masses, even when invading the

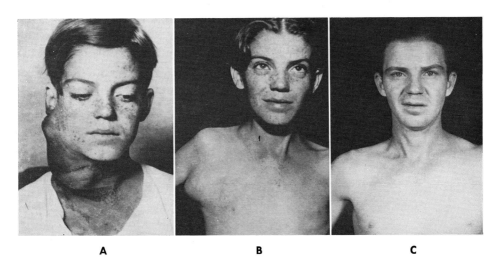

A **B** **C**

Fig. 774. A, Young boy with extensive cervical Hodgkin's disease. **B,** Several years later when axillary manifestation developed. **C,** Twenty-three years after initial treatment. Patient remains well thirty-three years after onset at 6 years of age. (**A** and **B,** Courtesy Dr. W. H. Cole, Asheville, N. C., and Dr. R. Elman, St. Louis, Mo.)

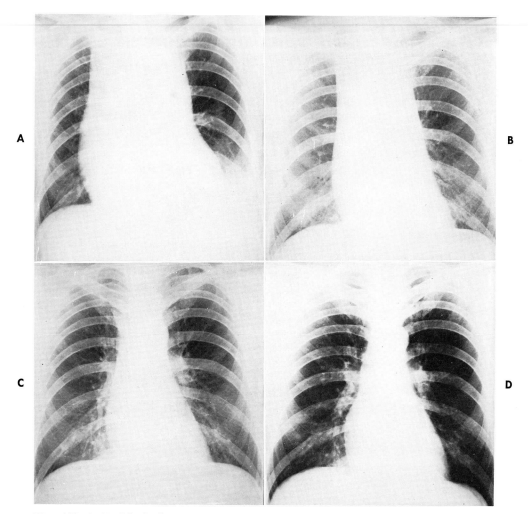

Fig. 775. **A,** Hodgkin's disease of mediastinum after roentgentherapy was started. **B,** Two weeks later. **C,** Four months after completion of treatment. **D,** Fifteen months after completion of treatment. Patient has remained without further manifestations of disease for over ten years.

pleura and lung, may totally regress (Fig. 775). The treatment of bone lesions contributes prompt alleviation of pain and reparative changes (Roussel et al.[120]). Early treatment of cases of paraplegia may be followed by motor return (Bataini and Ennuyer[11]). In the presence of pregnancy, radiotherapy should not be directed to the abdomen and pelvis, but irradiation of other areas is possible with adequate precautions (Smith et al.[130]). Rarely is there a situation that might force consideration of therapeutic abortion (Hartvigsen[58]; Peters and Middlemiss[110]). Young female patients with "active" Hodgkin's disease are often advised against becoming pregnant (Barry et al.[10]) on the assumption that the pregnancy may enhance the course of the disease. This point of view has been repeatedly disputed (Gilbert[47]).

Periods of remission during which the patient is apparently normal will result from the administration of radiations. However, prolongation of life will depend greatly upon the conscientious follow-up of the patients and effective radiotherapy of new areas of involvement as they become manifest. If, under treatment, the temperature becomes normal, the pruritus ceases with a regression of all nodes, and weight is regained, these signs are favorable. If, on the other hand, fever continues and the leukocyte count remains elevated or the weight further diminishes, then areas of active disease undoubtedly remain. Return of symptoms after a period of remission should lead to a thorough search for new areas of involvement.

Chemotherapy

Various drugs have had favorable effects in Hodgkin's disease, including the alkylating agents, the vinca alkaloids, actinomycin D, N-methyl hydrazine. The antimetabolites have been less effective (Karnofsky[81]). But chemotherapy has its effects on the neoplastic manifestations at the price of serious deleterious effects on normal vital tissues such as the bone marrow. Moreover, besides being unpredictable, the effects are neither complete nor lasting. It has been said that previous treatment hampers the response to chemotherapy (Frei and Gamble[40]). It is also true that previous chemotherapy damages importantly the possibilities of radiotherapy (Johnson and Brace[76]). In cases that are manageable by radiotherapy, we do not advocate the use of chemotherapy as a radiotherapeutic adjuvant. However, Buschke[23] advocates the combination in the management of spinal cord involvement by Hodgkin's disease. Chemotherapy is advocated in the palliative management of patients with advanced disease or when radiotherapy is no longer advisable (Newall[103]). Vincaleucoblastine gives excellent palliation (Bousser et al.[19]; Kenis[84]; Viala et al.[143]). Vinblastine has been tried in combination with chlorambucil (Lacher and Durant[86a]). As Aisenberg[4] has pointed out, the use of these drugs has not proved to increase survival. In addition, their enthusiastic and hopeful application may deprive the patient of adequate radiotherapeutic management and very long survival. *The drugs certainly do not enhance the effects of radiations, and they are not a curative agent.*

Prognosis

In 1965, there was in the United States a total of 3394 deaths from Hodgkin's disease, a crude rate of 1.8 per 100,000 population. The mortality rate has remained about the same in the past few decades.

The fact that Hodgkin's disease frequently affects young women and men usually arouses untoward emotions, haste, and inadequacies in its therapeutic management. It is pertinent to emphasize that adequate radiotherapy results often in long survivals (Gilbert and Rutishauser[50]), that *at least one patient out of every four may live in comfort for twenty-five years.* A five-year survival of over 50% and a fifteen-year survival of 40% are perfectly possible assuming adequate irradiation (Easson[31]). In recent years, the acknowledgement of these results and a wider application of Gilbert's precepts of extended irradiation to optimum dose levels has resulted in optimistic talk of complete cure of Hodgkin's disease (Easson[31]; Kaplan[79]; Smithers[133]). As adequately summed up by Jelliffe,[71] the use of insufficient doses of radiations and the reliance on chemotherapy alone must be strongly deprecated; they betray a pessimism engendered by lack of appreciation of our present possibilities in the treatment of Hodgkin's disease. Any claim of cure of Hodgkin's disease must reckon with the fact that such diagnosis is often made on benign adenopathies of young children, that nodes in patients with infectious mononucleosis and in patients receiving anticonvulsant drugs can be misdiagnosed for Hodgkin's disease, and that there are cases on record of as long as twenty-three years between manifestations of the disease (Regato[115]).

In general, the prognosis of patients with Hodgkin's disease correlates with the stage of the disease when first encountered (Peters et al.[109]). But, regardless of apparent stage, the presence of systemic symptoms, weight loss, pruritus, fever, chills, etc., is relatively unfavorable. Women have a relatively better prognosis than men (Papillon et al.[106]). Histologic evidence of nodular sclerosis and lymphocytic predominance is a favorable sign. Mediastinal involvement is often associated with the nodular sclerosing type and has a good prognosis (Burke et al.[22]). There seems to be no relationship of age to prognosis (Jenkin et al.[73]). Pregnancy has no adverse influence on prognosis (Hennessy and Rottino[59]). Musshoff et al.[101] reported a group of patients with bone involvement whose average survival was greater than that of patients presenting no bone involve-

Table 118. Median survival in each stage according to duration*

Stage	Before diagnosis	After diagnosis
I	6 mo	10 yr
IIA	10 mo	12 yr
IIB	6 mo	2 yr
III	7 mo	9.5 mo
All cases	6 mo	34 mo

*From Peters, M. V., et al.: Natural history of Hodgkin's disease as related to staging, Cancer 19:308-316, 1966.

ment. This paradoxical finding is supported by Stuhlberg and Ellis.[137]

Beyond early stage of development, favorable histopathology, and other hopeful circumstances, the long-time results depend primarily on the chronicity of the disease, the thoroughness of the radiotherapeutic approach, and painstaking and unrelenting follow-up for early treatment of new manifestations (Gilbert[45]; Hultberg[66]; Trubestein[138]; Hohl[61]). Cure is indeed a possibility, although difficult to define. As Peters et al.[109] pointed out, the extent of disease prior to treatment is the most dependable single influence in predicting the course of the disease. The results indicated in Table 118 represent an accurate appraisal of our present-day treatment, for the patients were precisely staged and adequately treated.

REFERENCES

1 Aisenberg, A. C.: Immunologic aspects of Hodgkin's disease, Medicine (Balt.) **43:**189-193, 1964.

2 Aisenberg, A. C.: Hodgkin's disease—prognosis, treatment and etiologic and immunologic considerations, New Eng. J. Med. **270:**508-514, 1964.

3 Aisenberg, A. C.: Studies of lymphocyte transfer reactions in Hodgkin's disease, J. Clin. Invest. **44:**555-564, 1965.

4 Aisenberg, A. C.: Current concepts; primary management of Hodgkin's disease, New Eng. J. Med. **278:**93-95, 1968.

5 Aisenberg, A. C., and Leskowitz, S.: Antibody formation in Hodgkin's disease, New Eng. J. Med. **268:**1269-1272, 1963.

6 Alison, R. E., and Bush, R. S.: Natural history of Hodgkin's disease as related to staging, Cancer **19:**308-316, 1966.

7 Allen, A. C.: Persistent "insect bites" (dermal eosinophilic granulomas) simulating lymphoblastomas, histiocytes and squamous cell carcinomas, Amer. J. Path. **24:**367-387, 1949.

8 Amiel, J. L., Bernard, J., Dreyfus, B., Laugier, A., Seligmann, M., and Pequignot, H.: Traitement actuel de la maladie de Hodgkin's et des reticulosarcome, Presse Med. **73:**353-356, 1965.

9 Azzam, S. A.: High incidence of Hodgkin's disease in children in Lebanon, Cancer Res. **26:**1202-1203, 1966.

10 Barry, R. M., Diamond, H. D., and Craver, L. F.: Influence of pregnancy on the course of Hodgkin's disease, Amer. J. Obstet. Gynec. **84:**445-454, 1962.

11 Bataini, J., and Ennuyer, A.: Les paraplegies hodgkiniennes, Ann. Radiol. (Paris) **1:**333-354, 1958.

12 Bayrd, E. D., Paulson, G. S., and Hargraves, M. M.: Hodgkin's specific cells in bone marrow aspirations; a brief review and report of two cases, Blood **9:**46-56, 1964.

13 Bichel, J.: Herpes zoster in Hodgkin's disease, Folia Clin. Int. (Barc.) **6:**304-306, 1956.

14 Bichel, J.: Long remissions in Hodgkin's disease, Acta Radiol. (Stockholm) **44:**325-336, 1955.

15 Bismuth, V., Bernageau, S., Desprez-Curely, J. P., and Bourdon, P.: La place de la lymphographie dans la maladie de Hodgkin, Sem. Hop. Paris **40:**2311-2322, 1964.

16 Boeck, C.: Multiple benign sarcoid of the skin, J. Cutan. Genitourin. Dis. **17:**543-550, 1899.

17 Bonenfant, J. L.: La lymph-reticulose medullaire chronique maligne avec syndrome hodgkinien (paragranuloma), Bull. Ass. Franc. Cancer **41:**296-315, 1954.

18 Bostick, W. L.: Evidence for the virus etiology of Hodgkin's disease, Ann. N. Y. Acad. Sci. **73:**307-334, 1958.

19 Bousser, J., Bilski-Pasquier, G., and Piquet, H.: The maintenance treatment of Hodgkin's disease with vincaleucoblastine. In Groupe Europeen de Chimiotherapie Anticancereuse: Antitumoral effects of Vinca rosea alkaloids; proceedings of the first symposium, Paris, 1965 (edited by S. Garattini and E. M. Sproston), Amsterdam, 1966, Excerpta Medica Foundation (International Congress series no. 106).

20 Bowdler, A. J., and Glick, I. W.: Autoimmune hemolytic anemia as the herald state of Hodgkin's disease, Ann. Intern. Med. **65:**761-767, 1966.

21 Brunschwig, A., and Kandel, E.: Correlation of the histologic changes and clinical symptoms in irradiated Hodgkin's disease and lymphoblastoma lymph nodes, Radiology **23:**315-326, 1934.

22 Burke, W. A., Burford, T. H., and Dorfman, R. F.: Hodgkin's disease of the mediastinum, Ann. Thorac. Surg. **3:**287-296, 1967.

23 Buschke, F.: Some reflections on the treatment and prognosis of Hodgkin's disease, Radiol. Clin. (Basel) **34:**285-309, 1965.

24 Contamin, A.: Les formes a debut purement mediastinal de la maladie de Hodgkin (A propos de 41 observations), Lyon, France, 1962, Imprimerie des Beaux-Arts.

25 Davidson, J. W.: Lymphography in malignant disease, Canad. Med. Ass. J. **97:**1282-1289, 1967.

26 Dawson, P. J., and Harrison, C. V.: A clinico-

pathological study of benign Hodgkin's disease, J. Clin. Path. **14**:219-231, 1961.

27 DeVore, J. W., and Doan, C. A.: Studies of Hodgkin's syndrome. XII. Hereditary and epidemiologic aspects, Ann. Intern. Med. **47**: 300-316, 1957.

28 Diamond, H. D.: Results of therapy in Hodgkin's disease, Ann. N. Y. Acad. Sci. **74**:357-362, 1958.

29 Di Pietro, S., and Pizzetti, F.: La prognosi istologica del granuloma maligno in base allo studio di 100 casi, Tumori **52**:451-463, 1966.

30 Dresser, R., and Spencer, J.: Hodgkin's disease and allied conditions of bone, Amer. J. Roentgen. **36**:809-815, 1936.

31 Easson, E. C.: Possibilities for the cure of Hodgkin's disease, Cancer **19**:345-350, 1966.

32 Easson, E. C., and Russell, M. H.: The cure of Hodgkin's disease, Brit. Med. J. **5347**: 1704-1707, 1963.

33 Ebstein, W.: Chronisches Rucksfallsfieber, ein neue Infectionskrankheit, Berlin. Klin. Wschr. **24**:837-842, 1887.

34 Ennuyer, A., Calle, R., Rosseau, S., and Bertoluzzi, M.: Les localisations oesophagiennes de la maladie de Hodgkin, Paris Med. **40**:164-167, 1950.

34a Enright, L. P., Trueblood, H. W., and Nelsen, T. S.: The surgical diagnosis of abdominal Hodgkin's disease, Surg. Gynec. Obstet. **130**:853-858, 1970.

35 Fairley, G. H., Patterson, M. J. L., and Scott, R. B.: Chemotherapy of Hodgkin's disease with cyclophosphamide, vinblastine and procarbazine, Brit. Med. J. **2**:75-78, 1966.

36 Falconer, E. H.: Blood picture in Hodgkin's disease, Calif. West. Med. **32**:83-87, 1930.

37 Farrell, W. J.: Lymphangiographic demonstration of lymphovenous communication after radiotherapy in Hodgkin's disease, Radiology **87**:630-634, 1966.

38 Fayos, J., Hendrix, R., Macdonald, V., and Lampe, I.: Hodgkin's disease; a review of radiotherapeutic experience, Amer. J. Roentgen. **93**:557-567, 1965.

39 Fisher, E. R., and Hazard, J. B.: Differentiation of megakaryocyte and Reed-Sternberg cell; with reference to the periodic-acid-Schiff reaction, Lab. Invest. **3**:261-269, 1954.

40 Frei, E., and Gamble, J. F.: Progress in the chemotherapy of Hodgkin's disease, Cancer **19**:378-384, 1966.

41 Fuller, L. M.: Results of large volume irradiation in the management of Hodgkin's disease and malignant lymphomas originating in the abdomen, Radiology **87**:1058-1064, 1966.

42 Gall, E. A., Morrison, H. R., and Scott, A. T.: The follicular type of malignant lymphoma, Ann. Intern. Med. **14**:2073-2090, 1941.

43 Garland, L. H.: Pulmonary sarcoidosis; the early roentgen findings, Radiology **48**:333-354, 1947.

44 Gilbert, R.: Le traitement de la granulomatose maligne par la radiotherapie, J. Radiol. Electr. **22**:577-585, 1938.

45 Gilbert, R.: Radiotherapy in Hodgkin's disease (malignant granulomatosis)—anatomic and clinical foundations; governing principles; results, Amer. J. Roentgen. **41**:198-241, 1939.

46 Gilbert, R.: Lymphogranulomatose (maladie de Hodgkin) ou granulomatose maligne. In Delherm, L.: Nouveau traité d'éléctro-radiothérapie, Paris, 1951, Masson et Cie.

47 Gilbert, R.: The problem of pregnancy in Hodgkin's disease, Acta Radiol. (Stockholm) **35**:71-75, 1951.

48 Gilbert, R.: La therapeutique actuelle de la granulomatose maligne (Hodgkin), J. Belg. Radiol. **39**:638-649, 1956.

49 Gilbert, R., and Babaiantz, L.: Notre méthode de roentgenthérapie de la lymphogranulomatose (Hodgkin); résultats éloignés, Acta Radiol. Electr. **17**:129, 1933.

50 Gilbert, R., and Rutishauser, E.: Lymphogranulomes (Hodgkin): deux cas de survies de trente ans après roentgenthérapie. Existe-t-il des formes abortives ou des états latents de la maladie? Oncologia (Basel) **9**:57-70, 1956.

51 Godden, J. O., Clagett, O. T., and Andersen, H. A.: Sensitivity to alcohol as a symptom of Hodgkin's disease, J.A.M.A. **160**:1274-1277, 1956.

52 Goldman, L. B.: Hodgkin's disease, J.A.M.A. **114**:1611-1616, 1940.

53 Goldman, L. B., and Victor, A. W.: Hodgkin's disease, New York J. Med. **45**:1313-1318, 1945.

54 Goldman, R.: Infraclavicular chest wall tumors in Hodgkin's disease, Calif. Med. **76**: 38-39, 1952.

55 Grand, C. G.: Tissue culture studies of cytoplasmic inclusion bodies in lymph nodes of Hodgkin's disease, Proc. Soc. Exp. Biol. Med. **56**:229-230, 1944.

56 Grossman, H., Winchester, P. H., Bragg, D. G., Tan, C., and Murphy, M. L.: Roentgenographic changes in childhood Hodgkin's disease, Amer. J. Roentgen. **108**:354-364, 1970.

57 Hanson, T. A. S.: Histological classification and survival in Hodgkin's disease; a study of 251 cases with special reference to nodular sclerosing Hodgkin's disease, Cancer **17**:1595-1603, 1964.

58 Hartvigsen, B.: Hodgkin's disease and pregnancy, Acta Radiol. (Stockholm) **44**:317-324, 1955.

59 Hennessy, M. P., and Rottino, A.: Hodgkin's disease in pregnancy, Amer. J. Obstet. Gynec. **87**:851-853, 1963.

60 Hoffbrand, B. I.: Hodgkin's disease, autoimmunity and the thymus, Brit. Med. J. **1**:1592-1594, 1965.

61 Hohl, K.: The present position of treatment and prognosis of Hodgkin's disease, Radiol. Clin. (Basel) **33**:273-286, 1964.

62 Hoster, H. A.: Studies in Hodgkin's disease syndrome; etiologic studies in Hodgkin's disease, Cancer Res. **7**:48, 1947.

63 Hoster, H. A.: Hodgkin's disease, Amer. J. Roentgen. **64**:913-918, 1950.

64 Hoster, H. A., Doan, C. A., and Schumacher, M.: Studies in Hodgkin's syndrome; relation-

ship of tubercle bacilli to Hodgkin's syndrome, J. Lab. Clin. Med. **20**:675-677, 1945.

65 Hoster, H. A., and Dratman, M. B.: Hodgkin's disease 1832-1947, Cancer Res. **8**:1-78, 1948.

66 Hultberg, S.: Pregnancy in Hodgkin's disease, Acta Radiol. (Stockholm) **41**:277-289, 1954.

67 Hyman, G. A., and Sommers, S. C.: The development of Hodgkin's disease and lymphoma during anticonvulsant therapy, Blood **28**:416-427, 1966.

68 Jackson, H., Jr., and Parker, F., Jr.: Hodgkin's disease; pathology, New Eng. J. Med. **231**:35-44, 1944.

69 Jackson, H., Jr., and Parker, F., Jr.: Hodgkin's disease; clinical diagnosis, New Eng. J. Med. **234**:37-41, 1946.

69a Jackson, H., Jr., and Parker, F., Jr.: Hodgkin's disease; treatment and prognosis, New Eng. J. Med. **234**:103-110, 1946.

70 James, A. H.: Hodgkin's disease with and without alcohol-induced pain, Quart. J. Med. **29**:47-66, 1960.

71 Jelliffe, A. M.: The present place of radiotherapy in the cure of Hodgkin's disease, Clin. Radiol. **16**:274-277, 1965.

72 Jelliffe, A. M., and Thomson, A. D.: The prognosis in Hodgkin's disease, Brit. J. Cancer **9**:21-36, 1955.

73 Jenkin, R. D. T., Peters, M. V., and Darte, J. M. M.: Hodgkin's disease in children, Amer. J. Roentgen. **100**:222-226, 1967.

74 Johnson, A. W.: Spontaneous regression of the glands in Hodgkin's disease, Brit. Med. J. **1**:916-917, 1954.

75 Johnson, R. E.: Modern approaches to the radiotherapy of lymphoma, Seminars Hemat. **6**:357-375, 1969.

76 Johnson, R. E., and Brace, K. C.: Radiation response of Hodgkin's disease recurrent after chemotherapy, Cancer **19**:368-370, 1966.

77 Johnson, R. E., Foley, H. T., Steckel, R. J., and Glenn, D. W.: Extended radiotherapy in advanced Hodgkin's disease; hematologic aspects, Arch. Intern. Med. (Chicago) **118**:70-74, 1966.

78 Kabakow, B., Mines, M. F., and King, F. H.: Hypercalcemia in Hodgkin's disease, New Eng. J. Med. **256**:59-62, 1957.

79 Kaplan, H. S.: Evidence for a tumoricidal dose level in the radiotherapy of Hodgkin's disease, Cancer Res. **26**:1221-1224, 1966.

80 Kaplan, H. S., and Rosenberg, S. A.: The treatment of Hodgkin's disease, Med. Clin. N. Amer. **50**:1591-1610, 1966.

81 Karnofsky, D. A.: Chemotherapy of Hodgkin's disease, Cancer **19**:371-377, 1966.

82 Kassel, R.: Etiological considerations in Hodgkin's disease, Ann. N. Y. Acad. Sci. **73**:335-343, 1958.

83 Keller, A. R., Kaplan, H. S., Lukes, R. J., and Rappaport, H.: Correlation of histopathology with other prognostic indicators in Hodgkin's disease, Cancer **22**:487-499, 1968.

84 Kenis, Y.: A comparative study of vinblastine and Natulan in the treatment of Hodgkin's disease; preliminary clinical observations and plan of the investigation. In Groupe Europeen de Chimiotherapie Anticancereuse: Antitumoral effects of Vinca rosea alkaloids; proceedings of the first symposium, Paris, 1965 (edited by S. Garattini and E. M. Sproston), Amsterdam, 1966, Excerpta Medica Foundation (International Congress series no. 106).

85 Klemperer, P.: The spleen in Hodgkin's disease, lymphosarcomatosis and leukemia, Amer. J. Med. Sci. **188**:593-596, 1934.

86 Lacher, M. J.: Role of surgery in Hodgkin's disease, New Eng. J. Med. **268**:289-292, 1963.

86a Lacher, M. J., and Durant, J. R.: Combined vinblastine and chlorambucil therapy of Hodgkin's disease, Ann. Intern. Med. **62**:468-476, 1965.

87 Laipply, T. C.: Lipomelanotic reticular hyperplasia of lymph nodes, Arch. Intern. Med. (Chicago) **81**:19-36, 1948.

88 Lee, B. J., Nelson, J. H., and Schwarz, G.: Evaluation of lymphangiography, inferior venacavography and intravenous pyelography in the clinical staging and management of Hodgkin's disease and lymphosarcoma, New Eng. J. Med. **271**:327-337, 1964.

89 Le Shan, L., Marvin, S., and Lyerly, O.: Some evidence of a relationship between Hodgkin's disease and intelligence, Arch. Gen. Psychiat. (Chicago) **1**:477-479, 1959.

90 L'esperance, E. S.: Pathogenicity of avian tubercle bacillus, J. Immun. **16**:27-36, 1929.

91 Lohmann, H. J.: Prognostic significance of histopathology in Hodgkin's granuloma, Acta Path. Microbiol. Scand. **64**:16-30, 1965.

92 Lukes, R. J.: Relationship of histologic features to clinical stages in Hodgkin's disease, Amer. J. Roentgen. **90**:944-955, 1963.

93 Lukes, R. J., and Butler, J. J.: The pathology and nomenclature of Hodgkin's disease, Cancer Res. **26**:1063-1081, 1966.

94 Lukes, R. J., Butler, J. J., and Hicks, E. B.: Le pronostic de la Hodgkin d'après la variété histologique et le stade clinique. Rôle des réactions de l'hôte, Nouv. Rev. Franc. Hemat. **6**:15-22, 1966.

95 MacMahon, B.: Epidemiology of Hodgkin's disease, Cancer Res. **26**:1189-1201, 1966.

96 Marchal, G., Bernard, J., Arvay, N., Bilski-Pasquier, G., Picard, J. D., Mathe, G., and Brule, G.: La lymphographie dans la maladie de Hodgkin (Étude de 45 cas), Nouv. Rev. Franc. Hemat. **2**:4-26, 1962.

97 Marcus, S. C.: Cancer illness among residents of Birmingham, Alabama (1948), United States Federal Security Agency, National Institutes of Health, P.H.S. pub. 216, Cancer morbidity series 8, Washington, D. C., 1952, National Cancer Institute.

98 Molander, D. W., and Pack, G. T., editors: Hodgkin's disease, Springfield, Ill., 1968, Charles C Thomas, Publisher.

99 Moolten, S. E.; Hodgkin's disease of the lung, Amer. J. Cancer **21**:253-294, 1934.

100 Motulsky, A. G., Weinberg, S., Saphir, O., and Rosenberg, E.: Lymph nodes in rheuma-

toid arthritis, Arch. Intern. Med. (Chicago) **90**:660-676, 1952.

101 Musshoff, K., Busch, M., and Kaminski, H.: Lymphogranulomatose (Morbus Hodgkin) mit Knochenbefall. Symptomatologie mit besonderer Berücksictigung des Röntgenbildes, Therapie und Prognose. Ein Bericht über 66 Fälle (Freiburger Krankengut 1948-1961), Fortschr. Roentgenstr. **101**:117-137, 1964.

102 Myles, T. J. M.: Hodgkin's disease and pregnancy, J. Obstet. Gynaec. Brit. Emp. **62**:884-891, 1955.

103 Newall, J.: The management of Hodgkin's disease, Clin. Radiol. **16**:40-50, 1965.

104 Oppenheim, A., and Pollack, R.: Boeck's sarcoid (sarcoidosis), Amer. J. Roentgen. **57**:28-35, 1947.

105 Papillon, J., Croizat, P., Revol, L., Chassard, J. L., Bothier, F., and Coste, J.: Les localisations osseuses de la lymphogranulomatose maligne, J. Radiol. Electr. **45**:109-116, 1964.

106 Papillon, J., Croizat, P., Revol, L., Chassard, J. L., Chassard, E., and Contamin, A.: Le pronostic de la maladie Hodgkin, J. Radiol. Electr. **47**:381-390, 1966.

107 Perttala, Y., and Svinhufvud, U.: Cavity formation in the lung in Hodgkin's disease; analysis of 453 cases, Ann. Med. Intern. Fenn. **54**:19-24, 1965.

108 Pel, P. K.: Zur symptomatologie der sogennanten Pseudo-leukamie, Berlin. Klin. Wschr. **22**:3, 1885.

109 Peters, M. V., Alison, R. E., and Bush, R. S.: Natural history of Hodgkin's disease as related to staging, Cancer **19**:308-316, 1966.

110 Peters, M. V., and Middlemiss, K. C. H.: A study of Hodgkin's disease treated by irradiation, Amer. J. Roentgen. **79**:114-121, 1958.

111 Pirofsky, B.: Autoimmune hemolytic anemia and neoplasia of the reticuloendothelium; with a hypothesis concerning etiologic relationships, Ann. Intern. Med. **68**:109-121, 1968.

112 Pitcock, J. A., Bauer, W. C., and McGavran, M. H.: Hodgkin's disease in children, Cancer **12**:1043-1051, 1959.

113 Rappaport, H., Winter, W. J., and Hicks, E. B.: Follicular lymphoma; a re-evaluation of its position in the scheme of malignant lymphoma, based on a survey of 253 cases, Cancer **9**:792-821, 1956.

114 Razis, D. V., Diamond, H. D., and Craver, L. F.: Familial Hodgkin's disease; its significance and implications, Ann. Intern. Med. **51**:933-971, 1959.

115 del Regato, J. A.: Reflections on the so-called lymphomas, Radiol. Clin. N. Amer. **6**:3-13, 1968.

116 del Regato, J. A., and Chahbazian, C. M.: Hodgkin's disease; radiation therapy. In Conn, H. F., editor: Current therapy, Philadelphia, 1969, W. B. Saunders Co., pp. 258-262.

117 Richman, S.: Roentgen manifestations in Hodgkin's disease of retroperitoneal lymph nodes, Radiology **50**:521-524, 1948.

118 Romeo, G., and Leonardi, R.: Sulla varietà ossea clinicamente primitiva del linfogranu-

loma maligno, Riv. Anat. Pat. Oncol. **11**:345-370, 1956.

119 Rosenberg, S. A.: Report of the Committee on the Staging of Hodgkin's Disease, Cancer Res. **26**:1310, 1966.

120 Roussel, J., Schoumacher, P., Pernot, M., Candela, A., Metz, R., and Kessler, Y.: Considérations sur les localisations osseuses de la maladie de Hodgkin, J. Radiol. Electr. **47**:482-485, 1966.

121 Rubin, P., and Kurohara, S. S.: Has prophylactic irradiation proved itself in the treatment of localized Hodgkin's disease? Radiology **87**:240-252, 1966.

122 Sagerman, R. H., Wolff, J. A., Sitarz, A., and Koon-Hung, L.: Radiation therapy for lymphoma in children, Radiology **86**:1096-1099, 1966.

123 Saltzstein, S. L., and Ackerman, L. V.: Lymphadenopathy induced by anticonvulsant drugs and mimicking clinically and pathologically malignant lymphomas, Cancer **12**:164-182, 1959.

124 Scheinmel, A., Roswit, B., and Lawrence, L. R.: Hodgkin's disease of the lung; roentgen appearance and therapeutic management, Radiology **54**:165-179, 1950.

125 Schier, W. W., Roth, A., Ostroff, G., and Schrift, M. H.: Hodgkin's disease and immunity, Amer. J. Med. **20**:94-99, 1956.

126 Scott, J. L.: The effect of nitrogen mustard and maintenance chlorambucil in the treatment of advanced Hodgkin's disease, Cancer Chemother. Rep. **27**:27-32, 1963.

127 Sherman, E. D.: Gastro-intestinal manifestations of lymphogranulomatosis (Hodgkin's disease), Arch. Intern. Med. (Chicago) **61**:60-82, 1938.

128 Slaughter, D. P., and Craver, L. F.: Hodgkin's disease, Amer. J. Roentgen. **47**:596-606, 1942.

129 Slaughter, D. P., Economous, S. G., and Southwick, H .W.: Surgical management of Hodgkin's disease, Ann. Surg. **148**:705-710, 1958.

130 Smith, B. W., Sheehy, T. W., and Rothberg, H.: Hodgkin's disease and pregnancy, Arch. Intern. Med. (Chicago) **102**:777-789, 1958.

131 Smith, M. J., and Stenstrom, K. W.: Compression of the spinal cord caused by Hodgkin's disease; case reports and treatment, Radiology **51**:77-84, 1948.

132 Smithers, D. W.: Hodgkin's disease, Brit. Med. J. **2**:263-268, 1967.

133 Smithers, D. W.: Factors influencing survival in patients with Hodgkin's disease, Clin. Radiol. **20**:124-132, 1969.

134 Solidoro, A., Guzmán, C., and Chang, A.: Relative increased incidence of childhood Hodgkin's disease in Peru, Cancer Res. **26**:1204-1208, 1966.

135 Spitz, S.: The histological effects of nitrogen mustards on human tumors and tissues, Cancer **1**:383-398, 1948.

136 Steiner, P. E.: Hodgkin's disease, Arch. Path. (Chicago) **36**:627-637, 1943.

136a Strum, S. B., Park, J. K., and Rappaport, H.: Observation of cells resembling Sternberg-

Reed cells in conditions other than Hodgkin's disease, Cancer **26**:176-190, 1970.

136b Strum, S. B., and Rappaport, H.: The significance of focal involvement of lymph nodes for the diagnosis and staging of Hodgkin's disease, Cancer **25**:1312-1317, 1970.

137 Stuhlberg, J., and Ellis, F. W.: Hodgkin's disease of bone; favorable prognostic significance, Amer. J. Roentgen. **93**:568-572, 1965.

138 Trübestein, H.: Beitrag zur Behandlung der Lymphogranulomatose, Strahlentherapie **99**:526-535, 1956.

139 Trübestein, H.: Der differenzierte histologische Befund der Lymphogranulomatose als Grundlage des Behandlungserfolges, Strahlentherapie **100**:62-71, 1956.

140 Trubowitz, S., Masek, B., and del Rosario, A.: Lymphocyte response to phytohemaglutinin in Hodgkin's disease; lymphatic leukemia and lymphosarcoma, Cancer **19**:2019-2023, 1966.

141 Uehlinger, E.: Ueber Knochen-lymphogranulomatose, Virchow Arch. Path. Anat. **228**:36-118, 1933 (extensive bibliography).

142 Ultmann, J. E.: Clinical features and diagnosis of Hodgkin's disease, Cancer **19**:297-307, 1966 (extensive bibliography).

143 Viala, J. J., Revol, L., and Croizat, P.: Two years' experience in Lyons with vincaleucoblastine, especially in Hodgkin's disease. In Groupe Europeen de Chimiotherapie Anticancereuse: Antitumoral effects of Vinca rosea alkaloids; proceedings of the first symposium, Paris, 1965 (edited by S. Garattini and E. M. Sproston), Amsterdam, 1966, Excerpta Medica Foundation (International Congress series no. 106).

144 Vieta, J. O., Friedell, H. L., and Craver, L. F.: A survey of Hodgkin's disease and lymphosarcoma in bone, Radiology **39**:1-15, 1942.

145 Vogel, J. M., Kimball, H. R., Foley, H. T., Wolff, S. M., and Perry, S.: Effect of extensive radiotherapy on the marrow granulocyte reserves of patients with Hodgkin's disease, Cancer **21**:798-804, 1968.

146 Wallace, S., Jackson, L., Schaffer, B., Gould, J., Greening, R., Weiss, A., and Kramer, S.: Lymphangiograms; their diagnostic and therapeutic potential, Radiology **76**:179, 1961.

147 Weil, A.: Spinal cord changes in lymphogranulomatosis, Arch. Neurol. Psychiat. (Chicago) **26**:1009-1026, 1931.

148 Wolpaw, S. E., Highley, C. S., and Hauser, H.: Intrathoracic Hodgkin's disease, Amer. J. Roentgen. **52**:374-387, 1944.

149 Woodard, H. Q., and Craver, L. F.: Serum phosphatase in lymphomatoid diseases, J. Clin. Invest. **19**:1-7, 1940.

150 Yang, Y. H., and Palmer, S. D.: The morphology of Reed-Sternberg cells in bone marrow, Amer. J. Clin. Path. **39**:115-120, 1963.

151 Yardumian, K., and Myers, L.: Primary Hodgkin's disease of the lung, Arch. Intern. Med. (Chicago) **86**:233-244, 1950.

Chapter 20

Leukemia

The leukemias are a group of diseases affecting primarily the lymphatic and reticuloendothelial systems and the bone marrow, resulting in overproduction of abnormal leukocytic elements at their site of origin, with or without an increase of these cells in the circulating blood and infiltration of various viscera (Amromin[4]). These leukemias are acute, subacute, or chronic. The essential abnormality resides in the leukemic cell and consists of an acquired inability of immature leukocytes to respond to forces normally regulating their proliferation and maturation (Furth[59]). Thus, leukemias clearly belong within the neoplastic diseases and may be considered as a form of cancer of the hemopoietic organs.

The predominant component cell betrays the origin of leukemias (Table 119). The granulocytic type may be subdivided into eosinophilic and basophilic types. Eosinophilic leukemia is thought to be merely a variant of the myelocytic type, and the basophilic leukemia is a doubtful entity, but plasma cell leukemia is a definite variety with an acute and a subacute variety (Moss and Ackerman[111]). Erythroleukemia (Di Guglielmo syndrome) is an acute leukemia closely related to myelocytic leukemia (Scott et al.[139]). Mast cell leukemia is the rarest of all types (Szweda et al.[149]).

Epidemiology

Leukemia is a relatively rare condition. *Chronic myelocytic leukemia* is most frequently found in individuals between 20 and 60 years of age, with the greatest number of cases occurring between the ages of 30 and 39 years. About two-thirds of all cases are found in male individuals. *Chronic lymphocytic leukemia* is prevalent between 45 and 60 years of age, and about three-fourths of all cases occur in men. This form of leukemia has a low incidence throughout the Orient (Dameshek and Gunz[41]; Wells and Lau[160]). *Acute leukemia* occurs most frequently in the first five years of life. It is most often lymphocytic and predominates in male infants (Dausset and Schwarzman[43]). Pierce et al.[119] found a peak at 2 to 3 years of age to be characteristic of acute lymphocytic leukemia, whereas no such peak age was present in other types; the age distribution was the same in Caucasian and Negro children. Cutler et al.[39] found a similar age distribution in over 10,000 cases of acute leukemia (Fig. 776). In children, leukemia is the most common form of cancer.

About two-thirds of monocytic leukemias are found in male individuals (Rappoport and Kugel[124]). Acute myelocytic and monocytic leukemias occur in children as well as in adults, but they are rarely found in patients over 50 years of age. Congenital leukemias (usually myelocytic) have been recorded (Bernhard et al.[14]) in frequent association with congenital abnormalities. No case has been recorded of transmission of the disease from a leukemic mother to her child (Ask-Upmark[10]). Several instances of leukemia in siblings have been reported. Andersen[6] studied a family in which five of eight siblings had leukemia in early childhood. Pearson et al.[117] collected ten instances of concordant leukemia in identical twins; this occurrence is greater than explained by chance but less than expected if strong genetic factors were operating. McPhedran et al.[99] reported ten members of two interrelated families who

Table 119. Classification of leukemia

Predominant component cell	Specific type of leukemia
Stem cell	Stem cell leukemia
Monocyte	Monocytic leukemia
Lymphocyte	Lymphocytic leukemia
Granulocyte	Granulocytic (myelocytic) leukemia
Erythroblast	Erythroleukemia
Plasma cell	Plasmacytic leukemia
Tissue mast cell	Mast cell leukemia

developed leukemia between 1948 and 1967. Most cases proved to be lymphocytic leukemia. Cytogenic studies from nineteen unaffected relatives showed no abnormalities. The findings suggested that the genetic factors predisposing to leukemia in some families may also determine the cell types. Certain cytogenic disorders

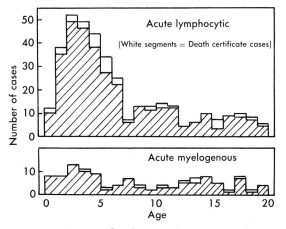

Fig. 776. Age distribution of patients under 20 years of age with acute lymphocytic and acute myelocytic leukemia—1940-1962. (From Cutler, S. J., et al.: Childhood leukemia in Connecticut, 1940-1962, Blood 30:1-25, 1967; by permission; WU neg. 69-6395.)

(Table 120) may predispose to leukemia (Fraumeni and Miller[57]).

The relative proportion of the various types of leukemia varies considerably from one series to another. Some of the differences may be explained by discrepancies in diagnosis, but they may be due also to the inclusion or not of pediatric material. In a series of 888 cases, Moore and Reinhard[108] found the following: 302 cases of chronic lymphocytic, 162 cases of acute lymphocytic, 246 cases of chronic myelocytic, fifty-three cases of acute myelocytic, and 125 cases of monocytic leukemia (Table 121). Plasmacytic leukemia is rare (Bichel et al.[16]).

The incidence of leukemia has been increasing in the United States. Since the rise has occurred primarily among elderly individuals, it has been suggested that it is due to aging of the population. It could also be due, in part, to improvement in diagnosis, but it is evident that the increase is a real one. Leukemia has been found to be two and one-half times less frequent among blacks than among whites (Pizzolato[121]). There are great difficulties involved in the epidemiologic studies of such a rare event as leukemia. Numerous possible leukemogenic influences could be

Table 120. Congenital cytogenetic disorders and leukemia-lymphoma*

Congenital disorder	*Cytogenetic defect*	*Associated leukemia-lymphoma*
Down's syndrome (mongolism)	Trisomy-21	Risk of leukemia known to be twentyfold or greater[158]
Klinefelter's syndrome (seminiferous tubule dysgenesis)	XXY or mosaic	Case reports 1 acute myelogenous leukemia[101] 1 chronic myelogenous leukemia[153] 1 acute lymphocytic leukemia[24] 2 reticulum cell sarcomas[11, 100] 1 acute undifferentiated leukemia[23]
D-trisomy (Patau's syndrome of multiple anomalies)	Trisomy in group 13-15	Case reports 1 congenital myeloblastic leukemia[135] 1 acute myelogenous leukemia[164]
Bloom's syndrome (low birth weight, stunted growth, sun-sensitive telangiectatic erythema of face)	Chromosome breakage and rearrangement of cultured blood cells	23 cases reviewed by Sawitsky et al.[134] 2 acute myelogenous leukemias 1 acute leukemia
Fanconi's syndrome (congenital pancytopenia with multiple anomalies	Chromosome breakage and rearrangement of cultured blood cells	2 case reports with acute monocytic leukemia[20]

*From Fraumeni, J. F., Jr., and Miller, R. W.: Epidemiology of human leukemia: recent observations, J. Nat. Cancer Inst. 38:593-605, 1967.

suspected in a rapidly changing society in which potential marrow depressants enjoy wide use, in industry as in medicine, and in which chemical pollutants are in abundance. Because ionizing radiations have been known to be capable of causing experimental leukemia and because of their wide use in diagnosis and in therapy, radiations have been justly suspected of contributing to the rise in the incidence of leukemia. Deaths from leukemia occur more frequently among radiologists than among other physicians (March[102, 103]).

The occurrence of leukemia among the survivors of the atomic destruction of Hiroshima and Nagasaki (1945) has been the subject of careful study (Lewis[95]; Kawabe[88]; Heyssel et al.[77]). The increase first manifested itself three years after the exposure (1948) and apparently reached its peak between 1950 and 1952 (Heyssel et al.[77]). The incidence is higher among those close to, than among those distant from, the "hypocenter." A curious sequence has been observed in the occurrence of type-specific leukemias (Bizzozero et al.[18]). In the early period (1946-1954), acute lymphocytic and chronic granulocytic leukemias were primarily observed in exposed persons under 30 years old. In the intermediate period (1955-1959), acute granulocytic leukemias developed in a relatively large number of individuals who were over 30 years old when exposed. Thus, age at the time of exposure, and possibly dose, are among the several factors that determine the type of leukemia. The latest period of observation (1960-1964) has only exhibited an absolute decline in the occur-

rence of leukemia. No significant increase in leukemia has been observed in the offspring of exposed survivors (Hoshino et al.[81]). The overall incidence of leukemia in Japan is about half that of western countries; the proportion of acute leukemia, particularly myelocytic, is relatively higher, whereas that of chronic lymphocytic leukemia is much lower (Moloney[107]; Wakezaka[157]).

There have been reports of an increased incidence of leukemia among patients irradiated for spondylitis (Court-Brown and Doll[33]). Since no such increase has been reported among the thousands of patients cured by radiotherapy of carcinoma of the cervix and other intensively irradiated radiocurable conditions, it must be assumed that, if real, this leukemogenic effect may result from relatively mild irradiation of the spinal marrow. A higher occurrence of leukemia has been reported among children irradiated in early life for an assumed enlargement of the thymus gland (Simpson et al.[144]). There is some evidence of increased occurrence of leukemia among children irradiated for other causes (Murray et al.[112]). No clear evidence has been offered that irradiation in utero resulting from diagnostic procedures has increased the occurrence of leukemia in these children (Stewart et al.[146]; Murray et al.[112]). The evidence is not clear enough to incriminate low-dosage exposures to radiations as the cause of leukemia (Gunz and Atkinson[67]). Kimball[89] stated that the accuracy of radiation-induced leukemia rates in human populations is open to serious question, particularly in what pertains to

Table 121. Age at onset and sex distribution of 888 cases of leukemia (1938-1952)*

Yr	Acute lymphocytic			Chronic lymphocytic			Acute myelocytic			Chronic myelocytic			Monocytic			Total
	M	F	T	M	F	T	M	F	T	M	F	T	M	F	T	
1-9	25	25	50	1	2	3	3	2	5	2	1	3	4	2	6	67
10-19	23	12	35	1	1	2	2	1	3	5	3	8	5	1	6	54
20-29	8	9	17	1	3	4	3	4	7	10	11	21	5	3	8	57
30-39	9	4	13	9	7	16	4	6	10	24	21	45	9	6	15	99
40-49	6	7	13	32	14	46	3	2	5	23	35	58	7	12	19	141
50-59	10	6	16	57	37	94	7	3	10	27	19	46	13	15	28	194
60-69	8	6	14	63	27	90	7	1	8	26	14	40	16	11	27	179
70+	2	2	4	37	10	47	5		5	15	10	25	10	6	16	97
Total	91	71	162	201	101	302	34	19	53	132	114	246	69	56	125	888

*From Moore, C. V., and Reinhard, E.: Personal communication, 1953.

either a threshold dose or a linear relationship between dose and response (Cronkite et al.[36]).

Nowell and Hungerford[115] described a minute acrocentric chromosome (named the Philadelphia chromosome) in the peripheral blood and bone marrow preparations of two children with chronic myelocytic leukemia. Fitzgerald et al.[54] demonstrated the Ph[1] chromosome in twelve other patients with chronic myelocytic leukemia. Although the chromosome is not found in every case, it is found in a great proportion of patients with remissions. Cohen[29] reported a case of autoimmune hemolytic anemia in a patient with the Ph[1] chromosome: four years later the patient developed chronic myelocytic leukemia with myelofibrosis. Chromosomal studies were done in a set of identical twins, one of whom had chronic myelocytic leukemia. A typical Ph[1] chromosome was found only in the diseased twin, indicating that the chromosomal abnormality is an acquired postzygotic one (Goh and Swisher[63]; Goh et al.[64]). Reisman and Trujillo[127] studied nine cases of chronic myelocytic leukemia in children and found the Ph[1] chromosome in diploid cells present in five who had the adult form of the disease but not present in the four other children with the infantile form of leukemia.

Avian and murine leukemias may be produced by viruses, and there are suggestions that human leukemias may be caused by viruses (Bryan et al.[26]) and, consequently, transmissible. However, separate studies have failed to demonstrate any clustering, in place or time, of human leukemia cases (Lock and Merrington[97]; Fraumeni et al.[56]). It has been suggested that the morphologic manifestations of leukemias are simply a defensive host reaction. Dameshek[40] believes it likely that chronic lymphocytic leukemia is an accumulative disease of lymphocytes rather than one due to excessive proliferation. In his view, the immunologically incompetent lymphocytes accumulate and eventually result in reduced immunity and death.

Pathology

Gross pathology

The pathologic alterations in all types of chronic leukemia tend to involve many systems, and if all the changes were tabulated, the abnormalities observed would be encyclopedic. The pathologic changes are mainly of two types: those that affect the blood-forming organs, particularly bone marrow, spleen, and lymph nodes, and those due to infiltration. The bone marrow is invariably hyperplastic and reddish gray in color. The degree of enlargement of lymph nodes, spleen, and liver varies with the different types of leukemia. In chronic lymphocytic leukemia, generalized lymphadenopathy is frequent. The extent of involvement of various lymph node groups varies, but it is common to see peripheral enlargement of all lymph node groups, and mediastinal and retroperitoneal lymph nodes are usually not enlarged at first but may show a minimal amount of replacement later. Moderate generalized lymph node enlargement is present terminally in myelocytic leukemia. The liver and spleen are invariably enlarged in chronic leukemia. Usually, but not invariably, the greatest prominence is in the myelocytic type (Kirshbaum and Preuss[90]). The enlarged spleen frequently shows perisplenitis with numerous adhesions. Infarcts of varying ages may be found in the granulocytic variety but are also observed in the lymphocytic variety. On section of the liver, diffuse infiltration manifested as grayish white areas measuring only a few millimeters will be seen in the myelocytic type, whereas in the lymphocytic variety these areas of infiltration are most prominent in the portal zone (Fig. 777). Cut section of the spleen shows this same type of infiltration and obliteration of architecture associated with various degrees of fibrosis. Leukemic infiltration is common in the kidneys and is invariably bilateral with enlargement of the organ.

Leukemic infiltration of the gastrointestinal tract is common in the lymphocytic variety and is most prominent in the stomach and ileum where lymphoid tissue is abundant (Fig. 778). The changes present may result in swelling of the folds of the stomach which resembles cerebral convolutions. In the ileum, there may at times be atrophy of the overlying mucosa followed by secondary ulceration of nodular areas. In a study of 264 patients with leukemia who came to autopsy, Cornes and Jones[32]

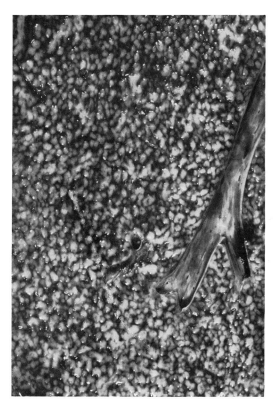

Fig. 777. Extensive infiltration of liver in chronic lymphocytic leukemia. Note limitation of grayish white leukemic infiltration to portal areas.

found thirty-nine to have leukemic lesions of the gastrointestinal tract. The proximal colon, stomach, and ileum were most commonly involved. Thirty-six patients had massive hemorrhage. Leukemic infiltration of the skin is present particularly in the lymphocytic form of leukemia.

Evidence of hemorrhagic tendencies as manifested by numerous ecchymoses and petechiae is common. Death may rarely occur from hemorrhage either into the gastrointestinal tract or into the brain. Fluid is commonly found in the pleural cavities and abdomen, and a terminal bronchopneumonia is a common complication. Leukemic infiltration of the kidneys associated with pyelonephritis may lead to kidney failure and death. Central nervous system involvement is not unusual, and leukemic infiltration in the brain is manifested by grayish nodules surrounded by areas of hemorrhage.

In *acute leukemia,* the gross findings vary only slightly, depending on the type of leukemia. In acute lymphocytic leukemia, there is a greater tendency to lymph node involvement than in the acute myelocytic and monocytic varieties. The liver is invariably enlarged in all cases. The spleen is also enlarged but not nearly so much as in the chronic forms of leukemia. It may

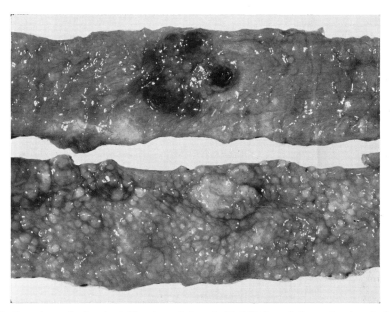

Fig. 778. Prominent leukemic infiltration of lymphoid follicles of ileum in chronic lymphocytic leukemia.

even be small in the acute monocytic variety. The bone marrow is hyperplastic in all cases. Evidence of bleeding phenomena may be present in all types, with petechiae, ecchymoses, and hemorrhages into the brain, gastrointestinal tract, lungs, and elsewhere.

In *chloroma,* a variant of acute myelocytic leukemia, green color in the tumor masses is usually present due probably to a lipochrome (Kandel[87]). According to Goodman and Iverson,[66] this pigment may be an intermediary product in the breakdown of hemoglobin to bilirubin. The pigmentation disappears an hour after death but can be made to reappear by hydrogen peroxide. With chloroma, there is invariably widespread invasion of many organs, and particularly striking are the retro-orbital tumor masses and the changes in the skull and thorax. The skull was involved in 73% of the patients reported by Rothschild,[130] with masses infiltrating into the dura, paranasal sinuses, orbit, nerves, scalp, and subcutaneous tissues. There are large yellowish green masses of tumor growing beneath the sternum, invading the pleura, muscles, and, at times, the myocardium. The kidneys usually show diffuse or nodular greenish tumor tissue, the spleen and liver are usually normal in size, and the bone marrow is hyperplastic. Rappaport[123] uses the term *granulocytic sarcoma* as a synonym for chloroma.

Microscopic pathology

The most important changes will be found in the bone marrow. In lymphocytic leukemia, there is a homogeneous replacement by lymphoid elements. In chronic myelocytic leukemia, the bone marrow shows an increase of myeloid elements with numerous eosinophilic myelocytes. There is a shift to younger forms and a striking decrease in the percentage of nucleated red cells. Proliferation of leukemic cells in the bone marrow may extend to the haversian canals and thence to the periosteum. Because of these infiltrative changes, pressure atrophy and rarefaction of trabeculae within the marrow with subsequent destruction of the cortex can occur.

The study of all types of leukemia reveals variable degrees of infiltration of various organs, depending upon the type of leukemia. In this infiltration, it is common to see destruction of normal tissue and replacement by masses of leukemic cells. These leukemic cells are often present in increased numbers within the blood vessels. Under high-power magnification, immature forms can be identified. In the lymphocytic variety, the infiltration is present where lymphatic tissue is most prominent and is consequently very diffuse predominantly in the submucosa of the gastrointestinal tract, particularly the stomach and ileum. In these areas, the normal follicles are erased and replaced by a homogeneous mass of lymphoid cells, many of them immature. The same process is present in the malpighian zones of the spleen. In the liver, there is a localization of the leukemic process around the portal areas in lymphocytic leukemia, but the infiltration is diffuse in chronic myelocytic leukemia. Lung involvement is found at autopsy in 30% of all patients (Falconer[50]). Leukemic infiltration of the skin is occasionally present (Fig. 780). Hemorrhagic phenomena are common, and there may be small areas of thrombosis. Extramedullary hemopoiesis in liver, spleen, and lymph nodes may be seen.

The central nervous system is often involved and occasionally also the cranial nerves, perineural spaces, meninges, and pial vessels. The areas of leukemic infiltration of the brain often show surrounding hemorrhage (Diamond[44]). The vascular lesions observed in the brain may be due to thrombosis of vessels by leukemic cells. Not too infrequently the walls of the vessels are invaded, and leukemic infiltration spreads out into the brain substance (Fried[58]). Schwab and Weiss[137] tabulated the neurologic findings in a large series of cases and found frequent cerebral invasion and cerebral hemorrhage. They also found frequent invasion of the cranial meninges and cranial nerves. Cranial nerve nuclei were involved in about one-sixth of the cases.

The practice of chemotherapy has modified greatly the pattern of pathologic changes identified at autopsy. Viola[156] emphasized the major role of infection as cause of death in patients with acute leukemia. Pneumonitis, bacteremia, and skin infections were most common. Gram-negative organisms may gain access to the circulation through ulcerations of the gastrointestinal tract. With the use of multiple therapeutic agents, fungal infections have increased. Prolla and Kirsner[122] studied 148 leukemic patients. Thirty-seven had gross lesions of the intestinal tract and twenty-seven had hemorrhagic necrosis of the intestine, and mycotic infections occurred in twenty-four. Other findings were appendicitis and perforation of the small and large intestine. In fifteen patients with acute leukemia, there were, at autopsy, ten cases of agranulocytic abscess infiltrates. Amromin and Solomon[5] reported necrotizing lesions of the gastrointestinal tract in sixty-three of 280 cases of leukemia. Other organs affected were the kidney, liver, testis, bowel, lung, central nervous system, and lymph nodes, indicating that the central nervous system was not the only reservoir of leukemia cells during remissions (Nies et al.[114]). Among the survivors of Hiroshima, the autopsy prevalence of myelofibrosis was four and one-half times greater than among the nonexposed individuals (Anderson et al.[7]).

Clinical evolution

The chronic forms of leukemia usually have an insidious onset, and it is difficult to establish exactly how long the disease has been present before the first symptom occurs.

In *chronic lymphocytic leukemia,* the outstanding first sign is the enlargement of the lymph nodes, particularly in the cervical region (Fig. 779). Because of this peripheral abnormality, this variety is probably diagnosed earlier than myelocytic leukemia. It is estimated, however, that the

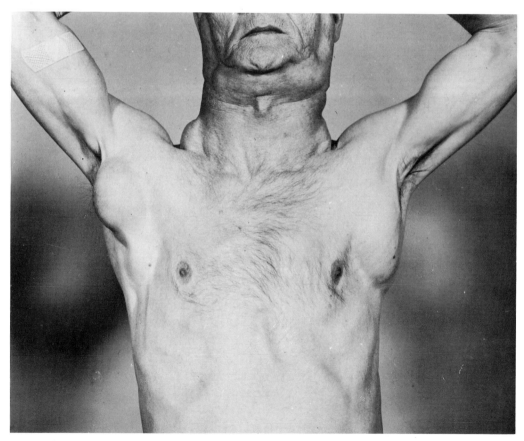

Fig. 779. Patient with chronic lymphocytic leukemia with voluminous but symmetrical adenopathy unlike that observed in generalized lymphosarcoma or Hodgkin's disease. (Courtesy Dr. A. Robert Kagan, Los Angeles, Calif.)

disease may progress from one to one and one-half years before it is recognized. The lymph nodes do not become very large, usually not more than 5 cm in diameter. In rare instances, there may not be a peripheral adenopathy. The spleen is usually enlarged several fingerbreadths below the costal margin. The white blood cell count may be normal or slightly depressed.

In *chronic myelocytic leukemia,* there is rarely any enlargement of the lymph nodes in the early stages, and the disease may be present for from two to five years before it is recognized. The outstanding symptom is the considerable enlargement of the spleen, which extends sometimes to the pubis and causes a sensation of heaviness and dragging. Tenderness of the sternum, usually limited to the gladiolus, is found in a majority of patients, but this is not pathognomonic of the myelocytic variety.

In later stages of both varieties of chronic leukemia, the symptomatology and the clinical findings are protean, with widespread involvement of multiple organs (Table 122). Anemia is usually manifested by pallor and is due to depressed or suboptimal erythropoiesis, hemorrhage, and frequently to hemolysis. There is also an increased metabolism, which, added to the anemia, produces tachycardia, weight loss,

intolerance to heat, perspiration, and dyspnea on exertion. If there is a latent cardiac disease in a patient verging on congestive failure or some asymptomatic narrowing of the coronary arteries, these two factors may cause congestive heart failure or angina pectoris. All these symptoms may gradually disappear with treatment. Neurologic complications may appear in chronic leukemia (Firkin and Moore[52]), including cerebral hemorrhage, cranial nerve paralysis (Schwab and Weiss[137]), increased intracranial pressure, meningitis, etc., sometimes accompanied by pyramidal signs. Priapism sometimes, but not always, accompanied by thrombi of the veins of the corpora cavernosa may also be present. Cases of leukemia may rarely begin with primary manifestations related to other organs such as the prostate (Flaherty et al.[55]) or female genitals (Hauptman and Taussig[72]). During the course of the disease, retinal hemorrhages, edema of the disk, sudden blindness, and leukemic retinitis can appear (Goldbach[65]).

Intense pain may result from infarction, particularly of the spleen. Involvement of other abdominal organs may simulate an acute abdominal condition. Leukemic infiltration of the skin may be present, particularly in the lymphocytic variety (Fig.

Table 122. Clinicopathologic correlation of lesions and symptoms in chronic leukemia

Pathology	Region	Symptoms
Lymph node enlargement	Mediastinum Retroperitoneal Elsewhere	Cough, dyspnea Gastrointestinal disturbances, distention, abdominal pain Pressure symptoms
Spleen	Enlargement Infarct	Dragging sensation Acute pain
Bone involvement	Bone marrow replacement Increased metabolism plus anemia Thrombopenia	Local bone pain (periosteal involvement), anemia, pallor, fatigue, palpitation, hemic murmurs Perspiration, easy fatigue, intolerance to heat, weight loss, increased appetite, increased pulse rate (not so marked as in hyperthyroidism), cardiac failure, angina pectoris Petechiae, purpura, hemorrhage
Gastrointestinal involvement	Stomach and ileum	Diarrhea, nausea, vomiting, occult blood (rarely, gross hemorrhage)
Nervous system (Schwab and Weiss[137])	Brain hemorrhage Cranial nerve nuclei	Paraplegias and pyramidial tract symptoms Cranial nerve paralysis
Kidneys (Merrill and Jackson[106])	Infiltration, nephrolithiasis (uric acid)	Renal colic, renal failure, pyuria
Lungs (Falconer[50])	Diffuse infiltration	Dyspnea

780). However, a considerably larger number of patients develop skin lesions entirely unrelated to the leukemia, probably due to lessened resistance to infections. Varied skin manifestations may be observed (Fairburn and Burgen[49]), and secondary infection often takes place. Skin lesions are particularly frequent in monocytic leukemia.

Infection and anemia are the principal causes of hospital admissions of patients with chronic lymphocytic leukemia. Aroesty and Furth[9] find that the frequency of infection and the occurrence of acquired hemolytic anemia suggest distorted and inadequate immune response. In the terminal phase of chronic myelocytic leukemia, there may be enlargement of lymph nodes, bleeding tendencies, and substantial increase in circulating leukocytes and in immature cells. In other words, the terminal phase of this form of chronic leukemia often reproduces the character of acute leukemia (Morrow et al.[110]). Few cases of

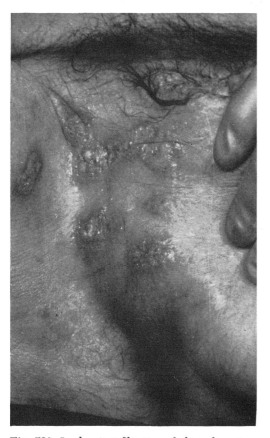

Fig. 780. Leukemic infiltration of skin of scrotum in patient with chronic lymphocytic leukemia.

chronic monocytic leukemia have been reported. Death often occurs in chronic leukemia because of infection, particularly bronchopneumonia, but may also result from sudden cerebral or gastrointestinal hemorrhage. Heart failure is not unusual as a cause of death.

Acute leukemia is mostly encountered in children. In most patients, there is a prodromal period of weakness and malaise followed by fever, tachycardia, and prostration. The onset is often sudden, and a diagnosis is seldom made before the disease has run at least half of its short course. About one-third of all patients have a history of hemorrhage after some minor operation such as a tonsillectomy or tooth extraction. Fever, pain in the bones and joints, petechiae, hemorrhages, and severe secondary infection are characteristic findings. Very often the laryngologist is consulted because of sore throat, enlarged tonsils, or changes in the oral and pharyngeal mucous membrane. Exclusive of peripheral blood and bone marrow studies, there are a few clinical findings that have a variable significance, but none of them is absolute. Enlargement of the spleen is invariably present in all types, but this is usually of moderate degree, and often the spleen is not even palpable. In the acute lymphocytic variety, the lymph nodes are generally enlarged, but patients have been seen without any enlargement. Monocytic leukemia frequently shows enlargement of the cervical lymph nodes, which may be tender because of coexisting oral infection with diffuse inflammation, ulceration, necrosis, and severe bleeding. Ulcerative lesions of the intestinal tract occur with high frequency. Pulmonary infiltration and hemorrhage may occur (Bodey et al.[21]). Neurologic complications may appear (Moore et al.[109]). Cases of meningeal leukemia have been increasingly reported (Nies et al.[114]; Hardisty and Norman[70]). In adult acute leukemia, localized abscesses are frequent. Spontaneous rupture of the spleen rarely occurs (Hynes et al.[83]).

Diagnosis

The clinical diagnosis of leukemia is usually easy. The patient may come to the physician for the first time because of bleeding following a tooth extraction. It is also common for the patient to discover a large mass in the upper abdominal quadrants. A thorough clinical examination, blood studies including supravital staining, and bone marrow aspiration are sometimes necessary to solve certain difficult cases. On routine physical examination of elderly patients, anemia with relative lymphocytosis or even with a normal differential count should awaken suspicion of chronic lymphocytic leukemia which may be proved by bone marrow biopsy.

Careful palpation of the neck, axillas, and inguinal and epitrochlear regions is always indicated. The enlarged spleen is usually easy to palpate and often can be percussed beneath the ribs. Its dimensions should be noted carefully. A light percussion may reveal the presence of sternal tenderness which is frequently found in myelocytic leukemia. Evidence of an abnormal tendency to bleed may be found in an examination of the eyegrounds, oral cavity, and skin. The examination should include a search for skin and neurologic manifestations. In chloroma, a variant of monocytic leukemia, the yellowish green appearance of the tumor masses, together with extreme anemia and exophthalmos, may suggest the diagnosis. In patients with polycythemia vera, a myelocytic leukemia may develop. Mast cell leukemia may present clinically as urticaria pigmentosa.

Roentgenologic examination

Roentgenologic examination of the chest is indicated in all patients with leukemia to detect possible mediastinal lymph node involvement and infiltration of the lung. Roentgenographic detection of bone involvement is seldom possible in chronic leukemia but is often present in acute leukemia (Willson[162]). Generalized osteoporosis is seldom seen, but areas of rarefaction are sometimes noted near the epiphysis, and this may lead to spontaneous fractures (Erb[48]). Thomas et al.[150] studied the pathologic changes in eighty-five consecutive patients with acute leukemia. Skeletal lesions occurred in the majority. Juxtaepiphyseal radiolucent bands occurred in 93% of the children but in only 10% of

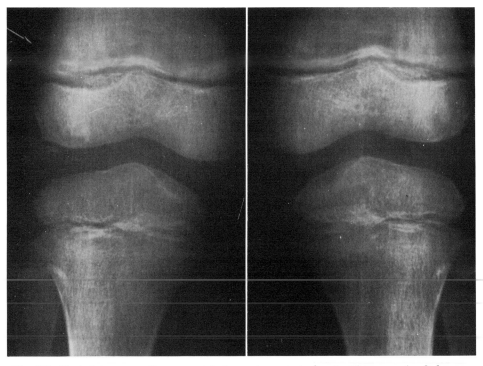

Fig. 781. Typical transverse line present in femur in acute leukemia. This area of radiolucency is caused by leukemic infiltration. (Courtesy Dr. Hugh Wilson, St. Louis, Mo.; WU neg. 60-7449.)

the adults (Fig. 781). Cortical or periosteal defects occurred in 50% of the children but in only 9% of the adults.

Bone changes are frequently observed in children. These changes are usually osteolytic but can be mixed in character. Baty and Vogt[13] described a narrow zone of diminished density proximal to the metaphysis in 70% of their cases of leukemia in children. There may also be subperiosteal proliferation in the juxta-articular portions of this bone that may suggest a primary malignant bone tumor (Apitz[8]). In chloroma, generalized osteoporosis may be present, particularly noticeable in the bones of the skull. A skeletal survey of children presenting bone pains or anemia may lead to a diagnosis of leukemia through the detection of bone lesions (Silverman[143]).

Laboratory examination

Although a clinical diagnosis of leukemia is frequently possible, the confirmation of this diagnosis will need the support of laboratory examination. In other instances, the diagnosis is possible only through specialized techniques in the laboratory. Quite often, the information received in this manner will also help in establishing a prognosis and in regulating the treatment. A fair proportion of patients with acute lymphocytic and myelocytic leukemia present subnormal white blood cell counts when first seen. The anemias coexisting with them are usually normocytic. Platelets are uniformly depressed in the acute form.

In leukemias, there is a frequent rise in the number of circulating leukocytes. However, the characteristic feature of this disease is the presence of immature cells that are not normally found in the circulating blood. Although immature cells have been seen in other diseases, blast cells in large numbers are present only with leukemia. In chronic lymphocytic leukemia, the rise in the number of circulating leukocytes seldom reaches the high values sometimes seen in the myelogenous variety. The total leukocyte count frequently varies between 100,000 and 200,000 per cubic millimeter. The overwhelming majority of these usually are adult lymphocytes presenting very little cytoplasm. Immature lymphocytes are observed but in a small proportion. In chronic granulocytic leukemia, the leukocytosis is usually high and may reach a million white cells per cubic millimeter. The majority of these cells are myelocytes. In addition, there are a great number of metamyelocytes, most of which are neutrophilic.

In acute monocytic leukemia, a rise in the leukocyte count is usually present, but in the lymphocytic and myelocytic varieties of acute leukemia, there may be a normal number of white cells or even leukopenia. On careful examination of the blood, however, an unusual number of immature leukocytes may be found. Some of the outstanding cytologic differences for the diagnosis of specific types of acute leukemia are given in Table 123. The differentiation frequently remains difficult, however, and usually special study will be necessary to establish the diagnosis.

A normal or subnormal number of circulating leukocytes may be found in leukemia. Although this is most common in the acute forms, it is also observed in the

Table 123. Cytologic differentiation of three varieties of acute leukemia*

Lymphocytic variety	Myelocytic variety	Monocytic variety
Predominant cell lymphoblast (50% to 90%) with round or oval nucleus and coarse, granular, or "stippled" chromatin and 1 or 2 nucleoli; chromatin arranged compactly about edges of nucleus and nucleoli; most other cells lymphocytes; few neutrophic leukocytes	30% to 60% of leukocytes immature; majority myeloblasts or undifferentiated myelocytes; round or oval nuclei with fine chromatin condensed around edges; several nucleoli; cytoplasm blue with few or no granules; neutrophilic polymorphonuclear leukocytes scarce; Auer bodies or mitotic figures may be found	Large numbers of monocytes (about 60%) with irregularly shaped nuclei and very fine reticular chromatin; nucleoli inconscpicuous; cytoplasm grayish blue with innumerable fine, dust-like granules, irregular cell boundaries; remaining cells lymphocytes and polymorphonuclear leukocytes, but few myelocytes, myeloblasts, or plasma cells

*Data from Wintrobe, M. M.: Clinical hematology, ed. 6, Philadelphia, 1967, Lea & Febiger.

chronic forms of the disease. This condition is sometimes given the contradictory title of *aleukemic leukemia* but is probably best designated subleukemic leukemia. Actually, many cases of leukemia pass through a stage of development during which there is no leukocytosis, and it is then that this diagnosis is usually made. Very rarely, however, except perhaps in some acute cases, do the number of circulating leukocytes remain normal or subnormal throughout the entire course of the disease. Here, again, the important factor is not the leukocytosis but the presence of immature cells. Bethell et al.[15] demonstrated that a subleukemic phase is present in more than half of patients with acute leukemia and in 11% of patients with chronic lymphocytic leukemia.

It should be emphasized that special staining techniques are of value for making the diagnosis of leukemia and differentiating the various types. The differential diagnosis between acute lymphocytic leukemia and acute myelocytic leukemia is of more than academic interest in view of their different responses to treatments. Supravital staining, according to the method of Sabin,[133] permits the study of living blood cells and is helpful for fine hematologic differentiation. This procedure, used in conjunction with the Romanowsky stains, is sometimes of considerable value in determining cell identity. It aids particularly in the identification of the monocyte. The peroxidase stain is of practical value only in relatively rare instances. The details of the hematologic techniques that are useful in the leukemias can be found in the excellent works of Custer,[37] Wintrobe,[163] and Blackfan and Diamond.[19]

The patient with chronic lymphocytic leukemia may develop hypogammaglobulinemia. In a series of forty patients with chronic lymphocytic leukemia, Hudson and Wilson[82] found 68% to have gamma globulin levels below the normal range. These patients also may develop agammaglobulinemia because of diffuse destruction or replacement of reticuloendothelial tissue by leukemic infiltration and plasma cell destruction.

In the acute leukemias, anemia is common. It may be present in patients with chronic lymphocytic and chronic myelocytic leukemia. This results from faster destruction of red blood cells than their production by the marrow (Bowie et al.[25]). Thrombocytopenia is most common with acute leukemia but may also be present with the chronic forms. It is particularly prevalent terminally in chronic lymphocytic leukemia when it is accompanied by hemolytic phenomena. Uric acid overproduction occurs consistently in patients with untreated chronic myelocytic leukemia but not in those with chronic lymphocytic leukemia (Krakoff and Balis[92]).

Biopsy

A *bone marrow biopsy* is frequently valuable for making a definite diagnosis, particularly in subleukemic leukemia. Aspiration of bone marrow (with a 15-gauge needle) is practicable. Bone marrow biopsies in multiple sites, particularly in children, may be helpful (Rheingold et al.[128]; Rubenstein[131]). The bone marrow should be placed preferably in Zenker's acetic fixative and stained with eosin methylene blue or Giemsa stain. In early chronic lymphocytic leukemia, the bone marrow may appear normal except for a few islands of adult lymphoid cells, but as the disease develops, a complete replacement occurs. In the granulocytic variety, there is distinct hyperplasia and overgrowth of normal bone marrow elements by immature cells of the myeloid series. Myelocytes are particularly prominent. After considerable irradiation, the bone marrow may reveal some degree of aplasia. In certain cases of chronic leukemia accompanied by anemia, it cannot be ascertained from the peripheral blood counts whether the anemia is due to replacement of the bone marrow by immature cells or whether the bone marrow itself is aplastic. In these instances, bone marrow study will determine whether radiation therapy is indicated. In acute leukemia, the bone marrow is invariably replaced by leukemic cells. In most instances, bone marrow examination will differentiate between disseminated neuroblastoma, lymphosarcoma, multiple myeloma, agnogenic myeloid metaplasia, pernicious anemia, and aplastic anemia. It must be emphasized that the interpretation of differential counts from the bone marrow using supravital staining technique requires the long experience of a well-qualified hematologist. Bone marrow biopsy may be very difficult of interpretation, particularly if it is poorly prepared.

The hematologist can frequently make the diagnosis of an obscure hematologic disorder by smears obtained by sternal or iliac puncture. The pathologist may help when there is spotty involvement of the marrow or when it is impossible to obtain a specimen by aspiration (Liao [95a]). Formal bone marrow biopsy may yield a diagnosis of leukemia, plasma cell myeloma, metastatic cancer, or myelosclerosis and myelofibrosis. If a dry tap occurs in the hands of an experienced hematologist, this is an indica-tion for formal bone marrow biopsy. We have often found that leukemic cells have packed the marrow and are held together in a web of reticulin, thus preventing their aspiration into a needle (Fig. 782).

A *lymph node* biopsy may be helpful in the diagnosis of leukemia. Nodes are enlarged in all types of leukemia and, on section, are homogeneous grayish white in appearance. Microscopically, a node may show complete obliteration of its structure by leukemic cells, with invasion of the capsule by cells in the pericapsular tissue. It is impossible to differentiate the small cell type of lymphosarcoma from lymphocytic leukemia. In myelocytic leukemia, individual cells are derived from the myeloid series, and large numbers of immature cells are often present. A diagnosis of reticulum cell sarcoma may be erroneously rendered on a node from myelocytic leukemia. This error is usually due to failure to recognize eosinophilic myelocytes. Studies of the imprints of the lymph node may be helpful (Libre and McFarland[96]; Garfinkel and Bennett[61]). In patients without hematologic signs of leukemia, an erroneous diagnosis of malignant lymphoma may be made on biopsy of the lymph nodes, and the eventual manifestations or leukemia may be explained as transformation (Regato[125]). It is not uncommon for the leukemic infiltration to be present between the germinal follicles, although in some instances the latter may be erased. In acute leukemias, a gingival biopsy may be sufficient to establish the diagnosis, but in chronic leukemias, the gingival changes are rarely specific (Wentz et al.[161]).

Differential diagnosis

A variety of pathologic conditions may be mistaken for leukemia, just as leukemia may be mistaken for some other condition.

Leukemia may be simulated by many conditions presenting leukocytosis that are designated as *leukemoid reactions*. Hill and Duncan[78] classify these reactions into:

1 Bone marrow irritation or stimulation (physical, chemical, or allergic)
2 Liberation leukocytosis (overwhelming demand by acute hemolysis, severe hemorrhage, septicemia, pernicious anemia in crisis)
3 Ectopic hemopoiesis

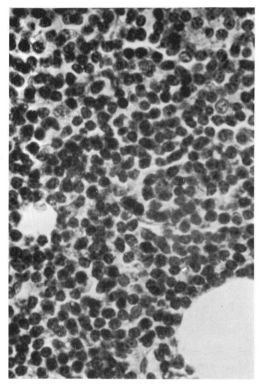

Fig. 782. Needle biopsy of iliac crest. Bone marrow is completely replaced with uniform cells of lymphoid series. There is an increase in reticulin. Patient was 65-year-old man with symptoms of weakness of eight months' duration. Physical examination showed petechiae over lower extremities, as well as enlarged liver and spleen and minimal lymphadenopathy. White blood count was 146,500; hemoglobin, 7.5 gm; platelets, 28,000; lymphocytes, 99%. Patient was given prednisone and chlorambucil with excellent clinical response. (×670; WU neg. 60-6019.)

By far the largest number of these leukemoid reactions are of the so-called bone marrow irritation type. Hill and Duncan[78] pointed out that in these cases all myeloid elements are present (myelocytes, myeloblasts, erythroblasts, and megakaryocytes), but the immature cells show no abnormal lobulation or granulation. The total white count in these leukemoid reactions may be over 75,000 with rather prominent eosinophilia and basophilia. Miliary tuberculosis, overwhelming infections such as osteomyelitis, severe reactions to intravenous medications, metastatic carcinoma of bones, and pyogenic infections may all stimulate this type of reaction. The differential character of leukemoid reactions and leukemias is summarized in Table 124.

Myelofibrosis and myelosclerosis is a disease in which the bone marrow is replaced by fibrous tissue and the bony trabeculae are prominent. There is variable extramedullary hemopoiesis, particularly in the reticuloendothelial system of the spleen, liver, and lymph nodes. Refractory anemia develops, and immature leukocytes may appear in the peripheral blood with or without leukocytosis. Myelofibrosis with myeloid metaplasia may be very difficult, or impossible, to differentiate from chronic myelocytic leukemia, particularly since myelofibrosis is observed in terminal stages of this leukemia (Krauss[93]).

A rare condition designated by Rappaport[123] as *malignant reticulohistiocytosis* is a systemic, progressive, irreversible, and invasive proliferation of morphologically atypical histiocytes and their undifferentiated precursors. We have seen this condition more frequently in children than in adults. There is often widespread involvement of hemopoietic organs with generalized lymph node enlargement, splenomegaly, hepatomegaly, and terminal hemorrhagic manifestations. Severe anemia, leukopenia, and thrombocytopenia are common. A frankly leukemic blood picture is uncommon (Cazal[28]; Marshall[104]; Scott and Robb-Smith[140]).

Agranulocytic angina may present leukopenia, tendency to hemorrhage, oral manifestations, and prostration, all of which may suggest a monocytic variety of acute leukemia. Agranulocytic angina, however, is more common in adults than in children, is not accompanied by severe anemia, and although a leukocytosis may be present, immature cells are rarely seen. In addition, the *platelet count is usually increased,* and the bone marrow biopsy does not show leukemic infiltration.

Infectious mononucleosis may be confused with lymphocytic leukemia because of its lymphadenopathy, leukocytosis, and enlarged spleen. This condition, however, is seldom accompanied by anemia and usually shows a positive sheep cell agglutination test that is never positive in leukemia unless horse serum has been recently given. The platelet count is invariably normal, and the lymph nodes show characteristic histologic changes (Custer and Smith[38]).

In children, *neuroblastomas of the suprarenal gland* may metastasize to the orbit and produce a characteristic exophthalmos and ecchymosis of the eyelids (p. 700). Such cases may be confused with chloroma, particularly because of accompanying anemia and poor general condition. A variety of other conditions such as mycosis fungoides, Mikulicz's disease, and certain forms of tuberculosis and syphilis may be confused with leukemias, but this rarely

Table 124. Differential character of leukemoid reactions and leukemia*

Leukemoid reactions	*True leukemia*
1. Immature as well as mature leukocytes show normal morphology	1. Leukocytes usually appear atypical, particularly immature ones
2. Myeloblasts may be present but usually are under 10%	2. Myeloblasts may be numerous, as high as 99+%
3. Immature red cells (normoblasts and erthroblasts) often increased in proportion to leukocyte immaturity	3. Immature red cells rarely increased in proportion to leukocyte immaturity
4. Platelets usually normal or increased	4. Platelets decreased, often severely, may be increased in chronic myelogenous form only
5. Anemia variable, depending on causal factors	5. Steadily progressing anemia, becoming extreme

*From Hill, J. M., and Duncan, C. N.: Leukemoid reactions, Amer. J. Med. Sci. 201:847-857, 1941.

occurs when the diagnosis relies on more information than a leukocyte count.

It must be pointed out that acute lymphocytic leukemia in children is frequently mistaken for *aplastic anemia* because of the normal or subnormal leukocyte count, thrombocytopenia, marked anemia, usually slight generalized lymphadenopathy, and enlarged spleen. The reticulocyte count in leukemia, in contrast to that in aplastic anemia, may be elevated, but a sternal bone marrow puncture usually resolves the diagnosis. However, in acute leukemias in children, articular manifestations may be diagnosed as septic in nature or suggesting inflammatory rheumatism. Rheumatic heart disease may be simulated by the presence of hemic murmurs, fever, and articular pains. Also, oral manifestations of acute leukemia in children may be confused with Ludwig's angina or diphtheria.

Treatment

Prior to 1947, there was no treatment for acute leukemia (Fig. 783). The observation of remissions with the use of folic acid

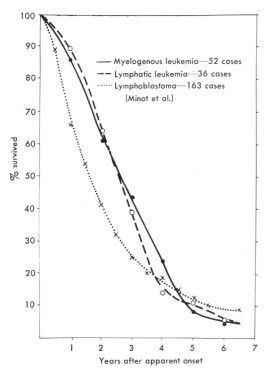

Fig. 783. Survival of untreated patients with leukemia. (From Shimkin, M. B.: Duration of life in untreated cancer, Cancer 4:1-7, 1951.)

antagonists, by Farber,[51] has led to an extensive investigation, to better understanding, and to significant improvement in the outlook for patients with leukemia, particularly children with acute forms of the disease. Radiotherapy can still be fruitfully used either for local irradiation of nodes, spleen, and mesenteric masses or as total body irradiation. Surgery is used for splenectomy in some patients with acute lymphocytic leukemia (Strumia et al.[147]). Blood and platelet transfusions and the use of antibiotics and other supportive measures are part of the often necessarily complicated care of these patients.

Chemotherapy

A variety of drugs have been found effective against leukemia. Among these, the most important are the *antimetabolites* (Methotrexate, 6-mercaptopurine, etc.), the polyfunctional *alkalating agents* (chlorambucil, vincristine, etc.), and the *adrenocorticosteroids* (prednisone). The mechanism of action of these drugs varies, and favorable response may imply a rather different form of action in one as in another variety of leukemia (Krakoff[91]). Differences in response are not necessarily related to differences in morphology, as testified by the better response in children with acute leukemia than in adults with similar acute leukemia.

Methotrexate, a folic acid analogue, when carefully administered, may induce remissions of variable duration in children with acute leukemia (Djerassi et al.[47]). It has not been possible to reduce the toxic effects of this drug without concomitant reduction of its antileukemic effects. A purine analogue, *6-mercaptopurine* is also effective in the treatment of acute leukemias and may prove useful in patients with acquired resistance to the previous administration of other agents.

Myleran, a compound synthesized by Haddow and Timmis,[68] has proved effective in the treatment of chronic myelocytic leukemia and closely related myeloproliferative diseases, being relatively free of side effects and producing rather consistent favorable results (Unugur et al.[154]). *Chlorambucil* is preferred in the treatment of chronic lymphocytic leukemia (Rundles et al.[132]). It affords a better-regulated response with less chance of bone marrow depression than other agents. *Cyclophosphamide*, another alkylating agent, is capable of causing remissions in acute leukemia in children (Pierce et al.[118]). *Vincristine sulfate*, a dimeric alkaloidal drug prepared from the *Vinca rosea* plant, has been found capable of inducing remissions in cases refractory to other antileukemic drugs (Heyn et al.[76]). *L-sarcolysin* has been found too toxic and insufficiently effective in acute leukemias (Holcomb et al.[80]). *L-asparaginase*, a proteolytic enzyme extracted from *Escherichia coli*, has proved to be another effective drug in the treatment of acute leukemias. However, it is not sufficiently effective to be used alone. Its association with other drugs may result in prohibitive toxicity (Oettgen et al.[115a]; Clarkson et al.[28a]; Tallal et al.[149a]).

The *adrenocorticosteroid hormones* have their greatest effectiveness in the treatment of frankly hemolytic anemias occurring in conjunction with chronic lymphocytic leukemia. Once the hemolysis has been arrested, the dose of steroid may be gradually reduced (Haut et al.[73]). The administration of *prednisone* alone results in a high proportion of remissions of relatively long duration (Vietti et al.[155]). A combination of vincristine and prednisone has been found capable of inducing remissions in at least four of five children with acute lymphocytic leukemia (George et al.[62]). This combination, associated with methotrexate and 6-mercaptopurine, is effective in acute myelocytic leukemias in the adult (Thompson et al.[151]). In acute leukemia associated with pregnancy, small doses of corticosteroids or antimetabolites may be used (Hoover and Schumacher[79]).

In leukemic meningitis, the intrathecal administration of methotrexate and *cystosine arabinoside* has been found helpful (Nies et al.[114]). Irradiation of the central nervous system, in association with chemotherapy, has been used with relative success (Mathé et al.[105]). In order to support the patient receiving these very toxic drugs until a remission is obtained, sustained transfusions of platelets, often on a daily basis, become necessary. Definite reduction of intracranial and gastrointestinal hemorrhages is thus achieved (Han et al.[70]). Patients with bone marrow aplasia

may be removed to pathogen-free rooms ("life islands"). Once a remission has taken place, methotrexate appears to be an efficient drug for maintenance therapy (Acute Leukemia Group B[1]).

Radiotherapy

For a long time, radiotherapy has been utilized in the palliative treatment of acute as well as chronic leukemias. The development of chemotherapy has shown its unquestionable superiority in acute leukemias, but irradiation remains a valuable adjunct in these cases. Radiotherapy remains most valuable in the management of chronic leukemias. In *acute leukemias* in children, radiotherapy may be utilized for the irradiation of the central nervous system where chemotherapeutic agents may not be effective. It has also been used to contribute to the palliation of hemorrhages of the bladder and small intestine as well as of bothersome cutaneous manifestations (Sharp et al.[142]). Total body irradiation has produced rare remissions, but it is best to use it in combination with chemotherapy rather than to rely on it alone. In the management of drug-resistant relapses, total body irradiation should be resorted to more often, however. In acute leukemias of the adult, radiotherapy is no more effective than chemotherapy insofar as inducing remissions and survival, but it may contribute also to the palliation of symptoms.

The management of *chronic leukemias* is best carried out with the adequate utilization of local and total body irradiation. Irradiation of the spleen, mesenteric masses, and voluminous adenopathies is most effective with relatively small doses, thus producing no ill effects (Parmentier et al.[116]). Total body irradiation is a safe and convenient means of management of the chronic leukemias, in which chemotherapy is of little or questionable value. Total body irradiation can be carried out easily and safely, within seriously controlled conditions, by means of roentgen rays of cobalt[60] teletherapy. The lack of available criteria to decide the length of treatments and the optimum moment to discontinue or to resume them has led us to experiment with weekly total body irradiation of patients with subacute or chronic myelocytic and lymphocytic leukemia. Some of our patients have been so treated for as long as seven years. They had long remissions during which a diagnosis of leukemia could not have been established. When they eventually died of leukemia, their bone marrow presented no signs of radiation injury. Djaldetti et al.[46] favor radiotherapy in the management of chronic lymphocytic leukemia with severe hemolytic anemia. Claims of "remissions" in patients with chronic lymphocytic leukemias require definition and long follow-up (Johnson et al.[86]). Management of these patients does not justify the exposure to toxicity of chemotherapeutic agents. Local and total body irradiation yields excellent palliation without the complications of chemotherapy.

The management of chronic myelocytic leukemia by means of radiotherapy carries definite advantages; total body irradiation may be supplemented by occasional irradiation of the spleen. When the acute phase presents itself, the patient may then receive the full impact of aggressive treatment with vincristine and prednisone. Such an attack is seldom possible in these patients if they have been treated by chemotherapy in the chronic phase of disease; by the time the acute manifestations appear, the patient is in a weak condition and an aggressive chemotherapeutic shift is seldom permissible.

Prognosis

The death rate from leukemia has been increasing in many countries. For the years 1962 and 1963, the age-adjusted death rate in the United States was 7.1 and 4.7 for males and females respectively, per 100,000 population. For the same years, the rates were 8.0 and 5.4 in Denmark, whereas they were only 3.5 and 2.7, respectively, in Japan and 3.4 and 3.0 in Chile. Deaths from leukemia occur more frequently among radiologists than among other physicians. In the United States, this differential was reduced in half in the decade 1949 to 1958 probably due to better measures of protection and reduction of exposure to radiations.

The use of chemotherapeutic agents and of the corticosteroid hormones has brought about a worthwhile improvement in the form of long remissions in children with acute leukemia. There has been an improvement in the survival of patients with acute leukemia. For those under 20 years of age in the state of Connecticut, the one-year survival was found to be 4% in 1940-1949, 14% in 1950-1954, and 29% in 1955-1959. The improvement was primarily due to longer survival of patients with acute lymphocytic leukemias (Cutler et al.[39]). From 1947 to 1966, 1445 patients with acute leukemia were treated at the Children's Hospital Medical Center of Boston, and fifteen lived for five years or more in good health (Farber[51]). Burchenal[27] collected a series of 157 cases of acute leukemia, with 103 patients living and well for five to seventeen years; one-half of those who survived five years are expected to survive for fifteen years.

Apparently healthy patients in whom chronic lymphocytic leukemia is unexpectedly discovered have the best prognosis. The median survival may extend from six to ten years (Boggs et al.[22]). Pronounced enlargement of the spleen or lymph nodes, significant leukocytosis, and the presence of anemia are all relatively unfavorable findings. Hemolytic phenomena with a positive Coombs test are also unfavorable. In chronic granulocytic leukemia, a more homogeneous group, the evaluation of results is simpler. Reinhard et al.[126] summarized their results of treatment in both chronic lymphocytic and granulocytic leukemia according to the life table method.

Tivey[152] concluded that the added effects of general medical care and specific therapy for leukemia have improved significantly the survival of the present-day patient, treated by total body irradiation, over the combined experience of those treated in the past twenty-five years. It is evident that whatever the approach, the patient benefits by the genuine interest of the hematologist, the chemotherapist, or the radiotherapist. It remains to be seen if the cooperative effort of these specialists may compound the benefits.

REFERENCES

1 Acute Leukemia Group B: Acute lymphocytic leukemia in children. Maintenance therapy with methotrexate administered intermittently, J.A.M.A. **207**:923-928, 1969.

2 Adams W. S., Valentine, W. N., Bassett, S.

H., and Lawrence, J. S.: The effect of cortisone and ACTH in leukemia, J. Lab. Clin. Med. **39**:570-581, 1952.

3 American Society of Clinical Pathologists: First report of the committee for clarification of the nomenclature of cells and diseases of the blood in blood-forming organs, Amer. J. Clin. Path. **18**:443-450, 1948.

4 Amromin, G. D.: Pathology of leukemia, New York, 1968, Hoeber Medical Division, Harper & Row, Publishers.

5 Amromin, G. D., and Solomon, R. D.: Necrotizing enteropathy, J.A.M.A. **182**:23-29, 1962.

6 Anderson, R. C.: Familial leukemia; a report of leukemia in five siblings with a brief review of the genetic aspects of this disease, Amer. J. Dis. Child. **81**:313-322, 1951.

7 Anderson, R. E., Hoshino, T., and Yamamoto, T.: Myelofibrosis with myeloid metaplasia in survivors of the atomic bomb in Hiroshima, Ann. Intern. Med. **60**:1-18, 1964.

8 Apitz, K.: Ueber Knochenveranderungen bei leukamie, Virchow Arch. Path. Anat. **302**:301-322, 1938.

9 Aroesty, J. M., and Furth, F. W.: Infection and chronic lymphocytic leukemia, New York J. Med. **62**:1946-1952, 1962.

10 Ask-Upmark, E.: Another follow-up study of children born of mothers with leukemia, Acta Med. Scand. **175**:391-394, 1964.

11 Augustine, J. R., and Jaworski, Z. F.: Unusual testicular histology in "true" Klinefelter's syndrome, Arch. Path. (Chicago) **66**:159-164, 1958.

12 Barnard, R. D.: Blood cholinesterase level and duration of life in the leukemias; with note on elevation of blood cholinesterase in certain "leukemoid" conditions, Med. Rec. **162**:16-22, 1949.

13 Baty, J. M., and Vogt, E. C.: Bone changes in leukemia in children, Amer. J. Roentgen. **34**:310-314, 1935.

14 Bernhard, W. G., Gore, I., and Kilby, R. A.: Congenital leukemia, Blood **6**:990-1001, 1951.

15 Bethell, F. H., Meyers, M. C., Bishop, R. C., and Spencer, H. H.: Advances in the treatment of leukemia, J. Michigan Med. Soc. **58**:614-622, 1959.

16 Bichel, J., Effersøe, P., Gormsen, H., and Horboe, N.: Leukemia cyelomatosis (plasma cell leukemia); a review with report of four cases, Acta Radiol. (Stockholm) **37**:196-207, 1952.

17 Bierman, H. R., Kelly, K. H., Petrakis, N. L., and Shimkin, M. B.: Leukemia; duration of life in children treated with corticotropin and cortisone, Calif. Med. **77**:238-241, 1952.

18 Bizzozero, O. J., Johnson, K. G., Ciocco, A., Kawasaki, S., and Toyoda, S.: Radiation-related leukemia in Hiroshima and Nagasaki 1946-1964. II. Observations on type-specific leukemia, survivorship, and clinical behavior, Ann. Intern. Med. **66**:522-530, 1967.

19 Blackfan, K. D., and Diamond, L. K.: Atlas of the blood in children, New York, 1944, Commonwealth Fund.

20 Bloom, G. E., Warner, S., Gerald, P. S., and Diamond, L. K.: Chromosome abnormalities in constitutional aplastic anemia, New Eng. J. Med. **274**:8-14, 1966.

21 Bodey, G. P., Powell, R. D., Hersh, E. M., Yeterian, A., and Freireich, E. J.: Pulmonary complications of acute leukemia, Cancer **19**:781-793, 1966.

22 Boggs, D. R., Sofferman, S. A., Wintrobe, M. M., and Cartwright, G. E.: Factors influencing duration of survival of patients with chronic lymphocytic leukemia, Amer. J. Med. **40**:243-254, 1966.

23 Borges, W. H., Nichlas, J. W., and Hamm, C. W.: Prezygotic determinants in acute leukemia, J. Pediat. **70**:180-184, 1967.

24 Bousser, J., and Tanzer, J.: Syndrome de Klinefelter et leucemie aiguë, a propos d'un cas, Nouv. Rev. Franc. Hemat. **3**:194-197, 1963.

25 Bowie, E. J. W., Kiely, J. M., Newlon, R. W., and Stickney, J. M.: The anemia of leukemia, J. Nucl. Med. **3**:423-435, 1962.

26 Bryan, W. R., Moloney, J. B., O'Connor, T. E., Fink, M. A., and Dalton, A. J.: Viral etiology of leukemia, Ann. Intern. Med. **62**:376-399, 1965.

27 Burchenal, J. H.: Long-term survivors in acute leukemia and Burkitt's tumor, Cancer **21**:595-599, 1968.

28 Cazal, P.: Aspects cliniques et hématologiques de la réticulose maligne, Acta Haemat. (Basel) **7**:65-85, 1952.

28a Clarkson, B., Krakoff, I., Burchenal, J., Karnofsky, D., Golbey, R., Dowling, M., Oettgen, H., and Lipton, A.: Clinical results of treatment with E. coli L-asparaginase in adults with leukemia, lymphoma, and solid tumors, Cancer **25**:279-305, 1970.

29 Cohen, S. M.: Chronic myelogenous leukemia with myelogenous leukemia with myelofibrosis, Arch. Intern. Med. (Chicago) **119**:620-625, 1967.

30 Cook, J. C., Krabbenhoft, K. L., and Leucutia, T.: Combined radiation and nitrogen mustard therapy in Hodgkin's disease as compared with radiation therapy alone, Amer. J. Roentgen. **82**:651-657, 1959.

31 Cooke, J. V.: The incidence of acute leukemia in children, J.A.M.A. **119**:547-550, 1942.

32 Cornes, J. S., and Jones, T. G.: Some important clinical and pathological features of leukemia lesions in the gastro-intestinal tract, Proc. Roy. Soc. Med. **55**:702-703, 1963.

33 Court-Brown, W. M., and Doll, R.: Leukemia and aplastic anemias in ankylosing spondylitis, London, 1957, Medical Research Council, Report 295, Her Majesty's Stationery Office.

34 Crail, H. W., Alt, H. L., and Nadler, W. H.: Myelofibrosis associated tuberculosis, Blood **3**:1426-1444, 1948.

35 Craver, L. F.: Value of early diagnosis of malignant lymphomas and leukemias, New York, 1952, The American Cancer Society, Inc.

36 Cronkite, E. P., Moloney, W., and Bond, V. P.: Radiation leukemogenesis, Amer. J. Med. **28**:673-682, 1960.

37 Custer, R. P.: An atlas of the blood and bone marrow, Philadelphia, 1949, W. B. Saunders Co.

38 Custer, R. P., and Smith, E. B.: The pathology of infectious mononucleosis, Blood **3**:830-857, 1948.

39 Cutler, S. J., Heise, H., and Eisenberg, H.: Childhood leukemia in Connecticut, 1940-1962, Blood **30**:1-25, 1967.

40 Dameshek, W.: Chronic lymphocytic leukemia —an accumulative disease of immunologically incompetent lymphocytes, Blood **29**:566-584, 1967.

41 Dameshek, W., and Gunz, G.: Leukemia, Philadelphia, 1958, Grune & Stratton, Inc.

42 D'Angio, G. J., Evans, A. E., and Mitus, A.: Roentgen therapy of certain complications of acute leukemia in childhood, Amer. J. Roentgen. **82**:541-553, 1959.

43 Dausset, J., and Schwarzman, V.: Influence of age and sex upon frequency and cytologic types of human leukemias, Blood **6**:976-989, 1951.

44 Diamond, I. B.: Leukemic changes in the brain, Arch. Neurol. Psychiat. (Chicago) **32**:118-142, 1934.

45 Di Guglielmo, G.: Les maladies erythremiques, Rev. Hemat. (Paris) **1**:355-398, 1946.

46 Djaldetti, M., de Vries, A., and Levie, B.: Hemolytic anemia in lymphocytic leukemia, Arch. Intern. Med. (Chicago) **110**:449-455, 1962.

47 Djerassi, I., Abir, E., Royer, G. L., and Treat, C. L.: Long-term remissions in childhood acute leukemia; use of infrequent infusions of methotrexate; supportive roles of platelet transfusions and citrovorum factor, Clin. Pediat. (Phila.) **5**:502-509, 1966.

48 Erb, I. H.: Bone changes in leukaemia. Part II. Pathology, Arch. Dis. Child. **9**:319-326, 1934.

49 Fairburn, E. A., and Burgen, A. S. V.: The skin lesions of monocytic leukaemia, Brit. J. Cancer **1**:352-362, 1947.

50 Falconer, C. F.: Leukemia and allied disorders, New York, 1938, The Macmillan Co.

51 Farber, S.: Chemotherapy in the treatment of leukemia and Wilms' tumor, J.A.M.A. **198**:154-164, 1966.

52 Firkin, B., and Moore, C. V.: Clinical manifestations of leukemia, Amer. J. Med. **28**:764-776, 1960.

53 Fisher, J. H., Welch, C. S., and Dameshek, W.: Splenectomy in leukemia and leukosarcoma, New Eng. J. Med. **246**:477-484, 1952.

54 Fitzgerald, P. H., Adams, A., and Gunz, F. W.: Chronic granulocytic leukemia and the Philadelphia chromosome, Blood **21**:183-196, 1963.

55 Flaherty, S. A., Cope, H. E., and Shecket, H. A.: Prostatic obstruction as the presenting symptom of acute monocytic leukemia, J. Urol. **44**:488-497, 1940.

56 Fraumeni, J. F., Jr., Ederer, F., and Handy, V. H.: Temporal—spatial distribution of childhood leukemia in New York State, Cancer **19**:996-1000, 1966.

57 Fraumeni, J. F., Jr., and Miller, R. W.: Epidemiology of human leukemia; recent observations, J. Nat. Cancer Inst. **38**:593-605, 1967.

58 Fried, B. M.: Leukemia and the central nervous system, Arch. Path. Lab. Med. **2**:23-40, 1926.

59 Furth, J.: Recent studies on the etiology and nature of leukemia, Blood **6**:964-975, 1951.

60 Gall, E. A., and Stout, H. H.: Histological lesion in lymph nodes in infectious mononucleosis, Amer. J. Path. **16**:433-448, 1940.

61 Garfinkel, L. S., and Bennett, D. E.: Extra medullary myeloblastic transformation in chronic myelocytic leukemia simulating a coexistent malignant lymphoma, Amer. J. Clin. Path. **51**:638-645, 1969.

62 George, P., Hernandez, K., Hustu, O., Borella, L., Holton, C., and Pinkel, D.: A study of "total therapy" of acute lymphocytic leukemia in children, J. Pediat. **72**:399-408, 1968.

63 Goh, K. O., and Swisher, S. N.: Identical twins and chronic myelocytic leukemia; chromosomal studies of a patient with chronic myelocytic leukemia and his normal identical twin, Arch. Intern. Med. (Chicago) **115**:475-478, 1965.

64 Goh, K., Swisher, S. N., and Herman, E. C.: Chronic myelocytic leukemia and identical twins; additional evidence of the Philadelphia chromosome as postzygotic abnormality, Arch. Intern. Med. (Chicago) **120**:213-219, 1967.

65 Goldbach, L. J.: Leukemic retinitis, Arch. Ophthal. (Chicago) **10**:808-817, 1933.

66 Goodman, E. G., and Iverson, L.: Chloroma— a clinico-pathologic study of two cases, Amer. J. Med. Sci. **211**:205-214, 1946.

67 Gunz, F. W., and Atkinson, H. R.: Medical radiations and leukaemia; a retrospective survey, Brit. Med. J. **1**:389-393, 1964.

68 Haddow, A., and Timmis, G. M.: Myleran in chronic myeloid leukemia; chemical constitution and biological action, Lancet **1**:207-208, 1953.

69 Han, T., Ezdinli, E. Z., and Sokal, J. E.: Complete remission in chronic lymphocytic leukemia and leukolymphosarcoma, Cancer **20**:243-253, 1967.

70 Han, T., Stutzman, L., Cohen, E., and Kim, U.: Effect of platelet transfusion on hemorrhage in patients with acute leukemia; an autopsy study, Cancer **19**:1937-1942, 1966.

71 Hardisty, R. M., and Norman, P. M.: Meningeal leukaemia, Arch. Dis. Child. **42**:441-447, 1967.

72 Hauptman, H., and Taussig, F. J.: Leucemic infiltration of the female internal genitalia as a cause of vaginal bleeding, Amer. J. Obstet. Gynec. **39**:70-77, 1940.

73 Haut, A., Altman, S. J., Wintrobe, M. M., and Cartwright, G. E.: The influence of chemotherapy on survival in acute leukemia; comparison of cases treated during 1954 to

1957 with those treated during 1947-1954, Blood 14:828-847, 1959.

74 Heller, E. L., Lewisohn, M. G., and Palin, W. E.: Aleukemic myelosis, Amer. J. Path. 23:327-365, 1947.

75 Hempelmann, L. H.: Epidemiological studies of leukemia in persons exposed to ionizing radiation, Cancer Res. 20:18-27, 1960 (extensive bibliography).

76 Heyn, R. M., Beatty, E. C., Hammond, D., Louis, J., Pierce, M., Murphy, M. L., and Severo, N.: Vincristine in the treatment of acute leukemia in children, Pediatrics 38: 82-91, 1966.

77 Heyssell, R., Brill, A. B., Woodbury, L. A., Nishimura, E. T., Ghose, T., Hoshino, T., and Yamasaki, M.: Leukemia in Hiroshima bomb survivors, Blood 15:313-331, 1960.

78 Hill, J. M., and Duncan, C. N.: Leukemoid reactions, Amer. J. Med. Sci. 201:847-857, 1941.

79 Hoover, B. A., II, and Schumacher, H. R.: Acute leukemia in pregnancy, Amer. J. Obstet. Gynec. 96:316-320, 1966.

80 Holcomb, T. M., Berry, D. H., Haggard, M. E., Sullivan, M. P., Watkins, W. L., and Windmiller, J.: L-sarcolysin (NSC-8806) therapy for acute leukemia in children, Cancer Chemother. Rep. 48:45-48, 1965.

81 Hoshino, T., Kato, H., Finch, S. C., and Hrubec, Z.: Leukemia in offspring of atomic bomb survivors, Blood 30:719-730, 1967.

82 Hudson, R. P., and Wilson, S. J.: Hypogammaglobulinemia and chronic lymphatic leukemia, Cancer 13:200-204, 1960.

83 Hynes, H. E., Silverstein, M. N., and Fawcett, K. J.: Spontaneous rupture of the spleen in acute leukemia, Cancer 17:1356-1360, 1964.

84 Johnson, R. E.: Evaluation of fractionated total-body irradiation in patients with leukemia and disseminated lymphomas, Radiology 86:1085-1089, 1966.

84a Johnson, R. E.: Total body irradiation of chronic lymphocytic leukemia; incidence and duration of remission, Cancer 25:523-530, 1970.

85 Johnson, R. E., Foley, H. T., Swain, R. W., and O'Conor, G. T.: Treatment of lymphosarcoma with fractionated total body irradiation, Cancer 20:482-485, 1967.

86 Johnson, R. E., Kagan, A. R., Gralnick, H. R., and Fass, L.: Radiation-induced remissions in chronic lymphocytic leukemia, Cancer 20:1382-1387, 1967.

87 Kandel, E. V.: Chloroma; review of the literature from 1926 to 1936 and report of three cases, Arch. Intern. Med. (Chicago) 59:691-704, 1937 (extensive bibliography).

88 Kawabe, Y.: The bone marrow of the A-bomb survivors with other than blood diseases, who lived more than 7 years after the exposure, Nagasaki Igakkai Zassi 33:310-325, 1958 (Japanese text).

89 Kimball, A. W.: Evaluation of data relating human leukemia and ionizing radiation, J. Nat. Cancer Inst. 21:383-391, 1958.

90 Kirshbaum, J. D., and Preuss, F. S.: Leu-

kemia; a clinical and pathologic study of one hundred and twenty-three fatal cases in a series of 14,400 necropsies, Arch. Intern. Med. (Chicago) 71:777-792, 1943.

91 Krakoff, I. H.: Mechanisms of drug action in leukemia, Amer. J. Med. 28:735-750, 1960.

92 Krakoff, I. H., and Balis, M. E.: Abnormalities of purine metabolism in human leukemia, Ann. N. Y. Acad. Sci. 113:1043-1052, 1964.

93 Krauss, S.: Chronic myelocytic leukemia with features simulating myelofibrosis with myeloid metaplasia, Cancer 19:1321-1332, 1966.

94 Kyle, R. A., Kiely, J. M., and Stickney, J. M.: Acquired hemolytic anemia in chronic lymphocytic leukemia and the lymphomas; survival and response to therapy in twenty-seven cases, Arch. Intern. Med. (Chicago) 104: 61-67, 1959.

95 Lewis, E. B.: Leukemia and ionizing radiation, Science 125:965-972, 1957 (extensive bibliography).

95a Liao, K. L.: Superiority of histologic sections of aspirated bone marrow in malignant lymphomas; a review of 1124 examinations, Cancer 1970 (in press).

96 Libre, E. P., and McFarland, W.: Chronic myelogenous leukemia, Arch. Intern. Med. (Chicago) 119:626-630, 1967.

97 Lock, S. P., and Merrington, M.: Leukaemia in Lewisham (1957-63), Brit. Med. J. 3: 759-760, 1967.

98 Loeb, V., Jr., Moore, C. V., and Dubach, R.: The physiologic evaluation and management of chronic bone marrow failure, Amer. J. Med. 15:499-517, 1953.

99 McPhedran, P., Heath, C. W., Jr., and Lee, J.: Patterns of familial leukemia; ten cases of leukemia in two interrelated families, Cancer 24:403-407, 1969.

100 MacSween, R. N. M.: Reticulum-cell sarcoma and rheumatoid arthritis in a patient with XY/XXY/XXXY Klinefelter's syndrome and normal intelligence, Lancet 1:460-461, 1965.

101 Mamunes, P., Lapidus, P. H., Abbott, J. A., and Roath, S.: Acute leukaemia and Klinefelter's syndrome, Lancet 2:26-27, 1961.

102 March, H. C.: Leukemia in radiologists in a 20-year period, Amer. J. Med. Sci. 220:282-286, 1950.

103 March, H. C.: Leukemia in radiologists; ten years later with a review of the pertinent evidence for radiation leukemia, Amer. J. Med. Sci. 242:137-149, 1961.

104 Marshall, A. H. E.: An outline of the cytology and pathology of the reticular tissue, Edinburgh/London, 1956, Oliver & Boyd, pp. 78-82.

105 Mathé, G., Schwarzenberg, L., Schneider, M., Schlumberger, J. R., Hayat, M., Amiel, J. L., Cattan, A., and Jasmin, C.: Acute lymphoblastic leukemia treated with a combination of prednisone, vincristine, and rubidomycin, Lancet 2:380-382, 1967.

106 Merrill, D., and Jackson, H., Jr.: The renal complications of leukemia, New Eng. J. Med. 228:271-276, 1943.

107 Moloney, W. C.: Leukemia in survivors of atomic bombing, New Eng. J. Med. **253**:88-90, 1955.

108 Moore, C. V., and Reinhard, E.: Personal communication, 1953.

109 Moore, E. W., Thomas, L. B., Shaw, R. K., and Freireich, E. J.: The central nervous system in acute leukemia, Arch. Intern. Med. (Chicago) **105**:451-468, 1960.

110 Morrow, G. W., Pease, G. L., Stroebel, C. F., and Bennett, W. A.: Terminal phase of chronic myelogenous leukemia, Cancer **18**:369-374, 1965.

111 Moss, W. T., and Ackerman, L. V.: Plasmacell leukemia, Blood **1**:396-406, 1946.

112 Murray, R., Hickel, P., and Hempelmann, L. H.: Leukemia in children exposed to ionizing radiation, New Eng. J. Med. **261**:585-589, 1959.

113 Nies, B. A., Bodey, G. P., Thomas, L. B., Brecher, G., and Freireich, E. J.: The persistence of extramedullary leukemic infiltrates during bone marrow remission of acute leukemia, Blood **26**:133-141, 1965.

114 Nies, B. A., Thomas, L. B., and Freireich, E. J.: Meningeal leukemia; a follow-up study, Cancer **18**:546-553, 1965.

115 Nowell, P. C., and Hungerford, D. A.: Chromosome changes in human leukemia and a tentative assessment of their significance, Ann. N. Y. Acad. Sci. **113**:654-662, 1964.

115a Oettgen, H. F., Stephenson, P. A., Schwartz, M. K., Leeper, R. D., Tallal, L., Tan, C. C., Clarkson, B. D., Golbey, R. B., Krakoff, I. H., Karnofsky, D. A., Murphy, M. L., and Burchenal, J. H.: Toxicity of E. coli L-asparaginase in man, Cancer **25**:253-278, 1970.

116 Parmentier, C., Schlienger, M., Hayat, M., Laugier, A., Schlumberger, J. R., Mathé, G., and Tubiana, M.: L'irradiation splénique dans les leucémies lymphocytaires chroniques décompensées, J. Radiol. Electr. **49**:187-198, 1968.

117 Pearson, H. A., Grello, F. W., and Cone, T. E., Jr.: Leukaemia in identical twins, New Eng. J. Med. **268**:1151-1156, 1963.

118 Pierce, M., Shore, N., Sitarz, A., Murphy, M. L., Louis, J., and Severo, N.: Cyclophosphamide therapy in acute leukemia of childhood; cooperative study conducted by members of Children's Cancer Cooperative Group A, Cancer **19**:1551-1560, 1966.

119 Pierce, M. I., Borges, W. H., Heyn, R., Wolff, J. A., and Gilbert, E. S.: Epidemiological factors and survival experience in 1770 children with acute leukemia; treated by members of Children's Study Group A between 1957 and 1964, Cancer **23**:1296-1304, 1969.

120 Piney, A.: Remissions in acute leukaemia; the role of blood transfusion in treatment, Acta Haemat. (Basel) **3**:1-16, 1950.

121 Pizzolato, P.: Leukemia in the Negro, J. Nat. Med. Ass. **41**:214-219, 1949.

122 Prolla, J. C., and Kirsner, J. B.: The gastrointestinal lesions and complications of the leukemias, Ann. Intern. Med. **61**:1084-1103, 1964.

123 Rappaport, H.: Tumors of the hematopoietic system. In Atlas of tumor pathology, Sect. 3, Fasc. 8, Washington, D. C., 1966, Armed Forces Institute of Pathology.

124 Rappoport, A. E., and Kugel, V. H.: Monocytic leukemia; a case report illustrating variations in the clinical picture, Blood **2**:332-355, 1947.

125 del Regato, J. A.: Reflections on the so-called lymphomas, Radiol. Clin. N. Amer. **6**:3-13, 1968.

126 Reinhard, E. H., Neely, C. L., and Samples, D. M.: Radioactive phosphorus in the treatment of chronic leukemias; long-term results over period of 15 years, Ann. Intern. Med. **50**:942-958, 1959.

127 Reisman, L. E., and Trujillo, L. E.: Chronic granulocytic leukemia of childhood; clinical and cytogenetic studies, J. Pediat. **62**:710-723, 1963.

128 Rheingold, J. J., Weifuse, L., and Dameshek, W.: Multiple sites for bone-marrow puncture, with particular reference to children, New Eng. J. Med. **240**:54-56, 1949.

129 Rosenthal, M. C., Saunders, R. H., Schwartz, L. I., Zannos, L., Santiago, E. P., and Dameshek, W.: The use of adrenocorticotropic hormone and cortisone in the treatment of leukemia and leukosarcoma, Blood **6**:804-823, 1951.

130 Rothschild, H.: Chlorome der Dura mater mit atypischen Symptomatologie, Deutsch. Z. Nervenheilk. **91**:57-76, 1926.

131 Rubinstein, M. A.: Aspiration of bone marrow from the iliac crest; comparison of iliac crest and sternal bone marrow studies, J.A.M.A. **137**:1281-1285, 1948.

132 Rundles, R. W., Grizzle, J., Bell, W. N., Corley, C. C., Frommeyer, W. B., Jr., Greenberg, B. G., Huguley, C. M., Jr., James, G. W., III, Jones, R., Jr., Larsen, W. E., Loeb, V., Leone, L. A., Palmer, J. G., Riser, W. H., Jr., and Wilson, S. J.: Comparison of chlorambucil and myleran in chronic lymphocytic and granulocytic leukemia, Amer. J. Med. **27**:424-432, 1959.

133 Sabin, F. R.: Studies of living human blood cells, Johns Hopkins Hosp. Bull. **32**:314-321, 1921.

134 Sawitsky, A., Bloom, D., and German, J.: Chromosomal breakage and acute leukemia in congenital telangiectatic erythema and stunted growth, Ann. Intern. Med. **65**:487-495, 1966.

135 Schade, H., Schoeller, L., and Schultz, K. W.: D-Trisomie (Pätau-Syndrom) mit kongenitaler myeloischer leukämie, Med. Welt **50**:2690-2692, 1962.

136 Schullenberger, C. C.: Evaluation of the comparative effectiveness of myleran and 6-MP in the management of patients with chronic myelocytic leukemia, Cancer Chemother. Rep. **16**:203-207, 1962.

137 Schwab, R. S., and Weiss, S.: The neurologic aspect of leukemia, Amer. J. Med. Sci. **189**:766-778, 1935.

138 Schwartz, S. O., and Schoolman, H. M.: The etiology of leukemia; the status of the virus as causative agent, Blood 14:279-294, 1959.

139 Scott, R. B., Ellison, R. R., and Ley, A. B.: A clinical study of twenty cases of erythroleukemia (di Guglielmo syndrome), Amer. J. Med. 37:162-171, 1964.

140 Scott, R. B., and Robb-Smith, A. H. T.: Histiocytic medullary reticulosis, Lancet 237: 194-198, 1939.

141 Segi, M., Kurihara, M., and Matsuyama, T.: Cancer mortality in Japan (1899-1962), Department of Public Health, Tohoku University School of Medicine, Sendai, Japan, 1965, pp. 14, 23, and 45.

142 Sharp, H. L., Nesbit, M. E., D'Angio, G. J., and Krivit, W.: Addition of local radiations after bone marrow remission in acute leukemia in children, Cancer 20:1403-1404, 1967.

143 Silverman, F. N.: The skeletal lesions in leukemia; clinical and roentgenographic observations in 103 infants and children with a review of the literature, Amer. J. Roentgen. 59: 819-844, 1948.

144 Simpson, C. L., Hempelmann, L. H., and Fuller, L. M.: Neoplasia in children treated with x-rays in infancy for thymic enlargement, Radiology 64:840-845, 1955.

145 Sinn, C. M., and Dick, F. W.: Monocytic leukemia, Amer. J. Med. 20:588-602, 1956.

146 Stewart, A., Webb, J., and Hewitt, D.: A survey of childhood malignancies, Brit. Med. J. 1:1495-1508, 1958.

147 Strumia, M. M., Strumia, P. V., and Bassert, D.: Splenectomy in leukemia; hematologic and clinical effects on 34 patients and review of 299 published cases, Cancer Res. 26:519-528, 1966.

148 Symposium on transplantation of bone marrow, Blood 13:266-301, 1958.

149 Szweda, J. A., Abraham, J. P., Fine, G., Nixon, R. K., and Rupe, C. E.: Systemic mast cell disease, Amer. J. Med. 32:227-239, 1962.

149a Tallal, L., Tan, C., Oettgen, H., Wollner, N., McCarthy, M., Helson, L., Burchenal, J., Karnofsky, D., and Murphy, M. L.: E. coli L-asparaginase in the treatment of leukemia and solid tumors in 131 children, Cancer 25: 306-320, 1970.

150 Thomas, L. B., Forkner, C. E., Jr., Frei, E., III, Besse, B. E., Jr., and Stabenau, J. R.: The skeletal lesions of acute leukemia, Cancer 14:608-621, 1961.

151 Thompson, I., Hall, T. C., and Moloney, W.

C.: Combination therapy of adult acute myelogenus leukemia; experience with the simultaneous use of vincristine, amethopterin, 6-mercaptopurine and prednisone, New Eng. J. Med. 273:1302-1307, 1965.

152 Tivey, H.: Prognosis for survival in the leukemias of childhood; review of the literature and the proposal of a simple method of reporting survival data for these diseases, Pediatrics 10:48-58, 1952.

153 Tough, I. M., Court Brown, W. M., Baikie, A. G., Buckton, K. E., Harnden, D. G., Jacobs, P. A., King, M. J., and McBride, J. A.: Cytogenetic studies in chronic myeloid leukaemia and acute leukaemia associated with mongolism, Lancet 1:411-417, 1961.

154 Unugur, A., Schulman, E., and Dameshek, W.: Treatment of chronic granulocytic leukemia with myleran, New Eng. J. Med. 256: 727-734, 1957.

155 Vietti, T. J., Sullivan, M. P., Berry, D. H., Haddy, T. B., Haggard, M. E., and Blattner, R. J.: The response of acute childhood leukemia to an initial and a second course of prednisone, J. Pediatrics 66:18-26, 1965.

156 Viola, M. V.: Acute leukemia and infection, J.A.M.A. 201:923-926, 1967.

157 Wakezaka, G.: A geographical pathological study of leukemia in Japan, J. Jap. Soc. Intern. Med. 17:225-231, 1966.

158 Wald, N., Borges, W. H., Li, C. C., Turner, J. H., and Harnois, M. C.: Leukaemia associated with mongolism, Lancet 1:1228, 1961.

159 Waters, W. J., and Lacson, P. S.: Mast cell leukemia presenting as urticaria pigmentosa, Pediatrics 19:1033-1042, 1957.

160 Wells, R., and Lau, K. S.: Incidence of leukaemia in Singapore, and rarity of chronic lymphocytic leukaemia in Chinese, Brit. Med. J. 1:759-763, 1960.

161 Wentz, F. M., Anday, G., and Orban, B.: Histopathologic changes in the gingiva in leukemia, J. Periodont. 20:119-128, 1949.

162 Willson, J. K. V.: The bone lesions of childhood leukemia, Radiology 72:672-681, 1959.

163 Wintrobe, M. M.: Clinical hematology, ed. 6, Philadelphia, 1967, Lea & Febiger.

164 Zuelzer, W. W., Thompson, R. L., and Mastrangelo, R.: Familial occurrence of somatic crossing over and related chromosome abnormalities in the pedigree of a patient with leukemia and partial D-trisomy, Abstract of Contributed Papers (No. 358), Third International Congress of Human Genetics, Chicago, Sept. 5-10, 1966.

Index